Geriatric Dosage Handbook

including

Monitoring,
Clinical Recommendations,
and OBRA Guidelines

2ⁿᵈ Edition *1995-96*

W9-CTJ-897

MAR 2 6 1996

LIBRARY
GREY NUNS HOSPITAL

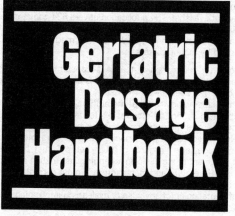

Geriatric Dosage Handbook

--- *including* ---

Monitoring, Clinical Recommendations, and OBRA Guidelines

2nd Edition *1995-96*

Todd P. Semla, PharmD
Assistant Professor of Pharmacy Practice
Department of Pharmacy Practice
Clinical Assistant Professor of Pharmacy Practice in Medicine, Section of Geriatric Medicine
University of Illinois at Chicago
Chicago, Illinois

Judith L. Beizer, PharmD
Associate Clinical Professor
College of Pharmacy and Allied Health Professions
St. John's University
Jamaica, New York

Martin D. Higbee, PharmD
Associate Professor of Clinical Pharmacy
Department of Pharmacy Practice
The University of Arizona
Tucson, Arizona

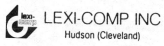
LEXI-COMP INC
Hudson (Cleveland)

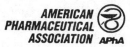
AMERICAN PHARMACEUTICAL ASSOCIATION APhA

HEALTH SCIENCES LIBRARY
EDMONTON GENERAL HOSPITAL

NOTICE

This handbook is intended to serve the user as a handy reference and not as a complete drug information resource. It does not include information on every therapeutic agent available. The publication covers 634 commonly used drugs and is specifically designed to present certain important aspects of drug data in a more concise format than is typically found in medical literature or product material supplied by manufacturers.

The nature of drug information is that it is constantly evolving because of ongoing research and clinical experience and is often subject to interpretation. While great care has been taken to ensure the accuracy of the information presented, the reader is advised that the authors, editors, reviewers, contributors, and publishers cannot be responsible for the continued currency of the information or for any errors or omissions in this book or for any consequences arising therefrom. Because of the dynamic nature of drug information, readers are advised that decisions regarding drug therapy must be based on the independent judgment of the clinician, changing information about a drug (eg, as reflected in the literature and manufacturer's most current product information), and changing medical practices. The editors are not responsible for any inaccuracy of quotation or for any false or misleading implication that may arise due to the text or formulas as used or due to the quotation of revisions no longer official.

The publishers have made every effort to trace the copyright holders for borrowed material. If they have inadvertently overlooked any, they will be pleased to make the necessary arrangements at the first opportunity.

The editors, authors, and contributors have written this book in their private capacities. No official support or endorsement by any federal or state agency or pharmaceutical company is intended or inferred.

If you have any suggestions or questions
regarding any information presented in this handbook,
please contact our drug information pharmacist at

1-800-837-LEXI

PHARM - EGH
HEALTH SCIENCES LIBRARY
EDMONTON GENERAL HOSPITAL
95-11702-09

Copyright © 1995 by Lexi-Comp Inc. All rights reserved.

Copyright © 1993, First Edition. Printed in Canada. No part of this publication may be reproduced, stored in a retrieval system, or transmitted, in any form or by any means, electronic, mechanical, photocopying, recording, or otherwise, without the prior written permission of the publisher.

This manual was produced using the FormuLex™ Program —
A complete publishing service of Lexi-Comp Inc.

Lexi-Comp Inc.
1100 Terex Road
Hudson, Ohio 44236-3771
(216) 650-6506

ISBN 0-916589-28-5

TABLE OF CONTENTS

PREFACE

The *Geriatric Dosage Handbook* is designed to be a practical and convenient guide to the dosing and usage of medications in the elderly population. As the percentage of the population over the age of 65 increases, most health care professionals will be faced with the challenge of the appropriate use of medications in the elderly.

Many physiologic changes occur with aging, some of which affect the pharmacokinetics and/or pharmacodynamics of medications. For the majority of drugs, exact dosing guidelines for geriatric patients have not been established and most references do not specifically address the use of the medications in the elderly. For practical purposes, it has been recommended to "start low, go slow." Our objective in producing this handbook is to refine this recommendation and provide the reader with specific considerations when using medications in older adults. Information has been compiled from the current literature and our clinical experiences, emphasizing choice of medication, dosing, changes in pharmacokinetics or pharmacodynamics, monitoring parameters, and adverse effects. References are listed at the end of drug monographs to support this information when it exists. Additional clinical drug information which is relevant to the practice of geriatric pharmacotherapy is also included in each monograph and in the appendices.

We hope this reference proves to be a valuable and practical source of clinical drug information for health care professionals caring for the elderly. We welcome comments to improve future editions.

ACKNOWLEDGMENTS

This handbook exists in its present form as a result of the concerted efforts of many individuals. The publisher and president of Lexi-Comp Inc, Robert D. Kerscher and the director of special projects, Laura C. Lawson, American Pharmaceutical Association (APhA) deserve much of the credit for bringing the concept of such a book to fruition.

Other members of the Lexi-Comp staff whose contributions were invaluable and whose patience with the editors' enumerable drafts, revisions, deletions, additions, and enhancements was inexhaustible include: Leonard L. Lance, BSPharm, pharmacy editor; Diane Harbart, MT (ASCP), medical editor; Lynn D. Coppinger, director of product development; Barbara F. Kerscher, production manager; Alexandra Hart, composition specialist; Jeanne Eads, Beth Daulbaugh, Julie Weekes, and Lisa Leukart, project managers; Jil Neuman, Jackie Mizer, and Tracey Reinecke, production assistants; Jeff J. Zaccagnini, Brian B. Vossler, and Jerry M. Reeves, sales managers; Edmund A. Harbart, vice-president, custom publishing division; and Jack L. Stones, vice-president, reference publishing division. The complex computer programming required for the typesetting of the book was provided by Jay L. Katzen, Dennis P. Smithers, David C. Marcus, Dale Jablonski, and Kenneth J. Hughes, system analysts, under the direction of Thury L. O'Connor, vice-president, and Alan R. Frasz, vice-president, information technologies.

Other APhA staff members whose contributions were important are Julian I. Graubart, Director Special Projects, Linda Sorin, Senior Director, Marketing, and James V. McGinnis, manager of art and production. A special thanks goes to Chris Lomax, PharmD, director of pharmacy, Children's Hospital, Los Angeles, who played a significant role in bringing APhA and Lexi-Comp together.

Much of the material contained in the book was a result of pharmacy contributors throughout the United States and Canada. Lexi-Comp has assisted many medical institutions to develop hospital-specific formulary manuals that contains clinical drug information as well as dosing. Working with these clinical pharmacists, hospital pharmacy and therapeutics committees, and hospital drug information centers, Lexi-Comp has developed an evolutionary drug database that reflects the practice of pharmacy in these major institutions.

In addition, the authors wish to thank their families, friends, and colleagues who supported them in their efforts to complete this handbook.

EDITORIAL ADVISORY PANEL

Judith A. Aberg, MD
Fellow
Department of Infectious Disease
Washington University School of Medicine
St Louis, Missouri

Lora L. Armstrong, RPh, BSPharm
Director of Drug Information Services
The University of Chicago Hospitals
Chicago, Illinois

Wayne R. DeMott, MD
Pathologists Chartered
Overland Park, Kansas

Morton P. Goldman, PharmD
Infectious Disease Pharmacist
Cleveland Clinic Foundation
Cleveland, Ohio

Harold J. Grady, PhD
Director of Clinical Chemistry
Truman Medical Center
Kansas City, Missouri

Larry D. Gray, PhD
Director of Microbiology
Bethesda Hospitals
Cincinnati, Ohio

Jane Hurlburt Hodding, PharmD
Supervisor, Children's Pharmacy
Memorial Miller Children's Hospital
Long Beach, California

Rebecca T. Horvat, PhD
Assistant Professor of Pathology and Laboratory Medicine
University of Kansas Medical Center
Kansas City, Kansas

Carlos M. Isada, MD
Department of Infectious Disease
Cleveland Clinic Foundation
Cleveland, Ohio

David S. Jacobs, MD
President, Pathologists Chartered
Overland Park, Kansas

Bernard L. Kasten, Jr., MD
Associate Director
Pathology and Laboratory Services
Bethesda Hospitals
Cincinnati, Ohio

Donna M. Kraus, PharmD
Associate Professor of Pharmacy Practice
Departments of Pharmacy Practice and Pediatrics
Clinical Pharmacist
Pediatric Intensive Care Unit
University of Illinois at Chicago
Chicago, Illinois

Charles Lacy, RPh, PharmD
Drug Information Pharmacist
Cedars-Sinai Medical Center
Los Angeles, California

Leonard L. Lance, RPh, BSPharm
Pharmacist
Lexi-Comp Inc.
Hudson, Ohio

Jerrold B. Leikin, MD
Associate Director
Emergency Services
Medical Director
Rush Poison Control Center
Rush Presbyterian-St. Luke's Medical Center
Chicago, Illinois

Eugene S. Olsowka, MD, PhD
Pathologist
Institute of Pathology
Saginaw, Michigan

Frank P. Paloucek, PharmD
Clinical Associate Professor
University of Illinois
Chicago, Illinois

Christopher J. Papasian, PhD
Director of Diagnostic Microbiology and Immunology Laboratories
Truman Medical Center
Kansas City, Missouri

Carol K. Taketomo, PharmD
Pharmacy Manager
Children's Hospital of Los Angeles
Los Angeles, California

Lowell L. Tilzer MD
Associate Medical Director
Community Blood Center of Greater Kansas City
Kansas City, Missouri

ABOUT THE AUTHORS

Todd P. Semla, MS, PharmD

Dr Semla received his Bachelor of Science in Pharmacy, his Master of Science in Clinical/Hospital Pharmacy, and his Doctor of Pharmacy degrees from the University of Iowa. After earning his doctorate, Dr Semla was awarded the American Society of Hospital Pharmacists Fellowship in Geriatric Pharmacotherapy which he completed at the University of Iowa.

Dr Semla has over 10 years experience in geriatric pharmacotherapy in a variety of clinical settings including ambulatory care, acute care and rehabilitation, and the nursing home. Since 1986, he has been on the faculty of the University of Illinois at Chicago College of Pharmacy where he is an Assistant Professor of Pharmacy Practice, a Clinical Assistant Professor of Pharmacy Practice in Medicine, Section of Geriatric Medicine in the College of Medicine, and the Pharmacotherapist for the Geriatric Assessment and Reactivation Unit and Geriatric Outpatient Assessment and Medicine Clinic at the University of Illinois Hospital and Clinics. He is also the Disciplinary Director for Pharmacy for the Illinois Geriatric Education Center.

Dr Semla's research interests include drug epidemiology in the elderly, Alzheimer's disease, and the effects of drugs on balance and postural control in the elderly. He has been an author of numerous publications in the geriatric, pharmacy and medical literature, and has presented original research at numerous professional meetings.

Dr Semla is an active member of several professional organizations including the American Geriatrics Society (AGS), the Illinois Geriatrics Society, the Gerontological Society of America (GSA), the International Society for Pharmacoepidemiology (ISPE), the American College of Clinical Pharmacy (ACCP), and the Illinois College of Clinical Pharmacy (ICCP).

Judith L. Beizer, PharmD

Dr Beizer received a bachelor's degree in pharmacy from the St Louis College of Pharmacy and then earned a doctor of pharmacy degree from the University of Tennessee. After pursuing a residency in clinical pharmacy at the Hospital of the University of Pennsylvania, she completed a fellowship in geriatric pharmacy at Montefiore Medical Center, Bronx, NY. During her fellowship, Dr Beizer was involved in a National Institute on Aging (NIA) grant concerning medication use and pharmacist intervention in community-dwelling elderly.

Dr Beizer is currently an Associate Clinical Professor at St John's University College of Pharmacy and Allied Health Professions, Jamaica, NY. As part of her duties, she serves as Clinical Coordinator for Pharmacy at The Parker Jewish Geriatric Institute, a long-term care facility in New Hyde Park, NY. At this facility she has expanded clinical pharmacy services and oversees students on rotation. Dr Beizer speaks regularly on the topic of medication use in the elderly and has published articles and abstracts on various issues in geriatric pharmacotherapy.

Dr Beizer is a member of several professional organizations, including the American Society of Hospital Pharmacists (ASHP), American Society of Consultant Pharmacists (ASCP), American College of Clinical Pharmacy (ACCP), and the Gerontological Society of America (GSA). She is a past chairperson of the ASHP Special Interest Group on Geriatric Pharmacy Practice.

Martin D. Higbee, PharmD

Dr Higbee received a bachelor's degree in pharmacy from The University of Utah in 1973. After a year of hospital pharmacy practice and clinical pharmacy experience received at The University of Utah, he entered the Doctor of Pharmacy degree program at The University of Texas at San Antonio. After graduation in 1977, he joined the University of Utah College of Pharmacy faculty. He became involved in the development of Salt Lake Veteran Administration Medical Center's Geriatric Treatment and Evaluation Unit. After the establishment of this unit, Dr Higbee created an ASHP accredited post-doctoral Geriatric Residency through the Veteran's Administration Medical Center and The

University of Utah College of Pharmacy. Dr Higbee was also on the editorial staff for the Eli Lily - AACP Geriatric Curriculum for Pharmacists project which created a geriatric textbook and curriculum for educators.

Dr Higbee joined the faculty at The University of Arizona in 1987. As part of his teaching responsibilities, he is the Clinical Pharmacist Consultant for the Veterans Administration Medical Center in Tucson, Arizona, where he is preceptor for doctor of pharmacy students taking their geriatric ambulatory care clinical experience rotation. Dr Higbee is also a nursing home consultant for local nursing homes in Arizona.

Dr Higbee regularly speaks locally and nationally on geriatric drug therapy topics and has published articles, chapters, and abstracts on various geriatric research and pharmacotherapy issues.

Dr Higbee is a member of numerous professional organizations, including American Society of Hospital Pharmacists (ASHP), American Pharmaceutical Association (APhA), American Society of Consultant Pharmacists (ASCP), American Association of Colleges of Pharmacy (AACP), and American College of Clinical Pharmacy (ACCP). He is a past chairman of the ASHP Special Interest Group on Geriatric Pharmacy Practice and past member of the AACP Task Force on Aging.

USE OF THE GERIATRIC DOSAGE HANDBOOK

The *Geriatric Dosage Handbook* is organized into a drug information section, an appendix, and a therapeutic category index.

The drug information section of the handbook, wherein all drugs are listed alphabetically, details information pertinent to each drug. Extensive cross-referencing is provided by brand name and synonyms.

Drug information is presented in a consistent format and will provide the following:

Generic Name	U.S. Adopted Name
Pronunciation Guide	
Related Information	Cross-reference to other pertinent drug information found in the Appendix
Brand Names	Common trade names
Synonyms	
Generic Available	Indicates if a generic form is available
Use	Information pertaining to appropriate use of the drug
Restrictions	According to DEA classification
Contraindications	Information pertaining to inappropriate use of the drug
Warnings	Hazardous conditions related to use of the drug and what to observe and parameters to monitor during therapy with the drug
Precautions	What to observe during therapy and disease states in which the drug should be cautiously used
Adverse Reactions	
Toxicology	
Drug Interactions	
Stability	
Overdosage	Comments and/or considerations are
Test Interactions	offered when appropriate
Patient Information	
Nursing Implications	
Monitoring Parameters	
Additional Information	
Mechanism of Action	How drugs work in the body to elicit a response
Pharmacodynamics	Dose response relationships including onset of action, time of peak action, and duration of action
Pharmacokinetics	Drug movement through the body over time which helps predict drug action. The magnitude of a drug's effect depends on the drug concentration at the site of action and deals with absorption, distribution, metabolism, and excretion.
Usual Dosage	The amount of the drug to be typically given or taken during therapy
Reference Range	Therapeutic and toxic serum concentrations listed when appropriate
Special Geriatric Considerations	Pertinent information specific to the elderly
Dosage Forms	Information with regard to form, strength, and availability of the drug
References	Sources used to verify included information

Appendix

The appendix offers a compilation of tables, guidelines, nomograms, and conversion information which can often be helpful when considering patient care.

Therapeutic Category Index

This index provides a useful listing of drugs by their therapeutic classification.

SAFE WRITING

Health professionals and their support personnel frequently produce handwritten copies of information they see in print; therefore, such information is subjected to even greater possibilities for error or misinterpretation on the part of others. Thus, particular care must be given to how drug names and strengths are expressed when creating written health care documents.

The following are a few examples of safe writing rules suggested by the Institute for Safe Medication Practices, Inc.*

1. There should be a space between a number and its units as it is easier to read. There should be no periods after the abbreviations mg or mL.

Correct	Incorrect
10 mg	10mg
100 mg	100mg

2. Never place a decimal and a zero after a whole number (2 mg is correct and 2.0 mg is incorrect). If the decimal point is not seen because it falls on a line or because individuals are working from copies where the decimal point is not seen, this causes a tenfold overdose.

3. Just the opposite is true for numbers less than one. Always place a zero before a naked decimal (0.5 mL is correct, .5 mL is **in**correct).

4. Never abbreviate the word unit. The handwritten U or u, looks like a 0 (zero), and may cause a tenfold overdose error to be made.

5. Q.D. is not a safe abbreviation for once daily, as when the Q is followed by a sloppy dot, it looks like QID which means four times daily.

6. O.D. is not a safe abbreviation for once daily, as it is properly interpreted as meaning "right eye" and has caused liquid medications such as saturated solution of potassium iodide and lugol's solution to be administered incorrectly. There is no safe abbreviation for once daily. It must be written out in full.

7. Do not use chemical names such as 6-mercaptopurine or 6-thioguanine, as 6 fold overdoses have been given when these were not recognized as chemical names. The proper names of these drugs are mercaptopurine or thioguanine.

8. Do not abbreviate drug names (5FC, 6MP, 5-ASA, MTX, HCTZ CPZ, PBZ, etc) as they are misinterpreted and cause error.

9. Do not use the apothecary system or symbols.

10. Do not abbreviate microgram as μg; instead use mcg as there is less likelihood of misinterpretation.

11. When writing an outpatient prescription, write a complete prescription. A complete prescription can prevent the prescriber, the pharmacist, and/or the patient from making a mistake and can eliminate the need for further clarification.

The legible prescriptions should contain:

a. patient's full name

b. for pediatric or geriatric patients: their age (or weight where applicable)

c. drug name, dosage form and strength; if a drug is new or rarely prescribed, print this information

d. number or amount to be dispensed

e. complete instructions for the patient, including the purpose of the medication

f. when there are recognized contraindications for a prescribed drug, indicate to the pharmacist that you are aware of this fact (ie, when prescribing a potassium salt for a patient receiving an ACE inhibitor, write "K serum leveling being monitored")

---

*From "Safe Writing" by Davis NM, PharmD and Cohen MR, MS, Lecturers and Consultants for Safe Medication Practices, 1143 Wright Drive, Huntingdon Valley, PA 19006. Phone: (215) 947-7566.

ALPHABETICAL
LISTING OF
DRUGS

Absorbine Jr.® Antifungal [OTC] *see* Tolnaftate *on page 705*

Absorbine® Antifungal [OTC] *see* Tolnaftate *on page 705*

Absorbine® Jock Itch [OTC] *see* Tolnaftate *on page 705*

Accupril® *see* Quinapril Hydrochloride *on page 616*

Accurbron® *see* Theophylline *on page 681*

Acebutolol Hydrochloride (a se byoo' toe lole)
Related Information
Beta-Blockers Comparison *on page 804-805*
Brand Names Sectral®
Generic Available No
Therapeutic Class Antiarrhythmic Agent, Class II; Beta-Adrenergic Blocker
Use Treatment of hypertension; ventricular arrhythmias; although not an approved indication, beta-adrenergic blockers generally reduce angina
Contraindications Hypersensitivity to beta-blocking agents, uncompensated congestive heart failure; cardiogenic shock; bradycardia or heart block; sinus node dysfunction; A-V conduction abnormalities. Although acebutolol primarily blocks beta$_1$-receptors, high doses can result in beta$_2$-receptor blockage. Therefore, use with caution in elderly with bronchospastic lung disease and renal dysfunction. **Note:** Geriatric patients often have decreased renal function.
Warnings Abrupt withdrawal of beta-blockers may result in an exaggerated cardiac beta-adrenergic responsiveness. Symptomatology has included reports of tachycardia, hypertension, ischemia, angina, myocardial infarction, and sudden death. It is recommended that patients be tapered gradually off of beta-blockers over a 2-week period rather than via abrupt discontinuation.
Precautions Diabetes mellitus (may mask signs/symptoms of hypoglycemia), renal function decline, myasthenia gravis, and severe peripheral vascular disease; use with caution in patients with bronchospasm disease or congestive heart failure, patients undergoing anesthesia, and hyperthyroidism
Adverse Reactions
Cardiovascular: Persistent bradycardia, torsade de pointes, ventricular arrhythmias, shortness of breath, heart block, hypotension, chest pain, edema, heart failure, Raynaud's phenomena, facial swelling
Central nervous system: Depression, confusion, dizziness, insomnia, lethargy, headache, nightmares, fatigue, cold extremities
Dermatologic: Rash, pruritus
Gastrointestinal: Constipation, diarrhea, nausea, dry mouth, gastritis, anorexia
Genitourinary: Impotence, decreased libido, urinary retention, urinary frequency
Neuromuscular & skeletal: Joint pain, muscle cramps
Ocular: Blurred vision, visual disturbance
Overdosage See Toxicology
Toxicology Sympathomimetics (eg, epinephrine or dopamine), glucagon or a pacemaker can be used to treat the toxic bradycardia, asystole, and/or hypotension. Initially, fluids may be the best treatment for toxic hypotension. Patients should remain supine; serum glucose and potassium should be measured. Use supportive measures: lavage, syrup of ipecac; atenolol may be removed by hemodialysis. I.V. glucose should be administered for hypoglycemia; seizures may be treated with phenytoin or diazepam intravenously; continuous monitoring of blood pressure and EKG is necessary. If PVCs occur, treat with lidocaine or phenytoin; avoid quinidine, procainamide, and disopyramide since these agents further depress myocardial function. Bronchospasm can be treated with theophylline on beta$_2$ agonists (epinephrine).
Drug Interactions
Pharmacologic action of beta-antagonists may be decreased by aluminum compounds, calcium salts, barbiturates, cholestyramine, colestipol, NSAIDs, penicillins (ampicillin), rifampin, salicylates, sulfinpyrazone, thyroid hormones; hypoglycemic effect of sulfonylureas may be blunted
Pharmacologic effect of beta-antagonists may be enhanced with concomitant use of calcium channel blockers, oral contraceptives, flecainide (bioavailability and effect of flecainide also enhanced), haloperidol (hypotensive effects of both drugs), H$_2$ antagonists (decreased metabolism), hydralazine (both drugs hypotensive effects increased), loop diuretics (increased serum levels of beta-blockers except atenolol), MAO inhibitors, phenothiazines, propafenone, quinidine, quinolones, thioamines; beta-blockers may decrease clearance of acetaminophen; beta-blockers may increase anticoagulant effects of warfarin (propranolol); benzodiazepine effects enhanced by the lipophilic beta-blockers (atenolol does not interact); significant and fatal increases in blood pressure have occurred after decrease in dose or discontinuation of clonidine in patients receiving both clonidine and beta-blockers together (reduce doses of each cautiously with small decreases); peripheral ischemia of ergot alkaloids enhanced by beta-blockers; beta-blockers increase serum concentration of lidocaine; beta-blockers increase hypotensive effect of prazosin
Mechanism of Action Competitively blocks beta$_1$-adrenergic receptors with little or no effect on beta$_2$-receptors except at high doses. Exhibits membrane stabilizing and

intrinsic sympathomimetic activity; low lipid solubility, therefore, little crosses blood-brain barrier.

Pharmacokinetics
Absorption: Oral: Well absorbed, 90%
Protein binding: 25%
Metabolism: Undergoes extensive first-pass
Bioavailability: Average, 40%
Half-life: 3-4 hours
Time to peak: 2-4 hours
Elimination: Primarily excreted by bile and intestinal wall 50% to 60%; renal excretion 30% to 40%; some hepatic elimination occurs

Usual Dosage Oral:
Geriatrics: Initial: 200-400 mg/day; dose reduction due to age-related decrease in Cl_{cr} will be necessary; do not exceed 800 mg/day

Adults: 400-800 mg/day in 2 divided doses; maximum: 1200 mg/day

Dosing adjustment in renal impairment:
Cl_{cr} 25-49 mL/minute/1.73 m^2: Reduce dose by 50%
Cl_{cr} <25 mL/minute/1.73 m^2: Reduce dose by 75%

Dosing adjustment in hepatic impairment: Use with caution

Monitoring Parameters Blood pressure, orthostatic hypotension, heart rate, CNS effects

Test Interactions Increased triglycerides, potassium, uric acid, cholesterol (S), glucose; decreased HDL

Patient Information Do not discontinue medication abruptly, sudden stopping of medication may precipitate or cause angina; consult pharmacist or physician before taking with other adrenergic drugs (eg, cold medications); notify physician if any of the following symptoms occur: difficult breathing, night cough, swelling of extremities, slow pulse, dizziness, lightheadedness, confusion, depression, skin rash, fever, sore throat, unusual bleeding or bruising; may produce drowsiness, dizziness, lightheadedness, blurred vision, confusion; use with caution while driving or performing tasks requiring alertness; may mask signs of hypoglycemia in diabetics; may be taken without regard to meals

Nursing Implications Advise against abrupt withdrawal

Special Geriatric Considerations Since bioavailability increased in elderly about twofold, geriatric patients may require lower maintenance doses, therefore, as serum and tissue concentrations increase beta$_1$ selectivity diminishes; due to alterations in the beta-adrenergic autonomic nervous system, beta-adrenergic blockade may result in less hemodynamic response than seen in younger adults. Studies indicate that despite decreased sensitivity to the chronotropic effects of beta blockade with age, there appears to be an increased myocardial sensitivity to the negative inotropic effect during stress (ie, exercise). Controlled trials have shown the overall response rate for propranolol to be only 20% to 50% in elderly populations. Therefore, all beta-adrenergic blocking drugs may result in a decreased response as compared to younger adults. Adjust dose for renal function in the elderly.

Dosage Forms Capsule: 200 mg, 400 mg

References
Kligman EW and Higbee MD, "Drug Therapy for Hypertension in the Elderly," *J Fam Pract*, 1989, 28(1):81-7.
Levison SP, "Treating Hypertension in the Elderly," *Clin Geriatr Med*, 1988, 4(1):1-12.
Vestal RE, Wood AJ, and Shand DG, "Reduced Beta-Adrenoceptor Sensitivity in the Elderly," *Clin Pharmacol Ther*, 1979, 26(2):181-6.
Yin FC, Raizes, GS, Guarnieri T, et al, "Age-Associated Decrease in Ventricular Response to Haemodynamic Stress During Beta-Adrenergic Blockade," *Br Heart J*, 1978, 40(12):1349-55.

Acephen® [OTC] *see* Acetaminophen *on this page*

Acetaminophen (a seet a min' oh fen)

Brand Names Acephen® [OTC]; Aceta® [OTC]; Anacin-3® [OTC]; Apacet® [OTC]; Banesin® [OTC]; Dapa® [OTC]; Datril® [OTC]; Dorcol® [OTC]; Feverall™ [OTC]; Genapap® [OTC]; Halenol® [OTC]; Neopap® [OTC]; Panadol® [OTC]; Tempra® [OTC]; Tylenol® [OTC]; Valadol® [OTC]

Synonyms APAP; N-Acetyl-P-Aminophenol; Paracetamol

Generic Available Yes

Therapeutic Class Analgesic, Non-narcotic; Antipyretic

Use Treatment of mild to moderate pain and fever; does not have antirheumatic effects

Contraindications Hypersensitivity to acetaminophen, G-6-PD deficiency

Warnings May cause severe hepatic toxicity with overdose; chronic daily doses of 5-8 g over several weeks or 3-4 g/day for 1 year have resulted in liver damage; use with caution in patients with alcoholic liver disease

Adverse Reactions
Dermatologic: Rash
Renal: Renal injury with chronic use
Miscellaneous: Hypersensitivity reactions (rare)

Overdosage Symptoms of overdose include hepatic necrosis, transient azotemia,

(Continued)

13

Acetaminophen (Continued)

renal tubular necrosis with acute toxicity, anemia, and GI disturbances with chronic toxicity

Toxicology Acetylcysteine 140 mg/kg orally (loading) followed by 70 mg/kg every 4 hours for 17 doses; therapy should be initiated based upon laboratory analysis suggesting high probability of hepatotoxic potential. Activated charcoal is very effective at binding acetaminophen; however, the dose of acetylcysteine may need to be increased. Intravenous acetylcysteine should be reserved for patients unable to take oral forms.

Drug Interactions
Decreased therapeutic effect: Rifampin
Increased hepatotoxicity with barbiturates, carbamazepine, hydantoins, sulfinpyrazone

Mechanism of Action Inhibits the synthesis of prostaglandins in the central nervous system and peripherally blocks pain impulse generation; produces antipyresis from inhibition of hypothalamic heat-regulating center

Pharmacokinetics
Protein binding: 20% to 50%
Metabolism: At normal therapeutic dosages the parent compound is metabolized in the liver to sulfate and glucuronide metabolites, while a small amount is metabolized by microsomal mixed function oxidases to a highly reactive intermediate (N-acetyl-imidoquinone) which is conjugated with glutathione and inactivated; at toxic doses (as little as 4 g in a single day) glutathione can become depleted, and conjugation becomes insufficient to meet the metabolic demand causing an increase in N-acetyl-imidoquinone concentration, which is thought to cause hepatic cell necrosis
Half-life: 1-3 hours; may be increased in the elderly, but this should not affect drug dosing
Time to peak serum concentration: Oral: 10-60 minutes after normal doses, but may be delayed in acute overdoses

Usual Dosage Geriatrics and Adults: Oral, rectal: 325-650 mg every 4-6 hours or 1000 mg 3-4 times/day; do **not** exceed 4 g/day

Dosing interval in renal impairment:
Cl$_{cr}$ 10-50 mL/minute: Administer every 6 hours
Cl$_{cr}$ <10 mL/minute: Administer every 8 hours (metabolites accumulate)
Moderately dialyzable (20% to 50%)

Dosing adjustment/comments in hepatic impairment: Appears to be well tolerated in cirrhosis; serum levels may need monitoring with long-term use

Monitoring Parameters Relief of pain or fever
Reference Range Toxic concentration with probable hepatotoxicity: >200 μg/mL at 4 hours or 50 μg/mL at 12 hours
Test Interactions Increased chloride, bilirubin, uric acid, glucose, ammonia (B), chloride (S), uric acid (S), alkaline phosphatase (S), chloride (S); decreased sodium, bicarbonate, calcium (S)
Patient Information Do not exceed recommended dosage; check cough and cold preparations for acetaminophen content
Nursing Implications Monitor patient for relief of pain and/or fever
Special Geriatric Considerations See Warnings and Usual Dosage
Dosage Forms
Caplet: 160 mg, 325 mg, 500 mg
Elixir: 120 mg/5 mL, 160 mg/5 mL, 167 mg/5 mL, 325 mg/5 mL
Liquid, oral: 160 mg/5 mL, 500 mg/15 mL
Suppository: 325 mg, 600 mg
Tablet: 325 mg, 500 mg, 650 mg

Acetaminophen and Codeine (a seet a min' oh fen)

Brand Names Capital® and Codeine; Phenaphen® With Codeine; Tylenol® With Codeine
Synonyms Codeine and Acetaminophen
Generic Available Yes
Therapeutic Class Analgesic, Narcotic
Use Relief of mild to moderate pain
Restrictions C-III
Contraindications Hypersensitivity to acetaminophen or codeine phosphate
Warnings Tablets contain metabisulfite which may cause allergic reactions; acetaminophen may cause hepatic damage in overdose or with chronic use of high doses
Precautions Use with caution in patients with hypersensitivity reactions to other phenanthrene derivative opioid agonists (morphine, hydrocodone, hydromorphone, levorphanol, oxycodone, oxymorphone) or respiratory disease or compromise
Adverse Reactions
Central nervous system: CNS depression, dizziness, drowsiness, sedation

Gastrointestinal: Constipation, nausea, vomiting
Ocular: Miosis
Respiratory: Respiratory depression
Miscellaneous: Physical and psychological dependence with prolonged use, biliary or urinary tract spasm

Overdosage Symptoms of overdose include hepatic necrosis, blood dyscrasias, respiratory depression

Toxicology Acetylcysteine 140 mg/kg orally (loading) followed by 70 mg/kg every 4 hours for 17 doses; therapy should begin after availability of serum acetaminophen level. Naloxone (2 mg I.V.) can also be used to reverse the toxic effects of the opiate (see caution with naloxone use.) Activated charcoal is effective at binding certain chemicals and this is especially true for acetaminophen; however, dose of acetylcysteine may need to be increased by 30% or charcoal should be removed first.

Drug Interactions Increased toxicity: CNS depressants, phenothiazines, tricyclic antidepressants, guanabenz, MAO inhibitors (may also → ↓ blood pressure)

Usual Dosage Doses should be titrated to appropriate analgesic effect
Geriatrics: 1 Tylenol® [#3] or 2 Tylenol® [#2] tablets every 4 hours; do not exceed 4g/ day acetaminophen
Adults: 1-2 tablets every 4 hours with a maximum of 12 tablets/24 hours

Monitoring Parameters Relief of pain, respiratory and mental status, blood pressure, bowel function

Patient Information May cause drowsiness; avoid alcoholic beverages; do not exceed recommended dose

Nursing Implications Observe patient for excessive sedation or confusion, respiratory depression, constipation

Special Geriatric Considerations The duration of action of codeine may be prolonged in the elderly; in addition, enhanced analgesia has been seen in elderly patients on therapeutic doses of narcotics; if one tablet/dose is used, it may be useful to add an additional 325 mg of acetaminophen to maximize analgesic effect

Dosage Forms
Capsule:
#2: Acetaminophen 325 mg and codeine phosphate 15 mg (C-III)
#3: Acetaminophen 325 mg and codeine phosphate 30 mg (C-III)
#4: Acetaminophen 325 mg and codeine phosphate 60 mg (C-III)
Elixir: Acetaminophen 120 mg and codeine phosphate 12 mg per 5 mL with alcohol 7% (C-V)
Suspension, oral, alcohol free: Acetaminophen 120 mg and codeine phosphate 12 mg per 5 mL (C-V)
Tablet: Acetaminophen 500 mg and codeine phosphate 30 mg (C-III); acetaminophen 650 mg and codeine phosphate 30 mg (C-III)
Tablet:
#1: Acetaminophen 300 mg and codeine phosphate 7.5 mg (C-III)
#2: Acetaminophen 300 mg and codeine phosphate 15 mg (C-III)
#3: Acetaminophen 300 mg and codeine phosphate 30 mg (C-III)
#4: Acetaminophen 300 mg and codeine phosphate 60 mg (C-III)

Acetaminophen and Hydrocodone *see* Hydrocodone and Acetaminophen *on page 350*

Acetaminophen and Oxycodone *see* Oxycodone and Acetaminophen *on page 528*

Aceta® [OTC] *see* Acetaminophen *on page 13*

Acetazolamide (a set a zole' a mide)
Related Information
Glaucoma Drug Therapy Comparison *on page 810*
Brand Names AK-Zol®; Dazamide®; Diamox®
Generic Available Yes
Therapeutic Class Anticonvulsant, Miscellaneous; Carbonic Anhydrase Inhibitor; Diuretic, Carbonic Anhydrase Inhibitor
Use Lower intraocular pressure to treat glaucoma, also as a diuretic, adjunct treatment of refractory seizure disorders and acute altitude sickness
Contraindications Hypersensitivity to acetazolamide or other sulfonamides; patients with hepatic or significant renal insufficiency; patients with decreased serum sodium and/or potassium; patients with adrenocortical insufficiency; severe pulmonary obstruction; long-term use in noncongestive angle-closure glaucoma
Warnings I.M. administration is painful because of the alkaline pH of the drug
Precautions Use with caution in patients with respiratory acidosis and diabetes mellitus; impairment of mental alertness and/or physical coordination may occur; electrolyte balance should be monitored
Adverse Reactions
Central nervous system: Fever, paresthesias, drowsiness, fatigue, malaise, confusion, convulsions

(Continued)

ALPHABETICAL LISTING OF DRUGS

Acetazolamide *(Continued)*

Dermatologic: Rash (including Stevens-Johnson syndrome, erythema multiforme, toxic epidermal necrolysis)

Endocrine & metabolic: Hyperchloremic metabolic acidosis in up to 55% of older patients, hypokalemia, elevation of blood glucose

Gastrointestinal: GI irritation, anorexia, dryness of the mouth, vomiting, constipation

Genitourinary: Urinary frequency

Hematologic: Bone marrow suppression

Neuromuscular & skeletal: Muscular weakness

Ocular: Myopia

Renal: Dysuria, renal calculi, glycosuria, hematuria

Toxicology For decontamination, lavage/activated charcoal with cathartic; hemodialysis may remove as much as 30% of dose

Drug Interactions

Increase lithium excretion and decreased excretion of amphetamines, quinidine, procainamide, flecainide, phenobarbital, and salicylates by alkalinization of the urine

Salicylates may also increase risk of metabolic acidosis

Hypokalemia may be compounded with concurrent use of diuretics or steroids

Primidone's absorption may be delayed

Digitalis toxicity may occur if hypokalemia is untreated

Stability Reconstituted solution may be stored under refrigeration (2°C to 8°C) for 24 hours (the product contains no preservative); discard unused solutions after 24 hours

Mechanism of Action Reversible inhibition of the enzyme carbonic anhydrase resulting in increased renal excretion of sodium, potassium, bicarbonate, and water; enzyme inhibition also decreases aqueous humor production, thus decreasing intraocular pressure

Pharmacodynamics

Onset of action: Lowering of intraocular pressure varies between 2 minutes with the I.V. form to 2 hours with the sustained release capsule

Peak effect:
I.V.: 15 minutes
Capsule, sustained release: 8-12 hours
Tablet: 1-4 hours

Duration:
I.V.: 4-5 hours
Capsule, sustained release: 18-24 hours
Tablet: 8-12 hours

Pharmacokinetics

Distribution: Into erythrocytes, kidneys and crosses the blood-brain barrier

Protein binding: 95% bound to serum proteins; increased plasma concentrations secondary to decreased clearance in older persons with decreased renal function; these changes increase the risk of hyperchloremic acidosis

Half-life: 2.4-5.8 hours

Elimination: 70% to 100% of the I.V. or tablet dose is excreted unchanged in the urine within 24 hours

Usual Dosage

Geriatrics: Oral: Initial: 250 mg once or twice daily; use lowest effective dose possible

Adults:
Glaucoma:
Oral: 250 mg 1-4 times/day or 500 mg sustained release capsule twice daily
I.M., I.V.: 250-500 mg, may repeat in 2-4 hours; standard doses may lead to excessive plasma concentrations
Edema: Oral, I.M., I.V.: 250-375 mg once daily
Epilepsy: Oral: 8-30 mg/kg/day in 1-4 divided doses
Altitude sickness: Oral: 250 mg every 6-12 hours

Dosing interval in renal impairment:
Cl_{cr} 10-50 mL/minute: Administer every 12 hours
Cl_{cr} <10 mL/minute: Avoid use → ineffective, may potentiate acidosis
Moderately dialyzable (20% to 50%)

Administration Reconstitute each 500 mg vial with 5 mL of sterile water for injection to yield a concentration of 100 mg/mL; may cause an alteration in taste, especially carbonated beverages; short-acting tablets may be crushed and suspended in cherry or chocolate syrup to disguise the bitter taste of the drug, do not use fruit juices, alternatively submerge tablet in 10 mL of hot water and add 10 mL honey or syrup

Monitoring Parameters Intraocular pressure, serum bicarbonate, sodium and potassium, periodic CBC with differential

Reference Range Total: 5-10 μg/mL; Free (unbound) 0.25-0.5 μg/mL

Test Interactions Increased chloride, bilirubin, uric acid, glucose, ammonia (B), chloride (S), uric acid (S), alkaline phosphatase (S), chloride (S); decreased sodium, bicarbonate, calcium (S)

Patient Information Report numbness or tingling of extremities to physician; do not crush, chew, or swallow contents of long-acting capsule, but may be opened and sprinkled on soft food; ability to perform tasks requiring mental alertness and/or physical coordination may be impaired; take with food

Additional Information Drug may cause substantial increase in blood glucose in some diabetic patients; sustained release capsule is not recommended for treatment of epilepsy

Special Geriatric Considerations Malaise and complaints of tiredness and myalgia are signs of excessive dosing and acidosis in the elderly

Dosage Forms
Capsule, sustained release: 500 mg
Injection: 500 mg
Tablet: 125 mg, 250 mg

References
Chapron DJ, Gomolin IH, and Sweeney KR, "Acetazolamide Blood Concentrations are Excessive in the Elderly: Propensity for Acidosis and Relationship to Renal Function," *J Clin Pharmacol*, 1989, 29(4):348-53.
Chapron DJ, Sweeney KR, Feig PU, et al, "Influence of Advanced Age on the Disposition of Acetazolamide," *Br J Clin Pharmacol*, 1985, 19:363-71.
Heller I, Halevy J, Cohen S, et al, "Significant Metabolic Acidosis Induced by Acetazolamide," *Arch Intern Med*, 1985, 145:1815-7.

Acetohexamide (a set oh hex' a mide)

Brand Names Dymelor®
Generic Available Yes
Therapeutic Class Antidiabetic Agent; Hypoglycemic Agent, Oral; Sulfonylurea Agent
Use Adjunct to diet for the management of mild to moderately severe, stable noninsulin-dependent (type II) diabetes mellitus
Contraindications Diabetes complicated by ketoacidosis, therapy of type I diabetes, hypersensitivity to sulfonylureas
Precautions Avoid alcohol or products containing alcohol; patients with liver disease or reduced renal function may have increased risk for symptomatic hypoglycemia
Adverse Reactions
Central nervous system: Headache
Endocrine & metabolic: Severe hypoglycemia, hyponatremia, syndrome of inappropriate antidiuretic hormone
Gastrointestinal: Nausea, vomiting, epigastric fullness, heartburn, diarrhea
Overdosage Symptoms of overdose include low blood sugar, tingling of lips and tongue, nausea, yawning, confusion, agitation, tachycardia, sweating, convulsions, stupor, and coma
Toxicology Hypoglycemia should be managed with 50 mL I.V. dextrose 50% followed immediately with a continuous infusion of 10% dextrose in water (administer at a rate sufficient enough to approach a serum glucose level of 100 mg/dL). The use of corticosteroids to treat the hypoglycemia is controversial, however, the addition of 100 mg of hydrocortisone to the dextrose infusion may prove helpful.
Drug Interactions Monitor patient closely; large number of drugs interact with sulfonylureas to enhance their hypoglycemic effects including oral anticoagulants, salicylates, NSAIDs, sulfonamides, phenylbutazone, insulin, clofibrate, fenfluramine, fluconazole, gemfibrozil, H_2 antagonists, methyldopa, tricyclic antidepressants, urinary acidifiers; decreased hypoglycemic effects by beta-blockers, cholestyramine, diazoxide, hydantoins, rifampin, thiazides, urinary alkalinizers
Mechanism of Action Believed to cause hypoglycemia by stimulating insulin release from the pancreatic beta cells; reduces glucose output from the liver (decreases gluconeogenesis); insulin sensitivity is increased at peripheral target sites (alters receptor sensitivity/receptor density); potentiates effects of ADH; may produce mild diuresis and significant uricosuric activity
Pharmacodynamics
Peak hypoglycemic effect: Within 8-10 hours
Duration: 12-24 hours (prolonged with renal impairment)
Pharmacokinetics
Protein binding: ~90% (ionic/nonionic)
Metabolism: In the liver to potent active metabolite
Half-life: 5-6 hours (parent compound has half-life of 0.8-2.4 hours)
Elimination: Urinary excretion <40% as unchanged drug; metabolite, hydroxyhexamide is more potent and is excreted less rapidly; ~80% to 95% of dose excreted in urine within 24 hours; ~15% is excreted in bile
Usual Dosage Geriatrics and Adults: Oral: 250 mg to 1.5 g/day in 1-2 divided doses; if daily dose is ≤1 g it should be as a single daily dose

Dosing adjustment in renal impairment: Cl_{cr} <50 mL/minute: Avoid use; prolonged hypoglycemia occurs in azotemic patients

Dosing adjustment in hepatic impairment: Initiate therapy at lower than recommended doses

Monitoring Parameters Fasting blood glucose, hemoglobin A_{1c} or fructosamine
Reference Range Fasting blood glucose: Geriatrics: 100-150 mg/dL; Adults: 80-140 mg/dL

(Continued)

Acetohexamide *(Continued)*

Test Interactions Decreased glucose, uric acid, decreased prothrombin time (S), decreased sodium (S)

Patient Information If nausea or stomach upset occurs, may be taken with food; avoid hypoglycemia, eat regularly, do not skip meals; keep sugar source with you

Nursing Implications Blood (preferred) and urine glucose concentrations should be monitored when therapy is started; normally takes 7 days to determine therapeutic response; patients who are anorexic or NPO may need to have their dose held to avoid hypoglycemia

Additional Information Produces a diuretic effect and increases the urinary excretion of uric acid

Special Geriatric Considerations Not considered a drug of choice in the elderly because of the potentially prolonged half-life of the more active metabolite; has not been specifically studied in the elderly; how "tightly" a geriatric patient's blood sugar of <150 mg/dL is now an acceptable end point. Such a decision should be based on the patient's functional and cognitive status, how well they recognize hypoglycemic or hyperglycemic symptoms, and how to respond to them, and their other disease states.

Dosage Forms Tablet: 250 mg, 500 mg

Acetophenazine Maleate *(a set oh fen' a zeen)*

Related Information

Antipsychotic Agents Comparison *on page 801*
Antipsychotic Medication Guidelines *on page 754*

Brand Names Tindal®

Generic Available No

Therapeutic Class Antipsychotic Agent

Use Management of manifestations of psychotic disorders; depressive neurosis; alcohol withdrawal; nausea and vomiting; Tourette's syndrome; Huntington's chorea; spasmodic torticollis and Reye's syndrome; nonpsychotic symptoms associated with dementia in elderly; see Special Geriatric Considerations

Contraindications Known hypersensitivity to acetophenazine; severe CNS depression, cross-sensitivity to other phenothiazines may exist; avoid use in patients with narrow-angle glaucoma, blood dyscrasias, severe liver or cardiac disease; subcortical brain damage; circulatory collapse; severe hypotension or hypertension

Warnings

Tardive dyskinesia: Prevalence rate may be 40% in elderly; elderly women especially at risk; embarrassment from dyskinesias may lead to greater social isolation; development of the syndrome and the irreversible nature are proportional to duration and total cumulative dose over time. May be reversible if diagnosed early in therapy; intermittent use of antipsychotics (not proven to be clinically effective) helps decrease total cumulative dose.

EPS: Extrapyramidal reactions are more common in elderly with up to 50% developing these reactions after age 60. These reactions may be more common in dementia patients. Drug-induced **Parkinson's syndrome** occurs often. Discontinuation usually resolves symptoms but may take weeks to months (12+) to clear. **Akathisia** is the most common EPS reaction in elderly. The symptoms of motor restlessness are difficult to diagnose in demented elderly; increased nervousness, assertiveness, restlessness with constant movement may indicate this adverse event. Consider decreasing dose of antipsychotic to treat as well as diagnose problem; usually see this reaction within 2-3 months of initiating antipsychotic drug.

Anticholinergic effects: These side effects most common with low potency antipsychotics (eg, thioridazine, chlorpromazine). CNS toxicity occurs more frequently and severely in elderly; increased confusion, memory loss, psychotic behavior, and agitation frequently occur as a consequence of anticholinergic effects to antipsychotic agents. Peripheral anticholinergic action troublesome to elderly; most peripheral anticholinergic effects last only 2-3 weeks; see Adverse Reactions.

Orthostatic hypotension: More common with low potency agents (eg, thioridazine, chlorpromazine, and clozapine) but of concern with all antipsychotic agents; orthostasis due to alpha-receptor blockade by antipsychotic agents. Elderly present many risk factors for orthostatic hypotension: blunted baroreceptor reflexes, decreased vascular tone, decreased vascular volume, and possible presence of cardiac diseases which result in decreased cardiac output.

Sedation: Common side effect with antipsychotic therapy; should not be used as a hypnotic unless insomnia is associated with target behavior symptoms treated with antipsychotic medications; see Special Geriatric Considerations. Anecdotal reports suggesting antipsychotic sedation in nonpsychotic patients is extremely unpleasant due to feelings of depersonalization, derealization, and dysphoria. Due to the long duration of action with antipsychotic drugs, these reactions may last up to 24 hours and result in decreased daytime function.

Cardiac toxicity: Life-threatening arrhythmias have occurred at therapeutic doses of antipsychotics. Thioridazine more commonly demonstrates EKG changes than other antipsychotics; suggested to use high potency antipsychotic agents (ie, haloperidol) in patients with cardiac conduction defects.

Precautions Use with caution in patients with severe cardiovascular disorder, seizures, and Parkinson's disease; benefits of therapy must be weighed against risks

Adverse Reactions

Cardiovascular: EKG changes, hypotension (especially orthostatic), tachycardia, arrhythmias, abnormal T waves with prolonged ventricular repolarization

Central nervous system: Drowsiness, restlessness, anxiety, extrapyramidal reactions, dystonic reactions, pseudoparkinsonian signs and symptoms, tardive dyskinesia, neuroleptic malignant syndrome, seizures, altered central temperature regulation

Dermatologic: Hyperpigmentation, pruritus, rash, contact dermatitis, photosensitivity (rare)

Endocrine & metabolic: Amenorrhea, galactorrhea, gynecomastia

Gastrointestinal: Dry mouth (problem for denture user), constipation, adynamic ileus, GI upset, weight gain

Genitourinary: Overflow incontinence, urinary retention, priapism, sexual dysfunction (up to 60%)

Hematologic: Agranulocytosis, leukopenia

Hepatic: Cholestatic jaundice

Ocular: Retinal pigmentation (more common than with chlorpromazine), blurred vision, decreased visual acuity (may be irreversible)

Sedation and extrapyramidal effects are more pronounced than anticholinergic and orthostatic effects

Overdosage Symptoms of overdose include deep sleep, coma, extrapyramidal symptoms, abnormal involuntary muscle movements, hypotension or hypertension; agitation, restlessness, fever, hypothermia or hyperthermia, seizures, cardiac arrhythmias, EKG changes

Toxicology Following initiation of essential overdose management, toxic symptom treatment and supportive treatment should be initiated. Hypotension usually responds to I.V. fluids or Trendelenburg positioning. If unresponsive to these measures the use of a parenteral inotrope may be required (eg, norepinephrine 0.1-0.2 mcg/kg/minute titrated to response). Do not use epinephrine. Seizures commonly respond to diazepam (I.V. 5-10 mg bolus every 15 minutes if needed up to a total of 30 mg) or to phenytoin or phenobarbital. Also critical cardiac arrhythmias often respond to I.V. phenytoin (15 mg/kg up to 1 g), while other antiarrhythmics can be used. Neuroleptics often cause extrapyramidal symptoms (eg, dystonic reactions) requiring management with diphenhydramine 1-2 mg/kg up to a maximum of 50 mg I.M. or I.V. slow push followed by a maintenance dose for 48-72 hours. When these reactions are unresponsive to diphenhydramine, benztropine mesylate I.V. 1-2 mg may be effective. These agents are generally effective within 2-5 minutes.

Drug Interactions

Alcohol may increase CNS sedation

Anticholinergic agents may decrease pharmacologic effects; increase anticholinergic side effects; may enhance tardive dyskinesia

Aluminum salts may decrease absorption of phenothiazines

Barbiturates may decrease phenothiazine serum concentrations

Bromocriptine may have decreased efficacy when administered with phenothiazines

Guanethidine's hypotensive effect is decreased by phenothiazines

Lithium administration with phenothiazines may increase disorientation

Meperidine and phenothiazine coadministration increases sedation and hypotension

Methyldopa administration with phenothiazine (trifluoperazine) may significantly increase blood pressure

Norepinephrine, epinephrine have decreased pressor effect when administered with chlorpromazine; therefore, be aware of possible decreased effectiveness or when any phenothiazine is used

Phenytoin serum concentrations may increase or decrease with phenothiazines; tricyclic antidepressants may have increased serum concentrations with concomitant administration with phenothiazines

Propranolol administered with phenothiazines may increase serum concentrations of both drugs

Valproic acid may have increased half-life when administered with phenothiazines (chlorpromazine)

Stability Protect from light; dispense in amber or opaque vials

Mechanism of Action Blocks postsynaptic mesolimbic dopaminergic D_1 and D_2 receptors in the brain; exhibits a strong alpha-adrenergic blocking and anticholinergic effect, depresses the release of hypothalamic and hypophyseal hormones; believed to depress the reticular activating system thus affecting basal metabolism, body temperature, wakefulness, vasomotor tone, and emesis

Pharmacokinetics

Absorption: Absorption may be affected by the inherent anticholinergic action on the gastrointestinal tissue causing variable absorption. Absorption from tablets is erratic with less variation seen with solutions.

Distribution: Widely distributed in tissues with CNS concentrations exceeding that of plasma due to their lipophilic characteristics

(Continued)

Acetophenazine Maleate *(Continued)*

Protein binding: Antipsychotic agents are bound 90% to 99% to plasma or proteins; highly bound to brain and lung tissue and other tissues with a high blood perfusion

Time to peak: 2-4 hours

Elimination: Occurs through hepatic metabolism (oxidation) where numerous active metabolites are produced; active metabolites excreted in urine; elimination half-lives of antipsychotics ranges from 20-40 hours which may be extended in elderly due to decline in oxidative hepatic reactions (phase I) with age. The biologic effect of a single dose persists for 24 hours. When the patient has accommodated to initial side effects (sedation), once daily dosing is possible due to the long half-life of antipsychotics.

Steady-state plasma levels are achieved in 4-7 days; therefore, if possible, do not make dose adjustments more than once in a 7-day period. Due to the long half-lives of antipsychotics, as needed (PRN) use is ineffective since repeated doses are necessary to achieve therapeutic tissue concentrations in the CNS.

Usual Dosage Oral:

Geriatrics (nonpsychotic patients; dementia behavior): Initial: 20 mg once daily; increase at 4- to 7-day intervals by 20 mg/day; increase dosing intervals (bid, tid, etc) as necessary to control response or side effects. For patients with sleep difficulty, administer 1 hour before bedtime; maximum daily dose: 140 mg; gradual increases (titration) may prevent some side effects or decrease their severity

Adults: 20 mg 3 times/day up to 60-120 mg/day

Not dialyzable (0% to 5%)

Monitoring Parameters Orthostatic blood pressures; tremors, gait changes, abnormal movement in trunk, neck, buccal area or extremities; monitor target behaviors for which the agent is given

Test Interactions Increased cholesterol (S), glucose; decreased uric acid (S)

Patient Information Do not take antacid within 1 hour of taking drug; may cause drowsiness, avoid alcohol; avoid excess sun exposure (use sun block); rise slowly from recumbent position; use of supportive stockings may help prevent orthostatic hypotension

Nursing Implications Observe for tremor and abnormal movement or posturing (extrapyramidal symptoms); increased confusion or psychotic behavior, constipation, urinary retention, abnormal gait

Special Geriatric Considerations See Warnings

Many elderly patients receive antipsychotic medications for inappropriate nonpsychotic behavior. Before initiating antipsychotic medication, the clinician should investigate any possible reversible cause; any stress or stress from any disease can cause acute "confusion" or worsening of baseline nonpsychotic behavior. Most commonly acute changes in behavior are due to increases in drug dose or addition of new drug to regimen; fluid electrolyte loss; infections; and changes in environment.

Any changes in disease status in any organ system can result in behavior changes.

Dosage Forms Tablet: 20 mg

Acetoxymethylprogesterone *see* Medroxyprogesterone Acetate *on page 437*

Acetylcholine Chloride (a se teel koe' leen)

Related Information

Glaucoma Drug Therapy Comparison *on page 810*

Brand Names Miochol®

Generic Available No

Therapeutic Class Cholinergic Agent, Ophthalmic; Ophthalmic Agent, Miotic

Use Produce complete miosis in cataract surgery, keratoplasty, iridectomy and other anterior segment surgery where rapid miosis is required

Contraindications Hypersensitivity to acetylcholine chloride; acute iritis and acute inflammatory disease of the anterior chamber

Warnings Open under aseptic conditions only

Precautions Systemic effects rarely occur, but can cause problems for patients with acute cardiac failure, bronchial asthma, peptic ulcer, hyperthyroidism, GI spasm, urinary trace obstruction, and Parkinson's disease. Retinal detachment may result in individuals with pre-existing retinal disease. An examination of the fundus is advised prior to treatment.

Adverse Reactions

Cardiovascular: Bradycardia, hypotension, flushing

Central nervous system: Headache

Ocular: Altered distance vision, decreased night vision, transient lenticular opacities

Respiratory: Breathing difficulty

Miscellaneous: Sweating

Toxicology Treatment includes flushing eyes with water or normal saline and supportive measures; if accidentally ingested, induce emesis or perform gastric lavage

Drug Interactions Decreased effect possible with flurbiprofen and suprofen, ophthalmic
Effects may be prolonged or enhanced in patients receiving tacrine

Stability Prepare solution immediately before use

Mechanism of Action Causes contraction of the sphincter muscles of the iris, resulting in miosis and contraction of the ciliary muscle, leading to accommodation

Pharmacodynamics
Onset of miosis: In seconds
Duration: ~10-20 minutes

Usual Dosage Geriatrics and Adults: Instill 0.5-2 mL of 1% injection (5-20 mg) instilled into anterior chamber before or after securing one or more sutures

Patient Information May sting on instillation; use caution while driving at night or performing hazardous tasks

Nursing Implications Discard any solution that is not used; open under aseptic conditions only

Special Geriatric Considerations See Usual Dosage and Patient Information

Dosage Forms Powder, intraocular ophthalmic: 20 mg (2 mL)

Acetylsalicylic Acid see Aspirin on page 58

Achromycin® see Tetracycline on page 678

Achromycin® V see Tetracycline on page 678

Aciclovir see Acyclovir on this page

Acidulated Phosphate Fluoride see Fluoride on page 299

A-Cillin® see Amoxicillin Trihydrate on page 49

Actagen® [OTC] see Triprolidine and Pseudoephedrine on page 723

Actifed® [OTC] see Triprolidine and Pseudoephedrine on page 723

Actigall™ see Ursodiol on page 727

Activated Dimethicone see Simethicone on page 645

Activated Ergosterol see Ergocalciferol on page 259

Activated Methylpolysiloxane see Simethicone on page 645

ACT® [OTC] see Fluoride on page 299

Acular® Ophthalmic see Ketorolac Tromethamine on page 392

ACV see Acyclovir on this page

Acycloguanosine see Acyclovir on this page

Acyclovir (ay sye' kloe ver)

Brand Names Zovirax®

Synonyms Aciclovir; ACV; Acycloguanosine

Generic Available No

Therapeutic Class Antiviral Agent, Oral; Antiviral Agent, Parenteral; Antiviral Agent, Topical

Use Treatment of initial and prophylaxis of recurrent mucosal and cutaneous herpes simplex (HSV-1 and HSV-2) infections; herpes simplex encephalitis; herpes zoster (shingles); genital herpes infection; and varicella-zoster infections in immunocompromised patients

Contraindications Hypersensitivity to acyclovir

Precautions Use with caution in patients with pre-existing renal disease or in those receiving other nephrotoxic drugs concurrently; maintain adequate and urine output during the first 2 hours after I.V. infusion; use with caution in patients with underlying neurologic abnormalities and in patients with serious renal, hepatic, or electrolyte abnormalities or substantial hypoxia

Adverse Reactions
Cardiovascular: Hypotension
Central nervous system: Headache, delirium, dizziness, seizures, insomnia
Dermatologic: Skin rash
Gastrointestinal: Nausea, vomiting
Hematologic: Bone marrow depression, anemia
Hepatic: Elevation of liver enzymes
Local: Phlebitis at injection site
Neuromuscular & skeletal: Tremulousness
Renal: Nephrotoxicity, dysuria
Miscellaneous: Sore throat, diaphoresis, thirst

Overdosage Symptoms of overdose include elevated serum creatinine, renal failure

Toxicology In the event of an overdose, sufficient urine flow must be maintained to avoid drug precipitation within the renal tubules. Hemodialysis has resulted in up to 60% reductions in serum acyclovir levels.

(Continued)

Acyclovir *(Continued)*

Drug Interactions

Probenecid increases acyclovir bioavailability, terminal half-life may be increased and renal clearance may be decreased

Zidovudine increases drowsiness and lethargy

Stability Incompatible with blood products and protein-containing solutions; reconstituted 50 mg/mL solution should be used within 12 hours; do not refrigerate reconstituted solutions as they may precipitate

Mechanism of Action Inhibits DNA synthesis and viral replication by competing with deoxyguanosine triphosphate for viral DNA polymerase and being incorporated into viral DNA

Pharmacokinetics

Absorption: Oral: 15% to 30%; food does not appear to affect absorption

Distribution: Widely throughout the body including brain, kidney, lungs, liver, spleen, muscle, uterus, vagina, and the CSF

Protein binding: <30%

Half-life (adults): Inversely affected by renal function; see table.

Creatinine Clearance (mL/min/1.73 m^2)	Half-life (hours)
>80	2.5
50–80	3
15–50	3.5
0	19.5

Time to peak: Peak serum levels appear within 1$^{1}/_{2}$ to 2 hours after an oral dose, and within 1 hour following intravenous administration

Elimination: Primary route of elimination is the kidney, following a small amount of hepatic metabolism; requires dosage adjustment with renal impairment, hemodialysis removes ~60% of the dose and to a much lesser extent by peritoneal dialysis

Usual Dosage Geriatrics and Adults:

Dosing weight should be based on the smaller of lean body weight or total body weight

Adult determination of lean body weight (LBW) in kg:

LBW males: 50 kg + (2.3 kg x inches >5 feet)

LBW females: 45 kg + (2.3 kg x inches >5 feet)

Treatment of herpes simplex virus infections:

I.V.:

Mucocutaneous HSV infection: 5 mg/kg/dose every 8 hours for 5-10 days

HSV encephalitis: 10 mg/kg/dose every 8 hours for 10 days

Oral:

Treatment: 200 mg every 4 hours while awake (5 times/day)

Prophylaxis: 200 mg 3-4 times/day or 400 mg twice daily

Topical: $^{1}/_{2}$" ribbon of ointment every 3 hours (6 times/day)

Treatment of varicella-zoster virus infections:

Oral:

800 mg/dose every 4 hours while awake (5 times/day) for 7-10 days or 1000 mg every 6 hours for 5 days

I.V.: 10 mg/kg/dose every 8 hours for 5-10 days

Prophylaxis in immunocompromised patients:

Varicella or herpes zoster in HIV-positive patients: Oral: 400 mg 5 times/day

Bone marrow transplant recipients: I.V.:

Patients who are HSV seropositive: 5 mg/kg/dose divided every 8 hours

Patients who are CMV seropositive: 10 mg/kg/dose divided every 8 hours; for clinically significant CMV infections, ganciclovir should be used in place of acyclovir

Dosing interval in renal impairment: See tables.

Administration Infuse over at least 1 hour; wear gloves when applying ointment

Monitoring Parameters Urinalysis, BUN, serum creatinine, liver enzymes, CBC

Reference Range

Level guidelines:

Pre: 0.1-1.6 μg/mL

Post: 3-10 μg/mL

Panic value: >50 μg/mL

Infusion time: 1 hour

Test Interactions Increased BUN, creatinine

Patient Information Contagious only when viral shedding is occurring; avoid sexual intercourse when lesions are visible; recurrences tend to appear within 3 months of original infection; acyclovir is **not** a cure

Parenteral Acyclovir Dosage in Renal Function Impairment

Creatinine Clearance (mL/min/1.73 m²)	% of Recommended Dose	Dosing Interval (h)
>50	100%	8
25–50	100%	12
10–25	100%	24
0–10	50%	24

Oral Acyclovir Dosage in Renal Function Impairment

Normal Dosage Regimen (5 times/day)	Creatinine Clearance (mL/min/1.73 m²)	Dose (mg)	Dosing Interval
200 mg q4h	>10 0–10	200 200	q4h, 5 times/day q12h
400 mg q12h	>10 0–10	400 200	q12h q12h
800 mg q4h	>25 10–25 0–10	800 800 800	q4h, 5 times/day q8h q12h

Nursing Implications Maintain adequate hydration of patient; check infusion site for phlebitis, rotate site to prevent phlebitis

Additional Information Appears to reduce the length and severity of chickenpox, but should be used unless patient is immunosuppressed; oral doses of 800 mg 5 times/day have been associated with a lower incidence of postherpetic neuralgias

Special Geriatric Considerations For herpes zoster, acyclovir should be started within 72 hours of the appearance of the rash to be effective; calculate creatinine clearance (see renal impairment dosing in Usual Dosage)

Dosage Forms
Capsule: 200 mg
Injection: 50 mg/mL (10 mL, 20 mL)
Ointment, topical: 5% (3 g, 15 g)
Suspension, oral: 200 mg/5 mL
Tablet: 800 mg

References
Dellamonica P, Carles M, Lokiec F, et al, "Preventing Recurrent Varicella and Herpes Zoster With Oral Acyclovir in HIV-Seropositive Patients," *Clin Pharm*, 1991, 10(4):301-2.
Huff JC, Bean B, Balfour HH Jr, et al, "Therapy of Herpes Zoster With Oral Acyclovir," *Am J Med*, 1988, 85(2A):84-9.
McKendrick MW, McGill JI, White JE, et al, "Oral Acyclovir in Acute Herpes Zoster," *Br Med J [Clin Res]*, 1986, 293:1529-32.
Morton P and Thomson AN, "Oral Acyclovir in the Treatment of Herpes Zoster in General Practice," *N Z Med J*, 1989, 102(863):93-5.

Adalat® see Nifedipine *on page 501*

Adalat® CC see Nifedipine *on page 501*

Adamantanamine Hydrochloride see Amantadine Hydrochloride *on page 34*

Adapin® see Doxepin Hydrochloride *on page 242*

Adenine Arabinoside see Vidarabine *on page 737*

Adrenalin® see Epinephrine *on page 256*

Adrenaline see Epinephrine *on page 256*

Adrin® see Nylidrin Hydrochloride *on page 512*

Adsorbocarpine® see Pilocarpine *on page 563*

Adsorbonac® [OTC] Ophthalmic see Sodium Chloride *on page 648*

Advil® [OTC] see Ibuprofen *on page 360*

AeroBid® see Flunisolide *on page 297*

Aerolate® see Theophylline *on page 681*

Aerolate III® see Theophylline *on page 681*

Aerolate JR® see Theophylline *on page 681*

ALPHABETICAL LISTING OF DRUGS

Aerolate SR® S *see* Theophylline *on page 681*

Aeroseb-Dex® *see* Dexamethasone *on page 207*

Aeroseb-HC® *see* Hydrocortisone *on page 351*

Afrinol® [OTC] *see* Pseudoephedrine *on page 609*

Afrin® Nasal Solution [OTC] *see* Oxymetazoline Hydrochloride *on page 530*

Aftate® [OTC] *see* Tolnaftate *on page 705*

Agoral® Plain [OTC] *see* Mineral Oil *on page 473*

A-hydroCort® *see* Hydrocortisone *on page 351*

Akarpine® *see* Pilocarpine *on page 563*

AK-Chlor® *see* Chloramphenicol *on page 148*

AK-Con® *see* Naphazoline Hydrochloride *on page 492*

AK-Dex® *see* Dexamethasone *on page 207*

AK-Dilate® Ophthalmic Solution *see* Phenylephrine Hydrochloride *on page 557*

AK-Homatropine® *see* Homatropine Hydrobromide *on page 343*

Akineton® *see* Biperiden Hydrochloride *on page 86*

AK-Nefrin® Ophthalmic Solution *see* Phenylephrine Hydrochloride *on page 557*

Akne-Mycin® *see* Erythromycin, Topical *on page 266*

AK-Pred® *see* Prednisolone *on page 584*

AK-Sulf® *see* Sodium Sulfacetamide *on page 651*

AK-Tate® *see* Prednisolone *on page 584*

AK-Trol® Ophthalmic *see* Neomycin, Polymyxin B, and Dexamethasone *on page 495*

AKWA Tears™ [OTC] *see* Ocular Lubricant *on page 515*

AK-Zol® *see* Acetazolamide *on page 15*

Alba-Dex® *see* Dexamethasone *on page 207*

Albalon® Liquifilm® *see* Naphazoline Hydrochloride *on page 492*

Albuterol (al byoo' ter ole)

Brand Names Proventil®; Ventolin®

Synonyms Salbutamol

Generic Available Yes

Therapeutic Class Adrenergic Agonist Agent; Beta-2-Adrenergic Agonist Agent; Bronchodilator

Use Bronchodilator in reversible airway obstruction due to asthma or COPD

Contraindications Hypersensitivity to albuterol, adrenergic amines or any ingredients

Warnings Use with caution in patients with unstable vasomotor symptoms, diabetes, hyperthyroidism, prostatic hypertrophy, or a history of seizures; also use caution in the elderly and those patients with cardiovascular disorders such as coronary artery disease, arrhythmias and hypertension

Precautions Excessive use may result in tolerance; deaths have been reported after excessive use; though the exact cause is unknown, cardiac arrest after a severe asthmatic crisis is suspected

Adverse Reactions
Cardiovascular: Tachycardia, palpitations, elevation or depression of blood pressure
Central nervous system: Nervousness, CNS stimulation, hyperactivity, insomnia
Gastrointestinal: GI upset
Neuromuscular & skeletal: Tremors (may be more common in the elderly)

Overdosage Symptoms of overdose include hypertension, tachycardia, seizures, angina, hypokalemia, and tachyarrhythmias

Toxicology Prudent use of a cardioselective beta-adrenergic blocker (eg, atenolol or metoprolol); keep in mind the potential for induction of bronchoconstriction in an asthmatic. Dialysis has not been shown to be of value in the treatment of an overdose with this agent.

Drug Interactions
Decreased therapeutic effect: Beta-adrenergic blockers (eg, propranolol)
Increased therapeutic effect: Inhaled ipratropium → ↑ duration of bronchodilation, nifedipine → ↑ FEV-1
Increased toxicity (cardiovascular): MAO inhibitors, tricyclic antidepressants, sympathomimetic agents (eg, amphetamine, dopamine, dobutamine), inhaled anesthetics (eg, enflurane)

Mechanism of Action Relaxes bronchial smooth muscle by action on beta$_2$-receptors with little effect on heart rate (minor beta$_1$ activity)

Pharmacodynamics
Peak bronchodilation effect: Within 0.5-2 hours
Duration: 3-4 hours

Pharmacokinetics
Metabolism: By the liver to an inactive sulfate, with 28% appearing in the urine as unchanged drug
Half-life:
Inhaled: 3.8 hours
Oral: 3.7-5 hours

Usual Dosage
Oral (see Special Geriatric Considerations):
Geriatrics: 2 mg 3-4 times/day; maximum: 8 mg 4 times/day
Adults: 2-4 mg 3-4 times/day; maximum: 8 mg 4 times/day; sustained release: 1-2 tablets every 12 hours

Inhalation: Geriatrics and Adults:
Nebulization: 2.5 mg 3-4 times/day (2.5 mg = 0.5 mL of the 0.5% inhalation solution) in 2.5 mL of normal saline; may be used more frequently in acute exacerbations
Metered dose inhaler: 2 puffs every 4-6 hours though some patients may be controlled on 1 puff every 4 hours; maximum: 12 puffs/day
Rotahaler®: 200 mcg inhaled every 4-6 hours using a Rotahaler® inhalation device

Monitoring Parameters Pulmonary function, blood pressure, pulse

Patient Information Do not exceed recommended dosage; rinse mouth with water following each inhalation to help with dry throat and mouth; follow specific instructions accompanying inhaler; if more than one inhalation is necessary, wait at least 1 full minute between inhalations. May cause nervousness, restlessness, insomnia – if these effects continue after dosage reduction, notify physician; also notify physician if palpitations, tachycardia, chest pain, muscle tremors, dizziness, headache, flushing or if breathing difficulty persists

Nursing Implications Before using, the inhaler must be shaken well; assess lung sounds, pulse, and blood pressure before administration and during peak of medication; observe patient for wheezing after administration, if this occurs, call physician

Special Geriatric Considerations Because of its minimal effect on beta₁-receptors and its relatively long duration of action, albuterol is a rational choice in the elderly when a beta agonist is indicated. Elderly patients may find it useful to utilize a spacer device when using a metered dose inhaler. The Ventolin® Rotahaler® is an alternative for patients who have difficulty using the metered dose inhaler. Oral use should be avoided due to adverse effects.

Dosage Forms
Aerosol: 90 mcg/actuation (17 g) (~200 inhalations)
Capsule, oral inhalation: 200 mcg
Solution, inhalation: 0.083% (3 mL unit dose); 0.5% (20 mL)
Syrup, as sulfate, alcohol and sugar free: 2 mg/5 mL (480 mL)
Tablet, as sulfate: 2 mg, 4 mg
Tablet, extended release: 4 mg

Alconefrin® Nasal Solution [OTC] see Phenylephrine Hydrochloride on page 557

Aldactazide® see Hydrochlorothiazide and Spironolactone on page 348

Aldactone® see Spironolactone on page 655

Aldomet® see Methyldopa on page 458

Aldoril® see Methyldopa and Hydrochlorothiazide on page 459

Aleve® [OTC] see Naproxen on page 493

Alimenazine Tartrate see Trimeprazine Tartrate on page 719

Alka-Mints® [OTC] see Calcium Salts (Oral) on page 111

Alkeran® see Melphalan on page 440

Aller-Chlor® [OTC] see Chlorpheniramine Maleate on page 152

Allerest® 12 Hour Nasal Solution [OTC] see Oxymetazoline Hydrochloride on page 530

Allerest® Eye Drops [OTC] see Naphazoline Hydrochloride on page 492

Allerfrin® [OTC] see Triprolidine and Pseudoephedrine on page 723

Allerhist® [OTC] see Brompheniramine and Phenylpropanolamine on page 94

AllerMax® [OTC] see Diphenhydramine Hydrochloride on page 228

Allerphed® [OTC] see Triprolidine and Pseudoephedrine on page 723

Allopurinol (al oh pure' i nole)

Related Information

Antacid Drug Interactions *on page 764*

Brand Names Lopurin™; Zurinol®; Zyloprim®

Generic Available Yes

Therapeutic Class Uric Acid Lowering Agent; Uricosuric Agent

Use Prevention of attack of gouty arthritis and nephropathy; also used to treat secondary hyperuricemia which may occur during treatment of tumors or leukemia; to prevent recurrent calcium oxalate calculi

Contraindications Do not use in patients with a previous severe allergy reaction

Precautions Reduce dosage in renal insufficiency, reinstate with caution in patients who have had a previous mild allergic reaction; monitor liver function and complete blood counts before initiating therapy and periodically during therapy

Adverse Reactions

Central nervous system: Neuritis, drowsiness, fever

Dermatologic: Pruritic maculopapular rash, exfoliative dermatitis

Gastrointestinal: GI irritation

Hematologic: Leukocytosis, leukopenia, thrombocytopenia, eosinophilia, bone marrow suppression

Hepatic: Hepatitis

Ocular: Cataracts

Renal: Renal impairment

Toxicology If significant amounts of allopurinol are thought to have been absorbed, it is a theoretical possibility that oxypurinol stones could be formed but no record of such occurrence in overdose exists. Alkalinization of the urine and forced diuresis can help prevent potential xanthine stone formation.

Drug Interactions

Decreased effect: Alcohol decreases effectiveness

Increased toxicity: Inhibits metabolism of azathioprine and mercaptopurine; use with ampicillin or amoxicillin may increase the incidence of skin rash; doses of allopurinol >600 mg/day may decrease theophylline clearance to result in toxicity; use with ACE inhibitors may increase the risk of hypersensitivity reactions; thiazide diuretics increase the incidence of hypersensitivity reactions to allopurinol

Stability Keep oral solution in refrigerator, remains stable for 56 days after preparation

Mechanism of Action Decreases the production of uric acid by inhibiting the action of xanthine oxidase, an enzyme that converts hypoxanthine to xanthine and xanthine to uric acid

Pharmacodynamics Decrease in serum uric acid occurs in 1-2 days with a nadir achieved in 1-3 weeks

Pharmacokinetics

Absorption: Oral: ~80% from GI tract

Protein binding: <1%

Metabolism: ~75% of the drug is metabolized to active metabolites, chiefly oxypurinol; allopurinol and oxypurinol are dialyzable

Half-life:

Parent: 1-3 hours

Oxypurinol: Normal renal function: 18-30 hours

Time to peak serum concentration: Within 2-4 hours

Usual Dosage Oral:

Geriatrics: Initial dose: 100 mg/day, increase until desired uric acid level is obtained

Adults: Daily doses >300 mg should be administered in divided doses

Gout: Average dose: 200-300 mg/day (mild); 400-600 mg/day (severe)

Maximum dose: 800 mg/day

Dosing interval in renal impairment: See table.

Myeloproliferative neoplastic disorders: 600-800 mg/day in 2-3 divided doses for prevention of acute uric acid nephropathy for 2-3 days starting 1-2 days before chemotherapy

Monitoring Parameters CBC, serum uric acid levels, I & O, hepatic and renal function, especially at start of therapy

Reference Range Uric acid, serum: Adults: Male: 3.4-7 mg/dL (SI: 202-416 μmol/L) or slightly more; Female: 2.4-6 mg/dL (SI: 143-357 μmol/L) or slightly more. Values above 7 mg/dL (SI: 416 μmol/L) are sometimes arbitrarily regarded as hyperuricemia, but there is no sharp line between normals on the one hand, and the serum uric acid of those with clinical gout. Normal ranges cannot be adjusted for purine ingestion, but high purine diet increases uric acid. Uric acid may be increased with body size, exercise, and stress.

Test Interactions Increased alkaline phosphatase, AST, ALT; decreased uric acid (S)

Patient Information Take after meals with plenty of fluid; discontinue the drug and contact physician at first sign of rash, painful urination, blood in the urine, irritation of the eyes, or swelling of the lips or mouth; may cause drowsiness

Nursing Implications Administer after meals; encourage fluid intake

Additional Information Skin rash occurs most often in patients taking diuretics concurrently; may predispose patient to ampicillin-induced rash

Adult Maintenance Doses of Allopurinol*

Creatinine Clearance (mL/min)	Maintenance Dose of Allopurinol (mg)
140	400 qd
120	350 qd
100	300 qd
80	250 qd
60	200 qd
40	150 qd
20	100 qd
10	100 q2d
0	100 q3d

*This table is based on a standard maintenance dose of 300 mg of allopurinol per day for a patient with a creatinine clearance of 100 mL/min.

Special Geriatric Considerations See Usual Dosage; adjust dose based on renal function

Dosage Forms Tablet: 100 mg, 300 mg

Almacone® II Suspension [OTC] *see* Aluminum Hydroxide, Magnesium Hydroxide and Simethicone *on page 31*

Alomide® *see* Lodoxamide Tromethamine *on page 415*

Alophen Pills® [OTC] *see* Phenolphthalein *on page 556*

Alphamul® [OTC] *see* Castor Oil *on page 124*

Alphatrex® *see* Betamethasone *on page 82*

Alpidine® *see* Apraclonidine Hydrochloride *on page 56*

Alplitest® *see* Tuberculin Purified Protein Derivative *on page 725*

Alprazolam (al pray' zoe lam)

Related Information
Anxiolytic/Hypnotic Use in Long-Term Care Facilities *on page 755-756*
Benzodiazepines Comparison *on page 802-803*

Brand Names Xanax®

Generic Available No

Therapeutic Class Antianxiety Agent; Benzodiazepine

Use Treatment of anxiety; adjunct in the treatment of depression; management of panic attacks

Restrictions C-IV

Contraindications Hypersensitivity to alprazolam or any component; there may be a cross-sensitivity with other benzodiazepines; severe uncontrolled pain, narrow-angle glaucoma, severe respiratory depression, pre-existing CNS depression

Warnings Withdrawal symptoms including seizures have occurred 18 hours to 3 days after abrupt discontinuation; when discontinuing therapy, decrease daily dose by no more than 0.5 mg every 3 days; reduce dose in patients with significant hepatic disease

Precautions Use with caution in patients with a history of drug dependence

Adverse Reactions
Central nervous system: Drowsiness, dizziness, confusion, sedation, ataxia, headache
Gastrointestinal: Dry mouth, constipation, diarrhea, nausea, vomiting
Neuromuscular & skeletal: Impaired coordination
Ocular: Blurred vision
Respiratory: Decreased respiratory rate, apnea, laryngospasm
Miscellaneous: Physical and psychological dependence with prolonged use

Overdosage Symptoms of overdose include somnolence, confusion, coma, and diminished reflexes

Toxicology Treatment for benzodiazepine overdose is supportive; rarely is mechanical ventilation required
Flumazenil has been shown to selectively block the binding of benzodiazepines to CNS receptors, resulting in a reversal of benzodiazepine-induced sedation; however, its use may not alter the course of overdose

Drug Interactions Benzodiazepines may increase digoxin concentrations and may decrease the effect of levodopa

(Continued)

Alprazolam *(Continued)*

Decreased metabolism: Cimetidine, fluoxetine

Increased metabolism: Rifampin

Increased toxicity: CNS depressants, alcohol

Mechanism of Action Benzodiazepines appear to potentiate the effects of GABA and other inhibitory neurotransmitters by binding to specific benzodiazepine-receptor sites in various areas of the CNS

Pharmacodynamics Studies have shown that the elderly are more sensitive to the effects of benzodiazepines as compared to younger adults

Pharmacokinetics

Absorption: Oral: Rapidly and well absorbed

Distribution: V_d: 0.9-1.2 L/kg

Protein binding: 80%

Metabolism: Extensive in the liver; major metabolite is inactive; alphahydroxyalprazolam (active)

Half-life: 12-15 hours

Time to peak serum concentration: Within 1-2 hours

Elimination: Metabolites and parent compound in the urine; elimination is prolonged in elderly men (half-life: 19.5 hours); elderly women had no significant change in alprazolam clearance

Usual Dosage Oral:

Geriatrics: Initial: 0.125-0.25 mg twice daily; increase by 0.125 mg/day as needed

Adults: 0.25-0.5 mg 2-3 times/day, titrate dose upward; maximum: 4 mg/day

Monitoring Parameters Respiratory and cardiovascular status, symptoms of anxiety, mental status

Test Interactions Increased alkaline phosphatase

Patient Information Avoid alcohol and other CNS depressants; may cause drowsiness; avoid activities needing good psychomotor coordination until CNS effects are known; may cause physical or psychological dependence; avoid abrupt discontinuation after prolonged use

Nursing Implications Assist with ambulation during initiation of therapy; monitor for alertness

Additional Information Not intended for management of anxieties and minor distresses associated with everyday life; treatment longer than 4 months should be reevaluated to determine the patient's need for the drug; when decreasing the dose or discontinuing alprazolam, decrease by no more than 0.5 mg every 3 days

Special Geriatric Considerations Due to short duration of action, it is considered to be a benzodiazepine of choice in the elderly; see Pharmacodynamics, Pharmacokinetics, and Additional Information

Dosage Forms Tablet: 0.25 mg, 0.5 mg, 1 mg, 2 mg

References

Greenblatt DJ, Divoll M, Abernethy DR, et al, "Alprazolam Kinetics in the Elderly: Relation to Antipyrine Disposition," *Arch Gen Psychiatry*, 1983, 40(3):287-90.

Reidenberg MM, Levy M, Warner H, et al, "Relationship Between Diazepam Dose, Plasma Level, Age, and Central Nervous System Depression," *Clin Pharmacol Ther*, 1978, 23(4):371-4.

AL-R® [OTC] *see* Chlorpheniramine Maleate *on page 152*

Altace™ *see* Ramipril *on page 621*

ALternaGEL® [OTC] *see* Aluminum Hydroxide *on this page*

Alu-Cap® [OTC] *see* Aluminum Hydroxide *on this page*

Aludrox® [OTC] *see* Aluminum Hydroxide and Magnesium Hydroxide *on next page*

Aluminum Hydroxide

Brand Names ALternaGEL® [OTC]; Alu-Cap® [OTC]; Alu-Tab® [OTC]; Amphojel® [OTC]; Dialume® [OTC]

Generic Available Yes

Therapeutic Class Antacid; Antidote, Hyperphosphatemia

Use Hyperacidity; hyperphosphatemia

Contraindications Hypersensitivity to aluminum salts or dry components

Warnings Hypophosphatemia may occur with prolonged administration or large doses; aluminum intoxication and osteomalacia may occur in patients with uremia

Precautions Use with caution in patients with congestive heart failure, renal failure, edema, cirrhosis, and low sodium diets, and patients who have recently suffered gastrointestinal hemorrhage; uremic patients not receiving dialysis may develop osteomalacia and osteoporosis due to phosphate depletion

Adverse Reactions

Central nervous system: Mental confusion, somnolence

Endocrine & metabolic: Hypermagnesemia, aluminum toxicity, osteomalacia, hypophosphatemia, dehydration

Gastrointestinal: Constipation, decreased bowel motility, fecal impaction, diarrhea

Miscellaneous: Hemorrhoids

Overdosage Symptoms of overdose include bone pain, malaise, muscular weakness, encephalopathy

Toxicology Deferoxamine, traditionally used as an iron chelator, has been shown to increase urinary aluminum output. Deferoxamine chelation of aluminum has resulted in improvements of clinical symptoms and bone histology. Deferoxamine, however, remains an experimental treatment for aluminum poisoning and has a significant potential for adverse effects.

Drug Interactions

Aluminum compounds decrease the pharmacologic effect of allopurinol, chloroquine, corticosteroids, diflunisol, digoxin, ethambutol, H_2 antagonists, iron compounds, isoniazid, penicillamine, phenothiazines, tetracyclines, thyroid hormones, triclopidine

Aluminum compounds increase the pharmacologic effect of benzodiazepines

Mechanism of Action Neutralize gastric acid and, therefore, increase pH of the stomach and duodenal bulb; with increased pH >4, the proteolytic activity of pepsin is diminished. Antacids also increase lower esophageal sphincter tone; aluminum ions inhibit gastric emptying by decreasing smooth muscle contraction

Pharmacodynamics Acid-neutralizing capacity varies from product to product; antacids ingested in a fasting state give reduced acidity for 30 minutes; if ingested 1 hour after meals, reduced acidity may be extended for 3 hours

Usual Dosage Geriatrics and Adults:

Oral: 500-1800 mg, 3-6 times/day, between meals and at bedtime

Suspension: 5-30 mL 3-6 times/day between meals and at bedtime

Monitoring Parameters Frequency of bowel movements, GI complaints (symptoms); phosphorous levels periodically when patient is on chronic therapy; when used as a phosphate binder, dose to achieve a serum phosphate concentration ≤4 mg/100 mL

Reference Range Aluminum normal range (serum): 0-6 ng/mL; dialysis patients may attain up to 40 ng/mL without symptoms of toxicity; >100 ng/mL possible CNS toxicity

Test Interactions Decreased phosphorus, inorganic (S)

Patient Information Dilute dose in water or juice, shake well; chew tablets thoroughly before swallowing with water; do not take oral drugs within 1-2 hours of administration; notify physician if relief is not obtained or if there are any signs to suggest bleeding from the GI tract

Nursing Implications Observe for constipation, fecal impaction, diarrhea, and hypophosphatemia

Additional Information Used primarily as a phosphate binder; dose should be followed with water

Special Geriatric Considerations Elderly, due to disease and/or drug therapy, may be predisposed to constipation and fecal impaction. Careful evaluation of possible drug interactions must be done. When used as an antacid in ulcer treatment, consider buffer capacity (mEq/mL) to calculate dose; consider renal insufficiency (<30 mL/minute) as predisposition to aluminum toxicity.

Dosage Forms

Capsule: 475 mg, 500 mg

Gel: 600 mg/5 mL (360 mL)

Suspension, oral: 320 mg/5 mL (500 mL), 675 mg/5 mL

Tablet: 300 mg, 500 mg, 600 mg

References

Bohannon AD and Lyles KW, "Drug-Induced Bone Disease," *Clin Geriatr Med*, 1994, 10(4):611-23.

Aluminum Hydroxide and Magnesium Hydroxide

Brand Names Aludrox® [OTC]; Camalox® [OTC]; Maalox® [OTC]; Maalox® Therapeutic Concentrate [OTC]; WinGel® [OTC]

Synonyms Magnesium Hydroxide and Aluminum Hydroxide

Generic Available Yes

Therapeutic Class Antacid

Use Antacid, hyperphosphatemia in renal failure

Contraindications Known hypersensitivity to aluminum hydroxide or magnesium hydroxide

Warnings Sodium content may be significant for patients with hypertension, renal failure, congestive heart failure; hypermagnesemia may result with renal insufficiency when >50 mEq of magnesium is administered daily; patients with Cl_{cr} <30 mL/minute are at risk for hypermagnesemia

Precautions Aluminum intoxication, osteomalacia, patients with GI hemorrhage; use with caution in patients on low sodium diets (patients with congestive heart failure, edema, hypertension), cirrhosis, and renal failure; magnesium intoxication may occur with renal insufficiency

Adverse Reactions

Central nervous system: Mental confusion

(Continued)

29

Aluminum Hydroxide and Magnesium Hydroxide
(Continued)

Endocrine & metabolic: Hypermagnesemia, aluminum intoxication, osteomalacia, hypophosphatemia, dehydration

Gastrointestinal: Constipation, diarrhea, fecal impaction

Overdosage

Aluminum: Osteomalacia (bone pain), malaise, weakness, and aluminum intoxication (encephalopathy) may occur in patients with renal insufficiency

Magnesium: CNS depression, confusion, hypotension, muscle weakness, blockage of peripheral neuromuscular transmission serum >4 mEq/L (4.8 mg/dL): deep tendon reflexes may be depressed; serum $\geq$10 mEq/L (12 mg/dL): deep tendon reflexes may disappear, respiratory paralysis may occur, heart block may occur

Toxicology Deferoxamine, traditionally used as an iron chelator, has been shown to increase urinary aluminum output. Deferoxamine chelation of aluminum has resulted in improvements of clinical symptoms and bone histology. Deferoxamine, however, remains an experimental treatment for aluminum poisoning and has a significant potential for adverse effects. Hypermagnesemia, toxic symptoms usually present with serum level >4 mEq/L; concurrent hypocalcemia, impaired clotting, somnolence, and disappearance of deep tendon reflexes. Serum level > 12 mEq/L may be fatal, serum level ~10 mEq/L may cause complete heart block; I.V. calcium (5-10 mEq) will reverse respiratory depression or heart block; peritoneal dialysis or hemodialysis may be needed.

Drug Interactions

Magnesium and aluminum combination compounds decrease the pharmacologic effect of benzodiazepines, captopril, glucocorticosteroids, fluoroquinolones, H_2 antagonists, hydantoins, iron compounds, ketoconazole, penicillamine, phenothiazines, salicylates, tetracyclines, ticlopidine; concomitant use with sodium polystyrene sulfonate may cause metabolic alkalosis in patients with renal insufficiency

Magnesium and aluminum combination compounds increase the pharmacologic effect of levodopa, quinidine, sulfonylureas, valproic acid

Mechanism of Action Neutralize gastric acid and, therefore, increase pH of the stomach and duodenal bulb; with increased pH above 4, the proteolytic activity of pepsin is diminished. Antacids also increase lower esophageal sphincter tone; aluminum ions inhibit gastric emptying by decreasing smooth muscle contraction.

Pharmacodynamics Acid-neutralizing capacity varies from product to product; see Appendix. Antacids ingested in a fasting state give reduced acidity for 30 minutes; if ingested 1 hour after meals, reduced acidity may be extended for 3 hours.

Usual Dosage Dosage depends upon disease condition being treated and specific agent used

Geriatrics and Adults: Oral:

Peptic ulcer disease: 144 mEq neutralizing capacity 1 and 3 hours after meals and as needed

Reflux esophagitis: 15-30 mL 20-40 minutes after meals and at bedtime

Phosphate binding: Dose titrated to achieve high normal serum phosphate concentrations; doses administered with meals

Monitoring Parameters Frequency of bowel movements and GI complaints (symptoms)

Aluminum: Monitor phosphorous levels periodically when patient is on chronic therapy; when used as a phosphate binder, dose to achieve a serum phosphate concentration $\leq$4 mg/100 mL; observe for complaints or bone pain, malaise, and muscular weakness

Magnesium: See Overdosage; observe for signs of mental confusion and increased somnolence

Reference Range

Aluminum: Normal range (serum): 0-6 ng/mL; dialysis patients may attain up to 40 ng/mL without symptoms of toxicity; >100 ng/mL possible CNS toxicity

Magnesium: Normal range (serum): 1.5-2.3 mg/dL (1.25-1.9 mEq/L); toxicity occurs with serum levels >4 mEq/L (4.8 mg/dL)

Test Interactions Decreased phosphorus, inorganic (S)

Patient Information Chew tablets thoroughly before swallowing with water; notify physician if relief is not obtained or if signs of bleeding from GI tract occur; if prescribed dose is exceeded in order to maintain symptom-free periods, advise physician

Nursing Implications Administer 1-2 hours apart from oral drugs; shake suspensions well; observe for constipation, fecal impaction, diarrhea, and hypophosphatemia; see Monitoring Parameters, Overdosage, and Reference Range

Additional Information Sodium content varies with product; check for each product if important for patient

Special Geriatric Considerations Elderly, due to disease or drug therapy, may be predisposed to diarrhea or constipation. Diarrhea may result in electrolyte imbalance. Decreased renal function (Cl_{cr} <30 mL/minute) may result in toxicity of aluminum or magnesium. Drug interactions must be considered. If possible, give antacid 1-2 hours apart from other drugs. When treating ulcers, consider buffer capacity (mEq/mL) antacid.

Dosage Forms
Suspension:
Aludrox®: Aluminum hydroxide 307 mg and magnesium hydroxide 103 mg per 5 mL
Maalox®: Aluminum hydroxide 225 mg and magnesium hydroxide 200 mg per 5 mL
Maalox® TC (high potency): Aluminum hydroxide 600 mg and magnesium hydroxide 300 mg per 5 mL
Tablet, chewable (Maalox®): Aluminum hydroxide 600 mg and magnesium hydroxide 300 mg
Various other products available with various proportions of aluminum and magnesium

References

Bohannon AD and Lyles KW "Drug-Induced Bone Disease," *Clin Geriatr Med*, 1994, 10(4):621-3.
Gams JG, "Clinical Significance of Magnesium: A Review," *Drug Intell Clin Pharm*, 1987, 21(3):240-6.
Peterson WL, Sturdevant RAL, Franki HD, et al, "Healing of Duodenal Ulcer With an Antacid Regimen," *N Engl J Med*, 1977, 297(7):341-5.

Aluminum Hydroxide, Magnesium Hydroxide and Simethicone

Brand Names Almacone® II Suspension [OTC]; Di-Gel® [OTC]; Gelusil® [OTC]; Maalox® Plus [OTC]; Mylanta® [OTC]; Mylanta®-II [OTC]

Generic Available Yes

Therapeutic Class Antacid; Antiflatulent

Use Temporary relief of hyperacidity associated with gas; may also be used for indications associated with other antacids

Contraindications Known hypersensitivity to aluminum hydroxide, magnesium hydroxide, or simethicone

Warnings Sodium content may be significant for patients with hypertension, renal failure, congestive heart failure; hypermagnesemia may result with renal insufficiency when >50 mEq of magnesium is administered daily; patients with Cl_{cr} <30 mL/minute are at risk for hypermagnesemia

Precautions Use with caution in patients with GI hemorrhage, patients on low sodium diets, patients with congestive heart failure, edema, hypertension, cirrhosis, and renal failure; magnesium intoxication may occur with renal insufficiency

Adverse Reactions
Central nervous system: Mental confusion, somnolence
Endocrine & metabolic: Dehydration or fluid restriction, hypermagnesemia, osteomalacia, hypophosphatemia
Gastrointestinal: Constipation, decreased bowel motility, fecal impaction, diarrhea

Overdosage
Aluminum: osteomalacia (bone pain), malaise, weakness, and aluminum intoxication (encephalopathy) may occur in patients with renal insufficiency
Magnesium: CNS depression, confusion, hypotension, muscle weakness, blockage of peripheral neuromuscular transmission serum >4 mEq/L (4.8 mg/dL): deep tendon reflexes may be depressed; serum ≥10 mEq/L (12 mg/dL): deep tendon reflexes may disappear, respiratory paralysis may occur, heart block may occur

Toxicology Deferoxamine, traditionally used as an iron chelator, has been shown to increase urinary aluminum output. Deferoxamine chelation of aluminum has resulted in improvements of clinical symptoms and bone histology. Deferoxamine, however, remains an experimental treatment for aluminum poisoning and has a significant potential for adverse effects. Hypermagnesemia, toxic symptoms usually present with serum level >4 mEq/L; concurrent hypocalcemia, impaired clotting, somnolence, and disappearance of deep tendon reflexes. Serum level >12 mEq/L may be fatal, serum level ~10 mEq/L may cause complete heart block; I.V. calcium (5-10 mEq) will reverse respiratory depression or heart block; peritoneal dialysis or hemodialysis may be needed.

Drug Interactions
Magnesium and aluminum combination compounds decrease the pharmacologic effect of benzodiazepines, captopril, glucocorticosteroids, fluoroquinolones, H_2 antagonists, hydantoins, iron compounds, ketoconazole, penicillamine, phenothiazines, salicylates, tetracyclines, ticlopidine; concomitant use with sodium polystyrene sulfonate may cause metabolic alkalosis in patients with renal insufficiency
Magnesium and aluminum combination compounds increase the pharmacologic effect of levodopa, quinidine, sulfonylureas, valproic acid

Mechanism of Action Neutralize gastric acid and, therefore, increase pH of the stomach and duodenal bulb; with increased pH >4, the proteolytic activity of pepsin is diminished. Antacids also increase lower esophageal sphincter tone; aluminum ions inhibit gastric emptying by decreasing smooth muscle contraction

Pharmacodynamics Acid-neutralizing capacity varies from product to product; antacids ingested in a fasting state give reduced acidity for 30 minutes; if ingested 1 hour after meals, reduced acidity may be extended for 3 hours

Usual Dosage Dosage depends upon disease condition being treated and specific agent used

(Continued)

31

Aluminum Hydroxide, Magnesium Hydroxide and Simethicone *(Continued)*

Geriatrics and Adults: Oral:

Peptic ulcer disease: 144 mEq neutralizing capacity 1 and 3 hours after meals and as needed

Reflux esophagitis: 15-30 mL 20-40 minutes after meals and at bedtime

Phosphate binding: Dose titrated to achieve high normal serum phosphate concentrations; doses administered with meals

Monitoring Parameters Frequency of bowel movements and GI complaints (symptoms)

Aluminum: Monitor phosphorous levels periodically when patient is on chronic therapy; when used as a phosphate binder, dose to achieve a serum phosphate concentration ≤4 mg/100 mL; observe for complaints or bone pain, malaise, and muscular weakness

Magnesium: See Overdosage; observe for signs of mental confusion and increased somnolence

Reference Range

Aluminum: Normal range (serum): 0-6 ng/mL; dialysis patients may attain up to 40 ng/mL without symptoms of toxicity; >100 ng/mL possible CNS toxicity

Magnesium: Normal range (serum): 1.5-2.3 mg/dL (1.25-1.9 mEq/L); toxicity occurs with serum levels >4 mEq/L (4.8 mg/dL)

Test Interactions Decreased phosphorus, inorganic (S)

Patient Information Dilute dose in water or juice; chew tablets thoroughly before swallowing with water; shake well; notify physician if relief is not obtained or if signs of bleeding from GI tract occur

Nursing Implications Administer 1-2 hours apart from oral drugs; see Monitoring Parameters, Overdosage, and Reference Range

Additional Information In order for simethicone to be effective, doses need to be 40-125 mg administered four times daily, not to exceed 500 mg daily; sodium content varies with product; check for each product if important for patient

Special Geriatric Considerations Elderly, due to disease or drug therapy, may be predisposed to diarrhea or constipation. Diarrhea may result in electrolyte imbalance. Decreased renal function (Cl$_{cr}$ <30 mL/minute) may result in toxicity of aluminum or magnesium. Drug interactions must be considered. If possible, give antacid 1-2 hours apart from other drugs. When treating ulcers, consider buffer capacity (mEq/mL) antacid.

Dosage Forms

Liquid:

Gelusil®; Mylanta®: Aluminum hydroxide 200 mg, magnesium hydroxide 200 mg and simethicone 25 mg per 5 mL

Maalox® Plus: Aluminum hydroxide 225 mg, magnesium hydroxide 200 mg and simethicone 25 mg per 5 mL (30 mL, 180 mL)

Mylanta®-II: Aluminum hydroxide 400 mg, magnesium hydroxide 400 mg and simethicone 40 mg per 5 mL (150 mL, 360 mL)

Tablet, chewable:

Mylanta®: Aluminum hydroxide 200 mg, magnesium hydroxide 200 mg and simethicone 20 mg

Mylanta®-II: Aluminum hydroxide 400 mg, magnesium hydroxide 400 mg and simethicone 40 mg

Various other products available which contain various proportions of aluminum hydroxide, magnesium hydroxide, and simethicone

References

Bohannon AD and Lyles KW "Drug-Induced Bone Disease," *Clin Geriatr Med*, 1994, 10(4):621-3.

Gams JG, "Clinical Significance of Magnesium: A Review," *Drug Intell Clin Pharm*, 1987, 21(3):240-6.

Peterson WL, Sturdevant RAL, Franki HD, et al, "Healing of Duodenal Ulcer With an Antacid Regimen," *N Engl J Med*, 1977, 297(7):341-5.

Aluminum Hydroxide, Magnesium Trisilicate, Sodium Bicarbonate and Alginic Acid

Brand Names Gaviscon® [OTC]; Gaviscon-2® [OTC]; Gaviscon® Extra Strength Relief Formula [OTC]

Generic Available No

Therapeutic Class Antacid

Use Temporary relief of hyperacidity

Unlabeled use: Gastroesophageal reflux

Contraindications Known hypersensitivity; not indicated for treatment of peptic ulcers

Warnings Sodium content may be significant for patients with hypertension, renal failure, congestive heart failure; hypermagnesemia may result with renal insufficiency when >50 mEq of magnesium is administered daily; patients with Cl$_{cr}$ <30 mL/minute are at risk for hypermagnesemia

Precautions Aluminum intoxication, osteomalacia, patients with GI hemorrhage; use with caution in patients on low sodium diets (patients with congestive heart failure, edema, hypertension), cirrhosis, and renal failure; magnesium intoxication may occur with renal insufficiency

Adverse Reactions
 Central nervous system: Mental confusion, somnolence
 Endocrine & metabolic: Dehydration or fluid restriction, hypermagnesemia, osteomalacia, hypophosphatemia
 Gastrointestinal: Constipation, decreased bowel motility, fecal impaction, diarrhea

Overdosage
 Aluminum: osteomalacia (bone pain), malaise, weakness, and aluminum intoxication (encephalopathy) may occur in patients with renal insufficiency
 Magnesium: CNS depression, confusion, hypotension, muscle weakness, blockage of peripheral neuromuscular transmission serum >4 mEq/L (4.8 mg/dL): deep tendon reflexes may be depressed; serum ≥10 mEq/L (12 mg/dL): deep tendon reflexes may disappear, respiratory paralysis may occur, heart block may occur; I.V. calcium (5-10 mEq) will reverse respiratory depression or heart block; in extreme cases, peritoneal dialysis or hemodialysis may be required

Drug Interactions
 Magnesium and aluminum combination compounds decrease the pharmacologic effect of benzodiazepines, captopril, glucocorticosteroids, fluoroquinolones, H_2 antagonists, hydantoins, iron compounds, ketoconazole, penicillamine, phenothiazines, salicylates, tetracyclines, ticlopidine; concomitant use with sodium polystyrene sulfonate may cause metabolic alkalosis in patients with renal insufficiency
 Magnesium and aluminum combination compounds increase the pharmacologic effect of levodopa, quinidine, sulfonylureas, valproic acid

Mechanism of Action Neutralize gastric acid and, therefore, increase pH of the stomach and duodenal bulb; with increased pH above 4, the proteolytic activity of pepsin is diminished. Antacids also increase lower esophageal sphincter tone; aluminum ions inhibit gastric emptying by decreasing smooth muscle contraction

Pharmacodynamics Acid-neutralizing capacity varies from product to product; antacids ingested in a fasting state give reduced acidity for 30 minutes; if ingested 1 hour after meals, reduced acidity may be extended for 3 hours

Usual Dosage Geriatrics and Adults: Oral: Chew 2-4 tablets 4 times/day

Monitoring Parameters Frequency of bowel movements and GI complaints (symptoms)
 Aluminum: Monitor phosphorous levels periodically when patient is on chronic therapy; when used as a phosphate binder, dose to achieve a serum phosphate concentration ≤4 mg/100 mL; observe for complaints or bone pain, malaise, and muscular weakness
 Magnesium: See Overdosage; observe for signs of mental confusion and increased somnolence

Reference Range
 Aluminum: Normal range (serum): 0-6 ng/mL; dialysis patients may attain up to 40 ng/mL without symptoms of toxicity; >100 ng/mL possible CNS toxicity
 Magnesium: Normal range (serum): 1.5-2.3 mg/dL (1.25-1.9 mEq/L); toxicity occurs with serum levels >4 mEq/L (4.8 mg/L)

Test Interactions Decreased phosphorus, inorganic (S)

Patient Information Chew tablets; do not swallow whole; can dilute liquid in water or juice; notify physician if relief is not obtained or if signs of bleeding from GI tract occur

Nursing Implications Administer 1-2 hours apart from oral drugs; observe for constipation, fecal impaction, diarrhea; see Monitoring Parameters, Overdosage, and References Range

Additional Information Sodium content varies with product; check for each product if important for patient

Special Geriatric Considerations Elderly, due to disease or drug therapy, may be predisposed to diarrhea or constipation. Diarrhea may result in electrolyte imbalance. Decreased renal function (Cl_{cr} <30 mL/minute) may result in toxicity of aluminum or magnesium. Drug interactions must be considered. If possible, give antacid 1-2 hours apart from other drugs. When treating ulcers, consider buffer capacity (mEq/mL) antacid.

Dosage Forms
 Liquid: Aluminum hydroxide 160 mg, magnesium trisilicate 40 mg, sodium alginate 400 mg, sodium bicarbonate 140 mg per 15 mL
 Tablet, chewable: Aluminum hydroxide dried gel 80 mg, magnesium trisilicate 20 mg, sodium bicarbonate 70 mg and alginic acid 200 mg

References
Bohannon AD and Lyles KW "Drug-Induced Bone Disease," *Clin Geriatr Med*, 1994, 10(4):621-3.
Gams JG, "Clinical Significance of Magnesium: A Review," *Drug Intell Clin Pharm*, 1987, 21(3):240-6.
Peterson WL, Sturdevant RAL, Franki HD, et al, "Healing of Duodenal Ulcer With an Antacid Regimen," *N Engl J Med*, 1977, 297(7):341-5.

Aluminum Phosphate

Brand Names Phosphaljel® [OTC]
Synonyms Aluminum Phosphate Gel
Generic Available No

(Continued)

Aluminum Phosphate *(Continued)*

Therapeutic Class Electrolyte Supplement, Oral
Use Increase fecal excretion of phosphates; no longer labeled for use as an antacid
Contraindications Known hypersensitivity to aluminum phosphate
Warnings Sodium content may be significant for patients with hypertension, renal failure, edema, cirrhosis, congestive heart failure, and those on low sodium diets
Precautions Aluminum intoxication, osteomalacia, patients with GI hemorrhage; caution in renal failure
Adverse Reactions
Endocrine & metabolic: Dehydration or fluid restriction
Gastrointestinal: Constipation, decreased bowel motility, fecal impaction
Miscellaneous: Hemorrhoids
Overdosage Symptoms of overdose include osteomalacia (bone pain), malaise, weakness, and in renal failure, encephalopathy
Toxicology Deferoxamine, traditionally used as an iron chelator, has been shown to increase urinary aluminum output. Deferoxamine chelation of aluminum has resulted in improvements of clinical symptoms and bone histology. Deferoxamine, however, remains an experimental treatment for aluminum poisoning and has a significant potential for adverse effects.
Drug Interactions
May decrease absorption of weak acidic drugs or increase absorption of weak basic drugs
Aluminum compounds decrease the pharmacologic effect of allopurinol, chloroquine, corticosteroids, diflunisol, digoxin, ethambutol, H_2 antagonists, iron compounds, isoniazid, penicillamine, phenothiazines, tetracyclines, thyroid hormones, triclopidine
Aluminum compounds increase the pharmacologic effect of benzodiazepines
Usual Dosage Geriatrics and Adults: Oral: 15-30 mL every 2 hours between meals
Monitoring Parameters Frequency of bowel movements and GI complaints (symptoms); observe for complaints of bone pain, malaise, and muscular weakness; phosphorous levels periodically when patient is on chronic therapy; when used as a phosphate binder, dose to achieve a serum phosphate concentration ≤4 mg/100 mL
Reference Range Normal range (serum): 0-6 ng/mL; dialysis patients may attain ≤40 ng/mL without symptoms of toxicity; >100 ng/mL possible CNS toxicity
Test Interactions Decreased phosphorus, inorganic (S)
Patient Information Dilute dose in water or juice, shake well; do not take within 1-2 hours of oral administration of other drugs unless instructed by physician, pharmacist, or nurse
Nursing Implications Observe for constipation, fecal impaction, and hypophosphatemia; see Monitoring Parameters
Additional Information Used primarily as a phosphate binder; dose should be followed with water
Special Geriatric Considerations Elderly, due to disease and/or drug therapy, may be predisposed to constipation and fecal impaction. Must consider renal insufficiency as predisposition to aluminum toxicity.
Dosage Forms Suspension: 233 mg/5 mL
References
Bohannon AD and Lyles KW "Drug-Induced Bone Disease," *Clin Geriatr Med*, 1994, 10(4):621-3.

Aluminum Phosphate Gel *see* Aluminum Phosphate *on previous page*
Aluminum Sucrose Sulfate, Basic *see* Sucralfate *on page 658*
Alupent® *see* Metaproterenol Sulfate *on page 449*
Alu-Tab® [OTC] *see* Aluminum Hydroxide *on page 28*

Amantadine Hydrochloride *(a man' ta deen)*
Brand Names Symmetrel®
Synonyms Adamantanamine Hydrochloride
Generic Available Yes
Therapeutic Class Anti-Parkinson's Agent; Antiviral Agent, Oral
Use Symptomatic and adjunct treatment of parkinsonism; also used in prophylaxis and treatment of influenza A viral infection; treatment of drug-induced extrapyramidal symptoms
Contraindications Hypersensitivity to amantadine hydrochloride or any component
Warnings Use with caution in patients with liver disease, a history of recurrent and eczematoid dermatitis, CHF, peripheral edema, uncontrolled psychosis or severe psychoneurosis, epilepsy or other seizures and in those receiving CNS stimulant drugs
Precautions May cause CNS effects or blurred vision; when treating Parkinson's disease, do not discontinue abruptly
Adverse Reactions
Cardiovascular: Orthostatic hypotension, edema, congestive heart failure

Central nervous system: Dizziness, confusion, headache, insomnia, difficulty in concentrating, anxiety, restlessness, irritability, hallucinations, psychosis

Dermatologic: Livedo reticularis

Gastrointestinal: Nausea, constipation, dry mouth

Genitourinary: Urinary retention

Overdosage Symptoms of overdose include nausea, vomiting, slurred speech, blurred vision, lethargy, hallucinations, seizures, myoclonic jerking

Toxicology Treatment should be directed at reducing the CNS stimulation and at maintaining cardiovascular function. Seizures can be treated with diazepam 5-10 mg I.V. every 15 minutes as needed; up to a total of 30 mg in an adult, while a lidocaine infusion may be required for the cardiac dysrhythmias. CNS toxicity can be treated with physostigmine 1-2 mg slow I.V. every 1-2 hours

Drug Interactions

Increased effect: Additive anticholinergic effects in patients receiving drugs with anticholinergic activity; additive CNS stimulant effect with CNS stimulants

Increased toxicity/levels with hydrochlorothiazide plus triamterene

Stability Protect from freezing

Mechanism of Action As an antiviral, blocks the uncoating of influenza A virus preventing penetration of virus into host; antiparkinsonian activity may be due to its blocking the reuptake of dopamine into presynaptic neurons and causing direct stimulation of postsynaptic receptors.

Pharmacodynamics Onset of action: Usually within 48 hours, antidyskinetic

Pharmacokinetics

Absorption: Well absorbed from GI tract

Distribution: Crosses the blood-brain barrier

Distribution: V_d:

Normal: 4.4 $\pm$0.2 L/kg

Renal failure: 5.1 $\pm$0.2 L/kg

Protein binding:

Normal renal function: ~67%

Hemodialysis patients: ~59%

Metabolism: Not appreciable, small amounts of an acetyl metabolite identified

Half-life:

Normal renal function: 2-7 hours

Elderly patients: 24-29 hours

Impaired renal function: 7-10 days

Hemodialysis patients: Usually within 8 days

Time to peak serum concentration: 1-4 hours

Elimination: 80% to 90% unchanged in urine by glomerular filtration and tubular secretion

Usual Dosage

Geriatrics: Dose based on renal function; some patients tolerate the drug better when it is given in 2 divided daily doses; see table.

Amantadine Dosing Guidelines in Renal Impairment

Cl_{cr} (mL/min/1.73 m^2)	Suggested Maintenance Regimen
>80	100 mg bid
60	200 mg/100 mg alternate days
50	100 mg/d
40	100 mg/d
30	200 mg 2 times/week*
20	100 mg 3 times/week
≤10	200 mg/100 mg alternating q7d†

*Loading dose of 200 mg recommended on the first day for Cl_{cr} <30 mL/minute.
†Includes patients maintained on 3 times/week hemodialysis.

Adults:

Parkinson's disease: 100 mg twice daily

Influenza A viral infection: 200 mg/day in 1-2 divided doses, start as soon as possible after onset of symptoms, continue for 24-48 hours after symptoms disappear

Prophylaxis: Minimum 10-day course of therapy following exposure or continue for 2-3 weeks after influenza A virus vaccine is given

Slightly dialyzable (5% to 20%)

Monitoring Parameters Renal function, Parkinson's symptoms, mental status, influenza symptoms, blood pressure

Patient Information Do not abruptly discontinue therapy, it may precipitate a parkinsonian crisis; may impair ability to perform activities requiring mental alertness or co-

(Continued)

Amantadine Hydrochloride *(Continued)*

ordination; take second dose of the day in the early afternoon to decrease the incidence of insomnia

Nursing Implications If insomnia occurs, the last daily dose should be taken in the early afternoon; assess parkinsonian symptoms prior to and throughout course of therapy

Additional Information In many patients, the therapeutic benefits of amantadine are limited to a few months

Special Geriatric Considerations Elderly patients may be more susceptible to the CNS effects of amantadine; using 2 divided daily doses may minimize this effect. The syrup may be used to administer doses <100 mg; studies have demonstrated that young adults on 200 mg/day achieve a plasma concentration of 300 ng/mL. To achieve this level (for influenza prophylaxis) in older adults, studies have suggested a dose of 100 mg or 1.4 mg/kg/day.

Dosage Forms
Capsule: 100 mg
Solution, oral: 50 mg/5 mL (473 mL)

References
Aoki FY and Sitar DS, "Amantadine Kinetics in Healthy Elderly Men: Implications for Influenza Prevention," *Clin Pharmacol Ther*, 1985, 37(2):137-44.

Aoki FY and Sitar DS, "Clinical Pharmacokinetics of Amantadine Hydrochloride," *Clin Pharmacokinet*, 1988, 14(1):35-51.

Somani SK, Degelau J, Cooper SL, et al, "Comparison of Pharmacokinetic and Safety Profiles of Amantadine 50- and 100-mg Daily Doses in Elderly Nursing Home Residents," *Pharmacotherapy*, 1991, 11(6):460-6.

Stange KC, Little DW, and Blatnik B, "Adverse Reactions to Amantadine Prophylaxis of Influenza in a Retirement Home," *J Am Geriatr Soc*, 1991, 33(7):700-5.

Ambien™ *see* Zolpidem Tartrate *on page 743*

Amcill® *see* Ampicillin *on page 51*

Amcort® *see* Triamcinolone *on page 710*

Amen® *see* Medroxyprogesterone Acetate *on page 437*

A-methaPred® *see* Methylprednisolone *on page 461*

Amethopterin *see* Methotrexate *on page 455*

Amfebutamone *see* Bupropion *on page 98*

Amikacin Sulfate *(am i kay' sin)*

Related Information
Aminoglycoside Dosing Guidelines *on page 753*
Drug Levels Commonly Monitored Guidelines *on page 771-772*

Brand Names Amikin®

Generic Available No

Therapeutic Class Antibiotic, Aminoglycoside

Use Treatment of documented gram-negative enteric infection resistant to gentamicin and tobramycin; documented infection of mycobacterial organisms susceptible to amikacin

Contraindications Hypersensitivity to amikacin sulfate or any component; cross-sensitivity may exist with other aminoglycosides

Warnings Aminoglycosides are associated with significant nephrotoxicity or ototoxicity; the ototoxicity is directly proportional to the amount of drug given and the duration of treatment; tinnitus or vertigo are indications of vestibular injury and impending bilateral irreversible damage; renal damage is usually reversible

Precautions Dose and/or frequency of administration must be modified in patients with renal impairment and elderly

Adverse Reactions Risk of hypomagnesemia if decrease in magnesium intake
Central nervous system: Confusion, delirium
Dermatologic: Rash
Hepatic: Hepatotoxicity with elevated LFTs
Neuromuscular & skeletal: Neuromuscular blockade
Otic: Ototoxicity
Renal: Nephrotoxicity
Miscellaneous: Drug fever

Overdosage Symptoms of overdose include ototoxicity, nephrotoxicity, and neuromuscular toxicity

Toxicology Treatment of choice following a single acute overdose appears to be the maintenance of good urine output of at least 3 mL/kg/hour. Dialysis is of questionable value in the enhancement of aminoglycoside elimination. If required, hemodialysis is preferred over peritoneal dialysis in patients with normal renal function. Careful hydration may be all that is required to promote diuresis and, therefore, the enhancement of the drug's elimination.

Drug Interactions Synergy with penicillins and cephalosporins, penicillins may inactivate *in vitro*; loop diuretics may potentiate the ototoxicity of the aminoglycosides

Increased/prolonged effect: Depolarizing and nondepolarizing neuromuscular block-ing agents

Increased toxicity: Concurrent use of amphotericin may increase nephrotoxicity

Stability Stable for 24 hours at room temperature when mixed in D_5W, $D_51/4NS$; $D_51/2NS$; NS; LR

Mechanism of Action Inhibits protein synthesis in susceptible bacteria by binding to ribosomal subunits

Pharmacokinetics

Absorption: I.M.: Aminoglycosides may be delayed in the bedridden patient

Half-life:

Adults: 2-3 hours

Anuria: 28-86 hours

Half-life and clearance are dependent on renal function primarily distributed into ex-tracellular fluid (highly hydrophilic); penetrates the blood-brain barrier when menin-ges are inflamed

Time to peak:

I.M.: Peak serum levels occur within 45-120 minutes

I.V.: Within 30 minutes

Elimination: 94% to 98% excreted unchanged in urine via glomerular filtration within 24 hours

Clearance (renal) may be reduced and half-life prolonged in geriatric patients

Usual Dosage I.M., I.V.:

Geriatrics: Initial: 15-20 mg/kg/day divided every 12-24 hours; occasionally every 8- or 48-hour dosing may be required; dosage adjustments should be based on serum concentrations and calculated pharmacokinetic parameters

Adults: 15-20 mg/kg/day divided every 8-12 hours

Dosing adjustment in renal impairment: Some patients may require larger or more frequent doses if serum levels document the need (ie, cystic fibrosis or febrile granulocytopenic patients). Give a loading dose of 5-7.5 mg/kg; subsequent dos-ages and frequency of administration are best determined by measurement of serum levels and assessment of renal insufficiency.

Dialyzable (50% to 100%)

Administration Administer I.M. injection in large muscle mass

Monitoring Parameters BUN, serum creatinine, serum peak and trough concentra-tions, hydration and urine output. In cases where extended treatment is warranted (>10 days), audiology testing should be considered.

Reference Range

Therapeutic:

Peak: 25-30 μg/mL

Trough: 4-8 μg/mL

Toxic:

Peak: >35 μg/mL

Trough: >10 μg/mL

Test Interactions Increased BUN, AST, ALT, alkaline phosphatase, bilirubin, creati-nine, LDH, protein; Decreased calcium, magnesium, potassium, sodium

Patient Information Report loss of hearing, ringing or roaring in the ears or feeling of fullness in head

Nursing Implications Aminoglycoside levels measured from blood taken from Silas-tic® central catheters can sometimes give falsely high readings; obtain culture for cul-ture and sensitivity before first dose; weigh patient and obtain baseline renal function before therapy begins; monitor vital signs, serum levels are reportedly lower in pa-tients with fever; give around-the-clock rather than 3 times/day, to promote less varia-tion in peak and trough serum levels

Additional Information Drug should be discontinued if signs of ototoxicity, nephro-toxicity, or hypersensitivity occurs; hearing should be tested before, during, and after treatment, when indicated; sodium content of 1 g: 29.9 mg (1.3 mEq)

Special Geriatric Considerations The aminoglycosides are important therapeutic in-terventions for infections due to susceptible organisms and as empiric therapy in seri-ously ill patients. Their use is not without risk of toxicity, however, these risks can be minimized if initial dosing is adjusted for estimated renal function and appropriate monitoring performed; see Warnings, Precautions, and Usual Dosage

Dosage Forms Injection: 50 mg/mL (2 mL); 250 mg/mL (2 mL, 4 mL)

References

Bauer LA and Blouin RA, "Influence of Age on Amikacin Pharmacokinetics in Patients Without Renal Disease. Comparison With Gentamicin and Tobramycin," *Eur J Clin Pharmacol*, 1983, 24(5):639-42.

Yasuhara H, Kobayashi S, Sakamoto K, et al, "Pharmacokinetics of Amikacin and Cephalothin in Bedridden Elderly Patients," *J Clin Pharmacol*, 1982, 22(8-9):403-9.

Amikin® see Amikacin Sulfate *on previous page*

Amiloride and Hydrochlorothiazide (a mill' oh ride)
Related Information
Amiloride Hydrochloride *on this page*
Hydrochlorothiazide *on page 347*
Brand Names Moduretic®
Synonyms Hydrochlorothiazide and Amiloride
Generic Available Yes
Therapeutic Class Diuretic, Combination
Use Antikaliuretic diuretic, antihypertensive
Contraindications Anuria, acute or chronic renal insufficiency; patients who are hypersensitive to this drug or to other sulfonamide-derived drugs
Precautions Should not be used in the presence of serum potassium levels >5.5 mEq/L
Adverse Reactions
Endocrine & metabolic: Hyperkalemia
Gastrointestinal: Nausea, diarrhea, GI pain
Usual Dosage Oral:
Geriatrics: Initial: ½ to 1 tablet daily
Adults: Start with 1 tablet daily, then may be increased to 2 tablets/day if needed; usually given in a single dose
Monitoring Parameters Blood pressure, serum electrolytes, renal function
Test Interactions Increased BUN, calcium, sodium, magnesium, chloride, uric acid
Patient Information Take with food in the morning
Special Geriatric Considerations Potassium excretion may be decreased in the elderly, increasing the risk of hyperkalemia with potassium-sparing diuretics such as amiloride.
Dosage Forms Tablet: Amiloride hydrochloride 5 mg and hydrochlorothiazide 50 mg

Amiloride Hydrochloride (a mill' oh ride)
Brand Names Midamor®
Generic Available Yes
Therapeutic Class Diuretic, Potassium Sparing
Use Counteract potassium loss induced by other diuretics in the treatment of hypertension or edematous conditions including congestive heart failure, hepatic cirrhosis and hypoaldosteronism; usually used in conjunction with a more potent diuretic such as thiazides or loop diuretics
Contraindications Hyperkalemia, potassium supplementation and impaired renal function, hypersensitivity to amiloride or any component
Warnings May cause hyperkalemia (serum levels >5.5 mEq/L) which, if uncorrected, is potentially fatal
Precautions Potassium excretion may be decreased in the elderly increasing the risk of hyperkalemia with the use of amiloride
Adverse Reactions
Central nervous system: Headache, lethargy
Dermatologic: Rash
Endocrine & metabolic: Hyperkalemia, gynecomastia, hyperchloremic metabolic acidosis, dehydration, hyponatremia
Gastrointestinal: Anorexia, nausea, vomiting, diarrhea
Toxicology Clinical signs are consistent with dehydration and electrolyte disturbance; severe hyperkalemia (>6.5 mEq/L). Ingestion of large amounts of potassium-sparing diuretics may result in life-threatening hyperkalemia. This can be treated with I.V. glucose (dextrose 25% in water), with concurrent I.V. sodium bicarbonate (1 mEq/kg up to 44 mEq/dose). If needed, Kayexalate® oral or rectal solutions in sorbitol may also be useful.
Drug Interactions
NSAIDs may reduce the therapeutic effect of amiloride; amiloride may reduce the inotropic effects of digoxin
Increased risk of hyperkalemia if given with other potassium-sparing diuretics, potassium preparations, or ACE inhibitors
Mechanism of Action Interferes with potassium/sodium exchange in the distal tubule
Pharmacokinetics
Absorption: Oral: ~50%
Distribution: V_d: 350-380 L
Half-life: 6-9 hours
Elimination: Excreted unchanged equally in urine and feces; renal clearance of amiloride is decreased in elderly
Usual Dosage
Geriatrics: Initial: 5 mg once daily or every other day
Adults: 5-10 mg/day (up to 20 mg)
Monitoring Parameters Blood pressure (standing, sitting/supine), serum electrolytes, renal function, weight, I & O
Test Interactions Increased potassium (S); decreased magnesium; transient renal and hepatic function tests have been noted

Patient Information Take in the morning with food or milk; avoid excessive ingestion of foods high in potassium or use of salt substitutes; report any muscle cramps, weakness, nausea, or dizziness

Nursing Implications Monitor I & O ratios and daily weight throughout therapy

Additional Information Medication should be discontinued if potassium level exceeds 6.5 mEq/L; combined with hydrochlorothiazide as Moduretic®; amiloride is considered an alternative to triamterene or spironolactone

Special Geriatric Considerations See Precautions

Dosage Forms Tablet: 5 mg

Aminobenzylpenicillin *see* Ampicillin *on page 51*

Aminoglycoside Dosing Guidelines *see page 753*

Aminohydroxypropylidine Diphosphonate *see* Pamidronate Disodium *on page 532*

Aminophyllin™ *see* Aminophylline *on this page*

Aminophylline (am in off' i lin)

Related Information

Drug Levels Commonly Monitored Guidelines *on page 771-772*

Brand Names Aminophyllin™; Phyllocontin®; Somophyllin®; Somophyllin®-DF; Truphylline®

Synonyms Theophylline Ethylenediamine

Generic Available Yes

Therapeutic Class Antiasthmatic; Bronchodilator; Theophylline Derivative

Use Bronchodilator in reversible airway obstruction due to asthma or COPD

Contraindications Uncontrolled arrhythmias, untreated seizure disorders, and hypersensitivity to xanthine or ethylenediamine; infection or irritation of the rectum or large colon when using suppositories

Precautions Use with caution in patients with peptic ulcer, hyperthyroidism, hypertension, and patients with compromised cardiac function

Adverse Reactions

Cardiovascular: Palpitation, sinus tachycardia, extrasystoles, hypotension, ventricular arrhythmias, flushing

Central nervous system: Irritability, restlessness, headache, insomnia, seizures, fever

Endocrine & metabolic: Hyperglycemia

Gastrointestinal: Nausea, vomiting, esophageal reflux, diarrhea, hematemesis, rectal bleeding, epigastric pain

Neuromuscular & skeletal: Tremors, muscle twitching

Renal: Diuresis, proteinuria

Respiratory: Tachypnea, respiratory arrest

Adverse reactions are uncommon at serum theophylline concentrations <20 mcg/mL

Overdosage Symptoms of overdose include tachycardia, extrasystoles, nausea, vomiting, anorexia, tonic-clonic seizures, insomnia, circulatory failure; agitation, irritability, headache

Toxicology If seizures have not occurred, induce vomiting; ipecac syrup is preferred. Do not induce emesis in the presence of impaired consciousness. Repeated doses of charcoal have been shown to be effective in enhancing the total body clearance of theophylline. Do not repeat charcoal doses if an ileus is present. Charcoal hemoperfusion may be considered if the serum theophylline level exceed 40 mcg/mL, the patient is unable to tolerate repeat oral charcoal administrations, or if severe toxic symptoms are present. Clearance with hemoperfusion is better than clearance from hemodialysis. Administer a cathartic, especially if sustained release agents were used. Phenobarbital administered prophylactically may prevent seizures.

Drug Interactions Changes in diet may affect the elimination of theophylline

Theophylline may decrease the effects of phenytoin, lithium, and neuromuscular blocking agents; theophylline increases the excretion of lithium; theophylline may have synergistic toxicity with sympathomimetics

Cimetidine, ranitidine, allopurinol, beta-blockers (nonspecific), erythromycin, influenza virus vaccine, corticosteroids, ephedrine, quinolones, thyroid hormones, oral contraceptives, amiodarone, troleandomycin, clindamycin, carbamazepine, isoniazid, loop diuretics, and lincomycin may increase theophylline concentrations

Cigarette and marijuana smoking, rifampin, barbiturates, hydantoins, ketoconazole, sulfinpyrazone, sympathomimetics, isoniazid, loop diuretics, carbamazepine, and aminoglutethimide may decrease theophylline concentrations

Tetracyclines enhance toxicity and benzodiazepine's action may be antagonized

Stability Do not use solutions if discolored or if crystals are present

Mechanism of Action Causes bronchodilatation, diuresis, CNS and cardiac stimulation, and gastric acid secretion by blocking phosphodiesterase which increases tissue concentrations of cyclic adenine monophosphate (cAMP) which in turn promotes catecholamine stimulation of lipolysis, glycogenolysis, and gluconeogenesis and in-

(Continued)

39

Aminophylline *(Continued)*

duces release of epinephrine from adrenal medulla cells. Other proposed mechanisms include inhibition of extracellular adenosine, stimulation of endogenous catecholamines, antagonism of PGE_2 and $PGE_{2\alpha}$, mobilization of intracellular calcium, and increased sensitivity of beta-adrenergic receptors in reactive airways.

Pharmacokinetics

Absorption: Oral: Depends upon dosage form; aminophylline is the ethylenediamine salt of theophylline, pharmacokinetic parameters are those of theophylline

Metabolism: In the liver

Half-life: Highly variable and dependent upon age, liver function, cardiac function, lung disease, and smoking history

Elimination: In urine as metabolites; see tables.

Aminophylline

Patient Group	Approximate Half–Life (h)
Geriatrics and Adults Nonsmoker Smoker	4–16 (8.7 avg) 4.4
Cardiac compromised, liver failure	20–30

Dosage Form	Time to Peak
Uncoated tablet	2 h
Enteric coated tablet	5 h
Chewable tablet	1–1.5 h
Extended release	4–7 h
Intravenous	<30 min

Usual Dosage Geriatrics and Adults (all dosages based upon **aminophylline**):

Treatment of acute bronchospasm:

Loading dose (in patients not currently receiving aminophylline or theophylline): 6 mg/kg (based on aminophylline) given I.V. over 20-30 minutes; administration rate should not exceed 25 mg/minute (aminophylline)

Approximate I.V. maintenance dosages are based upon **continuous infusions**; bolus dosing may be determined by multiplying the hourly infusion rate by 24 hours and dividing by the desired number of doses/day

Adults (healthy, nonsmoking): 0.7 mg/kg/hour

Older patients, patients with cor pulmonale, patients with congestive heart failure or liver failure: 0.25 mg/kg/hour

Oral:

Nonsustained release: 16-20 mg/kg/day in 4 divided doses

Sustained release: 9-13 mg/kg/day divided into 2-3 doses/day

Dosage should be adjusted according to serum level measurements during the first 12- to 24-hour period. Avoid using suppositories due to erratic, unreliable absorption. See table.

Guidelines for Drawing Theophylline Serum Levels

Dosage Form	Time to Draw Level
P.O. liquid, fast–release tab	Peak: 1 h post 4th dose Trough: just before 4th dose
P.O. slow–release product	Peak: 4 h post 3rd dose Trough: just before 3rd dose

Rectal: Geriatrics and Adults: 500 mg 3 times/day

Monitoring Parameters Heart rate, CNS effects (insomnia, irritability); respiratory rate (COPD patients often have resting controlled respiratory rates in low 20s)

Reference Range

Sample size: 0.5-1 mL serum (red top tube)

Therapeutic: 10-20 μg/mL; Toxic: >20 μg/mL some patients may have adequate clinical response with serum levels from 5-10 μg/mL

Timing of serum samples: If toxicity is suspected, draw a level any time during a continuous I.V. infusion, or 2 hours after an oral dose; if lack of therapeutic is effected, draw a trough immediately before the next oral dose or intermittent I.V. dose

Test Interactions May elevate uric acid levels

Patient Information Oral preparations should be taken with a full glass of water; avoid drinking or eating large quantities of caffeine-containing beverages or food; take at regular intervals; take sustained release tablets whole; do not chew beads; remain in bed for 15-20 minutes after inserting suppository; take with food if GI upset occurs; notify physician if nausea, vomiting, insomnia, nervousness, irritability, palpitations, seizures occur; do not change from one brand to another without consulting physician and pharmacist; do not change doses without consulting your physician

Nursing Implications Avoid I.M. injection, too painful; do not inject I.V. solution faster than 25 mg/minute; give oral and I.V. administration around-the-clock rather than 4 times/day, 3 times/day, etc (ie, 12-6-12-6, not 9-1-5-9) to promote less variation in peak and trough serum levels; do not crush sustained release drug products; do not crush enteric coated drug product; monitor vital signs, serum concentrations, and CNS effects (insomnia, irritability); encourage patient to drink adequate fluids (2 L/day) to decrease mucous viscosity in airways

Additional Information Elderly, acutely ill, and patients with severe respiratory problems, pulmonary edema, or liver dysfunction are at greater risk of toxicity because of reduced drug clearance; 100 mg aminophylline = 79 mg theophylline

Special Geriatric Considerations Although there is a great intersubject variability for half-lives of methylxanthines (2-10 hours). The elderly, as a group, have slower hepatic clearance. Therefore, use lower initial doses and monitor closely for response and adverse reactions. Additionally, elderly are at greater risk for toxicity due to concomitant disease (eg, congestive heart failure, arrhythmias), and drug use (eg, cimetidine, ciprofloxacin, etc); see Precautions and Drug Interactions

Dosage Forms
   Injection: 25 mg/mL (10 mL, 20 mL) – 250 mg (equivalent to 187 mg theophylline) per 10 mL; 500 mg (equivalent to 394 mg theophylline) per 20 mL
   Liquid, oral (dye free): 105 mg (equivalent to 90 mg theophylline) per 5 mL (240 mL)
   Suppository, rectal: 250 mg (equivalent to 198 mg theophylline) – 500 mg (equivalent to 395 mg theophylline)
   Tablet: 100 mg (equivalent to 79 mg theophylline) – 200 mg (equivalent to 158 mg theophylline) – 500 mg (equivalent to 395 mg theophylline)
   Tablet, controlled release: 225 mg (equivalent to 178 mg theophylline)

References
Kearney TE, Manoguerra AS, Curtis GP, et al, "Theophylline Toxicity and the Beta-Adrenergic System," *Ann Intern Med*, 1985, 102(6):766-9.

Mahler DA, Barlow PB, and Matthay RA, "Chronic Obstructive Pulmonary Disease," *Clin Geriatr Med*, 1986, 2(2):285-312.

Upton RA, "Pharmacokinetic Interactions Between Theophylline and Other Medication (Part II)," *Clin Pharmacokinet*, 1991, 20(2):135-50.

Aminosalicylic Acid (a mee noe sal i sill' ik)

Brand Names Pamisyl®
Synonyms PAS
Generic Available Yes
Therapeutic Class Antitubercular Agent; Nonsteroidal Anti-inflammatory Agent (NSAID), Oral
Use Treatment of tuberculosis with combination drugs
   Unlabeled use: Lipid lowering agent
Contraindications Hypersensitivity to aminosalicylic acid or its components
Precautions Use with caution in persons with reduced renal or hepatic function; patients with gastric ulcer, CHF, or sodium restriction
Adverse Reactions
   Cardiovascular: Vasculitis
   Central nervous system: Fever, encephalopathy
   Dermatologic: Skin eruptions
   Endocrine & metabolic: Goiter
   Gastrointestinal: Nausea, vomiting, diarrhea, abdominal pain
   Hematologic: Leukopenia, agranulocytosis, thrombocytopenia, blood dyscrasias
   Hepatic: Jaundice, hepatitis
   Miscellaneous: Infections, mononucleosis-like syndrome, hypersensitivity
Drug Interactions Decreased absorption of digoxin (oral dosing); vitamin B_{12} deficiency (give I.M. if needed)
Mechanism of Action Bacteriostatic against *Mycobacterium tuberculosis*
Pharmacokinetics
   Absorption: Sodium salt is readily absorbed in GI tract
   Distribution: Wide with high concentrations in pleural and caseous tissue; CSF concentrations are low
   Metabolism: Hepatic (>50% acetylation)
   Half-life: 1 hour
   Elimination: >80% excreted in urine as metabolites or free acid
   Excretion may be reduced and half-life prolonged in persons with hepatic or renal impairment
Usual Dosage Geriatrics and Adults: Oral: 14-16 g/day in 2-3 divided doses
Monitoring Parameters Signs and symptoms of resolving infection
Test Interactions May decrease serum cholesterol levels; false-positive urine glucose with copper reduction methods
   (Continued)

Aminosalicylic Acid *(Continued)*

Patient Information Take with food; may discolor urine red; do not take tablet if brown or purple in color; do not store in bathroom or kitchen as tablets will deteriorate in high humidity environments; notify physician of sore throat, bruising, bleeding, or skin rash

Nursing Implications Store in dry place; do not give tablets if discolored, give with meals

Special Geriatric Considerations See Precautions; elderly may require lower recommended dose

Dosage Forms Tablet: 500 mg

5-Aminosalicylic Acid *see* Mesalamine *on page 445*

Amiodarone Hydrochloride (a mee' oh da rone)

Brand Names Cordarone®

Generic Available No

Therapeutic Class Antiarrhythmic Agent, Class III

Use Management of resistant, life-threatening ventricular arrhythmias unresponsive to conventional therapy with less toxic agents; has also been used for treatment of supraventricular arrhythmias (atrial fibrillation, flutter, tachycardia) unresponsive to conventional therapy

Contraindications Hypersensitivity to amiodarone; severe sinus node dysfunction; marked sinus bradycardia; second and third degree A-V block; bradycardia-induced syncope, except if pacemaker is placed; thyroid disease

Warnings Not considered first-line antiarrhythmic due to high incidence of toxicity; 75% of patients experience adverse effects with large doses; exacerbation of arrhythmias (2% to 5%); discontinuation is required in 5% to 20% of patients; reserve for use in life-threatening arrhythmias refractory to other therapy; elevation of LFTs (AST/ALT), usually transient; discontinue if persistent

Precautions May be ineffective or cause arrhythmias in patients who have hypokalemia

Adverse Reactions Most patients develop adverse effects when administered chronically; gastrointestinal side effects are the most common

Patients ≥60 years of age may be at greater risk for adverse reactions

Cardiovascular: Atropine resistant bradycardia, heart block, sinus arrest, myocardial depression, congestive heart failure, paroxysmal ventricular tachycardia, hypotension; 10% to 20% of those who develop pulmonary toxicity die of cardiopulmonary adverse effects ammonia

Central nervous system: (5% to 14% incidence): Lack of coordination, fatigue, malaise, abnormal gait, ataxia, paresthesia, dizziness, headache, insomnia, nightmares, fever

Dermatologic: Slate blue discoloration of skin, photosensitivity (10%), rash

Endocrine & metabolic: Hypothyroidism (up to 11%) or less commonly hyperthyroidism; each 200 mg tablet contains 75 mg iodine; hyperglycemia, increased triglycerides; 49% of patients develop thyroid dysfunction, most have altered TFTs; amiodarone-induced hypothyroidism may be treated with thyroid supplement replacement; monitor serum T_4 and TSH with goal to achieve normal ranges of each

Gastrointestinal: Nausea, vomiting, anorexia, constipation

Hematologic: Coagulation abnormalities, thrombocytopenia

Hepatic: Increased liver enzymes, severe hepatic toxicity (potentially fatal), increased bilirubin, increased serum

Neuromuscular & skeletal: Tremors

Ocular: Corneal microdeposits (100% of patients), photophobia

Respiratory: Interstitial pneumonitis, hypersensitivity pneumonitis, pulmonary fibrosis (10% to 13% of patients); alveolar pneumonitis may present with cough, dyspnea, chest x-ray changes

Most patients develop adverse effects when administered chronically; gastrointestinal side effects are the most common

Patients ≥60 years of age may be at greater risk for adverse reactions

Overdosage Symptoms of overdose include sinus bradycardia and/or heart block, hypotension and Q-T prolongation; patients should be monitored for several days following ingestion; treat patient with general supportive measures

Toxicology Intoxication with amiodarone necessitates EKG monitoring. When bradycardia occurs, atropine may be given, however, atropine resistant bradycardia has been reported. In cases of difficult to treat amiodarone-induced bradycardia, injectable isoproterenol or a temporary pacemaker may be required; cholestyramine may enhance elimination

Drug Interactions

Amiodarone may increase plasma concentrations of digoxin and cardiac glycosides, flecainide, procainamide, quinidine, warfarin, theophylline, and phenytoin resulting in toxicities

Combined use with beta-blockers, digitalis, or calcium channel blockers may result in bradycardia, sinus arrest; use with class I antiarrhythmics → ventricular arrhythmias; amiodarone + general anesthetics may result in bradycardia, hypotension, heart block; cholestyramine may possibly decreased amiodarone serum levels

Mechanism of Action A class III antiarrhythmic agent which inhibits adrenergic stimulation, prolongs the action potential and refractory period in myocardial tissue; decreases A-V conduction and sinus node function. These effects may be due to selective blockade of tri-iodothyronine (T_3) in myocardium; also has weak calcium channel blocking activity; noncompetitive alpha- and beta-receptor antagonist; exhibits some anticholinergic activity

Pharmacodynamics

Onset of effect: 3 days to 3 weeks after starting therapy

Peak effect: 1 week to 5 months

Duration of effects after discontinuation of therapy: 7-50 days

Pharmacokinetics

Distribution: V_d: 66 L/kg (range: 18-148 L/kg)

Protein binding: 96%

Metabolism: In the liver, major metabolite N-desethylamiodarone (active); eliminated via biliary excretion; possible enterohepatic recirculation

Bioavailability: ~50% (range: 20% to 80%); maximum plasma concentration: 3-7 hours following oral administration

Half-life (oral chronic therapy): 40-55 days (range: 26-107 days)

Elimination: biphasic: 50% reduction of serum levels in 2.5-10 days; slow terminal elimination 26-107 days; steady-state levels achieved between 130-535 days with 265 days average; <1% excreted unchanged in urine

Usual Dosage Geriatrics and Adults: Ventricular arrhythmias: 800-1600 mg/day in 1-2 doses for 1-3 weeks, then 600-800 mg/day in 1-2 doses for 1 month; maintenance: 400-600 mg/day; lower doses are recommended for supraventricular arrhythmias. Administer with food if gastrointestinal side effects occur or when doses exceed 1000 mg/day; may be administered as a single daily dose once maintenance doses are achieved.

Not dialyzable

Monitoring Parameters Monitor heart rate and rhythm throughout therapy; monitor liver and thyroid function

Reference Range Therapeutic: 0.5-2.5 mg/L (SI: 1-4 µmol/L) (parent); desethyl metabolite is active and is present in equal concentration to parent drug

Test Interactions Thyroid function tests: Amiodarone partially inhibits the peripheral conversion of thyroxine (T_4) to tri-iodothyronine (T_3); serum T_4 and reverse tri-iodothyronine (RT_3) concentrations may be increased and serum T_3 may be decreased; most patients remain clinically euthyroid, however, clinical hypothyroidism or hyperthyroidism may occur

Patient Information Take with food; use sunscreen or stay out of sun to prevent burns; skin discoloration is reversible; photophobia may make sunglasses necessary

Nursing Implications Assess patient for signs of thyroid dysfunction, lethargy, edema of the hands, feet, weight loss, and pulmonary toxicity

Additional Information Onset of pharmacologic effects range from 5-30 days, full effect may take as long as 3 months; hospitalization required for initiation of therapy; response may require 1-2 weeks; CNS symptoms normally develops within 7 days, muscle weakness may present a great hazard for ambulation

Special Geriatric Considerations Information describing the clinical use and pharmacokinetics in elderly is lacking; however, elderly may be predisposed to toxicity. Half-life may be prolonged due to decreased clearance; monitor closely

Dosage Forms Tablet: 200 mg

References

Fenster PE and Nolan PE, "Antiarrhythmic Drugs," *Geriatric Pharmacology*, Bressler R and Katz MD, eds, New York, NY: McGraw-Hill, 1993, 6:105-49.

Amitone® **[OTC]** *see* Calcium Salts (Oral) *on page 111*

Amitriptyline and Perphenazine

Related Information

Amitriptyline Hydrochloride *on this page*

Perphenazine *on page 549*

Brand Names Etrafon®; Triavil®

Synonyms Perphenazine and Amitriptyline

Therapeutic Class Antidepressant, Tricyclic; Antipsychotic Agent

Adverse Reactions See individual agents

Special Geriatric Considerations Avoid use of combination products

Amitriptyline Hydrochloride (a mee trip' ti leen)

Related Information

Antidepressant Agents Comparison *on page 800*

Drug Levels Commonly Monitored Guidelines *on page 771-772*

Brand Names Elavil®; Endep®; Enovil®

Generic Available Yes

(Continued)

Amitriptyline Hydrochloride *(Continued)*

Therapeutic Class Antidepressant, Tricyclic

Use Treatment of various forms of depression, often in conjunction with psychotherapy; as an analgesic for certain chronic and neuropathic pain, migraine prophylaxis

Contraindications Hypersensitivity to amitriptyline (cross-sensitivity with other tricyclics may occur); narrow-angle glaucoma; patients receiving MAO inhibitor within past 14 days

Warnings To avoid cholinergic crisis, do not discontinue abruptly in patients receiving high doses chronically

Precautions Use with caution in patients with cardiac conduction disturbances, history of hyperthyroidism, renal or hepatic impairment, bipolar illness, benign prostatic hypertrophy; an EKG prior to initiation of therapy is advised

Adverse Reactions

Cardiovascular: Postural hypotension, arrhythmias, tachycardia, sudden death

Central nervous system: Sedation, fatigue, anxiety, confusion, insomnia, impaired cognitive function, seizures; extrapyramidal symptoms are possible, moderate to marked sedation can occur (tolerance to these effects usually occur)

Dermatologic: Photosensitivity

Endocrine and metabolic: Hypoglycemia, rarely SIADH

Gastrointestinal: Dry mouth, increased appetite and weight gain, constipation, decreased lower esophageal sphincter tone may cause GE reflux, paralytic ileus

Genitourinary: Urinary retention

Hematologic: Rarely agranulocytosis, leukopenia, eosinophilia

Hepatic: Increased liver enzymes, cholestatic jaundice

Neuromuscular & skeletal: Tremors, weakness

Ocular: Blurred vision, increased intraocular pressure

Miscellaneous: Allergic reactions

Anticholinergic effects may be pronounced; moderate to marked sedation can occur and is associated with falling

Overdosage Symptoms of overdose include agitation, confusion, hallucinations, urinary retention, hypothermia, hypotension, tachycardia

Toxicology Following initiation of essential overdose management, toxic symptoms should be treated. Ventricular arrhythmias often respond to phenytoin 15-20 mg/kg with concurrent systemic alkalinization (sodium bicarbonate 0.5-2 mEq/kg I.V.). Arrhythmias unresponsive to this therapy may respond to lidocaine 1 mg/kg I.V. followed by a titrated infusion. Physostigmine (1-2 mg I.V. slowly) may be indicated in reversing cardiac arrhythmias that are due to vagal blockade or for anticholinergic effects. Seizures usually respond to diazepam I.V. boluses (5-10 mg, up to 30 mg). If seizures are unresponsive or recur, phenytoin or phenobarbital may be required.

Drug Interactions

Amitriptyline may decrease the effects of guanethidine and may increase the effects of other CNS depressants, adrenergic agents (epinephrine, isoproterenol), anticholinergic agents and dicumarol

With MAO inhibitors, hyperpyrexia, tachycardia, hypertension, confusion, seizures, and death have been reported. Cimetidine, fluoxetine, methylphenidate, and haloperidol may decrease the metabolism and/or increase TCA levels and phenobarbital may increase the metabolism of amitriptyline; use with clonidine may result in hypertensive crisis.

Stability Keep oral solution in refrigerator, remains stable for 7 days after preparation; protect injection and Elavil® 10 mg tablets from light

Mechanism of Action Traditionally believed to increase the synaptic concentration of serotonin (5-HT) and or norepinephrine (NE) in the central nervous system by inhibition of their reuptake by the presynaptic neuronal membrane. However, additional receptor effects have been found including desensitization of adenyl cyclase, down regulation of beta-adrenergic receptors, and down regulation of serotonin receptors.

Pharmacodynamics Therapeutic effects begin in 7-21 days; NE <5-HT

Pharmacokinetics

Metabolism: In the liver to nortriptyline (active), hydroxy derivatives and conjugated derivatives

Half-life: Adults: 9-25 hours (15-hour average); half-life prolonged (mean: 21.7 hours)

Time to peak: Peak serum levels occur within 4 hours

Elimination: Renal excretion of 18% as unchanged drug; small amounts eliminated in feces by bile

Plasma levels increase with age and steady-state plasma levels are significantly increased in older patients compared to younger patients after equal doses

Usual Dosage Oral:

Geriatrics: Initial: 10-25 mg at bedtime; dose should be increased in 10-25 mg increments every week if tolerated; dose range: 25-150 mg/day

Adults: 30-100 mg/day single dose at bedtime or in divided doses; dose may be gradually increased up to 300 mg/day; once symptoms are controlled, decrease gradually to lowest effective dose

Nondialyzable

Monitoring Parameters Blood pressure, pulse; target symptoms

Reference Range
Therapeutic:
Amitriptyline and nortriptyline 100-250 ng/mL (SI: 360-900 nmol/L)
Nortriptyline 50-150 ng/mL (SI: 190-570 nmol/L)
Toxic: >0.5 µg/mL

Test Interactions Elevated glucose

Patient Information Avoid alcohol ingestion; do not discontinue medication abruptly; may cause urine to turn blue-green; may cause drowsiness, dry mouth, constipation, blurred vision; rise slowly to prevent dizziness

Nursing Implications Monitor blood pressure and pulse rate prior to and during initial therapy; evaluate mental status; monitor weight, may increase appetite and possibly a craving for sweets

Additional Information Plasma levels do not always correlate with clinical effectiveness; desired therapeutic effect (for depression) may take as long as 3-4 weeks, at that point dosage should be reduced to lowest effective level; when used for migraine headache prophylaxis, therapeutic effect may take as long as 6 weeks; a higher dosage may be required in a heavy smoker, because of increased metabolism

Special Geriatric Considerations The most anticholinergic and sedating of the antidepressants; pronounced effects on the cardiovascular system (hypotension), hence, many geropsychiatrists agree it is best to avoid in the elderly

Dosage Forms
Injection: 10 mg/mL (10 mL)
Tablet: 10 mg, 25 mg, 50 mg, 75 mg, 100 mg, 150 mg

References
Nies A, Robinson DS, Friedman MJ, et al, "Relationship Between Age and Tricyclic Antidepressant Plasma Levels," *Am J Psychiatry*, 1977, 134:790-3.
Schulz P, Turner-Tamiyasu K, Smith G, et al, "Amitriptyline Disposition in Young and Elderly Normal Men," *Clin Pharmacol Ther*, 1983, 33(3):360-6.

Amlodipine (am loe' di peen)

Related Information
Calcium Channel Blocking Agents Comparison *on page 806-807*

Brand Names Norvasc®

Generic Available No

Therapeutic Class Calcium Channel Blocker

Use Treatment of hypertension alone or in combination with antihypertensives; chronic stable angina alone or with other antianginal agents; vasospastic angina alone or in combination with other agents

Contraindications Hypersensitivity to amlodipine or any component or other calcium channel blocker; severe hypotension or second or third degree heart block

Warnings Use with caution in titrating dosages for impaired renal or hepatic function patients; use with caution in patients with congestive heart failure; may increase frequency, severity, duration of angina during initiation of therapy, increased intracranial pressure, idiopathic hypertrophic subaortic stenosis; do not abruptly withdraw therapy; use with caution in elderly due to greater propensity to hypotension

Precautions Sick sinus syndrome, severe left ventricular dysfunction, congestive heart failure, hepatic or renal impairment, hypertrophic cardiomyopathy (especially obstructive), concomitant therapy with beta-blockers or digoxin, edema

Adverse Reactions
Cardiovascular: Reductions in systemic blood pressure, flushing, tachycardia, palpitations
Central nervous system: Dizziness
Dermatologic: Acne
Gastrointestinal: Nausea, constipation

Overdosage Symptoms of overdose include hypotension

Toxicology Ipecac-induced emesis can hypothetically worsen calcium antagonist toxicity, since it can produce vagal stimulation. Supportive and symptomatic treatment, including I.V. fluids and Trendelenburg positioning, should be initiated as intoxication may cause hypotension. Although calcium (calcium chloride I.V. 1-2 g in adults with repeats as needed) has been used as an "antidote" for acute intoxications, there is limited experience to support its routine use and should be reserved for those cases where definite signs of myocardial depression are evident. Heart block may respond to isoproterenol, glucagon, atropine and/or calcium, although a temporary pacemaker may be required.

Drug Interactions Barbiturates, erythromycin, H_2 blockers, quinidine, beta-blockers, carbamazepines, fentanyl, digitalis glycosides

Mechanism of Action Inhibits calcium ion from entering "slow channels" or select voltage-sensitive areas of vascular smooth muscle and myocardium during depolarization, producing a relaxation of coronary vascular smooth muscle and coronary vasodilation; increases myocardial oxygen delivery in patients with vasospastic angina

Pharmacodynamics
Onset of action: 30-50 minutes

(Continued)

Amlodipine *(Continued)*

Peak effect: 6-12 hours
Duration: 24 hours

Pharmacokinetics
Absorption: Oral: Well absorbed; percent absorbed not determined to date
Protein binding: 93%
Metabolism: Hepatic, >90% to inactive compound
Bioavailability: 64% to 90%
Half-life: 30-50 hours
Elimination: Metabolite and parent drug excreted renally; 10% excreted unchanged in urine

Usual Dosage Oral:
Geriatrics: 2.5 mg once daily; increase by 2.5 mg increments at 7- to 14-day intervals; maximum recommended dose: 10 mg/day
Adults: 2.5-10 mg once daily

Monitoring Parameters Heart rate, blood pressure

Patient Information Do not discontinue abruptly; report any dizziness, shortness of breath, palpitations, or edema

Nursing Implications See Warnings, Precautions, Monitoring Parameters, Special Geriatric Considerations

Special Geriatric Considerations Elderly may experience a greater hypotensive response; constipation may be more of a problem in elderly; calcium channel blockers are no more effective in elderly than other therapies; however, they do not cause significant CNS effects which is an advantage over some antihypertensive agents.

Dosage Forms Tablet: 2.5 mg, 5 mg, 10 mg

Amobarbital *(am oh bar' bi tal)*

Related Information
Anxiolytic/Hypnotic Use in Long-Term Care Facilities *on page 755-756*

Brand Names Amytal®

Synonyms Amylobarbitone

Therapeutic Class Barbiturate; Hypnotic; Sedative

Restrictions C-II

Special Geriatric Considerations Use of this agent in the elderly is not recommended

Amobarbital and Secobarbital *(am oh bar' bi tal)*

Related Information
Anxiolytic/Hypnotic Use in Long-Term Care Facilities *on page 755-756*

Brand Names Tuinal®

Synonyms Secobarbital and Amobarbital

Therapeutic Class Barbiturate; Hypnotic

Restrictions C-II

Special Geriatric Considerations Use of this agent in the elderly is not recommended

Amonidrin® [OTC] *see* Guaifenesin *on page 331*

Amoxapine *(a mox' a peen)*

Related Information
Antidepressant Agents Comparison *on page 800*

Brand Names Asendin®

Generic Available Yes

Therapeutic Class Antidepressant

Use Treatment of neurotic and endogenous depression and mixed symptoms of anxiety and depression

Contraindications Hypersensitivity to amoxapine; cross-sensitivity with other tricyclics may occur; narrow-angle glaucoma; patients receiving MAO inhibitors within past 14 days

Warnings Do not discontinue abruptly in patients receiving high doses chronically

Precautions Use with caution in patients with seizures, cardiac conduction disturbances, cardiovascular diseases, urinary retention, hyperthyroidism, or those receiving thyroid replacement

Adverse Reactions Cardiac toxicities and risk of seizure are usually greater than anticholinergic effects
Cardiovascular: Cardiac toxicities, hypotension, arrhythmias
Central nervous system: Drowsiness, fever, dizziness, nervousness, insomnia, seizures, extrapyramidal effects, tardive dyskinesia, neuroleptic malignant syndrome
Dermatologic: Rash
Endocrine & metabolic: Amenorrhea, galactorrhea
Gastrointestinal: Constipation, dry mouth
Hematologic: Leukopenia
Ocular: Blurred vision

Overdosage Symptoms of overdose include grand mal convulsions, acidosis, coma, renal failure

Toxicology Following initiation of essential overdose management, toxic symptoms should be treated. Ventricular arrhythmias often respond to phenytoin 15-20 mg/kg with concurrent systemic alkalinization (sodium bicarbonate 0.5-2 mEq/kg I.V.). Arrhythmias unresponsive to this therapy may respond to lidocaine 1mg/kg I.V. followed by a titrated infusion. Physostigmine (1-2 mg I.V. slowly) may be indicated in reversing cardiac arrhythmias that are due to vagal blockade, or for anticholinergic effects. Seizures usually respond to diazepam I.V. boluses (5-10 mg, up to 30 mg). If seizures are unresponsive or recur, phenytoin or phenobarbital may be required.

Drug Interactions

May possibly decrease effects of clonidine and guanethidine

May increase effects of central nervous system depressants, adrenergic agents, anticholinergic agents; with monoamine oxidase inhibitors, hyperpyrexia, tachycardia, hypertension, seizures and death may occur

Fluoxetine may augment the effect of TCAs, delay starting TCA for 2-3 weeks after fluoxetine's discontinuation; similar interactions as with other tricyclics may occur

Mechanism of Action Traditionally believed to increase the synaptic concentration of serotonin and/or norepinephrine in the central nervous system by inhibition of their reuptake by the presynaptic neuronal membrane. However, additional receptor effects have been found including desensitization of adenyl cyclase, down regulation of beta-adrenergic receptors, and down regulation of serotonin receptors.

Pharmacodynamics Antidepressant effects usually occur after 1-3 weeks; NE >5-HT

Pharmacokinetics

Absorption: Oral: Rapidly and well absorbed

Distribution: V_d: 0.9-1.2 L/kg

Protein binding: 80%

Metabolism: Extensive in the liver

Half-life: 11-16 hours

Time to peak: Peak serum levels occur within 1-2 hours

Elimination: Excretion of metabolites and parent compound in urine

8-hydroxy metabolite is active, with a half-life: 30 hours

Usual Dosage Oral (once symptoms are controlled, decrease gradually to lowest effective dose):

Geriatrics: Initial: 25 mg at bedtime increased by 25 mg weekly for outpatients and every 3 days for inpatients if tolerated; usual dose: 50-150 mg/day, but doses up to 300 mg may be necessary

Adults: Initial: 25 mg 2-3 times/day, if tolerated, dosage may be increased to 100 mg 2-3 times/day; may be given in a single bedtime dose when dosage <300 mg/day
Maximum daily dose:
Outpatient: 400 mg
Inpatient: 600 mg

Monitoring Parameters Blood pressure, pulse; target symptoms

Reference Range Therapeutic: Amoxapine 20-100 ng/mL (SI: 64-319 nmol/L); 8-OH amoxapine 150-400 ng/mL (SI: 478-1275 nmol/L); both 200-500 ng/mL (SI: 637-1594 nmol/L)

Test Interactions Elevated glucose

Patient Information Dry mouth may be helped by sips of water, sugarless gum or hard candy; avoid alcohol; very important to maintain established dosage regimen; photosensitivity to sunlight can occur; rise slowly to prevent dizziness

Nursing Implications Monitor blood pressure and pulse rate prior to and during initial therapy; evaluate mental status; monitor weight, may increase appetite and possibly a craving for sweets; recognize signs of neuroleptic malignant syndrome and tardive dyskinesia

Additional Information May take up to 2 weeks for full therapeutic effects to be apparent; maintenance dose is usually given at bedtime to reduce daytime sedation; tolerance develops in 1-3 months in some patients, close medical follow-up is essential

Special Geriatric Considerations Has not been studied exclusively in the elderly; because of the risk for tardive dyskinesia and extrapyramidal side effects, amoxapine is not a drug of choice in the elderly; significant anticholinergic and orthostatic effects

Dosage Forms Tablet: 25 mg, 50 mg, 100 mg, 150 mg

Amoxicillin and Clavulanate Potassium see Amoxicillin and Clavulanic Acid on this page

Amoxicillin and Clavulanic Acid (a mox i sill' in & klav yoo lan' ick)
Brand Names Augmentin®
Synonyms Amoxicillin and Clavulanate Potassium
Generic Available No
Therapeutic Class Antibiotic, Penicillin
Use Treatment of otitis media, sinusitis, and infections caused by susceptible organisms involving the lower respiratory tract, skin and skin structure, and urinary tract

(Continued)

Amoxicillin and Clavulanic Acid *(Continued)*

Contraindications Known hypersensitivity to amoxicillin, clavulanic acid, or penicillin

Precautions In patients with renal impairment, doses and/or frequency of administration should be modified in response to the degree of renal impairment; high percentage of patients with infectious mononucleosis have developed rash during therapy with amoxicillin; use with caution in patients who are allergic to cephalosporins (anaphylactic reactions)

Adverse Reactions
Central nervous system: Seizures, fever
Dermatologic: Rash, urticaria; urticarial rash that appears after a few days of therapy may indicate hypersensitivity
Gastrointestinal: Nausea, vomiting, incidence of diarrhea is higher than with amoxicillin alone
Genitourinary: Vaginitis

Toxicology Many beta-lactam-containing antibiotics have the potential to cause neuromuscular hyperirritability or convulsive seizures. Hemodialysis may be helpful to aid in the removal of the drug from the blood, otherwise most treatment is supportive or symptom directed.

Drug Interactions Probenecid increased amoxicillin levels, allopurinol theoretically increased risk for amoxicillin rash

Stability Reconstituted oral suspension should be kept in refrigerator; discard unused suspension after 10 days

Mechanism of Action Amoxicillin interferes with bacterial cell wall synthesis during active multiplication causing cell death and resultant bactericidal activity against susceptible bacteria; clavulanic acid binds and inhibits beta-lactamases that inactivate amoxicillin resulting in amoxicillin having an expanded spectrum of activity

Pharmacokinetics
Absorption: Oral: Both amoxicillin and clavulanate are well absorbed
Metabolism: Clavulanic acid is metabolized in the liver
Half-life: Adults with normal renal function: Both agents are ~1 hour; amoxicillin pharmacokinetics are not affected by clavulanic acid
Time to peak: Peak levels of each appearing within 2 hours
Elimination: Amoxicillin excreted primarily unchanged in urine

Usual Dosage Geriatrics and Adults: Oral: Dose based on amoxicillin component; see amoxicillin

Dosing interval in renal impairment:
Cl_{cr} 10-50 mL/minute: Administer every 12 hours
Cl_{cr} <10 mL/minute: Administer every 24 hours
Moderately dialyzable (20% to 50%)

Test Interactions May interfere with urinary glucose determinations using Clinitest®

Patient Information Report diarrhea promptly; entire course of medication (10-14 days) should be taken to ensure eradication of organism; should be taken in equal intervals around-the-clock to maintain adequate blood levels; females should report onset of symptoms of candidal vaginitis

Nursing Implications Assess patient at beginning and throughout therapy for infection; observe for signs and symptoms of anaphylaxis; obtain specimens for C&S before the first dose; give around-the-clock rather than 3 times/day to promote less variation in peak and trough serum levels; do not give two 250 mg tablets as substitute for a 500 mg tablet, see Additional Information

Additional Information Urticarial rash that appears after a few days of therapy may indicate hypersensitivity; incidence of diarrhea is higher than with amoxicillin alone; both '250' and '500' tablets contain the same amount of clavulanic acid, thus two '250' tablets are not equivalent to one '500' tablet; clavulanic acid inhibits beta-lactamase destruction of amoxicillin

Special Geriatric Considerations Expanded coverage of this combination makes it a useful alternative when amoxicillin resistance is present and patients cannot tolerate alternative treatments; consider renal function (Cl_{cr} estimation) in elderly. Considered one of the drugs of choice in the outpatient treatment of community-acquired pneumonia in older adults.

Dosage Forms
Suspension, oral:
125: Amoxicillin trihydrate 125 mg and clavulanic acid 31.25 mg per 5 mL (75 mL, 150 mL)
250: Amoxicillin trihydrate 250 mg and clavulanic acid 62.5 mg per 5 mL (75 mL, 150 mL)
Tablet:
250: Amoxicillin trihydrate 250 mg and clavulanic acid 125 mg
500: Amoxicillin trihydrate 500 mg and clavulanic acid 125 mg
Chewable:
125: Amoxicillin trihydrate 125 mg and clavulanic acid 31.25 mg
250: Amoxicillin trihydrate 250 mg and clavulanic acid 62.5 mg

References
American Thoracic Society, "Guidelines for the Initial Management of Adults With Community-

Acquired Pneumonia: Diagnosis, Assessment of Severity, and Initial Antimicrobial Therapy," *Am Rev Respir Dis*, 1993, 148(5):1418-26.

Ancill RJ, Ballard JH, and Capewell MA, "Urinary Tract Infections in Geriatric Inpatients: A Comparative Study of Amoxicillin-Clavulanic Acid and Co-trimoxazole," *Curr Ther Res*, 1987, 41(4):444-8.

Amoxicillin Trihydrate (a mox i sill' in)

Brand Names A-Cillin®; Amoxil®; Larotid®; Polymox®; Trimox®; Utimox®; Wymox®

Synonyms Amoxycillin; *p*-Hydroxyampicillin

Generic Available Yes

Therapeutic Class Antibiotic, Penicillin

Use Treatment of otitis media, sinusitis, and infections caused by susceptible organisms involving the respiratory tract, skin, and urinary tract; prophylaxis of bacterial endocarditis

Contraindications Hypersensitivity to amoxicillin, penicillin, or any component

Precautions In patients with renal impairment, doses and/or frequency of administration should be modified in response to the degree of renal impairment; high percentage of patients with infectious mononucleosis have developed rash during therapy with amoxicillin; use with caution in patients with cephalosporin allergy (anaphylactic reaction)

Adverse Reactions

Central nervous system: Seizures, fever

Dermatologic: Rash (especially patients with mononucleosis)

Gastrointestinal: Diarrhea

Miscellaneous: Superinfection

Overdosage Symptoms of overdose include neuromuscular sensitivity, seizures

Toxicology Many beta-lactam-containing antibiotics have the potential to cause neuromuscular hyperirritability or convulsive seizures. Hemodialysis may be helpful to aid in the removal of the drug from the blood, otherwise most treatment is supportive or symptom directed.

Drug Interactions Probenecid increased amoxicillin levels, allopurinol theoretically increased risk for amoxicillin rash

Stability Oral suspension remains stable for 7 days at room temperature or 14 days if refrigerated

Mechanism of Action Interferes with bacterial cell wall synthesis during active multiplication causing cell death and resultant bactericidal activity against susceptible bacteria

Pharmacokinetics

Absorption: Oral: Rapid and nearly complete

Protein binding: 17% to 20%

Half-life (patients with Cl_{cr} <10 mL/minute): 7-21 hours

Time to peak:

Capsule: Peak levels occur within 2 hours

Suspension: 1 hour

Metabolism: Partial

Elimination: Renal excretion (80% as unchanged drug); ~30% removed by 3-hour hemodialysis

Usual Dosage Oral:

Geriatrics: Dosage may need to be adjusted based upon renal function

Adults: 250-500 mg every 8 hours; maximum dose: 2-3 g/day

Uncomplicated gonorrhea: 3 g plus probenecid 1 g in a single dose

Endocarditis prophylaxis: 3 g 1 hour before procedure and 1.5 g 6 hours later

Dosing interval in renal impairment:

Cl_{cr} 10-50 mL/minute: Administer every 12 hours

Cl_{cr} <10 mL/minute: Administer every 24 hours

Moderately dialyzable (20% to 50%)

Monitoring Parameters Signs and symptoms of infection (fever, urinary frequency or pain, etc) should begin to resolve after 1-2 days

Test Interactions Increased AST, ALT, protein

Patient Information Report diarrhea promptly; entire course of medication (10-14 days) should be taken to ensure eradication of organism; should be taken in equal intervals around-the-clock to maintain adequate blood levels

Nursing Implications Assess patient at beginning and throughout therapy for infection; observe for signs and symptoms of anaphylaxis; obtain specimens for C&S before the first dose; give around-the-clock rather than 3 times/day, etc (ie, 8-4-12, not 9-1-5) to promote less variation in peak and trough serum levels

Additional Information Food does not interfere with absorption; urticarial rash that appears after a few days of therapy may indicate hypersensitivity

Special Geriatric Considerations Resistance to amoxicillin has been a problem in patients on frequent antibiotics or in a nursing home. Alternative antibiotics may be necessary in these populations; consider renal function.

Dosage Forms

Capsule: 250 mg, 500 mg

(Continued)

Amoxicillin Trihydrate *(Continued)*

Suspension, oral: 125 mg/5 mL (5 mL unit dose, 80 mL, 100 mL, 150 mL, 200 mL); 250 mg/5 mL (5 mL unit dose, 80 mL, 100 mL, 150 mL, 200 mL)

Tablet, chewable: 125 mg, 250 mg

References

Dajani AS, Bisno AL, Chung KJ, et al, "Prevention of Bacterial Endocarditis. Recommendations by the American Heart Association," *JAMA*, 1990, 264(22):2919-22.

Hill S, Yeates M, Pathy J, et al, "A Controlled Trial of Norfloxacin and Amoxicillin in the Treatment of Uncomplicated Urinary Tract Infection in the Elderly," *J Antimicrob Chemother*, 1985, 15(4):505-6.

Amoxil® *see* Amoxicillin Trihydrate *on previous page*

Amoxycillin *see* Amoxicillin Trihydrate *on previous page*

Amphojel® [OTC] *see* Aluminum Hydroxide *on page 28*

Amphotericin B (am foe ter' i sin)

Brand Names Fungizone®

Generic Available Yes

Therapeutic Class Antifungal Agent, Systemic; Antifungal Agent, Topical

Use Treatment of severe systemic infections and meningitis caused by susceptible fungi; fungal peritonitis; irrigant for bladder fungal infections; and topically for cutaneous and mucocutaneous candidal infections

Contraindications Hypersensitivity to amphotericin or any component

Warnings I.V. amphotericin is used primarily for the treatment of patients with progressive and potentially fatal fungal infections; not to be used for common clinically inapparent forms of fungal disease

Precautions Because of the nephrotoxic potential of amphotericin, other nephrotoxic drugs should be avoided; BUN and serum creatinine levels should be determined every other day while therapy is increased and at least weekly thereafter

Adverse Reactions

Cardiovascular: Hypotension, hypertension, flushing

Central nervous system: Delirium, fever, headache, chills

Endocrine & metabolic: Hypokalemia, hypomagnesemia

Gastrointestinal: Nausea, vomiting

Hematologic: Bone marrow depression

Local: Phlebitis

Renal: Renal failure, renal tubular acidosis

Miscellaneous: Generalized pain

Adverse effects due to intrathecal amphotericin:

Cardiovascular: Headache

Central nervous system: Paresthesia, arachnoiditis, pain along lumbar nerves

Gastrointestinal: Nausea, vomiting

Genitourinary: Urinary retention

Ocular: Vision changes

Overdosage Symptoms of overdose include renal dysfunction, anemia, thrombocytopenia, granulocytopenia, fever, nausea, and vomiting

Drug Interactions

Nephrotoxic effects of other drugs (cyclosporine, aminoglycosides) may be enhanced

Corticosteroids may increase potassium depletion caused by amphotericin

May predispose patients receiving cardiac glycosides or skeletal muscle relaxants to toxicity secondary to hypokalemia

Stability Reconstitute only with sterile water without preservatives, not bacteriostatic water; benzyl alcohol, sodium chloride, or other electrolyte solutions may cause precipitation; for I.V. infusion, an in-line filter (>1 micron mean pore diameter) may be used; short-term exposure (<24 hours) to light during I.V. infusion does NOT appreciably affect potency

Mechanism of Action Binds to ergosterol altering cell membrane permeability in susceptible fungi and causing leakage of cell components with subsequent cell death

Pharmacokinetics

Distribution: Minimal amounts enter the aqueous humor, bile, CSF, amniotic fluid, pericardial fluid, pleural fluid and synovial fluid; poorly dialyzed

Protein binding: Plasma: 90%

Half-life:

Initial: 15-48 hours

Terminal phase: 15 days

Time to peak: I.V. infusions produce peak serum levels during the first hour after a 4- to 6-hour infusion

Usual Dosage Minimum dilution for amphotericin B infusions: 0.1 mg/mL

Geriatrics and Adults:

Test dose: I.V.: 1 mg infused over 20-30 minutes. If the test dose is tolerated, the initial therapeutic dose is 0.25 mg/kg. The daily dose can then be gradually increased, usually in 0.25 mg/kg increments on each subsequent day until the desired daily dose is reached.

Maintenance dose: I.V.: 0.25-1 mg/kg/day or 1.5 mg/kg every other day; do not exceed 1.5 mg/kg/day.

I.T.: 25-300 mcg every 48-72 hours; increase to 500 mcg as tolerated

Bladder irrigation: 50 mg/day in 1 L of sterile water irrigation solution instilled over 24 hours for 2-7 days or until cultures are clear

Dialysate: 1-2 mg/L of peritoneal dialysis fluid either with or without low-dose I.V. amphotericin B (a total dose of 2-10 mg/kg given over 7-14 days)

Topical: Apply to affected areas 2-4 times/day for 1-4 weeks depending on nature and severity of infection

Dosing adjustment in renal impairment: If renal dysfunction is due to the drug, the daily total can be decreased by 50% or the dose can be given every other day; I.V. therapy may take several months

Poorly dialyzed

Monitoring Parameters Monitor electrolytes, BUN, serum creatinine, LFTS, CBC regularly, I & O, signs of hypokalemia (muscle weakness, cramping, drowsiness, EKG changes, etc); if BUN exceeds 40 mg/dL or the serum creatinine exceeds 3 mg/dL, discontinue the drug or reduce the dose until renal function improves

Reference Range Therapeutic: 1-2 μg/mL (SI: 1-2.2 μmol/L)

Test Interactions Increased creatine phosphokinase [CPK] (S); decreased magnesium, potassium (S)

Patient Information Amphotericin cream may slightly discolor skin and stain clothing; personal hygiene is very important to help reduce the spread and recurrence of lesions; avoid covering topical applications with occlusive bandages; most skin lesions require 1-3 weeks of therapy

Nursing Implications May premedicate patients with acetaminophen and diphenhydramine 30 minutes prior to the amphotericin infusion. Meperidine (Demerol®) may help to reduce rigors. Dosage adjustments are not necessary with renal impairment. If renal dysfunction is due to the drug, the daily total can be decreased by 50% or the dose can be given every other day.

Special Geriatric Considerations The pharmacokinetics and dosing of amphotericin have not been studied in the elderly. It appears that use is similar to young adults; caution should be exercised and renal function and desired effect monitored closely

Dosage Forms
Cream: 3% (20 g)
Injection: 50 mg
Lotion: 3% (30 mL)
Ointment, topical: 3% (20 g)

References
Gallis HA, Drew RH, and Pickard WW, "Amphotericin B: 30 Years of Clinical Experience," *Rev Infect Dis*, 1990, 12(2):308-29.

Ampicillin (am pi sill' in)

Brand Names Amcill®; Amplin®; Omnipen®; Penamp®; Polycillin®; Principen®; Totacillin®

Synonyms Aminobenzylpenicillin

Generic Available Yes

Therapeutic Class Antibiotic, Penicillin

Use Treatment of susceptible bacterial infections

Contraindications Known hypersensitivity to ampicillin (penicillin)

Precautions Dosage adjustment may be necessary when Cl_{cr} <10-15 mL/minute; high percentage of patients with infectious mononucleosis have developed rash during therapy with ampicillin; use with caution in patients with cephalosporin allergy (anaphylactic reaction)

Adverse Reactions
Central nervous system: Penicillin encephalopathy
Dermatologic: Rash, itching
Gastrointestinal: Diarrhea, nausea, vomiting, stomach cramps and pain, pseudomembranous colitis
Miscellaneous: Superinfection

Overdosage Symptoms of overdose include neuromuscular sensitivity, seizures

Toxicology Many beta-lactam-containing antibiotics have the potential to cause neuromuscular hyperirritability or convulsive seizures. Hemodialysis may be helpful to aid in the removal of the drug from the blood, otherwise most treatment is supportive or symptom directed.

Drug Interactions Aminoglycosides (synergy possible), decreased elimination and increased serum concentrations with probenecid, allopurinol (rash)

Food/Drug Interactions Food decreases rate and extent of absorption; take on an empty stomach

Stability Oral suspension stable for 14 days under refrigeration; solutions for I.M. or direct I.V. should be used within 1 hour; solutions for I.V. infusion will be inactivated by dextrose at room temperature; if dextrose containing solutions are to be used, the resultant solution will only be stable for 2 hours versus 8 hours in the 0.9% sodium chloride injection.

(Continued)

Ampicillin *(Continued)*

Mechanism of Action Interferes with bacterial cell wall synthesis during active multiplication causing cell death and resultant bactericidal activity against susceptible bacteria

Pharmacokinetics
Absorption: Oral: 50%; not affected by age
Distribution: Into bile; penetration into CSF occurs with inflamed meninges only
Protein binding: 15% to 25%
Half-life:
Adults: 1-1.8 hours
Anuric patients: 8-20 hours
Time to peak: Oral: Peak serum levels appear within 1-2 hours
Elimination: ~90% of drug excreted unchanged in urine within 24 hours, ~40% is removed by hemodialysis
Clearance has been reported to be decreased and half-life prolonged in older patients

Usual Dosage Geriatrics and Adults (for geriatric patients, give usual adult dose unless renal function is markedly reduced):
I.M., I.V.: 8-12 g/day in 4-6 divided doses
Oral: 250-500 mg every 6 hours

Dosing interval in renal impairment:
Cl_{cr} 10-30 mL/minute: Administer every 6-12 hours
Cl_{cr} <10 mL/minute: Administer every 12 hours

Administration
Do not use D_5W as a diluent, D_5W has limited stability
Standard diluent: Dose/50 mL NS
Minimum volume: Concentration should not exceed 30 mg/mL; manufacturer may supply as either the anhydrous or the trihydrate form

Monitoring Parameters Signs and symptoms of infection (fever, urinary frequency or pain, etc) should begin to resolve after 1-2 days

Test Interactions Increased protein; urinary glucose (Benedict's solution, Clinitest®); increased AST, positive Coombs' [direct]

Patient Information Take on an empty stomach; complete full course of therapy; should be taken at equal intervals around-the-clock to maintain adequate blood levels; women should report onset of symptoms of candidal vaginitis

Nursing Implications Ampicillin and gentamicin should not be mixed in the same I.V. tubing or administered concurrently; do C&S before starting therapy; observe patient for signs and symptoms of hypersensitivity; keep resuscitation equipment, epinephrine, and antihistamine close by in the event of an anaphylactic reaction. Give on an empty stomach (ie, 1 hour prior to, or 2 hours after meals) to increase total absorption. Give around-the-clock rather than 4 times/day (ie, 12-6-12-6, not 9-1-5-9) to promote less variation in peak and trough serum levels. Dosage adjustment may be necessary when Cl_{cr} <10-15 mL/minute.

Additional Information Appearance of a rash should be carefully evaluated to differentiate a nonallergic ampicillin rash from a hypersensitivity reaction; ampicillin rash is dull red, macular or maculopapular, and only mildly pruritic; normally appears on pressure areas like knees, elbows, palms, or soles, and may spread in symmetric pattern over most of the body; incidence of ampicillin rash is higher in patients with viral infections, *Salmonella* infections, lymphocytic leukemia, or patients that have hyperuricemia

Sodium content of suspension (250 mg/5 mL, 5 mL): 10 mg (0.4 mEq)
Sodium content of 1 g: 66.7 mg (3 mEq)

Special Geriatric Considerations See Pharmacokinetics and Usual Dosage; adjust dose for renal function

Dosage Forms
Capsule, as anhydrous: 250 mg, 500 mg
Capsule, as trihydrate: 250 mg, 500 mg
Injection, as sodium: 125 mg, 250 mg, 500 mg, 1 g, 2 g, 10 g
Suspension, oral, as trihydrate: 125 mg/5 mL (5 mL unit dose, 80 mL, 100 mL, 150 mL, 200 mL); 250 mg/5 mL (5 mL unit dose, 80 mL, 100 mL, 150 mL, 200 mL); 500 mg/5 mL (5 mL unit dose, 100 mL)

References
Triggs EJ, Johnson JM, and Learoyd B, "Absorption and Disposition of Ampicillin in the Elderly," *Eur J Clin Pharmacol*, 1980, 18(2):195-8.

Ampicillin Sodium and Sulbactam Sodium

Brand Names Unasyn®
Synonyms Sulbactam and Ampicillin
Generic Available No
Therapeutic Class Antibiotic, Penicillin
Use Treatment of susceptible bacterial infections involved with skin and skin structure, intra-abdominal infections, gynecological infections; spectrum is that of ampicillin plus organisms producing beta-lactamases such as *S. aureus*, *H. influenzae*, *E. coli*, *Klebsiella*, *Acinetobacter*, *Enterobacter* and anaerobes

Contraindications Hypersensitivity to ampicillin, sulbactam or any component, or penicillins

Warnings Should not be administered to patients with mononucleosis

Precautions Use with caution in patients allergic to cephalosporins; a high percentage of patients with infectious mononucleosis have developed rash during therapy with ampicillin; modify dosage in patients with renal impairment whose Cl_{cr} is <10-15 mL/minute

Adverse Reactions

Cardiovascular: Chest pain, thrombophlebitis

Central nervous system: Fatigue, malaise, headache, chills

Dermatologic: Rash, itching

Gastrointestinal: Diarrhea, nausea, vomiting, enterocolitis, pseudomembranous colitis

Hematologic: Decreased WBC, neutrophils, platelets, hemoglobin, and hematocrit

Hepatic: Increased liver enzymes

Local: Pain at injection site (I.M.: 16%, I.V.: 3%)

Renal: Dysuria, increased BUN and creatinine

Miscellaneous: Candidiasis, hairy tongue, hypersensitivity reactions

Toxicology Many beta-lactam-containing antibiotics have the potential to cause neuromuscular hyperirritability or convulsive seizures. Hemodialysis may be helpful to aid in the removal of the drug from the blood, otherwise most treatment is supportive or symptom directed.

Drug Interactions Aminoglycosides, bacteriostatic agents, uricosuric agents (probenecid, indomethacin, sulfinpyrazone, and high dose aspirin >3-4 g/day), chlorpropamide, diuretics, pyrazinamide, diazoxide, alcohol, mecamylamine

Stability I.M. and direct I.V. administration: used within 1 hour after preparation; reconstitute with sterile water for injection or 0.5% or 2% lidocaine hydrochloride injection (I.M.); sodium chloride 0.9% (NS) is the diluent of choice for I.V. piggyback use, solutions made in NS are stable up to 72 hours when refrigerated whereas dextrose solutions (same concentration) are stable for only 4 hours

Mechanism of Action The addition of sulbactam, a beta-lactamase inhibitor, to ampicillin extends the spectrum of ampicillin to include beta-lactamase producing organisms; ampicillin acts by inhibiting bacterial cell wall synthesis during the stage of active multiplication

Pharmacokinetics

Protein binding:

Ampicillin: 28%

Sulbactam: 38%

Half-life: Ampicillin and sulbactam are similar: 1-1.8 hours and 1-1.3 hours, respectively

Time to peak: Peak serum concentrations of ampicillin and sulbactam are reached immediately

Elimination: ~75% to 85% of both drugs are excreted unchanged in the urine within 8 hours following administration

Reduced clearance and prolonged half-life in the elderly have been found for both compounds; age and renal function were negatively correlated with clearance

Usual Dosage Unasyn® (ampicillin/sulbactam) is a combination product; each 3 g vial contains 2 g of ampicillin and 1 g of sulbactam. Sulbactam has very little antibacterial activity by itself, but effectively extends the spectrum of ampicillin to include beta-lactamase producing strains that are resistant to ampicillin alone. Therefore, dosage recommendations for Unasyn® are based on the ampicillin component.

Geriatrics and Adults: I.M., I.V.: 1-2 g ampicillin every 6-8 hours; maximum: 8 g ampicillin/day, 4 g sulbactam/day

Dosing interval in renal impairment:

Cl_{cr} 15-29 mL/minute: Administer every 12 hours

Cl_{cr} 5-14 mL/minute: Administer every 24 hours

Monitoring Parameters Signs and symptoms of infection (fever, urinary frequency or pain, etc) should begin to resolve after 1-2 days; with prolonged therapy, monitor hematologic, renal, and hepatic function

Test Interactions False-positive urinary glucose levels (Benedict's solution, Clinitest®)

Patient Information Report sore throat, fever, fatigue, or diarrhea

Nursing Implications Do C&S before starting therapy; observe patient for signs and symptoms of hypersensitivity; keep resuscitation equipment, epinephrine, and antihistamine close by in the event of an anaphylactic reaction; observe for superinfection; for I.M. injection reconstitute with sterile water or 0.5% or 2% lidocaine hydrochloride. Reduce dose with decreased renal function.

Additional Information Appearance of a rash should be carefully evaluated to differentiate a nonallergic ampicillin rash from a hypersensitivity reaction; ampicillin rash is dull red, macular or maculopapular, and only mildly pruritic; normally appears on pressure areas like knees, elbows, palms, or soles, and may spread in symmetric pattern over most of the body; incidence of ampicillin rash is higher in patients with viral infections, *Salmonella* infections, lymphocytic leukemia, or patients that have hyperuricemia

(Continued)

Ampicillin Sodium and Sulbactam Sodium *(Continued)*

Special Geriatric Considerations See Pharmacokinetics and Usual Dosage; adjust dose for renal function

Dosage Forms Powder for injection:

1.5 g: Ampicillin sodium 1 g and sulbactam sodium 0.5 g

3 g: Ampicillin sodium 2 g and sulbactam sodium 1 g

References

Meyers BR, Wilkinson P, Mendelson MH, et al, "Pharmacokinetics of Ampicillin-Sulbactam in Healthy Elderly and Young Volunteers," *Antimicrob Agents Chemother*, 1991, 35(10):2098-101.

Rho SP, Jones A, Woo M, et al, "Single Dose Pharmacokinetics of Intravenous Ampicillin plus Sulbactam in Healthy Elderly and Young Subjects," *J Antimicrob Chemother*, 1989, 24(4):573-80.

Amplin® *see Ampicillin on page 51*

Amrinone Lactate *(am' ri none)*

Brand Names Inocor®

Generic Available No

Therapeutic Class Adrenergic Agonist Agent

Use Treatment of low cardiac output states (sepsis, congestive heart failure); adjunctive therapy of pulmonary hypertension

Contraindications Hypersensitivity to amrinone lactate or sulfites (contains 0.25 mg sodium metabisulfite)

Warnings Inotropic effects additive to other inotropic agents (digitalis, theophylline); use cautiously in patients with atrial and ventricular arrhythmias; may increase ventricular response since amrinone increases slightly atrioventricular condition; hypersensitivity may occur rapidly, within a few weeks of continued therapy

Precautions Monitor fluids and electrolytes; diuresis may result from improvement in cardiac output and may require dosage reduction of diuretics; do not use in valvular disease, idiopathic subaortic stenosis, or myocardial infarction; may cause arrhythmias; thrombocytopenia with continuous therapy; hepatotoxicity, hypovolemic patients (dehydrated diuresis) may have inadequate filling pressure

Adverse Reactions

Cardiovascular: Hypotension (1.3%), ventricular and supraventricular arrhythmias (3%) (may be related to infusion rate), chest pain (0.2%), pericarditis, vasculitis

Central nervous system: Fever (0.9%)

Gastrointestinal: Nausea, vomiting, abdominal pain, and anorexia

Hematologic: Thrombocytopenia (2.4% incidence) may be dose related; may be reversed with dose reduction within 4 weeks

Hepatic: Hepatotoxicity (0.2% incidence) discontinue amrinone if significant increase in liver enzymes with symptoms of idiosyncratic hypersensitivity reaction, ascites

Local: Burning at injection site

Neuromuscular & skeletal: Myositis

Respiratory: Pleuritis

Overdosage Symptoms of overdose include hypotension

Toxicology There is no specific antidote for amrinone intoxication. Overdosage with amrinone has caused severe hypotension by vasodilation, if this occurs general measures for circulatory support should be taken; decrease dose

Drug Interactions When furosemide is admixed with amrinone, a precipitate immediately forms; diuretics may cause significant hypovolemia and decrease filling pressure

Stability May be administered undiluted for I.V. bolus doses. For continuous infusion, dilute with 0.45% or 0.9% sodium chloride to final concentration of 1-3 mg/mL; use within 24 hours; do not directly dilute with dextrose-containing solutions, chemical interaction occurs; may be administered I.V. into running dextrose infusions. Furosemide forms a precipitate when injected in I.V. lines containing amrinone.

Mechanism of Action Inhibits myocardial cyclic adenosine monophosphate (cAMP) phosphodiesterase activity and increases cellular levels of cAMP resulting in a positive inotropic effect and increased cardiac output; also possesses systemic and pulmonary vasodilator effects resulting in pre- and afterload reduction; slightly increases atrioventricular conduction

Pharmacodynamics

Onset of action: I.V.: Following administration, hemodynamic actions occur within 2-5 minutes

Peak effects: Within 10 minutes

Duration: Dose dependent with low doses lasting ~30 minutes and higher doses lasting ~2 hours

Pharmacokinetics

Distribution: V_d: 1.2 L/kg

Protein binding: 10% to 49%

Metabolism: In the liver

Half-life:

Normal adult volunteers: 3.6 hours

Congestive heart failure: 5.8 hours, range: 3-15 hours
Elimination: Excreted (60% to 90% as metabolites) in urine within 24 hours; 10% to 40% excreted unchanged in urine

Usual Dosage Note: Dose should not exceed 10 mg/kg/24 hours
Geriatrics and Adults: 0.75 mcg/kg I.V. bolus over 2-3 minutes followed by maintenance infusion of 5-10 mcg/kg/minute

Monitoring Parameters Thrombocytopenia, hepatotoxicity, GI effects, blood pressure and heart rate every 5 minutes during infusion, CVP, PCWP, respiratory rate; monitor renal function and fluid electrolyte status (particularly potassium)

Reference Range 0.5-7 μg/mL

Patient Information Change position slowly because of postural hypotension

Nursing Implications Should be administered solely via an I.V. pump; patients should be carefully monitored for hemodynamic response (hypotension) and potential adverse effects (ie, thrombocytopenia, hepatotoxicity, and GI effects)

Additional Information Is normally prescribed for patients who have not responded well to therapy with digitalis, diuretics, and vasodilators; dosage is based on clinical response

Special Geriatric Considerations While amrinone is not specifically arrhythmogenic, elderly may be at high risk for ventricular and particularly atrial arrhythmias due to high incidence of arrhythmias in this population; also, elderly are often hypovolemic due to dehydration; therefore, monitor fluid status carefully (CVP line) in order to have effective falling pressure for maximal response; found to be as effective as dobutamine in elderly with heart failure in one study despite the decline in beta-adrenergic response with age

Dosage Forms Injection: 5 mg/mL (20 mL)

References
Rich MW, Woods WL, Davila-Roman VC, et al, "A Randomized Comparison of Intravenous Amrinone Versus Dobutamine in Older Patients With Decompensated Congestive Heart Failure," *JAGS*, 1995, 43:271-4.

Amylobarbitone *see* Amobarbital *on page 46*

Amytal® *see* Amobarbital *on page 46*

Anacin-3® [OTC] *see* Acetaminophen *on page 13*

Anacin® [OTC] *see* Aspirin *on page 58*

Anafranil® *see* Clomipramine Hydrochloride *on page 175*

Anaprox® *see* Naproxen *on page 493*

Anaspaz® *see* Hyoscyamine Sulfate *on page 359*

Ancef® *see* Cefazolin Sodium *on page 127*

Ancobon® *see* Flucytosine *on page 296*

Anergan® *see* Promethazine Hydrochloride *on page 599*

Anestacon® *see* Lidocaine Hydrochloride *on page 406*

Anexia® *see* Hydrocodone and Acetaminophen *on page 350*

Anigesic® *see* Salsalate *on page 637*

Anocol® *see* Chloramphenicol *on page 148*

Ansaid® *see* Flurbiprofen Sodium *on page 306*

Ansamycin *see* Rifabutin *on page 627*

Anspor® *see* Cephradine *on page 145*

Antacid Drug Interactions *see page 764*

Antidepressant Agents Comparison *see page 800*

Antidiuretic Hormone *see* Vasopressin *on page 732*

Antilirium® *see* Physostigmine *on page 562*

Antipsychotic Agents Comparison *see page 801*

Antipsychotic Medication Guidelines *see page 754*

Antispas® *see* Dicyclomine Hydrochloride *on page 215*

Anti-Tuss® [OTC] *see* Guaifenesin *on page 331*

Antivert® *see* Meclizine Hydrochloride *on page 434*

Antrizine® *see* Meclizine Hydrochloride *on page 434*

Anturane® *see* Sulfinpyrazone *on page 662*

Anxanil® *see* Hydroxyzine *on page 356*

Anxiolytic/Hypnotic Use in Long-Term Care Facilities *see page 755*

Apacet® [OTC] *see* Acetaminophen *on page 13*

APAP *see* Acetaminophen *on page 13*

Aplisol® *see* Tuberculin Purified Protein Derivative *on page 725*

APPG *see* Penicillin G Procaine, Aqueous *on page 541*

Apraclonidine Hydrochloride (a pra kloe' ni deen)
Brand Names Alpidine®; Iopidine®
Generic Available Yes
Therapeutic Class Alpha-2-Adrenergic Agonist Agent, Ophthalmic
Use
 0.5% solution: Short-term adjunctive therapy in patients on maximally tolerated medi-
 cal therapy who require additional IOP reduction
 1% solution: Prevention and treatment of postsurgical intraocular pressure elevation
Contraindications Known hypersensitivity to apraclonidine or clonidine; concurrent
 use of a monoamine oxidase inhibitor
Warnings Closely monitor patients who develop exaggerated reductions in intraocular
 pressure; use with caution in patients with cardiovascular disease and in patients
 with a history of vasovagal reactions
Precautions Efficacy as an adjunctive therapy may be limited in patients already using
 two aqueous suppressing drugs
Adverse Reactions
 Cardiovascular: Arrhythmias
 Central nervous system: Dizziness, depression, insomnia, lethargy, nervousness, par-
  esthesia, somnolence
 Dermatologic: Dermatitis
 Gastrointestinal: Dry mouth, nausea, constipation
 Ocular: Conjunctival blanching, mydriasis, upper lid elevation, burning, discomfort,
  itching, conjunctival microhemorrhage, blurred vision
 Respiratory: Dyspnea, rhinitis
 Miscellaneous: Allergic response, peripheral edema
Overdosage No cases of human ingestion reported; supportive treatment indicated
Drug Interactions Increased effect: Topical beta-blockers, pilocarpine → additive de-
 creased intraocular pressure; monoamine oxidase inhibitors (theoretical); may exacerbate effects of CNS depressants; tricyclic antidepressants have competitive effects
 (theoretical); additive effects possible with cardiovascular and other agents with hypotensive effects
Stability Store in tight, light-resistant containers
Mechanism of Action Apraclonidine is a potent alpha-adrenergic agent similar to
 clonidine; relatively selective for alpha$_2$-receptors but does retain some binding to
 alpha$_1$-receptors; appears to result in reduction of aqueous humor formation; more
 polar than clonidine which reduces its penetration through the blood-brain barrier and
 suggests that its pharmacological profile is characterized by peripheral rather than
 central effects
Pharmacodynamics
 Onset of action: 1 hour
 Maximum IOP: 3-5 hours
Pharmacokinetics Half-life: 8 hours
Usual Dosage Ophthalmic:
 0.5% solution: Instill 1-2 drops instilled in the affected eye(s) 3 times/day
 1% solution: Instill 1 drop in operative eye 1 hour prior to laser surgery, second drop
 in eye upon completion of procedure
Administration Wait 5 minutes between instillation of other ophthalmic agents to
 avoid washout of previous dose; after topical instillation, finger pressure should be
 applied to lacrimal sac to decrease drainage into the nose and throat and minimize
 possible systemic absorption
Monitoring Parameters Intraocular pressure, fundoscopic exam, visual field testing
Reference Range Steady-state concentration: Peak: 0.9 ng/mL; trough: 0.5 ng/mL
Patient Information May sting on instillation, do not touch dropper to eye; visual acuity may be decreased after administration; night vision may be decreased; distance
 vision may be altered; read package instructions for insertion
Nursing Implications See Administration and Patient Information
Special Geriatric Considerations Determine that the patient or caregiver can ade-
 quately administer ophthalmic medication dosage form
Dosage Forms Solution: 0.5% and 1% with benzalkonium chloride 0.01% (0.25 mL)

Apresazide® *see* Hydralazine and Hydrochlorothiazide *on page 345*

Apresoline® *see* Hydralazine Hydrochloride *on page 345*

Aprodine® [OTC] *see* Triprolidine and Pseudoephedrine *on page 723*

AquaMEPHYTON® *see* Vitamin K and Menadiol *on page 738*

Aquaphyllin® *see* Theophylline *on page 681*

Aquazide-H® *see* Hydrochlorothiazide *on page 347*

Aqueous Procaine Penicillin G *see* Penicillin G Procaine, Aqueous *on page 541*

Ara-A *see* Vidarabine *on page 737*

Arabinofuranosyladenine *see* Vidarabine *on page 737*

Aredia™ *see* Pamidronate Disodium *on page 532*

Argesic®-SA *see* Salsalate *on page 637*

8-Arginine Vasopressin *see* Vasopressin *on page 732*

Aristocort® Forte *see* Triamcinolone *on page 710*

Aristocort® Intralesional Suspension *see* Triamcinolone *on page 710*

Aristocort® Tablet *see* Triamcinolone *on page 710*

Aristospan® *see* Triamcinolone *on page 710*

Arlidin® *see* Nylidrin Hydrochloride *on page 512*

Arm-a-Med® Isoetharine *see* Isoetharine *on page 378*

Arm-a-Med® Isoproterenol *see* Isoproterenol *on page 380*

Arm-a-Med® Metaproterenol *see* Metaproterenol Sulfate *on page 449*

Armour® Thyroid *see* Thyroid *on page 691*

Arrestin® *see* Trimethobenzamide Hydrochloride *on page 720*

Artane® *see* Trihexyphenidyl Hydrochloride *on page 717*

Artha-G® *see* Salsalate *on page 637*

Arthropan® *see* Salicylates (Various Salts) *on page 633*

ASA *see* Aspirin *on next page*

A.S.A. [OTC] *see* Aspirin *on next page*

5-ASA *see* Mesalamine *on page 445*

Asacol® *see* Mesalamine *on page 445*

Ascorbic Acid (a skor' bik)

Brand Names Ascorbicap® [OTC]; Cecon® [OTC]; Cee-1000® T.D. [OTC]; Cetane® [OTC]; Cevalin® [OTC]; Ce-Vi-Sol® [OTC]; Cevita® [OTC]; C-Span® [OTC]; Flavor-cee® [OTC]; Vita-C® [OTC]

Synonyms Vitamin C

Generic Available Yes

Therapeutic Class Urinary Acidifying Agent; Vitamin, Water Soluble

Use Prevention and treatment of scurvy; urinary acidification; dietary supplementation; has been promoted in prevention and decreasing the severity of colds, wounds; urinary acidifier (4-12 g/day); idiopathic methemoglobinemia

Warnings Diabetics and patients prone to recurrent renal calculi should not take excessive doses for extended periods of time

Precautions Some products contain tartrazine and sulfites; avoid in sensitive patients

Adverse Reactions
Cardiovascular: Flushing
Central nervous system: Faintness, dizziness, headache, fatigue
Gastrointestinal: Nausea, vomiting, heartburn, diarrhea
Renal: Hyperoxaluria, large doses precipitate cystine, oxalate and urate renal stones

Overdosage Symptoms of overdose include renal calculi, nausea, gastritis, diarrhea

Toxicology Diuresis with forced fluids may be useful following a massive ingestion

Drug Interactions Iron, aspirin, estrogens, warfarin
Drug-lab tests: False-negative urine glucose determinations with doses >500 mg/day; occult blood tests may be falsely negative if vitamin C ingested within 48-72 hours of test

Stability Injectable form should be stored under refrigeration (2°C to 8°C); protect oral dosage forms from light; is rapidly oxidized when in solution in air and alkaline media

Mechanism of Action Vitamin C's biologic functions are not fully understood; it is necessary for collagen formation and tissue repair in the body; involved in some oxidation-reduction reactions as well as other metabolic reactions, such as synthesis of carnitine, steroids, and catecholamines; conversion of folic acid to folinic acid

Pharmacokinetics
Absorption: Oral: Readily absorbed with a wide distribution; absorption is an active process and is thought to be dose-dependent
Metabolism: In the liver by oxidation and sulfation
Elimination: In urine; there is an individual specific renal threshold for ascorbic acid; when blood levels are high, ascorbic acid is excreted in urine, whereas when the levels are subthreshold very little if any ascorbic acid is cleared into urine

Usual Dosage Geriatrics and Adults: Oral, I.M., I.V., S.C.:
Scurvy: 500-1000 mg/day for at least 2 weeks

(Continued)

57

Ascorbic Acid *(Continued)*

Urinary acidification: 4-12 g/day in 3-4 divided doses

RDA dietary supplement: 60 mg/day

Wound healing: 300-500 mg/day; larger amounts have been also recommended; maximum 7-10 days pre- and postoperatively

Burns: 1-2 g/day

Prevention and treatment of cold: 1-3 g/day

Monitoring Parameters Monitor for renal calculi; monitor pH of urine when acidifying

Reference Range None

Test Interactions False-positive urinary glucose with cupric sulfate reagent, false-negative urinary glucose with glucose oxidase method

Patient Information Do not use in large doses if diabetic or have a history of renal stones; do not exceed 3 g/day without physician's advice

Nursing Implications Avoid rapid I.V. injection; monitor urine pH when using as an acidifying agent

Additional Information Sodium content of 1 g of sodium ascorbate: ~5 mEq

Special Geriatric Considerations Minimum RDA for elderly is not established; vitamin C is provided mainly in citrus fruits and tomatoes; the elderly, however, avoid citrus fruits due to cost and difficulty preparing (peeling); daily replacement through a single multiple vitamins recommended; use of natural vitamin C or rose hips offers no advantages; acidity may produce GI complaints

Dosage Forms

Capsule, timed release: 500 mg

Crystals: 4 g/teaspoonful (1000 g)

Drops: 100 mg/mL (50 mL)

Injection: 100 mg/mL (2 mL, 10 mL); 250 mg/mL (30 mL, 50 mL)

Liquid: 35 mg/0.6 mL (50 mL)

Powder: 4 g/teaspoonful (1000 g)

Syrup: 500 mg/5 mL (5 mL, 10 mL, 120 mL, 480 mL)

Tablet: 50 mg, 100 mg, 250 mg, 500 mg, 1000 mg

Tablet:

Chewable: 100 mg, 250 mg, 500 mg

Timed release: 500 mg, 1500 mg

References
Myrianthopoulos M, "Dietary Treatment of Hyperlipidemia in the Elderly," *Clin Geriatr Med*, 1987, 3(2):343-59.

Ascorbicap® [OTC] *see* Ascorbic Acid *on previous page*

Ascriptin® [OTC] *see* Aspirin *on this page*

Asendin® *see* Amoxapine *on page 46*

Asmalix® *see* Theophylline *on page 681*

Aspergum® [OTC] *see* Aspirin *on this page*

Aspirin *(as' pir in)*

Brand Names Anacin® [OTC]; A.S.A. [OTC]; Ascriptin® [OTC]; Aspergum® [OTC]; Bayer® Aspirin [OTC]; Bufferin® [OTC]; Easprin®; Ecotrin® [OTC]; Empirin® [OTC]; Measurin® [OTC]; Synalgos® [OTC]; ZORprin®

Synonyms Acetylsalicylic Acid; ASA

Generic Available Yes

Therapeutic Class Analgesic, Non-narcotic; Anti-inflammatory Agent; Antiplatelet Agent; Antipyretic; Nonsteroidal Anti-inflammatory Agent (NSAID), Oral; Salicylate

Use Treatment of mild to moderate pain, inflammation and fever; management of rheumatoid arthritis, rheumatic fever, osteoarthritis, and gout (high dose); may be used as a prophylaxis of myocardial infarction and transient ischemic attacks (TIA)

Contraindications Bleeding disorders (factor VII or IX deficiencies), hypersensitivity to salicylates or other nonsteroidal anti-inflammatory drugs (NSAIDs); tartrazine dye and asthma

Warnings Tinnitus or impaired hearing may indicate toxicity; discontinue use 1 week prior to surgical procedures

Precautions Use with caution in patients with platelet and bleeding disorders, renal dysfunction, hepatic disease, history of salicylate-induced gastric irritation, peptic ulcer disease, erosive gastritis, bleeding disorders, hypoprothrombinemia, and vitamin K deficiency; use cautiously in asthmatics, especially those with aspirin intolerance and nasal polyps

Adverse Reactions

Central nervous system: Dizziness, mental confusion, CNS depression, fever, headache, lassitude

Dermatologic: Rash, urticaria, angioedema

Gastrointestinal: Nausea, vomiting, dyspepsia, epigastric discomfort, GI distress, ulcers, thirst

Hematologic: Occult bleeding, prolongation of bleeding time, leukopenia, thrombocytopenia, inhibition of platelet aggregation
Hepatic: Hepatotoxicity
Otic: Tinnitus
Respiratory: Bronchospasm, hyperventilation
Miscellaneous: Sweating

Overdosage 10-30 g; symptoms of overdose include tinnitus, headache, dizziness, confusion, metabolic acidosis, hyperpyrexia, hyperpnea, tachypnea, nausea, vomiting, irritability, disorientation, hallucinations, lethargy, stupor, dehydration, hyperventilation, hyperthermia, hyperactivity, depression leading to coma, respiratory failure, and collapse; laboratory abnormalities include hypokalemia, hypoglycemia or hyperglycemia with alterations in pH

Toxicology The "Done" nomogram is very helpful for estimating the severity of aspirin poisoning and directing treatment using serum salicylate levels. Treatment can also be based upon symptomatology; see table.

Aspirin or Other Salicylate Toxicity

Toxic Symptoms	Treatment
Overdose	Induce emesis with ipecac, and/or lavage with saline, followed with activated charcoal
Dehydration	I.V. fluids with KCl (no D_5W only)
Metabolic acidosis (must be treated)	Sodium bicarbonate
Hyperthermia	Cooling blankets or sponge baths
Coagulopathy/hemorrhage	Vitamin K I.V.
Hypoglycemia (with coma, seizures or change in mental status)	Dextrose 25 g I.V.
Seizures	Diazepam 5–10 mg I.V.

Drug Interactions
Aspirin may increase methotrexate serum levels and may displace valproic acid from binding sites which can result in toxicity; warfarin and aspirin → ↑ bleeding
NSAIDs and aspirin → ↑ GI adverse effects, possible decreased serum concentration of NSAIDs
Aspirin may antagonize effects of probenecid and sulfinpyrazone since salicylates in low dose (<2.4 g/day) antagonize uricosuric effect
Corticosteroids increased salicylate serum levels
Nizatidine increased serum salicylate levels
ACE inhibitors, anticoagulants, beta-blockers, heparin, loop diuretics, nitroglycerin, sulfinpyrazone, spironolactone, sulfonylureas, insulin, valproic acid

Stability Keep suppositories in refrigerator, do not freeze; hydrolysis of aspirin occurs upon exposure to water or moist air, resulting in salicylate and acetate, which possess a vinegar-like odor; do not use if a strong odor is present

Mechanism of Action Inhibits prostaglandin synthesis, acts on the hypothalamus heat-regulating center to reduce fever, blocks prostaglandin synthetase action which prevents formation of the platelet-aggregating substance thromboxane A_2; decreases pain receptor sensitivity. Other proposed mechanisms of action for salicylate anti-inflammatory action are lysosomal stabilization, kinin and leukotriene production, alteration of chemotactic factors, and inhibition of neutrophil activation. This latter mechanism may be the most significant pharmacologic action to reduce inflammation.

Pharmacokinetics
Absorption: From the stomach and small intestine
Distribution: Readily into most body fluids and tissues; aspirin is hydrolyzed to salicylate (active) by esterases in the GI mucosa, red blood cells, synovial fluid and blood
Plasma protein binding: Plasma protein bound (albumin) >90% at low concentrations and 76% at high concentrations (400 mcg/mL)
Metabolism: Metabolism of salicylate occurs primarily by hepatic microsomal enzymes
Half-life, aspirin: 15-20 minutes
Metabolic pathways are saturable such that salicylates half-life is dose-dependent ranging from 3 hours at lower doses (300-600 mg), 5-6 hours (after 1 g) and 15-30 hours with higher doses; in therapeutic anti-inflammatory doses, half-lives generally range from 6-12 hours
Time to peak: Peak plasma levels appear in ~1-2 hours
(Continued)

Aspirin *(Continued)*

Usual Dosage Geriatrics and Adults:

Analgesic and antipyretic: Oral, rectal: 325-1000 mg every 4-6 hours up to 4 g/day

Anti-inflammatory: Oral: Initial: 2.4-3.6 g/day in divided doses; usual maintenance: 3.6-5.4 g/day, monitor serum concentrations

TIA: Oral: 1.3 g/day in 2-4 divided doses; other studies have demonstrated equal efficacy with fewer side effects at a dose of 300 mg/day

Myocardial infarction, stroke, and atrial fibrillation prophylaxis: 81-325 mg/day

Dialyzable (50% to 100%)

Monitoring Parameters Serum concentrations, renal function; hearing changes or tinnitus; monitor for response (ie, pain, inflammation, range of motion, grip strength); observe for abnormal bleeding, bruising, weight gain

Reference Range

Sample size: 1.5-2 mL blood (purple top tube)

Timing of serum samples: Peak levels usually occur 2 hours after ingestion; the half-life increases with the dosage (eg, the half-life after 300 mg is 3 hours, and after 1 g is 5-6 hours, and after 8-10 g is 10-15 hours).

Salicylate serum concentrations correlate with the pharmacological actions and adverse effects observed. Anti-inflammatory therapeutic serum concentrations 15-30 mg/dL. See table.

Serum Salicylate: Clinical Correlations

Serum Salicylate Concentration (mg/dL)	Desired Effects	Adverse Effects/ Intoxication
~10	Antiplatelet Antipyresis Analgesia	GI intolerance and bleeding, hypersensitivity, hemostatic defects
15-30	Anti-inflammatory	Mild salicylism
25-40	Treatment of rheumatic fever	Nausea/vomiting, hyperventilation, salicylism, flushing, sweating, thirst, headache, diarrhea and tachycardia
>40-50		Respiratory alkalosis, hemorrhage, excitement, confusion, asterixis, pulmonary edema, convulsions, tetany, metabolic acidosis, fever, coma, cardiovascular collapse, renal and respiratory failure

Test Interactions False-negative results for glucose oxidase urinary glucose tests (Clinistix®); false-positives using the cupric sulfate method (Clinitest®); also, interferes with Gerhardt test (urinary ketone analysis), VMA determination; 5-HIAA, xylose tolerance test, and T_3 and T_4; increased PBI; increased uric acid

Patient Information Watch for bleeding gums or any signs of GI bleeding; take with food or milk to minimize GI distress, notify physician if ringing in ears or persistent GI pain occurs; do not crush or chew sustained release or enteric coated preparation; avoid other aspirin or salicylate containing products

Nursing Implications Administer with food or a full glass of water to minimize GI distress; do not crush sustained release tablets or enteric coated tablets; monitor for bleeding, bruising, tinnitus

Special Geriatric Considerations Elderly are a high-risk population for adverse effects from nonsteroidal anti-inflammatory agents. As much as 60% of elderly with GI complications to NSAIDs can develop peptic ulceration and/or hemorrhage asymptomatically. The concomitant use of H_2 blockers, omeprazole, and sucralfate is not effective as prophylaxis. Misoprostol is the only prophylactic agent proven effective. Also, concomitant disease and drug use contribute to the risk for GI adverse effects. Use lowest effective dose for shortest period possible. Consider renal function decline with age. Use of NSAIDs can compromise existing renal function especially when Cl_{cr} is ≤30 mL/minute. Tinnitus may be a difficult and unreliable indication of toxicity due to age-related hearing loss or eighth cranial nerve damage. CNS adverse effects such as confusion, agitation, and hallucination are generally seen in overdose or high dose situations, but elderly may demonstrate these adverse effects at lower doses than younger adults.

Dosage Forms

Capsule: 356.4 mg with caffeine 30 mg

Suppository, rectal: 120 mg, 200 mg, 300 mg, 600 mg

Tablet: 81 mg, 325 mg, 500 mg

Tablet:

With caffeine: 400 mg with caffeine 32 mg

Buffered: 325 mg with magnesium-aluminum hydroxide 150 mg
Chewable: 81 mg
Coated: 325 mg
Effervescent: 325 mg, 500 mg
Enteric coated: 81 mg, 325 mg, 500 mg
Sustained release: 650 mg, 800 mg

References

Clinch D, Banerjee AK, Ostrik G, "Absence of Abdominal Pain in Elderly Patients With Peptic Ulcer," *Age Ageing*, 1984, 13:120-3.

Clive DM and Stoff JS, "Renal Syndromes Associated With Nonsteroidal Anti-inflammatory Drugs," *N Engl J Med*, 1984, 310(9):563-72.

Knodel LC, "Preventing NSAID-Induced Ulcers: The Role of Misoprostol," *Consult Pharm*, 1989, 4:37-41.

Weissmann G, "Aspirin," *Sci Am*, 1991, 264(1):84-90.

Aspirin and Codeine (as' pir in)

Related Information
Aspirin *on page 58*
Codeine *on page 183*

Brand Names Empirin® With Codeine

Synonyms Codeine and Aspirin

Generic Available Yes

Therapeutic Class Analgesic, Narcotic

Use Relief of mild to moderate pain

Restrictions C-III

Contraindications Hypersensitivity to aspirin, codeine or any component

Precautions Use with caution in patients with impaired renal function, erosive gastritis, or peptic ulcer

Adverse Reactions
Central nervous system: CNS depression
Dermatologic: Rash, urticaria
Gastrointestinal: Nausea, vomiting, constipation
Hematologic: Occult bleeding
Hepatic: Hepatotoxicity
Respiratory: Respiratory depression, bronchospasm

Drug Interactions Refer to individual monographs for Aspirin and Codeine

Usual Dosage
Geriatrics: One #3 tablet (30 mg codeine) or two #2 tablets (15 mg codeine/each) every 4-6 hours as needed for pain
Adults: 1-2 tablets every 4-6 hours as needed for pain

Monitoring Parameters Pain relief, respiratory status, blood pressure, mental status

Test Interactions Urine glucose, urinary 5-HIAA, serum uric acid

Patient Information May cause drowsiness, avoid alcoholic beverages; check cough and cold preparations for aspirin content

Nursing Implications Observe patient for excessive sedation or confusion, respiratory depression, constipation

Special Geriatric Considerations The duration of action of codeine may be prolonged in the elderly; in addition, enhanced analgesia has been seen in elderly patients on therapeutic doses of narcotics; if one tablet/dose is used, it may be useful to add an addition 325 mg of aspirin to maximize analgesic effect

Dosage Forms Tablet:
#2: Aspirin 325 mg and codeine phosphate 15 mg
#3: Aspirin 325 mg and codeine phosphate 30 mg
#4: Aspirin 325 mg and codeine phosphate 60 mg

Aspirin and Oxycodone see Oxycodone and Aspirin *on page 529*

Asproject® see Salicylates (Various Salts) *on page 633*

Astemizole (a stem' mi zole)

Brand Names Hismanal®

Generic Available No

Therapeutic Class Antihistamine

Use Perennial and seasonal allergic rhinitis and other allergic symptoms including urticaria

Contraindications Hypersensitivity to astemizole or any component

Warnings Rare cases of severe cardiovascular events (cardiac arrest, arrhythmias) have been reported in the following situations: overdose (even as low as 20-30 mg/day), significant hepatic dysfunction, when used in combination with erythromycin, ketoconazole, or itraconazole

Adverse Reactions
Central nervous system: Not likely to cause drowsiness, dizziness, nervousness, headache. **Note:** Minimal sedation and anticholinergic effects are seen as compared to older antihistamines.

(Continued)

Astemizole *(Continued)*

Gastrointestinal: Appetite increase, dry mouth, weight increase

Overdosage Symptoms of overdose include sedation, apnea, diminished mental alertness, ventricular tachycardia, torsade de pointes

Toxicology There is no specific treatment for an antihistamine overdose, however most of its clinical toxicity is due to anticholinergic effects. Anticholinesterase inhibitors including physostigmine, neostigmine, pyridostigmine and edrophonium may be useful for the overdose with severe life-threatening symptoms. Physostigmine 1-2 mg I.V., slowly may be given to reverse the anticholinergic effects. Cases of ventricular arrhythmias following dosages above 200 mg have been reported, however, overdoses of up to 500 mg have been reported without ill effect. Patients should be carefully observed with EKG monitoring in cases of suspected overdose. Magnesium may be helpful for torsade de pointes or a lidocaine bolus followed by a titrated infusion.

Drug Interactions Increased toxicity: Erythromycin, other macrolide antibiotics, itraconazole, ketoconazole

Mechanism of Action Competes with histamine for H_1-receptor sites on effector cells in the gastrointestinal tract, blood vessels, and respiratory tract; binds to lung receptors significantly greater than it binds to cerebellar receptors, resulting in a reduced sedative potential

Pharmacokinetics

Distribution: Nonsedating action reportedly due to the drugs low lipid solubility and poor penetration through the blood-brain barrier

Protein binding: 97%

Metabolism: Undergoes exclusive first-pass metabolism

Half-life: 20 hours

Time to peak serum concentration: Oral: Long-acting, with steady-state plasma levels of parent compound and metabolites seen within 4-8 weeks following initiation of chronic therapy peak plasma levels appear in 1-4 hours following administration

Elimination: Eliminated by metabolism in the liver to active and inactive metabolites, which are thereby excreted in the feces and to a lesser degree in the urine

Usual Dosage Oral:

Geriatrics: 10 mg/day

Adults: 10 mg/day; to decrease time to steady-state, give 30 mg on first day, 20 mg on second day, then 10 mg/day in a single dose

Monitoring Parameters Relief of symptoms

Patient Information Take on an empty stomach, at least 2 hours after a meal or 1 hour before a meal. Because of its delayed onset, astemizole is useful for prophylaxis of allergic symptoms, rather than for acute relief. Do not exceed recommended doses.

Nursing Implications Give on an empty stomach

Additional Information Not likely to cause drowsiness

Special Geriatric Considerations Because of its low incidence of sedation and anticholinergic effects, astemizole would be a rational choice in the elderly when an antihistamine is indicated

Dosage Forms Tablet: 10 mg

AsthmaHaler® see Epinephrine *on page 256*

AsthmaNefrin® [OTC] see Epinephrine *on page 256*

Astramorph™ PF see Morphine Sulfate *on page 481*

Atabrine® see Quinacrine Hydrochloride *on page 615*

Atarax® see Hydroxyzine *on page 356*

Atenolol *(a ten' oh lole)*

Related Information

Beta-Blockers Comparison *on page 804-805*

Brand Names Tenormin®

Generic Available Yes

Therapeutic Class Antianginal Agent; Beta-Adrenergic Blocker

Use Treatment of hypertension, alone or in combination with other agents; also used in management of angina pectoris; selective inhibitor of $beta_1$-adrenergic receptors; postmyocardial infarction patients

Unlabeled use: Acute alcohol withdrawal, supraventricular and ventricular arrhythmias, and migraine headache prophylaxis; diastolic congestive heart failure

Contraindications Hypersensitivity to beta-blocking agents, pulmonary edema, cardiogenic shock, bradycardia, heart block, uncompensated congestive heart failure, sinus node dysfunction, A-V conduction abnormalities, diabetes mellitus. Although atenolol primarily blocks $beta_1$-receptors, high doses can result in $beta_2$-receptor blockade. Use with caution in elderly with bronchospastic lung disease and renal dysfunction. Geriatric patients often have decreased renal function, see Usual Dosage.

Warnings Abrupt withdrawal of beta-blockers may result in an exaggerated cardiac beta-adrenergic responsiveness. Symptomatology has included reports of tachycardia, hypertension, ischemia, angina, myocardial infarction, and sudden death. It is recommended that patients be tapered gradually off of beta-blockers over a 2-week period rather than via abrupt discontinuation.

Precautions Administer to congestive heart failure patients with caution; administer with caution to patients with bronchospastic disease, diabetes mellitus, hyperthyroidism, myasthenia gravis and renal function decline and severe peripheral vascular disease. Abrupt withdrawal of the drug should be avoided, drug should be discontinued over 2 weeks.

Adverse Reactions

Cardiovascular: Persistent bradycardia, hypotension, chest pain, edema, heart failure, second or third degree A-V block, Raynaud's phenomena

Central nervous system: Dizziness, fatigue, insomnia, lethargy, confusion, mental depression, headache, nightmares

Gastrointestinal: Constipation, diarrhea, nausea

Genitourinary: Impotence

Respiratory: Dyspnea have occurred when daily dosage exceeds 100 mg/day, wheezing

Miscellaneous: Cold extremities

Overdosage Symptoms of overdose include bradycardia, congestive heart failure, hypotension, bronchospasm, hypoglycemia; see Toxicology

Toxicology Sympathomimetics (eg, epinephrine or dopamine), glucagon or a pacemaker can be used to treat the toxic bradycardia, asystole, and/or hypotension. Initially, fluids may be the best treatment for toxic hypotension. Patients should remain supine; serum glucose and potassium should be measured. Use supportive measures: lavage, syrup of ipecac; atenolol may be removed by hemodialysis. I.V. glucose should be administered for hypoglycemia; seizures may be treated with phenytoin or diazepam intravenously; continuous monitoring of blood pressure and EKG is necessary. If PVCs occur, treat with lidocaine or phenytoin; avoid quinidine, procainamide, and disopyramide since these agents further depress myocardial function. Bronchospasm can be treated with theophylline on beta$_2$ agonists (epinephrine).

Drug Interactions

Pharmacologic action of beta-antagonists may be decreased by aluminum compounds, calcium salts, barbiturates, cholestyramine, colestipol, NSAIDs, penicillins (ampicillin), rifampin, salicylates, sulfinpyrazone, thyroid hormones; hypoglycemic effect of sulfonylureas may be blunted

Pharmacologic effect of beta-antagonists may be enhanced with concomitant use of calcium channel blockers, oral contraceptives, flecainide (bioavailability and effect of flecainide also enhanced), haloperidol (hypotensive effects of both drugs), H$_2$ antagonists (decreased metabolism), hydralazine (both drugs' hypotensive effects increased), loop diuretics (increased serum levels of beta-blockers except atenolol), MAO inhibitors, phenothiazines, propafenone, quinidine, quinolones, thioamines; beta-blockers may decrease clearance of acetaminophen; beta-blockers may increase anticoagulant effects of warfarin (propranolol); benzodiazepine effects enhanced by the lipophilic beta-blockers (atenolol does not interact)

Significant and fatal increases in blood pressure have occurred after decrease in dose or discontinuation of clonidine in patients receiving both clonidine and beta-blockers together (reduce doses of each cautiously with small decreases); peripheral ischemia of ergot alkaloids enhanced by beta-blockers; beta-blockers increase serum concentration of lidocaine; beta-blockers increase hypotensive effect of prazosin

Stability Dilutions in dextrose, sodium chloride, and sodium chloride and dextrose stable for 48 hours

Mechanism of Action Competitively blocks response to beta$_1$-adrenergic receptors with little or no effect on beta$_2$-receptors except at high doses; consider renal function, see Usual Dosage. Does not exhibit membrane stabilizing or intrinsic sympathomimetic activity; low lipid solubility, therefore, little crosses blood-brain barrier.

Pharmacokinetics

Absorption: Incompletely from GI tract (50%)

Distribution: Does **not** cross the blood-brain barrier

Protein binding: Low (3% to 15%)

Half-life: 6-9 hours (longest in patients with reduced renal function)

Time to peak: Oral: Peak serum concentrations occur within 2-4 hours

Elimination: 40% excreted as unchanged drug in urine, 50% in feces

Usual Dosage Geriatrics and Adults:

Oral: 50-100 mg/dose given daily; doses >100 mg/day are unlikely to produce further response; **geriatrics initial dose: 25 mg/day**

I.V.: For early treatment of myocardial infarction: 5 mg slow I.V. over 5 minutes; may repeat in 10 minutes; if both doses are tolerated, may start oral atenolol 50 mg every 12 hours;

Dosing interval in renal impairment:

Cl$_{cr}$ 15-35 mL/minute: Administer 50 mg/day maximum

Cl$_{cr}$ <15 mL/minute: Administer 50 mg every other day maximum

Postmyocardial infarction:

I.V.: Administer as soon as possible 5 mg over 5 minutes; follow with 5 mg I.V. 10 minutes later

(Continued)

Atenolol *(Continued)*

Oral: Follow with 100 mg/day or 50 mg twice daily for 6-9 days postmyocardial infarction

Moderately dialyzable (20% to 50%)

Monitoring Parameters Blood pressure, orthostatic hypotension, heart rate, CNS effects, EKG

Test Interactions Increased triglycerides, potassium, uric acid, cholesterol (S), glucose; decreased HDL

Patient Information Adhere to dosage regimen; watch for postural hypotension; do not discontinue medication abruptly, sudden stopping of medication may precipitate or cause angina; consult pharmacist or physician before taking with other adrenergic drugs (eg, cold medications); notify physician if any of the following symptoms occur: difficult breathing, night cough, swelling of extremities, slow pulse, dizziness, lightheadedness, confusion, depression, skin rash, fever, sore throat, unusual bleeding or bruising; may produce drowsiness, dizziness, lightheadedness, blurred vision, confusion; use with caution while driving or performing tasks requiring alertness; may mask signs of hypoglycemia in diabetics; may be taken without regard to meals

Nursing Implications Patient's therapeutic response may be evaluated by looking at blood pressure, apical and radial pulses, fluid I & O, daily weight, respirations, and circulation in extremities before and during therapy; monitor for CNS side effects; modify dosage in patients with renal insufficiency

Additional Information May potentiate hypoglycemia in a diabetic patient and mask signs and symptoms; patients who receive hemodialysis should receive 50 mg oral dose after each dialysis

Special Geriatric Considerations Due to alterations in the beta-adrenergic autonomic nervous system, beta-adrenergic blockade may result in less hemodynamic response than seen in younger adults. Studies indicate that despite decreased sensitivity to the chronotropic effects of beta blockade with age, there appears to be an increased myocardial sensitivity to the negative inotropic effect during stress (ie, exercise). Controlled trials have shown the overall response rate for propranolol to be only 20% to 50% in elderly populations. Therefore, all beta-adrenergic blocking drugs may result in a decreased response as compared to younger adults.

Dosage Forms
Injection: 0.5 mg/mL (10 mL)
Tablet: 50 mg, 100 mg

References
Aagaard GN, "Treatment of Hypertension in The Elderly," *Drug Treatment in the Elderly*, Vestal RE, ed, Boston, MA: ADIS Health Science Press, 1984, 77.

Ativan® *see* Lorazepam *on page 419*

Atovaquone

Brand Names Mepron™

Therapeutic Class Antiprotozoal

Use Acute oral treatment of mild to moderate *Pneumocystis carinii* pneumonia (PCP) in patients who are intolerant to co-trimoxazole

Contraindications Life-threatening allergic reaction to the drug or formulation

Warnings Has only been used in mild to moderate PCP; use with caution in elderly patients because of potentially impaired renal, hepatic, and cardiac function

Adverse Reactions
Central nervous system: Fever, insomnia, headache, anxiety, dizziness, asthenia
Dermatologic: Rash, pruritus
Endocrine & metabolic: Hypoglycemia, amylase, hyponatremia
Gastrointestinal: Nausea, diarrhea, vomiting, abdominal pain, anorexia, dyspepsia, oral *Monilia*, constipation
Hematologic: Leukopenia, neutropenia, anemia
Hepatic: Elevated liver enzymes (ALT, AST, alkaline phosphatase), and BUN
Renal: Elevated creatinine
Respiratory: Cough

Drug Interactions Possible increased toxicity with other highly protein bound drugs; however, serum concentrations of 15 mcg/mL of phenytoin failed to cause an interaction

Mechanism of Action Mechanism has not been fully elucidated; may inhibit electron transport in mitochondria inhibiting metabolic enzymes

Pharmacokinetics
Absorption: Decreased significantly in single doses >750 mg; increased threefold when administered with a high fat meal
Distribution: Enterohepatically recirculated
Protein binding: >99.9%
Bioavailability: ~30%
Half-life: 2.9 days
Elimination: In feces

Usual Dosage Geriatrics and Adults: Oral: 750 mg 3 times/day with food for 21 days

Patient Information Take only prescribed dose; take each dose with a meal, preferably one with high fat content

Nursing Implications Notify physician if patient is unable to eat significant amounts of food on an ongoing basis

Special Geriatric Considerations See Warnings; has not been extensively evaluated in patients >65 years of age

Dosage Forms Tablet, film coated: 250 mg

Atromid-S® see Clofibrate on page 174

Atropair® see Atropine Sulfate on this page

Atropine and Diphenoxylate see Diphenoxylate and Atropine on page 230

Atropine-Care® see Atropine Sulfate on this page

Atropine Sulfate (a' troe peen)

Brand Names Atropair®; Atropine-Care®; Atropisol®; Isopto® Atropine; I-Tropine®; Ocu-Tropine®

Generic Available Yes

Therapeutic Class Anticholinergic Agent; Anticholinergic Agent, Ophthalmic; Antidote, Organophosphate Poisoning; Antispasmodic Agent, Gastrointestinal; Bronchodilator; Ophthalmic Agent, Mydriatic

Use Preoperative medication to inhibit salivation and secretions; treatment of sinus bradycardia; management of peptic ulcer; treatment of exercise-induced bronchospasm; urinary incontinence; antidote for organophosphate pesticide poisoning; used to produce mydriasis and cycloplegia for examination of the retina and optic disk and accurate measurement of refractive errors; uveitis

Contraindications Hypersensitivity to atropine sulfate or any component; narrow-angle glaucoma; tachycardia; thyrotoxicosis; obstructive disease of the GI tract; obstructive uropathy, asthma

Precautions Use with caution in geriatric patients since they may be more sensitive to its effects. Low doses cause a paradoxical decrease in heart rates. Some commercial products contain sodium metabisulfite, which can cause allergic-type reactions. Heat prostration may occur in hot weather. Use with caution in patients with autonomic neuropathy, prostatic hypertrophy, hyperthyroidism, congestive heart failure, cardiac arrhythmias, chronic lung disease, biliary tract disease.

Adverse Reactions

Cardiovascular: Tachycardia, palpitations

Central nervous system: Fatigue, ataxia, delirium, headache, restlessness, ataxia.
  Note: The elderly may be at increased risk for confusion and hallucinations.

Dermatologic: Dry hot skin

Gastrointestinal: Impaired GI motility, dry mouth

Genitourinary: Difficult urination

Neuromuscular & skeletal: Tremors

Ocular: Mydriasis, blurred vision

Miscellaneous: Heat intolerance

Toxicology Anticholinergic toxicity is caused by strong binding of the drug to cholinergic receptors. Anticholinesterase inhibitors reduce acetylcholinesterase, the enzyme that breaks down acetylcholine and thereby allows acetylcholine to accumulate and compete for receptor binding with the offending anticholinergic. For anticholinergic overdose with severe life-threatening symptoms, physostigmine 1-2 mg S.C. or I.V., slowly may be given to reverse these effects.

Drug Interactions

Decreased effect of phenothiazines, levodopa, tacrine

Increased toxicity: Amantadine, tricyclic antidepressants, some antihistamines

Stability Store injection below 40°C, avoid freezing

Mechanism of Action Blocks the action of acetylcholine at parasympathetic sites in smooth muscle, secretory glands and the CNS; increases cardiac output, dries secretions, antagonizes histamine and serotonin

Pharmacokinetics

Absorption: Well absorbed from all dosage forms

Distribution: Wide throughout the body; crosses the blood-brain barrier

Metabolism: In the liver

Half-life: 2-3 hours

Elimination: Into urine of both metabolites and unchanged drug (30% to 50%)

Usual Dosage Geriatrics and Adults:

Preanesthetic: I.M., I.V., S.C.: 0.4-0.6 mg 30-60 minutes preop

Bradycardia: I.V.: 0.5-1 mg every 5 minutes, not to exceed a total of 2 mg

Ophthalmic, 1% solution: 1-2 drops before the procedure

Uveitis: 1-2 drops 4 times/day

Monitoring Parameters Blood pressure, pulse, mental status, anticholinergic effects

(Continued)

Atropine Sulfate (Continued)

Patient Information Maintain good oral hygiene habits, because lack of saliva may increase chance of cavities. Observe caution while driving or performing other tasks requiring alertness, as may cause drowsiness, dizziness, or blurred vision. Notify physician if skin rash, flushing or eye pain occurs, or if difficulty in urinating, constipation, or sensitivity to light becomes severe or persists.

Nursing Implications Observe for tachycardia if patient has cardiac problems; lack of saliva may increase chance of cavities, therefore, good oral hygiene should be promoted

Additional Information Because of its bothersome and potentially dangerous side effects, atropine is rarely used except as a preoperative agent or in the acute treatment of bradyarrhythmias

Special Geriatric Considerations Anticholinergic agents are generally not well tolerated in the elderly and their use should be avoided when possible. See Precautions, Adverse Reactions. In the elderly, anticholinergic agents should not be used as prophylaxis against extrapyramidal symptoms.

Dosage Forms

Injection: 0.1 mg/mL (5 mL, 10 mL); 0.3 mg/mL (1 mL, 30 mL); 0.4 mg/mL (1 mL, 20 mL, 30 mL); 0.5 mg/mL (1 mL, 5 mL, 30 mL); 0.8 mg/mL (0.5 mL, 1 mL); 1 mg/mL (1 mL, 10 mL)

Ophthalmic:

Ointment: 0.5%, 1% (3.5 g)

Solution: 0.5% (5 mL); 1% (2 mL); 2% (1 mL, 2 mL); 3% (5 mL)

Tablet: 0.4 mg

Tablet, soluble: 0.4 mg, 0.6 mg

References

Feinberg M, "The Problems of Anticholinergic Adverse Effects in Older Patients," *Drugs Aging*, 1993, 3(4):335-48.

Atropisol® *see* Atropine Sulfate *on previous page*

Atrovent® *see* Ipratropium Bromide *on page 376*

A/T/S® *see* Erythromycin, Topical *on page 266*

Attapulgite (at a pull' gite)

Brand Names Diar-Aid® [OTC]; Diasorb® [OTC]; Kaopectate® Advanced Formula® [OTC]; Rheaban® [OTC]

Generic Available Yes

Therapeutic Class Antidiarrheal

Use Symptomatic treatment of diarrhea

Restrictions See Warnings and Precautions

Contraindications Fecal impaction; constipation; ileus

Warnings Do not use with diarrhea associated with toxigenic bacteria or pseudomembranous colitis

Precautions Use with caution in patients >60 years of age due to fecal impaction potential; presence of high fever; do not use in patients predisposed to fecal impaction

Adverse Reactions Gastrointestinal: Constipation, fecal impaction

Overdosage May cause bowel impaction and intestinal obstruction

Drug Interactions Digoxin absorption may be decreased due to adsorbent action of attapulgite; caution should be used with concomitant administration of any drug due to attapulgite's adsorbent action

Mechanism of Action Controls diarrhea because of its adsorbent action

Pharmacokinetics Absorption: Not absorbed from GI tract

Usual Dosage Geriatrics and Adults: Oral: 1200-1500 mg after each loose bowel movement or every 2 hours; 15-30 mL up to 8 times/day, or up to 9000 mg/24 hours

Monitoring Parameters Monitor for reduction of stools per day and increased consistency; monitor for signs of fluid and electrolyte loss

Patient Information If diarrhea is not controlled in 48 hours, contact a physician

Nursing Implications Shake well before giving; re-evaluate cause of diarrhea if not controlled in 48 hours; diarrhea should also be treated by diet (ie, clear liquids, bland foods, and no dairy products for first 24-48 hours); monitor for signs of fluid and electrolyte loss

Special Geriatric Considerations Elderly often present bowel impaction with diarrhea. The use of adsorbents in the face of fecal impaction could aggravate this serious condition. Also, diarrhea causes fluid/electrolyte loss which elderly do not tolerate well. Use of adsorbents can cause further loss of fluid/electrolytes.

Dosage Forms Liquid, oral concentrate: 600 mg/15 mL

Attenuvax® *see* Measles Virus Vaccine, Live, Attenuated *on page 433*

Augmentin® *see* Amoxicillin and Clavulanic Acid *on page 47*

Auranofin (au rane' oh fin)

Brand Names Ridaura®
Generic Available No
Therapeutic Class Gold Compound
Use Management of active stage of classic or definite rheumatoid arthritis in patients that do not respond to or tolerate other agents; psoriatic arthritis; adjunctive or alternative therapy for pemphigus
Contraindications Renal disease, history of blood dyscrasias, congestive heart failure, exfoliative dermatitis, necrotizing enterocolitis, history of anaphylactic reactions
Warnings Therapy should be discontinued if platelet count falls below 100,000/mm^3; <4000 WBC, <1500 granulocytes/mm^3; explain the possibility of adverse reactions before initiating therapy; signs of gold toxicity include decrease in hemoglobin, leukopenia, granulocytes and platelets; proteinuria, hematuria, pruritus, stomatitis, persistent diarrhea, rash, metallic taste; diabetes mellitus and congestive heart failure should be in control before initiating therapy; use cautiously in patients with a history of blood dyscrasias, bone marrow depression, inflammatory bowel disease, allergic hemolytic anemias, drug allergy, or hypersensitivity, skin rash, history of renal or liver disease, uncontrolled hypertension, or compromised cerebral or cardiovascular circulation.
Precautions Use with caution in patients with impaired renal or hepatic function; NSAIDs and corticosteroids may be discontinued over time after initiating gold therapy; do not use with penicillamine, antimalarials, immunosuppressives, other than corticosteroids; for mild or minor adverse reactions, hold therapy until reaction resolves then may resume therapy at reduced doses; moderate to severe reaction requires discontinuation of gold therapy

Adverse Reactions
Central nervous system: Confusion, hallucination, seizures, fever, headache
Dermatologic: Dermatitis, pruritus, alopecia, gray-to-blue pigmentation
Gastrointestinal: Diarrhea (50%), loose stools, stomatitis, abdominal cramping, constipation, flatulence, dyspepsia, melena, GI bleeding, mouth ulcers, dysgeusia, dysphagia, metallic taste
Genitourinary: Vaginitis
Hematologic: Thrombocytopenia, aplastic anemia, eosinophilia
Hepatic: Hepatitis, increased LFTs, jaundice
Ocular: Iritis, corneal ulcers
Renal: Proteinuria, hematuria, nephrotic syndrome, glomerulitis
Respiratory: Bronchitis, interstitial pneumonitis, fibrosis
Miscellaneous: "Nitritoid" reactions include flushing, fainting, dizziness, sweating, nausea, vomiting, weakness

Overdosage Symptoms of overdose include hematuria, proteinuria, fever, nausea, vomiting, diarrhea
Toxicology For mild gold poisoning, dimercaprol 2.5 mg/kg 4 times/day for 2 days or for more severe forms of gold intoxication, dimercaprol 3 mg/kg every 4 hours for 2 days, should be initiated; then after 2 days, the initial dose should be repeated twice daily on the third day, and once daily thereafter for 10 days. Other chelating agents have been used with some success.
Drug Interactions Penicillamine, antimalarials, phenytoin, cytotoxic drugs, or immunosuppressive agents
Mechanism of Action The exact mechanism of action of gold is unknown; gold is taken up by macrophages which results in inhibition of phagocytosis and lysosomal membrane stabilization; other actions observed are decreased serum rheumatoid factor and alterations in immunoglobulins. Additionally, complement activation is decreased, prostaglandin synthesis is inhibited, and lysosomal enzyme activity is decreased.
Pharmacodynamics Therapeutic response may not be seen for 3-4 months after start of therapy
Pharmacokinetics
Absorption: Oral: ~15% to 33% (25% average) of gold in a dose
Protein binding: 60%
Half-life: 21-31 days (half-life dependent upon single or multiple dosing)
Time to peak: Peak blood gold concentrations are seen within 2 hours; peak serum levels: 1-2 hours
Elimination: 60% of absorbed gold is eliminated in urine while the remainder is eliminated in feces
Usual Dosage Geriatrics and Adults: Oral: 6 mg/day in 1-2 divided doses; after 6 months may be increased to 9 mg/day in 3 divided doses; if still no response after 3 months at 9 mg/day, discontinue drug; to start oral therapy after gold injections, discontinue parenteral gold and start oral gold at 6 mg/day either in divided doses or single daily dose
Monitoring Parameters Urinalysis, CBC with platelets done monthly; monitor for other side effects; see Adverse Reactions
Reference Range Gold: Normal: 0-0.1 μg/mL (SI: 0-0.0064 μmol/L); Therapeutic: 1-3 μg/mL (SI: 0.06-0.18 μmol/L); urine <0.1 μg/24 hours
(Continued)

Auranofin (Continued)

Test Interactions May enhance the response to a tuberculin skin test

Patient Information Minimize exposure to sunlight; report any signs of toxicity to physician (ie, pruritus, rash, sore mouth, indigestion, metallic taste); joint pain may take 1-2 months to start to subside

Nursing Implications Monitor urine for protein; CBC and platelets; monitor for mouth ulcers and skin reactions; may monitor serum levels

Additional Information Metallic taste may indicate stomatitis

Special Geriatric Considerations Tolerance to gold decreases with advanced age; use cautiously only after traditional therapy and other disease modifying antirheumatic drugs (DMARDs) have been attempted

Dosage Forms Capsule: 3 mg = 29% gold

Auro® Ear Drops [OTC] see Carbamide Peroxide on page 119

Aurothioglucose (aur oh thye oh gloo' kose)

Brand Names Solganal®

Generic Available No

Therapeutic Class Gold Compound

Use Adjunctive treatment in adult active rheumatoid arthritis; alternative or adjunct in treatment of pemphigus; for psoriatic patients who do not respond to NSAIDs

Contraindications Renal disease, history of blood dyscrasias, congestive heart failure, exfoliative dermatitis, hepatic disease, SLE, history of hypersensitivity to gold or any component

Warnings Explain the possibility of adverse reactions before initiating therapy; signs of gold toxicity include decrease in hemoglobin, leukopenia, granulocytes and platelets; proteinuria, hematuria, pruritus, stomatitis, persistent diarrhea, rash, metallic taste; diabetes mellitus and congestive heart failure should be in control before initiating therapy; use cautiously in patients with a history of blood dyscrasias, bone marrow depression, inflammatory bowel disease, allergic hemolytic anemias, drug allergy, or hypersensitivity, skin rash, history of renal or liver disease, uncontrolled hypertension, or compromised cerebral or cardiovascular circulation. Therapy should be discontinued if platelet count falls <100,000/mm^3; <4000 WBC, <1500 granulocytes/mm^3.

Precautions Use with caution in patients with impaired renal or hepatic function; NSAIDs and corticosteroids may be discontinued over time after initiating gold therapy; do not use with penicillamine, antimalarials, immunosuppressives, other than corticosteroids; for mild or minor adverse reactions, hold therapy until reaction resolves then may resume therapy at reduced doses; moderate to severe reaction requires discontinuation of gold therapy

Adverse Reactions

Central nervous system: Confusion, hallucinations, seizures, fever, headache

Dermatologic: Dermatitis, pruritus, alopecia, gray-to-blue pigmentation

Gastrointestinal: Stomatitis, flatulence, dyspepsia, melena, GI bleeding, mouth ulcers, dysgeusia, dysphagia, metallic taste

Genitourinary: Vaginitis

Hematologic: Thrombocytopenia, aplastic anemia, eosinophilia

Hepatic: Hepatitis, increased LFTs, jaundice

Ocular: Iritis, corneal ulcers

Renal: Proteinuria, hematuria, nephrotic syndrome, glomerulitis

Respiratory: Bronchitis, interstitial pneumonitis, fibrosis

Miscellaneous: "Nitritoid" reactions include flushing, fainting, dizziness, sweating, nausea, vomiting, weakness

Overdosage Symptoms of overdose include hematuria, proteinuria, fever, nausea, vomiting, diarrhea, thrombocytopenia, agranulocytosis, skin reaction (papulovesicular lesions, urticaria, pruritus, exfoliative dermatitis)

Toxicology For mild gold poisoning, dimercaprol 2.5 mg/kg 4 times/day for 2 days or for more severe forms of gold intoxication, dimercaprol 3-5 mg/kg every 4 hours for 2 days, should be initiated. Then after 2 days, the initial dose should be repeated twice daily on the third day, and once daily thereafter for 10 days. Other chelating agents have been used with some success.

Drug Interactions One report of increased phenytoin serum concentration with auranofin

Stability Protect from light and store at 15°C to 30°C

Mechanism of Action The exact mechanism of action of gold is unknown; gold is taken up by macrophages which results in inhibition of phagocytosis and lysosomal membrane stabilization; other actions observed are decreased serum rheumatoid factor and alterations in immunoglobulins. Additionally, complement activation is decreased, prostaglandin synthesis is inhibited, and lysosomal enzyme activity is decreased.

Pharmacodynamics Gold injections may result in decreased morning stiffness in 1-2 months; significant benefit may not be noted for 3-6 months

Pharmacokinetics

Absorption: I.M.: Erratic and slow

Protein binding: 95% to 99%

Metabolism: Unknown

Half-life: 3-27 days (single dose); 14-40 days (third dose); up to 168 days (11th dose)

Mean steady-state plasma levels: 1-5 mcg/mL

Time to peak: Peak serum levels occur within 4-6 hours

Elimination: Majority ultimately eliminated in urine and the remainder in feces; 70% renal excretion, 30% fecal

Usual Dosage Doses should initially be given at weekly intervals

Geriatrics and Adults: I.M.: 10 mg first week; 25 mg second and third week; then 50 mg/week until 800 mg to 1 g cumulative dose has been given; if improvement occurs without adverse reactions, give 25-50 mg every 2-3 weeks for 2-20 weeks; then every 3-4 weeks if patient remains stable; if no response after cumulative dose of 1 g, discontinue therapy

Monitoring Parameters Each visit, the patient should have urinalysis, CBC with platelets initially; then every 6 months on maintenance therapy; monitor for other adverse reactions; see Adverse Reactions

Reference Range Gold: Normal: 0-0.1 μg/mL (SI: 0-0.0064 μmol/L); Therapeutic: 1-3 μg/mL (SI: 0.06-0.18 μmol/L); urine <0.1 μg/24 hours

Patient Information Minimize exposure to sunlight; report any signs of toxicity to physician (ie, pruritus, rash, sore mouth, indigestion, metallic taste); joint pain may take 1-2 months to start to subside

Nursing Implications Deep I.M. injection into the upper outer quadrant of the gluteal region; addition of 0.1 mL of 1% lidocaine to each injection may reduce the discomfort with injection; vial should be thoroughly shaken before withdrawing a dose; explain the possibility of adverse reactions before initiating therapy; advise patients to report any symptoms of toxicity; monitor serum levels, CBC, platelets, urine protein; see Adverse Reactions, Warnings, Patient Information

Additional Information Patients with HLA-D locus histocompatibility antigens DRw2 and DRw3 may have genetic predisposition to toxic reactions

Special Geriatric Considerations Elderly have decreased tolerance to gold with age and may experience increased adverse effects; use cautiously only after traditional therapy and other disease modifying antirheumatic drugs (DMARDs) have been attempted

Dosage Forms Suspension, sterile: 50 mg/mL = 50% gold (10 mL)

Aventyl® Hydrochloride *see* Nortriptyline Hydrochloride *on page 511*

Axid® *see* Nizatidine *on page 508*

Ayr® [OTC] *see* Sodium Chloride *on page 648*

Azactam® *see* Aztreonam *on page 72*

Azatadine Maleate (a za' ta deen)

Brand Names Optimine®

Generic Available No

Therapeutic Class Antihistamine

Use Treatment of perennial and seasonal allergic rhinitis and chronic urticaria

Contraindications Hypersensitivity to azatadine or other components; patients receiving MAO inhibitors. Antihistamines should not be used to treat lower respiratory tract symptoms.

Warnings Use with caution in patient with narrow-angle glaucoma, stenosing peptic ulcer, urinary bladder obstruction, prostatic hypertrophy, asthmatic attacks. Antihistamines are more likely to cause dizziness, excessive sedation, syncope, toxic confusion states, and hypotension in the elderly.

Adverse Reactions

Central nervous system: Slight to moderate drowsiness, dizziness

Gastrointestinal: Nausea, vomiting, dry mouth

Ocular: Blurred vision

Respiratory: Thickening of bronchial secretions

Overdosage Symptoms of overdose include CNS depression or stimulation, dry mouth, flushed skin, fixed and dilated pupils, apnea

Toxicology There is no specific treatment for an antihistamine overdose, however, most of its clinical toxicity is due to anticholinergic effects. Anticholinesterase inhibitors may be useful by reducing acetylcholinesterase. Anticholinesterase inhibitors include physostigmine, neostigmine, pyridostigmine, and edrophonium. For anticholinergic overdose with severe life-threatening symptoms, physostigmine 1-2 mg I.V., slowly may be given to reverse these effects.

Drug Interactions Increased effect/toxicity: Procarbazine, CNS depressants, tricyclic antidepressants, alcohol, MAO inhibitors

Mechanism of Action Azatadine is a piperidine-derivative antihistamine; has both anticholinergic and antiserotonin activity; has been demonstrated to inhibit mediator release from human mast cells *in vitro*; mechanism of this action is suggested to prevent calcium entry into the mast cell through voltage-dependent calcium channels

Pharmacokinetics

Absorption: Oral: 90%

Distribution: Crosses the blood-brain barrier

(Continued)

Azatadine Maleate *(Continued)*

Protein binding: Minimally bound to plasma protein
Metabolism: Extensively conjugated in the liver
Half-life: 9 hours
Time to peak serum concentration: 4 hours after the dose
Elimination: 20% excreted unchanged in urine

Usual Dosage
Geriatrics: 1 mg once or twice daily
Adults: 1-2 mg twice daily

Monitoring Parameters Relief of symptoms, mental status

Patient Information May cause drowsiness; avoid CNS depressants and alcohol

Nursing Implications See Monitoring Parameters

Additional Information Azatadine offers no significant advantage over other antihistamines

Special Geriatric Considerations See Warnings, Additional Information

Dosage Forms Tablet: 1 mg

Azathioprine (ay za thye' oh preen)

Brand Names Imuran®

Generic Available No

Therapeutic Class Immunosuppressant Agent

Use Adjunct with other agents in prevention of rejection of renal transplants; also used in severe rheumatoid arthritis unresponsive to other agents; Crohn's disease, ulcerative colitis, multiple sclerosis

Contraindications Hypersensitivity to azathioprine or any component; patients with rheumatoid arthritis treated previously with alkylating agents may be at risk for secondary neoplasia

Warnings Chronic immunosuppression increases the risk of neoplasia; mutagenic potential; possible hematologic toxicities (leukopenia, thrombocytopenia); severe infections (fungal, bacterial, viral)

Precautions Use with caution in patients with liver disease, renal impairment, and those with cadaveric kidneys; reduce usual dosage 25% to 33% in patients receiving both allopurinol and azathioprine

Adverse Reactions
Cardiovascular: Hypotension
Central nervous system: Fever
Dermatologic: Alopecia, rash, maculopapular rash
Gastrointestinal: Nausea, vomiting, anorexia, diarrhea, aphthous stomatitis
Hematologic: Leukopenia, thrombocytopenia, bone marrow depression
Hepatic: Hepatotoxicity
Neuromuscular & skeletal: Arthralgias, which include myalgias, rigors
Ocular: Retinopathy
Respiratory: Dyspnea
Miscellaneous: Rare hypersensitivity reactions

Overdosage Symptoms of overdose include nausea, vomiting, diarrhea

Toxicology Following initiation of essential overdose management, symptomatic and supportive treatment should be instituted. Dialysis has been reported to remove significant amounts of the drug and its metabolites, and should be considered as a treatment option in those patients who deteriorate despite established forms of therapy.

Drug Interactions Allopurinol; reduce dose to $\frac{1}{4}$ to $\frac{1}{3}$ of usual dosage if allopurinol is given concurrently

Stability
Stability of parenteral admixture at room temperature (25°C) and refrigeration (4°C): 24 hours
Stable in neutral or acid solutions, but is hydrolyzed to mercaptopurine in alkaline solutions

Mechanism of Action Antagonizes purine metabolism and may inhibit synthesis of DNA, RNA, and proteins; may also interfere with cellular metabolism and inhibit mitosis

Pharmacokinetics
Protein binding: ~30%
Metabolism: Extensive by hepatic xanthine oxidase to 6-mercaptopurine (active)
Half-life:
Parent: 12 minutes
6-mercaptopurine: 0.7-3 hours
Elimination: Small amounts excreted as unchanged drug; metabolites eliminated eventually in urine

Usual Dosage
Rheumatoid arthritis: Oral:
Geriatrics: 1 mg/kg/day (50-100 mg); titrate gradually by 25 mg/day until response or toxicity (see dose adjustment for renal function)
Adults: 1 mg/kg/day for 6-8 weeks; increase by 0.5 mg/kg every 4 weeks until response or up to 2.5 mg/kg/day I.V. dose is equivalent to oral dose

Renal transplantation: Geriatrics and Adults: Oral, I.V.: Initial: 3-5 mg/kg/day; maintenance: 1-3 mg/kg/day

Dosing adjustment in renal impairment:
Cl_{cr} 10-50 mL/minute: Administer 75% of dose
Cl_{cr} <10 mL/minute: Administer 50% of dose
Slightly dialyzable (5% to 20%)

Monitoring Parameters Perform CBC with platelets weekly for first month, twice
monthly for second and third months, then monthly. Dose increases will require more
frequent monitoring; early sign of toxicity is WBC count dropping below 3000-4000/
mm^3

Test Interactions Increased AST, ALT, bilirubin, alkaline phosphatase, amylase (S),
prothrombin time (S); decreased uric acid, albumin

Patient Information Response in rheumatoid arthritis may not occur for up to 3
months; do not stop taking without the physician's approval, do not have any vaccinations before checking with your physician; check with your physician if you have a
persistent sore throat, unusual bleeding or bruising, fatigue, abdominal pain, pale
stools, darkened urine. May cause nausea, vomiting, fever, joint pain, and diarrhea;
notify physician if persistent.

Nursing Implications Hematologic status should be monitored during therapy; see
Monitoring Parameters

Additional Information Azathioprine is an imidazolyl derivative of 6-mercaptopurine.
If infection occurs, drug dosage should be reduced; NSAID therapy should be continued when beginning initial therapy with azathioprine in the treatment of rheumatoid
arthritis

Special Geriatric Considerations Toxicity to immunosuppressives is increased in elderly. Start with lowest recommended adult doses. Signs of infection, such as fever
and WBC rise, may not occur. Lethargy and confusion may be more prominent signs
of infection. Adjust dose for renal function in elderly.

Dosage Forms
Injection, as sodium: 5 mg/mL (20 mL)
Tablet, scored: 50 mg

References
Hutchins LF and Lipschitz DA, "Cancer, Clinical Pharmacology, and Aging," *Clin Geriatr Med*, 1987,
3(3):483-503.
Kaplan HG, "Use of Cancer Chemotherapy in the Elderly," *Drug Treatment in the Elderly*, Vestal RE,
ed, Boston, MA: ADIS Health Science Press, 1984, 338-49.

Azidothymidine *see* Zidovudine *on page 741*

Azithromycin
Brand Names Zithromax™
Generic Available No
Therapeutic Class Antibiotic, Macrolide
Use Treatment of adult patients (>16 years of age) with mild to moderate infections of
susceptible strains in upper and lower respiratory tract, skin and skin structure, and
sexually transmitted diseases due to nongonococcal urethritis and cervicitis due to
Chlamydia trachomatis

Contraindications Hypersensitivity to azithromycin, erythromycin, or other macrolide
antibiotics

Warnings Patients with a community acquired pneumonia due to *S. pneumoniae* or *H.
influenzae* should be stable enough for outpatient oral treatment. Patients who are
dehydrated, not eating, have respiratory, cardiac, or other chronic illnesses that may
be exacerbated by pneumonia should be hospitalized. Not for nosocomial pneumonia, patients with documented or suspected bacteremia, or in patients who are immunocompromised. Pseudomembranous colitis is possible with any broad spectrum
antibiotic, if suspected, stop the drug and pursue appropriate diagnostic work-up and
treatment. Patients treated for nongonococcal urethritis or cervicitis should have a se-
rological test for syphilis and gonococcal culture taken. Use caution in patients with
impaired hepatic or renal function. Cardiac effects have been reported with other
macrolides, but not with azithromycin.

Adverse Reactions All adverse reactions are reportedly reversible after discontinuation of the drug

Cardiovascular: Palpitations, chest pain
Central nervous system: Dizziness, headache, fatigue
Dermatologic: Allergy and rash, photosensitivity, angioedema
Gastrointestinal: Diarrhea (5%), nausea (3%), and abdominal pain (3%), dyspepsia,
flatulence, vomiting, melena
Genitourinary: Vaginitis, *Monilia*
Hematologic: Leukopenia, neutropenia, decreased platelet count, alkaline bilirubin,
blood glucose, LDH and phosphate; increased serum creatinine, phosphokinase,
potassium, ALT, GGT, and AST
Hepatic: Cholestatic jaundice
Renal: Nephritis, elevated BUN, creatinine

Overdosage Information is limited, GI symptoms such as nausea, vomiting

(Continued)
71

Azithromycin *(Continued)*

Toxicology Evacuation of unabsorbed drug when possible and other general support-ive measures

Drug Interactions Aluminum- and magnesium-containing antacids will decrease peak serum concentrations, but not the extent of absorption; other macrolide antibiotics such as erythromycin, have been shown to increase theophylline serum concentra-tions and enhance warfarin's anticoagulant effect. These findings have not been iden-tified with azithromycin, still careful monitoring is advised.

Mechanism of Action Inhibits microbial protein synthesis by binding to the 50S ribo-somal subunit

Pharmacokinetics

[Absorption: Oral: Rapidly absorbed from the GI tract

Distribution: Rapidly and widely distributed to body tissues and fluids; CSF concen-trations are minimal in the presence of noninflamed meninges; tissue concentra-tions, particularly in fibroblasts and phagocytes, are greater than those in plasma or serum; steady-state volume of distribution: 31.1 L/kg

Protein binding: Serum protein binding appears to be concentration-dependent, rang-ing from 51% at 0.02 mcg/mL to 7% at 2 mcg/mL

Half-life, terminal: Averages 68 hours in healthy young adults

Elimination: Biliary excretion of unchanged drug is the primary route of elimination, with ~6% of unchanged drug eliminated in the urine over a 1-week period

The long half-life and large volume of distribution are believed to be secondary to the high affinity for tissues. In elderly women, but not in elderly men, peak serum con-centrations were 30% to 50% greater compared to young adults; however, no signif-icant accumulation was noted.

Usual Dosage Geriatrics and Adults: Oral: 500 mg as a single loading dose on day 1 followed by 250 mg daily on days 2-5 (1.5 g total); the recommended dose for non-gonococcal urethritis and cervicitis due to *C. trachomatis* is a single 1 g dose

Monitoring Parameters Signs and symptoms of infection, mental status, appetite; hydration; cultures and sensitivity, if appropriate

Patient Information Complete full course of therapy; take on an empty stomach (1 hour before or 2 hours after meals); do not take with aluminum- or magnesium-containing antacids; notify physician if sore throat, unusual bleeding, or other infec-tions occur

Nursing Implications Monitor tolerance to medication; do not give concurrently with aluminum or magnesium antacids, see Drug Interactions; monitor respiratory, cardiac, and fluid status of nursing home patients being treated for pneumonia

Special Geriatric Considerations Dosage adjustment does not appear to be neces-sary in the elderly, see Usual Dosage and Pharmacokinetics; considered one of the drugs of choice in the treatment of outpatient treatment of community-acquired pneu-monia in older adults; see Warnings

Dosage Forms Capsule: 250 mg

References

American Thoracic Society, "Guidelines for the Initial Management of Adults With Community-Acquired Pneumonia: Diagnosis, Assessment of Severity, and Initial Antimicrobial Therapy," *Am Rev Respir Dis*, 1993, 148(5):1418-26.

Coates P, Daniel R, Houston AC, et al, "An Open Study to Compare the Pharmacokinetics, Safety, and Tolerability of a Multiple-Dose Regimen of Azithromycin in Young and Elderly Volunteers," *Eur J Clin Microbiol Infect Dis*, 1991, 10(10):850-2.

Peters DH, Friedel HA, and McTavish D, "Azithromycin: A Review of Its Antimicrobial Activity, Phar-macokinetic Properties and Clinical Efficacy," *Drugs*, 1992, 44(5):750-99.

Azmacort™ *see* Triamcinolone *on page 710*

Azo Gantrisin® *see* Sulfisoxazole and Phenazopyridine *on page 664*

Azo-Standard® *see* Phenazopyridine Hydrochloride *on page 552*

AZT *see* Zidovudine *on page 741*

Azthreonam *see* Aztreonam *on this page*

Aztreonam *(az' tree oh nam)*

Brand Names Azactam®

Synonyms Azthreonam

Generic Available No

Therapeutic Class Antibiotic, Miscellaneous

Use Treatment of patients with documented multidrug-resistant aerobic gram-negative infection in which beta-lactam therapy is contraindicated; used for urinary tract infec-tion, lower respiratory tract infections, septicemia, skin/skin structure infections, intra-abdominal infections and gynecological infections

Contraindications Hypersensitivity to aztreonam or any component

Warnings Check hypersensitivity to other beta-lactams; may have cross-allergenicity to penicillins and cephalosporins

Precautions Requires dosage reduction in renal impairment

Adverse Reactions

Cardiovascular: Thrombophlebitis, hypotension, transient EKG changes

Central nervous system: Seizures, confusion, insomnia, dizziness

Dermatologic: Rash, purpura, erythema multiforme, urticaria, petechiae, exfoliative dermatitis

Gastrointestinal: Diarrhea, nausea, vomiting, pseudomembranous colitis

Hematologic: Thrombocytopenia, eosinophilia, leukopenia, neutropenia

Hepatic: Elevation of liver enzymes, jaundice

Local: Pain at injection site

Toxicology If necessary, dialysis can reduce the drug concentration in the blood

Drug Interactions Avoid antibiotics that induce beta-lactamase production (cefoxitin, imipenem); probenecid and furosemide significantly increase aztreonam serum levels

Stability Reconstituted solutions are colorless to light yellow straw colored and may turn pink upon standing without affecting potency; use reconstituted solutions and I.V. solutions (in NS and D_5W) within 48 hours if kept at room temperature or 7 days if kept in refrigerator; reconstituted solutions are NOT for multiple-dose use; incompatible when mixed with nafcillin, metronidazole

Mechanism of Action Inhibits bacterial cell wall synthesis during active multiplication causing cell wall destruction

Pharmacokinetics

Absorption: I.M.: Well absorbed

Distribution: V_d (adults): 0.2 L/kg

Protein binding: 56%

Half-life: 1.3-2.2 hours (half-life prolonged in renal failure)

Time to peak: Peak serum concentrations appear within 60 minutes following a dose

Elimination: 60% to 70% excreted unchanged in urine and partially excreted in feces

In healthy older adults with normal renal function (mean Cl_{cr}: 99 mL/minute), there were no significant changes in pharmacokinetic parameters. However, in older adults with impaired renal function (mean Cl_{cr}: 24 mL/minute) serum concentrations were inversely related to Cl_{cr}

Usual Dosage

Geriatrics: Similar to adult dosing with appropriate adjustments for renal function (see below)

Adults:

Urinary tract infection: I.M., I.V.: 500 mg to 1 g every 8-12 hours

Moderately severe systemic infections: 1 g I.V. or I.M. or 2 g I.V. every 8-12 hours

Severe systemic or life-threatening infections (especially caused by *Pseudomonas aeruginosa*): I.V.: 2 g every 6-8 hours; maximum: 8 g/day

Dosing interval in renal impairment:

Cl_{cr} 10-30 mL/minute: Initial dose of 500 mg, 1 g, or 2 g, then reduce dose 50% given at the usual interval

Cl_{cr} <10 mL/minute: Initial dose of 500 mg, 1 g, or 2 g, then reduce dose 75% given at the usual interval

Moderately dialyzable (20% to 50%)

Administration I.V. route preferred for single doses >1 g or in patients with severe life-threatening infections; administer by IVP over 3-5 minutes or by intermittent infusion over 20-60 minutes at a final concentration not to exceed 20 mg/mL

Monitoring Parameters Resolution of signs and symptoms of infection, periodic liver function tests

Test Interactions Urine glucose (Clinitest®)

Nursing Implications See Administration

Additional Information Normally used with other antibiotics in life-threatening situations; member of new class of antibiotics called monobactams, with excellent gram-negative bacteria effectiveness, without ototoxicity or nephrotoxicity

Special Geriatric Considerations See Pharmacokinetics and Usual Dosage

Dosage Forms Injection: 500 mg (15 mL, 100 mL); 1 g (15 mL, 100 mL); 2 g (15 mL, 100 mL)

References

Creasey WA, Platt TB, Frantz M, et al, "Pharmacokinetics of Aztreonam in Elderly Male Volunteers," *Br J Clin Pharmacol*, 1985, 19:233-7.

Settler FR, Schramm M, Swabb EA, "Safety of Aztreonam and SQ 26,992 in Elderly Patients With Renal Insufficiency," *Rev Infect Dis*, 1985, (Suppl 4):5622.

Azulfidine® *see* Sulfasalazine *on page 661*

Azulfidine® EN-tabs® *see* Sulfasalazine *on page 661*

Bacampicillin Hydrochloride (ba kam pi sill' in)

Brand Names Spectrobid®

Synonyms Carampicillin Hydrochloride

Generic Available No

Therapeutic Class Antibiotic, Penicillin

Use Treatment of susceptible bacterial infections involving the urinary tract, skin structure, upper and lower respiratory tract; activity is identical to that of ampicillin

Contraindications Hypersensitivity to bacampicillin or any component or penicillins; patients with infectious mononucleosis

(Continued)

Bacampicillin Hydrochloride *(Continued)*

Precautions Use with caution in patients with severe renal impairment or a history of cephalosporin allergy; modify dosage in patients with renal insufficiency

Adverse Reactions
Dermatologic: Rash
Gastrointestinal: Nausea, diarrhea, pseudomembranous colitis
Hematologic: Agranulocytosis
Hepatic: Mild elevation in AST
Miscellaneous: Hypersensitivity reactions

Drug Interactions Increased levels with probenecid; allopurinol theoretically has an additive potential for amoxicillin/ampicillin rash

Stability Reconstituted suspension is stable for 10 days when stored in the refrigerator

Mechanism of Action Interferes with bacterial cell wall synthesis during active multiplication causing cell death and resultant bactericidal activity against susceptible bacteria

Pharmacokinetics
Protein binding: 15% to 25%
Bioavailability: 80% to 98%
Half-life: 65 minutes, prolonged in patients with impaired renal function
Bacampicillin is an inactive prodrug that is hydrolyzed to ampicillin; area under the serum concentration time curve is 40%, higher for bacampicillin than after equivalent ampicillin doses

Usual Dosage Geriatrics and Adults: Oral: 400-800 mg every 12 hours
Gonorrhea: 1.6 g bacampicillin plus 1 g probenecid as a single oral dose

Dosing interval in renal impairment:
Cl_{cr} 10-30 mL/minute to 10 mL/minute: Administer every 24 hours
Cl_{cr} <10 mL/minute: Administer every 36 hours

Monitoring Parameters Renal, hepatic and hematologic function tests

Test Interactions False-positive urine glucose with Clinitest®

Patient Information Take oral suspension 1 hour before or 2 hours after a meal; complete entire course of treatment unless instructed otherwise

Nursing Implications Assess patient at beginning and throughout therapy for infection; observe for signs and symptoms of anaphylaxis

Additional Information Each mg of bacampicillin is equivalent to 700 mcg of ampicillin; because it is a prodrug, no major advantages over ampicillin

Special Geriatric Considerations See Pharmacokinetics and Usual Dosage; adjust dose for renal function

Dosage Forms
Suspension, oral: 125 mg/5 mL equivalent to 87.5 mg of ampicillin/5 mL (70 mL, 100 mL, 140 mL, 200 mL)
Tablet: 400 mg equivalent to 280 mg ampicillin

Bacid® [OTC] *see Lactobacillus acidophilus* and *Lactobacillus bulgaricus on page 397*

Baclofen (bak' loe fen)

Brand Names Lioresal®
Generic Available No
Therapeutic Class Skeletal Muscle Relaxant
Use Treatment of reversible spasticity associated with multiple sclerosis or spinal cord lesions

Unlabeled use: Trigeminal neuralgia, tardive dyskinesia

Contraindications Hypersensitivity to baclofen or any component
Warnings Avoid abrupt withdrawal of the drug
Precautions Use with caution in patients with seizure disorder, impaired renal function

Adverse Reactions
Cardiovascular: Hypotension
Central nervous system: Drowsiness, fatigue, vertigo, dizziness, psychiatric disturbances, insomnia, slurred speech, headache, ataxia, hypotonia
Dermatologic: Rash
Gastrointestinal: Nausea, constipation, anorexia
Genitourinary: Urinary frequency, impotence

Overdosage Symptoms of overdose include vomiting, muscle hypotonia, salivation, drowsiness, coma, seizures, respiratory depression

Toxicology Following initiation of essential overdose management, symptomatic and supportive treatment should be instituted; atropine has been used to improve ventilation, heart rate, blood pressure, and core body temperature

Drug Interactions
Decreased effect: Lithium
Increased effect of opiate analgesics, benzodiazepines, hypertensive agents
Increased toxicity: CNS depressants (sedation), tricyclic antidepressants (short-term memory loss), clindamycin (neuromuscular blockade), guanabenz (sedation), MAO inhibitors (decreased blood pressure, CNS, and respiratory effects)

Mechanism of Action Inhibits the transmission of both monosynaptic and polysynaptic reflexes at the spinal cord level, possibly by hyperpolarization of primary afferent fiber terminals, with resultant relief of muscle spasticity

Pharmacodynamics
Onset of muscle relaxation effects: 3-4 days
Maximum clinical effects: Not seen for 5-10 days

Pharmacokinetics
Absorption: Oral: Rapid; absorption from the GI tract is thought to be dose dependent
Protein binding: 30%
Metabolized: Minimally in the liver
Half-life: 3.5 hours
Time to peak serum concentration: Within 2-3 hours
Elimination: 85% of oral dose excreted in urine and feces as unchanged drug

Usual Dosage Oral (the lowest effective dose is recommended; if benefits are not seen, withdraw the drug slowly):

Geriatrics: Initial: 5 mg 2-3 times/day, increasing gradually as needed
Adults: 5 mg 3 times/day, may increase 5 mg/dose every 3 days to a maximum of 80 mg/day

Monitoring Parameters Symptoms, blood pressure, mental status

Test Interactions Increased alkaline phosphatase, AST, glucose, ammonia (B); decreased bilirubin (S)

Patient Information Take with food or milk; abrupt withdrawal after prolonged use may cause anxiety, hallucinations, tachycardia or spasticity. Avoid alcohol and other CNS depressants. May cause drowsiness, dizziness, and fatigue.

Nursing Implications Epileptic patients should be closely monitored; supervise ambulation; avoid abrupt withdrawal of the drug

Additional Information Not indicated for muscle spasm associated with rheumatic disorders; not recommended in Parkinson's disease or stroke since the efficacy has not been established

Special Geriatric Considerations The elderly are more sensitive to the effects of baclofen and are more likely to experience adverse CNS effects at higher doses. Two cases of encephalopathy were reported after inadvertent high doses (50 mg/day and 90 mg/day) were given to elderly patients.

Dosage Forms Tablet: 10 mg, 20 mg

References
Abarbanel J, Herishanu Y, Frisher S, "Encephalopathy Associated With Baclofen," *Ann Neurol*, 1985, 17(6):617-8.

Bactocill® *see* Oxacillin Sodium *on page 521*

Bactrim™ *see* Co-trimoxazole *on page 189*

Bactrim™ DS *see* Co-trimoxazole *on page 189*

Bactroban® *see* Mupirocin *on page 482*

Baking Soda *see* Sodium Bicarbonate *on page 646*

Baldex® *see* Dexamethasone *on page 207*

Bancap HC® *see* Hydrocodone and Acetaminophen *on page 350*

Banesin® [OTC] *see* Acetaminophen *on page 13*

Banophen® [OTC] *see* Diphenhydramine Hydrochloride *on page 228*

Barbita® *see* Phenobarbital *on page 554*

Barophen® *see* Hyoscyamine, Atropine, Scopolamine and Phenobarbital *on page 357*

Bayer® Aspirin [OTC] *see* Aspirin *on page 58*

Baylocaine® *see* Lidocaine Hydrochloride *on page 406*

Beclomethasone Dipropionate (be kloe meth' a sone)

Brand Names Beclovent®; Beconase®; Beconase AQ®; Vancenase®; Vancenase® AQ; Vanceril®

Generic Available No

Therapeutic Class Anti-inflammatory Agent; Corticosteroid, Inhalant

Use
Oral inhalation: Treatment of bronchial asthma in patients who require chronic administration of corticosteroids
Nasal aerosol: Symptomatic treatment of seasonal or perennial rhinitis and nasal polyposis

Contraindications Status asthmaticus; hypersensitivity to the drug or fluorocarbons, oleic acid in the formulation

Warnings Not to be used in status asthmaticus

Precautions Avoid using higher than recommended dosages since suppression of hypothalamic, pituitary, or adrenal function may occur

(Continued)

Beclomethasone Dipropionate *(Continued)*

Adverse Reactions
Central nervous system: Headache

Gastrointestinal: Dry mouth

Local: Growth of *Candida* in the mouth, irritation and burning of the nasal mucosa, nasal ulceration

Respiratory: Cough, sneezing, pulmonary infiltrates, hoarseness, rhinorrhea, nasal stuffiness

Miscellaneous: Epistaxis

Overdosage Nasal: Irritation and burning of the nasal mucosa, sneezing, intranasal and pharyngeal *Candida* infections, nasal ulceration, epistaxis, rhinorrhea, nasal stuffiness, headache

Toxicology Nasal symptoms include irritation and burning of the nasal mucosa, sneezing, intranasal and pharyngeal *Candida* infections, nasal ulceration, epistaxis, rhinorrhea, nasal stuffiness, headache. When consumed in excessive quantities for prolonged periods, systemic hypercorticism and adrenal suppression may occur; in those cases, discontinuation and withdrawal of the corticosteroid should be done judiciously.

Stability Do not store near heat or open flame

Mechanism of Action Controls the rate of protein synthesis, depresses the migration of polymorphonuclear leukocytes, fibroblasts, reverses capillary permeability, and lysosomal stabilization at the cellular level to prevent or control inflammation

Pharmacokinetics
Absorption:

Oral: 90%

Inhalation: Readily, ~10% to 25% of an inhaled dose reaches the respiratory tract

Protein binding: 87%

Half-life: 15 hours (biphasic decay terminal decay is 15 hours, initial phase half-life: 3 hours); after inhalation, it is quickly hydrolyzed by pulmonary esterases prior to absorption

Metabolism/Elimination: With oral administration, hepatic metabolism and renal excretion occur

Usual Dosage
Inhalation: Geriatrics and Adults: 2-4 inhalations twice daily, not to exceed 20 inhalations/day

Aerosol inhalation (nasal): Adults: 2-4 sprays each nostril twice daily

Aqueous inhalation (nasal): 1-2 sprays each nostril twice daily

Patient Information Follow instructions that accompany product; inhaled beclomethasone makes many asthmatics cough, to reduce chance, inhale drug slowly or use prescribed inhaled bronchodilator 5 minutes before beclomethasone is used; keep inhaler clean and unobstructed, wash in warm water and dry thoroughly; notify physician if sore throat or sore mouth occurs; do not stop abruptly

Nursing Implications Take drug history of patients with perennial rhinitis, may be drug related; check mucous membranes for signs of fungal infection

Additional Information Not used in status asthmaticus; shake thoroughly before using; nasal inhalation and oral inhalation dosage forms are **not** to be used interchangeably

Special Geriatric Considerations Older patients may have difficulty with oral metered dose inhalers and may benefit from the use of a spacer or chamber device

Dosage Forms
Inhalation:

Nasal: 42 mcg/inhalation (16.8 g)

Oral: 42 mcg/inhalation (16.8 g)

Spray, aqueous, nasal: Each actuation delivers 42 mcg-200 metered doses (25 g)

Beclovent® *see* Beclomethasone Dipropionate *on previous page*

Beconase® *see* Beclomethasone Dipropionate *on previous page*

Beconase AQ® *see* Beclomethasone Dipropionate *on previous page*

Beef Regular Iletin® II *see* Insulin Preparations *on page 372*

Beepen-VK® *see* Penicillin V Potassium *on page 543*

Beldin® [OTC] *see* Diphenhydramine Hydrochloride *on page 228*

Belix® [OTC] *see* Diphenhydramine Hydrochloride *on page 228*

Bemote® *see* Dicyclomine Hydrochloride *on page 215*

Benadryl® [OTC] *see* Diphenhydramine Hydrochloride *on page 228*

Benazepril Hydrochloride (ben ay' ze prill)
Brand Names Lotensin®

Generic Available No

Therapeutic Class Angiotensin-Converting Enzyme (ACE) Inhibitors

Use Treatment of hypertension, either alone or in combination with other antihypertensive agents, particularly diuretics

Contraindications Hypersensitivity to benazepril or any component or any other angiotensin-converting enzyme inhibitor

Warnings ACE inhibitors prevent potassium excretion, approximately as much as amiloride or spironolactone; may cause neutropenia, agranulocytosis, angioedema, hepatic dysfunction, first-dose hypotension, proteinuria; use cautiously in elderly, may see exaggerated response

Precautions Use with caution and modify dosage in patients with renal impairment; use with caution in patients with collagen vascular disease, congestive heart failure, hypovolemia, valvular stenosis, hyperkalemia (>5.7 mEq/L), anesthesia

Adverse Reactions

Cardiovascular: Orthostatic blood pressure changes, angina, palpitations, chest pain, hypotension, syncope, flushing

Central nervous system: Nervousness, depression, anxiety, somnolence, fatigue, dizziness, headache, paresthesia, insomnia, asthenia

Dermatologic: Rash, pruritus, angioedema

Endocrine & metabolic: Hyperkalemia, hyponatremia

Gastrointestinal: Loss of taste perception, pancreatitis, dry mouth, constipation, nausea, vomiting, abdominal pain

Genitourinary: Impotence, decreased libido

Hematologic: Neutropenia, eosinophilia

Hepatic: Increased BUN, serum creatinine, hepatitis

Neuromuscular & skeletal: Myalgia, arthralgia, arthritis

Ocular: Blurred vision

Renal: Proteinuria, oliguria

Respiratory: Chronic cough (nonproductive, persistent; more often in women and seen in 5% to 29% of patients), asthma, bronchitis, bronchospasm, dyspnea, sinusitis

Miscellaneous: Sweating

Overdosage Symptoms of overdose include severe hypotension; supportive measures only; see Toxicology

Toxicology Following initiation of essential overdose management, toxic symptom treatment and supportive treatment should be initiated. Hypotension usually responds to I.V. fluids or Trendelenburg positioning. If unresponsive to these measures, the use of a parenteral inotrope may be required (eg, norepinephrine 0.1-0.2 mcg/kg/minute titrated to response). Seizures commonly respond to diazepam (I.V. 5-10 mg bolus every 15 minutes if needed up to a total of 30 mg) or to phenytoin or phenobarbital.

Drug Interactions

Benazepril and potassium-sparing diuretics → additive hyperkalemic effect

Benazepril and indomethacin or nonsteroidal anti-inflammatory agents → reduced antihypertensive response to benazepril

Allopurinol and benazepril → neutropenia

Antacids and ACE inhibitors → ↓ absorption of ACE inhibitors

Phenothiazines and ACE inhibitors → ↑ ACE inhibitor effect

Probenecid and ACE inhibitors (benazepril) → ↑ ACE inhibitors (benazepril) levels

Rifampin and ACE inhibitors (benazepril) → ↓ ACE inhibitor effect

Digoxin and ACE inhibitors → ↑ serum digoxin levels

Lithium and ACE inhibitors → ↑ lithium serum levels

Tetracycline and ACE inhibitors (benazepril) → ↓ tetracycline absorption (up to 37%)

Mechanism of Action Competitive inhibitor of angiotensin-converting enzyme (ACE); prevents conversion of angiotensin I to angiotensin II, a potent vasoconstrictor; results in lower levels of angiotensin II which causes an increase in plasma renin activity and a reduction in aldosterone secretion; a CNS mechanism may also be involved in hypotensive effect as angiotensin II increases adrenergic outflow from CNS; vasoactive kallikreins may be decreased in conversion to active hormones by ACE inhibitors, thus reducing blood pressure

Pharmacodynamics

Reduction in plasma angiotensin-converting enzyme activity:

Peak effect: 1-2 hours after oral administration of 2-20 mg dose

Duration of action: $>90\%$ inhibition for 24 hours has been observed after 5-20 mg oral dose

Reduction in blood pressure:

Single oral dose: Peak effect: 2-6 hours

With continuous therapy:

Maximum response: 2 weeks

Duration: 2 years

Pharmacokinetics

Absorption: Oral: Rapid, 37%; food does not alter significantly; metabolite (benazeprilat) itself unsuitable for oral administration due to poor absorption

Distribution: V_d: ~8.7 L

Protein binding: 96.7%; benazeprilat: 95.3%

(Continued)

Benazepril Hydrochloride (Continued)

Metabolism: Rapid and extensive in the liver to its active metabolite, benazeprilat, via enzymatic hydrolysis; undergoes significant first-pass metabolism and is completely eliminated from plasma in 4 hours

Half-life: Prolonged with renal impairment

Parent drug: 0.6 hours; prolonged with renal impairment

Metabolite elimination: 22 hours (from 24 hours after dosing onward) (average 10-11 hours with multiple dosing for benazeprilat the active metabolite)

Time to peak serum concentration:

Unchanged parent: 1-1.5 hours

Metabolite: 1.5-2 hours after fasting or 2-4 hours after a meal

Elimination: Nonrenal clearance (ie, biliary, metabolic) appears to contribute to the elimination of benazeprilat (11% to 12%), particularly in patients with severe renal impairment; hepatic clearance is the main elimination route of unchanged benazepril

Dialyzable: ~6% of metabolite removed by 4 hours of dialysis following 10 mg of benazepril administered 2 hours prior to procedure; parent compound was not found in the dialysate

Usual Dosage Oral: Patients taking diuretics should have them discontinued 2-3 days prior to starting benazepril; if they cannot be discontinued, then initial dose should be 5 mg; restart after blood pressure is stabilized if needed

Geriatrics: Initial: 10 mg/day in single or divided doses; usual range: 20-40 mg/day; adjust for renal function

Adults: 20-40 mg/day as a single dose or 2 divided doses

Dosing interval in renal impairment: Cl_{cr} <30 mL/minute: Administer 5 mg/day initially

Monitoring Parameters Serum potassium levels, BUN, serum creatinine, renal function, WBC

Patient Information Notify physician of persistent cough; do not stop therapy except under prescriber advice; notify physician if you develop sore throat, fever, swelling of hands, feet, face, eyes, lips, and tongue; difficult breathing, irregular heartbeats, chest pains, or cough. May cause dizziness, fainting, and lightheadedness, especially in first week of therapy, sit and stand up slowly; may cause changes in taste or rash; do not add a salt substitute (potassium) without advice of physician.

Nursing Implications May cause depression in some patients; discontinue if angioedema of the face, extremities, lips, tongue, or glottis occurs; watch for hypotensive effect within 1-3 hours of first dose or new higher dose; see Precautions, Warnings, Monitoring Parameters, and Special Geriatric Considerations

Special Geriatric Considerations Due to frequent decreases in glomerular filtration (also creatinine clearance) with aging, elderly patients may have exaggerated responses to ACE inhibitors; differences in clinical response due to hepatic changes are not observed. ACE inhibitors may be preferred agents in elderly patients with congestive heart failure and diabetes mellitus. Diabetic proteinuria is reduced and insulin sensitivity is enhanced. In general, the side effect profile is favorable in elderly and causes little or no CNS confusion; use lowest dose recommendations initially.

Dosage Forms Tablet: 5 mg, 10 mg, 20 mg, 40 mg

References

McAreavey D and Robertson JIS, "Angiotensin Converting Enzyme Inhibitors and Moderate Hypertension," *Drugs*, 1990, 40(3):326-45.

Benemid® see Probenecid on page 589

Bentyl® Hydrochloride see Dicyclomine Hydrochloride on page 215

Benylin® DM see Dextromethorphan on page 209

Benylin® Cough Syrup [OTC] see Diphenhydramine Hydrochloride on page 228

Benzathine Benzylpenicillin see Penicillin G Benzathine, Parenteral on page 539

Benzathine Penicillin G see Penicillin G Benzathine, Parenteral on page 539

Benzene Hexachloride see Lindane on page 407

Benzhexol Hydrochloride see Trihexyphenidyl Hydrochloride on page 717

Benzodiazepines Comparison see page 802

Benzonatate (ben zoe' na tate)

Brand Names Tessalon® Perles

Generic Available No

Therapeutic Class Antitussive; Local Anesthetic, Oral

Use Symptomatic relief of nonproductive cough

Contraindications Known hypersensitivity to benzonatate or related compounds

Precautions Release of benzonatate in the mouth can cause a temporary local anesthesia of the oral mucosa; capsules should be swallowed whole

Adverse Reactions

Central nervous system: Sedation, headache, dizziness

Gastrointestinal: GI upset, constipation, nausea

Miscellaneous: Nasal congestion, sensation of burning in the eyes

Overdosage Symptoms of overdose include restlessness, tremor, CNS stimulation

Toxicology The drug's local anesthetic activity can reduce the patient's gag reflex and, therefore, may contradict the use of ipecac following ingestion, this is especially true when the capsules are chewed. Gastric lavage may be indicated if initiated early on following an acute ingestion or in comatose patients. The remaining treatment is supportive and symptomatic. Treat convulsions with an I.V. short-acting barbiturate.

Mechanism of Action Tetracaine congener with antitussive properties; suppresses cough by topical anesthetic action on the respiratory stretch receptors

Pharmacodynamics

Onset of action: Therapeutic: Within 15-20 minutes

Duration: 3-8 hours

Usual Dosage Geriatrics and Adults: Oral: 100 mg 3 times/day, up to 600 mg/day

Monitoring Parameters Patient's chest sounds and respiratory pattern, mental status

Patient Information Swallow capsule whole; use of hard candy may increase saliva flow to aid in protecting pharyngeal mucosa

Nursing Implications Monitor patient's chest sounds and respiratory pattern; change patient position every 2 hours to prevent pooling of secretions in lung; capsules are not to be crushed

Special Geriatric Considerations No specific geriatric information is available about benzonatate; avoid use in patients with impaired gag reflex or who cannot swallow the capsule whole

Dosage Forms Capsule: 100 mg

Benzquinamide Hydrochloride (benz kwin' a mide)

Brand Names Emete-Con®

Generic Available No

Therapeutic Class Antiemetic

Use Antiemetic associated with anesthesia and surgery

Contraindications Hypersensitivity to benzquinamide hydrochloride or any component

Warnings May mask signs of intestinal obstruction and brain tumor

Precautions I.V. administration has been associated with hypertension and transient arrhythmias. I.M. is the preferred route

Adverse Reactions

Cardiovascular: Hypertension hypotension, cardiac arrhythmias, PVCs, PACF, atrial fibrillation

Central nervous system: Drowsiness (most common), insomnia, restlessness, headache, chills, shivering

Dermatologic: Hives, rash

Gastrointestinal: Anorexia, nausea, dry mouth

Neuromuscular & skeletal: Weakness, twitching, shaking, tremors

Ocular: Blurred vision

Miscellaneous: Sweating

Very large doses have produced extrapyramidal symptoms; hyperthermia, hiccups, flushing, salivation

Overdosage No specific antidote/supportive measures; see CNS stimulation and depressant symptoms in combination

Toxicology General supportive measures; no specific antidote. Not dialyzable since benzquinamide is moderately protein bound

Drug Interactions May increase action of pressor drugs

Stability Protect from light; do not reconstitute with NS, as a precipitate will result; when reconstituted as directed remains stable for 14 days at room temperature

Mechanism of Action Mechanism is unknown, but probably acts directly on the chemoreceptor trigger zone; has antiemetic, antihistaminic, anticholinergic, and mild sedative action

Pharmacodynamics

Onset of action: ~15 minutes

Duration: 3-4 hours

Pharmacokinetics

Absorption: I.M.: Rapid

Protein binding: 58%

Metabolism: Mainly by the liver

Time to peak: Peak blood levels occur 30 minutes after administration

Elimination: In urine, feces, and bile

(Continued)

Benzquinamide Hydrochloride *(Continued)*

Usual Dosage Geriatrics and Adults:
I.M.: 50 mg (0.5-1 mg/kg) may be repeated in 1 hour, then every 3-4 hours as needed
I.V.: 25 mg (0.2-0.4 mg/kg); not recommended route; restrict I.V. route to patients without any cardiovascular disease; see Precautions

Monitoring Parameters Monitor emetic episodes, monitor blood pressure, heart rate

Patient Information May cause drowsiness and dry mouth

Nursing Implications Reconstitute with 2.2 mL of sterile water; potent for 14 days at room temperature; do **not** reconstitute with normal saline (precipitate may develop); give either deep I.M. or by slow I.V. no faster than 25 mg/minute

Special Geriatric Considerations Due to higher incidence of cardiovascular disease in elderly, it would be best to avoid use if possible (see Precautions); since this agent has anticholinergic action (mild), be aware of possibility of CNS effects including confusion and delirium

Dosage Forms Injection: 50 mg

Benztropine Mesylate *(benz' troe peen)*

Brand Names Cogentin®

Generic Available Yes: Tablet

Therapeutic Class Anticholinergic Agent; Anti-Parkinson's Agent

Use Adjunctive treatment of all forms of parkinsonism; also used in treatment of drug-induced extrapyramidal effects (except tardive dyskinesia) and acute dystonic reactions

Contraindications Patients with narrow-angle glaucoma; hypersensitivity to any component; pyloric or duodenal obstruction, stenosing peptic ulcers; bladder neck obstructions; achalasia; myasthenia gravis

Precautions Use with caution in hot weather or during exercise. Elderly patients frequently develop increased sensitivity and require strict dosage regulation – side effects may be more severe in elderly patients with atherosclerotic changes. Use with caution in patients with tachycardia, cardiac arrhythmias, hypertension, hypotension, prostatic hypertrophy (especially in the elderly) or any tendency toward urinary retention, liver or kidney disorders and obstructive disease of the GI or GU tract. May exacerbate mental symptoms and precipitate a toxic psychosis when used to treat extrapyramidal reactions resulting from phenothiazines. When given in large doses or to susceptible patients, may cause weakness and inability to move particular muscle groups. Anticholinergic agents can aggravate tardive dyskinesia caused by neuroleptic agents.

Adverse Reactions
Cardiovascular: Tachycardia
Central nervous system: Drowsiness, nervousness, hallucinations, memory loss, coma (**the elderly may be at increased risk for confusion and hallucinations**)
Gastrointestinal: Nausea, vomiting, constipation, dryness of mouth
Genitourinary: Urinary hesitancy or retention
Ocular: Blurred vision, mydriasis
Miscellaneous: Heat intolerance

Overdosage Symptoms of overdose include CNS depression, confusion, nervousness, hallucinations, dizziness, blurred vision, nausea, vomiting, hyperthermia

Toxicology Anticholinergic toxicity is caused by strong binding of the drug to cholinergic receptors. Anticholinesterase inhibitors reduce acetylcholinesterase, the enzyme that breaks down acetylcholine and thereby allows acetylcholine to accumulate and compete for receptor binding with the offending anticholinergic. For anticholinergic overdose with severe life-threatening symptoms, physostigmine 1-2 mg S.C. or I.V., slowly may be given to reverse these effects.

Drug Interactions
Decreased effect of levodopa (decreased absorption)
Increased toxicity (central anticholinergic syndrome): Narcotic analgesics, phenothiazines, and other antipsychotics, tricyclic antidepressants, some antihistamines, quinidine, disopyramide

Mechanism of Action Thought to partially block striatal cholinergic receptors to help balance cholinergic and dopaminergic activity

Pharmacodynamics
Onset of action:
Parenteral dose: Within 15 minutes
Oral: Within 60 minutes
Duration: Activity can last from as little as 6 hours to as long as 48 hours

Usual Dosage Titrate dose in 0.5 mg increments at 5- to 6-day intervals
Geriatrics: Initial: 0.5 mg once or twice daily; increase by 0.5 mg as needed every 5-6 days; maximum: 6 mg/day

Adults:
Drug-induced extrapyramidal reaction: Oral, I.M., I.V.: 1-4 mg/dose 1-2 times/day
Acute dystonia: I.M., I.V.: 1-2 mg
Parkinsonism: Oral: 0.5-6 mg/day in 1-2 divided doses; if one dose is greater, give at bedtime

Monitoring Parameters Symptoms of EPS or Parkinson's, pulse, anticholinergic effects (ie, CNS, bowel, and bladder function)

Patient Information Take after meals or with food if GI upset occurs; do not discontinue drug abruptly; notify physician if adverse GI effects, rapid or pounding heartbeat, confusion, eye pain, rash, fever or heat intolerance occurs. Observe caution when performing hazardous tasks or those that require alertness such as driving, as may cause drowsiness. Avoid alcohol and other CNS depressants. May cause dry mouth – adequate fluid intake or hard sugar-free candy may relieve. Difficult urination or constipation may occur – notify physician if effects persist; may increase susceptibility to heat stroke.

Nursing Implications No significant difference in onset of I.M. or I.V. injection, therefore, there is usually no need to use the I.V. route. Improvement is sometimes noticeable a few minutes after injection. Do not discontinue drug abruptly.

Special Geriatric Considerations Anticholinergic agents are generally not well tolerated in the elderly and their use should be avoided when possible; see Precautions and Adverse Reactions. In the elderly, anticholinergic agents should not be used as prophylaxis against extrapyramidal symptoms.

Dosage Forms
Injection: 1 mg/mL (2 mL)
Tablet: 0.5 mg, 1 mg, 2 mg

References
Feinberg M, "The Problems of Anticholinergic Adverse Effects in Older Patients," *Drugs Aging*, 1993, 3(4):335-48.

Benzylpenicillin Benzathine *see* Penicillin G Benzathine, Parenteral *on page 539*

Benzylpenicillin Potassium *see* Penicillin G, Parenteral *on page 540*

Benzylpenicillin Sodium *see* Penicillin G, Parenteral *on page 540*

Bepridil (be' pri dil)
Related Information
Calcium Channel Blocking Agents Comparison *on page 806-807*
Brand Names Vascor®
Generic Available No
Therapeutic Class Antianginal Agent; Calcium Channel Blocker
Use Treatment of chronic stable angina, vasospastic angina, and unstable angina; due to side effect profile; see Adverse Reactions; primarily ventricular arrhythmias and agranulocytosis, this drug should be reserved for patients who have been intolerant of other antianginal therapy; bepridil may be used alone or in combination with nitrates or beta-blockers
Contraindications Sinus bradycardia; advanced heart block; ventricular tachycardia; cardiogenic shock, hypotension, congestive heart failure; hypersensitivity to verapamil or any component, hypersensitivity to calcium channel blockers and adenosine; atrial fibrillation or flutter associated with accessory conduction pathways; not to be given within a few hours of I.V. beta-blocking agents
Warnings Hypotension, congestive heart failure; cardiac conduction defects, PVCs, idiopathic hypertrophic subaortic stenosis; may cause platelet aggregation inhibition; do not abruptly withdraw (chest pain); hepatic dysfunction, renal function impairment, increased angina, increased intracranial pressure with cranial tumors; elderly may have greater hypotensive effect
Precautions Sick sinus syndrome, severe left ventricular dysfunction, congestive heart failure, hepatic or renal impairment, hypertrophic cardiomyopathy (especially obstructive), concomitant therapy with beta-blockers or digoxin, edema
Adverse Reactions
Cardiovascular: Hypertension, PVC, prolonged Q-T intervals, torsade de pointes, palpitations, bradycardia, tachycardia, syncope
Central nervous system: Fever, psychotic behavior, akathisia, dizziness, lightheadedness, drowsiness, nervousness, equilibrium disturbances, headache, paresthesia, insomnia, tinnitus, anxiety
Dermatologic: Skin rash and irritation
Gastrointestinal: GI upset, pharyngitis, gastritis, increased appetite, nausea, diarrhea, constipation, abdominal pain, dry mouth, flatulence, dysgeusia
Genitourinary: Impotence
Hematologic: Agranulocytosis
Neuromuscular & skeletal: Pain, myalgic asthenia, arthritis, hand tremor
Ocular: Blurred vision
Respiratory: Shortness of breath, wheezing, cough, respiratory infection, nasal congestion
Miscellaneous: Superinfection, peripheral edema, flu syndrome, sweating
Overdosage Symptoms of overdose include heartblock, hypotension, asystole, nausea, weakness, dizziness, drowsiness, confusion, and slurred speech; profound bradycardia and occasionally hyperglycemia; monitor potassium

(Continued)
81

Bepridil *(Continued)*

Toxicology Ipecac-induced emesis can hypothetically worsen calcium antagonist toxicity, since it can produce vagal stimulation. The potential for seizures precipitously following acute ingestion of large doses of a calcium antagonist may also contraindicate the use of ipecac. Supportive and symptomatic treatment, including I.V. fluids and Trendelenburg positioning, should be initiated as intoxication may cause hypotension. Although calcium (calcium chloride I.V. 1-2 g in adults over 5-10 minutes with repeats as needed) has been used as an "antidote" for acute intoxications, there is limited experience to support its routine use and should be reserved for those cases where definite signs of myocardial depression are evident. Heart block may respond to isoproterenol, glucagon, atropine and/or calcium although a temporary pacemaker may be required.

Drug Interactions Beta-blockers (increased cardiac and A-V conduction depression); fentanyl (increased volume requirements and hypotension); although this drug is new, other drug interactions not reported to the same degree as older agents; however, should be suspect of any drug interaction reported with other calcium channel blockers

Mechanism of Action Inhibits calcium ion from entering the "slow channels" or select voltage-sensitive areas of vascular smooth muscle and myocardium during depolarization; produces a relaxation of coronary vascular smooth muscle and coronary vasodilation; increases myocardial oxygen delivery in patients with vasospastic angina; this agent also inhibits fast sodium channels (inward) which may account for some of its side effects (eg, arrhythmias)

Pharmacodynamics Onset of action: Within 1 hour

Pharmacokinetics
Absorption: Oral: 95% to 100%
Metabolism/Bioavailability: Due to first-pass elimination, absolute bioavailability is ~60%
Half-life: ~24 hours
Time to peak: Peak levels attained within 2-3 hours
Elimination: Primarily by hepatic metabolism

Usual Dosage Geriatrics and Adults: Initial: 200 mg/day; adjust dosage after 10 days of administration; maximum daily dose: 400 mg; elderly require frequent monitoring due to side effect profile (cardiac); see Special Geriatric Considerations and Additional Information

Monitoring Parameters Heart rate, blood pressure, signs and symptoms of congestive heart failure

Reference Range Therapeutic: 1-2 ng/mL

Nursing Implications May cause cardiac arrhythmias if potassium is low

Additional Information This agent is not considered the drug of first choice for indications but is used for cases refractory to other calcium channel blockers

Special Geriatric Considerations Elderly may experience a greater hypotensive response; constipation may be more of a problem in elderly; calcium channel blockers are no more effective in elderly than other therapies, however, they do not cause significant CNS effects which is an advantage over some antihypertensive agents; see Additional Information

Dosage Forms Tablet: 200 mg, 300 mg, 400 mg

Berubigen® *see* Cyanocobalamin *on page 192*
Beta-2® *see* Isoetharine *on page 378*
Beta-Blockers Comparison *see page 804*
Betagan® *see* Levobunolol Hydrochloride *on page 401*

Betamethasone *(bay ta meth' a sone)*
Related Information
Antacid Drug Interactions *on page 764*
Corticosteroids Comparison, Topical *on page 809*
Brand Names Alphatrex®; Betatrex®; Beta-Val®; B-S-P®; Celestone®; Celestone® Soluspan®; Cel-U-Jec®; Dermabet®; Diprolene®; Diprolene® AF; Diprosone®; Maxivate®; Selestoject®; Uticort®; Valisone®
Synonyms Flubenisolone
Generic Available Yes
Therapeutic Class Anti-inflammatory Agent; Corticosteroid, Systemic; Corticosteroid, Topical (Medium/High Potency)
Use Inflammatory dermatoses such as seborrheic or atopic dermatitis, neurodermatitis, anogenital pruritus, psoriasis, inflammatory phase of xerosis, late phase of allergic dermatitis or irritant dermatitis
Contraindications Systemic fungal infections; hypersensitivity to betamethasone or any component
Precautions Use with caution in patients with hypothyroidism, cirrhosis, nonspecific ulcerative colitis and patients at increased risk for peptic ulcer disease; do not use oc-

clusive dressings on weeping or exudative lesions and general caution with occlusive dressings should be observed; discontinue if skin irritation or contact dermatitis should occur; do not use in patients with decreased skin circulation; avoid the use of high potency steroids on the face

Adverse Reactions

Cardiovascular: Hypertension, edema

Central nervous system: Convulsions, vertigo, confusion, headache, seizures, psychoses, pseudotumor cerebri

Dermatologic: Acne, hypopigmentation, skin atrophy, impaired wound healing

Endocrine & metabolic: Cushing's syndrome, pituitary-adrenal axis suppression, glucose intolerance, hypokalemia, alkalosis, postmenopausal bleeding, hot flashes

Gastrointestinal: Peptic ulcer, nausea, vomiting, pancreatitis

Local: Burning, itching, acne

Neuromuscular & skeletal: Muscle weakness, osteoporosis, fractures, aseptic necrosis of femoral and humeral heads, steroid myopathy

Ocular: Cataracts, glaucoma

Miscellaneous: Accelerated atherogenesis, sodium retention

Toxicology When consumed in excessive quantities, systemic hypercorticism and adrenal suppression may occur; in those cases, discontinuation and withdrawal of the corticosteroid should be done judiciously

Drug Interactions

Decreased effect with barbiturates, phenytoin, rifampin; decreased effect of salicylates, vaccines, toxoids, insulin, and oral hypoglycemics

Increased effect with estrogens

Increased hypokalemia when given with diuretics; could increase risk of digoxin toxicity

Mechanism of Action Controls the rate of protein synthesis, depresses the migration of polymorphonuclear leukocytes, fibroblasts, reverses capillary permeability, and lysosomal stabilization at the cellular level to prevent or control inflammation

Pharmacokinetics

Protein binding: 64%

Metabolism: Extensive in the liver

Half-life: 6.5 hours

Time to peak serum concentration: I.V.: Within 10-36 minutes

Elimination: <5% of dose excreted renally as unchanged drug

Usual Dosage

Geriatrics: Use the lowest effective dose

Adults:

Oral: 0.6-7.2 mg/day

I.M., I.V.: Betamethasone sodium phosphate: 0.6-9 mg/day divided every 12-24 hours

I.M.: Betamethasone sodium phosphate and betamethasone acetate: 0.5-9 mg/day ($\frac{1}{3}$ to $\frac{1}{2}$ of oral dose)

Intrabursal, intra-articular: 0.5-2 mL

Topical: Apply thin film 2-4 times/day

Monitoring Parameters Blood pressure, blood glucose, electrolytes

Test Interactions Increased amylase (S), chloride (S), cholesterol (S), glucose, protein, sodium (S); decreased calcium (S), chloride (S), potassium (S), thyroxine (S)

Patient Information Take with food or milk; take single daily dose in the morning; do not stop oral products abruptly; apply topical preparations in a thin layer

Nursing Implications Apply sparingly to areas; not for alternate day therapy; once daily doses should be given in the morning; not for use on broken skin or in areas of infection; do not apply to wet skin unless directed; do not apply to face or inguinal area; do not give injectable suspension I.V.

Additional Information

Alphatrex® = betamethasone dipropionate

Betatrex® = betamethasone valerate

Beta-Val® = betamethasone valerate

B-S-P® = betamethasone sodium phosphate

Celestone® = betamethasone

Celestone® Soluspan® = betamethasone sodium phosphate/betamethasone acetate

Diprolene® = betamethasone dipropionate

Diprosone® = betamethasone dipropionate

Maxivate® = betamethasone dipropionate

Selestoject® = betamethasone sodium phosphate

Uticort® = betamethasone benzoate

Valisone® = betamethasone valerate

Special Geriatric Considerations Because of the risk of adverse effects, systemic corticosteroids should be used cautiously in the elderly, in the smallest possible dose, and for the shortest possible time.

Dosage Forms

Betamethasone dipropionate salt (Diprosone®)

(Continued)

Betamethasone *(Continued)*
Aerosol: 0.1% (85 g)
Cream: 0.05% (15 g, 45 g)
Lotion: 0.05% (20 mL, 30 mL, 60 mL)
Ointment: 0.05% (15 g, 45 g)
Base (Celestone®)
Tablet: 0.6 mg
Syrup: 0.6 mg/5 mL (118 mL)
Benzoate salt (Uticort®)
Cream: 0.025% (60 g)
Gel: 0.025% (15 g, 60 g)
Lotion: 0.025% (60 mL)
Dipropionate salt, augmented (Diprolene®)
Cream: 0.05% (15 g, 45 g)
Gel: 0.05% (15 g, 45 g)
Lotion: 0.05% (30 mL, 60 mL)
Ointment, topical: 0.05% (15 g, 45 g)
Valerate salt (Betatrex®, Beta-Val®, Valisone®)
Cream: 0.1% (15 g, 45 g, 110 g, 430 g); 0.01% (15 g, 60 g)
Lotion: 0.1% (20 mL, 60 mL)
Ointment, topical: 0.1% (15 g, 45 g)
Sodium phosphate salt (Selestoject®)
Injection: 4 mg/mL (equivalent to 3 mg/mL) (5 mL)
Sodium phosphate and acetate salt (Celestone® Soluspan®)
Injection, suspension: 6 mg/mL (3 mg of betamethasone sodium phosphate and 3 mg of betamethasone acetate per mL) (5 mL)

Betapace® *see* Sotalol Hydrochloride *on page 654*
Betapen®-VK *see* Penicillin V Potassium *on page 543*
Betaseron® *see* Interferon Beta-1b *on page 374*
Betatrex® *see* Betamethasone *on page 82*
Beta-Val® *see* Betamethasone *on page 82*

Betaxolol Hydrochloride (be tax' oh lol)
Related Information
Beta-Blockers Comparison *on page 804-805*
Glaucoma Drug Therapy Comparison *on page 810*
Brand Names Betoptic®; Betoptic® S; Kerlone®
Generic Available No
Therapeutic Class Beta-Adrenergic Blocker; Beta-Adrenergic Blocker, Ophthalmic
Use Treatment of chronic open-angle glaucoma, ocular hypertension; management of hypertension
Contraindications Bronchial asthma, sinus bradycardia, second and third degree A-V block, cardiac failure, cardiogenic shock, hypersensitivity to betaxolol or any component
Precautions Use with caution in patients with cardiac failure or diabetes mellitus
Adverse Reactions
Cardiovascular: Bradycardia, palpitations, edema, congestive heart failure
Central nervous system: Headache, dizziness, fatigue, lethargy
Neuromuscular & skeletal: Exacerbation of myasthenia gravis
Ocular: Mild ocular stinging and discomfort, tearing, erythema, itching, keratitis, photophobia, decreased corneal sensitivity
Miscellaneous: Cold extremities
Overdosage Symptoms of overdose include bradycardia, hypotension, A-V block, CHF, bronchospasm, hypoglycemia
Toxicology Sympathomimetics (eg, epinephrine or dopamine), glucagon or a pacemaker can be used to treat the toxic bradycardia, asystole, and/or hypotension; initially, fluids may be the best treatment for toxic hypotension
Drug Interactions Increased toxicity (hypotension): Ophthalmic: Systemic beta-blockers, reserpine, carbonic anhydrase inhibitors
Stability Avoid freezing
Mechanism of Action Competitively blocks $beta_1$-receptors, with little or no effect on $beta_2$-receptors resulting in the inhibition of the chronotropic, inotropic, and vasodilator effects of beta-adrenergic stimulation. Ophthalmic reduces intraocular pressure by reducing the production of aqueous humor.
Pharmacodynamics
Onset of action:
Ophthalmic instillation: Within 30-60 minutes with maximal effects occurring within 2 hours
Oral: Blood pressure significantly decreases within 3 hours

Duration of action:
Ophthalmic instillation: 12 hours or longer
Oral: 25 hours

Pharmacokinetics
Absorption: Systemically absorbed from the eye
Metabolism: To multiple metabolites
Half-life: 12-22 hours
Elimination: Renal

Usual Dosage
Oral:
Geriatrics: Initial: 5 mg/day
Adults: 10 mg/day; may increase dose to 20 mg/day after 7-14 days if desired response is not achieved
Ophthalmic: Geriatrics and Adults: Instill 1 drop twice daily

Monitoring Parameters
Ophthalmic: Intraocular pressure
Systemic: Blood pressure, pulse

Patient Information May sting on instillation; do not touch dropper to eye; visual acuity may be decreased after administration; distance vision may be altered; assess patient's or caregiver's ability to administer; apply gentle pressure to lacrimal sac during and immediately following instillation (1 minute) to avoid systemic absorption; stop drug if breathing difficulty occurs

Nursing Implications Monitor for signs of congestive heart failure, hypotension, respiratory difficulty (bronchospasm); use cautiously in diabetics receiving hypoglycemic agents; teach proper instillation of eye drops; monitor blood pressure and heart rate

Additional Information Because of betaxolol's low lipid solubility, it is less likely to enter the CNS, decreasing the likelihood of CNS side effects

Special Geriatric Considerations Due to alterations in the beta-adrenergic autonomic nervous system, beta-adrenergic blockade may result in less hemodynamic response than seen in younger adults. Studies indicate that despite decreased sensitivity to the chronotropic effects of beta blockade with age, there appears to be an increased myocardial sensitivity to the negative inotropic effect during stress (ie, exercise). Controlled trials have shown the overall response rate for propranolol to be only 20% to 50% in elderly populations. Therefore, all beta-adrenergic blocking drugs may result in a decreased response as compared to younger adults.

Dosage Forms
Solution, ophthalmic (Betoptic®): 0.5% (2.5 mL, 5 mL, 10 mL)
Suspension, ophthalmic (Betoptic® S): 0.25% (2.5 mL, 10 mL, 15 mL)
Tablet (Kerlone®): 10 mg, 20 mg

Bethanechol Chloride (be than' e kole)

Brand Names Duvoid®; Myotonachol™; Urabeth®; Urecholine®
Generic Available Yes: Tablet
Therapeutic Class Cholinergic Agent
Use Nonobstructive urinary retention and retention due to neurogenic bladder; treatment and prevention of bladder dysfunction caused by phenothiazines; diagnosis of flaccid or atonic neurogenic bladder

Contraindications Hypersensitivity to bethanechol; do not use in patients with mechanical obstruction of the GI or GU tract or when the strength or integrity of the GI or bladder wall is in question. It is also contraindicated in patients with hyperthyroidism, peptic ulcer disease, latent or active asthma, epilepsy, parkinsonism, obstructive pulmonary disease, bradycardia, vasomotor instability, atrioventricular conduction defects, or hypotension

Warnings For S.C. injection only; do not give I.M. or I.V. since it may cause a severe cholinergic reaction

Precautions Potential for reflux infection if the sphincter fails to relax as bethanechol contracts the bladder; Myotonachol™ contains tartrazine

Adverse Reactions
Cardiovascular: Hypotension, cardiac arrest, flushed skin
Gastrointestinal: Abdominal cramps, diarrhea, nausea, vomiting, salivation
Respiratory: Bronchial constriction
Miscellaneous: Sweating, vasomotor response

Overdosage Symptoms of overdose include nausea, vomiting, abdominal cramps, diarrhea, involuntary defecation, flushed skin, hypotension, bronchospasm

Toxicology Atropine is the treatment of choice for intoxications manifesting with significant muscarinic symptoms. Atropine I.V. 0.6 mg every 3-60 minutes should be repeated to control symptoms and then continued as needed for 1-2 days following the acute ingestion. Epinephrine 0.1-1 mg S.C. may be useful in reversing severe cardiovascular or pulmonary sequels.

Drug Interactions
Decreased effect: Procainamide, quinidine
Increased toxicity: Ganglionic blockers (critical decrease in blood pressure)
Increased cholinergic effects: Anticholinesterase agents, tacrine

(Continued)

Bethanechol Chloride *(Continued)*

Mechanism of Action Stimulates cholinergic receptors in the smooth muscle of the urinary bladder and gastrointestinal tract resulting in increased peristalsis, increased GI and pancreatic secretions, bladder muscle contraction, and increased ureteral peristaltic waves

Pharmacodynamics
Onset of action:
Oral 30-90 minutes
S.C.: 5-15 minutes
Duration: Usually 1 hour

Pharmacokinetics Absorption: Oral: Variable

Usual Dosage Geriatrics (use lowest recommended dose) and Adults:
Oral: 10-50 mg 2-4 times/day
S.C.: 2.5-5 mg 3-4 times/day, up to 7.5-10 mg every 4 hours for neurogenic bladder

Monitoring Parameters Urinary output, blood pressure, pulse

Test Interactions Increased lipase, amylase (S), bilirubin, aminotransferase [ALT (SGPT)/AST (SGOT)] (S)

Patient Information Oral should be taken 1 hour before meals or 2 hours after meals to avoid nausea or vomiting; may cause abdominal discomfort, salivation, sweating or flushing – notify physician if these symptoms become pronounced. Rise slowly from sitting/lying down.

Nursing Implications Contraindicated for I.M. or I.V. use due to a likely severe cholinergic reaction; for S.C. injection only; observe closely for side effects; have bedpan readily available if administered for urinary retention

Additional Information Syringe containing atropine should be readily available for treatment of serious side effects

Special Geriatric Considerations Urinary incontinence in an elderly patient should be investigated. Bethanechol may be used for overflow incontinence (dribbling) but clinical efficacy is variable; see Contraindications, Precautions, and Adverse Reactions

Dosage Forms
Injection: 5 mg/mL (1 mL)
Tablet: 5 mg, 10 mg, 25 mg, 50 mg

References
Romanowski GL, Shimp LA, Balson AB, et al, "Urinary Incontinence in the Elderly: Etiology and Treatment," *Drug Intell Clin Pharm*, 1988, 22(7-8):525-33.

Betoptic® *see* Betaxolol Hydrochloride *on page 84*

Betoptic® S *see* Betaxolol Hydrochloride *on page 84*

Biaxin™ Filmtabs® *see* Clarithromycin *on page 170*

Bicillin® *see* Penicillin G Benzathine, Parenteral *on page 539*

Bicillin® C-R *see* Penicillin G Benzathine and Procaine Combined *on page 539*

Bicillin® C-R 900/300 *see* Penicillin G Benzathine and Procaine Combined *on page 539*

Bicillin® L-A *see* Penicillin G Benzathine, Parenteral *on page 539*

Bicitra® *see* Sodium Citrate and Citric Acid *on page 649*

Bio-Gan® *see* Trimethobenzamide Hydrochloride *on page 720*

Biozyme-C® *see* Collagenase *on page 187*

Biperiden Hydrochloride *(bye per' i den)*

Brand Names Akineton®

Generic Available No

Therapeutic Class Anti-Parkinson's Agent

Use Treatment of all forms of parkinsonism including drug-induced type (extrapyramidal symptoms)

Contraindications Hypersensitivity to any component; narrow-angle glaucoma, pyloric or duodenal obstruction; stenosing peptic ulcers; bladder neck obstructions; achalasia; myasthenia gravis

Precautions Use with caution in hot weather or during exercise. Elderly patients frequently develop increased sensitivity and require strict dosage regulation – side effects may be more severe in elderly patients with atherosclerotic changes. Use with caution in patients with tachycardia, cardiac arrhythmias, hypertension, hypotension, prostatic hypertrophy (especially in the elderly) or any tendency toward urinary retention, liver or kidney disorders and obstructive disease of the GI or GU tract. May exacerbate mental symptoms and precipitate a toxic psychosis when used to treat extrapyramidal reactions resulting from phenothiazines. When given in large doses or to susceptible patients, may cause weakness and inability to move particular muscle groups. Anticholinergic agents can aggravate tardive dyskinesia caused by neuroleptic agents.

Adverse Reactions
Cardiovascular: Tachycardia
Central nervous system: Coma, nervousness, memory loss, drowsiness (**the elderly may be at increased risk for confusion and hallucinations**)
Gastrointestinal: Nausea, vomiting, constipation, dryness of mouth
Genitourinary: Urinary retention
Ocular: Blurred vision, mydriasis
Miscellaneous: Heat intolerance

Overdosage Symptoms of overdose include CNS depression, confusion, nervousness, hallucinations, dizziness, blurred vision, nausea, vomiting, hyperthermia

Toxicology Anticholinergic toxicity is caused by strong binding of the drug to cholinergic receptors; anticholinesterase inhibitors reduce acetylcholinesterase, the enzyme that breaks down acetylcholine and thereby allows acetylcholine to accumulate and compete for receptor binding with the offending anticholinergic. For anticholinergic overdose with severe life-threatening symptoms, physostigmine 1-2 mg S.C. or I.V., slowly may be given to reverse these effects.

Drug Interactions
Decreased effect of levodopa (decreased absorption); decreased effect with tacrine
Increased toxicity (central anticholinergic syndrome): Narcotic analgesics, phenothiazines, and other antipsychotics, tricyclic antidepressants, some antihistamines, quinidine, disopyramide

Mechanism of Action Thought to partially block striatal cholinergic receptors to help balance cholinergic and dopaminergic activity

Pharmacokinetics
Bioavailability: 29%
Half-life: 18.4-24.3 hours
Time to peak serum concentration: 1-1.5 hours

Usual Dosage
Geriatrics: Oral: Initial: 2 mg 1-2 times/day

Adults:
Parkinsonism: Oral: 2 mg 3-4 times/day; maximum: 16 mg/day
Drug-induced extrapyramidal reaction:
Oral: 2 mg 1-3 times/day
I.M., I.V.: 2 mg every 30 minutes until symptoms resolved; maximum: 8 mg/day

Monitoring Parameters Symptoms of EPS or Parkinson's, pulse, anticholinergic effects (ie, CNS, bowel, and bladder function)

Patient Information Take after meals or with food if GI upset occurs; do not discontinue drug abruptly; notify physician if adverse GI effects, rapid or pounding heartbeat, confusion, eye pain, rash, fever or heat intolerance occurs. Observe caution when performing hazardous tasks or those that require alertness such as driving, as may cause drowsiness. Avoid alcohol and other CNS depressants. May cause dry mouth – adequate fluid intake or hard sugar-free candy may relieve. Difficult urination or constipation may occur – notify physician if effects persist; may increase susceptibility to heat stroke.

Nursing Implications No significant difference in onset of I.M. or I.V. injection, therefore, there is usually no need to use the I.V. route. Improvement is sometimes noticeable a few minutes after injection. Do not discontinue drug abruptly.

Special Geriatric Considerations Anticholinergic agents are generally not well tolerated in the elderly and their use should be avoided when possible. See Precautions, Adverse Reactions. In the elderly, anticholinergic agents should not be used as prophylaxis against extrapyramidal symptoms.

Dosage Forms
Injection, as lactate: 5 mg/mL (1 mL)
Tablet, as hydrochloride: 2 mg

References
Feinberg M, "The Problems of Anticholinergic Adverse Effects in Older Patients," *Drugs Aging*, 1993, 3(4):335-48.

Biphenabid *see Probucol on page 589*
Bisac-Evac® [OTC] *see Bisacodyl on this page*

Bisacodyl (bis a koe' dill)
Brand Names Bisac-Evac® [OTC]; Bisacodyl Uniserts®; Bisco-Lax® [OTC]; Carter's Little Pills® [OTC]; Clysodrast®; Dacodyl® [OTC]; Deficol® [OTC]; Dulcolax® [OTC]; Fleet® Laxative [OTC]; Theralax® [OTC]
Generic Available Yes
Therapeutic Class Laxative, Stimulant
Use Treatment of constipation; colonic evacuation prior to procedures or examination
Contraindications Do not use in patients with abdominal pain, obstruction, nausea, or vomiting; appendicitis, acute surgical abdomen
Warnings Excessive use may lead to fluid and electrolyte imbalance
Precautions Drug is habit-forming and may result in laxative dependence and loss of
(Continued)

Bisacodyl *(Continued)*

normal bowel function with prolonged use; rectal bleeding and failure to respond to therapy may require further evaluation; discoloration of urine may occur

Adverse Reactions
Endocrine & metabolic: Electrolyte and fluid imbalance (metabolic acidosis or alkalosis, hypocalcemia)
Gastrointestinal: Abdominal cramps, nausea, vomiting, diarrhea, griping, bloating
Miscellaneous: Rectal burning, sweating

Overdosage Symptoms of overdose include diarrhea, abdominal pain, nausea, vomiting, fluid/electrolyte loss, hypotension, lethargy, fatigue

Drug Interactions Milk and antacids will cause early release of drug in stomach rather than in small intestine

Mechanism of Action Stimulates peristalsis by directly irritating the smooth muscle of the intestine, possibly the colonic intramural plexus; alters water and electrolyte secretion producing net intestinal fluid accumulation and laxation

Pharmacodynamics Onset of action:
Oral: Within 6-10 hours
Rectal: 15-60 minutes

Pharmacokinetics
Absorption: Oral, rectal: <5% absorbed systemically
Metabolism: In the liver with conjugated metabolites
Elimination: Excreted in bile and urine

Usual Dosage
Geriatrics:
Oral: Initial: 5 mg/day
Rectal: 5-10 mg/day

Adults:
Oral: 10-15 mg/day as a single dose
Rectal: 10 mg/day as a single dose

Monitoring Parameters Monitor stools daily or weekly; fluid/electrolyte status

Patient Information Swallow tablets whole, do **not** crush or chew; do not take antacid or milk within 2 hours of taking drug; patients should assure proper dietary fiber and fluid intake with adequate exercise if medically appropriate; do not use if abdominal pain, nausea, or vomiting are present; laxative use should be used for a short period of time (<1 week); prolonged use may result in abuse, dependence, as well as fluid and electrolyte loss; notify physician if bleeding occurs or if constipation is not relieved

Nursing Implications Administer tablets 2 hours prior to or 4 hours after antacids; increased pH may dissolve the enteric coating leading to GI distress; do not crush enteric coated drug product

Special Geriatric Considerations The chronic use of stimulant cathartics is inappropriate and should be avoided; although constipation is a common complaint from elderly, such complaints require evaluation; short term use of stimulants is best; if prophylaxis is desired, this can be accomplished with bulk agents (psyllium), stool softeners, and hyperosmotic agents (sorbitol 70%); stool softeners are unnecessary if stools are well hydrated, soft, or "mushy"

Dosage Forms
Enema: 10 mg/30 mL
Powder, as tannex: 2.5 g
Suppository, rectal: 5 mg, 10 mg
Tablet, enteric coated: 5 mg

Bisacodyl Uniserts® *see Bisacodyl on previous page*

Bisco-Lax® [OTC] *see Bisacodyl on previous page*

Bismatrol® [OTC] *see Bismuth on this page*

Bismuth *(bis' muth)*

Brand Names Bismatrol® [OTC]; Devrom® [OTC]; Pepto-Bismol® [OTC]; Pink Bismuth® [OTC]

Synonyms Bismuth Subgallate; Bismuth Subsalicylate

Generic Available Yes

Therapeutic Class Antidiarrheal

Use Symptomatic treatment of mild, nonspecific diarrhea; indigestion, nausea, control of traveler's diarrhea (enterotoxigenic *Escherichia coli*)

Unlabeled use: Adjunctive therapy in *H. pylori* infections associated with PUD

Contraindications Do not use in patients with known hypersensitivity to salicylates; history of severe GI bleeding; history of coagulopathy

Warnings See Precautions; do not use prior to radiologic examinations of GI tract; bismuth is radiopaque

Precautions Subsalicylate should be used with caution if patient is taking aspirin, additive toxicity; use with caution in anticoagulated patients; use in debilitated, immobile patients may lead to bowel impaction

Adverse Reactions Gastrointestinal: Impaction may occur in debilitated patients

Overdosage Symptoms of overdose include tinnitus (subsalicylate), fever

Toxicology It is unusual to develop toxicity from short-term administrations of bismuth salts, and most toxic symptoms occur following subacute or chronic intoxications. Chelation with dimercaprol in doses of 3 mg/kg or penicillamine 100 mg/kg/day for 5 days can hasten recovery from bismuth-induced encephalopathy. When associated with methemoglobinemia, bismuth intoxications should be treated with methylene blue 1-2 mg/kg in a 1% sterile aqueous solution I.V. push over 4-6 minutes. This may be repeated within 60 minutes if necessary, up to a total dose of 7 mg/kg. Seizures usually respond to I.V. diazepam.

Drug Interactions Aspirin, tetracycline, corticosteroids, methotrexate

Mechanism of Action Bismuth subsalicylate exhibits both antisecretory and antimicrobial action. This agent may provide some anti-inflammatory action as well. The salicylate moiety provides antisecretory effect and the bismuth exhibits antimicrobial directly against bacterial and viral gastrointestinal pathogens. Bismuth has some antacid properties.

Pharmacokinetics Absorption: Oral: Undergoes chemical dissociation to various bismuth salts; bismuth is minimally absorbed across the GI tract while the salt (eg, salicylate) may be readily (>90%) absorbed; 2 tablets yield 204 mg salicylate; 30 mL of suspension yields 258 mg

Usual Dosage Geriatrics and Adults: Oral:

Nonspecific diarrhea: Subsalicylate: 2 tablets or 30 mL every 30 minutes to 1 hour as needed up to 8 doses/24 hours

Prevention of traveler's diarrhea: 2.1 g/day or 2 tablets 4 times/day before meals and at bedtime for up to 3 weeks of high risk; suspension also used (4.2 g/day)

Subgallate: 1-2 tablets 3 times/day with meals

Monitoring Parameters Signs/symptoms of nausea, diarrhea, tinnitus, CNS toxic effects, GI bleeding

Reference Range Mild toxicity, serum concentration $\geq$30 mg/dL; severe, >50 mg/dL

Test Interactions Increased uric acid

Patient Information Chew tablet well or shake suspension well before using; may darken stools; if diarrhea persists for more than 2 days, consult a physician; tinnitus may indicate toxicity and use should be discontinued

Nursing Implications Seek causes for diarrhea; monitor for tinnitus; may aggravate or cause gout attack; may enhance bleeding if used with anticoagulants

Special Geriatric Considerations Tinnitus and CNS side effects (confusion, dizziness, high tone deafness, delirium, psychosis) may be difficult to assess in some elderly. Limit use of this agent in elderly.

Dosage Forms
Suspension, as subsalicylate: 262 mg/15 mL (240 mL)
Tablet, chewable, as subsalicylate: 262 mg
Tablet, chewable, as subgallate: 200 mg

Bismuth Subgallate see Bismuth on previous page

Bismuth Subsalicylate see Bismuth on previous page

Bisoprolol Fumarate (bis oh' proe lol)
Related Information
Beta-Blockers Comparison on page 804-805
Brand Names Zebeta®
Therapeutic Class Beta-Adrenergic Blocker
Use Treatment of hypertension, alone or in combination with other agents

Unlabeled use: Angina pectoris, supraventricular arrhythmias, PVCs

Contraindications Hypersensitivity to beta-blocking agents, uncompensated congestive heart failure; cardiogenic shock; bradycardia or heart block; sinus node dysfunction; A-V conduction abnormalities. Although bisoprolol primarily blocks beta$_1$-receptors, high doses can result in beta$_2$-receptor blockage. Therefore, use with caution in elderly with bronchospastic lung disease and renal dysfunction. **Note:** Geriatric patients often have decreased renal function.

Warnings Use with caution in patients with inadequate myocardial function; abrupt withdrawal of beta-blockers may result in an exaggerated cardiac beta-adrenergic responsiveness. Symptomatology has included reports of tachycardia, hypertension, ischemia, angina, myocardial infarction, and sudden death. It is recommended that patients be tapered gradually off of beta-blockers over a 2-week period rather than via abrupt discontinuation.

Precautions Diabetes mellitus (may mask signs/symptoms of hypoglycemia), renal function decline, myasthenia gravis, and severe peripheral vascular disease; use with caution in patients with bronchospasm disease or congestive heart failure, patients undergoing anesthesia, and hyperthyroidism

Adverse Reactions
Cardiovascular: Persistent bradycardia, hypotension, chest pain, edema, heart failure, Raynaud's phenomena, heart block

(Continued)

Bisoprolol Fumarate *(Continued)*

Central nervous system: Fatigue, dizziness, insomnia, lethargy, nightmares, depression, confusion, headache

Dermatologic: Rash, pruritus

Gastrointestinal: Constipation, diarrhea, nausea, dry mouth, anorexia

Genitourinary: Impotence, urinary retention

Respiratory: Shortness of breath

Miscellaneous: Cold extremities, blurred vision, facial swelling, muscle cramps

Overdosage Symptoms of overdose include severe hypotension, bradycardia, heart failure and bronchospasm, hypoglycemia

Toxicology Sympathomimetics (eg, epinephrine or dopamine), glucagon or a pacemaker can be used to treat the toxic bradycardia, asystole, and/or hypotension. Initially, fluids may be the best treatment for toxic hypotension. Patients should remain supine; serum glucose and potassium should be measured. Use supportive measures: lavage, syrup of ipecac; not significantly dialyzable. I.V. glucose should be administered for hypoglycemia; seizures may be treated with phenytoin or diazepam intravenously; continuous monitoring of blood pressure and EKG is necessary. If PVCs occur, treat with lidocaine or phenytoin; avoid quinidine, procainamide, and disopyramide since these agents further depress myocardial function. Bronchospasm can be treated with theophylline on beta$_2$ agonists (epinephrine).

Drug Interactions

Pharmacologic action of beta-antagonists may be decreased by aluminum compounds, calcium salts, barbiturates, cholestyramine, colestipol, NSAIDs, penicillins (ampicillin), rifampin, salicylates, sulfinpyrazone, thyroid hormones; hypoglycemic effect of sulfonylureas may be blunted

Pharmacologic effect of beta-antagonists may be enhanced with concomitant use of calcium channel blockers, oral contraceptives, flecainide (bioavailability and effect of flecainide also enhanced), haloperidol (hypotensive effects of both drugs), H$_2$ antagonists (decreased metabolism), hydralazine (both drugs hypotensive effects increased), loop diuretics (increased serum levels of beta-blockers except atenolol), MAO inhibitors, phenothiazines, propafenone, quinidine, quinolones, thioamines; beta-blockers may decrease clearance of acetaminophen; beta-blockers may increase anticoagulant effects of warfarin (propranolol); benzodiazepine effects enhanced by the lipophilic beta-blockers (atenolol does not interact)

Significant and fatal increases in blood pressure have occurred after decrease in dose or discontinuation of clonidine in patients receiving both clonidine and beta-blockers together (reduce doses of each cautiously with small decreases); peripheral ischemia of ergot alkaloids enhanced by beta-blockers; beta-blockers increase serum concentration of lidocaine; beta-blockers increase hypotensive effect of prazosin

Mechanism of Action Selective inhibitor of beta$_1$-adrenergic receptors; competitively blocks beta$_1$-receptors, with little or no effect on beta$_2$-receptors at doses <10 mg; low lipid solubility, therefore, little crosses the blood-brain barrier

Pharmacokinetics

Absorption: Rapid and almost complete from GI tract ($\geq$90%)

Distribution: Wide to body tissues; highest concentrations in heart, liver, lungs, and saliva; crosses the blood-brain barrier to a limited extent

Protein binding: 26% to 33%

Metabolism: Significant first-pass metabolism; metabolized in the liver

Half-life: 9-12 hours

Time to peak serum concentration: 1.7-3 hours

Elimination: ~50% unchanged in urine, <2% excreted in feces

Usual Dosage Oral:

Geriatrics: Initial dose: 2.5 mg/day; may be increased by 2.5-5 mg/day; maximum recommended dose: 20 mg/day

Adults: 5 mg once daily, may be increased to 10 mg, and then up to 20 mg once daily, if necessary; may be given without regard to meals

Dosing adjustment in renal/hepatic impairment: Cl$_{cr}$ <40 mL/minute: Initial: 2.5 mg/day; increase cautiously

Not dialyzable

Monitoring Parameters Blood pressure, EKG, orthostatic hypotension, heart rate, CNS effects

Test Interactions Increased thyroxine (S), cholesterol (S), glucose; increased triglycerides, uric acid; decreased HDL

Patient Information Adhere to dosage regimen; watch for postural hypotension; do not discontinue medication abruptly, sudden stopping of medication may precipitate or cause angina; consult pharmacist or physician before taking with other adrenergic drugs (eg, cold medications); notify physician if any of the following symptoms occur: difficult breathing, night cough, swelling of extremities, slow pulse, dizziness, lightheadedness, confusion, depression, skin rash, fever, sore throat, unusual bleeding or bruising; may produce drowsiness, dizziness, lightheadedness, blurred vision, confusion; use with caution while driving or performing tasks requiring alertness; may mask signs of hypoglycemia in diabetics; may be taken without regard to meals

Nursing Implications Patient's therapeutic response may be evaluated by looking at blood pressure, apical and radial pulses, fluid I & O, daily weight, respirations, and circulation in extremities before and during therapy; monitor for CNS side effects; modify dosage in patients with renal insufficiency

Additional Information May potentiate hypoglycemia in a diabetic patient and mask signs and symptoms

Special Geriatric Considerations Due to alterations in the beta-adrenergic autonomic nervous system, beta-adrenergic blockade may result in less hemodynamic response than seen in younger adults. Studies indicate that despite decreased sensitivity to the chronotropic effects of beta blockade with age, there appears to be an increased myocardial sensitivity to the negative inotropic effect during stress (ie, exercise). Controlled trials have shown the overall response rate for propranolol to be only 20% to 50% in elderly populations. Therefore, all beta-adrenergic blocking drugs may result in a decreased response as compared to younger adults.

Dosage Forms Tablet: 5 mg, 10 mg

References

Aagaard GN, "Treatment of Hypertension in The Elderly," *Drug Treatment in the Elderly*, Vestal RE, ed, Boston, MA: ADIS Health Science Press, 1984, 77.

Bitolterol Mesylate (bye tole' ter ole)

Brand Names Tornalate®

Generic Available No

Therapeutic Class Beta-2-Adrenergic Agonist Agent; Bronchodilator

Use Prevent and treat bronchial asthma and bronchospasm

Contraindications Known hypersensitivity to bitolterol

Warnings Use with caution in patients with unstable vasomotor symptoms, diabetes, hyperthyroidism, prostatic hypertrophy or a history of seizures; also use caution in the elderly and those patients with cardiovascular disorders such as coronary artery disease, arrhythmias, and hypertension

Precautions Excessive use may result in tolerance; deaths have been reported after excessive use; though the exact cause is unknown, cardiac arrest after a severe asthmatic crisis is suspected

Adverse Reactions

Cardiovascular: Tachycardia, palpitations, hypertension

Central nervous system: CNS stimulation, nervousness, hyperactivity, insomnia, dizziness, headache

Gastrointestinal: Nausea, vomiting, GI upset, bad taste

Neuromuscular & skeletal: Tremors (may be more common in the elderly)

Overdosage Symptoms of overdose include tremor, dizziness, nervousness, headache, nausea, coughing, seizures, angina, hypertension

Toxicology In cases of overdose, supportive therapy should be instituted, and prudent use of a cardioselective beta-adrenergic blocker (eg, atenolol or metoprolol) should be considered, keeping in mind the potential for induction of bronchoconstriction in an asthmatic individual. Dialysis has not been shown to be of value in the treatment of an overdose with this agent.

Drug Interactions

Decreased therapeutic effect: Beta-adrenergic blockers (eg, propranolol)

Increased therapeutic effect: Inhaled ipratropium → ↑ duration of bronchodilation, nifedipine → ↑ FEV-1

Increased toxicity (cardiovascular): MAO inhibitors, tricyclic antidepressants, sympathomimetic agents (eg, amphetamine, dopamine, dobutamine), inhaled anesthetics (eg, enflurane)

Mechanism of Action Selectively stimulates $beta_2$-adrenergic receptors in the lungs producing bronchial smooth muscle relaxation; minor $beta_1$ activity

Pharmacodynamics

Onset of action: 3-4 minutes

Duration: 4-8 hours

Pharmacokinetics

Metabolism: Bitolterol, a prodrug, is hydrolyzed to colterol (active) following inhalation

Half-life: 3 hours

Time to peak plasma colterol concentration: Inhalation: Within 1 hour

Elimination: In urine and feces

Usual Dosage Geriatrics and Adults:

Bronchospasm: 2 inhalations at an interval of at least 1-3 minutes, followed by a third inhalation if needed

Prevention of bronchospasm: 2 inhalations every 8 hours; do not exceed 3 inhalations every 6 hours or 2 inhalations every 4 hours

Monitoring Parameters Pulmonary function, blood pressure, pulse

Patient Information Do not exceed recommended dosage; rinse mouth with water following each inhalation to help with dry throat and mouth. Follow specific instructions accompanying inhaler; if more than one inhalation is necessary, wait at least 1 full minute between inhalations. May cause nervousness, restlessness, insomnia – if

(Continued)

Bitolterol Mesylate *(Continued)*

these effects continue after dosage reduction, notify physician. Also notify physician if palpitations, tachycardia, chest pain, muscle tremors, dizziness, headache, flushing or if breathing difficulty persists.

Nursing Implications Before using, the inhaler must be shaken well; assess lung sounds, pulse, and blood pressure before administration and during peak of medication; observe patient for wheezing after administration, if this occurs, call physician

Special Geriatric Considerations Elderly patients may find it useful to utilize a spacer device when using a metered dose inhaler; difficulty in using the inhaler often limits its effectiveness; see Adverse Reactions

Dosage Forms Aerosol, oral: 370 mcg/metered spray

Black Draught® [OTC] *see* Senna *on page 641*

Bleph®-10 *see* Sodium Sulfacetamide *on page 651*

Blephamide® *see* Sodium Sulfacetamide and Prednisolone Acetate *on page 652*

Blocadren® *see* Timolol Maleate *on page 697*

Bonine® [OTC] *see* Meclizine Hydrochloride *on page 434*

Breatheasy® *see* Epinephrine *on page 256*

Breonesin® [OTC] *see* Guaifenesin *on page 331*

Brethaire® *see* Terbutaline Sulfate *on page 673*

Brethine® *see* Terbutaline Sulfate *on page 673*

Bretylium Tosylate *(bre til' ee um)*

Brand Names Bretylol®

Generic Available Yes

Therapeutic Class Antiarrhythmic Agent, Class III

Use Treatment and prophylaxis of ventricular tachycardia and fibrillation which have failed to respond to traditional first-line therapies; also used in the treatment of other serious ventricular arrhythmias resistant to lidocaine

Contraindications Digitalis intoxication-induced arrhythmias

Warnings Hypotension to which tolerance develops over days of use; transient hypertension; transient aggravation of existing arrhythmia; use caution or avoid use in patients with fixed cardiac output, aortic stenosis, pulmonary hypertension; see Precautions and Adverse Reactions

Precautions Hypotension (50% in supine position), patients with fixed cardiac output (severe pulmonary hypertension or aortic stenosis) may experience severe hypotension due to decrease in peripheral resistance without ability to increase cardiac output; reduce dose in renal failure patients

Adverse Reactions

Cardiovascular: Hypotension (incidence 50% to 75%), transient initial hypertension, increase in PVCs, bradycardia, flushing, syncope

Central nervous system: Vertigo, confusion, anxiety, paranoid reactions, lethargy, emotional lability, hyperthermia

Dermatologic: Rash

Gastrointestinal: Nausea, vomiting, rarely diarrhea, abdominal pain

Local: Muscle atrophy and necrosis with repeated I.M. injections at same site

Ocular: Conjunctivitis

Renal: Renal impairment

Respiratory: Nasal congestion, nasal stuffiness, shortness of breath

Miscellaneous: Hiccups, diaphoresis

Overdosage Underdosing occurs more frequently than overdose; overdose results in significant hypertension followed by severe hypotension; see Toxicology

Toxicology Administration of short-acting hypotensive agent, nitroprusside (Nipride®), should be used for the hypertensive response; do not use long-acting hypotensive agents which may enhance hypotensive action of bretylium; hypotension should be treated with fluid administration and pressor agents such as dopamine or norepinephrine

Drug Interactions

Other antiarrhythmic agents may potentiate or antagonize cardiac effects, toxic effects may be additive

Pressor effects of catecholamines may be enhanced by bretylium

May potentiate digitalis toxicity due to initial release of norepinephrine

Stability The premix infusion should be stored at room temperature and protected from freezing; compatible solutions for dilution: D_5W for injection, D_5W in 0.45% NS; D_5W in 0.9% NS; 5% D_5W in lactated Ringer's, 0.9% NS; 5% sodium bicarbonate; 20% mannitol; lactated Ringer's; D_5W with potassium chloride 40 mEq/L; calcium chloride 54.4 mEq/L in D_5W

Mechanism of Action Class II antiarrhythmic; after an initial release of norepinephrine at the peripheral adrenergic nerve terminals, inhibits further release by postganglionic nerve endings in response to sympathetic nerve stimulation and inhibits reuptake into postganglionic adrenergic neurons; this action apparently increases ventricular fibrillation threshold, increases refractory period and action potential duration, and increases pacemaker tissue firing rate and ventricular conduction velocity

Pharmacodynamics
Onset of action:
I.V.: Antiarrhythmic effects seen within 6-20 minutes following administration
I.M.: May require 2 hours following administration
Peak effects: Within 6-9 hours
Duration: 6-24 hours

Pharmacokinetics
Absorption: I.M.: Well absorbed; suppression of ventricular fibrillation and tachycardia may not begin for 20 minutes to 2 hours
Protein binding: 1% to 6%
Metabolism: Not metabolized
Half-life: 7-8 hours; will increase 2-4 times with renal impairment/failure
Elimination: 70% to 80% (of I.M. dose) unchanged in urine over the first 24 hours with 10% over following 3 days

Usual Dosage Geriatrics and Adults (intended for short-term use only):
Immediate life-threatening ventricular arrhythmias; ventricular fibrillation; unstable ventricular tachycardia. **Note**: Patients should undergo defibrillation/cardioversion before and after bretylium doses as necessary. Adjust dose for renal function in elderly.
Initial dose: I.V.: 5 mg/kg (undiluted) over 1 minute; if arrhythmias persist, give 10 mg/kg (undiluted) over 1 minute and repeat as necessary (usually at 15- to 30-minute intervals) up to a total dose of 30 mg/kg
Other life-threatening ventricular arrhythmias:
Initial dose: I.M., I.V.: 5-10 mg/kg, may repeat every 1-2 hours if arrhythmias persist; give I.V. dose (diluted) over 10-30 minutes
Maintenance dose:
I.M.: 5-10 mg/kg every 6-8 hours
I.V. (diluted): 5-10 mg/kg every 6 hours
I.V. infusion (diluted): 1-2 mg/minute (little experience with doses >40 mg/kg/day)

Dosing adjustment in renal impairment:
Cl_{cr} 10-50 mL/minute: Administer 25% to 50% of dose
Cl_{cr} <10 mL/minute: Avoid use
Moderately dialyzable (20% to 50%)

Monitoring Parameters EKG and blood pressure throughout therapy is absolutely essential

Reference Range None clearly established

Patient Information Anticipate vomiting

Nursing Implications I.M. injection should not exceed 5 mL volume in any one site; give around-the-clock rather than 4 times/day, 3 times/day, etc (ie, 12-6-12-6, not 9-1-5-9) to promote less variation in peak and trough serum levels

Additional Information Subtherapeutic doses may cause hypotension

Special Geriatric Considerations See Precautions and Adverse Reactions; since renal function may be decreased, calculate or measure Cl_{cr} to guide dosing; see Usual Dosage; may have prolonged half-life with aging; adjust dose for renal function in elderly

Dosage Forms Injection: 50 mg/mL (10 mL) in ampuls, vials, and syringes

References
Fenster PE and Nolan PE, "Antiarrhythmic Drugs," *Geriatric Pharmacology*, Bressler R and Katz MD, eds, New York, NY: McGraw-Hill, 1993, 6:105-49.

Bretylol® see Bretylium Tosylate on previous page

Brevibloc® see Esmolol Hydrochloride on page 266

Bricanyl® see Terbutaline Sulfate on page 673

Bromaline® [OTC] see Brompheniramine and Phenylpropanolamine on next page

Bromanate® [OTC] see Brompheniramine and Phenylpropanolamine on next page

Bromarest® [OTC] see Brompheniramine Maleate on page 95

Bromatapp® [OTC] see Brompheniramine and Phenylpropanolamine on next page

Brombay® [OTC] see Brompheniramine Maleate on page 95

Bromocriptine Mesylate (broe moe krip' teen)
Brand Names Parlodel®
Generic Available No
Therapeutic Class Anti-Parkinson's Agent; Ergot Alkaloid
(Continued)

Bromocriptine Mesylate *(Continued)*

Use Treatment of parkinsonism in patients unresponsive or allergic to levodopa; also used in conditions associated with hyperprolactinemia and acromegaly

Contraindications Hypersensitivity to bromocriptine or any component, severe ischemic heart disease or peripheral vascular disorders

Precautions Use with caution in impaired renal or hepatic function

Adverse Reactions
Cardiovascular: Hypotension, hypertension, syncope
Central nervous system: Dizziness, drowsiness, fatigue, insomnia, headache, hallucinations, nightmares
Gastrointestinal: Nausea, vomiting, anorexia, abdominal cramps

Note: Incidence of adverse effects is high, especially at beginning of treatment and with dosages >20 mg/day

Overdosage Symptoms of overdose include nausea, vomiting, hypotension

Toxicology When unresponsive to I.V. fluids or Trendelenburg positioning, patient often responds to norepinephrine infusions started at 0.1-0.2 mcg/kg/minute followed by a titrated infusion

Drug Interactions
Decreased effect: Phenothiazines, haloperidol, reserpine, metoclopramide, methyldopa
Increased toxicity: Ergot alkaloids, hypotensive agents

Mechanism of Action Semisynthetic ergot alkaloid derivative with dopaminergic properties; inhibits prolactin secretion; can improve symptoms of Parkinson's disease by directly stimulating dopamine receptors in the corpus striatum

Pharmacokinetics
Protein binding: 90% to 96%
Metabolism: Majority metabolized in the liver
Half-life:
Biphasic: 6-8 hours
Terminal phase: 50 hours
Time to peak serum concentration: Oral: Within 1-2 hours
Elimination: In bile, with only 2% to 6% being excreted unchanged in urine

Usual Dosage Geriatrics and Adults: Oral:
Parkinsonism: 1.25 mg twice daily, increase by 1.25-2.5 mg/day in 2- to 4-week intervals; usual dose range: 30-90 mg/day in 3 divided doses, though elderly patients can usually be managed on lower doses

Hyperprolactinemia: 2.5 mg 2-3 times/day

Acromegaly: Initial: 1.25-2.5 mg, increasing as necessary every 3-7 days; usual dose: 20-30 mg/day

Monitoring Parameters Monitor blood pressure closely as well as hepatic, hematopoietic, and cardiovascular function

Test Interactions Increased BUN, AST, ALT, CPK, alkaline phosphatase, uric acid

Patient Information Take with food or milk to minimize nausea; drowsiness commonly occurs upon initiation of therapy; limit use of alcohol; avoid exposure to cold

Nursing Implications Raise bed rails and institute safety measures; aid patient with ambulation; may cause postural hypotension and drowsiness; incidence of side effects is high (68%) with nausea the most common

Additional Information Usually used with levodopa or levodopa/carbidopa to treat Parkinson's disease; when adding bromocriptine, the dose of levodopa/carbidopa can usually and should be decreased

Special Geriatric Considerations See Adverse Reactions and Usual Dosage

Dosage Forms
Capsule: 5 mg
Tablet: 2.5 mg

References
Koller WC, Silver DE, and Lieberman A, "An Algorithm for the Management of Parkinson's Disease," *Neurology*, 1994, 44(12):S1-52.

Brompheniramine and Phenylpropanolamine
(brome fen ir' a meen)

Related Information
Brompheniramine Maleate *on next page*
Phenylpropanolamine Hydrochloride *on page 559*

Brand Names Allerhist® [OTC]; Bromaline® [OTC]; Bromanate® [OTC]; Bromatapp® [OTC]; Bromphen® [OTC]; Dimaphen® [OTC]; Dimetapp® [OTC]; Myphetapp® [OTC]; Tamine® [OTC]

Therapeutic Class Antihistamine/Decongestant Combination

Adverse Reactions
Cardiovascular: Palpitations
Central nervous system: Excitability, drowsiness, dizziness, headache
Dermatologic: Rash

Gastrointestinal: Anorexia, nausea, dry mouth
Hematologic: Leukopenia
Usual Dosage Geriatrics and Adults: Oral:
Elixir: 10 mL
Tablet: 1 tablet every 4-6 hours
Sustained release: 1 tablet every 12 hours
Special Geriatric Considerations See Warnings and Precautions for individual agents; use cautiously in patients with cardiovascular disease
Dosage Forms
Elixir: Brompheniramine maleate 2 mg and phenylpropanolamine hydrochloride 12.5 mg per 5 mL with 2.3% alcohol (120 mL)
Tablet, immediate release: Brompheniramine maleate 4 mg and phenylpropanolamine hydrochloride 25 mg
Tablet, sustained release: Brompheniramine maleate 12 mg and phenylpropanolamine hydrochloride 75 mg

Brompheniramine Maleate (brome fen ir' a meen)

Brand Names Bromarest® [OTC]; Brombay® [OTC]; Bromphen® [OTC]; Brotane® [OTC]; Chlorphed® [OTC]; Codimal-A®; Cophene-B®; Dehist®; Diamine T.D.® [OTC]; Dimetane® [OTC]; Histaject®; Nasahist B®; ND-Stat®; Oraminic® II; Sinusol-B®; Veltane®
Synonyms Parabromdylamine
Generic Available Yes
Therapeutic Class Antihistamine
Use Perennial and seasonal allergic rhinitis and other allergic symptoms including urticaria
Contraindications Narrow-angle glaucoma, bladder neck obstruction, symptomatic prostatic hypertrophy, asthmatic attacks, and stenosing peptic ulcer, hypersensitivity to brompheniramine or any component
Warnings Antihistamines are more likely to cause dizziness, excessive sedation, syncope, toxic confusional states, and hypotension in the elderly.
Precautions Use with caution in patients with heart disease, hypertension, thyroid disease, and asthma
Adverse Reactions
Central nervous system: Paradoxical excitability, drowsiness, dizziness, confusion
Dermatologic: Rash
Gastrointestinal: Nausea, anorexia, dry mouth

Compared with other first generation antihistamines, brompheniramine is relatively nonsedating

Overdosage Symptoms of overdose include dry mouth, flushed skin, dilated pupils, CNS depression
Toxicology There is no specific treatment for an antihistamine overdose, however, most of its clinical toxicity is due to anticholinergic effects. Anticholinesterase inhibitors may be useful by reducing acetylcholinesterase. Anticholinesterase inhibitors include physostigmine, neostigmine, pyridostigmine and edrophonium. For anticholinergic overdose with severe life-threatening symptoms, physostigmine 1-2 mg I.V., slowly may be given to reverse these effects.
Drug Interactions Increased toxicity: CNS depressants, MAO inhibitors, alcohol, tricyclic antidepressants
Stability Solutions may crystallize if stored below 0°C, crystals will dissolve when warmed
Mechanism of Action Competes with histamine for H_1-receptor sites on effector cells in the gastrointestinal tract, blood vessels, and respiratory tract
Pharmacodynamics
Onset of action: Maximal clinical effects seen within 3-9 hours
Duration of action varies with formulation
Pharmacokinetics
Metabolism: Extensive by the liver
Half-life: 12-34 hours
Time to peak serum concentration: Oral: Within 2-5 hours
Elimination: In urine as inactive metabolites; 2% fecal elimination
Usual Dosage
Oral:
Geriatrics: Initial: 4 mg once or twice daily. **Note:** Duration of action may be 36 hours or more, even when serum concentrations are low.
Adults: 4 mg every 4-6 hours or 8 mg of sustained release form every 8-12 hours or 12 mg of sustained release every 12 hours; maximum: 24 mg/day

I.M., I.V., S.C.: Adults: 5-20 mg every 4-12 hours; maximum: 40 mg/24 hours
Monitoring Parameters Relief of symptoms
Patient Information May cause drowsiness; avoid alcohol; take with food or milk; swallow whole; do not crush or chew sustained release products
(Continued)

95

Brompheniramine Maleate *(Continued)*

Nursing Implications Raise bed rails, institute safety measures, aid patient with ambulation

Additional Information Causes less drowsiness than some conventional antihistamines

Special Geriatric Considerations See Contraindications, Warnings, and Usual Dosage; anticholinergic action may cause significant confusional symptoms

Dosage Forms
Elixir: 2 mg/5 mL with 3% alcohol (120 mL, 480 mL, 4000 mL)
Injection: 10 mg/mL (10 mL)
Tablet: 4 mg, 8 mg
Tablet, sustained release: 8 mg, 12 mg

Bromphen® [OTC] *see* Brompheniramine and Phenylpropanolamine *on page 94*

Bromphen® [OTC] *see* Brompheniramine Maleate *on previous page*

Bronitin® *see* Epinephrine *on page 256*

Bronkaid® Mist [OTC] *see* Epinephrine *on page 256*

Bronkodyl® *see* Theophylline *on page 681*

Bronkometer® *see* Isoetharine *on page 378*

Bronkosol® *see* Isoetharine *on page 378*

Brotane® [OTC] *see* Brompheniramine Maleate *on previous page*

B-S-P® *see* Betamethasone *on page 82*

Bufferin® [OTC] *see* Aspirin *on page 58*

Bumetanide *(byoo met' a nide)*

Brand Names Bumex®

Generic Available No

Therapeutic Class Diuretic, Loop

Use Management of edema associated with congestive heart failure or hepatic or renal disease including nephrotic syndrome; used alone or in combination with antihypertensives in the treatment of hypertension

Contraindications Hypersensitivity to bumetanide or any component; allergy to sulfonamides may result in cross-hypersensitivity to bumetanide; anuria or increasing azotemia

Warnings Loop diuretics are potent diuretics; excess amounts can lead to profound diuresis with fluid and electrolyte loss; close medical supervision and dose evaluation is required, particularly in the elderly

Adverse Reactions
Cardiovascular: Hypotension
Central nervous system: Dizziness, headache, encephalopathy
Dermatologic: Rash, photosensitivity
Endocrine & metabolic: Hyperglycemia, hypokalemia, hypochloremia, hyponatremia
Gastrointestinal: Cramps, nausea, vomiting
Genitourinary: Azotemia
Hepatic: Alteration of liver function test results
Neuromuscular & skeletal: Weakness
Otic: Impaired hearing
Renal: Decreased uric acid excretion, increased serum creatinine

Overdosage Symptoms of overdose include electrolyte depletion, volume depletion

Toxicology Treatment is primarily symptomatic and supportive; hypotension responds to fluids and Trendelenburg position; replace electrolytes as necessary

Drug Interactions
Decreased effect: Indomethacin, other NSAIDs
Increased hypotensive effect: Other antihypertensives
Increased level of lithium
Increased risk of ototoxicity: Aminoglycosides, other loop diuretics, vancomycin
When given with digoxin, diuretic-induced hypokalemia increases the risk of digoxin toxicity

Stability I.V. infusion solutions should be used within 24 hours after preparation

Mechanism of Action Inhibits reabsorption of sodium and chloride in the ascending loop of Henle and distal renal tubule, interfering with the chloride-binding cotransport system, thus causing increased excretion of water, sodium, chloride, magnesium, and calcium

Pharmacodynamics
Onset of action:
Oral, I.M.: 30-60 minutes
I.V.: Within a few minutes

Duration: 6 hours
Pharmacokinetics
Distribution: V_d: 13-25 L/kg
Protein binding: 95%
Metabolism: Partial in the liver
Half-life: 1-1.5 hours
Elimination: Majority of unchanged drug and metabolites excreted in urine
Usual Dosage
Geriatrics: Initial: Oral: 0.5 mg once daily, increase as necessary

Adults:
Oral: 0.5-2 mg/dose (maximum: 10 mg/day) 1-2 times/day
I.M., I.V.: 0.5-1 mg/dose (maximum: 10 mg/day)
Monitoring Parameters Blood pressure (standing and sitting/supine), serum electrolytes, renal function; in high doses, monitor auditory function, I & O, weight
Test Interactions Increased BUN, creatinine, ammonia (B), amylase (S), glucose, uric acid (S); decreased sodium, calcium, chloride, potassium
Patient Information May be taken with food or milk; get up slowly from a lying or sitting position to minimize dizziness, lightheadedness or fainting; also use extra care when exercising, standing for long periods of time and during hot weather; take in the morning; may cause increased sensitivity to sunlight
Nursing Implications Give I.V. slowly, over 1-2 minutes; be alert to complaints about hearing difficulty; check patient for orthostasis; see Monitoring Parameters
Additional Information Can be used in furosemide-allergic patients; 1 mg = 40 mg furosemide
Special Geriatric Considerations See Warnings; severe loss of sodium and/or increases in BUN can cause confusion; for any change in mental status in patients on bumetanide, monitor electrolytes and renal function
Dosage Forms
Injection: 0.25 mg/mL (2 mL, 4 mL, 10 mL)
Tablet: 0.5 mg, 1 mg, 2 mg

Bumex® see Bumetanide *on previous page*

Buprenex® see Buprenorphine Hydrochloride *on this page*

Buprenorphine Hydrochloride (byoo pre nor' feen)
Related Information
Pharmacokinetics of Narcotic Agonist Analgesics *on page 812*
Brand Names Buprenex®
Generic Available No
Therapeutic Class Analgesic, Narcotic
Use Management of moderate to severe pain
Restrictions C-V
Contraindications Hypersensitivity to buprenorphine or any component
Warnings If used in narcotic dependent patients, may cause withdrawal effects
Precautions Use with caution in severe impairment of hepatic, pulmonary, or renal function
Adverse Reactions
Cardiovascular: Hypotension
Central nervous system: Vertigo, confusion, sedation, dizziness, headache
Gastrointestinal: Nausea
Respiratory: Respiratory depression
Overdosage Symptoms of overdose include CNS depression, pinpoint pupils, hypotension, bradycardia
Toxicology Treatment of an overdose includes support of the patient's airway, establishment of an I.V. line, and administration of naloxone 2 mg I.V. with repeat administration as necessary up to a total of 10 mg
Drug Interactions Increased toxicity: CNS depressants, barbiturate anesthetics, benzodiazepines
Stability Protect from excessive heat or light
Mechanism of Action Opiate agonist/antagonist that produces analgesia by binding to kappa and mu opiate receptors in the CNS
Pharmacodynamics Onset of analgesia: Within 10-30 minutes
Pharmacokinetics
Absorption: I.M.: 30% to 40%
Distribution: V_d: 97-187 L/kg
Protein binding: Highly protein bound
Metabolism: Mainly in the liver; undergoes extensive first-pass metabolism
Half-life: 2.2-3 hours
Elimination: 70% in feces via bile and 20% in urine as unchanged drug
Usual Dosage I.M., slow I.V.:
Geriatrics: 0.15 mg every 6 hours
Adults: 0.3-0.6 mg every 6 hours as needed
Monitoring Parameters Pain relief, respiratory and mental status, blood pressure

(Continued)

Buprenorphine Hydrochloride *(Continued)*
Test Interactions Increased amylase, lipase

Patient Information May cause drowsiness and/or dizziness

Nursing Implications Monitor respiratory status during therapy; gradual withdrawal of drug is necessary to avoid withdrawal symptoms

Additional Information 0.3 mg = 10 mg morphine or 75 mg meperidine, has longer duration of action than either; may precipitate abstinence syndrome in narcotic-dependent patients; therefore, use buprenorphine before starting a patient on a narcotic. Long-term use is not recommended.

Special Geriatric Considerations One postmarketing study found that elderly patients were more likely to suffer from confusion and drowsiness after buprenorphine as compared to younger patients

Dosage Forms Injection: 0.3 mg/mL

References

Harcus AH, Ward AE, and Smith DW, "Buprenorphine: Experience in an Elderly Population of 975 Patients During a Year's Monitored Release," *Br J Clin Pract*, 1980, 34(5):144-6.

Bupropion (byoo proe' pee on)
Related Information

Antidepressant Agents Comparison *on page 800*

Brand Names Wellbutrin®

Synonyms Amfebutamone

Generic Available No

Therapeutic Class Antidepressant

Use Treatment of depression

Contraindications Seizure disorder, prior diagnosis of bulimia or anorexia nervosa, known hypersensitivity to bupropion, concurrent use of a monoamine oxidase (MAO) inhibitor

Precautions Estimated seizure potential is increased many fold in doses in the 450-600 mg/day dosage; giving a single dose of 150 mg or less will lessen the seizure potential; recent myocardial infarction or unstable heart disease

Adverse Reactions

Central nervous system: Agitation, insomnia, fever, headache, psychosis, confusion, anxiety, restlessness, seizures, chills, akathisia

Gastrointestinal: Nausea, vomiting, weight loss

Genitourinary: Impotence

Neuromuscular & skeletal: Tremors

Ocular: Blurred vision

Overdosage Symptoms of overdose include labored breathing, salivation, arched back, ataxia, convulsions

Toxicology Hospitalize patient if still conscious, induce vomiting, administer activated charcoal every 6 hours for two times and obtain baseline labs, obtain EKG and EEG over the next 48 hours; maintain hydration. In patients who are comatose, stuporous, or seizing, perform gastric lavage after adequate airway has been established via intubation. Treat seizures with I.V. benzodiazepines and supportive therapies; dialysis may be of limited value after drug absorption because of slow tissue to plasma diffusion.

Drug Interactions Carbamazepine, phenytoin, cimetidine, phenobarbital (bupropion may enhance metabolism), enhanced acute toxicity with phenelzine; levodopa increases nausea and agitation; risk of seizure activity following abrupt withdrawal of benzodiazepines

Mechanism of Action Bupropion is an antidepressant structurally different from all other previously marketed antidepressants; like other antidepressants the mechanism of bupropion's activity is not fully understood; the drug is a weak blocker of serotonin and norepinephrine re-uptake, inhibits neuronal dopamine re-uptake and is not a monoamine oxidase A or B inhibitor

Pharmacodynamics May take up to 4 weeks or longer until full effect is seen

Pharmacokinetics

Absorption: Rapidly from the GI tract

Distribution: V_d: 1.4-3.2 L/kg

Protein binding: 82% to 88%; has not been studied in the elderly

Metabolism: Extensive in the liver to multiple metabolites (whose elimination may be decreased by liver or renal dysfunction)

Bioavailability, oral: 5%

Half-life: 14 hours

Time to peak: Oral: Peak plasma levels occur within 2 hours

Usual Dosage Oral:

Geriatrics: Initial: 50-100 mg/day, increase by 50-100 mg every 3-4 days as tolerated; there is evidence that the elderly respond at 150 mg/day in divided doses, but some may require a higher dose

Adults: 100 mg 3 times/day; begin at 100 mg twice daily; may increase to a maximum dose of 450 mg/day

Monitoring Parameters Signs and symptoms of depression; mood; weight; blood pressure

Patient Information Take in equally divided doses 3-4 times/day to minimize the risk of seizures; avoid alcohol; may impair driving or other motor or cognitive skills and judgment

Nursing Implications Monitor body weight; be aware that drug may cause seizures

Additional Information Use in patients with renal or hepatic impairment increases the possibilities of possible toxic effects

Special Geriatric Considerations Limited data is available about the use of bupropion in the elderly; two studies have found it equally effective when compared to imipramine. Its side effect profile (minimal anticholinergic and blood pressure effects) may make it useful in persons who do not tolerate traditional cyclic antidepressants; see Usual Dosage.

Dosage Forms Tablet: 75 mg, 100 mg

References

Branconnier RJ, Cole JO, Ghazvinian S, et al, "Clinical Pharmacology of Bupropion and Imipramine in Elderly Depressives," *J Clin Psychiatry*, 1983, 44(5 Pt 2):130-3.

Hayes PE and Kristoff CA, "Adverse Reactions to Five New Antidepressants," *Clin Pharm*, 1986, 5:471-80.

Kane JM, Cole K, Sarantakos S, et al, "Safety and Efficacy of Bupropion in Elderly Patients: Preliminary Observations," *J Clin Psychiatry*, 1983, 44(5 Pt 2):134-6.

BuSpar® *see* Buspirone Hydrochloride *on this page*

Buspirone Hydrochloride (byoo spye' rone)

Related Information
Anxiolytic/Hypnotic Use in Long-Term Care Facilities *on page 755-756*

Brand Names BuSpar®

Generic Available No

Therapeutic Class Antianxiety Agent

Use Management of anxiety
Unlabeled use: Panic attacks

Contraindications Hypersensitivity to buspirone or any component

Warnings Use in hepatic or renal impairment is not recommended

Precautions Causes less sedation than other anxiolytics, but patients should be cautioned about driving until they are certain buspirone does not affect them adversely; avoid alcoholic beverages

Adverse Reactions
Central nervous system: Sedation, disorientation, excitement, dizziness, fever, headache, encephalopathy, ataxia
Dermatologic: Rash, urticaria
Gastrointestinal: Nausea, vomiting, diarrhea, flatulence
Hematologic: Leukopenia, eosinophilia

Overdosage Symptoms of overdose include dizziness, drowsiness, pinpoint pupils, nausea, vomiting

Toxicology There is no known antidote for buspirone and most therapies are supportive and symptomatic in nature

Drug Interactions
Increased effect: Cimetidine
Increased toxicity: MAO inhibitors, CNS depressants, alcohol, increased haloperidol concentrations

Food/Drug Interactions Food may decrease the absorption of buspirone, but it may also decrease the first-pass metabolism, thereby increasing the bioavailability of buspirone

Mechanism of Action Selectively antagonizes CNS serotonin 5-HT$_1$A receptors without affecting benzodiazepine-GABA receptors; may down-regulate postsynaptic 5-HT$_2$ receptors as do antidepressants

Pharmacodynamics Onset of action: Decrease in anxiety is seen after one week of therapy, but it may take several weeks for the full effects to be seen

Pharmacokinetics Studies in the elderly found no significant changes in pharmacokinetic parameters
Protein binding: 95%
Metabolism: In the liver by oxidation and undergoes extensive first-pass metabolism
Half-life: 2-3 hours; range: 2-11 hours
Time to peak serum concentration: Within 40-60 minutes

Usual Dosage Oral:
Geriatrics: Initial: 5 mg twice daily, increase by 5 mg/day every 2-3 days as needed up to 20-30 mg/day; maximum daily dose: 60 mg/day; see Additional Information

Adults: 15 mg/day (5 mg 3 times/day); increase by 5 mg/day every 2-3 days, as needed to a maximum of 60 mg/day; see Additional Information

Dosage should be decreased in patients with severe hepatic insufficiency; anuric patients should be dosed at 25% to 50% of the usual dose

(Continued)

Buspirone Hydrochloride *(Continued)*

Monitoring Parameters Mental status, symptoms of anxiety

Test Interactions Increased AST, ALT

Patient Information May cause drowsiness or dizziness; take with food; report any change in senses (ie, smelling, hearing, vision); cautious use with alcohol is recommended; takes 2-3 weeks to see the full effect of this medication

Nursing Implications See Monitoring Parameters

Additional Information Has shown little potential for abuse; not effective when used PRN

Special Geriatric Considerations Because buspirone is less sedating than other anxiolytics, it may be a useful agent in geriatric patients when an anxiolytic is indicated

Dosage Forms Tablet: 5 mg, 10 mg

References

Gammans RE, Westrick ML, Shea JP, et al, "Pharmacokinetics of Buspirone in Elderly Subjects," *J Clin Pharmacol*, 1989, 29(1):72-8.

Busulfan *(byoo sul' fan)*

Brand Names Myleran®

Generic Available No

Therapeutic Class Antineoplastic Agent, Alkylating Agent

Use Chronic myelogenous leukemia and marrow-ablative conditioning regimens prior to bone marrow transplantation

Contraindications Hypersensitivity to busulfan or any component; failure to respond to previous courses

Warnings The U.S. Food and Drug Administration (FDA) currently recommends that procedures for proper handling and disposal of antineoplastic agents be considered. May cause severe and serious bone marrow suppression (pancytopenia) that may be more prolonged than that produced by other alkylating agents. May take 1 month to 2 years to recover bone marrow function after discontinuing therapy; bronchopulmonary dysplasia (busulfan lung) with fibrosis occurs rarely; carcinogenic potential has been described as with other alkylating agents

Precautions May induce severe bone marrow hypoplasia; reduce or discontinue dosage at first sign, as reflected by an abnormal decrease in any of the formed elements of the blood; use with caution in patients recently given other myelosuppressive drugs or radiation treatment

Adverse Reactions

Central nervous system: Dizziness, seizures

Dermatologic: Hyperpigmentation

Endocrine & metabolic: Addison-like syndrome, hyperuricemia

Gastrointestinal: Nausea, vomiting

Hematologic: Leukopenia, thrombocytopenia, anemia

Hepatic: Hepatic dysfunction, increased LFTs

Ocular: Blurred vision

Renal: Hemorrhagic cystitis

Respiratory: Pulmonary fibrosis

Overdosage Symptoms of overdose include leukopenia, thrombocytopenia, pancytopenia (rare)

Toxicology Initiate general supportive measures; monitor hematologic status closely; transfusions as needed

Drug Interactions Thioguanine (esophageal varices formed with long-term use); increased myelosuppression when used concomitantly with other immunosuppressives

Mechanism of Action Interferes with the normal function of DNA by alkylation and cross-linking the strands of DNA

Pharmacokinetics

Absorption: Oral: Rapidly and well absorbed

Metabolism: Extensive in the liver 10% to 50%

Time to peak:

I.V.: Peak plasma levels occur within 5 minutes

Oral: Within 4 hours

Elimination: In urine as metabolites within 24 hours

Usual Dosage Oral (refer to individual protocols):

Geriatrics: Start with lowest recommended doses for adults

Adults: 4-8 mg/day for remission induction of CML

Maintenance dose: Controversial, range from 1-4 mg/day to 2 mg/week

Monitoring Parameters Decrease in leukocytes not seen in first 10-15 days of therapy. Leukocyte count may increase during initiation of therapy and does not reflect resistance to therapy. Do not increase dose if WBC count increases during initiation of therapy. Monitor CBC and platelets weekly. Once remission is achieved, monitoring intervals may be increased according to protocol with physician discretion. Observe for signs of bleeding, bruising, infection, or pulmonary disease; see Additional Information

Test Interactions Increased potassium (S)

Patient Information Watch for signs of bleeding, bruising, coughing, difficulty breathing, fever, joint pain, or flank pain. May cause darkening of skin, dizziness, fatigue, mental confusion, nausea, vomiting, anorexia. Take medication the same time each day. Excellent oral hygiene is needed to minimize oral discomfort

Nursing Implications Avoid I.M. injection if platelet count falls <100,000/mm³; see Monitoring Parameters

Additional Information Use with caution in patients recently given other myelosuppressive drugs or radiation treatment

Myelosuppressive effects:
WBC: Moderate
Platelets: Moderate
Onset (days): 7
Nadir (days): 14-21
Recovery (days): 28

Special Geriatric Considerations Toxicity to immunosuppressives is increased in elderly. Start with lowest recommended adult doses; see Usual Dosage. Signs of infection, such as fever and rise in WBCs, may not occur. Lethargy and confusion may be more prominent signs of infection.

Dosage Forms Tablet: 2 mg

References
Heard BE and Cooke RA, "Busulphan Lung," *Thorax*, 1968, 23(2):187-93.
Hutchins LF and Lipschitz DA, "Cancer, Clinical Pharmacology, and Aging," *Clin Geriatr Med*, 1987, 3(3):483-503.
Kaplan HG, "Use of Cancer Chemotherapy in the Elderly," *Drug Treatment in the Elderly*, Vestal RE, ed, Boston, MA: ADIS Health Science Press, 1984, 338-49.

Butabarbital Sodium (byoo ta bar' bi tal)
Related Information
Anxiolytic/Hypnotic Use in Long-Term Care Facilities *on page 755-756*
Brand Names Butalan®; Buticaps®; Butisol Sodium®
Therapeutic Class Barbiturate; Hypnotic; Sedative
Restrictions C-III
Special Geriatric Considerations Use of this agent in the elderly is not recommended

Butalan® *see* Butabarbital Sodium *on this page*

Buticaps® *see* Butabarbital Sodium *on this page*

Butisol Sodium® *see* Butabarbital Sodium *on this page*

Butorphanol Tartrate (byoo tor' fa nole)
Related Information
Pharmacokinetics of Narcotic Agonist Analgesics *on page 812*
Brand Names Stadol®; Stadol® NS
Generic Available No
Therapeutic Class Analgesic, Narcotic
Use Management of moderate to severe pain; nasal butorphanol is being studies in the treatment of migraine headache pain
Contraindications Hypersensitivity to butorphanol or any component; avoid use in opiate-dependent patients who have not been detoxified, may precipitate opiate withdrawal
Warnings Use with caution in hepatic or renal disease, may elevate CSF pressure, may increase cardiac workload
Precautions May cause CNS effects, such as drowsiness
Adverse Reactions
Cardiovascular: Hypotension
Central nervous system: CNS depression, headache
Gastrointestinal: Anorexia, nausea, vomiting, constipation, dry mouth
Respiratory: Respiratory depression
Overdosage Symptoms of overdose include respiratory depression, cardiac and CNS depression
Toxicology Treatment of an overdose includes support of the patient's airway, establishment of an I.V. line and administration of naloxone 2 mg I.V. with repeat administration as necessary up to a total of 10 mg.
Drug Interactions Increased toxicity: CNS depressants, barbiturate anesthetics
Stability Store at room temperature, protect from freezing
Mechanism of Action Mixed narcotic agonist-antagonist with central analgesic actions; binds to opiate receptors in the CNS, causing inhibition of ascending pain pathways, altering the perception of and response to pain; produces generalized CNS depression
Pharmacodynamics Peak effect:
I.M.: Within 30-60 minutes
I.V.: Within 4-5 minutes

(Continued)

Butorphanol Tartrate *(Continued)*
Nasal: 1-2 hours

Pharmacokinetics Plasma concentrations after a single dose were not significantly different between elderly and young subjects
Absorption: I.M.: Rapidly and well absorbed
Protein binding: 80%
Metabolism: In the liver
Half-life:
  Geriatrics: 5.5 hours
  Adults: 2.5-4 hours
Elimination: Primarily in urine

Usual Dosage
Geriatrics:
  I.M., I.V.: 0.5-2 mg every 6-8 hours, increase as necessary
  Nasal: 1 mg (1 spray in one nostril); after 90-120 minutes, assess whether a second dose is needed; may repeat in 3-4 hours

Adults:
  I.M.: 1-4 mg every 3-4 hours as needed
  I.V.: 0.5-2 mg every 3-4 hours as needed
  Nasal: 1 mg (1 spray in one nostril); after 60-90 minutes, assess whether a second dose is needed; may repeat in 3-4 hours

Dosing adjustment in renal impairment:
Cl_{cr} 10-50 mL/minute: Administer 75% of dose
Cl_{cr} <10 mL/minute: Administer 50% of dose

Monitoring Parameters Pain relief, respiratory and mental status, blood pressure

Patient Information May cause drowsiness, avoid alcohol; follow instructions for use of nasal spray

Nursing Implications Observe for excessive sedation or confusion, respiratory depression; raise bed rails, aid with ambulation

Special Geriatric Considerations See Pharmacokinetics and Usual Dosage; adjust dose for renal function in elderly

Dosage Forms
Injection: 1 mg/mL, 2 mg/mL
Spray, nasal: 10 mg/mL (2.5 mL) [14-15 doses]

References
Ramsey R, Higbee M, Maesner J, et al, "Influence of Age on the Pharmacokinetics of Butorphanol," *Acute Care*, 1986, 12(Suppl 1):8-16.

BW-430C *see* Lamotrigine *on page 398*

Byclomine® *see* Dicyclomine Hydrochloride *on page 215*

Cafergot® *see* Ergotamine *on page 261*

Calan® *see* Verapamil Hydrochloride *on page 735*

Calan® SR *see* Verapamil Hydrochloride *on page 735*

Cal Carb-HD® [OTC] *see* Calcium Salts (Oral) *on page 111*

Calci-Chew™ [OTC] *see* Calcium Salts (Oral) *on page 111*

Calciday-667® [OTC] *see* Calcium Salts (Oral) *on page 111*

Calcifediol (kal si fe dye' ole)
Brand Names Calderol®
Synonyms 25-HCC; 25-Hydroxyvitamin D_3
Generic Available No
Therapeutic Class Vitamin D Analog
Use Treatment and management of metabolic bone disease associated with chronic renal failure

Contraindications Hypercalcemia, known hypersensitivity to calcifediol, vitamin D toxicity, malabsorption syndrome, hypervitaminosis D, decreased renal function

Warnings Must give concomitant calcium supplementation; maintain adequate fluid intake; calcium-phosphate product (serum calcium times phosphorus) must not exceed 70; avoid hypercalcemia; renal function impairment with secondary hyperparathyroidism

Precautions Use with caution in coronary artery disease, decreased renal function, renal stones, and elderly

Adverse Reactions
Cardiovascular: Hypotension, cardiac arrhythmias
Central nervous system: Irritability, headache, somnolence, convulsions
Dermatologic: Pruritus
Endocrine & metabolic: Metastatic calcification, polydipsia
Gastrointestinal: Anorexia, weight loss, pancreatitis, nausea, vomiting, dry mouth, constipation, metallic taste

102

Hematologic: Anemia
Hepatic: Elevated AST/ALT
Neuromuscular & skeletal: Muscle pain, bone pain, weakness
Ocular: Conjunctivitis, photophobia
Renal: Polyuria, renal damage

Overdosage Symptoms of overdose include hypercalcemia, hypercalciuria

Toxicology Following withdrawal of the drug, treatment consists of bed rest, liberal intake of fluids, reduced calcium intake, and cathartic administration. Severe hypercalcemia requires I.V. hydration and forced diuresis with I.V. furosemide (20-40 mg I.V. every 4-6 hours for adults). Urine output should be monitored and maintained at >3 mL/kg/hour. I.V. saline can quickly and significantly increase excretion of calcium into the urine. Calcitonin, cholestyramine, prednisone, sodium EDTA and mithramycin have all been used successfully to treat the more resistant cases of vitamin D-induced hypercalcemia.

Drug Interactions
Vitamin D may increase absorption of magnesium from magnesium compounds; hypercalcemia may be precipitated by vitamin D and, therefore, may increase cardiac arrhythmias in patients taking digitalis glycosides and verapamil; hypoparathyroid patients may develop hypercalcemia when using thiazide diuretics
Phenytoin and barbiturates decrease half-life of vitamin D; mineral oil with prolonged use decreases vitamin D absorption; cholestyramine reduces absorption of vitamin D

Stability Store in light-resistant container

Mechanism of Action Vitamin D analog that (along with calcitonin and parathyroid hormone) regulates serum calcium homeostasis by promoting absorption of calcium and phosphorus in the small intestine; promotes renal tubule resorption of phosphate; increases rate of accretion and resorption in bone minerals

Pharmacodynamics Maximal calcemic effects: Seen in 4 weeks with daily administration

Pharmacokinetics
Absorption: Rapid from the small intestine
Half-life: 12-22 days
Time to peak: Oral: Peak serum levels occur within 4 hours
Elimination: In bile and feces, stored in liver and fat depots, muscle, skin, and bones

Usual Dosage Daily supplement for elderly (800 IU): 20 mcg
Geriatrics and Adults: Hepatic osteodystrophy: 20-100 mcg/day or every other day; titrate to obtain normal serum calcium/phosphate levels; increase dose at 4-week intervals; see Additional Information

Monitoring Parameters Urine output; obtain serum calcium levels twice weekly during titration phase; if hypercalcemia is encountered, discontinue agent until calcium concentrations return to normal

Reference Range Calcium (serum) 9-10 mg/dL (4.5-5 mEq/L); phosphate 2.5-5 mg/dL

Test Interactions Increased calcium (S), cholesterol (S)

Patient Information Do not take more than the recommended amount. While taking this medication, your physician may want you to follow a special diet or take a calcium supplement. Follow this diet closely. Avoid taking magnesium supplements or magnesium containing antacids. Early symptoms of hypercalcemia include weakness, fatigue, somnolence, headache, anorexia, dry mouth, metallic taste, nausea, vomiting, cramps, diarrhea, muscle pain, bone pain, and irritability.

Nursing Implications Monitor calcium and phosphate levels closely; monitor symptoms of hypercalcemia; see Adverse Reactions

Additional Information 1000 mcg = 40,000 units of vitamin D activity; this product not generally recommended for daily supplementation due to dosage forms, strengths, and cost

Special Geriatric Considerations Recommended daily allowances (RDA) have not been developed for persons >65 years of age; vitamin D, folate, and B_{12} (cyanocobalamin) have decreased absorption with age, but the clinical significance is yet unknown. Calorie requirements decrease with age and therefore, nutrient density must be increased to ensure adequate nutrient intake, including vitamins and minerals. Therefore, the use of a daily supplement with a multiple vitamin with minerals is recommended. Elderly consume less vitamin D, absorption may be decreased, and many elderly have decreased sun exposure; therefore, elderly should receive supplementation with 800 units (20 mcg)/day. This is a recommendation of particular need to those with high risk for osteoporosis.

Dosage Forms Capsule: 20 mcg, 50 mcg

References
Letsou AP and Price LS, "Health Aging and Nutrition: An Overview," *Clin Geriatr Med*, 1987, 3(2):253-60.

Myrianthopoulos M, "Dietary Treatment of Hyperlipidemia in the Elderly," *Clin Geriatr Med*, 1987, 3(2):343-59.

Riggs BL and Melton LJ, "The Prevention and Treatment of Osteoporosis," *N Engl J Med*, 1992, 327(9):620-7.

ALPHABETICAL LISTING OF DRUGS

Calciferol™ *see* Ergocalciferol *on page 259*

Calcijex™ *see* Calcitriol *on next page*

Calcimar® *see* Calcitonin *on this page*

Calci-Mix™ [OTC] *see* Calcium Salts (Oral) *on page 111*

Calciparine® *see* Heparin *on page 340*

Calcipotriene
Brand Names Dovonex®
Therapeutic Class Antipsoriatic Agent, Topical
Use Treatment of moderate plaque psoriasis
Contraindications Hypersensitivity to any of the components; hypercalcemia or evidence of vitamin D toxicity; do not use on the face
Warnings Apply directly to skin lesions; warn patient not to exceed the ordered dose. In clinical studies, skin-related adverse effects were more severe in the elderly compared to younger adults.
Precautions May cause irritation of lesions and surrounding uninvolved skin; transient, reversible hypercalcemia has occurred with the use of calcipotriene
Adverse Reactions
Dermatologic: Burning, stinging, pruritus, erythema, facial dermatitis, worsening of psoriasis, skin atrophy, hyperpigmentation
Endocrine & metabolic: Hypercalcemia
Toxicology Topically applied calcipotriene can be absorbed in sufficient amounts to produce systemic effects
Mechanism of Action Synthetic vitamin D_3 analog which regulates skin cell production and proliferation
Pharmacokinetics
Absorption: ~6% when applied to psoriasis plaque
Metabolism: Within 24 hours most of the drug is converted to inactive metabolites by the liver
Usual Dosage Geriatrics and Adults: Apply to skin lesions twice daily; rub in gently and completely
Monitoring Parameters Healing of lesions, serum calcium levels
Patient Information Apply only to affected areas; do not exceed the ordered dose; avoid contact with face or eyes; wash hands after application; report any local adverse effects
Special Geriatric Considerations See Warnings
Dosage Forms Ointment, topical: 0.005% (30 g, 60 g, 100 g)

Calcitonin (kal si toe' nin)
Brand Names Calcimar®; Cibacalcin®
Synonyms Calcitonin (Human); Calcitonin (Salmon)
Generic Available No
Therapeutic Class Antidote, Hypercalcemia
Use
Calcitonin (salmon): Treatment of Paget's disease of bone and as adjunctive therapy for hypercalcemia; also used in postmenopausal osteoporosis
Calcitonin (human): Treatment of Paget's disease of bone
Contraindications Hypersensitivity to salmon protein or gelatin diluent
Precautions A skin test should be performed prior to initiating therapy with salmon calcitonin; the skin test is 0.1 mL of 10 IU dilution of calcitonin (must be prepared) injected intradermally; observe injection site for 15 minutes for wheal or significant erythema
Adverse Reactions
Cardiovascular: Flushing of the face, swelling
Central nervous system: Dizziness, headache, parasthesia, chills
Dermatologic: Rash, urticaria
Gastrointestinal: Nausea, vomiting, diarrhea, anorexia
Local: Pain and swelling at the injection site
Neuromuscular & skeletal: Weakness
Renal: Diuresis
Respiratory: Shortness of breath, nasal congestion
Overdosage Symptoms of overdose include hypocalcemia, hypocalcemic tetany
Stability Refrigeration is recommended for salmon calcitonin, stable for up to 2 weeks at room temperature; normal saline has been recommended for the dilution to prepare a skin test; protect from light; calcitonin human may be stored at room temperature
Mechanism of Action Structurally similar to human calcitonin; regulates serum calcium concentration along with vitamin D and parathyroid hormone; acts on bone to decrease osteoclast activity, in the kidney to decrease tubular reabsorption of sodium and calcium, and in the GI tract to increase the absorption of calcium
Pharmacokinetics
Hypercalcemia:
Onset of reduction in calcium: 2 hours

Duration of effect: 6-8 hours
Metabolism: Rapidly by the kidneys
Half-life: S.C.: 1.2 hours
Elimination: As inactive metabolites in urine
Usual Dosage Geriatrics and Adults:
Hepatic osteodystrophy: 20-100 mcg/kg/day or every other day, titrate to obtain normal serum calcium/phosphate levels

Calcitonin salmon:
Skin test: 1 unit/0.1 mL intracutaneously
Paget's disease: I.M., S.C.: 100 units/day
Postmenopause osteoporosis: I.M., S.C.: 100 units/day
Hypercalcemia: I.M., S.C.: 4 units/kg every 12 hours, may increase to maximum of 8 units/kg every 6 hours

Calcitonin human: Paget's disease: I.M., S.C.: 0.5 mg/day; some patients require as little as 0.25 mg or 0.5 mg 2-3 times/week; severe cases may require 0.5 mg twice daily
Administration I.M. route is preferred
Monitoring Parameters Serum alkaline phosphatase, 24-hour urinary hydroxyproline before and every 3 months; symptom response (pain, fracture); serum calcium and electrolytes
Reference Range Therapeutic: <19 pg/mL (SI: 19 ng/L) basal, depending on the assay
Test Interactions Decreased calcium (S)
Patient Information Keep in refrigerator; take at bedtime to minimize nausea and flushing
Nursing Implications Keep in refrigerator when volume exceeds 2 mL; skin test should be performed prior to administration of salmon calcitonin
Special Geriatric Considerations Long-term studies are needed to determine whether calcitonin's effects on bone density and fracture rates are beneficial; calcitonin may also be effective in steroid-induced osteoporosis and other states associat-. ed with high bone turnover
Dosage Forms Injection: 0.5 mg/vial
References
Bauwens SF, "Osteomalacia and Osteoporosis," *Pharmacotherapy: A Pathophysiologic Approach*, 2nd ed, DiPiro JT, Talbert RL, Hayes PE, et al, eds, New York, NY, 1992, 1293-1312.

Calcitonin (Human) see Calcitonin on previous page

Calcitonin (Salmon) see Calcitonin on previous page

Calcitriol (kal si trye' ole)
Related Information
Antacid Drug Interactions *on page 764*
Brand Names Calcijex™; Rocaltrol®
Synonyms 1,25 dihydroxycholecalciferol
Generic Available No
Therapeutic Class Vitamin D Analog
Use Management of hypocalcemia in patients on chronic renal dialysis; reduce elevated parathyroid hormone levels; decrease severity of psoriatic lesions in psoriatic vulgaris
Contraindications Hypercalcemia; vitamin D toxicity; abnormal sensitivity to the effects of vitamin D; malabsorption syndrome; decreased function
Warnings Must give concomitant calcium supplementation; maintain adequate fluid intake; calcium-phosphate product (serum calcium times phosphorus) must not exceed 70; avoid hypercalcemia; renal function impairment with secondary hyperparathyroidism
Precautions Use with caution in coronary artery disease, decreased renal function, renal stones, and elderly
Adverse Reactions
Cardiovascular: Increased blood pressure, cardiac arrhythmias
Central nervous system: Somnolence, headache, hyperthermia
Dermatologic: Pruritus
Endocrine & metabolic: Hypercholesterolemia, hypercalcemia
Gastrointestinal: Nausea, vomiting, constipation, anorexia, weight loss, dry mouth, pancreatitis, metallic taste
Genitourinary: Nocturia, uremia, albuminuria
Hepatic: Increased liver enzymes
Neuromuscular & skeletal: Myalgia, bone pain, weakness
Ocular: Calcific conjunctivitis, photophobia
Renal: Polyuria, polydipsia
Respiratory: Rhinorrhea
Overdosage Symptoms of overdose include hypercalcemia, hypercalciuria
Toxicology Following withdrawal of the drug, treatment consists of bed rest, liberal in-
(Continued)

Calcitriol *(Continued)*

take of fluids, reduced calcium intake, and cathartic administration. Severe hypercalcemia requires I.V. hydration and forced diuresis with I.V. furosemide (20-40 mg I.V. every 4-6 hours for adults). Urine output should be monitored and maintained at >3 mL/kg/hour. I.V. saline can quickly and significantly increase excretion of calcium into the urine. Calcitonin, cholestyramine, prednisone, sodium EDTA and mithramycin have all been used successfully to treat the more resistant cases of vitamin D-induced hypercalcemia.

Drug Interactions
Vitamin D may increase absorption of magnesium from magnesium compounds; hypercalcemia may be precipitated by vitamin D and, therefore, may increase cardiac arrhythmias in patients taking digitalis glycosides and verapamil; hypoparathyroid patients may develop hypercalcemia when using thiazide diuretics

Phenytoin and barbiturates decrease half-life of vitamin D; mineral oil with prolonged use decreases vitamin D absorption; cholestyramine reduces absorption of vitamin D

Stability Store in tight, light-resistant container

Mechanism of Action Promotes absorption of calcium in the intestines and retention at the kidneys thereby increasing calcium levels in the serum; decreases excessive serum phosphatase levels, parathyroid hormone levels, and decreases bone resorption; increases renal tubule phosphate resorption

Pharmacodynamics
Onset of action: ~2-6 hours
Duration: 3-5 days
Maximum calcemic effects: 2-4 weeks after daily administration

Pharmacokinetics
Absorption: Oral: Rapid
Metabolism: Primarily to 1,24,25-trihydroxycholecalciferol and 1,24,25-trihydroxy ergocalciferol
Half-life: 1.5 days
Elimination: Principally in bile and feces, and 4% to 6% excreted in urine; stored primarily in liver but also in skin, fat, bone, and muscle

Usual Dosage Geriatrics and Adults: Individualize dosage to maintain calcium levels of 9-10 mg/dL (adjust for low albumin)

Renal failure: Oral: 0.25 mcg/day or every other day (may require 0.5-1 mcg/day); increase doses by 0.25 mcg/day at 4- to 8-week intervals; obtain serum calcium concentrations twice weekly during titration phase; see Additional Information

Unlabeled use:
Renal failure: I.V.: 0.5 mcg (0.01 mcg/kg) 3 times/week; most doses in the range of 0.5-3 mcg (0.01-0.05 mcg/kg) 3 times/week
Hypoparathyroidism/pseudohypoparathyroidism: Oral: 0.5-2 mcg/day, administer in the morning; see Additional Information

Monitoring Parameters Monitor renal function, serum calcium and phosphate concentrations; if hypercalcemia is encountered, discontinue agent until serum calcium returns to normal

Reference Range Calcium (serum) 9-10 mg/dL (4.5-5 mEq/L) but do not include the I.V. dosages; phosphate 2.5-5 mg/dL

Test Interactions Increased calcium, cholesterol, magnesium, BUN, AST, ALT, calcium (S), cholesterol (S); decreased alkaline phosphatase

Patient Information Do not take more than the recommended amount. While taking this medication, your physician may want you to follow a special diet or take a calcium supplement. Follow this diet closely. Avoid taking magnesium supplements or magnesium containing antacids. Early symptoms of hypercalcemia include weakness, fatigue, somnolence, headache, anorexia, dry mouth, metallic taste, nausea, vomiting, cramps, diarrhea, muscle pain, bone pain and irritability.

Nursing Implications Monitor calcium and phosphate levels closely; monitor symptoms of hypercalcemia; see Adverse Reactions

Additional Information Calcitriol degrades upon prolonged exposure to light; not used as a daily supplement due to dosage forms, strengths, and cost (1 mcg = 40,000 units)

Special Geriatric Considerations Recommended daily allowances (RDA) have not been developed for persons >65 years of age; vitamin D, folate, and B₁₂ (cyanocobalamin) have decreased absorption with age, but the clinical significance is yet unknown. Calorie requirements decrease with age and therefore, nutrient density must be increased to ensure adequate nutrient intake, including vitamins and minerals. Therefore, the use of a daily supplement with a multiple vitamin with minerals is recommended. Elderly consume less vitamin D, absorption may be decreased, and many elderly have decreased sun exposure; therefore, elderly should receive supplementation with 800 units of vitamin D (20 mcg)/day. This is a recommendation of particular need to those with high risk for osteoporosis.

Dosage Forms
Capsule: 0.25 mcg, 0.5 mcg

Injection: 1 mcg/mL, 2 mcg/mL

References

Letsou AP and Price LS, "Health Aging and Nutrition: An Overview," *Clin Geriatr Med*, 1987, 3(2):253-60.

Myrianthopoulos M, "Dietary Treatment of Hyperlipidemia in the Elderly," *Clin Geriatr Med*, 1987, 3(2):343-59.

Riggs BL and Melton LJ, "The Prevention and Treatment of Osteoporosis," *N Engl J Med*, 1992, 327(9):620-7.

Calcium Acetate

Brand Names Phos-Ex®; PhosLo®

Generic Available No

Therapeutic Class Calcium Salt

Use Control of hyperphosphatemia in end stage renal failure and does not promote aluminum absorption; calcium acetate binds phosphorus in the GI tract better than other calcium salts due to its lower solubility and subsequent reduction in calcium or phosphorus absorption

Contraindications Hypercalcemia, renal calculi, hypophosphatemia, ventricular fibrillation. In ventricular fibrillation during cardiac resuscitation, and in patients with risk of digitalis toxicity, renal or cardiac disease

Warnings Use with caution in patients on digitalis, because hypercalcemia may precipitate cardiac arrhythmias. Always start at low-dose and do not increase without careful monitoring of serum calcium; estimate of daily dietary calcium intake should be made initially and the intake adjusted as needed. Use with caution in patients with CHF, renal failure. No other calcium supplements should be given concurrently; progressive hypercalcemia due to overdose may be severe as to require emergency measures; chronic hypercalcemia may lead to vascular calcification, and other soft tissue calcification. The serum calcium level should be monitored twice weekly during the early dose adjustment period.

Precautions Use caution when administering to patients with renal failure; hypercalcemia and hypercalciuria may develop at therapeutic doses over long periods of time; hypoparathyroidism may induce hypercalcemia and hypercalciuria, especially when patients receive high doses of vitamin D; administer cautiously to a digitalized patient, may precipitate arrhythmias

Adverse Reactions

Central nervous system: Mood and mental changes

Endocrine & metabolic: Metastatic calcinosis, milk-alkali syndrome

Gastrointestinal: Constipation, flatulence, laxative effect, acid rebound, dyspepsia, nausea, vomiting, GI hemorrhage, fecal impaction

Hematologic: Hypophosphatemia, hypercalcemia (with prolonged use), hypomagnesemia

Renal: Renal calculi, renal dysfunction, polyuria, hypercalciuria

Overdosage Symptoms of overdose include lethargy, nausea, vomiting, anorexia, constipation, abdominal pain, dry mouth, thirst, polyuria; severe hypercalcemia: Confusion, delirium, stupor, coma

Toxicology Following withdrawal of the drug, treatment consists of bed rest, liberal intake of fluids, reduced calcium intake, and cathartic administration. Severe hypercalcemia requires I.V. hydration and forced diuresis with I.V. furosemide (20-40 mg I.V. every 4-6 hours for adults). Urine output should be monitored and maintained at >3 mL/kg/hour. I.V. saline can quickly and significantly increase excretion of calcium into urine. Calcitonin, cholestyramine, prednisone, sodium EDTA, biphosphonates, and mithramycin have all been used successfully to treat the more resistant cases of vitamin D-induced hypercalcemia.

Drug Interactions

Calcium may antagonize the effects of verapamil; renders tetracycline antibiotics inactive (orally)

Thiazide diuretics may induce hypercalcemia

Decreased atenolol absorption

Iron salts, quinolones have decreased absorption

Polystyrene sulfonate has decreased binding of potassium and may precipitate metabolic alkalosis

Stability Admixture incompatibilities: Carbonates, phosphates, sulfates, tartrates

Mechanism of Action Moderates nerve and muscle performance via action potential excitation threshold regulation; combines with dietary phosphate to form insoluble calcium phosphate which is excreted in feces

Pharmacokinetics Calcium is absorbed in soluble, ionized form; solubility of calcium is increased in an acid environment (except calcium lactate); therefore, administer with meals to maximize acidity and solubility to enhance absorption

Absorption: From the GI tract, requires vitamin D

Elimination: Mainly in feces as unabsorbed calcium with 20% eliminated by the kidneys

Usual Dosage Geriatrics and Adults: Oral: 2 tablets with each meal; dosage may be increased to bring serum phosphate value to <6 mg/dL; most patients require 3-4 tablets with each meal

(Continued)

Calcium Acetate *(Continued)*

Administration Tablets must be taken with meals to be effective

Monitoring Parameters Plasma and urine concentrations; plasma phosphate, EKG in hyperkalemic states

Reference Range Serum calcium: 9-10.4 mg/dL; due to a poor correlation between the serum ionized calcium (free) and total serum calcium, particularly in states of low albumin or acid/base imbalances, direct measurement of ionized calcium is recommended. In low albumin states, the corrected **total** serum calcium may be estimated by this equation (assuming a normal albumin of 4 g/dL); corrected total calcium = total serum calcium + 0.8 (4 - measured serum albumin)

Test Interactions Increased calcium (S); decreased magnesium; decreased phosphorus

Patient Information Take with food; do not take calcium supplements within 1-2 hours of taking other medicine by mouth or eating large amounts of fiber-rich foods; do not drink large amounts of alcohol or caffeine-containing beverages or use tobacco if calcium causes dyspepsia

Nursing Implications See Adverse Reactions, Additional Information, Overdosage, and Special Geriatric Considerations

Additional Information

Doses for calcium supplementation are given in elemental calcium; calcium salts vary in their amount of elemental calcium

Calcium carbonate (40% elemental calcium)
Calcium gluconate (9% elemental calcium)
Calcium lactate (13% elemental calcium)
Calcium citrate (21% elemental calcium)
Dibasic calcium phosphate (23% elemental calcium)
Calcium acetate (25% elemental calcium)
Tricalcium phosphate (39% elemental calcium)

All calcium preparations should be administered in divided doses to maximize calcium absorption; no more than 300-350 mg of elemental calcium should be given at a time. Women receiving estrogen therapy require 900-1000 mg total daily elemental calcium intake. Women not receiving estrogens require 1500 mg elemental calcium daily to maintain calcium balance.

12.7 mEq/g; 250 mg/g elemental calcium (25% elemental calcium)

Special Geriatric Considerations Constipation and gas can be significant in elderly, but are usually mild; see Warnings

Dosage Forms Elemental calcium listed in brackets
Capsule: 500 mg [125 mg]
Tablet: 250 mg [62.5 mg], 667 mg [169 mg], 1000 mg [250 mg]

Calcium Carbonate *see* Calcium Salts (Oral) *on page 111*

Calcium Carbonate and Simethicone *see* Calcium Salts (Oral) *on page 111*

Calcium Channel Blocking Agents Comparison *see page 806*

Calcium Citrate *see* Calcium Salts (Oral) *on page 111*

Calcium Glubionate *see* Calcium Salts (Oral) *on page 111*

Calcium Gluconate *see* Calcium Salts (Oral) *on page 111*

Calcium Gluconate (Parenteral)

Brand Names Kalcinate®

Generic Available Yes

Therapeutic Class Calcium Salt

Use Treatment and prevention of hypocalcemia, treatment of tetany, cardiac disturbances of hyperkalemia, cardiac resuscitation when epinephrine fails to improve myocardial contractions, or calcium channel blocker toxicity

Contraindications In ventricular fibrillation during cardiac resuscitation, and in patients with risk of digitalis toxicity, renal or cardiac disease; hypercalcemia, renal calculi, hypophosphatemia

Warnings May produce cardiac arrest

Precautions Use caution when administering to patients with renal failure; avoid too rapid I.V. administration; use with caution in digitalized patients, respiratory failure or acidosis; avoid extravasation; hypercalcemia and hypercalciuria may develop at therapeutic doses over long periods of time; hypoparathyroidism may induce hypercalcemia and hypercalciuria, especially when patients receive high doses of vitamin D; administer cautiously to a digitalized patient, may precipitate arrhythmias

Adverse Reactions

Cardiovascular: Vasodilatation, hypotension, bradycardia, cardiac arrhythmias, ventricular fibrillation

Central nervous system: Lethargy, mental confusion, coma, mania, headache

Dermatologic: Erythema, tissue necrosis

Endocrine & metabolic: Decrease serum magnesium, hypercalcemia, hypophosphatemia

Gastrointestinal: Vomiting, constipation (not proven), dyspepsia, flatulence

Hepatic: Elevated serum amylase

Neuromuscular & skeletal: Muscle weakness

Renal: Hypercalciuria

Overdosage Symptoms of overdose include hypercalcemia, mild hypercalcemia: Lethargy, nausea, vomiting, anorexia, constipation, abdominal pain, dry mouth, thirst, polyuria; severe hypercalcemia: Confusion, delirium, stupor, coma

Drug Interactions

Calcium may antagonize the effects of verapamil; renders tetracycline antibiotics inactive (orally)

Thiazide diuretics may induce hypercalcemia

Decreased atenolol absorption

Iron salts, quinolone have decreased absorption

Polystyrene sulfonate has decreased binding of potassium and may precipitate metabolic alkalosis

Stability Admixture incompatibilities: carbonates, phosphates, sulfates, tartrates; store at room temperature; do not use if precipitate occurs

Mechanism of Action Moderates nerve and muscle performance via action potential excitation threshold regulation; may prevent negative calcium balance when used as a supplement orally

Usual Dosage Geriatrics and Adults (dosage is in terms of elemental calcium): I.V.:

Hypocalcemia: 2-15 g/24 hours as a continuous infusion or in divided doses

Hypocalcemia secondary to citrated blood infusion; give 0.45 mEq **elemental** calcium for each 100 mL citrated blood infused

Calcium antagonist toxicity, magnesium intoxication; cardiac arrest in the presence of hyperkalemia or hypocalcemia: 1-3 g

Tetany: 1-3 g may be administered until therapeutic response occurs

Cardiac resuscitation: 500-800 mg/dose (5-8 mL) every 10 minutes

Exchange transfusion: 300 mg/100 mL of citrated blood exchanged

Monitoring Parameters EKG, plasma and urine calcium concentrations

Reference Range Mild hypercalcemia: >10.5 mg/dL; severe hypercalcemia: >12 mg/dL; serum calcium: 9-10.4 mg/dL; due to a poor correlation between the serum ionized calcium (free) and total serum calcium, particularly in states of low albumin or acid/base imbalances, direct measurement of ionized calcium is recommended. In low albumin states, the corrected **total** serum calcium may be estimated by this equation (assuming a normal albumin of 4 g/dL); corrected total calcium = total serum calcium + 0.8 (4 - measured serum albumin)

Test Interactions Increased calcium (S); decreased magnesium; decreased phosphorus

Nursing Implications I.M. injections should be administered in the gluteal region in adults, usually in volumes <5 mL; do not use scalp veins or small hand or foot veins for I.V. administration; generally, I.V. infusion rates should not exceed 0.7-1.5 mEq/minute (1.5-3.3 mL/minute); stop the infusion if the patient complains of pain or discomfort. Warm to body temperature; administer slowly, usually no faster than 1.5-3.3 mL/minute, do not inject into the myocardium when using calcium during advanced cardiac life support; see Adverse Reactions, Overdosage, Additional Information, and Special Geriatric Considerations

Additional Information 1 g calcium gluconate = 90 mg elemental calcium = 4.8 mEq calcium;

Doses for calcium supplementation are given in elemental calcium; calcium salts vary in their amount of elemental calcium

Calcium carbonate (40% elemental calcium)
Calcium gluconate (9% elemental calcium)
Calcium lactate (13% elemental calcium)
Calcium citrate (21% elemental calcium)
Dibasic calcium phosphate (23% elemental calcium)
Calcium acetate (25% elemental calcium)
Tricalcium phosphate (39% elemental calcium)

All calcium preparations should be administered in divided doses to maximize calcium absorption; no more than 300-350 mg of elemental calcium should be given at a time. Women receiving estrogen therapy require 900-1000 mg total daily elemental calcium intake. Women not receiving estrogens require 1500 mg elemental calcium daily to maintain calcium balance.

Special Geriatric Considerations Constipation and gas can be significant in elderly, but are usually mild; see Warnings

Dosage Forms Injection: 100 mg/mL (10 mL)

References

Bauwens SF, Drinka PJ, Boh LE, "Pathogenesis and Management of Primary Osteoporosis," *Clin Pharm*, 1986, 5:639-59.

Heaney RP, Recker RR, and Saville PD, "Menopausal Changes in Calcium Balance Performance," *J Lab Clin Med*, 1978, 92(6):953-63.

(Continued)

Calcium Gluconate (Parenteral) *(Continued)*

Recker RR, "Calcium Absorption and Achlorhydria," *N Engl J Med*, 1985, 313(2):70-3.

Calcium Lactate *see* Calcium Salts (Oral) *on next page*

Calcium Phosphate, Tribasic *see* Calcium Salts (Oral) *on next page*

Calcium Polycarbophil *(pol ee kar' boe fil)*

Brand Names Equalactin® Chewable Tablet [OTC]; Fiberall® Chewable Tablet [OTC]; FiberCon® Tablet [OTC]; Fiber-Lax® Tablet [OTC]; FiberNorm® [OTC]; Mitrolan® Chewable Tablet [OTC]

Generic Available Yes

Therapeutic Class Antidiarrheal; Laxative, Bulk-Producing

Use Treatment of constipation or acute nonspecific diarrhea by restoring a more normal moisture level and providing bulk in the patient's intestinal tract; polycarbophil is indicated for constipation in diarrhea associated with irritable bowel syndrome and diverticulosis; calcium polycarbophil is supplied as the approved substitute whenever a bulk-forming laxative is ordered in a tablet, capsule, wafer, or other oral solid dosage form

Contraindications Hypersensitivity to any component; do not use if patient is experiencing nausea, vomiting, appendicitis, fecal impaction, acute surgical abdomen, intestinal obstruction, undiagnosed abdominal pain

Warnings Laxatives used excessively may lead to fluid/electrolyte imbalance; stimulant cathartics may lead to abuse or dependency with chronic use (laxative abuse syndrome); cathartic colon, which may present as ulcerative colitis, occurs with chronic use of stimulant cathartics; melanosis coli is a dark pigmentation of the colonic mucosa from chronic use of anthraquinone derivatives

Precautions Habit-forming and may result in laxative dependence and loss of normal bowel function with prolonged use; rectal bleeding or failure to respond requires further evaluation for possibly serious medical problems

Adverse Reactions
Cardiovascular: Palpitations
Central nervous system: Dizziness, faintness
Gastrointestinal: Nausea, vomiting, diarrhea, abdominal cramps, bloating, flatulence, perianal irritation
Neuromuscular & skeletal: Weakness
Miscellaneous: Sweating

Overdosage Symptoms of overdose include abdominal pain, diarrhea, flatulence, possible impaction

Drug Interactions Decreased effect of oral anticoagulants, digoxin, potassium-sparing diuretics, salicylates, tetracyclines

Mechanism of Action Calcium polycarbophil is a hydrophilic agent which retains free water within the intestinal lumen and indirectly opposes dehydrating forces of the bowel, promoting formed stools; in diarrhea, it absorbs free fecal water, forming a gel and produces formed stools

Pharmacodynamics
Onset of action: 12-24 hours; can be up to 72 hours
Site of action: Small and large intestines

Usual Dosage Geriatrics and Adults: Oral: 1 g 4 times/day, up to 6 g/day; for severe diarrhea, repeat doses every 30 minutes; do not exceed 6 g/day

Administration When using as a laxative, patient should drink with adequate fluids (8 oz of water or other fluids) with each dose

Monitoring Parameters Monitor for diarrhea, abdominal pain, bowel obstruction, or impaction

Test Interactions Decreased potassium (S)

Patient Information Must be mixed in a glass of water or juice; drink a full glass of liquid with each dose; must drink fluids throughout the day to be effective and avoid impaction; report bleeding or failure to respond to physician, pharmacist, or nurse; do not use for acute constipation

Nursing Implications Bulk laxatives increase stool frequency; watch for signs of fluid/electrolyte loss; see Warnings and Contraindications

Additional Information Each calcium polycarbophil tablet contains ~100 mg of absorbable elemental calcium; chewable tablets are available

Special Geriatric Considerations Elderly may have insufficient fluid intake which may predispose them to fecal impaction and bowel obstruction; bloating and flatulence may be a problem when used short term; use cautiously in patients with a history of bowel impaction/obstruction

Dosage Forms Tablet:
Chewable:
Equalactin®, Mitrolan®: 500 mg
Fiberall®: 1250 mg
Sodium free:
FiberCon®: 500 mg
Fiber-Lax®, FiberNorm®: 625 mg

Calcium Salts (Oral)

Brand Names Alka-Mints® [OTC]; Amitone® [OTC]; Cal Carb-HD® [OTC]; Calci-Chew™ [OTC]; Calciday-667® [OTC]; Calci-Mix™ [OTC]; Cal-Plus® [OTC]; Caltrate® 600 [OTC]; Caltrate, Jr.® [OTC]; Chooz® [OTC]; Citracal® [OTC]; Dicarbosil® [OTC]; Equilet® [OTC]; Florical® [OTC]; Gencalc® 600 [OTC]; Mallamint® [OTC]; Neo-Calglucon® [OTC]; Nephro-Calci® [OTC]; Os-Cal® 500 [OTC]; Oyst-Cal 500 [OTC]; Oystercal® 500; Posture® [OTC]; Rolaids® Calcium Rich [OTC]; Titralac® Plus Liquid [OTC]; Tums® [OTC]; Tums® E-X Extra Strength Tablet [OTC]; Tums® Extra Strength Liquid [OTC]

Synonyms Calcium Carbonate; Calcium Carbonate and Simethicone; Calcium Citrate; Calcium Glubionate; Calcium Gluconate; Calcium Lactate; Calcium Phosphate, Tribasic

Generic Available Yes

Therapeutic Class Antacid; Antidote, Hyperphosphatemia; Calcium Salt

Use Antacid and calcium supplement

Contraindications Hypercalcemia, renal calculi, hypophosphatemia, ventricular fibrillation. In ventricular fibrillation during cardiac resuscitation, and in patients with risk of digitalis toxicity, renal or cardiac disease

Precautions Use caution when administering to patients with renal failure; hypercalcemia and hypercalciuria may develop at therapeutic doses over long periods of time; hypoparathyroidism may induce hypercalcemia and hypercalciuria, especially when patients receive high doses of vitamin D; administer cautiously to a digitalized patient, may precipitate arrhythmias

Adverse Reactions

Central nervous system: Mental confusion, headache, mood changes

Endocrine & metabolic: Hypercalcemia, milk-alkali syndrome (doses >2 g/day), hypophosphatemia, hypercalcinosis, hypomagnesemia

Gastrointestinal: Constipation (not proven), nausea, vomiting, dyspepsia, flatulence, laxative effect, acid rebound, fecal impaction, GI hemorrhage

Renal: Hypercalciuria, renal calculi, renal dysfunction, polyuria

Overdosage Symptoms of overdose include hypercalcemia, lethargy, nausea, vomiting, coma; following withdrawal of the drug, treatment consists of bed rest, liberal intake of fluids, reduced calcium intake, and cathartic administration.

Toxicology Severe hypercalcemia requires I.V. hydration and forced diuresis with I.V. furosemide (20-40 mg I.V. every 4-6 hours for adults). Urine output should be monitored and maintained at >3 mL/kg/hour. I.V. saline can quickly and significantly increase excretion of calcium into urine. Calcitonin, cholestyramine, prednisone, sodium EDTA, biphosphonates, and mithramycin have all been used successfully to treat the more resistant cases of vitamin D-induced hypercalcemia.

Drug Interactions

Calcium may antagonize the effects of verapamil; renders tetracycline antibiotics inactive (orally)

Thiazide diuretics may induce hypercalcemia

Decreased atenolol absorption

Iron salts, quinolones have decreased absorption

Stability Admixture incompatibilities: carbonates, phosphates, sulfates, tartrates

Mechanism of Action Moderates nerve and muscle performance via action potential excitation threshold regulation; may prevent negative calcium balance when used as dietary supplement as treatment or for osteoporosis; calcium carbonate is used as an antacid for acute dyspepsia

Pharmacokinetics Calcium is absorbed in soluble, ionized form; solubility of calcium is increased in an acid environment (except calcium lactate); therefore, administer with meals to maximize acidity and solubility to enhance absorption

Usual Dosage Geriatrics and Adults: Oral (dosage is in terms of elemental calcium):
Dietary supplement: 500 mg to 2 g, 2-4 times/day; see Additional Information

Osteoporosis/bone loss: 1000-1500 mg in divided doses/day; see Additional Information

Antacid: Calcium carbonate: 0.5-2 g divided in 2-6 doses/day

Recommended daily allowance: 800 mg/day

Monitoring Parameters Plasma and urine calcium concentrations; EKG if hypercalcemic

Reference Range Mild hypercalcemia: >10.5 mg/dL; severe hypercalcemia: >12 mg/dL; serum calcium: 9-10.4 mg/dL; due to a poor correlation between the serum ionized calcium (free) and total serum calcium, particularly in states of low albumin or acid/base imbalances, direct measurement of ionized calcium is recommended. In low albumin states, the corrected **total** serum calcium may be estimated by this equation (assuming a normal albumin of 4 g/dL); corrected total calcium = total serum calcium + 0.8·(4 - measured serum albumin)

Test Interactions Increased calcium (S); decreased magnesium; decreased phosphorus

Patient Information Do not take calcium supplements within 1-2 hours of taking other medicine by mouth or eating large amounts of fiber-rich foods; do not drink large amounts of alcohol or caffeine-containing beverages or use tobacco; take with meals

(Continued)

Calcium Salts (Oral) *(Continued)*

Nursing Implications See Adverse Reactions, Additional Information, Overdosage, and Special Geriatric Considerations

Additional Information Doses for calcium supplementation are given in elemental calcium; calcium salts vary in their amount of elemental calcium

Calcium carbonate (40% elemental calcium)
Calcium gluconate (9% elemental calcium)
Calcium lactate (13% elemental calcium)
Calcium citrate (21% elemental calcium)
Dibasic calcium phosphate (23% elemental calcium)
Calcium acetate (25% elemental calcium)
Tricalcium phosphate (39% elemental calcium)

All calcium preparations should be administered in divided doses to maximize calcium absorption; no more than 300-350 mg of elemental calcium should be given at a time. Women receiving estrogen therapy require 900-1000 mg total daily elemental calcium intake. Women not receiving estrogens require 1500 mg elemental calcium daily to maintain calcium balance.

Special Geriatric Considerations Constipation and gas can be significant in elderly but are usually mild and may be eliminated by switching to another salt form. Calcium carbonate has been associated with the highest incidence of side effects, probably due to its high calcium content. Calcium carbonate absorption is impaired in achlorhydria. Since achlorhydria is common in elderly, calcium carbonate may not be the ideal calcium supplement for dietary or treatment use. Administration with food helps this problem.

Dosage Forms Elemental calcium listed in brackets
Calcium carbonate:
Capsule: 1500 mg [600 mg]
  Calci-Mix™: 1250 mg [500 mg]
  Florical®: 364 mg [145.6 mg] with sodium fluoride 8.3 mg
Liquid (Tums® Extra Strength): 1000 mg/5 mL (360 mL)
Lozenge (Mylanta® Soothing Antacids): 600 mg [240 mg]
Powder (Cal Carb-HD®): 6.5 g/packet [2.6 g]
Suspension, oral: 1250 mg/5 mL [500 mg]
Tablet: 650 mg [260 mg], 1500 mg [600 mg]
  Calciday-667®: 667 mg [267 mg]
  Os-Cal® 500, Oyst-Cal® 500, Oystercal® 500: 1250 mg [500 mg]
  Cal-Plus®, Caltrate® 600, Gencalc® 600, Nephro-Calci®: 1500 mg [600 mg]
  Chewable:
    Alka-Mints®: 850 mg [340 mg]
    Amitone®: 350 mg [140 mg]
    Caltrate, Jr.®: 750 mg [300 mg]
    Calci-Chew™, Os-Cal®: 750 mg [300 mg]
    Chooz®, Dicarbosil®, Equilet®, Tums®: 500 mg [200 mg]
    Mallamint®: 420 mg [168 mg]
    Rolaids® Calcium Rich: 550 mg [220 mg]
    Tums® E-X Extra Strength: 750 mg [300 mg]
    Tums® Ultra®: 1000 mg [400 mg]
  Florical®: 364 mg [145.6 mg] with sodium fluoride 8.3 mg

Calcium carbonate and simethicone (Titralac® Plus Liquid):
Liquid: Calcium carbonate 500 mg [200 mg] and simethicone 20 mg per 5 mL

Calcium citrate (Citracal®):
Tablet: 950 mg [200 mg]
Tablet, effervescent: 2376 mg [500 mg]

Calcium glubionate (Neo-Calglucon®):
Syrup: 1.8 g/5 mL [115 mg/5 mL] (480 mL)

Calcium gluconate:
Tablet: 500 mg [45 mg], 650 mg [58.5 mg], 975 mg [87.75 mg], 1 g [90 mg]

Calcium lactate:
Tablet: 325 mg [42.25 mg], 650 mg [84.5 mg]

Calcium phosphate, tribasic (Posture®):
Tablet, sugar free: 1565.2 mg [600 mg]

References

Bauwens SF, Drinka PJ, Boh LE, "Pathogenesis and Management of Primary Osteoporosis," *Clin Pharm*, 1986, 5:639-59.
Heaney RP, Recker RR, and Saville PD, "Menopausal Changes in Calcium Balance Performance," *J Lab Clin Med*, 1978, 92(6):953-63.
Recker RR, "Calcium Absorption and Achlorhydria," *N Engl J Med*, 1985, 313(2):70-3.

CaldeCORT® *see* Hydrocortisone *on page 351*

Calderol® *see* Calcifediol *on page 102*

Calm-X® [OTC] *see* Dimenhydrinate *on page 227*

Cal-Plus® [OTC] *see* Calcium Salts (Oral) *on page 111*

Caltrate® 600 [OTC] *see* Calcium Salts (Oral) *on page 111*

Caltrate, Jr.® [OTC] *see* Calcium Salts (Oral) *on page 111*

Camalox® [OTC] *see* Aluminum Hydroxide and Magnesium Hydroxide *on page 29*

Cankaid® Oral [OTC] *see* Carbamide Peroxide *on page 119*

Capastat® Sulfate *see* Capreomycin Sulfate *on this page*

Capital® and Codeine *see* Acetaminophen and Codeine *on page 14*

Capoten® *see* Captopril *on next page*

Capozide® *see* Captopril and Hydrochlorothiazide *on page 116*

Capreomycin Sulfate (kap ree oh̲ mye' sin)
Brand Names Capastat® Sulfate
Generic Available No
Therapeutic Class Antibiotic, Miscellaneous; Antitubercular Agent
Use In conjunction with at least one other antituberculosis agent in the treatment of tuberculosis
Contraindications Known hypersensitivity to capreomycin sulfate
Warnings The use of capreomycin in patients with renal insufficiency or pre-existing auditory impairment must be undertaken with great caution, and the risk of additional eighth nerve impairment or renal injury should be weighed against the benefits to be derived from therapy. Since other parenteral antituberculous agents (eg, streptomycin) also have similar and sometimes irreversible toxic effects, particularly on eighth cranial nerve and renal function, simultaneous administration of these agents with capreomycin is not recommended. Use with nonantituberculous drugs (ie, aminoglycoside antibiotics) having ototoxic or nephrotoxic potential should be undertaken only with great caution.
Adverse Reactions
  Dermatologic: Rash
  Hematologic: Eosinophilia, leukocytosis, thrombocytopenia
  Local: Pain induration, bleeding at injection site
  Otic: Ototoxicity, tinnitus
  Renal: Nephrotoxicity
Overdosage Symptoms of overdose include renal failure, ototoxicity, thrombocytopenia treatment is supportive
Drug Interactions Aminoglycosides increased risk for nephrotoxicity or respiratory paralysis; increased effect/duration of nondepolarizing neuromuscular blocking agents
Mechanism of Action Capreomycin is a cyclic polypeptide antimicrobial. It is administered as a mixture of capreomycin IA and capreomycin IB. The mechanism of action of capreomycin is not well understood. Mycobacterial species that have become resistant to other agents are usually still sensitive to the action of capreomycin. However, significant cross-resistance with viomycin, kanamycin, and neomycin occurs.
Pharmacokinetics
  Absorption: Oral: Poor absorption necessitates parenteral administration
  Half-life: Dependent upon renal function and varies with creatinine clearance; 4-6 hours
  Time to peak: I.M.: Peak serum concentrations occur 1 hour
  Elimination: Essentially excreted unchanged in the urine; no significant accumulation after ≥30 day of 1 g/day dosing in patients with normal renal function
Usual Dosage I.M.:
  Geriatrics: Usual adult dose with adjustments for dosing in renal impairment; see table on next page.

  Adults: 15 mg/kg/day up to 1 g/day for 60-120 days
Administration Give by deep I.M. injection into large muscle mass
Monitoring Parameters Check hearing with audiometry and assess vestibular function regularly. Monitor BUN, creatinine, and potassium throughout the course of treatment
Test Interactions Decreased potassium (S), increased BUN, leukocytosis, decreased platelets
Patient Information Report hearing loss to physician immediately; do not discontinue without notifying physician
Nursing Implications See Administration
Special Geriatric Considerations Has not been studied in the elderly. I.M. administration may limit use due to painful injection or lack of sites in patients with decreased muscle mass; adjust dose for renal function
Dosage Forms Injection: 100 mg/mL (10 mL)

Capreomycin Sulfate

Cl_cr (mL/min)	Dose (mg/kg) for each dosing interval		
	24 h	48 h	72 h
0	1.29	2.58	3.87
10	2.43	4.87	7.3
20	3.58	7.16	10.7
30	4.72	9.45	14.2
40	5.87	11.7	
50	7.01	14	
60	8.16		
80	10.4		
100	12.7		
110	13.9		

Capsaicin (kap say' sin)

Brand Names Zostrix® [OTC]; Zostrix®-HP
Generic Available No
Therapeutic Class Analgesic, Topical; Topical Skin Product
Use

Zostrix®: Temporary relief of pain (neuralgia) following herpes zoster infections
Zostrix®-HP: Relief of neuralgias such as diabetic neuropathy and postsurgical pain

Unlabeled use: Psoriasis, vitiligo, intractable pruritus, phantom limb pain, migraine headaches (intranasally)

Adverse Reactions Local: Transient burning on application
Mechanism of Action Renders the skin insensitive to pain by depleting and preventing reaccumulation of substance P in peripheral sensory neurons. Substance P is thought to be the primary chemomediator of pain impulses from the periphery to the central nervous system.
Usual Dosage Geriatrics and Adults: Apply to affected area up to 3-4 times/day
Monitoring Parameters Relief of pain
Patient Information Wash hands immediately after application; for external use only; avoid contact with eyes; do not use on broken or irritated skin; transient burning may occur upon application but should disappear after a few days; if symptoms get worse or persist longer than 28 days, or clear up and recur, discontinue use and consult physician
Nursing Implications Wash hands immediately after application
Additional Information If used less than 3 times/day, this product may not be effective
Special Geriatric Considerations Capsaicin products are available over-the-counter. Counsel patients about the appropriate use of these products.
Dosage Forms Cream: 0.025% (45 g, 90 g); 0.075% (30 g, 60 g)
References

Cordell GA and Araujo OE, "Capsaicin: Identification, Nomenclature, and Pharmacotherapy," *Ann Pharmacother*, 1993, 27(3):330-6.

Captopril (kap' toe pril)

Related Information

Antacid Drug Interactions *on page 764*
Brand Names Capoten®
Generic Available No
Therapeutic Class Angiotensin-Converting Enzyme (ACE) Inhibitors
Use Management of hypertension and treatment of congestive heart failure; increase circulation in Raynaud's phenomenon; idiopathic edema; diabetic nephropathy

Unlabeled use: Hypertensive crisis, diabetic nephropathy, rheumatoid arthritis, diagnosis of anatomic renal artery stenosis, hypertension secondary to scleroderma renal crisis, diagnosis of aldosteronism, idiopathic edema, Bartter's syndrome, postmyocardial infarction for prevention of ventricular failure

Contraindications Hypersensitivity to captopril or any component or any ACE inhibitor
Warnings Neutropenia, agranulocytosis, angioedema, decreased renal function (hypertension, renal artery stenosis, congestive heart failure), hepatic dysfunction (elimination, activation), proteinuria, first-dose hypotension (hypovolemia, CHF, dehydrated patients at risk, eg, diuretic use, elderly), elderly (due to renal function changes)

Precautions Use with caution and modify dosage in patients with renal impairment; use with caution in patients with collagen vascular disease, congestive heart failure, hypovolemia, valvular stenosis, hyperkalemia (>5.7 mEq/L), anesthesia

Adverse Reactions

Cardiovascular: Hypotension, tachycardia, arrhythmias, orthostatic blood pressure, angina, palpitations, chest pain, syncope, congestive heart failure, Raynaud's syndrome, flushing, vasculitis

Central nervous system: Nervousness, depression, confusion, somnolence, fatigue, dizziness, headache, paresthesias, insomnia

Dermatologic: Rash, photosensitivity, pruritus, angioedema

Endocrine & metabolic: Hyperkalemia, hyponatremia

Gastrointestinal: Pancreatitis, constipation, anorexia, nausea, gastritis, dysgeusia, dry mouth, peptic ulcer, weight loss, vomiting, diarrhea, abdominal pain

Genitourinary: Impotence, urinary frequency

Hematologic: Neutropenia, agranulocytosis, pancytopenia, thrombocytopenia

Hepatic: Increased BUN, serum creatinine, hepatitis

Neuromuscular & skeletal: Myalgia, arthralgia, arthritis

Ocular: Blurred vision

Renal: Proteinuria, oliguria, renal insufficiency, nephrotic syndrome, interstitial nephritis

Respiratory: Chronic cough (nonproductive, persistent; more often in women and seen in 15% to 30% of patients), bronchospasm, dyspnea

Miscellaneous: Loss of taste perception, sweating

Overdosage Symptoms of overdose include severe hypotension

Toxicology Following initiation of essential overdose management, toxic symptom treatment and supportive treatment should be initiated. Hypotension usually responds to I.V. fluids or Trendelenburg positioning. If unresponsive to these measures, the use of a parenteral inotrope may be required (eg, norepinephrine 0.1-0.2 mcg/kg/minute titrated to response). Seizures commonly respond to diazepam (I.V. 5-10 mg bolus in adults every 15 minutes if needed up to a total of 30 mg) or to phenytoin or phenobarbital.

Drug Interactions

Captopril and potassium-sparing diuretics → additive hyperkalemic effect

Captopril and indomethacin or nonsteroidal anti-inflammatory agents → reduced antihypertensive response to captopril

Allopurinol and captopril → neutropenia

Antacids and ACE inhibitors → ↓ absorption of ACE inhibitors

Phenothiazines and ACE inhibitors → ↑ ACE inhibitor effect

Probenecid and ACE inhibitors (captopril) → ↑ ACE inhibitors (captopril) levels

Rifampin and ACE inhibitors (captopril) → ↓ ACE inhibitor effect

Digoxin and ACE inhibitors → ↑ serum digoxin levels

Lithium and ACE inhibitors → ↑ lithium serum levels

Tetracycline and ACE inhibitors (captopril) → ↓ tetracycline absorption (up to 37%)

Capsaicin may cause or exacerbate coughing with ACE inhibitors

Food decreases captopril absorption, see Additional Information

Stability All solutions made must be stored in glass bottles; syrup is stable for 7 days at 4°C and 22°C; distilled water is stable at 7 days at 22°C and 14 days at 4°C; distilled water with sodium bicarbonate is stable 14 days at 22°C and 56 days at 4°C

Mechanism of Action Competitive inhibitor of angiotensin-converting enzyme (ACE); prevents conversion of angiotensin I to angiotensin II, a potent vasoconstrictor; results in lower levels of angiotensin II which causes an increase in plasma renin activity and a reduction in aldosterone secretion; a CNS mechanism may also be involved in hypotensive effect as angiotensin II increases adrenergic outflow from CNS; vasoactive kallikreins may be decreased in conversion to active hormones by ACE inhibitors, thus reducing blood pressure

Pharmacodynamics

Onset of action: Oral: Maximal decrease in blood pressure in 60-90 minutes after dose

Duration: Dose related; may require several weeks of therapy before full hypotensive effect is seen

Pharmacokinetics

Absorption: Oral: 60% to 75%

Distribution: V_d: 7 L/kg

Protein binding: 25% to 30%

Metabolism: 50%

Half-life:

Normal adults: Dependent upon renal and cardiac function: 1.9 hours

Impaired renal function: 3.5-32 hours

Anuria: 20-40 hours

Time to peak: Peak serum levels occur within 1-2 hours

Elimination: 95% excreted in urine in 24 hours; 40% to 50% excreted unchanged urine

Usual Dosage Note: Dosage must be titrated according to patient's response; use lowest effective dose; see Additional Information and Administration

(Continued)

115

Captopril *(Continued)*

Geriatrics and Adults: Oral: Initial: 12.5-25 mg/dose given every 8-12 hours; increase by 12.5-25 mg/dose to maximum of 450 mg/day; increase doses at 1- to 2-week intervals

Congestive heart failure: Initial dose: 6.25-12.5 mg 2 times/day

Diabetic nephropathy: 25 mg 3 times/day

Note: Smaller dosages (6.25-12.5 mg) given every 8-12 hours are indicated in patients with renal dysfunction; renal function and leukocyte count should be carefully monitored during therapy; increase at intervals of 1-2 weeks

Moderately dialyzable (20% to 50%)

Administration Tablets may be used to make a solution of captopril; see Stability

Monitoring Parameters Serum potassium levels, BUN, serum creatinine, renal function, WBC

Test Interactions Increased BUN, creatinine, potassium, positive Coombs' [direct]; decreased cholesterol (S); may cause false-positive results in urine acetone determinations using sodium nitroprusside reagent

Patient Information Administer 1 hour before meals; do not stop therapy except under prescriber advice; notify physician if you develop sore throat, fever, swelling of hands, feet, face, eyes, lips, and tongue; difficult breathing, irregular heartbeats, chest pains, or cough. May cause dizziness, fainting, and lightheadedness, especially in first week of therapy, sit and stand up slowly; may cause changes in taste or rash; do not add a salt substitute (potassium) without advice of physician

Nursing Implications Watch for hypotensive effect within 1-3 hours of first dose or new higher dose; see Precautions, Warnings, Monitoring Parameters, and Special Geriatric Considerations

Additional Information Many patients complain of transient cough during early therapy; food decreases absorption of captopril 30% to 40%; administer captopril 1 hour before meals; clinical significance not known; therefore, observe for loss of effect. Newer data demonstrates that lower doses of ACE inhibitors are effective and toxic reactions are decreased

Special Geriatric Considerations Due to frequent decreases in glomerular filtration (also creatinine clearance) with aging, elderly patients may have exaggerated responses to ACE inhibitors; differences in clinical response due to hepatic changes are not observed. ACE inhibitors may be preferred agents in elderly patients with congestive heart failure and diabetes mellitus. Diabetic proteinuria is reduced and insulin sensitivity is enhanced. In general, the side effect profile is favorable in elderly and causes little or no CNS confusion; use lowest dose recommendations initially.

Dosage Forms Tablet: 12.5 mg, 25 mg, 50 mg, 100 mg

Extemporaneous Preparation(s) See Stability

References
Lewis EJ, Hunsicker LG, Bain RP, et al, "The Effect of Angiotensin-Converting Enzyme Inhibition on Diabetic Nephropathy," *N Engl J Med*, 1993, 329(20):1456-62.

McAreavey D and Robertson JIS, "Angiotensin Converting Enzyme Inhibitors and Moderate Hypertension," *Drugs*, 1990, 40(3):326-45.

Captopril and Hydrochlorothiazide

Related Information
Captopril *on page 114*
Hydrochlorothiazide *on page 347*

Brand Names Capozide®

Generic Available No

Therapeutic Class Antihypertensive, Combination

Special Geriatric Considerations Combination products are not recommended for first-line treatment and divided doses of diuretics may increase the incidence of nocturia in the elderly

Dosage Forms Tablet:
25/15: Captopril 25 mg and hydrochlorothiazide 15 mg
25/25: Captopril 25 mg and hydrochlorothiazide 25 mg
50/15: Captopril 50 mg and hydrochlorothiazide 15 mg
50/25: Captopril 50 mg and hydrochlorothiazide 25 mg

Carafate® *see* Sucralfate *on page 658*

Carampicillin Hydrochloride *see* Bacampicillin Hydrochloride *on page 73*

Carbachol *(kar' ba kole)*

Related Information
Glaucoma Drug Therapy Comparison *on page 810*

Brand Names Isopto® Carbachol; Miostat®

Synonyms Carbacholine; Carbamylcholine Chloride

Generic Available No

Therapeutic Class Cholinergic Agent, Ophthalmic; Ophthalmic Agent, Miotic

Use Lower intraocular pressure in the treatment of glaucoma; to cause miosis during surgery

Contraindications Acute iritis, acute inflammatory disease of the anterior chamber, hypersensitivity to carbachol or any component

Precautions Use with caution in patients undergoing general anesthesia and in presence of corneal abrasion

Adverse Reactions
Cardiovascular: Syncope, arrhythmias, flushing
Central nervous system: Headache
Gastrointestinal: Salivation, GI cramps, vomiting, diarrhea
Genitourinary: Increased bladder tone
Local: Ciliary spasm with temporary decrease of visual acuity
Ocular: Corneal clouding, persistent bullous keratopathy, postoperative keratitis, retinal detachment, transient ciliary and conjunctival injection
Respiratory: Asthma
Miscellaneous: Sweating

Overdosage Symptoms of overdose include miosis, flushing, vomiting, bradycardia, bronchospasm, involuntary urination; flush eyes with water or normal saline; if accidentally ingested, induce emesis or perform gastric lavage

Toxicology Atropine is the treatment of choice for intoxications manifesting with significant muscarinic symptoms. Atropine I.V. 2-4 mg every 3-60 minutes should be repeated to control symptoms and then continued as needed for 1-2 days following the acute ingestion. Epinephrine 0.1-1 mg S.C. may be useful in reversing severe cardiovascular or pulmonary sequel.

Mechanism of Action Synthetic direct-acting cholinergic agent that causes miosis by stimulating muscarinic receptors in the eye

Pharmacodynamics
Onset of miosis:
Ophthalmic: Within 10-20 minutes
Intraocular: Within 2-5 minutes
Duration of action:
Ophthalmic: Reductions in intraocular pressure persist for 4-8 hours
Intraocular: Lasts 24 hours

Usual Dosage Geriatrics and Adults:
Intraocular: 0.5 mL instilled in anterior chamber before or after securing sutures
Ophthalmic: Instill 1-2 drops up to 4 times/day

Administration Finger pressure should be applied on the lacrimal sac for 1-2 minutes following topical instillation; remove excess around the eye with a tissue

Patient Information May sting on instillation; may cause headache, altered distance vision, and decreased night vision; do not touch dropper to eye

Nursing Implications Instillation for miosis prior to eye surgery should be gentle and parallel to the iris face and tangential to the pupil border; discard unused portion; see Administration

Special Geriatric Considerations Assess patient's ability to self-administer; see Usual Dosage

Dosage Forms Solution:
Intraocular: 0.01% (1.5 mL)
Ophthalmic: 0.75% (15 mL, 30 mL); 1.5% (15 mL, 30 mL); 2.25% (15 mL); 3% (15 mL, 30 mL)

Carbacholine see Carbachol on previous page

Carbamazepine (kar ba maz' e peen)
Related Information
Drug Levels Commonly Monitored Guidelines on page 771-772
Brand Names Epitol®; Tegretol®
Generic Available Yes: Tablet
Therapeutic Class Anticonvulsant, Miscellaneous
Use Prophylaxis of generalized tonic-clonic, partial (especially complex partial), and mixed partial (treatment of choice) or generalized seizure disorder; may be used to relieve pain in trigeminal neuralgia or diabetic neuropathy

Unlabeled use: Has been used to treat bipolar disorders and other schizoaffective disorders; resistant schizophrenia, alcohol withdrawal, restless leg syndrome, and psychotic behavior associated with dementia

Contraindications Hypersensitivity to carbamazepine or any component; may have cross-sensitivity with tricyclic antidepressants; should not be used in any patient with bone marrow depression, MAO inhibitor use, or history of bone marrow depression

Warnings Potentially fatal blood cell abnormalities have been reported following treatment; early detection of hematologic change is important; advise patients of early signs and symptoms which are fever, sore throat, mouth ulcers, infections, easy bruising, petechial or purpuric hemorrhage; use with caution in glaucoma due to mild anticholinergic action; may cause confusion or activate latent psychosis; elderly at risk for confusion or agitation

(Continued)

117

Carbamazepine *(Continued)*

Precautions MAO inhibitors should be discontinued for a minimum of 14 days before carbamazepine is begun; administer with caution to patients with history of cardiac damage or hepatic disease; may cause drowsiness, dizziness, or blurred vision

Adverse Reactions

Cardiovascular: Edema, congestive heart failure, syncope, hypertension, hypotension, thrombophlebitis, arrhythmias

Central nervous system: Sedation, dizziness, slurred speech, difficulty concentrating, fatigue, ataxia

Dermatologic: Rash (but does not necessarily mean the drug should not be stopped), pruritus, alopecia, urticaria, Stevens-Johnson syndrome, exfoliative dermatitis, toxic epidermal necrolysis

Endocrine & metabolic: Hyponatremia, SIADH

Gastrointestinal: Nausea, gastric distress, abdominal pain, diarrhea, constipation, anorexia, dry mouth, glossitis, stomatitis

Genitourinary: Urinary retention

Hematologic: Neutropenia (can be transient), aplastic anemia (1 in 200,000 patients), agranulocytosis, thrombocytopenia; leukopenia is the most frequent hematologic effect

Hepatic: Hepatitis

Neuromuscular & skeletal: Arthralgias, leg cramps

Ocular: Nystagmus, diplopia

Respiratory: Dyspnea

Overdosage Symptoms of overdose include dizziness, ataxia, drowsiness, nausea, vomiting, tremor, agitation, nystagmus, urinary retention, tachycardia, hypotension, hypertension, shock, dysrhythmias, coma, seizures, twitches, respiratory depression, neuromuscular disturbances

Toxicology Activated charcoal (50-100 g initially; ≥ 12 g/hour with nasogastric tube) is effective at binding carbamazepine; monitor EKG, blood pressure, body temperature, pupillary reflexes, bladder function for several days following ingestion; provide general supportive care

Drug Interactions

Erythromycin, isoniazid, propoxyphene, verapamil, danazol, nicotinamide, diltiazem, and cimetidine may inhibit hepatic metabolism of carbamazepine with resultant increase of carbamazepine serum concentrations and toxicity

Carbamazepine may induce the metabolism of warfarin, doxycycline, oral contraceptives, phenytoin, theophylline, benzodiazepines, ethosuximide, valproic acid, corticosteroids and thyroid hormones

May increase metabolism of acetaminophen increasing the possibility of hepatotoxicity and decreasing its analgesic/antipyretic activity

Barbiturates and primidone may decrease serum concentrations of carbamazepine

Lithium may have increased CNS toxicity; valproic acid levels may decrease

Mechanism of Action May depress activity in the nucleus ventralis of the thalamus or decrease synaptic transmission or to decrease summation of temporal stimulation leading to neural discharge by limiting influx of sodium ions across cell membrane or other unknown mechanisms; stimulates the release of ADH and potentiates its action in promoting reabsorption of water; chemically related to tricyclic antidepressants; in addition to anticonvulsant effects, carbamazepine has anticholinergic, antineuralgic, antidiuretic, muscle relaxant, and antiarrhythmic properties

Pharmacokinetics

Absorption: Slow from GI tract

Distribution: V_d (adults): 0.59-2 L/kg

Protein binding 75% to 90%

Metabolism: Induces liver enzymes to increase its own metabolism and shortens half-life over time; metabolized in liver to active epoxide metabolite

Bioavailability: 85% oral

Half-life:

Initial: 18-55 hours

Multiple dosing: 12-17 hours

Time to peak: Unpredictable peak levels occur within 4-8 hours

Elimination: 1% to 3% excreted unchanged in urine

Usual Dosage Oral (dosage must be adjusted according to patient's response and serum concentrations):

Geriatrics and Adults: 200 mg twice daily to start, increase by 200 mg/day at 2- to 3-week intervals until therapeutic levels achieved and autoinduction adjustment of its own metabolism; usual dose: 800-1200 mg/day in 2-4 divided doses; some patients have required up to 1.6-2.4 g/day; most common chronic dose range: 7-15 mg/kg/day; must give at least twice daily due to autoinduction

Monitoring Parameters CBC, blood levels and response

Reference Range Therapeutic: 6-12 μg/mL (SI: 25-51 μmol/L). Patients who require higher levels (8-12 μg/mL (SI: 34-51 μmol/L)) should be watched closely; trough levels >4 μg/mL are often needed. Side effects including CNS effects occur commonly at higher dosage levels. If other anticonvulsants are given therapeutic range is 4-8 µg/mL (SI: 17-34 µmol/L).

Test Interactions Increased BUN, AST, ALT, bilirubin, alkaline phosphatase (S); decreased calcium, T_3, T_4, sodium (S)

Patient Information Take with food, may cause drowsiness, periodic blood test monitoring required; notify physician if you observe bleeding, bruising, jaundice, abdominal pain, pale stools, mental disturbances, fever, chills, sore throat, or mouth ulcers

Nursing Implications Observe patient for excessive sedation

Additional Information Suspension dosage form must be given on a 3-4 times/day schedule versus tablets which can be given 2-4 times/day; may cause a rash, but does not necessarily mean the drug should be stopped

Special Geriatric Considerations See Adverse Reactions; elderly may have increase risk of SIADH-like syndrome

Dosage Forms
Suspension: 100 mg/5 mL (450 mL)
Tablet: 200 mg
Tablet, chewable: 100 mg

Carbamide Peroxide (kar' ba mide per ox' ide)

Brand Names Auro® Ear Drops [OTC]; Cankaid® Oral [OTC]; Debrox® Otic [OTC]; Gly-Oxide® Oral [OTC]; Murine® Ear Drops [OTC]; Orajel® Brace-Aid Rinse [OTC]; Proxigel® Oral [OTC]

Synonyms Urea Peroxide

Generic Available Yes

Therapeutic Class Anti-infective Agent, Oral; Otic Agent, Cerumenolytic

Use
Oral: Relief of minor inflammation of gums, oral mucosal surfaces and lips including canker sores and dental irritation
Otic: Emulsify and disperse ear wax

Contraindications Otic preparation should not be used in patients with a perforated tympanic membrane; ear drainage, ear pain or rash in the ear; dizziness

Warnings With prolonged use of oral carbamide peroxide, there is a potential for overgrowth of opportunistic organisms; damage to periodontal tissues; delayed wound healing

Adverse Reactions
Central nervous system: Dizziness
Dermatologic: Rash
Local: Irritation, tenderness, pain, redness

Stability Store in tight, light-resistant containers; oral gel should be stored under refrigeration

Mechanism of Action Carbamide peroxide releases hydrogen peroxide which serves as a source of nascent oxygen upon contact with catalase; deodorant action is probably due to inhibition of odor-causing bacteria; softens impacted cerumen due to its foaming action

Usual Dosage Geriatrics and Adults:
Oral (should not be used for >7 days):
Gel: Massage on affected area 4 times/day
Solution: Apply several drops undiluted to affected area of the mouth 4 times/day and at bedtime for up to 7 days, expectorate after 2-3 minutes; as an adjunct to oral hygiene after brushing, swish 10 drops for 2-3 minutes, then expectorate
Otic (should not be used for longer than 4 days): Instill 5-10 drops twice daily for up to 4 days; keep drops in ear for several minutes by keeping head tilted or placing cotton in ear

Administration See Usual Dosage

Patient Information Contact physician if dizziness or otic redness, rash, irritation, tenderness, pain, drainage, or discharge develop; do not drink or rinse mouth for 5 minutes after oral use of gel

Nursing Implications Patient may complain of foaming

Additional Information Otic preparation should not be used for >4 days; oral preparation should not be used for longer than 7 days

Special Geriatric Considerations Avoid contact with hearing aids

Dosage Forms
Gel, oral (Proxigel®): 11% (36 g)
Solution:
Oral (Cankaid®, Gly-Oxide®, Orajel® Brace-Aid Rinse): 10% in glycerin (15 mL, 22.5 mL, 30 mL, 60 mL)
Otic (Auro® Ear Drops, Debrox®, Murine® Ear Drops): 6.5% in glycerin (15 mL, 30 mL)

Carbamylcholine Chloride see Carbachol on page 116

Carbenicillin (kar ben i sill' in)
Brand Names Geocillin®; Geopen®; Pyopen®
Synonyms Carbenicillin Disodium; Carbenicillin Indanyl Sodium; Carindacillin
Generic Available No
Therapeutic Class Antibiotic, Penicillin
Use Treatment of serious infections caused by susceptible gram-negative aerobic bacilli or mixed aerobic-anaerobic bacterial infections and/or urinary tract infections excluding those secondary to *Klebsiella* sp and *Serratia marcescens*
Contraindications Hypersensitivity to carbenicillin or any component or penicillins
Warnings Oral carbenicillin should be limited to treatment of urinary tract infections and prostatitis
Precautions Do not use in patients with severe renal impairment (Cl_{cr} <10 mL/minute); use with caution in patients with history of cephalosporin allergy; dosage modification required in patients with impaired renal and/or hepatic function; because of its high sodium content (5 mEq/g), use with caution in patients with hypertension, congestive heart failure, or cephalosporin allergy
Adverse Reactions
Dermatologic: Rash, urticaria, pruritus
Endocrine & metabolic: Hypokalemia
Gastrointestinal: Nausea, vomiting, diarrhea, abdominal cramps
Hematologic: Eosinophilia, hemolytic anemia, neutropenia, thrombocytopenia
Hepatic: Elevation in liver enzymes
Miscellaneous: Furry tongue
Overdosage Symptoms of overdose include neuromuscular hypersensitivity, convulsions
Toxicology Many beta-lactam-containing antibiotics have the potential to cause neuromuscular hyperirritability or convulsive seizures. Hemodialysis may be helpful to aid in the removal of the drug from the blood, otherwise most treatment is supportive or symptom directed.
Drug Interactions Probenecid significantly prolongs half-life; decreased effect with administration of aminoglycosides within 1 hour, may inactivate both drugs
Mechanism of Action Interferes with bacterial cell wall synthesis during active multiplication
Pharmacokinetics
Absorption: Oral: 30% to 40%
Distribution: Into bile, low concentrations attained in CSF
Protein binding: 50%
Half-life: 60-90 minutes and is prolonged to 10-20 hours with renal insufficiency
Time to peak: Peak carbenicillin levels occur within 30-120 minutes; in patients with normal renal function, serum concentrations of carbenicillin following oral absorption are inadequate for the treatment of systemic infections
Elimination: ~80% to 99% of dose excreted unchanged in urine
Usual Dosage Geriatrics and Adults: Oral: 1-2 tablets (382-764 mg) every 6 hours
Prostatitis: 2 tablets every 6 hours
Dosing interval in renal impairment:
Cl_{cr} 10-50 mL/minute: Administer every 12-24 hours
Cl_{cr} <10 mL/minute: Administer every 24-48 hours
Moderately dialyzable (20% to 50%)
Monitoring Parameters Signs and symptoms of infection (fever, urinary frequency, dysuria, etc)
Reference Range Therapeutic: Not established; Toxic: >250 μg/mL (SI: >660 μmol/L)
Test Interactions False-positive urine or serum proteins; false-positive urine glucose (Clinitest®)
Patient Information Tablets have a bitter taste, can be taken with food; complete full course of treatment; notify physician of edema, difficulty breathing, bruising, or bleeding
Nursing Implications Watch for increased edema, rales, or signs of congestion, bruising, or bleeding; give around-the-clock to promote less variation in peak and trough serum levels
Special Geriatric Considerations Has not been studied in the elderly; see Usual Dosage; adjust for renal function in the elderly
Dosage Forms Tablet, as indanyl sodium: 382 mg

Carbenicillin Disodium *see* Carbenicillin *on this page*

Carbenicillin Indanyl Sodium *see* Carbenicillin *on this page*

Carbidopa (kar bi doe' pa)
Brand Names Lodosyn®
Therapeutic Class Anti-Parkinson's Agent
Additional Information Usually used in combination with levodopa (Sinemet®); plain carbidopa tablets are available from Merck Sharp & Dohme to physicians for use in patients requiring individual titration of carbidopa and levodopa
Dosage Forms Tablet: 25 mg

Carbidopa and Levodopa see Levodopa and Carbidopa on page 402

Cardene® see Nicardipine Hydrochloride on page 500

Cardilate® see Erythrityl Tetranitrate on page 262

Cardioquin® see Quinidine on page 618

Cardizem® see Diltiazem on page 226

Cardizem® CD see Diltiazem on page 226

Cardizem® SR see Diltiazem on page 226

Cardura® see Doxazosin on page 241

Carfin® see Warfarin Sodium on page 739

Carindacillin see Carbenicillin on previous page

Carisoprodate see Carisoprodol on this page

Carisoprodol (kar eye soe proe' dole)

Brand Names Rela®; Sodol®; Soma®; Soma® Compound; Soprodol®; Soridol®

Synonyms Carisoprodate; Isobamate

Generic Available Yes

Therapeutic Class Skeletal Muscle Relaxant

Use Relief of discomfort associated with acute, painful musculoskeletal conditions

Contraindications Acute intermittent porphyria, hypersensitivity to carisoprodol, meprobamate or any component

Warnings Use with caution in addiction-prone individuals; abrupt withdrawal has caused mild symptoms in some patients and psychological dependence has been reported, though rare. Idiosyncratic reactions may occur rarely within minutes or hours of the first dose; symptoms include weakness, transient quadriplegia, dizziness, ataxia, temporary loss of vision, diplopia, agitation, euphoria, disorientation; symptoms subside in a few hours; use with caution in renal and hepatic dysfunction

Adverse Reactions
Cardiovascular: Tachycardia, orthostatic hypotension, facial flushing, syncope
Central nervous system: Sedation, dizziness, fatigue, vertigo, agitation, headache, insomnia, ataxia
Gastrointestinal: Nausea, vomiting
Neuromuscular & skeletal: Tremors
Miscellaneous: Cross-hypersensitivity with meprobamate has been reported

Overdosage Symptoms of overdose include CNS depression, stupor, coma, shock, respiratory depression

Toxicology Treatment is supportive following attempts to enhance drug elimination; hypotension should be treated with I.V. fluids and/or Trendelenburg positioning; carisoprodol is dialyzable

Drug Interactions Increased toxicity: Alcohol, CNS depressants, phenothiazines, clindamycin, MAO inhibitors

Mechanism of Action Precise mechanism is not yet clear, but many effects have been ascribed to its central depressant actions

Pharmacodynamics
Onset of action: Within 30 minutes
Duration: 4-6 hours

Pharmacokinetics
Metabolism: By the liver
Half-life: 8 hours
Elimination: Excreted by kidneys

Usual Dosage
Geriatrics: See Special Geriatric Considerations
Adults: Oral: 350 mg 3-4 times/day; take last dose at bedtime; compound: 1-2 tablets 4 times/day
Dosing adjustment in hepatic impairment: Dosage may need to be decreased in patients with severe hepatic dysfunction

Monitoring Parameters Relief of pain and/or muscle spasm, mental status

Patient Information May cause drowsiness or dizziness; avoid alcohol and other CNS depressants; because of the risk of postural hypotension, rise slowly from sitting or lying down

Nursing Implications Raise bed rails, institute safety measures, assist with ambulation

Special Geriatric Considerations There are no data on the use of skeletal muscle relaxants in the elderly; because of the risk of orthostatic hypotension and CNS depression, avoid or use with caution in the elderly; not considered a drug of choice in the elderly

Dosage Forms Tablet:
Rela®, Sodol®, Soma®, Soprodol®, Soridol®: 350 mg
Soma® Compound: Carisoprodol 200 mg and aspirin 325 mg

(Continued)

121

Carisoprodol *(Continued)*

Soma® Compound with codeine: Carisoprodol 200 mg, aspirin 325 mg, and codeine phosphate 16 mg

Carteolol Hydrochloride

Related Information

Beta-Blockers Comparison *on page 804-805*

Brand Names Cartrol®; Ocupress®

Generic Available No

Therapeutic Class Beta-Adrenergic Blocker; Beta-Adrenergic Blocker, Ophthalmic

Use Management of hypertension; treatment of chronic open-angle glaucoma and intraocular hypertension

Contraindications Uncompensated congestive heart failure, cardiogenic shock, bradycardia or heart block, asthma or any other bronchospastic disorder; diabetes mellitus, or hypersensitivity to beta-blocking agents

Warnings Abrupt withdrawal of beta-blockers may result in an exaggerated cardiac beta-adrenergic responsiveness. Symptomatology has included reports of tachycardia, hypertension, ischemia, angina, myocardial infarction, and sudden death. It is recommended that patients be tapered gradually off of beta-blockers over a 2-week period rather than via abrupt discontinuation.

Precautions Administer to congestive heart failure patients with caution; administer with caution to patients with bronchospastic disease, diabetes mellitus, hyperthyroidism, myasthenia gravis and renal function decline and severe peripheral vascular disease. Abrupt withdrawal of the drug should be avoided, drug should be discontinued over 2 weeks.

Adverse Reactions

Cardiovascular: Mesenteric arterial thrombosis, A-V block, persistent bradycardia, hypotension, chest pain, edema, heart failure, Raynaud's phenomena

Central nervous system: Fatigue, dizziness, headache, insomnia, lethargy, nightmares, depression, confusion

Dermatologic: Purpura

Gastrointestinal: Ischemic colitis, constipation, nausea, diarrhea

Genitourinary: Impotence

Hematologic: Thrombocytopenia

Respiratory: Bronchospasm

Miscellaneous: Cold extremities

Overdosage Symptoms of overdose include bradycardia, congestive heart failure, hypotension, bronchospasm, hypoglycemia; see Toxicology

Toxicology Sympathomimetics (eg, epinephrine or dopamine), glucagon or a pacemaker can be used to treat the toxic bradycardia, asystole, and/or hypotension. Initially, fluids may be the best treatment for toxic hypotension. Patients should remain supine; serum glucose and potassium should be measured. Use supportive measures: lavage, syrup of ipecac; I.V. glucose should be administered for hypoglycemia; seizures may be treated with phenytoin or diazepam intravenously; continuous monitoring of blood pressure and EKG is necessary. If PVCs occur, treat with lidocaine or phenytoin; avoid quinidine, procainamide, and disopyramide since these agents further depress myocardial function. Bronchospasm can be treated with theophylline on beta$_2$ agonists (epinephrine).

Drug Interactions

Phenobarbital, rifampin may decrease beta-blocker bioavailability and may decrease its activity

Cimetidine may reduce beta-blocker clearance and increase its effects

Aluminum-containing antacid may reduce GI absorption of beta-blockers; nonsteroidal anti-inflammatory agents, sulfinpyrazone, flecainide, MAO inhibitors, phenothiazines, aluminum compounds, calcium, cholestyramine, colestipol, haloperidol, H$_2$ blockers, loop diuretics, ciprofloxacan, quinidine, ergot alkaloids, salicylates, sympathomimetics, thyroid hormones, insulins, lidocaine, calcium channel blockers, catecholamine depleting drugs, clonidine, disopyramide, prazosin, theophylline

Mechanism of Action Blocks both beta$_1$- and beta$_2$-receptors and has mild intrinsic sympathomimetic activity; has negative inotropic and chronotropic effects and can significantly slow A-V nodal conduction; low lipid solubility will decrease CNS side effects

Pharmacodynamics Ophthalmic: 22% to 25% reduction of IOP given twice daily

Onset: Not known

Maximum effect: Not described

Duration: 12 hours

Pharmacokinetics

Absorption: Well absorbed, 80%

Protein binding: 25% to 30%

Bioavailability: Oral: 85%

Half-life: 6 hours

Elimination: 50% to 70% excreted unchanged in urine

Usual Dosage Geriatrics and Adults:
   Oral: 2.5 mg as a single daily dose, with a maintenance dose normally 2.5-5 mg once daily; maximum daily dose: 10 mg; doses >10 mg do not increase response and may in fact decrease effect
   Ophthalmic: Instill 1 drop in affected eye(s) twice daily; see Additional Information

   Dosing interval in renal impairment:
   Cl_{cr} >60 mL/min/1.73 m^2: Administer every 24 hours
   Cl_{cr} 20-60 mL/min/1.73 m^2: Administer every 48 hours
   Cl_{cr} <20 mL/min/1.73 m^2: Administer every 72 hours

Monitoring Parameters Blood pressure, orthostatic hypotension, heart rate, CNS effects

Patient Information Do not discontinue medication abruptly, sudden stopping of medication may precipitate or cause angina; consult pharmacist or physician before taking with other adrenergic drugs (eg, cold medications); notify physician if any of the following symptoms occur: difficult breathing, night cough, swelling of extremities, slow pulse, dizziness, lightheadedness, confusion, depression, skin rash, fever, sore throat, unusual bleeding or bruising; may produce drowsiness, dizziness, lightheadedness, blurred vision, confusion; use with caution while driving or performing tasks requiring alertness; may mask signs of hypoglycemia in diabetics; may be taken without regard to meals

Nursing Implications Advise against abrupt withdrawal; monitor orthostatic blood pressures, apical and peripheral pulse and mental status changes (ie, confusion, depression)

Additional Information Since bioavailability increased in elderly about twofold, geriatric patients may require lower maintenance doses, therefore, as serum and tissue concentrations increase beta$_1$ selectivity diminishes; when treating glaucoma/intraocular hypertension, if the desired IOP is not achieved, consider adding concomitant therapy with pilocarpine, dipivefrin, etc

Special Geriatric Considerations Due to alterations in the beta-adrenergic autonomic nervous system, beta-adrenergic blockade may result in less hemodynamic response than seen in younger adults. Studies indicate that despite decreased sensitivity to the chronotropic effects of beta blockade with age, there appears to be an increased myocardial sensitivity to the negative inotropic effect during stress (ie, exercise). Controlled trials have shown the overall response rate for propranolol to be only 20% to 50% in elderly populations. Therefore, all beta-adrenergic blocking drugs may result in a decreased response as compared to younger adults; adjust dose for renal function in elderly.

Dosage Forms
   Solution, ophthalmic: 1% (5 mL, 10 mL)
   Tablet: 2.5 mg, 5 mg

Carter's Little Pills® [OTC] *see Bisacodyl on page 87*

Cartrol® *see Carteolol Hydrochloride on previous page*

Casanthranol and Docusate *see Docusate and Casanthranol on page 237*

Cascara Sagrada (kas kar' a)
Generic Available Yes
Therapeutic Class Laxative, Stimulant
Use Temporary relief of constipation; sometimes used with milk of magnesia ("black and white" mixture)
Contraindications Nausea, vomiting, abdominal pain, fecal impaction, intestinal obstruction, GI bleeding, appendicitis, congestive heart failure; hypersensitivity to cascara sagrada or any component
Warnings Laxatives used excessively may lead to fluid/electrolyte imbalance; stimulant cathartics may lead to abuse or dependency with chronic use (laxative abuse syndrome); cathartic colon, which may present as ulcerative colitis, occurs with chronic use of stimulant cathartics; melanosis coli is a dark pigmentation of the colonic mucosa from chronic use of anthraquinone derivatives
Precautions Habit-forming and may result in laxative dependence and loss of normal bowel function with prolonged use; rectal bleeding or failure to respond requires further evaluation for possibly serious medical problems
Adverse Reactions
   Central nervous system: Faintness
   Endocrine & metabolic: Electrolyte and fluid imbalance
   Gastrointestinal: Abdominal cramps, nausea, diarrhea, bloating, flatulence
   Miscellaneous: Sweating, discolors urine reddish pink or brown, perianal irritation
Overdosage Symptoms of overdose include hypokalemia, hypocalcemia, metabolic acidosis or alkalosis, abdominal pain, diarrhea, malabsorption, weight loss and protein-losing enteropathy
Stability Protect from light and heat
Mechanism of Action Direct chemical irritation of the intestinal mucosa resulting in
(Continued)

Cascara Sagrada *(Continued)*

an increased rate of colonic motility; stimulation of the myenteric plexus and change in fluid and electrolyte secretion of the gastrointestinal mucosa

Pharmacodynamics Onset of action: 6-10 hours

Pharmacokinetics
Absorption: Oral: Small amount from small intestine
Metabolism: In the liver

Usual Dosage Geriatrics and Adults: Oral:
Aromatic fluid extract: 5 mL/day (range 2-6 mL) as needed at bedtime
Tablet: 1 tablet (325 mg) at bedtime as needed; avoid chronic use
Black and white cocktail (M.O.M./cascara): 5 mL cascara sagrada fluid extract with 25 mL milk of magnesia (total 30 mL) at bedtime as needed

Monitoring Parameters Monitor stools per day, consistency, occult or gross blood; also with chronic use, monitor serum electrolytes; monitor for dehydration and hypotension

Test Interactions Decreased calcium (S), decreased potassium (S)

Patient Information Should not be used regularly for more than 1 week; may discolor urine or feces (yellow-brown); do not use in presence of nausea, vomiting, or abdominal pain; stimulant laxative use should be limited; notify physician if unrelieved by laxative, rectal bleeding occurs, or signs of electrolyte imbalance develop (dizziness, weakness, muscle cramps); take with a full glass of water

Nursing Implications See Warnings, Precautions, Monitoring Parameters, Additional Information, and Special Geriatric Considerations

Additional Information Cascara sagrada fluid extract is five times more potent than cascara sagrada aromatic fluid extract and contains 18% alcohol

Special Geriatric Considerations Elderly are often predisposed to constipation due to disease, immobility, drugs, low residue diets, and a decreased "thirst reflex" with age. Avoid stimulant cathartic use on a chronic basis if possible. Use osmotic, lubricant, stool softeners, and bulk agents as prophylaxis. Patients should be instructed for proper dietary fiber and fluid intake as well as regular exercise. Monitor closely for fluid/electrolyte imbalance, CNS signs of fluid/electrolyte loss, and hypotension.

Dosage Forms
Aromatic fluid extract: 120 mL, 473 mL (contains 18% alcohol)
Tablet: 325 mg

Castor Oil (kas' tor)

Brand Names Alphamul® [OTC]; Emulsoil® [OTC]; Fleet® Flavored Castor Oil [OTC]; Neoloid® [OTC]; Purge® [OTC]

Synonyms Oleum Ricini

Generic Available Yes

Therapeutic Class Laxative, Stimulant

Use Preparation for rectal or bowel examination or surgery; occasionally used to relieve constipation; also applied to skin as emollient and protectant

Contraindications Known hypersensitivity to castor oil; nausea, vomiting, abdominal pain, fecal impaction, GI bleeding, appendicitis, congestive heart failure, dehydration

Warnings Castor oil induces a strong purgative action and therefore should not be used for routine treatment of constipation

Precautions Use only when a prompt and thorough catharsis is desired

Adverse Reactions
Cardiovascular: Hypotension
Central nervous system: Dizziness
Endocrine & metabolic: Electrolyte disturbance
Gastrointestinal: Abdominal cramps, nausea, diarrhea

Overdosage Symptoms of overdose include diarrhea, abdominal cramps, nausea, vomiting, hypotension, dizziness

Stability Protect from heat (castor oil emulsion should be protected from freezing)

Mechanism of Action Acts primarily in the small intestine; hydrolyzed to ricinoleic acid which stimulates secretory processes, decreases glucose absorption, therefore reduces net absorption of fluid and electrolytes and stimulates peristalsis

Pharmacodynamics Onset of action: Oral: 2-6 hours after dose

Usual Dosage
Geriatrics and Adults: 15-60 mL as a single dose
Adults: Emulsified castor oil: 30-60 mL/dose

Monitoring Parameters Monitor number of stools per day; consistency, fluid status, and blood pressure if fluid loss is excessive

Patient Information Laxative use should be short term (< 7 days); discontinue use when bowel regularity returns; notify physician if constipation is unrelieved, blood appears in stool, or if dizziness, muscle weakness, or cramping is experienced; take with full glass of water or juice; maintain adequate fluid intake

Nursing Implications Do not administer at bedtime because of rapid onset of action; see Monitoring Parameters

Additional Information Chill or give with juice or carbonated beverage to improve palatability

Special Geriatric Considerations See Warnings. Strong and chronic purging may cause severe fluid and electrolyte loss which may affect mental function (CNS).

Dosage Forms
Emulsion, castor oil: 36.4%, 60%, 67%, 95%
Liquid, castor oil: 95%, 100%

Cataflam® see Diclofenac Sodium on page 212

Catapres® see Clonidine on page 177

Catapres-TTS® see Clonidine on page 177

Ceclor® see Cefaclor on this page

Cecon® [OTC] see Ascorbic Acid on page 57

Cee-1000® T.D. [OTC] see Ascorbic Acid on page 57

Cefaclor (sef' a klor)
Brand Names Ceclor®
Generic Available No
Therapeutic Class Antibiotic, Cephalosporin (Second Generation)
Use Treatment of otitis media, sinusitis, and infections caused by susceptible organisms involving the respiratory tract, skin and skin structure, bone and joint, and urinary tract and gynecologic as well as septicemia
Contraindications Hypersensitivity to cefaclor or any component or cephalosporins
Warnings Prolonged use may result in superinfection
Precautions Use with caution in patients with impaired renal function and a history of colitis; modify dosage in patients with severe renal impairment; use with caution in patients with penicillin allergy (anaphylactic reactions, pruritic rash)
Adverse Reactions
Dermatologic: Rash, urticaria, pruritus, Stevens-Johnson syndrome
Gastrointestinal: Nausea, vomiting, diarrhea, pseudomembranous colitis
Hematologic: Eosinophilia, hemolytic anemia, neutropenia
Hepatic: Cholestatic jaundice, slight elevation of AST, ALT
Neuromuscular & skeletal: Arthralgia
Overdosage Symptoms of overdose include neuromuscular hypersensitivity, convulsions
Toxicology Many beta-lactam-containing antibiotics have the potential to cause neuromuscular hyperirritability or convulsive seizures. Hemodialysis may be helpful to aid in the removal of the drug from the blood, otherwise most treatment is supportive or symptom directed.
Drug Interactions Probenecid prolongs half-life and decreases clearance
Stability Refrigerate suspension after reconstitution; discard after 14 days
Mechanism of Action Interferes with bacterial cell wall synthesis during active multiplication causing cell death and resultant bactericidal activity against susceptible bacteria
Pharmacokinetics
Absorption: Oral: Acid stable, well absorbed
Half-life: 30-60 minutes (prolonged with renal impairment)
Time to peak: Peak serum levels occur within 30-60 minutes
Elimination: Most of a dose (80%) is excreted unchanged in urine
Usual Dosage Geriatrics and Adults: Oral: 250-500 mg every 8 hours or daily dose can be given in 2 divided doses
Dosage adjustment in renal impairment: Cl_{cr} <50 mL/minute: Administer 50% of dose in 2 divided doses
Moderately dialyzable (20% to 50%)
Monitoring Parameters Signs and symptoms of infections, including mental status
Test Interactions Positive Coombs' [direct], false-positive urine glucose (Clinitest®), false ↑ serum or urine creatinine
Patient Information Complete full course of therapy; may take with food or milk
Special Geriatric Considerations Has not been studied in the elderly, see Usual Dosage; adjust dose for renal function in elderly; considered one of the drugs of choice in the outpatient treatment of community-acquired pneumonia in older adults
Dosage Forms
Capsule: 250 mg, 500 mg
Suspension, oral: 125 mg/5 mL (75 mL, 150 mL); 187 mg/5 mL (50 mL, 100 mL); 250 mg/5 mL (75 mL, 150 mL); 375 mg/5 mL (50 mL, 100 mL)
References
American Thoracic Society, "Guidelines for the Initial Management of Adults With Community-Acquired Pneumonia: Diagnosis, Assessment of Severity, and Initial Antimicrobial Therapy," Am Rev Respir Dis, 1993, 148(5):1418-26.

Cefadroxil Monohydrate (sef a drox' ill)
Brand Names Duricef®; Ultracef®
Generic Available No
Therapeutic Class Antibiotic, Cephalosporin (First Generation)
(Continued)

Cefadroxil Monohydrate *(Continued)*

Use Treatment of susceptible bacterial infections, including those caused by group A beta-hemolytic *Streptococcus*

Contraindications Hypersensitivity to cefadroxil and/or cephalosporins

Precautions Use with caution in patients allergic to penicillin; reduce dose for decreased renal function; prolonged use may result in superinfection

Adverse Reactions
Dermatologic: Maculopapular and erythematous rash
Gastrointestinal: Dyspepsia, diarrhea, pseudomembranous colitis, nausea, vomiting
Hematologic: Neutropenia
Miscellaneous: Superinfection

Overdosage Symptoms of overdose include neuromuscular hypersensitivity, convulsions

Drug Interactions Increased levels with probenecid

Stability Refrigerate suspension after reconstitution; discard after 14 days

Mechanism of Action Interferes with bacterial cell wall synthesis during active multiplication causing cell death and resultant bactericidal activity against susceptible bacteria

Pharmacokinetics
Absorption: Oral: Rapidly and well absorbed from GI tract
Distribution: V_d: 0.31 L/kg
Protein binding: 20%
Half-life: 1-2 hours; in renal failure, the half-life increases to 20-24 hours
Time to peak: Peak serum levels occur within 70-90 minutes
Elimination: >90% of dose excreted unchanged in urine within 8 hours
Effects of aging on the pharmacokinetics of cefadroxil are not well studied; only older patients with impaired renal function have been studied

Usual Dosage Oral:
Geriatrics: Usual adult dosage with adjustments for patients with renal impairment

Dosing interval (for 500 mg dose) in renal impairment (following an initial 1 g dose):
Cl_{cr} >50 mL/minute: No adjustment necessary
Cl_{cr} 25-50 mL/minute: Administer every 12 hours
Cl_{cr} 10-25 mL/minute: Administer every 24 hours
Cl_{cr} 0-10 mL/minute: Administer every 36 hours

Adults: 1-2 g/day in 2 divided doses

Monitoring Parameters Signs and symptoms of infection, including mental status

Test Interactions Positive Coombs' [direct], glucose, protein; decreased glucose

Patient Information Complete full course of therapy; can be taken with food or milk; report persistent diarrhea to physician

Nursing Implications Give around-the-clock to promote less variation in peak and trough serum levels

Special Geriatric Considerations See Pharmacokinetics and Usual Dosage; adjust dose for renal function in elderly

Dosage Forms
Capsule: 500 mg
Suspension, oral: 125 mg, 250 mg, 500 mg (5 mL)
Tablet: 1 g

References
Cutler RE, Blair AD, and Kelly MR, "Cefadroxil Kinetics in Patients With Renal Insufficiency," *Clin Pharmacol Ther*, 1979, 25(5 Pt 1):514-21.

Cefadyl® see Cephapirin Sodium *on page 144*

Cefamandole Nafate *(sef a man' dole)*

Brand Names Mandol®

Generic Available No

Therapeutic Class Antibiotic, Cephalosporin (Second Generation)

Use Treatment of susceptible bacterial infection; mainly respiratory tract, skin and skin structure, bone and joint, urinary tract and gynecologic as well as septicemia

Contraindications Hypersensitivity to cefamandole nafate or any component and cephalosporins

Precautions Use with caution in patients allergic to penicillins; reduce dose for decreased renal function; increased tendency for bleeding

Adverse Reactions
Central nervous system: CNS irritation, seizures, fever
Dermatologic: Rash, urticaria
Gastrointestinal: Diarrhea, abdominal cramps, pseudomembranous colitis
Hematologic: Leukopenia, thrombocytopenia, positive Coombs' test, eosinophilia, hypoprothrombinemia
Hepatic: Transient elevation of liver enzymes, cholestatic jaundice
Local: Pain at injection site
Miscellaneous: Superinfection

Overdosage Symptoms of overdose include neuromuscular hypersensitivity, convulsions

Toxicology Many beta-lactam-containing antibiotics have the potential to cause neuromuscular hyperirritability or convulsive seizures. Hemodialysis may be helpful to aid in the removal of the drug from the blood, otherwise most treatment is supportive or symptom directed.

Drug Interactions

Disulfiram-like reaction has been reported when taken within 72 hours of alcohol consumption

The hypoprothrombinemic effects of anticoagulants and heparin may be increased

Probenecid will increase and prolong cefamandole plasma levels

May potentiate aminoglycoside nephrotoxicity

Stability After reconstitution CO_2 gas is liberated which allows solution to be withdrawn without injecting air; solution is stable for 24 hours at room temperature and 96 hours when refrigerated; for I.V. infusion in NS and D_5W is stable for 24 hours at room temperature; 1 week when refrigerated or 26 weeks when frozen

Mechanism of Action Interferes with bacterial cell wall synthesis during active multiplication causing cell death and resultant bactericidal activity against susceptible bacteria

Pharmacokinetics

Distribution: Well throughout the body, except the CSF poor penetration even with inflamed meninges; extensive enterohepatic circulation; high concentrations in the bile

Protein binding: 56% to 78%

Half-life: 30-60 minutes

Time to peak:

I.M.: Peak serum levels within 1-2 hours

I.V.: Within 10 minutes

Elimination: Majority of drug excreted unchanged in urine

Cefamandole's pharmacokinetics were not altered in older men with "normal" renal function (S_{cr} ≤1.5 mg/dL)

Usual Dosage I.M., I.V.:

Geriatrics: Usual adult dose with adjustments for renal impairment when appropriate

Adults: 4-12 g/24 hours divided every 4-6 hours 500-1000 mg every 4-8 hours

Dosing interval in renal impairment:

Cl_{cr} 50-80 mL/minute: 1-2 g every 6 hours

Cl_{cr} 25-50 mL/minute: 1-2 g every 8 hours

Cl_{cr} 10-25 mL/minute: 1 g every 8 hours

Cl_{cr} 2-10 mL/minute: 1 g every 12 hours

Cl_{cr} <2 mL/minute: 0.5-0.75 g every 12 hours

Moderately dialyzable (20% to 50%)

Monitoring Parameters Signs and symptoms of infection, including mental status

Test Interactions Increased alkaline phosphatase, AST, ALT, BUN, creatinine, prothrombin time (S), glucose, protein; decreased glucose; positive Coombs' [direct]

Patient Information Avoid alcoholic beverages; report signs of bleeding, bruising, or superinfection

Nursing Implications Watch for signs of bruising or bleeding

Additional Information Sodium content of 1 g: 3.3 mEq

Special Geriatric Considerations See Pharmacokinetics and Usual Dosage; the risk of coagulation abnormalities (increased PT) limits the use of cefamandole in the elderly; adjust dose for renal function in elderly

Dosage Forms Injection: 500 mg, 1 g, 2 g

References

Mellin HE, Welling PG, and Madsen PO, "Pharmacokinetics of Cefamandole in Patients With Normal and Impaired Renal Function," *Antimicrob Agents Chemother*, 1977, 11:262-6.

Cefanex® see Cephalexin Monohydrate on page 142

Cefazolin Sodium (sef a' zoe lin)

Brand Names Ancef®; Kefzol®; Zolicef®

Generic Available Yes

Therapeutic Class Antibiotic, Cephalosporin (First Generation)

Use Treatment of gram-positive bacilli and cocci (except enterococcus); some gram-negative bacilli including *E. coli*, *Proteus*, and *Klebsiella* may be susceptible

Contraindications Hypersensitivity to cefazolin sodium or any component, cephalosporins

Precautions Modify dosage in patients with renal impairment; use with caution in patients with penicillin allergy

Adverse Reactions

Central nervous system: CNS irritation, seizures, confusion, fever

Dermatologic: Rash, urticaria

Gastrointestinal: Diarrhea

(Continued)

Cefazolin Sodium (Continued)

Hematologic: Leukopenia, thrombocytopenia, neutropenia

Hepatic: Transient elevation of liver enzymes, cholestatic jaundice

Overdosage Symptoms of overdose include neuromuscular hypersensitivity, convulsions

Toxicology Many beta-lactam-containing antibiotics have the potential to cause neuromuscular hyperirritability or convulsive seizures. Hemodialysis may be helpful to aid in the removal of the drug from the blood, otherwise most treatment is supportive or symptom directed.

Drug Interactions

Furosemide may be a possible additive to nephrotoxicity

Probenecid may decrease cephalosporin elimination

May potentiate aminoglycoside-induced nephrotoxicity

Stability Reconstituted solution is stable for 24 hours at room temperature and 96 hours when refrigerated; for I.V. infusion in NS or D_5W solution is stable for 24 hours at room temperature, 96 hours when refrigerated or 12 weeks when frozen; after freezing, thawed solution is stable for 48 hours at room temperature or 10 days when refrigerated

Mechanism of Action Interferes with bacterial cell wall synthesis during active multiplication causing cell death and resultant bactericidal activity against susceptible bacteria

Pharmacokinetics

Distribution: V_d: No change

Protein binding: 74% to 86%

Metabolism: Hepatic metabolism is minimal

Half-life: 90-150 minutes (prolonged with renal impairment); mean half-life was twice as long, 3.5 hours, and mean total clearance was reduced by 50% in older adults compared to younger adults

CSF penetration is poor

Time to peak:

I.M.: Peak serum levels occur within 30 minutes to 2 hours

I.V.: Within 5 minutes

Elimination: 80% to 100% excreted unchanged in urine

Usual Dosage I.M., I.V.:

Geriatrics: Usual adult dose with adjustments for renal function when appropriate

Adults: 1-2 g every 8 hours

Dosing interval in renal impairment:

Cefazolin Sodium

Cl_{cr} (mL/min)	Dose (mg) for each dosing interval
≥55	250–1000 q6–8h
35–54	250–1000 ≥8h
11–34	125–500 q12h
≤10	125–500 q24h

Moderately dialyzable (20% to 50%)

Monitoring Parameters Signs and symptoms of infection; WBC, mental status

Test Interactions False-positive urine glucose using Clinitest®, positive Coombs' [direct], false ↑ serum or urine creatinine

Nursing Implications Give around-the-clock rather than 3 times/day (ie, 8-4-12) to promote less variation in peak and trough serum levels; dosage modification required in renal insufficiency

Additional Information Sodium content of 1 g: 47 mg (2 mEq)

Special Geriatric Considerations See Pharmacokinetics and Usual Dosage; adjust dose for renal function

Dosage Forms

Infusion:, premixed (frozen): 500 mg in D_5W (50 mL); 1 g in D_5W (50 mL)

Injection: 250 mg, 500 mg, 1 g, 5 g, 10 g, 20 g

References

Simon VC, Malerczyk V, Tenschert B, et al, "Die Geriatrische Pharmakologie von Cefazolin, Cefradin, und Sulfisomidin," *Arzneim Forsch*, 1976, 26(7):1377-82.

Cefixime (sef ix' eem)

Brand Names Suprax®

Generic Available No

Therapeutic Class Antibiotic, Cephalosporin (Third Generation)

Use Treatment of urinary tract infections, otitis media, respiratory infections due to susceptible organisms; documented poor compliance with other oral antimicrobials; outpatient therapy of serious soft tissue or skeletal infections due to susceptible organisms; single dose for *N. gonorrheae*

Contraindications Hypersensitivity to cefixime or cephalosporins

Warnings Prolonged use may result in superinfection

Precautions Modify dosage in patients with renal impairment; use with caution in patients hypersensitive to penicillin, and patients with a history of colitis

Adverse Reactions
Central nervous system: Fever, headache, dizziness, malaise, somnolence
Dermatologic: Skin rash
Gastrointestinal: Nausea, diarrhea, abdominal pain, flatulence, dyspepsia, pseudomembranous colitis
Hematologic: Transient thrombocytopenia, leukopenia, eosinophilia, and decreased hemoglobin and hematocrit
Hepatic: Transient elevation of liver enzymes
Renal: Transient elevation of BUN or creatinine

Overdosage Symptoms of overdose include neuromuscular hypersensitivity, convulsions

Drug Interactions
Probenecid may prolong cefixime's half-life and increase serum concentration
Salicylates may decrease peak serum concentrations and AUC

Stability Reconstituted oral solution may be kept at room temperature without potency loss for 14 days; **do not refrigerate**

Mechanism of Action Interferes with bacterial cell wall synthesis during active multiplication causing cell death and resultant bactericidal activity against susceptible bacteria

Pharmacokinetics
Absorption: Oral: 40% to 50%
Protein binding: 65%
Half-life:
Normal renal function: 3-4 hours
Renal failure: Up to 11.5 hours
Time to peak: Peak serum levels occur within 2-6 hours
Elimination: 50% of absorbed dose is excreted as active drug in urine and 10% in bile
Decreased clearance and prolonged half-life have been reported in older adults

Usual Dosage Oral:
Geriatrics: Usual adult dose with adjustments for renal function when appropriate

Adults: 400 mg/day in 1-2 divided doses
N. gonorrheae: Single 400 mg dose followed with doxycycline is recommended

Dosing adjustment in renal impairment:
Cl_{cr} 21-60 mL/minute or renal hemodialysis: Administer 75% of the standard dose
Cl_{cr} ≤20 mL/minute or continuous ambulatory peritoneal dialysis: Administer 50% of the standard dose
10% removed by hemodialysis

Monitoring Parameters With prolonged therapy, monitor renal and hepatic function periodically; signs and symptoms of infection

Test Interactions False-positive reaction for urine glucose using Clinitest®

Patient Information Complete full course of therapy; can be taken with food or milk; report persistent diarrhea

Nursing Implications Modify dosage in patients with renal impairment

Additional Information Otitis media should be treated with the suspension since it results in higher peak blood levels than the tablet

Special Geriatric Considerations See Pharmacokinetics and Usual Dosage; adjust dose for renal function

Dosage Forms
Suspension, oral: 100 mg/5 mL (50 mL, 100 mL)
Tablet: 200 mg, 400 mg

References
Faulkner RD, Bohaycheck W, Lanc RA, et al, "Pharmacokinetics of Cefixime in Young and Elderly," *J Antimicrob Chemother*, 1988, 21(6):787-94.

Cefizox® *see* Ceftizoxime *on page 139*

Cefmetazole Sodium (sef met' a zole)
Brand Names Zefazone®
Generic Available No
Therapeutic Class Antibiotic, Cephalosporin (Second Generation)
Use Second generation cephalosporin with an antibacterial spectrum similar to cefoxitin, useful on many aerobic and anaerobic gram-positive and gram-negative bacteria; prophylaxis for vaginal or abdominal hysterectomy, cesarean section, colorectal surgery, cholecystectomy (high-risk patients)
Contraindications Hypersensitivity to cefmetazole or any component, cephalosporins
Precautions Use with caution in patients with impaired renal or impaired function; patients with a history of gastrointestinal disease (colitis) or penicillin allergy
(Continued)

Cefmetazole Sodium (Continued)

Adverse Reactions
Cardiovascular: Hypotension, shock
Central nervous system: Fever, headache
Dermatologic: Rash
Endocrine & metabolic: Hot flashes
Gastrointestinal: Diarrhea, nausea, vomiting, epigastric pain, pseudomembranous colitis
Genitourinary: Vaginitis
Hematologic: Bleeding
Local: Pain at injection site, phlebitis
Respiratory: Dyspnea, respiratory distress
Miscellaneous: candidiasis, epistaxis

Overdosage Symptoms of overdose include neuromuscular hypersensitivity, convulsions

Toxicology Many beta-lactam-containing antibiotics have the potential to cause neuromuscular hyperirritability or convulsive seizures. Hemodialysis may be helpful to aid in the removal of the drug from the blood, otherwise most treatment is supportive or symptom directed.

Drug Interactions
Probenecid may prolong cephalosporin half-life
May potentiate aminoglycoside nephrotoxicity

Stability Reconstituted solution and I.V. infusion in NS or D_5W solution are stable for 24 hours at room temperature, 7 days when refrigerated, or 6 weeks when frozen; after freezing, thawed solution is stable for 24 hours at room temperature or 7 days when refrigerated

Mechanism of Action Interferes with bacterial cell wall synthesis during active multiplication causing cell death and resultant bactericidal activity against susceptible bacteria

Pharmacokinetics
Protein binding: 65%
Metabolism: <15%
Half-life: 72 minutes
Elimination: Renal

Usual Dosage Geriatrics and Adults: I.V.:
Infections: 2 g every 6-12 hours for 5-14 days
Prophylaxis: 1-2 g 30-90 minutes before surgery
Dosing interval in renal impairment: See table.

Cefmetazole Sodium

Cl_{cr} (mL/min/1.73 m²)	Dose (g) for each dosing interval
50–90	1–2 q12h
30–49	1–2 q16h
10–29	1–2 q24h
<10	1–2 q48h

Monitoring Parameters Signs and symptoms of infection including mental status and prothrombin times

Test Interactions Positive Coombs' [direct], falsely elevated urinary 17-ketosteroid values

Patient Information Do not drink alcohol for at least 24 hours after receiving dose; report persistent diarrhea; females should report symptoms of vaginitis

Nursing Implications Do not admix with aminoglycosides in same bottle/bag

Additional Information Sodium content of 1 g: 2 mEq

Special Geriatric Considerations Cefmetazole has not been studied in the elderly; see Usual Dosage; adjust dose for renal function

Dosage Forms Injection: 1 g, 2 g

References
Donowitz GR and Mandell GL, "Beta-Lactam Antibiotics," *N Engl J Med*, 1988, 318(7):419-26.

Cefobid® *see* Cefoperazone Sodium *on next page*

Cefonicid Sodium (se fon' i sid)
Brand Names Monocid®
Generic Available No
Therapeutic Class Antibiotic, Cephalosporin (Second Generation)

Use Treatment of susceptible bacterial infection; mainly respiratory tract, skin and skin structure, bone and joint, urinary tract and gynecologic as well as septicemia; second generation cephalosporin

Contraindications Hypersensitivity to cefonicid sodium or any component and cephalosporins

Precautions Use with caution in patients allergic to penicillin; reduce dose for decreased renal function

Adverse Reactions
    Central nervous system: Fever, headache
    Dermatologic: Skin rash
    Gastrointestinal: Nausea, diarrhea, abdominal pain, pseudomembranous colitis
    Hematologic: Increased platelets and eosinophils
    Hepatic: Transient elevations in liver enzymes
    Local: Pain at injection site
    Renal: Transient increase in BUN or creatinine

Overdosage Symptoms of overdose include neuromuscular hypersensitivity, convulsions

Toxicology Many beta-lactam-containing antibiotics have the potential to cause neuromuscular hyperirritability or convulsive seizures. Hemodialysis may be helpful to aid in the removal of the drug from the blood, otherwise most treatment is supportive or symptom directed.

Drug Interactions
    Probenecid may prolong half-life and increase serum levels
    May potentiate aminoglycoside nephrotoxicity

Stability Reconstituted solution and I.V. infusion in NS or D_5W solution are stable for 24 hours at room temperature or 72 hours if refrigerated

Mechanism of Action Interferes with bacterial cell wall synthesis during active multiplication causing cell death and resultant bactericidal activity against susceptible bacteria

Usual Dosage Geriatrics and Adults: I.M., I.V.: 0.5-2 g every 24 hours
    Prophylaxis: Preop: 1 g/hour
    Dosing interval in renal impairment: See table.

Cefonicid Sodium

Cl_{cr} (mL/min/1.73 m^2)	Dose (mg/kg) for each dosing interval
60–79	10–25 q24h
40–59	8–20 q24h
20–39	4–15 q24h
10–19	4–15 q48h
5–9	4–15 q3–5d
<5	3–4 q3–5d

Administration I.M. injection into relatively large muscle and aspirate; dose of 2 g should be divided in half and given into two separate sites

Monitoring Parameters Signs and symptoms of infection including mental status

Test Interactions False-positive urine glucose using Clinitest®, positive Coombs' [direct], false elevation of serum or urine creatinine

Nursing Implications See Administration

Special Geriatric Considerations Adjust dose for renal function (estimated Cl_{cr}); see Usual Dosage. I.M. administration should be avoided in patients with limited muscle mass.

Dosage Forms Injection: 500 mg, 1 g

Cefoperazone Sodium (sef oh per' a zone)
Brand Names Cefobid®
Generic Available No
Therapeutic Class Antibiotic, Cephalosporin (Third Generation)
Use Treatment of susceptible bacterial infection; mainly respiratory tract, skin and skin structure, bone and joint, urinary tract and gynecologic as well as septicemia
Contraindications Hypersensitivity to cefoperazone or any component, cephalosporins
Precautions Use with caution in patients allergic to penicillin, increased tendency for bleeding
Adverse Reactions
    Dermatologic: Maculopapular and erythematous rash
    Gastrointestinal: Dyspepsia, diarrhea, pseudomembranous colitis, nausea
    Hematologic: Increased risk of bleeding
(Continued)

Cefoperazone Sodium (Continued)

Local: Bleeding (increased PT), pain, and induration at injection site

Overdosage Symptoms of overdose include neuromuscular hypersensitivity, convulsions

Toxicology Many beta-lactam-containing antibiotics have the potential to cause neuromuscular hyperirritability or convulsive seizures. Hemodialysis may be helpful to aid in the removal of the drug from the blood, otherwise most treatment is supportive or symptom directed.

Drug Interactions May have synergy with aminoglycosides and theoretically increase risk of nephrotoxicity; disulfiram-like reactions have been reported when alcohol was ingested within 72 hours after administration

Stability Reconstituted solution and I.V. infusion in NS or D$_5$W solution is stable for 24 hours at room temperature, 5 days when refrigerated or 3 weeks when frozen; after freezing, thawed solution is stable for 48 hours at room temperature or 10 days when refrigerated

Mechanism of Action Interferes with bacterial cell wall synthesis during active multiplication causing cell death and resultant bactericidal activity against susceptible bacteria

Pharmacokinetics

Half-life: 2 hours (half-life higher with hepatic disease or biliary obstruction); mean half-life in the elderly has been reported to be as long as 10.5 hours and appears to be affected by both renal dysfunction and nonrenal clearance

Time to peak serum concentration:

I.M.: Within 1-2 hours

I.V.: Within 15-20 minutes

Serum levels following I.V. administration are 2-3 times serum levels following I.M. administration

Elimination: Primarily via hepatobiliary pathway, 25% is eliminated renally

Usual Dosage Geriatrics and Adults: I.M., I.V.: 2-4 g/day in divided doses every 12 hours (up to 12 g/day)

Dosing adjustment in hepatic impairment: Reduce dose 50% in patients with advanced cirrhosis

Monitoring Parameters Signs and symptoms of infection including mental status

Test Interactions Prothrombin time (S), false-positive urine glucose with cupric sulfate solution (Clinitest®), positive Coombs' [direct]

Patient Information Report bleeding or bruising; avoid alcoholic beverages during and 72 hours after completion of therapy

Nursing Implications Monitor for coagulation abnormalities; may need to reduce dose in hepatic disease or biliary obstruction

Additional Information Sodium content of 1 g: 1.5 mEq

Special Geriatric Considerations See Pharmacokinetics and Usual Dosage

Dosage Forms Injection: 2 g

References

Deeter RG, Weinstein MP, Swanson KA, et al, "Crossover Assessment of Serum Bactericidal Activity and Pharmacokinetics of Five Broad-Spectrum Cephalosporins in the Elderly," *Antimicrob Agents Chemother*, 1990, 34(6):1007-13.

Meyers BR, Mendelson MN, Deeter RG, et al, "Pharmacokinetics of Cefoperazone in Ambulatory Elderly Volunteers Compared With Young Adults," *Antimicrob Agents Chemother*, 1987, 31(6):925-9.

Naber K, Adam D, Schalkhauser K, et al, "Pharmacokinetics of Cefoperazone in Geriatric Patients and Concentrations in Different Tissues of the Urinary Tract," *Excerpta Medica*, 1982, 114.

Cefotan® *see Cefotetan Disodium* *on next page*

Cefotaxime Sodium (sef oh taks' eem)

Brand Names Claforan®

Generic Available No

Therapeutic Class Antibiotic, Cephalosporin (Third Generation)

Use Treatment of documented or suspected infections including *N. gonorrhoeae* and meningitis due to susceptible organisms

Contraindications Hypersensitivity to cefotaxime or any component, cephalosporins

Warnings Prolonged use may result in superinfection

Precautions Use with caution in patients with impaired renal function or history of colitis; modify dosage in patients with renal impairment; use with caution in patients with penicillin allergy

Adverse Reactions

Central nervous system: Fever, headache, agitation, confusion

Dermatologic: Rash, pruritus

Gastrointestinal: Pseudomembranous colitis, diarrhea, nausea, vomiting

Hematologic: Transient neutropenia, thrombocytopenia

Hepatic: Transient elevation of liver enzymes

Local: Phlebitis, pain at injection site

Renal: Transient elevations of BUN or creatinine

Overdosage Symptoms of overdose include neuromuscular hypersensitivity, convulsions

Toxicology Many beta-lactam-containing antibiotics have the potential to cause neuromuscular hyperirritability or convulsive seizures. Hemodialysis may be helpful to aid in the removal of the drug from the blood, otherwise most treatment is supportive or symptom directed.

Drug Interactions
Probenecid may prolong cephalosporin half-life
May have synergy with aminoglycosides and theoretically increase risk of nephrotoxicity

Stability Reconstituted solution is stable for 24 hours at room temperature and 10 days when refrigerated; for I.V. infusion in NS or D_5W solution is stable for 24 hours at room temperature, 5 days when refrigerated or 13 weeks when frozen; after freezing, thawed solution is stable for 24 hours at room temperature or 10 days when refrigerated

Mechanism of Action Interferes with bacterial cell wall synthesis during active multiplication by binding to penicillin binding proteins, causing cell death and resultant bactericidal activity against susceptible bacteria

Pharmacokinetics
Protein binding: 31% to 50%
Metabolism: Partially in the liver to active metabolite, desacetylcefotaxime
Half-life:
Cefotaxime: 1-1.5 hours (prolonged with renal and/or hepatic impairment)
Desacetylcefotaxime: 1.5-1.9 hours (prolonged with renal impairment)
Time to peak serum concentration:
I.M.: Within 30 minutes
I.V.: Within ~5 minutes
In patients 60-80 years of age, the serum half-life was prolonged, the clearance decreased, and AUC increased for cefotaxime and less so for its desacetyl metabolite. A significantly greater increase in half-life and decrease in clearance in patients >80 years of age has been reported.

Usual Dosage Geriatrics and Adults: I.M., I.V.:
Uncomplicated gonorrhea: I.M.: Single 1 g dose
Uncomplicated infection: 1 g every 12 hours
Moderate to severe infection: 1-2 g every 6-8 hours
Life-threatening infection: 2 g/dose every 4 hours; maximum dose: 12 g/day

Dosing adjustment in renal impairment: Cl_{cr} <20 mL/minute: Reduce dose 50%
Moderately dialyzable (20% to 50%)

Administration Cefotaxime can be administered IVP over 3-5 minutes, or I.V. retrograde or I.V. intermittent infusion over 15-30 minutes; final concentration for I.V. administration should not exceed 100 mg/mL; I.M. dosing should be in a large muscle mass (ie, gluteus maximus)

Monitoring Parameters Signs and symptoms of infection including mental status

Test Interactions Positive Coombs' [direct]

Nursing Implications See Administration

Special Geriatric Considerations See Pharmacokinetics and Usual Dosage; adjust dose for renal function

Dosage Forms
Infusion, premixed (frozen): 1 g in D_5W (50 mL); 2 g in D_5W (50 mL)
Injection: 1 g, 2 g, 10 g

References
Deeter RG, Weinstein MP, Swanson KA, et al,"Crossover Assessment of Serum Bactericidal Activity and Pharmacokinetics of Five Broad-Spectrum Cephalosporins in the Elderly," *Antimicrob Agents Chemother*, 1990, 34(6):1007-13.
Ludwig E, Székely É, Csiba A, et al,"Pharmacokinetics of Cefotaxime and Desacetylcefotaxime in Elderly Patients," *Drugs*, 1988, 35(Suppl 2):51-6.

Cefotetan Disodium (sef' oh tee tan)

Brand Names Cefotan®

Generic Available No

Therapeutic Class Antibiotic, Cephalosporin (Second Generation)

Use Treatment of susceptible bacterial infection; mainly respiratory tract, skin and skin structure, bone and joint, urinary tract and gynecologic as well as septicemia

Contraindications Hypersensitivity to cefotetan or any component, cephalosporins

Precautions Use with caution in patients with a history of penicillin allergy

Adverse Reactions
Central nervous system: Fever
Dermatologic: Rash, pruritus, urticaria
Gastrointestinal: Diarrhea, nausea, vomiting, pseudomembranous colitis, abdominal pain
Hematologic: Prolongation of bleeding time or prothrombin time, neutropenia, thrombocytopenia, eosinophilia, agranulocytosis, hemolytic anemia

(Continued)

Cefotetan Disodium *(Continued)*

Local: Phlebitis

Miscellaneous: Super infection

Overdosage Symptoms of overdose include neuromuscular hypersensitivity, convulsions

Toxicology Many beta-lactam-containing antibiotics have the potential to cause neuromuscular hyperirritability or convulsive seizures. Hemodialysis may be helpful to aid in the removal of the drug from the blood, otherwise most treatment is supportive or symptom directed.

Drug Interactions

Probenecid may prolong cephalosporin half-life

Alcohol (disulfiram-like reaction)

May have synergy with aminoglycosides and theoretically increase risk of nephrotoxicity

Stability Reconstituted solution is stable for 24 hours at room temperature and 96 hours when refrigerated; for I.V. infusion in NS or D_5W solution and after freezing, thawed solution is stable for 24 hours at room temperature or 96 hours when refrigerated; frozen solution is stable for 12 weeks

Mechanism of Action Interferes with bacterial cell wall synthesis during active multiplication causing cell death and resultant bactericidal activity against susceptible bacteria

Pharmacokinetics

Protein binding: 76% to 90%

Half-life: 3-5 hours

Time to peak: I.M.: Peak plasma levels occur within 1.5-3 hours

Elimination: Primarily excreted unchanged in urine with 20% excreted in bile

Usual Dosage I.M., I.V.:

Geriatrics: Usual adult dose adjusted for renal function

Adults: 1-6 g/day in divided doses every 12 hours, 1-2 g may be given every 24 hours for urinary tract infection

Dosing interval in renal impairment:

Cl_{cr} 10-30 mL/minute: Administer every 24 hours

Cl_{cr} <10 mL/minute: Administer every 48 hours

Slightly dialyzable (5% to 20%)

Administration I.M. doses should be given in a large muscle mass (ie, gluteus maximus)

Monitoring Parameters Signs and symptoms of infection including mental status

Test Interactions Increased alkaline phosphatase, AST, ALT, BUN, creatinine, glucose, protein; decreased glucose; positive Coombs' test

Patient Information Avoid alcoholic beverages during and for 72 hours after completion of therapy

Nursing Implications Give around-the-clock to promote less variation in peak and trough serum levels; reduce dose in patients with impaired renal function; see Administration

Additional Information Sodium content of 1 g: 3.5 mEq

Special Geriatric Considerations Cefotetan has not been studied in the elderly; see Usual Dosage; adjust dose for renal function in elderly

Dosage Forms Injection: 1 g, 2 g

Cefoxitin Sodium *(se fox' i tin)*

Brand Names Mefoxin®

Generic Available No

Therapeutic Class Antibiotic, Cephalosporin (Second Generation)

Use Less active against staphylococci and streptococci than first generation cephalosporins, but active against anaerobes including *Bacteroides fragilis*; active against gram-negative enteric bacilli including *E. coli*, *Klebsiella*, and *Proteus*

Contraindications Hypersensitivity to cefoxitin or any component, cephalosporins

Warnings Prolonged use may result in superinfection

Precautions Use with caution in patients with history of colitis; cefoxitin may increase resistance of organisms by inducing beta-lactamase; use with caution and modify dosage in patients with renal impairment; use with caution in patients with a history of penicillin allergy

Adverse Reactions

Cardiovascular: Thrombophlebitis

Central nervous system: Fever

Dermatologic: Rash, exfoliative dermatitis

Gastrointestinal: Nausea, vomiting, pseudomembranous colitis, diarrhea

Hematologic: Transient leukopenia, thrombocytopenia, anemia, eosinophilia

Hepatic: Transient elevation in serum AST concentration

Local: Pain at injection site

Renal: Elevations in BUN or serum creatinine

Overdosage Symptoms of overdose include neuromuscular hypersensitivity, convulsions

Toxicology Many beta-lactam-containing antibiotics have the potential to cause neuro-muscular hyperirritability or convulsive seizures. Hemodialysis may be helpful to aid in the removal of the drug from the blood, otherwise most treatment is supportive or symptom directed.

Drug Interactions
Probenecid prolongs half-life and elevates serum concentrations
Theoretically increases risk of nephrotoxicity with other nephrotoxic drugs

Stability Reconstituted solution is stable for 24 hours at room temperature and 48 hours when refrigerated; for I.V. infusion in NS or D_5W solution is stable for 24 hours at room temperature, 1 week when refrigerated or 26 weeks when frozen; after freezing, thawed solution is stable for 24 hours at room temperature or 5 days when refrigerated

Mechanism of Action Interferes with bacterial cell wall synthesis during active multiplication causing cell death and resultant bactericidal activity against susceptible bacteria

Pharmacokinetics
Protein binding: 65% to 79%
Half-life: 45-60 minutes, increases significantly with renal insufficiency
Time to peak serum concentration:
I.M.: Within 20-30 minutes
I.V.: Within 5 minutes
Elimination: Rapidly excreted as unchanged drug (85%) in urine; poorly penetrates into CSF even with inflammation of the meninges
Compared to younger patients (<55 years), older patients (66-94 years) have been reported to have a reduced total body clearance, prolonged half-life, increased volume of distribution, and reduced protein binding

Usual Dosage I.M., I.V.:
Geriatrics: Usual adult dose adjusted for estimated Cl_{cr}
Adults: 1-2 g every 6-8 hours (I.M. injection is painful)

Dosing interval in renal impairment:
Cl_{cr} 30-50 mL/minute: Administer every 8-12 hours
Cl_{cr} 10-30 mL/minute: Administer every 12-24 hours
Cl_{cr} 5-9 mL/minute: Administer 500 mg every 12-24 hours
Cl_{cr} <5 mL/minute: Administer 500 mg every 24-48 hours
Moderately dialyzable (20% to 50%)

Administration I.M. dose should be administered in a large muscle mass (ie, gluteus maximus)

Monitoring Parameters Monitor renal function periodically when used in combination with other nephrotoxic drugs

Test Interactions Positive Coombs' [direct]; false-positive urine glucose (Clinitest®), false ↑ in serum or urine creatinine

Nursing Implications Give around-the-clock rather than 4 times/day, 3 times/day, etc (ie, 12-6-12-6, not 9-1-5-9) to promote less variation in peak and trough serum levels; modify dosage in patients with renal insufficiency; see Usual Dosage and Administration

Additional Information Sodium content of 1 g: 53 mg (2.3 mEq)

Special Geriatric Considerations See Pharmacokinetics and Usual Dosage; adjust dose for renal function in elderly

Dosage Forms
Infusion, premixed (frozen): 1 g in D_5W (50 mL): 2 g in D_5W (50 mL)
Injection: 1 g, 2 g, 10 g

References
Garcia MJ, Garcia A, Nieto MJ, et al, "Disposition of Cefoxitin in the Elderly," *Int J Clin Pharmacol Ther Toxicol*, 1980, 18(11):503-9.

Cefpodoxime Proxetil (sef pode ox' eem)

Brand Names Vantin®
Generic Available No
Therapeutic Class Antibiotic, Cephalosporin (Second Generation)
Use Treatment of susceptible acute, community-acquired pneumonia caused by *S. pneumoniae* or nonbeta-lactamase producing *H. influenzae*; acute uncomplicated gonorrhea caused by *N. gonorrhoeae*; uncomplicated skin and skin structure infections caused by *S. aureus* or *S. pyogenes*; acute otitis media caused by *S. pneumoniae, H. influenzae,* or *M. catarrhalis*; pharyngitis or tonsillitis; and uncomplicated urinary tract infections caused by *E. coli, Klebsiella,* and *Proteus*
Contraindications Hypersensitivity to cefpodoxime or cephalosporins
Warnings Modify dosage in patients with severe renal impairment; prolonged use may result in superinfection; hypersensitivity to penicillins
Adverse Reactions
Central nervous system: Headache
Dermatologic: Rash
Gastrointestinal: Nausea (3.8%), vomiting, abdominal pain, diarrhea (7.1%), pseudomembranous colitis

(Continued)

135

Cefpodoxime Proxetil (Continued)

Genitourinary: Vaginal fungal infections (3.3%)

Hematologic: Eosinophilia; leukocytosis; thrombocytosis; decrease in hemoglobin, hematocrit; leukopenia; prolonged PT and PTT

Hepatic: Transient elevation in AST, ALT, bilirubin

Renal: Increase in BUN and creatinine

Overdosage Symptoms of overdose include neuromuscular hypersensitivity, convulsions

Toxicology Many beta-lactam-containing antibiotics have the potential to cause neuromuscular hyperirritability or convulsive seizures. Hemodialysis may be helpful to aid in the removal of the drug from the blood, otherwise most treatment is supportive or symptom directed.

Drug Interactions

Antacids and H_2-receptor antagonists (reduce absorption and serum concentration of cefpodoxime)

Probenecid (inhibits renal excretion of cefpodoxime)

Stability After mixing, keep suspension in refrigerator, shake well before using; discard unused portion after 14 days

Mechanism of Action Interferes with bacterial cell wall synthesis during active multiplication, causing cell wall death and resultant bactericidal activity against susceptible bacteria

Pharmacokinetics

Absorption: Oral: Rapidly and well absorbed, acid stable; enhanced in the presence of food or low gastric pH

Distribution: Good tissue penetration, including lung and tonsils; penetrates into pleural fluid

Protein binding: 18% to 23%

Metabolism: Oral: De-esterified in the GI tract to the active metabolite, cefpodoxime

Bioavailability: Oral: 50%

Half-life: 2.2 hours (prolonged with renal impairment); elderly: 3.65 hours

Peak levels: Within 2-3 hours

Elimination: Plasma clearance: ~200-300 mL/minute; primarily eliminated by the kidney with 80% of dose excreted unchanged in urine in 24 hours

Usual Dosage Adults: Oral: 100-400 mg every 12 hours

Uncomplicated gonorrhea: 200 mg as a single dose

Dosing adjustment in renal impairment: Cl_{cr} <30 mL/minute: Administer every 24 hours

Hemodialysis patients: Dose 3 times/week following dialysis

Monitoring Parameters Signs and symptoms of infection

Test Interactions Positive Coombs' [direct]

Patient Information Take with food; chilling improves flavor (do not freeze); report persistent diarrhea; entire course of medication (10-14 days) should be taken to ensure eradication of organism; should be taken in equal intervals around-the-clock to maintain adequate blood levels; females should report symptoms of vaginitis

Nursing Implications Assess patient at beginning and throughout therapy for infection; give around-the-clock to promote less variation in peak and trough serum levels

Additional Information Dose adjustment is not necessary in patients with cirrhosis

Special Geriatric Considerations Considered one of the drugs of choice for outpatient treatment of community-acquired pneumonia in older adults; dosage adjustment is not necessary unless renal impairment; see Usual Dosage and Pharmacokinetics

Dosage Forms

Granules for oral suspension (lemon creme flavor): 50 mg/5 mL (100 mL); 100 mg/5 mL (100 mL)

Tablet, film coated: 100 mg, 200 mg

References

American Thoracic Society, "Guidelines for the Initial Management of Adults With Community-Acquired Pneumonia: Diagnosis, Assessment of Severity, and Initial Antimicrobial Therapy," Am Rev Respir Dis, 1993, 148(5):1418-26.

Backhouse C, Wade A, Williamson P, et al, "Multiple Dose Pharmacokinetics of Cefpodoxime in Young Adult and Elderly Patients," J Antimicrob Chemother, 1990, 26(Supp E):29-34.

Cefprozil

Brand Names Cefzil®

Generic Available No

Therapeutic Class Antibiotic, Cephalosporin (Second Generation)

Use Treatment of otitis media, sinusitis, and infections caused by susceptible organisms involving the respiratory tract, skin and skin structure

Contraindications Known hypersensitivity to cefprozil or any cephalosporin

Warnings Cross-allergenicity with penicillin 5% to 16%; serum sickness-like reactions and seizures (in patients with severe renal impairment) have been reported with some cephalosporins

Precautions Dose adjustment required in patients with impaired renal function; pseudomembranous colitis, superinfection

Adverse Reactions

Central nervous system: Dizziness, fatigue, confusion, tonic-clonic seizures, headache

Dermatologic: Stevens-Johnson syndrome, erythema multiforme, toxic epidermal necrolysis

Gastrointestinal: Cholestasis, nausea, vomiting, diarrhea

Hematologic: Anemia (hemolytic, aplastic), hemorrhage, hematological disorders

Hepatic: Elevated liver enzymes, total bilirubin, alkaline phosphatase, hepatic dysfunction

Renal: Renal dysfunction

Miscellaneous: Hypersensitivity reactions

Toxicology Many beta-lactam-containing antibiotics have the potential to cause neuromuscular hyperirritability or seizures. Hemodialysis may be helpful in the removal of the drug from the blood, otherwise most treatment should be supportive or symptom directed; seizures should be treated with anticonvulsant therapy such as 5-10 mg I.V. diazepam.

Drug Interactions Probenecid (elevated plasma levels and risk of toxicity)

Stability The reconstituted suspension should be refrigerated and any unused portion discarded after 14 days

Mechanism of Action Interferes with bacterial cell wall synthesis during active multiplication causing cell death and resultant bactericidal activity against susceptible bacteria

Pharmacokinetics A mixture of cis- (90%) and trans- (10%) isomers; well absorbed from the GI tract (90%); food does not delay or reduce absorption; distribution is to most body tissues including the aqueous humor, bone, soft tissues, and the CSF. Elimination is primarily renal with 60% to 70% of the drug excreted in the urine in 24 hours; hepatic dysfunction does not appear to significantly alter elimination. Significantly greater peak concentrations and area under the curve is found in patients with Cl_{cr} <30 mL/minute; also, the half-life is prolonged 1.7 vs 5.9 hours and renal clearance reduced 198 mL/minute vs 18.8 mL/minute compared to patients with normal renal function.

Usual Dosage

Geriatrics and Adults: Duration of treatment ≥10 days:

Upper respiratory tract infections; 500 mg every 24 hours

Lower respiratory tract infections: 500 mg every 12 hours

Uncomplicated skin and skin structure infections: 250-500 mg every 12 hours or 500 mg every 24 hours

Adults: 250-500 mg every 12-24 hours for 10 days

Dosing adjustment in renal impairment: Cl_{cr} 0-30 mL/minute: Administer 50% of standard dose at the standard interval

Hemodialysis patients: Give dose at the completion of hemodialysis

Monitoring Parameters Culture and sensitivity; response to treatment (fever, WBC, mental status, appetite)

Test Interactions Positive Coombs' (direct), false-positive urine glucose therapy with Clinitest® tablets, Benedict's or Fehling's solution; false-positive test for proteinuria; false-elevated urinary 17-ketosteroid values

Patient Information Complete full course of therapy; take at regular intervals; may take with food or milk; report persistent diarrhea; chilling suspension improves flavor (do not freeze)

Special Geriatric Considerations Has not been studied exclusively in the elderly; adjust dose for estimated renal function; see Usual Dosage

Dosage Forms

Powder for oral suspension: 125 mg/5 mL (50 mL, 100 mL); 250 mg/5 mL (50 mL, 100 mL)

Tablet: 250 mg, 500 mg

References

Shukla UA, Pittman KA, and Barbhaiya RH, "Pharmacokinetic Interactions of Cefprozil With Food, Propantheline, Metoclopramide, and Probenecid in Healthy Volunteers," *J Clin Pharmacol*, 1992, 32(8):725-31.

Shyu WC, Pittman KA, Wilber RB, et al, "Pharmacokinetics of Cefprozil in Healthy Subjects and Patients With Hepatic Impairment," *J Clin Pharmacol*, 1991, 31(4):372-6.

Ceftazidime (sef' tay zi deem)

Brand Names Ceptaz™; Fortaz®; Tazidime®

Generic Available No

Therapeutic Class Antibiotic, Cephalosporin (Third Generation)

Use Treatment of documented susceptible *Pseudomonas aeruginosa* infection; *Pseudomonas* infection in patient at risk of developing aminoglycoside-induced nephrotoxicity and/or ototoxicity; empiric therapy of a febrile, granulocytopenic patient

Contraindications Hypersensitivity to ceftazidime or any component, cephalosporins

Warnings Prolonged use may result in superinfection

Precautions Use with caution and modify dosage in patients with impaired renal function; use with caution in patients with history of colitis or penicillin allergy

(Continued)

Ceftazidime *(Continued)*

Adverse Reactions
Central nervous system: Fever, headache
Dermatologic: Rash
Gastrointestinal: Nausea, vomiting, pseudomembranous colitis
Hematologic: Eosinophilia, thrombocytosis, transient leukopenia, hemolytic anemia
Hepatic: Transient elevation in liver enzymes
Local: Phlebitis
Renal: BUN and creatinine increases
Miscellaneous: Candidiasis

Overdosage Symptoms of overdose include neuromuscular hypersensitivity, convulsions

Toxicology Many beta-lactam-containing antibiotics have the potential to cause neuromuscular hyperirritability or convulsive seizures. Hemodialysis may be helpful to aid in the removal of the drug from the blood, otherwise most treatment is supportive or symptom directed.

Drug Interactions Aminoglycosides: *in vitro* studies indicate additive or synergistic effect against some strains of *Enterobacteriaceae* and *Pseudomonas aeruginosa*, and theoretically may increase risk of nephrotoxicity; increased levels with probenecid

Stability Reconstituted solution and I.V. infusion in NS or D_5W solution is stable for 24 hours at room temperature, 10 days when refrigerated or 12 weeks when frozen; after freezing, thawed solution is stable for 24 hours at room temperature or 4 days when refrigerated; 96 hours under refrigeration, after mixing

Mechanism of Action Interferes with bacterial cell wall synthesis during active multiplication causing cell death and resultant bactericidal activity against susceptible bacteria

Pharmacokinetics
Distribution: Widely throughout the body including bone, bile, skin, CSF (diffuses into CSF with higher concentrations when the meninges are inflamed) endometrium, heart, pleural and lymphatic fluids
Protein binding: 17%, <10% protein binding in the elderly; in the elderly half-life increased, volume of distribution decreased, and AUC increased
Half-life: 1-2 hours (prolonged with renal impairment)
Time to peak: I.M.: Peak serum levels occur within 60 minutes
Elimination: By glomerular filtration with 80% to 90% of the dose excreted as unchanged drug within 24 hours

Usual Dosage I.M., I.V.:
Geriatric patients with normal renal function should be dosed every 12 hours

Adults: 1-2 g every 8-12 hours (250-500 mg every 12 hours for urinary tract infections)

Dosing interval in renal impairment:
Cl_{cr} 30-50 mL/minute: Administer every 12 hours
Cl_{cr} 10-30 mL/minute: Administer every 24 hours
Cl_{cr} <10 mL/minute: Administer every 48 hours
Dialyzable (50% to 100%)

Dosing in hemodialysis: 1 g loading dose, then 1 g after each dialysis session. Neurotoxicity and convulsions have been reported in dialysis patients receiving 2-3 g every 12 hours.

Administration Any carbon dioxide bubbles that may be present in the withdrawn solution should be expelled prior to injection. Ceftazidime can be administered IVP over 3-5 minutes, or I.V. retrograde or I.V. intermittent infusion over 15-30 minutes; final concentration for I.V. administration should not exceed 100 mg/mL; can be reconstituted for I.M. administration with 0.5% or 1% lidocaine if volume tolerated.

Monitoring Parameters Serum creatinine with concurrent use of an aminoglycoside; a change in renal function necessitates a change in dose; signs of infection such as fever, WBC, mental status

Test Interactions Positive Coombs' [direct], false-positive urine glucose (Clinitest®)

Additional Information Sodium content of 1 g: 54 mg (2.3 mEq). For most elderly; weak third generation cephalosporin strongest against anaerobes and gram-positive bacteria; *Pseudomonas* sp.

Special Geriatric Considerations Changes in renal function associated with aging and corresponding alterations in pharmacokinetics result in every 12-hour dosing being an adequate dosing interval

Dosage Forms
Infusion, premixed (frozen): 500 mg in D_5W (50 mL); 1 g in $D_{1.4}W$ (50 mL); 2 g in $D_{3.2}W$ (50 mL); 1 g in NS (50 mL); 2 g in NS (100 mL)
Injection: 500 mg, 1 g, 2 g, 6 g, 10 g

References
Sirgo MA and Norris S, "Ceftazidime in the Elderly: Appropriateness of Twice-Daily Dosing," *DICP Ann Pharmacother*, 1991, 25(3):284-8.
Slaker RA and Danielson B, "Neurotoxicity Associated With Ceftazidime Therapy in Geriatric Patients With Renal Dysfunction," *Pharmacotherapy*, 1991, 11(4):351-2.

Ceftin® see Cefuroxime *on page 141*

Ceftizoxime (sef ti zox' eem)
Brand Names Cefizox®
Generic Available No
Therapeutic Class Antibiotic, Cephalosporin (Third Generation)
Use Treatment of susceptible bacterial infection; mainly respiratory tract, skin and skin structure, bone and joint, urinary tract and gynecologic as well as septicemia
Contraindications Hypersensitivity to ceftizoxime or any component, cephalosporins
Precautions Use with caution in patients allergic to penicillin; reduce dosage in patients with decreased renal function
Adverse Reactions
Central nervous system: Fever, headache
Dermatologic: Rash, pruritus
Gastrointestinal: Pseudomembranous colitis, diarrhea, nausea, vomiting
Hematologic: Transient neutropenia, thrombocytopenia
Hepatic: Transient elevation of liver enzymes
Local: Burning at the injection site, phlebitis
Renal: Transient elevations in BUN or serum creatinine
Overdosage Symptoms of overdose include neuromuscular hypersensitivity, convulsions
Toxicology Many beta-lactam-containing antibiotics have the potential to cause neuromuscular hyperirritability or convulsive seizures. Hemodialysis may be helpful to aid in the removal of the drug from the blood, otherwise most treatment is supportive or symptom directed.
Drug Interactions Increased levels with probenecid; concurrent use with an aminoglycoside may increase risk of nephrotoxicity
Stability Reconstituted solution is stable for 24 hours at room temperature and 96 hours when refrigerated; for I.V. infusion in NS or D_5W solution is stable for 24 hours at room temperature, 96 hours when refrigerated or 12 weeks when frozen; after freezing, thawed solution is stable for 24 hours at room temperature or 10 days when refrigerated
Mechanism of Action Interferes with bacterial cell wall synthesis during active multiplication causing cell death and resultant bactericidal activity against susceptible bacteria
Pharmacokinetics
Distribution: V_d: 0.35-0.5 L/kg
Protein binding: 30%
Half-life: 1.6 hours (half-life increases to 25 hours when Cl_{cr} fall <10 mL/minute)
Time to peak: I.M.: Peak serum levels occur within 30-60 minutes
Elimination: Excreted unchanged in urine
One study has reported the pharmacokinetics of ceftizoxime in the elderly. Following a single 2 g I.V. dose the mean serum half-life was 3.5 hours; mean V_{dss}: 14.2 L/1.73 m^2; mean clearance: 62.5 mL/minute/1.73 m^2
Usual Dosage Geriatrics and Adults: I.M., I.V.: 1-2 g every 8-12 hours, up to 2 g every 4 hours or 4 g every 8 hours for life-threatening infections

Dosing interval in renal impairment:
Cl_{cr} 50-79 mL/minute: Administer 500-1500 mg every 8 hours
Cl_{cr} 5-49 mL/minute: Administer 250-1000 mg every 12 hours
Cl_{cr} 0-4 mL/minute (dialysis): Administer 250-1000 mg every 24-48 hours
Moderately dialyzable (20% to 50%)
Administration Give I.M. injections in a large muscle mass (ie, gluteus maximus)
Monitoring Parameters Signs and symptoms of infection including mental status
Test Interactions Increased alkaline phosphatase, AST, ALT, BUN, creatinine, glucose, protein, positive Coombs' reaction [direct]; decreased glucose; tests have been reported, false-positive urinary glucose determinations
Nursing Implications Give around-the-clock to promote less variation in peak and trough serum levels; see Administration
Additional Information Sodium content of 1 g: 60 mg (2.6 mEq)
Special Geriatric Considerations See Pharmacokinetics and Usual Dosage; adjust dose for renal function in elderly
References
Deeter RG, Weinstein MP, Swanson KA, et al, "Crossover Assessment of Serum Bactericidal Activity and Pharmacokinetics of Five Broad-Spectrum Cephalosporins in the Elderly," *Antimicrob Agents Chemother*, 1990, 34(6):1007-13.

Ceftriaxone Sodium (sef try ax' one)
Brand Names Rocephin®
Generic Available No
Therapeutic Class Antibiotic, Cephalosporin (Third Generation)
Use Treatment of documented infection due to susceptible organisms including the lower respiratory tract, skin and skin structure, bone and joint, intra-abdominal, urinary tract, meningitis, septicemia, and gonorrhea
(Continued)

Ceftriaxone Sodium *(Continued)*

Contraindications Hypersensitivity to ceftriaxone sodium or any component, cephalosporins

Warnings Prolonged use may result in superinfection

Precautions Use with caution in patients with gallbladder, biliary tract, liver, pancreatic disease, or history of colitis; use with caution in patients allergic to penicillin

Adverse Reactions

Dermatologic: Rash

Gastrointestinal: Diarrhea, nausea, vomiting, colitis, sludging in the gallbladder

Hematologic: Eosinophilia; thrombocytosis; leukopenia; anemia; increased prothrombin time

Hepatic: Jaundice, transient elevation in liver enzymes, cholelithiasis

Local: Pain at injection site

Renal: Increased BUN

Overdosage Symptoms of overdose include neuromuscular hypersensitivity, convulsions

Toxicology Many beta-lactam-containing antibiotics have the potential to cause neuromuscular hyperirritability or convulsive seizures. Hemodialysis may be helpful to aid in the removal of the drug from the blood, otherwise most treatment is supportive or symptom directed.

Drug Interactions Increased levels with probenecid; may have synergy with the aminoglycosides and theoretically increase the risk of nephrotoxicity; alcohol (disulfiram-like reaction)

Stability Reconstituted solution (100 mg/mL) is stable for 3 days at room temperature and 3 days when refrigerated; for I.V. infusion in NS or D_5W solution is stable for 3 days at room temperature, 10 days when refrigerated or 26 weeks when frozen; after freezing, thawed solution is stable for 3 days at room temperature or 10 days when refrigerated

Mechanism of Action Interferes with bacterial cell wall synthesis during active multiplication causing cell death and resultant bactericidal activity against susceptible bacteria

Pharmacokinetics

Distribution: Widely throughout the body including gallbladder, lungs, bone, bile, CSF (diffuses into the CSF at higher concentrations when the meninges are inflamed)

Protein binding: 85% to 95%

Half-life: 5-9 hours (with normal renal and hepatic function)

Time to peak:

I.M.: Peak serum levels occur within 1-2 hours

I.V.: Within minutes

Elimination: Excreted unchanged in urine (33% to 65%) by glomerular filtration and in feces

Studies of ceftriaxone in the elderly have found a prolonged serum half-life (15 hours) and a reduced total clearance with or without a change in the volume of distribution. The change in renal clearance has been correlated to a reduction in Cl_{cr}. An increased free fraction was also found in one study suggesting a reduction in protein binding.

Usual Dosage Geriatrics and Adults: I.M., I.V.: 1-2 g every 12-24 hours depending on the type and severity of the infection; usual dose: 1-2 g every 24 hours; maximum dose: 4 g/day

Dosing adjustment in renal or hepatic impairment: Not necessary

Uncomplicated gonorrhea: Single 250 mg I.M. dose

Administration Give I.M. doses in a large muscle mass (ie, maximus gluteus)

Monitoring Parameters Signs and symptoms of infection including mental status

Test Interactions False-positive urine glucose with Clinitest®

Nursing Implications Give around-the-clock to promote less variation in peak and trough serum levels; see Administration

Additional Information Sodium content of 1 g: 2.6 mEq

Special Geriatric Considerations See Pharmacokinetics and Usual Dosage; no adjustment for renal function necessary

Dosage Forms

Infusion, premixed (frozen): 1 g in $D_{3.8}W$ (50 mL); 2 g in $D_{24}W$ (50 mL)

Injection: 250 mg, 500 mg, 1 g, 2 g, 10 g

References

Deeter RG, Weinstein MP, Swanson KA, et al, "Crossover Assessment of Serum Bactericidal Activity and Pharmacokinetics of Five Broad-Spectrum Cephalosporins in the Elderly," *Antimicrob Agents Chemother*, 1990, 34(6):1007-13.

Hayton WL and Stoeckel K, "Age-Associated Changes in Ceftriaxone Pharmacokinetics," *Clin Pharmacokinet*, 1986, 11(1):76-82.

Luderer JR, Patel IH, Durkin J, et al, "Age and Ceftriaxone Kinetics," *Clin Pharmacol Ther*, 1984, 35(1):19-25.

Richards DM, Heel RC, Brogden RN, et al, "Ceftriaxone: A Review of Its Antibacterial Activity, Pharmacological Properties and Therapeutic Use," *Drugs*, 1984, 27(6):469-527.

Cefuroxime (se fyoor ox' eem)

Brand Names Ceftin®; Kefurox®; Zinacef®

Generic Available No

Therapeutic Class Antibiotic, Cephalosporin (Second Generation)

Use Infections caused by staphylococci, group B streptococci, *H. influenzae* (type A and B), *E. coli*, *Enterobacter*, *Salmonella*, and *Klebsiella*; treatment of susceptible infections of the lower respiratory tract, otitis media, urinary tract, skin and soft tissue, bone and joint, sepsis and gonorrhea

Contraindications Hypersensitivity to cefuroxime or any component, cephalosporins

Warnings Prolonged use may result in superinfection

Precautions Use with caution and modify dosage in patients with renal impairment; use with caution in patients with history of colitis; use with caution in patients allergic to penicillin

Adverse Reactions

Cardiovascular: Thrombophlebitis

Central nervous system: Dizziness, fever, headache

Dermatologic: Rash

Gastrointestinal: Nausea, vomiting, diarrhea, stomach cramps, GI bleeding, pseudomembranous colitis

Genitourinary: Vaginitis

Hematologic: Transient neutropenia and leukopenia, decreased hemoglobin and hematocrit, eosinophilia

Hepatic: Transient increase in liver enzymes

Local: Pain at the injection site

Renal: Transient elevation in creatinine or BUN

Overdosage Symptoms of overdose include neuromuscular hypersensitivity, convulsions

Toxicology Many beta-lactam-containing antibiotics have the potential to cause neuromuscular hyperirritability or convulsive seizures. Hemodialysis may be helpful to aid in the removal of the drug from the blood, otherwise most treatment is supportive or symptom directed.

Drug Interactions Concomitant administration with an aminoglycoside may result in synergy and theoretically increase the risk of nephrotoxicity; probenecid increases serum levels of cefuroxime

Stability Reconstituted solution is stable for 24 hours at room temperature and 48 hours when refrigerated; for I.V. infusion in NS or D_5W solution is stable for 24 hours at room temperature, 7 days when refrigerated or 26 weeks when frozen; after freezing, thawed solution is stable for 24 hours at room temperature or 21 days when refrigerated

Mechanism of Action Interferes with bacterial cell wall synthesis during active multiplication causing cell death and resultant bactericidal activity against susceptible bacteria

Pharmacokinetics

Absorption: Increased when given with or shortly after food

Protein binding: 33% to 50%

Bioavailability: Oral cefuroxime axetil: 37% to 52%

Half-life (adults): 1-2 hours (prolonged in renal impairment)

The serum half-life of cefuroxime is prolonged in the elderly due to decreased renal function; mean half-life: 2-4 hours

Time to peak:

I.M.: Peak plasma levels occur within 15-60 minutes

I.V.: 2-3 minutes

Elimination: Primarily excreted 66% to 100% as unchanged drug in urine by both glomerular filtration and tubular secretion; can be removed by dialysis

Usual Dosage Geriatrics and Adults:

Oral: 125-500 mg twice daily, depending on severity of infection

I.M., I.V.: 750-1.5 g every 6 hours; maximum: 6 g/24 hours

Dosing interval in renal impairment:

Cl_{cr} >20 mL/minute: Administer 750-1500 mg every 8 hours

Cl_{cr} 10-20 mL/minute: Administer 750 mg every 12 hours

Cl_{cr} <10 mL/minute: Administer 750 mg every 24 hours

Hemodialysis patients: Give doses following dialysis

Administration Tablets can be crushed and given with soft foods to mask the bitter taste; I.M. doses should be given deep into a large muscle (ie, gluteus maximus)

Monitoring Parameters Signs and symptoms of infection including mental status

Test Interactions Positive Coombs' [direct]; false-positive urine glucose with Clinitest®

Patient Information Complete full course of therapy, do not skip doses; can be taken with food or milk; notify physician if severe diarrhea occurs

Nursing Implications Give around-the-clock to promote less variation in peak and trough serum levels; see Administration

Additional Information Sodium content of 1 g: 54.2 mg (2.4 mEq)

Special Geriatric Considerations See Pharmacokinetics and Usual Dosage; adjust

(Continued)

Cefuroxime *(Continued)*

dose for renal function in elderly; consider one of the drugs of choice for outpatient treatment of community-acquired pneumonia in the older adult

Dosage Forms
Infusion, premixed (frozen): 750 mg in $D_{2.8}W$ (50 mL); 1.5 g in water (50 mL)
Injection, as cefuroxime sodium: 750 mg, 1.5 g, 7.5 g
Tablet, as cefuroxime axetil: 125 mg, 250 mg, 500 mg

References
American Thoracic Society, "Guidelines for the Initial Management of Adults With Community-Acquired Pneumonia: Diagnosis Assessment of Severity and Initial Antimicrobial Therapy," *Am Rev Respir Dis*, 1993, 148(5):1418-26.
Broekhuysen J, Deger F, Douchamps J, et al, "Pharmacokinetic Study of Cefuroxime in the Elderly," *Br J Clin Pharmacol*, 1981, 21(6):801-5.
Douglas JG, Bax RP, and Munro JF, "The Pharmacokinetics of Cefuroxime in the Elderly," *J Antimicrob Chemother*, 1980, 6(4):543-9.

Cefzil® *see* Cefprozil *on page 136*

Celestone® *see* Betamethasone *on page 82*

Celestone® Soluspan® *see* Betamethasone *on page 82*

Celontin® *see* Methsuximide *on page 457*

Cel-U-Jec® *see* Betamethasone *on page 82*

Cenafed® [OTC] *see* Pseudoephedrine *on page 609*

Cenafed® Plus [OTC] *see* Triprolidine and Pseudoephedrine *on page 723*

Cena-K® *see* Potassium Chloride *on page 576*

Cenocort® *see* Triamcinolone *on page 710*

Cenocort® Forte *see* Triamcinolone *on page 710*

Centrax® *see* Prazepam *on page 581*

Cephalexin Monohydrate *(sef a lex' in)*

Brand Names Cefanex®; C-Lexin®; Entacef®; Keflet®; Keflex®; Keftab®
Generic Available Yes
Therapeutic Class Antibiotic, Cephalosporin (First Generation)
Use Treatment of susceptible bacterial infections, including those caused by group A beta-hemolytic *Streptococcus, Staphylococcus, Klebsiella pneumoniae, E. coli, Proteus mirabilis,* and *Shigella*
Contraindications Hypersensitivity to cephalexin or any component, cephalosporins
Warnings Prolonged use may result in superinfection
Precautions Use with caution and modify dosage in patients with renal impairment; use with caution in patients with history of colitis; use with caution in patients with penicillin allergy
Adverse Reactions
Central nervous system: Dizziness, fatigue, headache
Dermatologic: Rash
Gastrointestinal: Nausea, vomiting, pseudomembranous colitis, abdominal cramps
Hematologic: Transient neutropenia, anemia, positive Coombs' test
Hepatic: Transient elevation in liver enzymes
Overdosage Symptoms of overdose include neuromuscular hypersensitivity, convulsions
Toxicology Many beta-lactam-containing antibiotics have the potential to cause neuromuscular hyperirritability or convulsive seizures. Hemodialysis may be helpful to aid in the removal of the drug from the blood, otherwise most treatment is supportive or symptom directed.
Drug Interactions Increased levels with probenecid; theoretical synergy and increased risk of nephrotoxicity with aminoglycosides
Stability Refrigerate suspension after reconstitution; discard after 14 days
Mechanism of Action Interferes with bacterial cell wall synthesis during active multiplication causing cell death and resultant bactericidal activity against susceptible bacteria
Pharmacokinetics
Half-life: 0.5-1.2 hours (prolonged with renal impairment)
Protein binding: 6% to 15%
Time to peak: Oral: Peak serum levels occur within 60 minutes
Elimination: 80% to 100% of dose excreted as unchanged drug in urine within 8 hours
Usual Dosage Geriatrics and Adults: Oral: 250-1000 mg every 6 hours
Dosing interval in renal impairment:
Cl_{cr} 10-40 mL/minute: Administer every 8-12 hours
Cl_{cr} 5-10 mL/minute: Administer every 12 hours
Cl_{cr} <5 mL/minute: Administer every 12-24 hours

Moderately dialyzable (20% to 50%)

Monitoring Parameters Signs and symptoms of infection

Test Interactions False-positive urine glucose with Clinitest®; positive Coombs' test [direct]; false ↑ serum or urine creatinine

Patient Information Complete full course of therapy; may take with food or milk if GI upset occurs; notify physician if severe diarrhea occurs

Nursing Implications Give on an empty stomach (ie, 1 hour prior to, or 2 hours after meals) to increase total absorption; give around-the-clock rather than 4 times/day to promote less variation in peak and trough serum levels

Special Geriatric Considerations See Usual Dosage; adjust dose for renal function

Dosage Forms

Capsule: 250 mg, 500 mg

Suspension, oral: 125 mg/5 mL (5 mL unit dose, 60 mL, 100 mL, 200 mL); 250 mg/5 mL (5 mL unit dose, 100 mL, 200 mL)

Tablet: 250 mg, 500 mg, 1 g

Tablet, as hydrochloride: 250 mg, 500 mg

Cephalothin Sodium (sef a' loe thin)

Brand Names Keflin®

Generic Available Yes

Therapeutic Class Antibiotic, Cephalosporin (First Generation)

Use Treatment of susceptible bacterial infections, including those caused by group A beta-hemolytic *Streptococcus*

Contraindications Hypersensitivity to cephalothin, cephalosporins

Warnings Prolonged use might result in superinfection

Precautions Modify dosage according to renal function; use with caution in patients with penicillin allergy

Adverse Reactions

Dermatologic: Maculopapular and erythematous rash

Gastrointestinal: Dyspepsia, diarrhea, pseudomembranous colitis, nausea, vomiting

Local: Bleeding, pain, and induration at injection site

Overdosage Symptoms of overdose include neuromuscular hypersensitivity, convulsions

Toxicology Many beta-lactam-containing antibiotics have the potential to cause neuromuscular hyperirritability or convulsive seizures. Hemodialysis may be helpful to aid in the removal of the drug from the blood, otherwise most treatment is supportive or symptom directed.

Drug Interactions Increased levels with probenecid; concomitant administration with an aminoglycoside may result in synergy and theoretically increase the risk of nephrotoxicity

Stability Reconstituted solution is stable for 12-24 hours at room temperature and 96 hours when refrigerated; for I.V. infusion in NS or D_5W solution is stable for 24 hours at room temperature, 96 hours when refrigerated or 12 weeks when frozen; after freezing, thawed solution is stable for 24 hours at room temperature or 96 hours when refrigerated

Mechanism of Action Interferes with bacterial cell wall synthesis during active multiplication causing cell death and resultant bactericidal activity against susceptible bacteria

Pharmacokinetics

Protein binding: 65% to 80%; does not penetrate the CSF unless the meninges are inflamed

Metabolism: Partially deacetylated in the liver and kidney

Half-life: 30-60 minutes

Time to peak:

I.M.: Within 30 minutes

I.V.: Peak serum levels occur within 15 minutes

Elimination: 50% to 75% of dose appears as unchanged drug in urine

In a small number (4) of bedridden elderly, the half-life and volume of distribution were increased and the total clearance decreased compared to younger healthy volunteers

Usual Dosage Geriatrics and Adults: I.M., I.V.: 500 mg to 2 g every 4-6 hours

Dosing interval in renal impairment: See table.

Cephalothin Sodium

Cl_{cr} (mL/min)	Maximum dose (g) for each dosing interval
50–80	2 q6h
25–50	1.5 q6h
10–25	1 q6h
2–10	0.5 q6h
<2	0.5 q8h

ALPHABETICAL LISTING OF DRUGS

Cephalothin Sodium *(Continued)*

Monitoring Parameters Signs and symptoms of infection including mental status
Test Interactions Increased creatinine (S), prothrombin time (S), glucose; positive Coombs' [direct], increased protein; decreased glucose
Nursing Implications Give I.M. dose deep into large muscle mass (ie, gluteus maximus) to decrease pain and induration
Additional Information Sodium content of 1 g: 2.8 mEq
Special Geriatric Considerations See Pharmacokinetics and Usual Dosage; adjust dose for renal function in elderly
Dosage Forms Powder for injection: 1 g, 2 g, 4 g, 20 g
References
Yasuhara H, Kobayashi S, Sakamoto K, et al, "Pharmacokinetics of Amikacin and Cephalothin in Bedridden Elderly Patients," *J Clin Pharmacol*, 1982, 22(8-9):403-9.

Cephapirin Sodium (sef a pye' rin)
Brand Names Cefadyl®
Generic Available No
Therapeutic Class Antibiotic, Cephalosporin (First Generation)
Use Treatment of infections when caused by susceptible strains in serious respiratory, genitourinary, gastrointestinal, skin and soft-tissue, bone and joint infections; septicemia; endocarditis
Contraindications Hypersensitivity to cephapirin or any component, cephalosporins
Warnings Prolonged use might result in superinfection
Precautions Modify dose according to renal function; use with caution in patients with penicillin allergy
Adverse Reactions
Central nervous system: CNS irritation, seizures, fever
Dermatologic: Rash, urticaria
Gastrointestinal: Diarrhea, pseudomembranous colitis
Hematologic: Leukopenia, thrombocytopenia, positive Coombs' test
Hepatic: Transient elevation of liver enzymes
Overdosage Symptoms of overdose include neuromuscular hypersensitivity, convulsions
Toxicology Many beta-lactam-containing antibiotics have the potential to cause neuromuscular hyperirritability or convulsive seizures. Hemodialysis may be helpful to aid in the removal of the drug from the blood, otherwise most treatment is supportive or symptom directed.
Drug Interactions Decreased elimination and increased serum concentration with probenecid; theoretic synergy and increased risk for nephrotoxicity with aminoglycosides
Stability Reconstituted solution is stable for 24 hours at room temperature and 10 days when refrigerated; for I.V. infusion in NS or D_5W solution is stable for 24 hours at room temperature, 10 days when refrigerated or 14 days when frozen; after freezing, thawed solution is stable for 12 hours at room temperature or 10 days when refrigerated
Mechanism of Action Interferes with bacterial cell wall synthesis during active multiplication causing cell death and resultant bactericidal activity against susceptible bacteria
Pharmacokinetics
Protein binding: 22% to 25%
Metabolism: Partially in the liver, kidney and plasma
Half-life: 36-60 minutes
Time to peak serum concentration:
I.M.: Within 30 minutes
I.V.: Within 5 minutes
Elimination: Metabolites (50% active) excreted in urine; 60% to 85% is excreted as unchanged drug in urine
Usual Dosage Geriatrics and Adults: I.M., I.V.: 1 g every 6 hours up to 12 g/day
Dosing interval in renal impairment: Cl_{cr} <10 mL/minute: Administer every 12 hours
Hemodialysis patients: 7.5-15 mg/kg just prior to dialysis and every 12 hours thereafter
Administration Give I.M. doses deep into a large muscle mass (ie, gluteus maximus)
Monitoring Parameters Signs and symptoms of infection including mental status
Test Interactions Positive Coombs' [direct]; increased glucose, protein; decreased glucose
Nursing Implications See Administration
Special Geriatric Considerations Cephapirin has not been studied in the elderly; see Usual Dosage; adjust dose for renal function
Dosage Forms Injection: 1 g, 2 g

144

Cephradine (sef' ra deen)

Brand Names Anspor®; Ro-Ceph®; Velosef®

Generic Available Yes

Therapeutic Class Antibiotic, Cephalosporin (First Generation)

Use Treatment of susceptible bacterial infections, including those caused by group A beta-hemolytic *Streptococcus*

Contraindications Hypersensitivity to cephradine or any component, cephalosporins

Warnings Prolonged use may result in superinfection

Precautions Modify dose according to renal function; use with caution in patients with penicillin allergy

Adverse Reactions

Dermatologic: Rash

Gastrointestinal: Nausea, vomiting, diarrhea, pseudomembranous colitis

Renal: Increased BUN and creatinine

Overdosage Symptoms of overdose include neuromuscular hypersensitivity, convulsions

Toxicology Many beta-lactam-containing antibiotics have the potential to cause neuromuscular hyperirritability or convulsive seizures. Hemodialysis may be helpful to aid in the removal of the drug from the blood, otherwise most treatment is supportive or symptom directed.

Drug Interactions Decreased elimination and increased serum concentrations with probenecid; theoretical synergy and increased risk of nephrotoxicity with aminoglycosides

Stability Reconstituted solution is stable for 2 hours at room temperature and 24 hours when refrigerated; for I.V. infusion in NS or D_5W solution is stable for 10 hours at room temperature, 48 hours when refrigerated or 6 weeks when frozen; after freezing, thawed solution is stable for 10 hours at room temperature or 48 hours when refrigerated

Mechanism of Action Interferes with bacterial cell wall synthesis during active multiplication causing cell death and resultant bactericidal activity against susceptible bacteria

Pharmacokinetics

Absorption: Oral: Faster than I.M. absorption, yet well absorbed from all routes

Protein binding: 18% to 20%

Half-life: 1-2 hours

Time to peak: Oral, I.M.: Peak serum concentrations occur within 60-120 minutes

Elimination: ~80% to 90% of drug recovered in urine as unchanged drug within 6 hours

Usual Dosage Geriatrics and Adults: Oral, I.M., I.V.: 2-4 g/day in 4 equally divided doses up to 8 g/day

Dosing adjustment in renal impairment:

Cl_{cr} >20 mL/minute: Administer 500 mg every 6 hours

Cl_{cr} 5-20 mL/minute: Administer 250 mg every 6 hours

Cl_{cr} <5 mL/minute: Administer 250 mg every 12 hours

Hemodialysis patients: 250 mg at the start of dialysis, then 250 mg at 12 and 36-48 hours later

Administration I.M. doses should be given deep into a large muscle mass (ie, gluteus maximus)

Monitoring Parameters Signs and symptoms of infection including mental status

Test Interactions Positive Coombs' [direct]; increased glucose, protein; decreased glucose

Patient Information Complete full course of therapy, do not miss doses; may be taken with food or milk; call physician if severe diarrhea occurs

Nursing Implications See Administration

Special Geriatric Considerations Cephradine has not been studied in the elderly; see Usual Dosage; adjust dose for renal function in elderly

Dosage Forms

Capsule: 250 mg, 500 mg

Powder for injection: 250 mg, 500 mg, 1 g, 2 g vials

Suspension, oral: 125 mg/5 mL (100 mL); 250 mg/5 mL (200 mL)

Tablet: 1 g

Cetane® [OTC] *see* Ascorbic Acid *on page 57*

Cetapred® *see* Sodium Sulfacetamide and Prednisolone Acetate *on page 652*

Cevalin® [OTC] *see* Ascorbic Acid *on page 57*

Ce-Vi-Sol® [OTC] *see* Ascorbic Acid *on page 57*

Cevita® [OTC] *see* Ascorbic Acid *on page 57*

Cheracol® *see* Guaifenesin and Codeine *on page 332*

Chlo-Amine® [OTC] *see* Chlorpheniramine Maleate *on page 152*

Chloracol® *see* Chloramphenicol *on page 148*

Chloral *see* Chloral Hydrate *on this page*

Chloral Hydrate (klor al hye' drate)

Related Information
Anxiolytic/Hypnotic Use in Long-Term Care Facilities *on page 755-756*

Brand Names Noctec®; Somnos®

Synonyms Chloral; Hydrated Chloral; Trichloroacetaldehyde Monohydrate

Generic Available Yes

Therapeutic Class Hypnotic; Sedative

Use Short-term sedative and hypnotic (<2 weeks), sedative/hypnotic for dental and diagnostic procedures; sedative prior to EEG evaluations

Restrictions C-IV

Contraindications Hypersensitivity to chloral hydrate or any component; hepatic or renal impairment; gastritis or ulcers; severe cardiac disease

Warnings Trichloroethanol (TCE), a metabolite of chloral hydrate, is a carcinogen in mice; there is no data in humans

Precautions Use with caution in patients with porphyria

Adverse Reactions
Central nervous system: Disorientation, sedation, ataxia, excitement (paradoxical), dizziness, fever, headache, "hangover" effect
Dermatologic: Rash, urticaria
Gastrointestinal: Gastric irritation, nausea, vomiting, diarrhea, flatulence
Hematologic: Leukopenia, eosinophilia
Miscellaneous: Physical and psychological dependence may occur with prolonged use of large doses

Overdosage Symptoms of overdose include hypotension, respiratory depression, coma, hypothermia, cardiac arrhythmias

Toxicology Treatment is supportive and symptomatic; lidocaine or propranolol may be used for ventricular dysrhythmias, while isoproterenol or atropine may be required for torsade de pointes; activated charcoal may prevent drug absorption

Drug Interactions
Increased effect of warfarin, CNS depressants, alcohol
Increased toxicity with alcohol (flushing, tachycardia, etc), furosemide,® intravenous (flushing, diaphoresis, and blood pressure changes)

Stability Sensitive to light; exposure to air causes volatilization; store in light-resistant, airtight container

Mechanism of Action Central nervous system depressant effects are due to its active metabolite trichloroethanol, mechanism unknown

Pharmacodynamics
Peak effect: Within 30-60 minutes
Duration: 4-8 hours

Pharmacokinetics
Absorption: Oral, rectal: Well absorbed
Protein binding: Trichloroacetic acid is highly protein bound and displaces other acidic drugs
Metabolism: Rapid to trichloroethanol; variable amounts metabolized in liver and kidney to trichloroacetic acid (inactive)
Half-life: Trichloroethanol: 8-11 hours
Elimination: Metabolites excreted in urine; small amounts excreted in feces via bile

Usual Dosage
Geriatrics: Hypnotic: Initial: Oral: 250 mg at bedtime

Adults:
Sedation, anxiety: Oral, rectal: 250 mg 3 times/day
Hypnotic: Oral, rectal: 500-1000 mg at bedtime or 30 minutes prior to procedure, not to exceed 2 g/24 hours

Dosing adjustment/comments in renal impairment: Cl_{cr} <50 mL/minute: Avoid use
Dialyzable (50% to 100%)

Dosing adjustment/comments in hepatic impairment: Avoid use in patients with severe hepatic impairment

Administration Do not crush capsule; contains drug in liquid form

Monitoring Parameters Mental status, vital signs

Test Interactions False-positive urine glucose using Clinitest® method; may interfere with fluorometric urine catecholamine and urinary 17-hydroxycorticosteroid tests

Patient Information Take capsule with a full glass of water or fruit juice; swallow capsules whole, do not chew; avoid alcohol and other CNS depressants; avoid activities needing good psychomotor coordination until CNS effects are known; drug may cause physical or psychological dependence; avoid abrupt discontinuation after prolonged use; if taking at home prior to a diagnostic procedure, have someone else transport you

Nursing Implications Gastric irritation may be minimized by diluting dose in water or other oral liquid

Additional Information Tolerance to hypnotic effect develops, therefore, not recommended for use >2 weeks; taper dosage to avoid withdrawal with prolonged use

Special Geriatric Considerations Chloral hydrate is considered a second line hypnotic agent in the elderly; interpretive guidelines from the Health Care Financing Administration (HCFA) discourage the use of chloral hydrate in residents of long-term care facilities

Dosage Forms
Capsule: 250 mg, 500 mg
Suppository: 325 mg, 500 mg, 650 mg
Syrup: 250 mg/5 mL, 500 mg/5 mL

Chlorambucil (klor am' byoo sil)

Brand Names Leukeran®

Generic Available No

Therapeutic Class Antineoplastic Agent, Alkylating Agent (Nitrogen Mustard)

Use Management of chronic lymphocytic leukemia, Hodgkin's and non-Hodgkin's lymphoma; management of nephrotic syndrome unresponsive to conventional therapy; breast and ovarian carcinoma; Waldenström macroglobulinemia, testicular carcinoma, thrombocythemia, choriocarcinoma; rheumatoid arthritis; idiopathic membranous nephropathy

Contraindications Hypersensitivity to chlorambucil or any component, or previous resistance, severe bone marrow depression; cross-hypersensitivity with other alkylating agents may occur

Warnings The U.S. Food and Drug Administration (FDA) currently recommends that procedures for proper handling and disposal of antineoplastic agents be considered. Can severely suppress bone marrow function; affects human fertility; carcinogenic in humans and probably mutagenic and teratogenic as well; chromosomal damage has been documented; secondary AML may be associated with chronic therapy

Precautions Use with caution in patients with seizure disorder and bone marrow suppression; reduce initial dosage if patient has received radiation therapy, myelosuppressive drugs or has a depressed baseline leukocyte or platelet count within the previous 4 weeks

Adverse Reactions
Central nervous system: Confusion, ataxia, seizures
Dermatologic: Rash
Endocrine & metabolic: Hyperuricemia
Gastrointestinal: Nausea, vomiting, oral ulcers
Genitourinary: Oligospermia
Hematologic: Leukopenia, thrombocytopenia, anemia
Hepatic: Hepatotoxicity with jaundice
Neuromuscular & skeletal: Peripheral neuropathy, tremors, muscle twitching, weakness
Respiratory: Pulmonary fibrosis
Miscellaneous: Drug fever

Overdosage Symptoms of overdose include vomiting, ataxia, coma, seizures, agitation, tremor, confusion, pancytopenia

Toxicology There are no known antidotes for chlorambucil intoxication, and treatment is mainly supportive, directed at decontaminating the GI tract and controlling symptoms; blood products may be used to treat the hematologic toxicity

Drug Interactions Bone marrow suppression may be enhanced with other antineoplastic agents

Stability Protect from light

Mechanism of Action Interferes with DNA replication and RNA transcription by alkylation and cross-linking the strands of DNA (bifunctional alkylating agent)

Pharmacokinetics
Absorption: Oral: Well absorbed
Protein binding (mostly albumin): ~99%
Metabolism: In the liver to an active metabolite
Half-life: 6 minutes
Time to peak: Peak plasma levels occur in 1 hour

(Continued)

Chlorambucil *(Continued)*

Elimination: 60% excreted in urine within 24 hours principally as metabolites

Usual Dosage Oral (refer to individual protocols):

Geriatrics: Use lowest recommended doses for adults; usual dose for elderly is 2-4 mg/day, particularly for use in treatment of rheumatoid arthritis

Adults: General short courses: 0.1-0.2 mg/kg/day or 4-8 mg/m^2/day for 2-3 weeks for remission induction, then adjust dose on basis of blood counts; maintenance therapy: 0.03-0.1 mg/kg/day

Nephrotic syndrome: 0.1-0.2 mg/kg/day every day for 5-15 weeks with low dose prednisone

CLL: Biweekly regimen: Initial: 0.4 mg/kg dose is increased by 0.1 mg/kg every 2 weeks until a response occurs and/or myelosuppression occurs; monthly regimen: Initial: 0.4 mg/kg, increase dose by 0.2 mg/kg every 4 weeks until a response occurs and/or myelosuppression occurs

Malignant lymphomas: Non-Hodgkin's lymphoma: 0.1 mg/kg/day; Hodgkin's: 0.2 mg/kg/day

Not dialyzable

Monitoring Parameters Monitor WBC and platelet counts closely (weekly); observe for CNS side effects/toxicity

Test Interactions Increased potassium (S)

Patient Information Any signs of infection (fever, chills, sore throat), easy bruising or bleeding, shortness of breath, black tarry stools, yellow discoloration of skin or eyes, bloody or dark urine, joint pain, swelling, or painful or burning urination should be brought to physician's attention. Nausea, vomiting or hair loss sometimes occurs. Food may delay absorption; take on empty stomach; avoid alcohol, prolonged sun exposure. May cause loss of appetite.

Nursing Implications See Monitoring Parameters, Patient Information, and Additional Information

Additional Information

Myelosuppressive effects:

WBC: Moderate

Platelets: Moderate

Onset (days): 7

Nadir (days): 10-14

Recovery (days): 28

Special Geriatric Considerations Toxicity to immunosuppressives is increased in elderly. Start with lowest recommended adult doses; see Usual Dosage. Signs of infection, such as fever and rise in WBCs, may not occur. Lethargy and confusion may be more prominent signs of infection.

Dosage Forms Tablet, sugar coated: 2 mg

References

Hutchins LF and Lipschitz DA, "Cancer, Clinical Pharmacology, and Aging," *Clin Geriatr Med*, 1987, 3(3):483-503.

Kaplan HG, "Use of Cancer Chemotherapy in the Elderly," *Drug Treatment in the Elderly*, Vestal RE, ed, Boston, MA: ADIS Health Science Press, 1984, 338-49.

Chloramphenicol *(klor am fen' i kole)*

Brand Names AK-Chlor®; Anocol®; Chloracol®; Chlorofair®; Chloromycetin®; Chloroptic®; Econochlor®; I-Chlor®; Ocu-Chlor®; Ophthochlor®; Spectro-Chlor®

Generic Available Yes

Therapeutic Class Antibiotic, Miscellaneous; Antibiotic, Ophthalmic; Antibiotic, Otic

Use Treatment of serious infections due to organisms resistant to other less toxic antibiotics or when its penetrability into the site of infection is clinically superior to other antibiotics to which the organism is sensitive; useful in infections caused by *Bacteroides, H. influenzae, Neisseria meningitidis, Salmonella,* and *Rickettsia*

Contraindications Hypersensitivity to chloramphenicol or any component

Warnings Serious and fatal blood dyscrasias have occurred after both short-term and prolonged therapy; should not be used when less potentially toxic agents are effective; prolonged use may result in superinfection; use with care in patients with glucose 6-phosphate dehydrogenase deficiency

Precautions Reduce dose with impaired liver function

Adverse Reactions

Central nervous system: Nightmares, headache, mental depression, confusion, delirium

Dermatologic: Rash

Gastrointestinal: Diarrhea, stomatitis, enterocolitis, unpleasant taste, nausea, vomiting

Hematologic: Bone marrow depression, aplastic anemia

Neuromuscular & skeletal: Peripheral neuropathy

Ocular: Optic neuritis

Overdosage Symptoms of overdose include anemia, metabolic acidosis, hypotension, hypothermia

Drug Interactions

Chloramphenicol inhibits the metabolism and may increase the effects of chlorpropamide, tolbutamide, phenytoin, phenobarbital, oral anticoagulants, cyclophosphamide

Phenobarbital and rifampin may decrease concentration of chloramphenicol

Acetaminophen may increase chloramphenicol serum concentrations

Response to iron and vitamin B_{12} may be decreased; avoid concomitant use with other drugs that may cause bone marrow depression

Stability Refrigerate ophthalmic solution; constituted solutions remain stable for 30 days; use only clear solutions; frozen solutions remain stable for 6 months

Mechanism of Action Reversibly binds to 50S ribosomal subunits of susceptible organisms preventing amino acids from being transferred to growing peptide chains thus inhibiting protein synthesis

Pharmacokinetics

Absorption: Oral: 75% to 100%

Chloramphenicol palmitate is hydrolyzed in the GI tract to the base; chloramphenicol sodium succinate must be hydrolyzed by esterases to active base

Protein binding: 60%

Metabolism: Extensive metabolism in the liver (90%) to inactive metabolites, principally by glucuronidation

Half-life: 1.6-3.3 hours (increased with hepatic insufficiency)

Time to peak: Oral: Peak serum levels occur within 30 minutes to 3 hours

Elimination: 5% to 15% excreted as unchanged drug in urine and 4% excreted in bile

Usual Dosage Geriatrics and Adults:

Ophthalmic: Apply 1-2 drops or small amount of ointment every 3-6 hours; increase interval between applications after 48 hours

Topical: Gently rub into the affected area 3-4 times/day

Meningitis: Oral, I.V.: 50 mg/kg/day in divided doses every 6 hours; maximum daily dose: 4 g/day

Slightly dialyzable (5% to 20%)

Monitoring Parameters Complete blood count with reticulocyte count should be done before therapy and then weekly; periodic liver and renal function; see Reference Levels

Reference Range

Sample size: 0.5-2 mL blood (red top tube) or 0.1-1 mL serum (separated)

Therapeutic: 15-20 μg/mL; Toxic: >40 μg/mL

Timing of serum samples: Draw levels 1.5 hours and 3 hours after I.V. dose or oral dose

Test Interactions Increased iron (B), prothrombin time (S); decreased urea nitrogen (B)

Patient Information Take on empty stomach; take with food if GI upset, at evenly spaced intervals (every 6 hours around-the-clock); notify physician if fever, sore throat, unusual bruising or bleeding, or decreased energy are experienced

Nursing Implications Give around-the-clock rather than 4 times/day to promote less variation in peak and trough serum levels; see Monitoring Parameters

Additional Information Sodium content of 1 g (injection): 51.8 mg (2.25 mEq)

Special Geriatric Considerations Chloramphenicol has not been studied in the elderly; it is not necessary to adjust the dose based upon the decrease in renal function associated with age. Chloramphenicol should be reserved for serious infections and the oral form avoided.

Dosage Forms

Capsule: 250 mg, 500 mg

Cream: 1% (30 g)

Injection, as sodium succinate: 100 mg/mL

Ointment, ophthalmic: 1% (3.5 g)

Powder for solution, ophthalmic: 25 mg/vial

Solution:

Ophthalmic: 0.5% (7.5 mL)

Otic: 0.5% (15 mL)

References

Nahata MC and Powell DA, "Bioavailability and Clearance of Chloramphenicol After Intravenous Chloramphenicol Succinate," *Clin Pharmacol Ther*, 1981, 30(3):368-72.

Yoshikawa TT, "Antimicrobial Therapy for the Elderly Patient," *J Am Geriatr Soc*, 1990, 38(12):1353-72.

Chlorate® [OTC] *see* Chlorpheniramine Maleate *on page 152*

Chlordiazepoxide (klor dye az e pox' ide)

Related Information

Anxiolytic/Hypnotic Use in Long-Term Care Facilities *on page 755-756*

Benzodiazepines Comparison *on page 802-803*

Brand Names Libritabs®; Librium®

Synonyms Methaminodiazepoxide Hydrochloride

(Continued)

Chlordiazepoxide (Continued)

Generic Available Yes

Therapeutic Class Benzodiazepine; Hypnotic; Sedative

Use Management of anxiety and as a preoperative sedative, symptoms of alcohol withdrawal

Restrictions C-IV

Contraindications Hypersensitivity to chlordiazepoxide or any component, may be cross-sensitive with other benzodiazepines; pre-existing CNS depression, severe uncontrolled pain, narrow-angle glaucoma, severe respiratory depression

Precautions Use with caution in patients with liver dysfunction or a history of drug dependence

Adverse Reactions
Cardiovascular: Hypotension, tachycardia, edema
Central nervous system: Drowsiness, ataxia, confusion, mental impairment
Dermatologic: Skin eruptions
Gastrointestinal: Nausea, constipation
Hematologic: Blood dyscrasias
Neuromuscular & skeletal: Reflex slowing
Miscellaneous: Drug dependence, **falls in the elderly**

Overdosage Symptoms of overdose include hypotension, respiratory depression, coma, hypothermia, cardiac arrhythmias

Toxicology Treatment for benzodiazepine overdose is supportive; rarely is mechanical ventilation required; flumazenil has been shown to selectively block the binding of benzodiazepines to CNS receptors, resulting in a reversal of benzodiazepine-induced CNS depression; respiratory depression may not be reversed

Drug Interactions
Decreased metabolism: Cimetidine, fluoxetine
Increased metabolism: Rifampin
Increased toxicity: CNS depressants, alcohol

Stability Refrigerate injection; protect from light

Mechanism of Action Benzodiazepines appear to potentiate the effects of GABA and other inhibitory neurotransmitters by binding to specific benzodiazepine-receptor sites in various areas of the CNS

Pharmacodynamics Studies have shown that the elderly are more sensitive to the effects of benzodiazepines as compared to younger adults

Pharmacokinetics
Absorption: I.M.: Slow and erratic
Distribution: V_d: 3.3 L/kg
Protein binding: 90% to 98%
Metabolism: Extensive in the liver to desmethyldiazepam (active and long-acting)
Half-life: 6.6-25 hours; increased in elderly and in severe liver disease
Time to peak serum concentration:
Oral: Within 2 hours
I.M.: Results in lower peak plasma levels than oral administration
Elimination: Very little excreted in urine as unchanged drug

Usual Dosage
Geriatrics: Anxiety: Oral: 5 mg 2-4 times/day

Adults:
Anxiety: Oral: 15-100 mg divided 3-4 times/day
Alcohol withdrawal symptoms: Oral, I.V.: 50-100 mg to start, dose may be repeated in 2-4 hours as necessary to a maximum of 300 mg/24 hours

Dosing adjustment in renal impairment: Cl_{cr} <10 mL/minute: 50% of dose
Not dialyzable (0% to 5%)

Administration I.V. form is a powder and should be reconstituted with 5 mL of sterile water or saline prior to administration; do not use diluent provided with ampul for I.V. administration

Monitoring Parameters Respiratory, cardiovascular and mental status; check for orthostasis

Reference Range Therapeutic: 0.1-3 μg/mL (SI: 0-10 μmol/L); Toxic: >23 μg/mL (SI: >77 μmol/L)

Patient Information Avoid alcohol and other CNS depressants; may cause drowsiness; avoid activities needing good psychomotor coordination until CNS effects are known; may cause physical or psychological dependence; avoid abrupt discontinuation after prolonged use

Nursing Implications Up to 300 mg may be given I.M. or I.V. during a 6-hour period, but not more than this in any 24-hour period (see Administration); assist patient with ambulation during initiation of therapy

Special Geriatric Considerations See Pharmacodynamics and Pharmacokinetics; due to its long-acting metabolite, chlordiazepoxide is not considered a drug of choice in the elderly; long-acting benzodiazepines have been associated with falls in the elderly; interpretive guidelines from the Health Care Financing Administration (HCFA) discourage the use of this agent in residents of long-term care facilities

Dosage Forms
Capsule: 5 mg, 10 mg, 25 mg
Injection: 100 mg/ampul
Tablet: 5 mg, 10 mg, 25 mg

References
Hicks R, Dysken MW, Davis JM, et al, "The Pharmacokinetics of Psychotropic Medication in the Elderly: A Review," *J Clin Psychiatry*, 1981, 42(10):374-85.
Reidenberg MM, Levy M, Warner H, et al, "Relationship Between Diazepam Dose, Plasma Level, Age, and Central Nervous System Depression," *Clin Pharmacol Ther*, 1978, 23(4):371-4.

Chlorhexidine Gluconate (klor hex' i deen)

Brand Names Hibiclens® [OTC]; Peridex®
Generic Available No
Therapeutic Class Antibiotic, Oral Rinse; Antibiotic, Topical
Use Skin cleanser for surgical scrub, cleanser for skin wounds, germicidal hand rinse, and as antibacterial dental rinse; chlorhexidine is active against gram-positive and gram-negative organisms, facultative anaerobes, aerobes, and yeast
Contraindications Known hypersensitivity to chlorhexidine gluconate
Adverse Reactions Staining of oral surfaces (mucosa, teeth, dorsum of tongue) may be visible as soon as one week after therapy begins and is more pronounced when there is a heavy accumulation of unremoved plaque and when teeth fillings have rough surfaces. Stain does not have a clinically adverse effect but because removal may not be possible, patient with frontal restoration should be advised of the potential permanency of the stain. Inform patient that reduced taste perception during treatment is reversible with discontinuation of chlorhexidine.
Usual Dosage Geriatrics and Adults: Oral rinse (Peridex®):
Precede use of solution by flossing and brushing teeth, completely rinse toothpaste from mouth; swish 15 mL undiluted oral rinse around in mouth for 30 seconds, then expectorate. Caution patient not to swallow the medicine; avoid eating for 2-3 hours after treatment. (The cap on bottle of oral rinse is a measure for 15 mL.)
When used as a treatment of gingivitis, the regimen begins with oral prophylaxis. Patient treats mouth with 15 mL chlorhexidine; swish for 30 seconds, then expectorate. This is repeated twice daily (morning and evening). Patient should have a re-evaluation followed by a dental prophylaxis every 6 months.
Patient Information Do not swallow, do not rinse after use; may cause reduced taste perception which is reversible; keep out of eyes and ears; may discolor teeth
Special Geriatric Considerations See Usual Dosage
Dosage Forms
Liquid, topical, with isopropyl alcohol 4%:
Dyna-Hex® Skin Cleanser: 2% (120 mL, 240 mL, 480 mL, 960 mL, 4000 mL); 4% (120 mL, 240 mL, 480 mL, 4000 mL)
Exidine® skin cleanser, Hibiclens® skin cleanser: 4% (15 mL, 120 mL, 240 mL, 480 mL, 960 mL, 4000 mL)
Rinse:
Oral (mint flavor) (Peridex®): 0.12% with alcohol 11.6% (480 mL)
Topical (Hibistat® hand rinse): 0.5% with isopropyl alcohol 70% (120 mL, 240 mL)
Sponge/Brush (Hibiclens®): 4% with isopropyl alcohol 4% (22 mL)
Wipes (Hibistat®): 0.5% (50s)

Chlorobenzoxazoline *see Chlorzoxazone on page 160*

Chlorofair® *see Chloramphenicol on page 148*

Chloromycetin® *see Chloramphenicol on page 148*

Chloroptic® *see Chloramphenicol on page 148*

Chlorothiazide (klor oh thye' a zide)

Brand Names Diuril®
Generic Available Yes: Tablet
Therapeutic Class Diuretic, Thiazide
Use Management of mild to moderate hypertension, or edema associated with congestive heart failure, or nephrotic syndrome in patients unable to take oral hydrochlorothiazide, when a thiazide is the diuretic of choice
Contraindications Hypersensitivity to chlorothiazide or any component; cross-sensitivity with other thiazides or sulfonamides; do not use in anuric patients.
Warnings The injection must not be administered S.C. or I.M.; I.V. chlorothiazide should only be used in emergency situations or when the patient is unable to take the oral form
Precautions May cause hyperbilirubinemia, fluid and electrolyte imbalance, hyperglycemia, hyperuricemia
Adverse Reactions
Cardiovascular: Hypotension
Dermatologic: Rash, photosensitivity
Endocrine & metabolic: Hypokalemia, hypochloremic alkalosis, hyperglycemia, hyperlipidemia, hyponatremia, hyperuricemia
(Continued)

Chlorothiazide *(Continued)*

Genitourinary: Prerenal azotemia

Hematologic: Rarely blood dyscrasias

Overdosage Symptoms of overdose include electrolyte depletion, volume depletion

Toxicology Treatment is primarily symptomatic and supportive; hypotension responds to fluids and Trendelenburg position; replace electrolytes as necessary

Drug Interactions

Decreased effect: NSAIDs; when given with digoxin, diuretic-induced hypokalemia increases the risk of digoxin toxicity

Decreased effect of oral hypoglycemics; decreased absorption with cholestyramine and colestipol

Increased effect with furosemide and other loop diuretics

Increased toxicity/levels of lithium

Stability Reconstituted solution is stable for 24 hours at room temperature; precipitation will occur in <24 hours in pH is <7.4

Mechanism of Action Inhibits sodium reabsorption in the distal tubules causing increased excretion of sodium and water as well as potassium and hydrogen ions

Pharmacodynamics

Onset of action: Oral: Diuresis: 2 hours

Duration:

Oral: 6-12 hours

I.V.: Diuretic action: ~2 hours

Pharmacokinetics

Absorption: Oral: Poor

Half-life: 1-2 hours

Time to peak serum concentration: Within 4 hours

Usual Dosage

Geriatrics: Oral: 500 mg once daily or 1 g 3 times/week

Adults: Oral, I.V.: 500 mg to 2 g/day divided in 1-2 doses

Administration I.V. must be prepared with at least 15 mL of diluent

Monitoring Parameters Blood pressure (standing and sitting/supine), serum electrolytes, renal function, I & O, weight

Test Interactions Increased ammonia (B), amylase (S), calcium (S), chloride (S), cholesterol (S), glucose, uric acid (S); decreased chloride (S), magnesium, potassium (S), sodium (S)

Patient Information Take in the morning; may cause increased sensitivity to sunlight; rise slowly from lying down or sitting

Nursing Implications Injection must **not** be administered S.C. or I.M., see Monitoring Parameters; check patient for orthostasis

Additional Information Sodium content of 500 mg injection: 57.5 mg (2 mEq)

Special Geriatric Considerations Chlorothiazide is minimally effective in patients with a Cl_{cr} <30 mL/minute; this may limit the usefulness of chlorothiazide in the elderly

Dosage Forms

Injection, as sodium: 25 mg/mL (20 mL)

Suspension: 250 mg/5 mL (237 mL)

Tablet: 250 mg, 500 mg

Chlorphed®-LA Nasal Solution [OTC] *see* Oxymetazoline Hydrochloride *on page 530*

Chlorphed® [OTC] *see* Brompheniramine Maleate *on page 95*

Chlorpheniramine Maleate *(klor fen ir' a meen)*

Brand Names Aller-Chlor® [OTC]; AL-R® [OTC]; Chlo-Amine® [OTC]; Chlorate® [OTC]; Chlor-Pro® [OTC]; Chlor-Trimeton® [OTC]; Kloromin® [OTC]; Phenetron®; Telachlor®; Teldrin® [OTC]

Generic Available Yes

Therapeutic Class Antihistamine

Use Perennial and seasonal allergic rhinitis and other allergic symptoms including urticaria

Contraindications Hypersensitivity to chlorpheniramine maleate or any component; narrow-angle glaucoma, bladder neck obstruction, symptomatic prostate hypertrophy, asthmatic attacks, and stenosing peptic ulcer

Warnings Antihistamines are more likely to cause dizziness, excessive sedation, syncope, toxic confusional states, and hypotension in the elderly

Precautions Use with caution in patients with heart disease, hypertension, thyroid disease, and asthma

Adverse Reactions

Central nervous system: Drowsiness, headache, paradoxical excitability

Dermatologic: Dermatitis

Gastrointestinal: Nausea, dry mouth

Ocular: Diplopia

Genitourinary: Polyuria, urinary retention

Neuromuscular & skeletal: Weakness

Respiratory: Thick bronchial secretions

Overdosage Symptoms of overdose include dry mouth, flushed skin, dilated pupils, CNS depression

Toxicology There is no specific treatment for an antihistamine overdose, however, most of its clinical toxicity is due to anticholinergic effects. Anticholinesterase inhibitors may be useful by reducing acetylcholinesterase. Anticholinesterase inhibitors include physostigmine, neostigmine, pyridostigmine and edrophonium. For anticholinergic overdose with severe life-threatening symptoms, physostigmine 1-2 mg I.V., slowly may be given to reverse these effects.

Drug Interactions Increased toxicity (CNS depression): CNS depressants, monoamine oxidase inhibitors, alcohol, tricyclic antidepressants, phenothiazines

Stability Injectable form should be protected from light

Mechanism of Action Competes with histamine for H_1-receptor sites on effector cells in the gastrointestinal tract, blood vessels, and respiratory tract

Pharmacokinetics

Protein binding: 69% to 72%

Metabolism: In the liver

Half-life: 20-24 hours; one study found no significant difference in the half-life in elderly subjects though there was wide interindividual variation

Elimination: Metabolites and parent drug (3% to 4%) excreted in urine; 35% of total within 48 hours

Usual Dosage

Oral:

Geriatrics: 4 mg once or twice daily or 8 mg sustained release at bedtime. **Note:** Duration of action may be 36 hours or more even when serum concentrations are low.

Adults: 4 mg every 4-6 hours, not to exceed 24 mg/day or sustained release 8-12 mg every 12 hours

I.M., I.V., S.C.: Adults: 5-20 mg every 4-12 hours; maximum: 40 mg/24 hours

Administration Do not crush sustained release tablet

Monitoring Parameters Relief of symptoms

Patient Information May cause drowsiness; avoid CNS depressants and alcohol; swallow whole, do not crush or chew

Nursing Implications Raise bed rails, institute safety measures, assist with ambulation

Additional Information Chlorpheniramine is available in various combinations. These include acetaminophen; phenylephrine; phenylpropanolamine; pseudoephedrine; phenylephrine and phenyltoloxamine; phenylpropanolamine and acetaminophen; pseudoephedrine and iodine; phenyltoloxamine, phenylpropanolamine, and phenylephrine.

Special Geriatric Considerations See Contraindications, Warnings, and Usual Dosage; anticholinergic action may cause significant confusional symptoms

Dosage Forms

Capsule: 12 mg

Capsule, timed release: 8 mg, 12 g

Injection: 10 mg/mL (1 mL, 30 mL); 100 mg/mL (2 mL)

Syrup: 2 mg/5 mL (120 mL, 473 mL)

Tablet: 4 mg, 8 mg, 12 mg

Tablet:

Chewable: 2 mg

Timed release: 8 mg, 12 mg

References

Simons KJ, Martin TJ, Watson WT, et al, "Pharmacokinetics and Pharmacodynamics of Terfenadine and Chlorpheniramine in the Elderly," *J Allergy Clin Immunol*, 1990, 85(3):540-7.

Chlorpromazine Hydrochloride (klor proe' ma zeen)

Related Information

Antacid Drug Interactions *on page 764*

Antipsychotic Agents Comparison *on page 801*

Antipsychotic Medication Guidelines *on page 754*

Brand Names Ormazine; Thorazine®

Generic Available Yes

Therapeutic Class Antiemetic; Antipsychotic Agent; Phenothiazine Derivative

Use Treatment of nausea and vomiting; psychoses; Tourette's syndrome; mania; intractable hiccups (adults); behavioral problems in nonpsychotic symptoms associated with dementia in elderly; Huntington's chorea; spasmodic torticollis; see Special Geriatric Considerations

Contraindications Hypersensitivity to chlorpromazine hydrochloride or any component; cross-sensitivity with other phenothiazines may exist; avoid use in patients with narrow-angle glaucoma, bone marrow depression, severe liver or cardiac disease; subcortical brain damage; circulatory collapse; severe hypotension or hypertension

(Continued)

Chlorpromazine Hydrochloride *(Continued)*

Warnings Significant hypotension may occur, especially when the drug is adminis
tered parenterally; extended release capsules and injection contain benzyl alcohol; in
jection also contains sulfites which may cause allergic reaction

Tardive dyskinesia: Prevalence rate may be 40% in elderly; elderly women especiall
at risk; embarrassment from dyskinesias may lead to greater social isolation; deve
opment of the syndrome and the irreversible nature are proportional to duration an
total cumulative dose over time. May be reversible if diagnosed early in therapy; in
termittent use of antipsychotics (not proven use) helps decrease total cumulativ
dose.

EPS: Extrapyramidal reactions are more common in elderly with up to 50% developin
these reactions after age 60. These reactions may be more common in dementi
patients. Drug-induced **Parkinson's syndrome** occurs often. Discontinuation usu
ally resolves symptoms but may take weeks to months (12+) to clear. **Akathisia** i
the most common EPS reaction in elderly. The symptoms of motor restlessness ar
difficult to diagnose in demented elderly; increased nervousness, assertiveness
restlessness with constant movement may indicate this adverse event. Conside
decreasing dose if antipsychotic to treat as well as diagnose problem; usually se
this reaction within 2-3 months of initiating antipsychotic drug.

Anticholinergic effects: These side effects most common with low potency antipsy
chotics (eg, thioridazine, chlorpromazine). CNS toxicity occurs more frequently an
severely in elderly; increased confusion, memory loss, psychotic behavior, and ag
tation frequently occur as a consequence of anticholinergic effects to antipsychoti
agents. Peripheral anticholinergic action troublesome to elderly; most peripheral an
ticholinergic effects last only 2-3 weeks; see Adverse Reactions.

Orthostatic hypotension: More common with low potency agents (eg, thioridazine
chlorpromazine, and clozapine) but of concern with all antipsychotic agents
orthostasis due to alpha-receptor blockade by antipsychotic agents. Elderly pres
ent many risk factors for orthostatic hypotension: blunted baroreceptor reflexes, de
creased vascular tone, decreased vascular volume, and possible presence of card
ac diseases which result in decreased cardiac output.

Sedation: Common side effect with antipsychotic therapy; should not be used as
hypnotic unless insomnia is associated with target behavior symptoms treated wit
antipsychotic medications; see Special Geriatric Considerations. Anecdotal report
suggesting antipsychotic sedation in nonpsychotic patients is extremely unpleas
ant due to feelings of depersonalization, derealization, and dysphoria. Due to th
long duration of action with antipsychotic drugs, these reactions may last up to 2
hours and result in decreased daytime function.

Cardiac toxicity: Life-threatening arrhythmias have occurred at therapeutic doses
antipsychotics. Thioridazine more commonly demonstrates EKG changes tha
other antipsychotics; suggested to use high potency antipsychotic agents (ie
haloperidol) in patients with cardiac conduction defects.

Precautions Use with caution in patients with cardiovascular disease, seizures, an
Parkinson's disease; benefits of therapy must be weighed against risks

Adverse Reactions

Cardiovascular: Hypotension (especially with I.V. use), orthostatic hypotension
tachycardia, arrhythmias, abnormal T waves with prolonged ventricular repolariza
tion

Central nervous system: Sedation, drowsiness, restlessness, anxiety, extrapyramida
reactions, pseudoparkinsonian signs and symptoms, tardive dyskinesia, neurolep
tic malignant syndrome, seizures, altered central temperature regulation

Dermatologic: Hyperpigmentation, pruritus, rash, photosensitivity

Endocrine & metabolic: Amenorrhea, galactorrhea, gynecomastia

Gastrointestinal: GI upset, dry mouth (problem for denture users), constipation, ady
namic ileus, weight gain

Genitourinary: Urinary retention, overflow incontinence, priapism, sexual dysfunctior
(up to 60%), impotence

Hematologic: Agranulocytosis, leukopenia (usually in patients with large doses fo
prolonged periods), thrombocytopenia, hemolytic anemia, eosinophilia

Hepatic: Cholestatic jaundice (rare)

Ocular: Retinal pigmentation, blurred vision

Miscellaneous: Anaphylactoid reactions

Overdosage Symptoms of overdose include deep sleep, coma, extrapyramidal symp
toms, abnormal involuntary muscle movements, hypotension or hypertension; agita
tion, restlessness, fever, hypothermia or hyperthermia, seizures, cardiac arrhythmias
EKG changes

Toxicology Following initiation of essential overdose management, toxic symptom
treatment and supportive treatment should be initiated. Hypotension usually re
sponds to I.V. fluids or Trendelenburg positioning. If unresponsive to these measures
the use of a parenteral inotrope may be required (eg, norepinephrine 0.1-0.2 mcg/kg
minute titrated to response). Do not use epinephrine. Seizures commonly respond to

diazepam (I.V. 5-10 mg bolus every 15 minutes if needed up to a total of 30 mg) or to phenytoin or phenobarbital. Also critical cardiac arrhythmias often respond to I.V. phenytoin (15 mg/kg up to 1 g), while other antiarrhythmics can be used. Neuroleptics often cause extrapyramidal symptoms (eg, dystonic reactions) requiring management with diphenhydramine 1-2 mg/kg up to a maximum of 50 mg I.V. slow push followed by a maintenance dose for 48-72 hours. When these reactions are unresponsive to diphenhydramine, benztropine mesylate I.V. 1-2 mg may be effective. These agents are generally effective within 2-5 minutes.

Drug Interactions
Alcohol may increase CNS sedation
Anticholinergic agents may decrease pharmacologic effects; increase anticholinergic side effects; may enhance tardive dyskinesia
Aluminum salts may decrease absorption of phenothiazines
Barbiturates may decrease phenothiazine serum concentrations
Bromocriptine may have decreased efficacy when administered with phenothiazines
Guanethidine's hypotensive effect is decreased by phenothiazines
Lithium administration with phenothiazines may increase disorientation
Meperidine and phenothiazine coadministration increases sedation and hypotension
Methyldopa administration with phenothiazine (trifluoperazine) may significantly increase blood pressure
Norepinephrine, epinephrine have decreased pressor effect when administered with chlorpromazine; therefore, be aware of possible decreased effectiveness or when any phenothiazine is used
Phenytoin serum concentrations may increase or decrease with phenothiazines; tricyclic antidepressants may have increased serum concentrations with concomitant administration with phenothiazines
Propranolol administered with phenothiazines may increase serum concentrations of both drugs
Valproic acid may have increased half-life when administered with phenothiazines (chlorpromazine)

Stability Slightly yellowed solution does not indicate potency loss, but a markedly discolored solution should be discarded; diluted injection (1 mg/mL) with NS and stored in 5 mL vials remain stable for 30 days; protect all dosage forms from light, clear or slightly yellow solutions may be used; should be dispensed in amber or opaque vials/bottles. Solutions may be diluted or mixed with fruit juices or other liquids but must be administered immediately after mixing; do not prepare bulk dilutions or store bulk dilutions.

Mechanism of Action Blocks postsynaptic mesolimbic dopaminergic D_1 and D_2 receptors in the brain; exhibits a strong alpha-adrenergic blocking and anticholinergic effect, depresses the release of hypothalamic and hypophyseal hormones; believed to depress the reticular activating system thus affecting basal metabolism, body temperature, wakefulness, vasomotor tone, and emesis

Pharmacokinetics
Metabolism: Extensive in the liver to active and inactive metabolites
Half-life:
Biphasic: 30 hours
Phase 1 half-life: 2 hours
Elimination: <1% excreted as unchanged drug in urine within 24 hours

Usual Dosage
Geriatrics (nonpsychotic patient; dementia behavior): Initial: 10-25 mg 1-2 times/day; increase at 4- to 7-day intervals by 10-25 mg/day. Increase dose intervals (bid, tid, etc) as necessary to control behavior response or side effects; maximum daily dose: 800 mg; gradual increases (titration) may prevent some side effects or decrease their severity.

Adults:
Psychosis:
Oral: Range: 30-800 mg/day in 1-4 divided doses, initiate at lower doses and titrate as needed; usual dose is 200 mg/day; some patients may require 1-2 g/day
I.M., I.V.: Initial: 25 mg, may repeat (25-50 mg) in 1-4 hours, gradually increase to a maximum of 400 mg/dose every 4-6 hours until patient controlled; usual dose 300-800 mg/day
Nausea and vomiting:
Oral: 10-25 mg every 4-6 hours
I.M., I.V.: 25-50 mg every 4-6 hours
Rectal: 25-100 mg every 6-8 hours

Not dialyzable (0% to 5%)

Monitoring Parameters Orthostatic blood pressures; tremors, gait changes, abnormal movement in trunk, neck, buccal area or extremities; monitor target behaviors for which the agent is given

Reference Range Therapeutic: 30-300 ng/mL (SI: 157-942 nmol/L); Toxic: >750 ng/mL (SI: >2355 nmol/L); serum concentrations not often obtained since dose is titrated to best response, also correlation to response is controversial

(Continued)

Chlorpromazine Hydrochloride (Continued)

Test Interactions False-positives for phenylketonuria, amylase, uroporphyrins, urobilinogen; possible false-negative pregnancy urinary test

Patient Information Oral concentrate must be diluted in 2-4 oz of liquid (water, fruit juice, carbonated drinks, milk, or pudding); do not take antacid within 1 hour of taking drug; avoid alcohol; avoid excess sun exposure (use sun block); may cause drowsiness, rise slowly from recumbent position; use of supportive stockings may help prevent orthostatic hypotension

Nursing Implications Dilute oral concentrate with water or juice before administration; avoid skin contact with oral suspension or solution; may cause contact dermatitis; monitor orthostatic blood pressures 3-5 days after initiation of therapy or a dose increase; observe for tremor and abnormal movement or posturing (extrapyramidal symptoms); watch for hypotension when administering I.M. or I.V.

Special Geriatric Considerations See Warnings

Many elderly patients receive antipsychotic medications for inappropriate nonpsychotic behavior. Before initiating antipsychotic medication, the clinician should investigate any possible reversible cause; any stress or stress from any disease can cause acute "confusion" or worsening of baseline nonpsychotic behavior. Most commonly acute changes in behavior are due to increases in drug dose or addition of new drug to regimen; fluid electrolyte loss; infections; and changes in environment.

Any changes in disease status in any organ system can result in behavior changes.

Dosage Forms

Capsule, sustained action: 30 mg, 75 mg, 150 mg, 200 mg, 300 mg

Concentrate: 30 mg/mL (120 mL); 100 mg/mL (60 mL, 240 mL)

Injection: 25 mg/mL (1 mL, 2 mL, 10 mL)

Suppository: 25 mg, 100 mg

Syrup: 10 mg/5 mL (120 mL)

Tablet: 10 mg, 25 mg, 50 mg, 100 mg, 200 mg

Chlorpropamide (klor proe' pa mide)

Brand Names Diabinese®

Generic Available Yes

Therapeutic Class Antidiabetic Agent; Hypoglycemic Agent, Oral; Sulfonylurea Agent

Use Adjunct to diet for the management of mild to moderately severe, stable noninsulin-dependent (type II) diabetes mellitus

Unlabeled use: Nephrogenic diabetes insipidus

Contraindications Cross-sensitivity may exist with other hypoglycemics or sulfonamides; do not use with type I diabetes, or with severe renal, hepatic, thyroid, or other endocrine disease, diabetes complicated by ketoacidosis; patients with reduced renal function, dietary noncompliance or irregular meals, alcohol abusers

Precautions Patients should be properly instructed in the early detection and treatment of hypoglycemia

Adverse Reactions

Cardiovascular: Edema

Central nervous system: Headache, dizziness

Dermatologic: Rash, hives, photosensitivity

Endocrine & metabolic: Hypoglycemia, hyponatremia, SIADH

Gastrointestinal: Anorexia, nausea, vomiting, diarrhea, constipation, heartburn, epigastric fullness

Hematologic: Aplastic anemia, hemolytic anemia, bone marrow depression, agranulocytosis

Hepatic: Jaundice

Overdosage Symptoms of overdose include low blood glucose levels, tingling of lips and tongue, tachycardia, convulsions, stupor, coma

Toxicology Intoxications with sulfonylureas can cause hypoglycemia and are best managed with glucose administration (oral for milder hypoglycemia or by injection in more severe forms)

Drug Interactions

Decreased chlorpropamide effectiveness with thiazides, hydantoins (eg, phenytoin), and beta-adrenergic blockers

Increased toxicity: Increased alcohol-associated disulfiram reactions; increased oral anticoagulant effect; salicylates → ↑ chlorpropamide effect → ↓ blood glucose; MAO inhibitors increased hypoglycemic response; sulfonamides → ↓ sulfonylureas clearance

Mechanism of Action Stimulates insulin release from the pancreatic beta cells; reduces glucose output from the liver; insulin sensitivity is increased at peripheral target sites

Pharmacodynamics

Peak clinical effect: Oral: Within 6-8 hours

Duration: May exceed 60 hours in the elderly

Pharmacokinetics

Distribution: V_d: 0.13-0.23 L/kg, increased in older diabetics

Protein binding: 88% to 99%

Metabolism: Extensive (~80%) in the liver; clearance decreased in older patients with diabetes

Half-life: 30-42 hours, prolonged in the elderly or with renal disease; in older diabetics: 99 hours

Time to peak: Peak serum levels occur within 3-4 hours

Elimination: 10% to 30% excreted in urine as unchanged drug

Usual Dosage Oral (dosage is variable and should be individualized based upon the patient's response):

Geriatrics: Initial: 100 mg once daily; increase by 50-125 mg/day at 3- to 5-day intervals; maximum daily dose: 750 mg

Adults: 250 mg once daily; subsequent dosages may be increased or decreased by 50-125 mg/day at 3- to 5-day intervals; maximum daily dose: 750 mg

Monitoring Parameters Fasting blood glucose, Hgb A_{1c} or fructosamine levels

Reference Range Glucose: Adults: 60-115 mg/dL; elderly fasting blood glucose: 100-150 mg/dL

Test Interactions Positive Coombs' [direct]; decreased cholesterol (S), decreased prothrombin time (S), decreased sodium (S)

Patient Information Avoid hypoglycemia, eat regularly, do not skip meals; carry a quick source of sugar with you

Nursing Implications Patients who are anorexic or NPO may need to hold the dose to avoid hypoglycemia

Additional Information Long half-life may complicate recovery from excess effects

Special Geriatric Considerations Because of chlorpropamide's long half-life, duration of action, drug interactions, and the increased risk for hypoglycemia, it is not considered a hypoglycemic agent of choice in the elderly; see Pharmacokinetics and Pharmacodynamics. How "tightly" a geriatric patient's blood glucose should be controlled is controversial; however, a fasting blood sugar of <150 mg/dL is now an acceptable end point. Such a decision should be based on the patient's functional and cognitive status, how well they recognize hypoglycemic or hyperglycemic symptoms, and how to respond to them, and their other disease states.

Dosage Forms Tablet: 100 mg, 250 mg

References

Arrigoni L, Fundak G, Horn J, et al, "Chlorpropamide Pharmacokinetics in Young Healthy Adults and Older Diabetic Patients," *Clin Pharm*, 1987, 6(2):162-4.

Chlor-Pro® [OTC] *see* Chlorpheniramine Maleate *on page 152*

Chlorprothixene (klor proe thix' een)

Related Information

Antipsychotic Agents Comparison *on page 801*

Antipsychotic Medication Guidelines *on page 754*

Brand Names Taractan®

Generic Available No

Therapeutic Class Antipsychotic Agent; Thioxanthene Derivative

Use Management of manifestations of psychotic disorders; depressive neurosis; alcohol withdrawal; nausea and vomiting; nonpsychotic symptoms associated with dementia in elderly, Tourette's syndrome; Huntington's chorea; spasmodic torticollis and Reye's syndrome; see Special Geriatric Considerations

Contraindications Circulatory collapse, hypersensitivity to chlorprothixene or any component; may cross react with thiothixene; comatose states due to central depressant drugs; severe CNS depression; subcortical brain damage; severe hypotension or hypertension; avoid use in patients with narrow-angle glaucoma, blood dyscrasias, severe liver or cardiac disease

Warnings

Tardive dyskinesia: Prevalence rate may be 40% in elderly; elderly women especially at risk; embarrassment from dyskinesias may lead to greater social isolation; development of the syndrome and the irreversible nature are proportional to duration and total cumulative dose over time. May be reversible if diagnosed early in therapy; intermittent use of antipsychotics (not proven use) helps decrease total cumulative dose.

EPS: Extrapyramidal reactions are more common in elderly with up to 50% developing these reactions after age 60. These reactions may be more common in dementia patients. Drug-induced **Parkinson's syndrome** occurs often. Discontinuation usually resolves symptoms but may take weeks to months (12+) to clear. **Akathisia** is the most common EPS reaction in elderly. The symptoms of motor restlessness are difficult to diagnose in demented elderly; increased nervousness, assertiveness, restlessness with constant movement may indicate this adverse event. Consider decreasing dose if antipsychotic to treat as well as diagnose problem; usually see this reaction within 2-3 months of initiating antipsychotic drug.

Anticholinergic effects: These side effects most common with low potency antipsychotics (eg, thioridazine, chlorpromazine). CNS toxicity occurs more frequently and

(Continued)

157

Chlorprothixene *(Continued)*

severely in elderly; increased confusion, memory loss, psychotic behavior, and agitation frequently occur as a consequence of anticholinergic effects to antipsychotic agents. Peripheral anticholinergic action troublesome to elderly; most peripheral anticholinergic effects last only 2-3 weeks; see Adverse Reactions.

Orthostatic hypotension: More common with low potency agents (eg, thioridazine, chlorpromazine, and clozapine) but of concern with all antipsychotic agents; orthostasis due to alpha-receptor blockade by antipsychotic agents. Elderly present many risk factors for orthostatic hypotension: blunted baroreceptor reflexes, decreased vascular tone, decreased vascular volume, and possible presence of cardiac diseases which result in decreased cardiac output.

Sedation: Common side effect with antipsychotic therapy; should not be used as a hypnotic unless insomnia is associated with target behavior symptoms treated with antipsychotic medications; see Special Geriatric Considerations. Anecdotal reports suggesting antipsychotic sedation in nonpsychotic patients is extremely unpleasant due to feelings of depersonalization, derealization, and dysphoria. Due to the long duration of action with antipsychotic drugs, these reactions may last up to 24 hours and result in decreased daytime function.

Cardiac toxicity: Life-threatening arrhythmias have occurred at therapeutic doses of antipsychotics. Thioridazine more commonly demonstrates EKG changes than other antipsychotics; suggested to use high potency antipsychotic agents (ie, haloperidol) in patients with cardiac conduction defects.

Adverse Reactions

Cardiovascular: EKG changes, hypotension (especially orthostatic), tachycardia, arrhythmias, abnormal T waves with prolonged ventricular repolarization

Central nervous system: Drowsiness, restlessness, anxiety, extrapyramidal reactions, dystonic reactions, pseudoparkinsonian signs and symptoms, tardive dyskinesia, neuroleptic malignant syndrome, seizures, altered central temperature regulation

Dermatologic: Hyperpigmentation, pruritus, rash, contact dermatitis, photosensitivity (rare)

Endocrine & metabolic: Amenorrhea, galactorrhea, gynecomastia

Gastrointestinal: Dry mouth (problem for denture user), constipation, adynamic ileus, GI upset, weight gain

Genitourinary: Urinary retention, overflow incontinence, priapism, sexual dysfunction (up to 60%)

Hematologic: Agranulocytosis, leukopenia (usually in patients with large doses for prolonged periods)

Hepatic: Cholestatic jaundice

Ocular: Retinal pigmentation (more common than with chlorpromazine), blurred vision, decreased visual acuity (may be irreversible)

Sedation and anticholinergic effects are more pronounced than extrapyramidal effects

Overdosage Symptoms of overdose include deep sleep, coma, extrapyramidal symptoms, abnormal involuntary muscle movements, hypotension or hypertension; agitation, restlessness, fever, hypothermia or hyperthermia, seizures, cardiac arrhythmias, EKG changes

Toxicology Following initiation of essential overdose management, toxic symptom treatment and supportive treatment should be initiated. Hypotension usually responds to I.V. fluids or Trendelenburg positioning. If unresponsive to these measures the use of a parenteral inotrope may be required (eg, norepinephrine 0.1-0.2 mcg/kg/minute titrated to response). Do not use epinephrine. Seizures commonly respond to diazepam (I.V. 5-10 mg bolus in adults every 15 minutes if needed up to a total of 30 mg) or to phenytoin or phenobarbital. Also critical cardiac arrhythmias often respond to I.V. phenytoin (15 mg/kg up to 1 g), while other antiarrhythmics can be used. Neuroleptics often cause extrapyramidal symptoms (eg, dystonic reactions) requiring management with diphenhydramine 1-2 mg/kg up to a maximum of 50 mg I.M. or I.V. slow push followed by a maintenance dose for 48-72 hours. When these reactions are unresponsive to diphenhydramine, benztropine mesylate I.V. 1-2 mg may be effective. These agents are generally effective within 2-5 minutes.

Drug Interactions Guanethidine's hypotensive effect may be decreased by thioxanthenes

Stability Protect all dosage forms from light, clear or slightly yellow solutions may be used; should be dispensed in amber or opaque vials/bottles. Solutions may be diluted or mixed with fruit juices or other liquids but must be administered immediately after mixing; do not prepare bulk dilutions or store bulk dilutions.

Mechanism of Action Blocks postsynaptic mesolimbic dopaminergic D_1 and D_2 receptors in the brain; exhibits a strong alpha-adrenergic blocking and anticholinergic effect, depresses the release of hypothalamic and hypophyseal hormones; believed to depress the reticular activating system thus affecting basal metabolism, body temperature, wakefulness, vasomotor tone, and emesis

Pharmacokinetics

Absorption: Oral absorption results in peak concentrations between 2-4 hours. Absorption may be affected by the inherent anticholinergic action on the gastrointestinal tissue causing variable absorption. Absorption from tablets is erratic with less variation seen with solutions.

Distribution: Widely distributed in tissues with CNS concentrations exceeding that of plasma due to their lipophilic characteristics.

Protein binding: Antipsychotic agents are bound 90% to 99% to plasma proteins; highly bound to brain and lung tissue and other tissues with a high blood perfusion.

Elimination: Elimination occurs through hepatic metabolism (oxidation) where numerous active metabolites are produced; active metabolites excreted in urine; elimination half-lives of antipsychotics ranges from 20-40 hours which may be extended in elderly due to decline in oxidative hepatic reactions (phase I) with age. The biologic effect of a single dose persists for 24 hours. When the patient has accommodated to initial side effects (sedation), once daily dosing is possible due to the long half-life of antipsychotics.

Steady-state plasma levels are achieved in 4-7 days; therefore, if possible, do not make dose adjustments more than once in a 7-day period. Due to the long half-lives of antipsychotics, as needed (PRN) use is ineffective since repeated doses are necessary to achieve therapeutic tissue concentrations in the CNS.

Usual Dosage
Geriatrics (nonpsychotic patient; dementia behavior): 10 mg 1-2 times/day; increase dose 10 mg/day at 4- to 7-day intervals; increase dosing intervals (bid, tid, etc) as necessary to control response or side effects; maximum daily dose: 300 mg; gradual increases (titration) may prevent some side effects or decrease their severity

Adults:
Oral: 25-50 mg 3-4 times/day, to be increased as needed; doses exceeding 600 mg/day are rarely required
I.M.: 25-50 mg up to 3-4 times/day

Not dialyzable (0% to 5%)

Monitoring Parameters Orthostatic blood pressures; tremors, gait changes, abnormal movement in trunk, neck, buccal area or extremities; monitor target behaviors for which the agent is given

Test Interactions Increased cholesterol (S), glucose; decreased uric acid (S)

Patient Information Do not take antacid within 1 hour of taking drug; avoid alcohol; avoid excess sun exposure (use sun block); may cause drowsiness, rise slowly from recumbent position; use of supportive stockings may help prevent orthostatic hypotension

Nursing Implications Avoid skin contact with oral suspension or solution; may cause contact dermatitis; monitor orthostatic blood pressures 3-5 days after initiation of therapy or a dose increase; observe for tremor and abnormal movement or posturing (extrapyramidal symptoms)

Special Geriatric Considerations See Warnings
Many elderly patients receive antipsychotic medications for inappropriate nonpsychotic behavior. Before initiating antipsychotic medication, the clinician should investigate any possible reversible cause; any stress or stress from any disease can cause acute "confusion" or worsening of baseline nonpsychotic behavior. Most commonly acute changes in behavior are due to increases in drug dose or addition of new drug to regimen; fluid electrolyte loss; infections; and changes in environment. Any changes in disease status in any organ system can result in behavior changes.

Dosage Forms
Injection: 12.5 mg/mL (2 mL)
Tablet: 10 mg, 25 mg, 50 mg, 100 mg

Chlorthalidone (klor thal' i done)

Brand Names Hygroton®

Generic Available Yes

Therapeutic Class Diuretic, Miscellaneous

Use Management of mild to moderate hypertension, used alone or in combination with other agents; treatment of edema associated with congestive heart failure, or nephrotic syndrome

Contraindications Hypersensitivity to chlorthalidone or any component, cross-sensitivity with other thiazides or sulfonamides; do not use in anuric patients

Precautions Use with caution in hypokalemia, renal disease, hepatic disease, gout, lupus, erythematosus, diabetes mellitus

Adverse Reactions
Cardiovascular: Hypotension
Dermatologic: Photosensitivity, rash
Endocrine & metabolic: Fluid and electrolyte imbalances (hypokalemia, hypocalcemia, hypomagnesemia, hyponatremia), hyperglycemia
Genitourinary: Prerenal azotemia, polyuria
Hematologic: Rarely blood dyscrasias

Overdosage Symptoms of overdose include electrolyte depletion, volume depletion

Toxicology Treatment is primarily symptomatic and supportive; hypotension responds to fluids and Trendelenburg position; replace electrolytes as necessary

(Continued)

Chlorthalidone *(Continued)*

Drug Interactions

Decreased effect of oral hypoglycemics; decreased absorption with cholestyramine and colestipol

Decreased effect: NSAIDs; when given with digoxin, diuretic-induced hypokalemia increases the risk of digoxin toxicity

Increased effect with furosemide and other loop diuretics

Increased toxicity/levels of lithium

Mechanism of Action Inhibits sodium reabsorption in the distal tubules causing increased excretion of sodium and water as well as potassium and hydrogen ions

Pharmacodynamics

Peak clinical effect: Within 2-6 hours

Duration: 24-72 hours

Pharmacokinetics

Absorption: 65%

Metabolism: In the liver

Half-life: 35-55 hours and may be prolonged with renal impairment; (anuria): 81 hours

Elimination: ~50% to 65% of dose excreted unchanged in urine

Usual Dosage Oral:

Geriatrics: Initial: 12.5-25 mg/day or every other day; there is little advantage to using doses >25 mg/day

Adults: 25-100 mg/day or 100 mg 3 times/week

Monitoring Parameters Blood pressure (standing and sitting/supine), serum electrolytes, renal function, I & O, weight

Test Interactions Increased creatine phosphokinase [CPK] (S), ammonia (B), amylase (S), calcium (S), chloride (S), cholesterol (S), glucose, increased acid (S), decreased chloride (S), magnesium, potassium (S), sodium (S)

Patient Information Take in the morning; may cause increased sensitivity to sunlight; rise slowly from lying down or sitting

Nursing Implications Administer in the morning, see Monitoring Parameters; check patient for orthostasis

Special Geriatric Considerations Recent studies have found chlorthalidone effective in the treatment of isolated systolic hypertension in the elderly

Dosage Forms Tablet: 25 mg, 50 mg, 100 mg

References

Hulley SB, Furberg CD, Gurland B, et al, "Systolic Hypertension in the Elderly Program (SHEP): Antihypertensive Efficacy of Chlorthalidone," *Am J Cardiol*, 1985, 56(15):913-20.

SHEP Cooperative Research Group, "Prevention of Stroke by Antihypertensive Drug Treatment in Older Persons With Isolated Systolic Hypertension," *JAMA*, 1991, 265(24):3255-64.

Chlor-Trimeton® [OTC] *see* Chlorpheniramine Maleate *on page 152*

Chlorzoxazone *(klor zox' a zone)*

Brand Names Paraflex®; Parafon Forte™ DSC; Strifon® Forte DSC

Synonyms Chlorobenzoxazoline

Generic Available Yes

Therapeutic Class Centrally Acting Skeletal Muscle Relaxant; Skeletal Muscle Relaxant

Use Symptomatic treatment of muscle spasm and pain associated with acute musculoskeletal conditions

Contraindications Known hypersensitivity to chlorzoxazone; impaired liver function

Precautions If signs or symptoms of impaired liver dysfunction occur, discontinue drug

Adverse Reactions

Central nervous system: Drowsiness, dizziness, lightheadedness, paresthesia, headache

Dermatologic: Rash, urticaria

Gastrointestinal: Nausea, vomiting, diarrhea, GI bleeding

Hematologic: Anemia, granulocytopenia

Hepatic: Hepatitis

Overdosage Symptoms of overdose include nausea, vomiting, diarrhea, drowsiness, dizziness, headache, absent tendon reflexes, hypotension

Toxicology Treatment is supportive following attempts to enhance drug elimination. Hypotension should be treated with I.V. fluids and/or Trendelenburg positioning. Dialysis and hemoperfusion and osmotic diuresis have all been useful in reducing serum drug concentrations. The patient should be observed for possible relapses due to incomplete gastric emptying.

Drug Interactions Increased effect/CNS toxicity: Alcohol, CNS depressants

Mechanism of Action Acts on the spinal cord and subcortical levels by depressing polysynaptic reflexes. This results in reduced skeletal muscle spasm, relief of pain, and increased mobility of involved muscles.

Pharmacodynamics

Onset of action: 60 minutes

Duration: 3-4 hours

Pharmacokinetics
Absorption: Oral: Readily absorbed
Metabolism: Extensive in the liver by glucuronidation
Elimination: In urine as conjugates

Usual Dosage Oral:
Geriatrics: Initial: 250 g 2-4 times/day; increase as necessary to 750 g 3-4 times/day
Adults: 250-500 mg 3-4 times/day up to 750 mg 3-4 times/day

Monitoring Parameters Liver function tests, relief of symptoms, mental status

Patient Information Avoid alcohol and CNS depressants; may cause drowsiness, dizziness, or lightheadedness; urine may turn orange or purple-red; take with food or milk

Nursing Implications Give with food or milk if GI complaints occur; may discolor urine

Additional Information Not useful in the chronic spasticity associated with stroke or Parkinson's disease

Special Geriatric Considerations There are no data on the use of skeletal muscle relaxants in the elderly. Start dosing low and increase as necessary. Chlorzoxazone has a relatively short half-life and no anticholinergic effects, so it is a rational choice when a skeletal muscle relaxant is indicated in older patients.

Dosage Forms
Caplet (Parafon Forte™ DSC): 500 mg
Capsule (Blanex®, Lobac®, Miflex®, Mus-Lac®, Skelex®): 250 mg with acetaminophen 300 mg
Tablet:
Paraflex®: 250 mg
Chlorofon-F®, Pargen® Fortified, Polyflex: 250 mg with acetaminophen 300 mg

Cholac® *see Lactulose on page 397*

Cholecalciferol

Brand Names Delta-D®
Synonyms D_3
Generic Available No
Therapeutic Class Vitamin D Analog
Use Dietary supplement, treatment of vitamin D deficiency or prophylaxis of deficiency

Unlabeled use: Hypocalcemic tetany, hypoparathyroidism

Contraindications Hypercalcemia, hypersensitivity to cholecalciferol or any component; malabsorption syndrome; evidence of vitamin D toxicity, decreased renal function

Warnings Administer with extreme caution in patients with impaired renal function, heart disease, renal stones, or arteriosclerosis; maintain adequate fluid intake, calcium-phosphate product must not exceed 70%; avoid hypercalcemia; must administer with supplemental calcium; use caution in patients with renal impairment and hyperparathyroidism

Precautions Use with caution in coronary artery disease and elderly

Adverse Reactions
Cardiovascular: Hypertension, arrhythmias
Central nervous system: Drowsiness, irritability, headache, somnolence, seizures
Endocrine & metabolic: Acidosis
Gastrointestinal: Nausea, vomiting, anorexia, dry mouth, constipation, weight loss, metallic taste
Hematologic: Anemia
Hepatic: Elevated AST/ALT
Neuromuscular & skeletal: Muscle and bone pain, weakness, metastatic calcifications
Ocular: Photophobia
Renal: Polyuria, polydipsia, nephrocalcinosis, renal damage

Overdosage Symptoms of overdose include hypercalcemia, anorexia, nausea, weakness, constipation, diarrhea, mental confusion, tinnitus, ataxia, depression, hallucinations, syncope, coma; polyuria, polydipsia, nocturia, hypercalciuria, irreversible renal insufficiency or proteinuria, azotemia; will spread tissue calcifications, hypertension

Toxicology Following withdrawal of the drug, treatment consists of bed rest, liberal intake of fluids, reduced calcium intake, and cathartic administration. Severe hypercalcemia requires I.V. hydration and forced diuresis with I.V. furosemide (20-40 mg I.V. every 4-6 hours). Urine output should be monitored and maintained at >3 mL/kg/hour. I.V. saline can quickly and significantly increase excretion of calcium into the urine. Calcitonin, cholestyramine, prednisone, sodium EDTA, and mithramycin have all been used successfully to treat the more resistant cases of vitamin D-induced hypercalcemia.

Drug Interactions
Vitamin D may increase absorption of magnesium from magnesium compounds; hypercalcemia may be precipitated by vitamin D and, therefore, may increase cardiac arrhythmias in patients taking digitalis glycosides and verapamil; hypoparathyroid patients may develop hypercalcemia when using thiazide diuretics

(Continued)

Cholecalciferol *(Continued)*

Phenytoin and barbiturates decrease half-life of vitamin D; mineral oil with prolonged use decreases vitamin D absorption; cholestyramine reduces absorption of vitamin D

Usual Dosage Geriatrics and Adults: Oral: 400-1000 units/day; general supplementation: 400 units; see Additional Information

Monitoring Parameters Monitor renal function, serum calcium, and phosphate concentrations; if hypercalcemia is encountered, discontinue agent until serum calcium returns to normal

Reference Range Calcium (serum) 9-10 mg/dL (4.5-5 mEq/L); phosphate 2.5-5 mg/dL

Test Interactions Increases calcium (S), cholesterol (S); false increased serum cholesterol levels with the Zlavkis-Zak reaction

Patient Information Do not take more than the recommended amount. While taking this medication, your physician may want you to follow a special diet or take a calcium supplement. Follow this diet closely. Avoid taking magnesium supplements or magnesium-containing antacids. Early symptoms of hypercalcemia include weakness, fatigue, somnolence, headache, anorexia, dry mouth, metallic taste, nausea, vomiting, cramps, diarrhea, muscle pain, bone pain, and irritability.

Additional Information 1 mg of cholecalciferol = 40,000 units of vitamin D activity

Special Geriatric Considerations Recommended daily allowances (RDA) have not been developed for persons >65 years of age; vitamin D, folate, and B$_{12}$ (cyanocobalamin) have decreased absorption with age, but the clinical significance is yet unknown. Calorie requirements decrease with age and, therefore, nutrient density must be increased to ensure adequate nutrient intake, including vitamins and minerals. Therefore, the use of a daily supplement with a multiple vitamin with minerals is recommended. Elderly consume less vitamin D, absorption may be decreased and many elderly have decreased sun exposure; therefore, elderly should receive supplementation with 800 units (20 mcg)/day. This is a recommendation of particular need to those with high risk for osteoporosis.

Dosage Forms Tablet: 400 units, 1000 units

References

Letsou AP and Price LS, "Health Aging and Nutrition: An Overview," *Clin Geriatr Med*, 1987, 3(2):253-60.

Myrianthopoulos M, "Dietary Treatment of Hyperlipidemia in the Elderly," *Clin Geriatr Med*, 1987, 3(2):343-59.

Riggs BL and Melton LJ, "The Prevention and Treatment of Osteoporosis," *N Engl J Med*, 1992, 327(9):620-7.

Choledyl® *see* Oxtriphylline *on page 525*

Cholera Vaccine (kol' er a)

Related Information

Immunization Guidelines *on page 759-762*

Therapeutic Class Vaccine, Inactivated Bacteria

Use Primary immunization for cholera prophylaxis for individuals traveling or living in endemic or epidemic countries

Contraindications Acute respiratory or other active infections, immune deficiency states, known hypersensitivity to cholera vaccine

Warnings Do not inject I.V.; do not give I.M. to persons with thrombocytopenia, coagulation defects, or receiving anticoagulants; hypersensitivity to vaccine, have epinephrine 1:1000 available to treat anaphylactic reactions

Precautions Aspirate syringe before delivering I.M. or S.C. dose to avoid accidental I.V. administration

Adverse Reactions

Central nervous system: Malaise, fever, headache

Local: Pain, swelling, tenderness, erythema, and induration at injection site; may persist for 1-2 days

Drug Interactions Yellow fever vaccine; do not give within 3 weeks of yellow fever vaccination

Stability Refrigerate at 2°C to 8°C (36°F to 46°F), avoid freezing

Mechanism of Action A sterile suspension of equal parts of phenol inactivated Ogawa and Inaba serotypes of *Vibrio cholerae*; 50% effective; protection lasts 3-6 months

Usual Dosage Geriatrics and Adults: I.M., S.C.: 0.5 mL in 2 doses one week to 1 month or more apart; give boosters (0.5 mL) 6 months apart

Patient Information Local reactions can occur up to 2 days; avoid food and water which may be contaminated

Nursing Implications Defer immunization in individuals with moderate or severe febrile illness; do not give I.V.; administer I.M., S.C., or intradermally

Special Geriatric Considerations Review history of elderly to assure no drug or disease is contraindicated with use of vaccine

Dosage Forms Injection: 8 billion killed organisms/mL (1.5 mL, 20 mL)

Cholestyramine Resin (koe less' tir a meen)

Brand Names Cholybar®; Questran®

Therapeutic Class Antilipemic Agent

Use Adjunct in the management of primary hypercholesterolemia; pruritus associated with elevated levels of bile acids; diarrhea associated with excess fecal bile acids; binding toxicologic agents; pseudomembraneous colitis

Contraindications Avoid using in complete biliary obstruction

Warnings Questran® Light contains aspartame; caution patients with phenylketonuria

Precautions Use with caution in patients with constipation

Adverse Reactions

Dermatologic: Rash

Endocrine & metabolic: Hyperchloremic acidosis

Gastrointestinal: Constipation, nausea, vomiting, abdominal distention and pain, malabsorption of fat-soluble vitamins, bowel obstruction

Local: Irritation of perianal area, skin, or tongue

Renal: Increased urinary calcium excretion

Overdosage Symptoms of overdose include GI obstruction

Drug Interactions May decrease oral absorption of digitalis glycosides, warfarin, thyroid hormones, thiazide diuretics, propranolol, phenobarbital, acetaminophen, corticosteroids, amiodarone, methotrexate, naproxen, piroxicam, and other drugs by binding to the drug in the intestine; compounded effect with other drugs that cause constipation

Mechanism of Action Forms a nonabsorbable complex with bile acids in the intestine, releasing chloride ions in the process; inhibits enterohepatic reuptake of intestinal bile salts and thereby increases the fecal loss of bile salt-bound low density lipoprotein cholesterol

Pharmacodynamics Peak effects: Within 21 days

Pharmacokinetics

Absorption: Not absorbed from GI tract

Elimination: In feces as an insoluble complex with bile acids

Usual Dosage Geriatrics and Adults: Oral (dosages are expressed in terms of anhydrous resin): 3-4 g 3-4 times/day to a maximum of 16-32 g/day in 2-4 divided doses

Monitoring Parameters Bowel function, plasma cholesterol (LDL and VLDL fractions)

Test Interactions Increased prothrombin time (S); decreased cholesterol (S), iron (B)

Patient Information Take before meals; mix with liquids, pulpy fruits, or soups; chew bars thoroughly and follow with fluids (at least 4 fluid oz); do not take concurrently with other medications; take 1 hour before or 4-6 hours after other medications; adhere to prescribed diet

Nursing Implications Do not administer the powder in its dry form; just prior to administration, mix with fluid or with applesauce; administer warfarin at least 1-2 hours prior to, or 6 hours after cholestyramine because cholestyramine may bind warfarin and decrease its total absorption. **Note:** Cholestyramine itself may cause hypoprothrombinemia in patients with impaired enterohepatic circulation; can be very constipating, monitor for bowel function to prevent fecal impaction.

Additional Information Overdose may result in GI obstruction; Questran® Light contains aspartame

Special Geriatric Considerations The definition of and, therefore, when to treat hyperlipidemia in the elderly is a controversial issue. The National Cholesterol Education Program recommends that all adults 20 years of age and older maintain a plasma cholesterol level <200 mg/dL. By this definition, 60% of all elderly would be considered to have an elevated plasma cholesterol. However, plasma cholesterol has been shown to be a less reliable predictor of coronary heart disease in the elderly. Therefore, it is the authors' belief that pharmacologic treatment be reserved for those who are unable to obtain a desirable plasma cholesterol level by diet alone and for whom the benefits of treatment are believed to outweigh the potential adverse effects, drug interactions, and cost of treatment.

Dosage Forms

Bar, chewable (caramel or raspberry flavor): 4 g (25s)

Powder: 4 g of resin/9 g of powder (9 g, 378 g)

Powder, for oral suspension, with aspartame: 4 g of resin/5 g of powder (5 g, 210 g)

References

Leaf DA, "Lipid Disorders: Applying New Guidelines to Your Older Patients," *Geriatrics*, 1994, 49(5):35-41.

Choline Magnesium Salicylate (koe' leen)

Brand Names Trilisate®

Generic Available No

Therapeutic Class Analgesic, Non-narcotic; Anti-inflammatory Agent; Nonsteroidal Anti-inflammatory Agent (NSAID), Oral; Salicylate

Use Treatment of mild to moderate pain, inflammation and fever; management of rheumatic fever, rheumatoid arthritis, osteoarthritis, and gout

Contraindications Bleeding disorders (factor VII or IX deficiencies), hypersensitivity to salicylates or other nonsteroidal anti-inflammatory drugs (NSAIDs); tartrazine dye and asthma

(Continued)

Choline Magnesium Salicylate *(Continued)*

Warnings Tinnitus or impaired hearing may indicate toxicity; discontinue use 1 week prior to surgical procedures

Precautions Use with caution in patients with platelet and bleeding disorders, renal dysfunction, hepatic disease, history of salicylate-induced gastric irritation, peptic ulcer disease, erosive gastritis, bleeding disorders, hypoprothrombinemia, and vitamin K deficiency; use cautiously in asthmatics, especially those with aspirin intolerance and nasal polyps

Adverse Reactions

Central nervous system: Dizziness, mental confusion, CNS depression, headache, lassitude, fever

Dermatologic: Rash, urticaria, angioedema

Gastrointestinal: Nausea, vomiting, GI distress, ulcers, thirst

Hematologic: Bleeding, inhibition of platelet aggregation, leukopenia, thrombocytopenia

Hepatic: Hepatotoxicity

Otic: Tinnitus

Respiratory: Pulmonary edema, bronchospasm, hyperventilation

Miscellaneous: Sweating

Overdosage 10-30 g; symptoms of overdose include tinnitus, headache, dizziness, confusion, metabolic acidosis, hyperpyrexia, hyperpnea, tachypnea, nausea, vomiting, irritability, disorientation, hallucinations, lethargy, stupor, dehydration, hyperventilation, hyperthermia, hyperactivity, depression leading to coma, respiratory failure, and collapse; laboratory abnormalities include hypokalemia, hypoglycemia or hyperglycemia with alterations in pH

Toxicology The "Done" nomogram is very helpful for estimating the severity of aspirin poisoning and directing treatment using serum salicylate levels. Treatment can also be based upon symptomatology; see table.

Aspirin or Other Salicylate Toxicity

Toxic Symptoms	Treatment
Overdose	Induce emesis with ipecac, and/or lavage with saline, followed with activated charcoal
Dehydration	I.V. fluids with KCl (no D_5W only)
Metabolic acidosis (must be treated)	Sodium bicarbonate
Hyperthermia	Cooling blankets or sponge baths
Coagulopathy/hemorrhage	Vitamin K I.V.
Hypoglycemia (with coma, seizures or change in mental status)	Dextrose 25 g I.V.
Seizures	Diazepam 5–10 mg I.V.

Drug Interactions

Antacids + Trilisate® → decreased salicylate concentration

Warfarin + Trilisate® → possible increased hypoprothrombinemic effect; ammonium chloride, vitamin C (high dose), methionine, antacids, urinary alkalinizers, carbonic anhydrase inhibitors, corticosteroids, nizatidine, alcohol, ACE inhibitors, beta-blockers, loop diuretics, methotrexate, probenecid, sulfinpyrazine, spironolactone

Mechanism of Action Inhibits prostaglandin synthesis, acts on the hypothalamus heat-regulating center to reduce fever; decreases pain receptor sensitivity. Other proposed mechanisms of action for salicylate anti-inflammatory action are lysosomal stabilization, kinin and leukotriene production, alteration of chemotactic factors, and inhibition of neutrophil activation. This latter mechanism may be the most significant pharmacologic action to reduce inflammation.

Pharmacokinetics

Absorption: From the stomach and small intestine

Distribution: Readily into most body fluids and tissues

Half-life: Dose-dependent ranging from 2-3 hours at low doses to 30 hours at high doses

Time to peak: Peak plasma levels appear in ~2 hours

Usual Dosage Geriatrics and Adults (based on **total salicylate content**): Oral: 500 mg to 1.5 g 1-3 times/day

Monitoring Parameters Serum concentrations, renal function; hearing changes or tinnitus; monitor for response (ie, pain, inflammation, range of motion, grip strength); observe for abnormal bleeding, bruising, weight gain

Reference Range

Salicylate blood levels for anti-inflammatory effect: 150-300 μg/mL (15-30 mg/dL)

Analgesia and antipyretic effect: 30-50 μg/mL (3-5 mg/dL)

Test Interactions False-negative results for glucose oxidase urinary glucose tests (Clinistix®); false-positives using the cupric sulfate method (Clinitest®); also, interferes with Gerhardt test (urinary ketone analysis), VMA determination; 5-HIAA, xylose tolerance test, and T_3 and T_4; increased PBI; increased uric acid

Patient Information Do not take with antacids; watch for any signs of bleeding (stool); take with food to minimize GI distress; report ringing in ears, persistent GI pain to physician or pharmacist

Nursing Implications Liquid may be mixed with fruit juice just before drinking; do not administer with antacids; see Monitoring Parameters, Reference Range, and Special Geriatric Considerations

Additional Information Salicylate salts do not inhibit platelet aggregation and, therefore, should not be substituted for aspirin in the prophylaxis of thrombosis; use caution in patients with renal failure or reduced renal function (ie, elderly – magnesium accumulation)

Special Geriatric Considerations Elderly are a high-risk population for adverse effects from nonsteroidal anti-inflammatory agents. As much as 60% of elderly can develop peptic ulceration and/or hemorrhage asymptomatically. The concomitant use of H_2 blockers, omeprazole, and sucralfate is not effective as prophylaxis. Misoprostol is the only prophylactic agent proven effective. Also, concomitant disease and drug use contribute to the risk for GI adverse effects. Avoid use of multiple drugs (OTCs) which contain salicylates (eg, bismuth subsalicylate with other salicylates). Use lowest effective dose for shortest time period possible. Consider renal function decline with age. Use of NSAIDs can compromise existing renal function especially when Cl_{cr} is $\leq$30 mL/minute. Tinnitus may be a difficult and unreliable indication of toxicity due to age-related hearing loss or eighth cranial nerve damage. CNS adverse effects such as confusion, agitation, and hallucination are generally seen in overdose or high dose situations, but elderly may demonstrate these adverse effects at lower doses than younger adults.

Dosage Forms See table.

Choline Magnesium Salicylate

Brand Name	Dosage Form	Total Salicylate	Choline Salicylate	Magnesium Salicylate
Trilisate®	Liquid	500 mg/5 mL	293 mg/5 mL	362 mg/5 mL
Trilisate 500®	Tablet	500 mg	293 mg	362 mg
Trilisate 750®	Tablet	750 mg	440 mg	544 mg
Trilisate 1000®	Tablet	1000 mg	587 mg	725 mg

References
Weissmann G, "Aspirin," *Sci Am*, 1991, 264(1):84-90.

Choline Salicylate see Salicylates (Various Salts) on page 633

Choline Theophyllinate see Oxtriphylline on page 525

Cholybar® see Cholestyramine Resin on page 163

Chooz® [OTC] see Calcium Salts (Oral) on page 111

Chronulac® see Lactulose on page 397

Cibacalcin® see Calcitonin on page 104

Cibalith-S® see Lithium on page 413

Ciloxan™ see Ciprofloxacin Hydrochloride on page 168

Cimetidine (sye met' i deen)
Related Information
Antacid Drug Interactions on page 764
Brand Names Tagamet®
Generic Available No
Therapeutic Class Histamine-2 Antagonist
Use Short-term treatment of active duodenal ulcers and benign gastric ulcers; long-term prophylaxis of duodenal ulcer; gastric hypersecretory states; gastroesophageal reflux; prevention of upper GI bleeding in critically ill patients

Unlabeled use: Prevent aspiration pneumonitis, hyperparathyroidism, tinea capitis, herpes virus infection, hirsutism, chronic idiopathic urticaria, dermatologic symptoms of anaphylaxis, acetaminophen overdose, and dyspepsia

Contraindications Hypersensitivity to cimetidine or any component or other H_2 antagonists

Warnings Adjust dosages in renal/hepatic impairment; decline in renal function with age

(Continued)

Cimetidine *(Continued)*

Precautions Gastric malignancy may be masked

Adverse Reactions

Cardiovascular: Bradycardia, hypotension, cardiac arrhythmias

Central nervous system: Dizziness, mental confusion, agitation, headache, phytobezoar formation, depression, psychosis, hallucinations, anxiety

Dermatologic: Rash, exfoliative dermatitis, alopecia, epidermal necrolysis

Endocrine & metabolic: Gynecomastia

Gastrointestinal: Mild diarrhea, pancreatitis

Genitourinary: Urinary retention

Hematologic: Neutropenia, agranulocytosis, thrombocytopenia

Hepatic: Elevated AST and ALT

Neuromuscular & skeletal: Peripheral neuropathy, myalgia, arthralgia, polymyositis

Renal: Rare reversible nephritis, elevated creatinine

Respiratory: Bronchospasm

Overdosage No experience with intentional overdose; reported ingestions of 20 g have had transient side effects seen with recommended doses; animal data have shown respiratory failure, tachycardia, muscle tremors, vomiting, restlessness, hypotension, salivation, emesis, and diarrhea

Toxicology Treatment is primarily symptomatic and supportive

Drug Interactions

Decreased elimination of lidocaine, theophylline, caffeine, calcium channel blockers, labetalol, carbamazepine, metoprolol, moricizine, pentoxifylline, phenytoin, propafenone, chloroquine sulfonylureas, metronidazole, triamterene, procainamide, quinidine and propranolol; inhibition of warfarin metabolism, tricyclic antidepressant metabolism, diazepam elimination and cyclosporine elimination; antacids may reduce the absorption of cimetidine

Increased absorption with cisapride

Stability I.V. infusion solution with NS or D_5W solution is stable for 48 hours at room temperature; do not refrigerate the injection since precipitation may occur

Mechanism of Action Competitive inhibition of histamine at H_2 receptors of the gastric parietal cells resulting in reduced gastric acid secretion; gastric volume and hydrogen ion concentration reduced

Pharmacodynamics 400 mg twice daily and 300 mg 4 times/day suppress nocturnal acid secretion 47% to 83% over a 6- to 8-hour interval; 800 mg at bedtime decreases acid secretion 85% over 8 hours; 1600 mg at bedtime gives 100% reduction over 8 hours

Pharmacokinetics

Protein binding: 13% to 25%

Bioavailability: 60% to 70%

Half-life: Adults with normal renal function: 2 hours

Time to peak: Oral: Peak serum levels appear within 1-2 hours

Elimination: Principally as unchanged drug by the kidney; some excretion in bile and feces

Usual Dosage Geriatrics and Adults (see Additional Information and Special Geriatric Considerations):

Short-term treatment of active ulcers:

Oral: 300 mg 4 times/day or 800 mg at bedtime or 400 mg twice daily for up to 8 weeks

I.M., I.V.: 300 mg every 6 hours or 37.5 mg/hour by continuous infusion; I.V. dosage should be adjusted to maintain an intragastric pH ≥5

Duodenal ulcer prophylaxis: Oral: 400-800 mg at bedtime

Gastric hypersecretory conditions: Oral, I.M., I.V.: 300-600 mg every 6 hours; dosage not to exceed 2.4 g/day

Dosing interval in renal impairment:

Cl_{cr} >40 mL/minute: Administer 300 mg every 6 hours

Cl_{cr} 20-40 mL/minute: Administer 300 mg every 8 hours

Cl_{cr} 0-20 mL/minute: Administer 300 mg every 12 hours

Monitoring Parameters Signs and symptoms of peptic ulcer disease, occult blood with GI bleeding, gastric pH where necessary; monitor renal function to correct dose; monitor for side effects

Reference Range Therapeutic: >1 μg/mL (SI: 4 μmol/L); mental confusion reported with levels >1.25 μg/mL

Test Interactions Increased creatinine, AST, ALT

Patient Information Take with or immediately after meals; inform pharmacist and physician (nurse, practitioner) of any concomitant drug therapy; stagger doses with antacids

Nursing Implications Give with meals so that the peak effect occurs at the proper time (peak inhibition of gastric acid secretion occurs at 1 and 3 hours after dosing in fasting subjects and ~2 hours in nonfasting subjects; this correlates well with the time food is no longer in the stomach offering a buffering effect); modify dosage in patients with renal impairment

Additional Information All presently available H_2 blockers have equivalent healing properties for both DU and GU when dose at equivalent doses; practitioners should realize that when H_2 blocker doses are adjusted for renal function, it is **not** a "dose reduction" that results in less than therapeutic tissue concentration. Therapeutic concentrations are maintained with doses adjusted for renal function. When prophylaxing for gastric ulcers, must use full therapeutic dose; prophylaxis for DU can be reduced as indicated

Special Geriatric Considerations H_2 blockers are the preferred drugs for treating PUD in elderly due to cost and ease of administration. These agents are no less or more effective than any other therapy. The preferred agents, due to side effects and drug interaction profile and pharmacokinetics are ranitidine, famotidine, and nizatidine. Treatment for PUD in elderly is recommended for 12 weeks since their lesions are larger and, therefore, take longer to heal. Always adjust dose based upon creatinine clearance.

Dosage Forms
Infusion: 300 mg in 50 mL NS
Injection: 150 mg/mL (2 mL)
Liquid, oral: 300 mg/5 mL (5 mL, 240 mL)
Tablet: 200 mg, 300 mg, 400 mg, 800 mg

References
Fennerty MD and Higbee M, "Drug Therapy of Gastrointestinal Disease," *Geriatric Pharmacology*, Bressler R and Katz MD, eds, New York, NY: McGraw-Hill, 1993, 585-608.
Somogyi A and Gugler R, "Clinical Pharmacokinetics of Cimetidine," *Clin Pharmacokinet*, 1983, 8(6):463-95.
Somogyi A and Muirhead M, "Pharmacokinetic Interactions of Cimetidine 1987," *Clin Pharmacokinet*, 1987, 12(5):321-66.

Cinobac® *see* Cinoxacin *on this page*
Cinonide® *see* Triamcinolone *on page 710*

Cinoxacin (sin ox' a sin)
Brand Names Cinobac®
Generic Available No
Therapeutic Class Antibiotic, Quinolone
Use Urinary tract infections caused by susceptible pathogens: *E. coli*, *P. mirabilis*, *P. vulgaris*, *K. pneumoniae*, *Klebsiella* sp, and *Enterobacter* sp
Contraindications History of convulsive disorders, hypersensitivity to cinoxacin or any component or other quinolones and nalidixic acid
Warnings Dose should be adjusted in patients with renal impairment; use with caution in patients with a history of hepatic disease
Adverse Reactions
Central nervous system: Dizziness, insomnia, confusion, headache
Gastrointestinal: Nausea, vomiting, abdominal pain, diarrhea, heartburn, dysgeusia, flatulence, anorexia
Hematologic: Thrombocytopenia
Ocular: Photophobia
Otic: Tinnitus
Drug Interactions Probenecid will decrease renal secretion and increase serum concentrations
Mechanism of Action Inhibits microbial synthesis of DNA with resultant problems in protein synthesis
Pharmacokinetics
Absorption: Oral: Rapid and complete; food decreases peak levels by 30% but not total amount absorbed; peak serum levels occur within 2-3 hours
Distribution: Concentrates in prostate tissue
Protein binding: 60% to 80%
Half-life: 1.5 hours
Elimination: Prolonged in renal impairment, ~60% excreted as unchanged drug in urine
Usual Dosage
Geriatrics: Usual adult dose adjusted for renal function when appropriate
Adults: 1 g/day in 2-4 doses
Dosing adjustment in renal impairment following an initial 500 mg dose:
Cl_{cr} >80 mL/minute/1.73 m^2: Administer 500 mg every 12 hours
Cl_{cr} 50-80 mL/minute/1.73 m^2: Administer 250 mg every 8 hours
Cl_{cr} 20-50 mL/minute/1.73 m^2: Administer 250 mg every 12 hours
Cl_{cr} <20 mL/minute/1.73 m^2: Administer 250 mg every 24 hours
Monitoring Parameters Signs and symptoms of infection; cultures and sensitivities
Test Interactions BUN, AST, ALT, serum creatinine and alkaline phosphatase have been reported to be elevated; hematocrit/hemoglobin have been reported to be reduced
Patient Information Complete entire course of therapy; may be taken with food or milk; may cause dizziness, use caution when driving or performing other tasks that require alertness; eyes may be sensitive to light

(Continued)
167

Cinoxacin (Continued)

Special Geriatric Considerations See Usual Dosage; adjust dose for renal function in elderly

Dosage Forms Capsule: 250 mg, 500 mg

Cin-Quin® see Quinidine on page 618

Cipro™ see Ciprofloxacin Hydrochloride on this page

Ciprofloxacin Hydrochloride (sip roe flox' a sin)

Brand Names Ciloxan™; Cipro™; Cipro™ IV

Generic Available No

Therapeutic Class Antibiotic, Ophthalmic; Antibiotic, Quinolone

Use Treatment of documented or suspected pseudomonal infection in home care patients; documented multi-drug resistant gram-negative organisms; documented infectious diarrhea due to *Campylobacter jejuni*, *Shigella*, or *Salmonella*; osteomyelitis caused by susceptible organisms in which parenteral therapy is not feasible; used ophthalmically for superficial ocular infections due to strains of microorganisms susceptible to ciprofloxacin

Contraindications Hypersensitivity to ciprofloxacin, any component or other quinolones, and nalidixic acid

Warnings Prolonged use may result in superinfection; use with caution in patients with seizure disorders or renal impairment; modify dosage in patients with renal impairment

Precautions CNS stimulation may occur which may lead to tremor, restlessness, confusion and very rarely to hallucinations or convulsive seizures; use with caution in patients with known or suspected CNS disorders; phototoxicity

Adverse Reactions

Central nervous system: Restlessness, dizziness, confusion, seizures, headache, hallucinations, psychosis

Dermatologic: Rash

Gastrointestinal: Nausea, diarrhea, pseudomembranous colitis, vomiting, GI bleeding

Genitourinary: Vaginitis

Hematologic: Anemia

Hepatic: Increased liver enzymes

Neuromuscular & skeletal: Arthralgia, tremors

Renal: Acute renal failure, increased serum creatinine and BUN

Toxicology For acute overdose, empty stomach contents by inducing vomiting or gastric lavage; observe and treat the patient symptomatically; maintain fluid status

Drug Interactions Antacids, iron salts, sucralfate, and zinc salts may reduce absorption by up to 98%, if given at the same time; increased toxicity/serum levels of theophylline, cyclosporine, nitrofurantoin, anticoagulants, caffeine; increased toxicity/levels of ciprofloxacin with azlocillin, cimetidine, probenecid

Food/Drug Interactions Calcium-containing foods (milk, yogurt) may decrease absorption, best to avoid concomitant ingestion

Stability Stable up to 14 days at refrigerated or room temperature when diluted with NS, USP or D_5W, USP; protect from freezing

Mechanism of Action Inhibits DNA-gyrase in susceptible organisms; inhibits relaxation of supercoiled DNA and promotes breakage of double-stranded DNA

Pharmacokinetics

Protein binding: 16% to 43%

Metabolism: Partially in the liver to active metabolites

Bioavailability: Oral: 50% to 85%; in elderly, the bioavailability has been reported to be increased (70% to 80%), serum half-life is prolonged (4.8-6.8 hours) secondary to reduced renal clearance

Half-life (patients with normal renal function): 3-5 hours

Time to peak: Oral: Peak serum levels occur within 0.5-2 hours

Elimination: 30% to 50% of dose excreted as unchanged drug in urine; 20% to 40% of a dose is excreted in feces primarily from biliary excretion

Only small amounts of ciprofloxacin are removed by dialysis (<10%)

Usual Dosage

Geriatrics: Normal adult dose adjusted for renal function

Adults:

Oral: 250-750 mg every 12 hours, depending on severity of infection and susceptibility

Ophthalmic: 1-2 drops every 2 hours while awake for 2 days, then 1-2 drops every 4 hours for 5 days

I.V.: 200-400 mg every 12 hours depending on severity of infection

Dosing adjustment in renal impairment:

Cl_{cr} >50 mL/minute (oral); ≥30 mL/minute (I.V.): Unchanged

Cl_{cr} 30-50 mL/minute: Administer 250-500 mg (oral) every 12 hours

Cl_{cr} 5-29 mL/minute: Administer 250-500 mg (oral) every 18 hours; 200-400 mg every 18-24 hours (I.V.)

Hemodialysis or peritoneal dialysis: 250-500 mg every 24 hours (after dialysis) Only small amounts of ciprofloxacin are removed by dialysis (<10%)

Monitoring Parameters Patients receiving concurrent ciprofloxacin and theophylline should have serum levels of theophylline monitored; patients receiving concurrent warfarin should have prothrombin time or INR monitored; patients receiving cyclosporine should be watched for nephrotoxicity and have their cyclosporine levels monitored

Reference Range Therapeutic: 2.6-3 μg/mL; Toxic: >5 μg/mL

Patient Information May be taken with food to minimize upset stomach; avoid antacid use; drink fluid liberally; instruct patient on use of ophthalmic product

Nursing Implications Hold antacids for 3-4 hours after giving; give around-the-clock rather than 2 times/day (ie, 9 and 9, not 9 and 5) to promote less variation in peak and trough serum levels; encourage fluids

Special Geriatric Considerations See Pharmacokinetics and Usual Dosage; ciprofloxacin should not be used as first-line therapy unless the culture and sensitivity findings show resistance to usual therapy; the interactions with caffeine and theophylline can result in serious toxicity in the elderly; adjust dose for renal function

Dosage Forms

Injection, I.V.: 200 mg (20 mL vials) (1%); 100 mL (5% dextrose containers); 400 mg (40 mL vials) (1%); 200 mL (5% dextrose containers)

Solution, ophthalmic: 3.5 mg/mL (2.5 mL, 5 mL)

Tablet: 250 mg, 500 mg, 750 mg

References

Bayer A, Gajewska A, Stephens M, et al, "Pharmacokinetics of Ciprofloxacin in the Elderly," *Respiration*, 1987, 51(4):292-5.

Campoli-Richards DM, Monk JP, Price A, et al, "Ciprofloxacin: A Review of Its Antibacterial Activity, Pharmacokinetic Properties and Therapeutic Use," *Drugs*, 1988, 35(4):373-447.

Guay DRP, Awni WM, Peterson PK, et al, "Single and Multiple Dose Pharmacokinetics of Oral Ciprofloxacin in Elderly Patients," *Int J Clin Pharmacol Ther Toxicol*, 1988, 26(6):279-84.

Nilsson-Ehle I and Ljungberg B, "Quinolone Disposition in the Elderly: Practical Implications," *Drugs Aging*, 1991, 1(4):279-88.

Cipro™ IV *see* Ciprofloxacin Hydrochloride *on previous page*

Cisapride (sis' a pride)

Brand Names Propulsid®

Therapeutic Class Antiemetic; Cholinergic Agent

Use Treatment of nocturnal symptoms of gastroesophageal reflux disease (GERD), also demonstrated effectiveness for gastroparesis, refractory constipation, and nonulcer dyspepsia

Contraindications Hypersensitivity to cisapride or any of its components; GI hemorrhage, mechanical obstruction, GI perforation, or other situations when GI motility stimulation is dangerous

Precautions Steady-state serum concentrations are often higher in geriatric patients due to increased elimination half-life, however, adverse effect rate is no greater than in younger adults

Adverse Reactions

Central nervous system: Headache, insomnia, anxiety, nervousness, migraine headache

Dermatological: Rash, pruritus

Gastrointestinal: Diarrhea, abdominal pain, nausea, constipation, flatulence, dyspepsia

Hematologic: Thrombocytopenia, pancytopenia, leukopenia, granulocytopenia, increased LFTs, aplastic anemia

Neuromuscular & skeletal: Tremors

Respiratory: Rhinitis, sinusitis, coughing, upper respiratory tract infection

Miscellaneous: Pain, fever, increased incidence of viral infection

Overdosage Acute toxicity may present with tremors, seizures, dyspnea, ptosis, catalepsy, catatonia, hypotonia, loss of righting reflex, diarrhea, retching, borborygmi, stool and urinary frequency, and flatulence

Toxicology Treat with gastric lavage or activated charcoal; general supportive measures

Drug Interactions

Decreased effect with atropine or other anticholinergics

Increased effect/toxicity of Coumadin® (warfarin), absorption of cimetidine, and ranitidine increased

Increased serum concentrations observed with alcohol and benzodiazepines

Mechanism of Action Enhances the release of acetylcholine at the myenteric plexus. *In vitro* studies have shown cisapride to have serotonin-4 receptor agonistic properties which may increase gastrointestinal motility and cardiac rate; increases lower esophageal sphincter pressure and lower esophageal peristalsis; accelerates gastric emptying of both liquids and solids.

Pharmacokinetics

Onset of effect: 0.5-1 hour

Bioavailability: 35% to 40%

(Continued)

ALPHABETICAL LISTING OF DRUGS

Cisapride *(Continued)*

Protein binding: 97.5% to 98%
Metabolism: Extensive to norcisapride, which is eliminated in urine and feces
Half-life: 6-12 hours
Elimination: <10% of dose excreted into feces and urine

Usual Dosage Geriatrics and Adults: Oral: Initial: 10 mg 4 times/day at least 15 minutes before meals and at bedtime; in some patients the dosage will need to be increased to 20 mg to obtain a satisfactory result

Monitoring Parameters Symptoms of relief or GERD, abdominal complaints, diarrhea; see Adverse Reactions

Patient Information May enhance effects of alcohol and benzodiazepines; take 15-30 minutes before meals

Special Geriatric Considerations Steady-state serum concentrations are higher than those in younger adults; however, the therapeutic dose and pharmacologic effects are the same as those in younger adults

Dosage Forms Tablet, scored: 10 mg

Citracal® [OTC] *see* Calcium Salts (Oral) *on page 111*
Citrate of Magnesia *see* Magnesium Citrate *on page 426*
Citroma® [OTC] *see* Magnesium Citrate *on page 426*
Citro-Nesia™ [OTC] *see* Magnesium Citrate *on page 426*
CI-719 *see* Gemfibrozil *on page 319*
Cla *see* Clarithromycin *on this page*
Claforan® *see* Cefotaxime Sodium *on page 132*

Clarithromycin (kla rith' roe mye sin)

Brand Names Biaxin™ Filmtabs®
Synonyms Cla
Generic Available No
Therapeutic Class Antibiotic, Macrolide
Use Treatment against most respiratory pathogens (eg, *S. pyogenes, S. pneumoniae, S. agalactiae, S. viridans, M. catarrhalis, C. trachomatis, Legionella* spp., *Mycoplasma pneumoniae, S. aureus*). Clarithromycin is highly active (MICs ≤0.25 mcg/mL) against *H. influenzae*, the combination of clarithromycin and its metabolite demonstrate an additive effect. Additionally, clarithromycin has shown activity against *C. pneumoniae* (including strain TWAR) and *M. avium* infection.
Contraindications Hypersensitivity to clarithromycin, erythromycin, or any macrolide antibiotic
Warnings In presence of severe renal impairment with or without coexisting hepatic impairment, decreased dosage or prolonged dosing interval may be appropriate; antibiotic associated colitis has been reported with use of clarithromycin; elderly patients experienced increased incidents of adverse effects due to known age-related decreases in renal function
Adverse Reactions The incidence of adverse GI effects (diarrhea, nausea, vomiting, dyspepsia, abdominal pain) is lower (13%) compared to erythromycin-treated patients (32%)

Cardiovascular: Ventricular tachycardia, torsade de pointes
Central nervous system: Headache
Gastrointestinal: Diarrhea, flatulence, nausea, abdominal pain, abnormal taste, dyspepsia
Hematologic: Decreased white blood cell count, elevated prothrombin time
Hepatic: Elevated AST, alkaline phosphatase, and bilirubin
Renal: Elevated BUN and serum creatinine

Overdosage Symptoms of overdose include nausea, vomiting, diarrhea, prostration, reversible pancreatitis, hearing loss with or without tinnitus or vertigo
Toxicology General and supportive care only
Drug Interactions Increased levels: Clarithromycin has been shown to increase serum **theophylline** levels by as much as 20%. **Carbamazepine** levels have been shown to increase after a single dose of clarithromycin. While other drug interactions (digoxin, anticoagulants, ergotamine, triazolam) known to occur with erythromycin have not been reported in clinical trials with clarithromycin, concurrent use of these drugs should be monitored closely.
Mechanism of Action Exerts its antibacterial action by binding to 50S ribosomal subunit resulting in inhibition of protein synthesis. The 14-OH metabolite of clarithromycin is twice as active as the parent compound.
Pharmacokinetics
Absorption: Highly stable in the presence of gastric acid (unlike erythromycin)
Distribution: Widely into most body tissues with the exception of the CNS
Metabolism: Partially converted to the microbiologically active metabolite, 14-OH clarithromycin

170

Bioavailability: 50% (250 mg tablet)
Half-life, elimination: 3-4 hours with a 250 mg dose; 5-7 hours with a 500 mg dose; 7.7 hours in healthy elderly
Time to peak serum concentration: Oral: 2-4 hours
Elimination: Following 250 mg or 500 mg doses every 12 hours, ~20% to 30% of unchanged parent drug is excreted in urine

Usual Dosage Geriatrics and Adults: Oral: Usual dose: 250-500 mg every 12 hours for 7-14 days

Upper respiratory tract: 250-500 mg every 12 hours for 10-14 days
Pharyngitis/tonsillitis: 250 mg every 12 hours for 10 days
Acute maxillary sinusitis: 500 mg every 12 hours for 14 days

Lower respiratory tract: 250-500 mg every 12 hours for 7-14 days
Acute exacerbation of chronic bronchitis due to:
M. catarrhalis and S. pneumoniae: 250 mg every 12 hours for 7-14 days
H. influenzae: 500 mg every 12 hours for 7-14 days
Pneumonia due to M. pneumoniae and S. pneumoniae: 250 mg every 12 hours for 7-14 days

Uncomplicated skin and skin structure: 250 mg every 12 hours for 7-14 days

Dosing adjustment in severe renal impairment: Decreased doses or prolonged dosing intervals are recommended

Patient Information May be taken with meals; finish all medication; do not skip doses

Nursing Implications Clarithromycin may be given with or without meals; give every 12 hours rather than twice daily to avoid peak and trough variation

Special Geriatric Considerations Considered one of the drugs of choice in the outpatient treatment of community-acquired pneumonia in older adults. After doses of 500 mg every 12 hours for 5 days, 12 healthy elderly had significantly increased C_{max} and C_{min}, elimination half-lives of clarithromycin and 14-OH clarithromycin compared to 12 healthy young subjects. These changes were attributed to a significant decrease in renal clearance; at a dose of 1000 mg twice daily, 100% of 13 older adults experienced an adverse event compared to only 10% taking 500 mg twice daily; see Usual Dosage and Pharmacokinetics.

Dosage Forms Tablet, film coated: 250 mg, 500 mg

References
American Thoracic Society, "Guidelines for the Initial Management of Adults With Community-Acquired Pneumonia: Diagnosis, Assessment of Severity, and Initial Antimicrobial Therapy," *Am Rev Respir Dis*, 1993, 148(5):1418-26.
Chu SY, Wilson DS, Guay DR, et al, "Clarithromycin Pharmacokinetics in Healthy Young and Elderly Volunteers," *J Clin Pharmacol*, 1992, 32(11):1045-9.
Wallace RJ Jr, Brown BA, and Griffith DE, "Drug Intolerance to High-Dose Clarithromycin Among Elderly Patients," *Diagn Microbiol Infect Dis*, 1993, 16(3):215-21.

Claritin® *see* Loratadine *on page 418*

Clear Eyes® [OTC] *see* Naphazoline Hydrochloride *on page 492*

Clemastine Fumarate (klem' as teen)

Brand Names Tavist®
Generic Available No
Therapeutic Class Antihistamine
Use Perennial and seasonal allergic rhinitis and other allergic symptoms including urticaria
Contraindications Narrow-angle glaucoma, bladder neck obstruction, symptomatic prostate hypertrophy, asthmatic attacks, and stenosing peptic ulcer, hypersensitivity to clemastine or any component
Warnings Antihistamines are more likely to cause dizziness, excessive sedation, syncope, toxic confusional states, and hypotension in the elderly.
Precautions Use with caution in patients with heart disease, hypertension, thyroid disease, and asthma.
Adverse Reactions
Central nervous system: Sedation, paradoxical excitation
Gastrointestinal: Nausea, dry mouth
Ocular: Diplopia
Renal: Polyuria
Respiratory: Thick bronchial secretions
Overdosage Symptoms of overdose include dry mouth, flushed skin, dilated pupils, CNS depression
Toxicology There is no specific treatment for an antihistamine overdose, however, most of its clinical toxicity is due to anticholinergic effects. Anticholinesterase inhibitors may be useful by reducing acetylcholinesterase. Anticholinesterase inhibitors include physostigmine, neostigmine, pyridostigmine and edrophonium. For anticholinergic overdose with severe life-threatening symptoms, physostigmine 1-2 mg I.V., slowly may be given to reverse these effects.
Drug Interactions Increased toxicity (CNS depression): CNS depressants, MAO inhibitors, alcohol, tricyclic antidepressants, phenothiazines

(Continued)

Clemastine Fumarate *(Continued)*

Mechanism of Action Competes with histamine for H_1-receptor sites on effector cells in the gastrointestinal tract, blood vessels, and respiratory tract

Pharmacodynamics
Peak therapeutic effect: Within 5-7 hours
Duration of action: 10-12 hours; some patients experience therapeutic effects for 24 hours

Pharmacokinetics
Absorption: Almost 100% from GI tract
Metabolism: In the liver
Elimination: In urine

Usual Dosage Oral:
Geriatrics: 1.34 mg once or twice daily
Adults: 1.34 mg twice daily to 2.68 mg 3 times/day; do not exceed 8.04 mg/day

Monitoring Parameters Relief of symptoms

Patient Information May cause drowsiness; avoid CNS depressants and alcohol

Nursing Implications Monitor for relief of symptoms, side effects

Additional Information 1.34 mg of clemastine fumarate = 1 mg clemastine base. Clemastine offers no significant benefit over other antihistamines except that it may be dosed twice daily (in adults) as compared to other antihistamines with more frequent dosing.

Special Geriatric Considerations See Contraindications and Warnings

Dosage Forms
Syrup: 0.67 mg/5 mL with 5.5% alcohol (120 mL)
Tablet: 1.34 mg, 2.68 mg

Cleocin HCl® *see* Clindamycin *on this page*

Cleocin Phosphate® *see* Clindamycin *on this page*

Cleocin T® *see* Clindamycin *on this page*

C-Lexin® *see* Cephalexin Monohydrate *on page 142*

Clindamycin *(klin da mye' sin)*

Brand Names Cleocin HCl®; Cleocin Phosphate®; Cleocin T®

Generic Available Yes: Injection

Therapeutic Class Acne Products; Antibiotic, Anaerobic; Antibiotic, Miscellaneous

Use Treatment of aerobic and anaerobic streptococci (except enterococci), most staphylococci, *Bacteroides* sp. and *Actinomyces*; used topically in treatment of severe acne

Contraindications Hypersensitivity to clindamycin or any component; previous pseudomembranous colitis, hepatic impairment; do not use for the treatment of minor bacterial or viral infections

Warnings Can cause severe and possibly fatal colitis; characterized by severe persistent diarrhea, severe abdominal cramps and possibly, the passage of blood and mucus; discontinue drug if significant diarrhea occurs

Precautions Dosage adjustment may be necessary in patients with severe hepatic dysfunction; no change necessary with renal insufficiency; diarrhea may not be well tolerated in the frail elderly because of fluid and electrolyte loss; superinfection with prolonged therapy

Adverse Reactions
Cardiovascular: Thrombophlebitis, hypotension
Dermatologic: Urticaria, rash, Stevens-Johnson syndrome
Gastrointestinal: Diarrhea, nausea, vomiting, pseudomembranous colitis
Hematologic: Eosinophilia, granulocytopenia, thrombocytopenia, neutropenia
Hepatic: Elevation of liver enzymes
Local: Sterile abscess at I.M. injection site, polyarthritis
Renal: Rare renal dysfunction

Drug Interactions Increased duration of neuromuscular blockade from tubocurarine, pancuronium; erythromycin (*in vitro* antagonism)

Stability Do **not** refrigerate the reconstituted oral solution because it will thicken; oral solution stable for 2 weeks at room temperature following reconstitution; I.V. infusion solution in NS or D_5W solution is stable for 24 hours at room temperature

Mechanism of Action Reversibly binds to 50S ribosomal subunits preventing peptide bond formation thus inhibiting bacterial protein synthesis; bacteriostatic or bactericidal depending on drug concentration, infection site, and organism

Pharmacokinetics
Absorption: Topical: ~10% absorbed systemically
Distribution: No significant levels seen in CSF, even with inflamed meninges
Protein binding: 94%
Bioavailability: Oral: ~90%
Half-life: 1.6-5.3 hours, average: 2-3 hours

Time to peak:
Oral: Peak serum levels occur within 60 minutes
I.M.: Within 1-3 hours
Elimination: Most of the drug is eliminated by hepatic metabolism; 10% of an oral dose is excreted in urine and 3.6% is excreted in feces as active drug and metabolites
No significant levels are seen in CSF, even with inflamed meninges

Usual Dosage
Geriatrics and Adults:
Oral: 150-450 mg/dose every 6-8 hours; maximum dose: 1.8 g/day
I.M., I.V.: 1.2-1.8 g/day in 2-3 divided doses; maximum dose: 3.6 g/day

Adults:
Topical: Apply twice daily
Pneumonitis carinii pneumonia:
Oral: 300-450 mg 4 times/day with primaquine
I.M., I.V.: 1200-2400 mg/day with pyrimethamine
I.V.: 600 mg 4 times/day with primaquine
Vaginal: One full applicator (100 mg) inserted intravaginally once daily before bedtime for 7 consecutive days

Dosing interval in renal impairment: No change necessary

Administration Administer oral dosage form with a full glass of water to minimize esophageal ulceration. Give around-the-clock rather than 4 times/day, 3 times/day, etc (ie, 12-6-12-6, not 9-1-5-9) to promote less variation in peak and trough serum levels.

Monitoring Parameters Observe for changes in bowel frequency; during prolonged therapy monitor CBC, liver and renal function tests periodically

Patient Information Report any severe diarrhea immediately and do not take antidiarrheal medication; take each oral dose with a full glass of water; finish all medication; do not skip doses; should not engage in sexual intercourse during treatment with vaginal product; avoid contact of topical gel/solution with eyes, abraded skin, or mucous membranes

Nursing Implications See Administration

Special Geriatric Considerations Clindamycin has not been studied in the elderly; however, since it is eliminated principally by nonrenal mechanisms, major alteration in its pharmacokinetics are not expected; see Precautions

Dosage Forms
Capsule, as hydrochloride: 75 mg, 150 mg, 300 mg
Infusion: 300 mg in D_5W (50 mL); 600 mg in D_5W (50 mL)
Injection, as phosphate: 150 mg/mL (2 mL, 4 mL, 6 mL, 60 mL)
Solution, topical, as hydrochloride: 1% (30 mL, 60 mL)
Suspension, oral, as phosphate: 75 mg/5 mL (100 mL)

References
Yoshikawa TT, "Antimicrobial Therapy for the Elderly Patient," *J Am Geriatr Soc*, 1990, 38(12):1353-72.

Clinoril® *see* Sulindac *on page 664*

Clofazimine Palmitate (kloe fa' zi meen)
Brand Names Lamprene®
Generic Available No
Therapeutic Class Antibiotic, Miscellaneous
Use Treatment of dapsone-resistant leprosy; multibacillary dapsone-sensitive leprosy; erythema nodosum leprosum; *Mycobacterium avium* - intracellular (MAI) infections
Contraindications Hypersensitivity to clofazimine or any component
Warnings Use with caution in patients with GI problems; well tolerated when administered in dosages ≤100 mg/day; dosages >100 mg/day should be used for as short a duration as possible; skin discoloration may lead to depression; two suicides have been reported
Adverse Reactions
Central nervous system: Dizziness, drowsiness
Dermatologic: Pink to brownish black discoloration of the skin and conjunctiva, dry skin, rash, pruritus
Endocrine & metabolic: Increased blood glucose
Gastrointestinal: Constipation, abdominal pain, diarrhea, nausea, vomiting, bowel obstruction, GI bleeding
Ocular: Irritation of the eyes
Toxicology Following GI decontamination, treatment is supportive
Drug Interactions Decreased effect with dapsone (unconfirmed)
Mechanism of Action Binds preferentially to mycobacterial DNA to inhibit mycobacterial growth; also has some anti-inflammatory activity through an unknown mechanism
Pharmacokinetics
Absorption: Oral: 45% to 70% of dose absorbed slowly
(Continued)

Clofazimine Palmitate *(Continued)*

Distribution: Remains in tissues for prolonged periods
Metabolism: Partially in the liver to two metabolites
Half-life:
  Terminal: 8 days
  Tissue: 70 days
Elimination: Mainly in feces; only negligible amounts excreted unchanged in urine; small amounts excreted in sputum, saliva, and sweat

Usual Dosage Geriatrics and Adults: Oral:
Dapsone-resistant leprosy: 100 mg/day in combination with one or more antileprosy drugs for 3 years; then alone 100 mg/day
Dapsone-sensitive multibacillary leprosy: 100 mg/day in combination with 2 or more antileprosy drugs for at least 2 years and continue until negative skin smears are obtained, then institute single drug therapy with appropriate agent
Erythema nodosum leprosum: 100-200 mg/day for up to 3 months or longer then taper dose to 100 mg/day when possible
Pyoderma gangrenosum: 300-400 mg/day for up to 12 months

  Dosing adjustment in hepatic impairment: Should be considered in severe hepatic dysfunction
Monitoring Parameters GI complaints
Test Interactions Increased ESR, increased glucose (S), increased albumin, increased bilirubin, increased AST
Patient Information Drug may cause a pink to brownish-black discoloration of the skin, conjunctiva, tears, sweat, urine, feces, and nasal secretions; although reversible, may take months to years to disappear after therapy is complete; take with meals
Special Geriatric Considerations No specific studies in the elderly; use with caution in diabetics; see Adverse Reactions
Dosage Forms Capsule: 50 mg, 100 mg

Clofibrate *(kloe fye' brate)*
Brand Names Atromid-S®
Generic Available Yes
Therapeutic Class Antilipemic Agent
Use Adjunct to dietary therapy in the management of hyperlipidemias associated with high triglyceride levels (type III hyperlipidemia); primarily lowers triglycerides and very low density lipoprotein
Contraindications Hypersensitivity to clofibrate or any component, severe hepatic or renal impairment, primary biliary cirrhosis
Warnings Clofibrate has been shown to be tumorigenic in toxicity studies using rats; discontinue if lipid response is not obtained; no evidence substantiates a beneficial effect on cardiovascular mortality
Adverse Reactions The most frequent is nausea which usually decreases with continued therapy or reduction in dosage

Central nervous system: Fatigue, drowsiness, dizziness
Dermatologic: Skin rash, alopecia, dry skin, dry and brittle hair, urticaria, pruritus
Gastrointestinal: Nausea, vomiting, diarrhea, gastritis, weight gain, flatulence, abdominal pain
Genitourinary: Impotence
Hematologic: Leukopenia, eosinophilia, anemia
Hepatic: Hepatomegaly, increased liver function test
Neuromuscular & skeletal: Myalgia, weakness
Renal: Rhabdomyolysis-induced renal failure
Miscellaneous: Flulike symptoms

Drug Interactions
May potentiate the anticoagulant effects of warfarin; insulin and sulfonylureas effects may be increased
Probenecid may increase the effects of clofibrate
Mechanism of Action Mechanism is unclear but thought to reduce cholesterol synthesis and triglyceride hepatic-vascular transference
Pharmacokinetics
Absorption: Occurs completely
Distribution: V_d: 5.5 L/kg
Protein binding: 95%
Metabolism: In the liver to an inactive glucuronide ester
Intestinal transformation is required to activate the drug
Half-life: 6-24 hours, increases significantly with reduced renal function
Anuria: 110 hours
Time to peak: Peak serum levels occur within 3-6 hours
Elimination: 40% to 70% excreted in urine
Usual Dosage Geriatrics and Adults: Oral: 500 mg 4 times/day

  Dosing interval in renal impairment:
  Cl_{cr} 15-50 mL/minute: Administer every 12-18 hours

Cl_{cr} <10 mL/minute: Avoid use

Monitoring Parameters Serum lipid profile; triglycerides and fractionated cholesterol

Test Interactions Increased creatine phosphokinase [CPK] (S); decreased alkaline phosphatase (S), cholesterol (S), glucose (S), uric acid (S)

Patient Information May be taken with food if stomach upset occurs; contact your physician if severe stomach pain with nausea and vomiting occurs, fever or chills, chest pain, irregular heart rhythm, shortness of breath, weight gain, decreased urination, blood in urine, leg swelling; adhere to prescribed diet

Special Geriatric Considerations The definition of and, therefore, when to treat hyperlipidemia in the elderly is a controversial issue. The National Cholesterol Education Program recommends that all adults 20 years of age and older maintain a plasma cholesterol level <200 mg/dL. By this definition, 60% of all elderly would be considered to have an elevated plasma cholesterol. However, plasma cholesterol has been shown to be a less reliable predictor of coronary heart disease in the elderly. Therefore, it is the authors' belief that pharmacologic treatment be reserved for those who are unable to obtain a desirable plasma cholesterol level by diet alone and for whom the benefits of treatment are believed to outweigh the potential adverse effects, drug interactions, and cost of treatment. Adjust dose for renal function.

Dosage Forms Capsule: 500 mg

Clomipramine Hydrochloride (kloe mi' pra meen)

Related Information

Antidepressant Agents Comparison *on page 800*

Brand Names Anafranil®

Generic Available No

Therapeutic Class Antidepressant, Tricyclic

Use Treatment of obsessive-compulsive disorder (OCD)

Unlabeled use: May also relieve depression, panic attacks, and chronic pain

Contraindications Patients in acute recovery stage of recent myocardial infarction; not to be used within 14 days of MAO inhibitors

Warnings Seizures are likely and are dose-related; can be additive when coadministered with other drugs that can lower the seizure threshold; use with caution in patients with asthma, bladder outlet destruction, angle-closure glaucoma

Adverse Reactions

Cardiovascular: Orthostatic hypotension, tachycardia

Central nervous system: Seizures, drowsiness, dizziness, confusion, headache, delirium, hyperthermia, asthenia, aggressive reaction

Dermatologic: Rash, dry skin

Gastrointestinal: Dry mouth, constipation, nausea, vomiting, increased appetite, weight gain

Genitourinary: Urinary retention, ejaculation failure

Hematologic: Agranulocytosis, anemia

Hepatic: Hepatitis

Ocular: Increased intraocular pressure, blurred vision

Otic: Vestibular disorder

Overdosage Symptoms of overdose include agitation, confusion, hallucinations, hyperthermia, CNS depression, dry mucous membranes, arrhythmias

Toxicology Following initiation of essential overdose management, toxic symptoms should be treated

Ventricular arrhythmias often respond to systemic alkalinization (sodium bicarbonate 0.5-2 mEq/kg I.V.) and/or phenytoin 15-20 mg/kg. Arrhythmias unresponsive to this therapy may respond to lidocaine 1 mg/kg I.V. followed by a titrated infusion. Physostigmine (1-2 mg I.V. slowly for adults) may be indicated in reversing cardiac arrhythmias that are life-threatening.

Seizures usually respond to diazepam I.V. boluses (5-10 mg for adults up to 30 mg). If seizures are unresponsive or recur, phenytoin or phenobarbital may be required.

Drug Interactions

Decreased effect with barbiturates, carbamazepine, phenytoin

Increased effect of alcohol, CNS depressants, anticholinergics, sympathomimetics

Increased toxicity: MAO inhibitors (increased temperature, seizures, coma, and death); antipsychotics (increased risk of hyperthermia)

Mechanism of Action Clomipramine appears to affect serotonin uptake while its active metabolite, desmethylclomipramine, affects norepinephrine uptake

Pharmacodynamics Onset of action: 1-3 weeks; 5 HT >NE

Pharmacokinetics

Absorption: Oral: Rapid

Metabolism: Extensive first-pass; metabolized to desmethylclomipramine (active) in the liver

Half-life: 20-30 hours

Usual Dosage Geriatrics and Adults: Oral: Initial: 25 mg/day and gradually increase, as tolerated, to 100 mg/day the first 2 weeks, may then be increased to a total of 250 mg/day maximum

(Continued)

175

Clomipramine Hydrochloride *(Continued)*

Monitoring Parameters Signs and symptoms of disorder, plasma concentrations, blood pressure

Reference Range Therapeutic plasma level: 80-100 ng/mL

Test Interactions Elevated glucose

Patient Information May cause seizures; caution should be used in activities that require alertness like driving, operating machinery, or swimming; effect of drug may take several weeks to appear; avoid alcohol; do not discontinue abruptly; may cause dry mouth, constipation, blurred vision

Special Geriatric Considerations Not approved as an antidepressant, clomipramine's anticholinergic and hypotensive effects limit its use versus other preferred antidepressants; elderly patients were found to have higher dose-normalized plasma concentrations as a result of decreased demethylation (decreased 50%) and hydroxylation (25%)

Dosage Forms Capsule: 25 mg, 50 mg, 75 mg

References

Bocksberger JP, Gex-Fabry M, Gauthey L, et al, "Clomipramine Therapy in the Geriatric Hospital: Experience With Therapeutic Drug Monitoring," *Ther Drug Monit*, 1994, 16(2):113-9.

Clonazepam (kloe na' ze pam)

Related Information

Anxiolytic/Hypnotic Use in Long-Term Care Facilities *on page 755-756*

Benzodiazepines Comparison *on page 802-803*

Brand Names Klonopin™

Generic Available No

Therapeutic Class Anticonvulsant, Benzodiazepine

Use Prophylaxis of absence (petit mal), petit mal variant (Lennox-Gastaut), akinetic, and myoclonic seizures

Unlabeled use: Restless legs syndrome, neuralgia (chronic pain syndromes), multifocal tic disorder, parkinsonian dysarthria, acute manic episodes in bipolar disorder, and adjunct therapy for schizophrenia

Restrictions C-IV

Contraindications Hypersensitivity to clonazepam, any component, or other benzodiazepines; severe liver disease, acute narrow-angle glaucoma

Precautions Use with caution in patients with chronic respiratory disease or impaired renal function; abrupt discontinuance may precipitate withdrawal symptoms, status epilepticus or seizures; use cautiously in depressed patients

Adverse Reactions

Cardiovascular: Hypotension

Central nervous system: Drowsiness, changes in behavior or personality, ataxia, vertigo, confusion, hallucinations, depression, disorientation, memory impairment, decreased concentration, headache, hypotonia, choreiform movements, staggering, falling

Dermatologic: Rash

Gastrointestinal: Nausea, dry mouth, vomiting, diarrhea, constipation, anorexia, hypersalivation

Hematologic: Thrombocytopenia, anemia, leukopenia, eosinophilia

Neuromuscular & skeletal: Tremors

Ocular: Nystagmus, blurred vision

Respiratory: Bronchial hypersecretion, respiratory depression, apnea

Miscellaneous: Physical and psychological dependence

Overdosage Symptoms of overdose include somnolence, confusion, ataxia, diminished reflexes, or coma

Toxicology Treatment for benzodiazepine overdose is supportive. Rarely is mechanical ventilation required. Flumazenil (Romazicon™) has been shown to selectively block the binding of benzodiazepines to CNS receptors, resulting in a reversal of benzodiazepine-induced CNS depression.

Drug Interactions Benzodiazepines may increase digoxin concentrations and may decrease the effect of levodopa; probenecid may increase onset of action and prolong the effect of benzodiazepine

Decreased metabolism: Cimetidine, fluoxetine

Increased metabolism: Rifampin

Increased toxicity: CNS depressants, alcohol

Mechanism of Action Suppresses the spike-and-wave discharge in absence seizures by depressing nerve transmission in the motor cortex

Pharmacodynamics

Onset of action: 20-60 minutes

Duration: 12 hours

Pharmacokinetics

Absorption: Oral: Well absorbed

Distribution: V_d: 1.5-4.4 L/kg

Protein binding 85%

Metabolism: Extensive

Half-life: 19-50 hours

Elimination: Metabolites excreted as glucuronide or sulfate conjugates; less than 2% excreted unchanged in urine

Usual Dosage Geriatrics and Adults: Oral: Initial daily dose not to exceed 1.5 mg given in 3 divided doses; may increase by 0.5-1 mg every third day until seizures are controlled or adverse effects seen; usual maintenance dose: 0.05-0.2 mg/kg; do not exceed 20 mg/day

Monitoring Parameters Monitor blood pressure, respiratory rate, motor coordination, mental status

Reference Range

Sample size: 2 mL serum or plasma (green top tube)

Therapeutic levels: 20-80 ng/mL; Toxic concentration: >80 ng/mL

Timing of serum samples: Peak serum levels occur 1-3 hours after oral ingestion; half-life: 20-40 hours; therefore, steady-state occurs in 5-7 days

Patient Information May cause drowsiness, dizziness, confusion. Avoid alcohol; use with caution when driving or performing tasks requiring alertness

Nursing Implications Observe patient for excess sedation, respiratory depression, orthostasis

Additional Information Ethosuximide or valproic acid may be preferred for treatment of absence (petit mal) seizures; clonazepam-induced behavioral disturbances may be more frequent in mentally handicapped patients; up to 30% of patients have demonstrated a loss of anticonvulsant control within several months which requires a dosage adjustment

Special Geriatric Considerations Hepatic clearance may be decreased allowing accumulation of active drug. Observe for signs of CNS and pulmonary toxicity; see Adverse Reactions

Dosage Forms Tablet: 0.5 mg, 1 mg, 2 mg

Clonidine (kloe' ni deen)

Brand Names Catapres®; Catapres-TTS®

Generic Available Yes: Tablet

Therapeutic Class Alpha-Adrenergic Agonist

Use Management of mild to moderate hypertension; either used alone or in combination with other antihypertensives; not recommended for first-line therapy for hypertension; unlabeled uses: heroin withdrawal, smoking cessation therapy, prophylaxis of migraines, glaucoma, paralytic ileus, diabetic diarrhea, vasomotor symptoms of menopause, postherpetic neuralgia, ulcerative colitis

Contraindications Hypersensitivity to clonidine hydrochloride or any component

Warnings Do not abruptly discontinue; rapid increase in blood pressure, and symptoms of sympathetic overactivity (such as increased heart rate, tremor, agitation, anxiety, insomnia, sweating, palpitations) may occur; if need to discontinue, taper dose gradually over more than 1 week

Precautions Dosage modification may be required in patients with renal impairment; use with caution in cerebrovascular disease, coronary insufficiency, renal impairment, sinus node dysfunction; use with caution in patients unable to comply with the therapeutic regimen because of the risk of rebound hypertension

Adverse Reactions

Cardiovascular: Raynaud's phenomenon, hypotension, bradycardia, palpitation, tachycardia, congestive heart failure

Central nervous system: Drowsiness, headache, dizziness, fatigue, insomnia, anxiety, nightmares, hallucinations, delirium, nervousness, depression

Dermatologic: Rash

Endocrine & metabolic: Sodium and water retention, parotid pain

Gastrointestinal: Constipation, anorexia, dry mouth

Local: Skin reactions with patch

Overdosage Symptoms of overdose include bradycardia, CNS depression, hypothermia, diarrhea, respiratory depression, apnea

Toxicology Treatment is primarily supportive and symptomatic. Hypotension usually responds to I.V. fluids or Trendelenburg positioning. If unresponsive to these measures the use of a parenteral vasoconstrictor may be required (eg, norepinephrine 0.1-0.2 mcg/kg/minute titrated to response). Naloxone may be utilized in treating the hypotension, CNS depression and/or apnea and should be given I.V. 0.4-2 mg, with repeats as needed. Atropine 15 mcg/kg I.V. may be needed for symptomatic bradycardia.

Drug Interactions

Beta-blockers may potentiate bradycardia in patients receiving clonidine and may increase the rebound hypertension seen with clonidine withdrawal; discontinue beta-blocker several days before clonidine is tapered off

Other hypotensive agents may potentiate hypotensive effects

Tricyclic antidepressants antagonize hypotensive effects of clonidine

(Continued)

Clonidine *(Continued)*

Mechanism of Action Stimulates alpha$_2$-adrenoreceptors in the brain stem, thus activating an inhibitory neuron, resulting in reduced sympathetic outflow, producing a decrease in vasomotor tone and heart rate

Pharmacodynamics
Onset of action: Oral: 30-60 minutes
Peak effect: Within 2-4 hours
Duration: 6-10 hours

Pharmacokinetics
Distribution: V$_d$: 2.1 L/kg
Metabolism: Hepatic to inactive metabolites; enterohepatic recirculation
Bioavailability: Oral: 75% to 95%
Half-life:
Normal renal function: 6-20 hours
Renal impairment: 18-41 hours
Elimination: 65% excreted in urine (32% unchanged and 22% excreted in feces)

Usual Dosage
Geriatrics: Oral: Initial: 0.1 mg once daily at bedtime; increase gradually as needed

Adults: Oral: Initial: 0.1 mg twice daily, usual maintenance dose: 0.2-1.2 mg/day in 2 divided doses; maximum recommended dose: 2.4 mg/day

Unlabeled route of administration: Sublingual clonidine 0.1-0.2 mg twice daily may be effective in patients unable to take oral medication

Clonidine tolerance test (test of growth hormone release from the pituitary): 0.1 mg/m^2 or 4 mcg/kg as a single dose

Transdermal: Initial: Catapres-TTS® 1 every week; maximum: 2 Catapres-TTS® every week
Conversion from oral to transdermal:
Day 1: Place Catapres-TTS® 1; administer 100% of oral dose
Day 2: Administer 50% of oral dose
Day 3: Administer 25% of oral dose
Always start with Catapres-TTS® 1 unless the patient was on a large oral dose
Not dialyzable (0% to 5%)

Administration Catapres-TTS® comes in 2 parts - the small patch containing the drug and an overlay to keep the patch in place for 1 week; both parts should be used for maximum efficacy; it may be useful to note on the patch which day it should be changed

Monitoring Parameters Blood pressure, standing and sitting/supine; mental status

Reference Range Therapeutic: 1-2 ng/mL (SI: 4.4-8.7 nmol/L)

Test Interactions Increased sodium (S); decreased catecholamines (U)

Patient Information Do not stop drug except on instruction of physician; check daily to be sure patch present; may cause drowsiness

Nursing Implications Patches should be applied weekly at bedtime to a clean, hairless area of the upper outer arm or chest; rotate patch sites weekly; see Administration

Special Geriatric Considerations Because of its potential CNS adverse effects, clonidine may not be considered a drug of choice in the elderly. If the decision is to use clonidine, adjust dose based on response and adverse reactions.

Dosage Forms
Patch, transdermal: 1, 2, and 3 (0.1mg, 0.2 mg, 0.3 mg/day for 7-day duration)
Tablet, as hydrochloride: 0.1 mg, 0.2 mg, 0.3 mg

Clonidine and Chlorthalidone

Related Information
Chlorthalidone *on page 159*
Clonidine *on previous page*

Brand Names Combipres®

Generic Available Yes

Therapeutic Class Antihypertensive, Combination

Special Geriatric Considerations Combination products are not recommended for first-line treatment and divided doses of diuretics may increase the incidence of nocturia in the elderly

Dosage Forms Tablet:
0.1: Clonidine 0.1 mg and chlorthalidone 15 mg
0.2: Clonidine 0.2 mg and chlorthalidone 15 mg
0.3: Clonidine 0.3 mg and chlorthalidone 15 mg

ClorazeCaps® *see* Clorazepate Dipotassium *on this page*

Clorazepate Dipotassium *(klor az' e pate)*

Related Information
Anxiolytic/Hypnotic Use in Long-Term Care Facilities *on page 755-756*

Benzodiazepines Comparison *on page 802-803*

Brand Names ClorazeCaps®; ClorazeTabs®; Gen-XENE®; Tranxene®

Generic Available Yes

Therapeutic Class Anticonvulsant, Benzodiazepine; Benzodiazepine; Sedative

Use Treatment of generalized anxiety and panic disorders; management of alcohol withdrawal; adjunct anticonvulsant in management of partial seizures

Restrictions C-IV

Contraindications Hypersensitivity to clorazepate dipotassium or any component; cross-sensitivity with other benzodiazepines may exist; avoid using in patients with pre-existing CNS depression, severe uncontrolled pain, or narrow-angle glaucoma

Precautions Use with caution in patients with hepatic or renal disease, or a history of drug dependence; abrupt discontinuation may cause withdrawal symptoms or seizures

Adverse Reactions
Cardiovascular: Hypotension
Central nervous system: Drowsiness, dizziness, confusion, amnesia, headache, depression, ataxia
Dermatologic: Rash
Gastrointestinal: Nausea, dry mouth
Ocular: Blurred vision
Miscellaneous: Physical and psychological dependence with long-term use; long-term use may also be associated with renal or hepatic injury and reduced hematocrit

Overdosage Symptoms of overdose include somnolence, confusion, ataxia, diminished reflexes, coma

Toxicology Treatment for benzodiazepine overdose is supportive; rarely is mechanical ventilation required; flumazenil has been shown to selectively block the binding of benzodiazepines to CNS receptors, resulting in a reversal of benzodiazepine-induced CNS depression, but not respiratory depression

Drug Interactions
Decreased metabolism: Cimetidine, fluoxetine
Increased metabolism: Rifampin
Increased toxicity: CNS depressants, alcohol

Stability Unstable in water

Mechanism of Action Benzodiazepines appear to potentiate the effects of GABA and other inhibitory neurotransmitters by binding to specific benzodiazepine-receptor sites in various areas of the CNS

Pharmacodynamics Studies have shown that the elderly are more sensitive to the effects of benzodiazepines as compared to younger adults

Pharmacokinetics
Absorption: Rapidly decarboxylated to desmethyldiazepam (active) in acidic stomach prior to absorption
Metabolism: In the liver to oxazepam (active)
Half-life: Adults:
Desmethyldiazepam: 48-96 hours
Oxazepam: 6-8 hours
Time to peak serum concentration: Oral: Within 1 hour
Elimination: Metabolites excreted primarily in urine

Usual Dosage Oral:
Geriatrics: Anxiety: 7.5 mg 1-2 times/day

Adults:
Anxiety: 7.5-15 mg 2-4 times/day, or given as single dose of 15-22.5 mg at bedtime
Alcohol withdrawal: Initial: 30 mg, then 15 mg 2-4 times/day on first day; maximum daily dose: 90 mg; gradually decrease dose over subsequent days

Monitoring Parameters Respiratory, cardiovascular, and mental status

Reference Range Therapeutic: 0.12-1 μg/mL (SI: 0.36-3.01 μmol/L)

Patient Information Avoid alcohol and other CNS depressants; may cause drowsiness; avoid activities needing good psychomotor coordination until CNS effects are known; may cause physical or psychological dependence; avoid abrupt discontinuation after prolonged use

Nursing Implications Assist patient with ambulation during initiation of therapy; monitor for alertness

Additional Information Clorazepate offers no advantage over the other benzodiazepines

Special Geriatric Considerations See Pharmacodynamics; due to its long-acting metabolite, clorazepate is not considered a drug of choice in the elderly; long-acting benzodiazepines have been associated with falls in the elderly; interpretive guidelines from the Health Care Financing Administration (HCFA) discourage the use of this agent in residents of long-term care facilities

Dosage Forms
Capsule: 3.75 mg, 7.5 mg, 15 mg
Tablet: 3.75 mg, 7.5 mg, 15 mg
Tablet, single dose: 11.25 mg, 22.5 mg

ClorazeTabs® *see* Clorazepate Dipotassium *on page 178*

Clotrimazole (kloe trim' a zole)

Brand Names Gyne-Lotrimin® [OTC]; Lotrimin®; Mycelex®; Mycelex®-G

Generic Available Yes

Therapeutic Class Antifungal Agent, Oral Nonabsorbed; Antifungal Agent, Topical; Antifungal Agent, Vaginal

Use Treatment of susceptible fungal infections, including oropharyngeal candidiasis, dermatophytoses, superficial mycoses, and cutaneous candidiasis, as well as vulvovaginal candidiasis; limited data suggests that the use of clotrimazole troches may be effective for prophylaxis against oropharyngeal candidiasis in neutropenic patients

Contraindications Hypersensitivity to clotrimazole or any component

Precautions Clotrimazole troches should not be used for treatment of systemic fungal infection

Adverse Reactions

Gastrointestinal: Nausea and vomiting may occur in patients on clotrimazole troches

Hepatic: Abnormal liver function tests

Local: Mild burning, irritation, stinging to skin or vaginal area

Mechanism of Action Binds to phospholipids in the fungal cell membrane altering cell wall permeability resulting in loss of essential intracellular elements

Pharmacokinetics

Absorption: Through intact skin is negligible, when administered topically; following oral topical administration, salivary levels occur within 3 hours following 30 minutes of dissolution time in the mouth; high vaginal levels occur following vaginal cream administration within 8-24 hours and within 1-2 days following vaginal tablet administration

Elimination: As metabolites via bile

Usual Dosage Geriatrics and Adults:

Oral: 10 mg troche dissolved slowly 5 times/day for 14 days

Topical: Apply twice daily

Vaginal: 100 mg/day for 7 days or 200 mg/day for 3 days or 500 mg single dose or 5 g (= 1 applicatorful) of 1% vaginal cream daily for 7-14 days

Monitoring Parameters Periodic liver function tests during oral therapy with clotrimazole lozenges

Patient Information May cause irritation to the skin; avoid contact with the eyes; lozenge (troche) must be dissolved slowly in the mouth

Nursing Implications Give around-the-clock rather than 4 times/day, 3 times/day, etc (ie, 12-6-12-6, not 9-1-5-9) to promote less variation in peak and trough serum levels

Special Geriatric Considerations Localized fungal infections frequently follow broad spectrum antimicrobial therapy; specifically, oral and vaginal infections due to Candida

Dosage Forms

Cream:

Topical: 1% (15 g, 30 g, 45 g, 90 g)

Vaginal: 1% (45 g, 90 g)

Lotion: 1% (30 mL)

Solution, topical: 1% (10 mL, 30 mL)

Tablet, vaginal: 100 mg (7's); 500 mg (1's)

Cloxacillin Sodium (klox a sill' in)

Brand Names Cloxapen®; Tegopen®

Generic Available Yes

Therapeutic Class Antibiotic, Penicillin

Use Treatment of susceptible bacterial infections, notably penicillinase-producing staphylococci (not methicillin-resistant) causing respiratory tract, skin and skin structure, bone and joint, urinary tract infections, endocarditis, septicemia, and meningitis

Contraindications Hypersensitivity to cloxacillin or any component, or penicillins

Precautions Use with caution in patients allergic to cephalosporins

Adverse Reactions

Central nervous system: Fever

Dermatologic: Rash

Gastrointestinal: Nausea, vomiting, diarrhea

Hematologic: Eosinophilia, leukopenia, neutropenia, thrombocytopenia, agranulocytosis

Hepatic: Serum sickness-like reactions, hepatotoxicity

Renal: Hematuria

Overdosage Symptoms of overdose include neuromuscular hypersensitivity, convulsions

Toxicology Many beta-lactam-containing antibiotics have the potential to cause neuromuscular hyperirritability or convulsive seizures. Hemodialysis may be helpful to aid in the removal of the drug from the blood, otherwise most treatment is supportive or symptom directed.

Drug Interactions
Increased levels with probenecid
Cloxacillin has been reported to decrease effect of warfarin in a small number of patients

Stability Refrigerate oral solution after reconstitution; discard after 14 days; stable for 3 days at room temperature

Mechanism of Action Interferes with bacterial cell wall synthesis during active multiplication causing cell death and resultant bactericidal activity against susceptible bacteria

Pharmacokinetics
Absorption: Oral: ~50%
Protein binding: 90% to 98%
Metabolism: Significant in the liver to active and inactive metabolites
Half-life: 30-90 minutes (prolonged with renal impairment); reported to be longer in the elderly, but is not considered clinically significant
Time to peak: Oral: Peak serum levels occur within 0.5-2 hours
Elimination: In urine and through bile

Usual Dosage Geriatrics and Adults: Oral: 250-500 mg every 6 hours
Not dialyzable (0% to 5%)

Monitoring Parameters Signs and symptoms of infection; mental status, WBC; PT for patients on warfarin

Test Interactions False-positive urine and serum proteins

Patient Information Complete full course of therapy; contact your physician or pharmacist if not improving or diarrhea develops

Nursing Implications Administer 1 hour before or 2 hours after meals

Special Geriatric Considerations See Pharmacokinetics and Usual Dosage; dosage change for renal function is not necessary

Dosage Forms
Capsule: 250 mg, 500 mg
Suspension, oral: 125 mg/5 mL (100 mL, 200 mL)

References
Bluhm G, Jacobson B, Julander I, et al, "Antibiotic Prophylaxis in Pacemaker Surgery - A Prospective Study," *Scand J Thorac Cardiovasc Surg*, 1984, 18(3):227-34.

Cloxapen® see Cloxacillin Sodium *on previous page*

Clozapine (kloe' za peen)
Related Information
Antipsychotic Agents Comparison *on page 801*
Antipsychotic Medication Guidelines *on page 754*

Brand Names Clozaril®
Generic Available No
Therapeutic Class Antipsychotic Agent

Use Management of severely ill schizophrenic patients who fail to respond to standard antipsychotic therapy; not recommended at this time for nonpsychotic symptoms associated with dementia or other diseases in elderly

Contraindications In patients with WBC of 3500 cells/mm^3 or lower before therapy; if WBC falls to <3000 cells/mm^3 during therapy the drug should be withheld until signs and symptoms of infection disappear and WBC rise above 3000 cells/mm^3 or granulocytes decrease (ANC) falls <500/mm^2

Warnings Significant risk of agranulocytosis, potentially life-threatening; therefore, reserve clozapine for use in severely ill schizophrenic patients who fail therapy with standard antipsychotic therapy either because of insufficient effectiveness or inability to achieve effective dose due to intolerable ADRs; before initiating clozapine therapy, it is strongly recommended to attempt at least two trials, each with different standard antipsychotic agents at an adequate dose for an adequate period of time. Patients treated with clozapine must have a baseline WBC with differential, repeated weekly throughout treatment and for 4 weeks after discontinuing clozapine. No established risk factors have been established, however, a higher number of patients with Jewish background developed agranulocytosis in US studies. The numbers were disproportionate to other ethnic groups; also caution should be used with women and elderly since these two groups have a higher incidence of agranulocytosis occurring with the use of antipsychotic therapy

Seizures: Occurs with high doses
Cardiovascular disease: Use with caution; see changes seen with other antipsychotic agents; see Adverse Reactions
Orthostatic hypotension: May occur, especially during initiation and rapid dose increases
Neuroleptic malignant syndrome (NMS): A potentially serious and fatal symptom complex associated with antipsychotic therapy. However, no cases of NMS due to clozapine alone have been reported to date. There has been reports with patients treated concomitantly with lithium or other CNS active agents

(Continued)

Clozapine *(Continued)*

Tardive dyskinesia: No cases of tardive dyskinesia have been reported. However, it cannot be concluded that clozapine does not cause this symptom complex until more clinical use of this agent has been evaluated

Precautions Fever, transient elevations (>100.4°F) occur in the first 3 weeks of therapy; if fever persists, may need to stop therapy; evaluate for infection and agranulocytosis; if fever is high consider NMS; see Warnings

Anticholinergic: May cause increased confusion in elderly; consider effects on bladder, bowel, and in patients with cardiovascular disease

CNS: Severe sedation may impair mental and physical abilities; especially in first few days of therapy; use gradual dose increases

Use with caution in patients with renal, hepatic, or cardiac disease due to limited experience with clozapine

Adverse Reactions

Cardiovascular: Hypotension, tachycardia, EKG changes, syncope

Central nervous system: Seizures, headache, dizziness, agitation, fatigue, insomnia, drowsiness, visual disturbances, fever, akathisia

Dermatologic: Rash

Gastrointestinal: Hypersalivation, dry mouth, nausea, vomiting, constipation, heartburn, abdominal discomfort, diarrhea, weight gain

Genitourinary: Incontinence

Hematologic: Agranulocytosis

Neuromuscular & skeletal: Tremors

Miscellaneous: Sweating

Overdosage Symptoms of overdose include altered states of consciousness, tachycardia, hypotension, hypersalivation, respiratory depression

Toxicology Following initiation of essential overdose management, toxic symptom treatment and supportive treatment should be initiated. Hypotension usually responds to I.V. fluids or Trendelenburg positioning. If unresponsive to these measures the use of a parenteral inotrope may be required (eg, norepinephrine 0.1-0.2 mcg/kg/minute titrated to response). Do not use epinephrine. Seizures commonly respond to diazepam (I.V. 5-10 mg bolus every 15 minutes if needed up to a total of 30 mg) or to phenytoin or phenobarbital. Also critical cardiac arrhythmias often respond to I.V. phenytoin (15 mg/kg up to 1 g), while other antiarrhythmics can be used. Neuroleptics often cause extrapyramidal symptoms (eg, dystonic reactions) requiring management with diphenhydramine 1-2 mg/kg up to a maximum of 50 mg I.M. or I.V. slow push followed by a maintenance dose for 48-72 hours. When these reactions are unresponsive to diphenhydramine, benztropine mesylate I.V. 1-2 mg may be effective. These agents are generally effective within 2-5 minutes.

Drug Interactions

Anticholinergic: Enhanced anticholinergic effect by clozapine

Antihypertensives: Augment hypotensive effect

CNS active drugs: Enhances CNS pharmacologic effects or CNS active drugs

Bone marrow suppressants: Clozapine may act synergistically with other bone marrow suppressing drugs

Protein binding: Clozapine highly bound to serum protein; use cautiously with other highly protein bound drugs (eg, warfarin, phenytoin, phenobarbital, etc)

Stability Dispensed in "clozapine patient system" packaging

Mechanism of Action Clozapine is a weak dopamine$_1$ and dopamine$_2$ receptor blocker; in addition, it blocks the serotonin$_2$, alpha-adrenergic, and histamine H$_1$ central nervous system receptors; clozapine appears to be preferentially more active in the limbic system than in striatal areas. Its low affinity for D$_1$ and D$_2$ receptors in striatal area may explain its relatively low EPS side effects. Clozapine, as does other antipsychotics, increases delta and theta activity but slows dominant alpha frequencies on EEG. REM sleep is increased.

Pharmacokinetics

Absorption: Well absorbed

Protein binding: 95% bound to serum proteins

Metabolism: Undergoes extensive metabolism primarily to unconjugated forms

Bioavailability: Food does not appear to affect bioavailability

Half-life, elimination: (mean): 12 hours (range: 4-66 hours)

Time to peak: Occurs on an average of 2.5 hours after administration (range 1-6 hours)

Elimination: In urine

Usual Dosage Oral:

Geriatrics: Experience in elderly is limited; initial dose should be 25 mg/day; increase as tolerated by 25 mg/day to desired response; maximum daily dose in elderly should probably be 450 mg; dose titration to 300-450 mg/day may be attained in 2 weeks if tolerated; however, elderly may require slower titration and daily increases may not be tolerated

Adults: 25 mg once or twice daily initially and increased, as tolerated to a target dose of 300-450 mg/day, but may require doses as high as 600-900 mg/day

Monitoring Parameters CBC (WBC); orthostatic blood pressures; tremors, gait changes, abnormal movement in trunk, neck, buccal area or extremities; monitor target behaviors for which the agent is given

Patient Information Report any lethargy, fever, sore throat, flu-like symptoms or any other signs or symptoms of infection; may cause drowsiness, orthostatic hypotension; inform patient of importance of weekly blood tests

Nursing Implications Benign, self-limiting temperature elevations sometimes occur during the first 3 weeks of treatment; monitor orthostatic blood pressures; observe for signs of infection; observe for motor abnormalities

Additional Information Medication should not be stopped abruptly; taper off over 1-2 weeks; WBC testing should occur weekly for the duration of therapy and for 4 weeks after discontinuation of clozapine

Special Geriatric Considerations Not recommended for use in nonpsychotic patients; see Warnings

Many elderly patients receive antipsychotic medications for inappropriate nonpsychotic behavior. Before initiating antipsychotic medication, the clinician should investigate any possible reversible cause; any stress or stress from any disease can cause acute "confusion" or worsening of baseline nonpsychotic behavior. Most commonly acute changes in behavior are due to increases in drug dose or addition of new drug to regimen; fluid electrolyte loss; infections, and/or changes in environment

Any changes in disease status in any organ system can result in behavior changes.

Dosage Forms Tablet: 25 mg, 100 mg

References

Drug Facts and Comparisons, New York, NY: JB Lippincott, 1990, 265E-F.

Peabody CA, Warner MD, Whiteford HA, et al, "Neuroleptics and the Elderly," *J Am Geriatr Soc*, 1987, 35(3):233-8.

Risse SC and Barnes R, "Pharmacologic Treatment of Agitation Associated With Dementia," *J Am Geriatr Soc*, 1986, 34(5):368-76.

Saltz BL, Woerner MG, Kane JM, et al, "Prospective Study of Tardive Dyskinesia Incidence in the Elderly," *JAMA*, 1991, 266(17):2402-6.

Seifert RD, "Therapeutic Drug Monitoring: Psychotropic Drugs," *J Pharm Pract*, 1984, 6:403-16.

Clozaril® *see* Clozapine *on page 181*

Clysodrast® *see* Bisacodyl *on page 87*

Cobex® *see* Cyanocobalamin *on page 192*

Codeine (koe' deen)

Related Information
  Narcotic Agonist Comparative Pharmacology *on page 811*
  Pharmacokinetics of Narcotic Agonist Analgesics *on page 812*

Synonyms Codeine Phosphate; Codeine Sulfate; Methylmorphine

Generic Available Yes

Therapeutic Class Analgesic, Narcotic; Antitussive

Use Treatment of mild to moderate pain; antitussive in lower doses

Restrictions C-II

Contraindications Hypersensitivity to codeine or any component

Warnings Some preparations contain sulfites which may cause allergic reactions

Precautions Use with caution in patients with hypersensitivity reactions to other phenanthrene derivative opioid agonists (morphine, hydrocodone, hydromorphone, levorphanol, oxycodone, oxymorphone); respiratory diseases including asthma, emphysema, COPD; or severe liver or renal insufficiency

Adverse Reactions
  Cardiovascular: Palpitations, hypotension, bradycardia, peripheral vasodilation
  Central nervous system: CNS depression, increased intracranial pressure
  Dermatologic: Pruritus
  Endocrine & metabolic: Antidiuretic hormone release
  Gastrointestinal: Nausea, vomiting, constipation
  Ocular: Miosis
  Respiratory: Respiratory depression
  Miscellaneous: Physical and psychological dependence, biliary or urinary tract spasm, histamine release

Overdosage Symptoms of overdose include CNS and respiratory depression, gastrointestinal cramping, constipation

Toxicology Treatment of an overdose includes support of patient's airway, establishment of an I.V. line, and naloxone 2 mg I.V. with repeat administration as necessary up to a total of 10 mg

Drug Interactions Increased toxicity: CNS depressants, phenothiazines, tricyclic antidepressants, alcohol

Stability Store injection between 15°C to 30°C, avoid freezing; do not use if injection is discolored or contains a precipitate

Mechanism of Action Binds to opiate receptors in the CNS, causing inhibition of ascending pain pathways, altering the perception of and response to pain; causes

(Continued)

Codeine *(Continued)*

cough supression by direct central action in the medulla; produces generalized CNS depression

Pharmacodynamics
Onset of action:
Oral: 30-60 minutes
I.M.: 10-30 minutes
Peak action:
Oral: 60-90 minutes
I.M.: 30-60 minutes
Duration of action: 4-6 hours; may be increased in the elderly; enhanced analgesia has been seen in elderly patients on therapeutic doses of narcotics

Pharmacokinetics
Absorption: Oral: Adequate
Protein binding: 7%
Metabolism: Hepatic metabolism to morphine (active)
Half-life: 2.5-3.5 hours
Elimination: 3% to 16% excreted in urine as unchanged drug, norcodeine and free and conjugated morphine

Usual Dosage Doses should be titrated to appropriate analgesic effect; when changing routes of administration, note that oral dose is 66% as effective as parenteral dose

Analgesic: Oral, I.M., S.C.: Geriatrics and Adults: Usual: 30 mg/dose; range: 15-60 mg every 4-6 hours as needed; maximum: 360 mg/24 hours

Antitussive: Oral (for nonproductive cough): Adults: 10-20 mg/dose every 4-6 hours as needed; maximum: 120 mg/day

Dosing adjustment in renal impairment:
Cl_{cr} 10-50 mL/minute: Administer 75% of dose
Cl_{cr} <10 mL/minute: Administer 50% of dose

Dosing adjustment in hepatic impairment: Probably necessary in hepatic insufficiency

Monitoring Parameters Pain relief, respiratory and mental status, blood pressure
Reference Range Therapeutic: Not established; Toxic: >1.1 μg/mL
Test Interactions Increased aminotransferase [ALT (SGPT)/AST (SGOT)] (S)
Patient Information Avoid alcohol, may cause drowsiness; may cause GI upset, can take with food
Nursing Implications Observe patient for excessive sedation or confusion, respiratory depression, constipation
Additional Information May be habit-forming; dextromethorphan has equivalent antitussive activity but has much lower toxicity in accidental overdose
Special Geriatric Considerations The elderly may be particularly susceptible to CNS depression and confusion as well as the constipating effects of narcotics; see Pharmacodynamics

Dosage Forms
Injection, as phosphate: 30 mg/mL (1 mL, 2 mL); 60 mg/mL (1 mL, 2 mL)
Syrup: 10 mg/5 mL, 60 mg/5 mL
Tablet, as sulfate: 15 mg, 30 mg, 60 mg
Tablet, as phosphate, soluble: 15 mg, 30 mg, 60 mg
Tablet, as sulfate, soluble: 15 mg, 30 mg, 60 mg

References
Ferrell BA, "Pain Management in Elderly People," *J Am Geriatr Soc*, 1991, 39(1):64-73.
Kaiko RF, Wallenstein SL, Rogers AG, et al, "Narcotics in the Elderly," *Med Clin North Am*, 1982, 66(5):1079-89.

Codeine and Acetaminophen *see* Acetaminophen and Codeine *on page 14*

Codeine and Aspirin *see* Aspirin and Codeine *on page 61*

Codeine and Guaifenesin *see* Guaifenesin and Codeine *on page 332*

Codeine Phosphate *see* Codeine *on previous page*

Codeine Sulfate *see* Codeine *on previous page*

Codimal-A® *see* Brompheniramine Maleate *on page 95*

Codoxy® *see* Oxycodone and Aspirin *on page 529*

Cogentin® *see* Benztropine Mesylate *on page 80*

Co-Gesic® *see* Hydrocodone and Acetaminophen *on page 350*

Cognex® *see* Tacrine Hydrochloride *on page 668*

Colace® [OTC] *see* Docusate *on page 236*

Colax® [OTC] *see* Docusate and Phenolphthalein *on page 238*

ColBENEMID® *see* Colchicine and Probenecid *on page 186*

Colchicine (kol' chi seen)

Generic Available Yes: Tablet

Therapeutic Class Anti-inflammatory Agent; Uricosuric Agent

Use Treat acute gouty arthritis attacks and to prevent recurrences of such attacks; management of familial Mediterranean fever

Contraindications Hypersensitivity to colchicine or any component; severe renal, GI disease, cardiac disorders, or blood dyscrasias

Warnings Use cautiously in patients with hepatic dysfunction; elderly and debilitated patients are at risk for adverse effects

Precautions Severe local irritation can occur following S.C. or I.M. administration; GI side effects may cause difficulty in patients with peptic ulcer disease or spastic colon; colchicine-induced myoneuropathy after misdiagnosed as polymyositis or uremic neuropathy; reversible vitamin B_{12} malabsorption

Adverse Reactions

Central nervous system: Peripheral neuritis

Dermatologic: Rash, alopecia, purpura

Gastrointestinal: Nausea, vomiting, diarrhea, abdominal pain

Genitourinary: Azoospermia

Hematologic: Agranulocytosis, aplastic anemia, bone marrow suppression

Hepatic: Hepatotoxicity, elevate alkaline phosphatase and AST

Neuromuscular & skeletal: Myopathy

Overdosage Symptoms of overdose include burning in throat, watery to bloody diarrhea, nausea, vomiting, abdominal pain, hypotension, anuria, cardiovascular collapse, delirium, convulsions, shock, S-T segment elevation, muscle weakness, paralysis, respiratory failure, hepatic damage; by 5th day, leukopenia, thrombocytopenia, coagulopathy, alopecia, stomatitis

Toxicology Gastric lavage, treat for shock; hemodialysis or peritoneal dialysis effective; atropine and morphine relieve abdominal pain; use respiratory assistance as needed; give general supportive care; deaths occur with 65 mg orally or 7 mg I.V.

Drug Interactions May decrease platelet counts; may cause false-positive results when testing urine for blood or hemoglobin

Stability Protect tablets from light; I.V. colchicine is incompatible with dextrose or I.V. solutions with preservatives

Mechanism of Action Decreases leukocyte motility, decreases phagocytosis in joints, and lactic acid production, thereby reducing the deposition of urate crystals that perpetuates the inflammatory response; interferes with kinin formation and reduces phagocytosis thereby decreasing inflammatory response

Pharmacodynamics Articular pain and swelling decrease within 12 hours; attack resolved in 1-2 days

Pharmacokinetics

Distribution: Partially deacetylated in the liver

Protein binding: 10% to 31%

Half-life: 12-30 minutes

Time to peak: Oral: Peak serum levels occur within 30-120 minutes then decline for 2 hours before increasing again due to enterohepatic recycling

Elimination: Primarily in feces via bile; 10% to 20% eliminated unchanged in urine

Usual Dosage Geriatrics and Adults:

Prophylaxis of familial Mediterranean fever: Oral: 1-2 mg/day in 2-3 divided doses

Gout:

Oral: Acute attacks: Initial: 0.5-1.2 mg, then 0.5-0.6 mg every 1-2 hours or 1-1.2 mg every 1-2 hours until relief or GI side effects occur; maximum total dose: 8 mg/day; wait 3 days before initiating a second course

I.V.: Initial: 1-3 mg, then 0.5 mg every 6 hours until response, not to exceed 4 mg/day; if pain recurs, it may be necessary to administer a daily dose of 1 to 2 mg for several days, however, do not give more colchicine by any route for at least 7 days after a full course of I.V. therapy (4 mg), transfer to oral colchicine in a dose similar to that being given I.V.

Prophylaxis of recurrent attacks: Oral:

Less than 1 attack per year: 0.5-0.6 mg/day for 3-4 days/week

More than 1 attack per year: 0.5-0.6 mg/day

Severe cases: 1-1.8 mg/day

Dosing interval in renal impairment: Cl_{cr} <10 mL/minute: Decrease dose by 50%

Not dialyzable (0% to 5%)

Test Interactions May cause false-positive results in urine tests for erythrocytes or hemoglobin

Patient Information Discontinue if nausea or vomiting occur; avoid alcohol; if taking for acute attack, discontinue as soon as pain resolves; do not exceed 8 mg/day orally; notify physician if sore throat, persistent abdominal pain, nausea, diarrhea, fever, bleeding, bruising, tiredness, weakness, numbness, or tingling occur

Nursing Implications Injection should be made over 2-5 minutes into tubing of free-flowing I.V. with compatible fluid; **incompatible with dextrose**; see Adverse Reactions; monitor for response; CBC, LFTs, renal function

(Continued)

Colchicine *(Continued)*

Special Geriatric Considerations Colchicine appears to be more toxic in elderly, particularly in the presence of renal, gastrointestinal, or cardiac disease. The most predictable oral side effects are (gastrointestinal) vomiting, abdominal pain, and nausea. If colchicine is stopped at this point, other more severe adverse effects may be avoided, such as bone marrow suppression, peripheral neuritis, etc.

Dosage Forms
Injection: 0.5 mg/mL (2 mL)
Tablet: 0.5 mg, 0.6 mg, 0.65 mg

References
Levy M, Spino M, and Read SE, "Colchicine: A State-of-the-Art Review," *Pharmacotherapy*, 1991, 11(3):196-211.

Colchicine and Probenecid

Related Information
Colchicine *on previous page*
Probenecid *on page 589*

Brand Names ColBENEMID®

Synonyms Probenecid and Colchicine

Generic Available Yes

Therapeutic Class Uricosuric Agent

Use Treatment of chronic gouty arthritis when complicated by frequent, recurrent acute attacks of gout

Usual Dosage Geriatrics and Adults: Oral: 1 tablet daily for 1 week; then 1 tablet twice daily thereafter

Special Geriatric Considerations See monographs for individual agents

Dosage Forms Tablet: Colchicine 0.5 mg and probenecid 0.5 g

Colestid® *see* Colestipol Hydrochloride *on this page*

Colestipol Hydrochloride *(koe les' ti pole)*

Brand Names Colestid®

Therapeutic Class Antilipemic Agent

Use Adjunct in the management of primary hypercholesterolemia; to relieve pruritus associated with elevated levels of bile acids, possibly used to decrease plasma half-life of digoxin as an adjunct in the treatment of toxicity

Contraindications Hypersensitivity to colestipol or any component; avoid using in complete biliary obstruction

Precautions Patients with high triglycerides, GI dysfunction (constipation); may be associated with increased bleeding tendency as a result of hypothrombinemia secondary to vitamin K deficiency; may cause depletion of vitamins A, D, and E

Adverse Reactions
Central nervous system: Dizziness, headache, anxiety, vertigo, drowsiness, fatigue
Dermatologic: Urticaria, dermatitis
Endocrine & metabolic: Increased serum phosphorous and chloride with decrease of sodium and potassium
Gastrointestinal: Constipation, abdominal pain and distention, belching, flatulence, nausea, vomiting, diarrhea, anorexia, peptic ulceration
Hepatic: Transient increases in serum AST (SGOT) and alkaline phosphatase concentrations
Neuromuscular & skeletal: Muscle and joint pain, arthritis, weakness
Respiratory: Shortness of breath

Overdosage Symptoms of overdose include GI obstruction, nausea, GI distress

Toxicology Treatment is supportive

Drug Interactions Since colestipol is an anion-exchange resin, it is capable of binding to a number of drugs (especially tetracycline, penicillin G, chlorothiazide, digoxin, and propranolol) in the GI tract and may delay or reduce their absorption; may prevent absorption of vitamin A, D, E, and K; oral supplements of vitamin A and D may be necessary

Mechanism of Action Binds with bile acids to form an insoluble complex that is eliminated in the feces; it thereby increases the fecal loss of bile acid-bound low density lipoprotein cholesterol

Pharmacokinetics Absorption: Oral: Not absorbed

Usual Dosage Geriatrics and Adults: 5-30 g/day in divided doses 2-4 times/day

Administration Dry powder should be added to at least 90 mL of liquid and stirred until completely mixed; other drugs should be administered at least 1 hour before or 4 hours after colestipol

Monitoring Parameters Serum lipid profile; plasma cholesterol (LDL and VLDL fractions); observe for gastrointestinal side effects

Test Interactions Increased prothrombin time (S); decreased cholesterol (S)

Patient Information Mix in liquids, cereals, soda, soup, or pulpy fruits; add at least 90 mL of liquid; do not take dry; stir well, powder will not dissolve; rinse glass with small amount of liquid to ensure full dose is taken

Nursing Implications See Administration

Special Geriatric Considerations The definition of and, therefore, when to treat hyperlipidemia in the elderly is a controversial issue. The National Cholesterol Education Program recommends that all adults 20 years of age and older maintain a plasma cholesterol level <200 mg/dL. By this definition, 60% of all elderly would be considered to have an elevated plasma cholesterol. However, plasma cholesterol has been shown to be a less reliable predictor of coronary heart disease in the elderly. Therefore, it is the authors' belief that pharmacologic treatment should be reserved for those who are unable to obtain a desirable plasma cholesterol level by diet alone and for whom the benefits of treatment are believed to outweigh the potential adverse effects, drug interactions, and cost of treatment.

Dosage Forms Granules: 5 g packet, 300 g, 500 g

Collagenase (kol' la je nase)
Brand Names Biozyme-C®; Santyl®
Generic Available No
Therapeutic Class Enzyme, Topical Debridement
Use Promotes debridement of necrotic tissue in dermal ulcers and severe burns
Contraindications Known hypersensitivity to collagenase
Warnings For external use only; avoid contact with eyes
Precautions Monitor patients for signs or symptoms of systemic bacterial infections; apply collagenase only to lesion, slight erythema has occurred in surrounding tissue
Adverse Reactions Local: Pain and burning may occur at site of application
Toxicology Action of enzyme may be stopped by applying Burow's solution
Drug Interactions Decreased effect: Enzymatic activity is inhibited by detergents, benzalkonium chloride, hexachlorophene, nitrofurazone, tincture of iodine, and heavy metal ions (silver and mercury)
Mechanism of Action Collagenase is an enzyme derived from the fermentation of *Clostridium histolyticum* and differs from other proteolytic enzymes in that its enzymatic action has a high specificity for native and denatured collagen. Collagenase will not attack collagen in healthy tissue or newly formed granulation tissue. In addition, it does not act on fat, fibrin, keratin, or muscle.
Usual Dosage Topical: Apply once daily (or more frequently if the dressing becomes soiled)
Administration Prior to application, cleanse lesion of debris and digested material; when infection is present, neomycin-bacitracin-polymyxin B may be used with collagenase; excess ointment should be removed each time the dressing is changed; treatment should be discontinued when debridement is complete and granulation tissue is well established
Monitoring Parameters Healing of ulcer
Patient Information For external use only; avoid contact with eyes
Nursing Implications Do not introduce into major body cavities; monitor debilitated patients for systemic bacterial infections; see Administration
Special Geriatric Considerations Preventive skin care should be instituted in all older patients at high risk for decubitus ulcers; collagenase is indicated in stage 3 and 4 decubitus ulcers
Dosage Forms Ointment, topical: 250 units/g (15 g, 30 g)
References
Chamberlain TM, Cali TS, Cuzzell J, et al, "Assessment and Management of Pressure Sores in Long-Term Care Facilities," *Consult Pharm*, 1992, 7(12)1328-40.

Collyrium Fresh® [OTC] *see* Tetrahydrozoline Hydrochloride *on page 680*

Combipres® *see* Clonidine and Chlorthalidone *on page 178*

Comfort® [OTC] *see* Naphazoline Hydrochloride *on page 492*

Compazine® *see* Prochlorperazine *on page 592*

Compound E *see* Cortisone Acetate *on next page*

Compound F *see* Hydrocortisone *on page 351*

Compound S *see* Zidovudine *on page 741*

Compoz® [OTC] *see* Diphenhydramine Hydrochloride *on page 228*

Constant-T® *see* Theophylline *on page 681*

Constilac® *see* Lactulose *on page 397*

Constulose® *see* Lactulose *on page 397*

Control® [OTC] *see* Phenylpropanolamine Hydrochloride *on page 559*

Cophene-B® *see* Brompheniramine Maleate *on page 95*

Cordarone® *see* Amiodarone Hydrochloride *on page 42*

Corgard® *see* Nadolol *on page 485*

ALPHABETICAL LISTING OF DRUGS

Correctol® [OTC] *see* Docusate and Phenolphthalein *on page 238*

Cortaid® [OTC] *see* Hydrocortisone *on page 351*

Cortalone® *see* Prednisolone *on page 584*

Cortan® *see* Prednisone *on page 586*

Cort-Dome® *see* Hydrocortisone *on page 351*

Cortef® *see* Hydrocortisone *on page 351*

Corticosteroids Comparison, Systemic *see page 808*

Corticosteroids Comparison, Topical *see page 809*

Cortifoam® *see* Hydrocortisone *on page 351*

Cortisol *see* Hydrocortisone *on page 351*

Cortisone Acetate (kor' ti sone)
Related Information
Antacid Drug Interactions *on page 764*
Corticosteroids Comparison, Systemic *on page 808*
Brand Names Cortone® Acetate
Synonyms Compound E
Generic Available Yes
Therapeutic Class Adrenal Corticosteroid; Anti-inflammatory Agent; Corticosteroid, Systemic
Use Management of adrenocortical insufficiency
Contraindications Serious infections, except septic shock or tuberculous meningitis, idiopathic thrombocytopenia purpura (I.M. use), administration of live virus vaccines
Precautions Use with caution in patients with hypothyroidism, cirrhosis, hypertension, congestive heart failure, ulcerative colitis, thromboembolic disorders, osteoporosis, convulsive disorders, peptic ulcer, diabetes mellitus, myasthenia gravis
Adverse Reactions
Cardiovascular: Edema, hypertension, accelerated atherogenesis
Central nervous system: Vertigo, seizures, headache, psychosis, pseudotumor cerebri
Dermatologic: Acne, skin atrophy, impaired wound healing, hirsutism
Endocrine & metabolic: Cushing's syndrome, pituitary-adrenal axis suppression, growth suppression, glucose intolerance, hypokalemia, alkalosis, hot flashes, postmenopausal bleeding
Gastrointestinal: Peptic ulcer, nausea, vomiting, pancreatitis
Neuromuscular & skeletal: Muscle weakness, osteoporosis, fractures, aseptic necrosis of femoral and humeral heads, steroid myopathy
Ocular: Cataracts, glaucoma
Miscellaneous: Increased susceptibility to infections
Toxicology When consumed in excessive quantities for prolonged periods, systemic hypercorticism and adrenal suppression may occur; in those cases, discontinuation and withdrawal of the corticosteroid should be done judiciously
Drug Interactions
Steroids decrease the effect of anticholinesterases, isoniazid, salicylates, insulin, oral hypoglycemics
Decreased effect: Barbiturates, phenytoin, rifampin
Increased effect (hypokalemia) of potassium-depleting diuretics
Increased risk of digoxin toxicity (due to hypokalemia)
Increased effect: Estrogens, ketoconazole
Mechanism of Action Decreases inflammation by suppression of migration of polymorphonuclear leukocytes and reversal of increased capillary permeability; suppresses immune response with pharmacologic doses
Pharmacodynamics
Peak effect:
Oral: Within 2 hours
I.M.: Within 20-48 hours
Duration of action: 30-36 hours
Pharmacokinetics
Absorption: Slow
Distribution: To muscles, liver, skin, intestines, and kidneys
Metabolism: In the liver to inactive metabolites
Half-life: 30 minutes; biologic half-life: 8-12 hours
Elimination: In bile and urine
Usual Dosage Oral, I.M. (depends upon the condition being treated and the response of the patient) (see Additional Information):
Geriatrics: Use lowest effective dose
Adults: 20-300 mg/day
Monitoring Parameters Blood pressure, blood glucose, electrolytes, symptoms of fluid retention

Test Interactions Increased amylase (S), chloride (S), cholesterol (S), glucose, protein, sodium (S); decreased calcium (S), chloride (S), potassium (S), thyroxine (S)

Patient Information Take with food or milk; take single daily doses in the morning; do not stop abruptly

Nursing Implications I.M. use only; shake vial before measuring out dose; withdraw gradually following long-term therapy

Additional Information Approximately 80% the potency of cortisol; the adrenal cortex secretes 12-15/m^2 of cortisol daily; the maximum activity of the adrenal cortex is between 2 AM and 8 AM and it is minimal between 4 PM and midnight; if possible, administer glucocorticoids before 9 AM to minimize adrenocortical suppression; prolonged therapy (>5 days) of pharmacologic doses of corticosteroids may lead to hypothalamic-pituitary-adrenal suppression, the degree of adrenal suppression varies with the degree and duration of glucocorticoid therapy; this must be taken into consideration when taking patients off steroids; supplemental doses may be warranted during times of stress in the course of withdrawal therapy

Special Geriatric Considerations Because of the risk of adverse effects, systemic corticosteroids should be used cautiously in the elderly, in the smallest possible dose, and for the shortest possible time.

Dosage Forms
Injection: 25 mg/mL (10 mL, 20 mL); 50 mg/mL (10 mL)
Tablet: 5 mg, 10 mg, 25 mg

Cortone® Acetate *see* Cortisone Acetate *on previous page*

Cortril® *see* Hydrocortisone *on page 351*

Cotrim® *see* Co-trimoxazole *on this page*

Cotrim® DS *see* Co-trimoxazole *on this page*

Co-trimoxazole (ko-tri mox' a zole)

Brand Names Bactrim™; Bactrim™ DS; Cotrim®; Cotrim® DS; Septra®; Septra® DS; Sulfamethoprim®; Sulfatrim®; Sulfatrim® DS; Sulfoxaprim®; Sulfoxaprim® DS; Trisulfam®; Uroplus® DS; Uroplus® SS

Synonyms SMX-TMP; Sulfamethoxazole and Trimethoprim; TMP-SMX; Trimethoprim and Sulfamethoxazole

Generic Available Yes

Therapeutic Class Antibiotic, Sulfonamide Derivative

Use Oral treatment of urinary tract infections; acute exacerbations of chronic bronchitis in adults; prophylaxis of *Pneumocystis carinii* pneumonitis (PCP); I.V. treatment of documented PCP, empiric treatment of highly suspected PCP in immune compromised patients; treatment of documented or suspected shigellosis, typhoid fever, or *Nocardia asteroides* infection in patients who are NPO

Contraindications Hypersensitivity to any sulfa drug or any component; porphyria; megaloblastic anemia due to folate deficiency

Warnings Fatalities associated with sulfonamides, although rare, have occurred due to severe reactions including Stevens-Johnson syndrome, toxic epidermal necrolysis, hepatic necrosis, agranulocytosis, aplastic anemia and other blood dyscrasias; discontinue use at first sign of rash or any sign of adverse reaction

Precautions Use with caution in patients with G-6-PD deficiency, impaired renal or hepatic function; adjust dosage in patients with renal impairment

Adverse Reactions
Central nervous system: Confusion, depression, hallucinations, seizures, fever, ataxia
Dermatologic: Rash, erythema multiforme, Stevens-Johnson syndrome, epidermal necrolysis, photosensitivity, urticaria
Gastrointestinal: Nausea, vomiting, glossitis, stomatitis, diarrhea, pseudomembranous colitis
Hematologic: Thrombocytopenia, megaloblastic anemia, granulocytopenia, aplastic anemia, hemolysis (with G-6-PD deficiency)
Hepatic: Hepatitis
Renal: Interstitial nephritis, increased serum creatinine due to trimethoprim's interference with creatinine's tubular secretion
Miscellaneous: Serum sickness

Overdosage Symptoms of overdose include anorexia, nausea, vomiting, dizziness, headache, loss of consciousness, toxic fever, acidosis, acute hemolytic anemia, hepatic jaundice, toxic neuritis

Drug Interactions
Decreased effect of cyclosporines
Increased effect of sulfonylureas and oral anticoagulants
Increased toxicity/levels of phenytoin
Increased toxicity by displacing methotrexate from protein binding sites
Increased nephrotoxicity of cyclosporines

Stability Do not refrigerate injection; is less soluble in more alkaline pH; protect from light; stability of parenteral admixture at room temperature (25°C): 5 mL/125 mL D$_5$W = 6 hours; 5 mL/100 mL D$_5$W = 4 hours; 5 mL/75 mL D$_5$W = 2 hours

(Continued)

Co-trimoxazole (Continued)

Mechanism of Action Sulfamethoxazole interferes with bacterial folic acid synthesis and growth via inhibition of dihydrofolic acid formation from para-aminobenzoic acid; trimethoprim inhibits dihydrofolic acid reduction to tetrahydrofolate resulting in sequential inhibition of enzymes of the folic acid pathway

Pharmacokinetics

Absorption: Oral: Almost completely, 90% to 100%

Protein binding:

SMX: 68%

TMP: 45%

Metabolism:

SMX is N-acetylated and glucuronidated

TMP is metabolized to oxide and hydroxylated metabolites

Half-life:

SMX: 9 hours

TMP: 6-17 hours, both are prolonged in renal failure

Time to peak: Peak serum levels occur within 1-4 hours

Elimination: Both are excreted in urine as metabolites and unchanged drug

Effects of aging on the pharmacokinetics of both agents has been variable; increase in half-life and decreases in clearance have been associated with reduced creatinine clearance

Usual Dosage Geriatrics and Adults (dosage recommendations are based on the trimethoprim component):

Urinary tract infection, chronic bronchitis: Oral: 1 double strength tablet every 12 hours for 10-14 days

Sepsis: I.V.: 20 TMP/kg/day divided every 6 hours

Pneumocystis carinii:

Prophylaxis: Oral, I.V.: 10 mg TMP/kg/day divided every 12 hours for 3 days/week

Treatment: I.V.: 20 mg TMP/kg/day divided every 6 hours

Dosing interval/adjustment in renal impairment:

Cl_{cr} 30-50 mL/minute: Administer every 12-18 hours or reduce dose by 25%

Cl_{cr} 15-30 mL/minute: Administer every 18-24 hours or reduce dose by 50%

Cl_{cr} <15 mL/minute: Not recommended

Administration Infuse over 60-90 minutes, must dilute well before giving; not for I.M. injection

Monitoring Parameters Signs and symptoms of infection including mental status

Test Interactions False-positive urine glucose tests that use Benedict's method

Patient Information Take oral medication with 8 oz of water on an empty stomach (1 hour before or 2 hours after meals) for best absorption; report any skin rashes immediately; complete full course of therapy

Nursing Implications Maintain adequate fluid intake to prevent crystalluria; see Administration

Additional Information Injection vehicle contains benzyl alcohol and sodium metabisulfite; the 5:1 ratio (SMX to TMP) remains constant in all dosage forms

Do not use NS as a diluent; injection vehicle contains benzyl alcohol and sodium metabisulfite

Special Geriatric Considerations Elderly patients appear at greater risk for more severe adverse reactions; see Pharmacokinetics and Usual Dosage; adjust dose based on renal function

Dosage Forms

Injection: Sulfamethoxazole 80 mg and trimethoprim 16 mg per mL (5 mL, 10 mL, 20 mL, 30 mL, 50 mL)

Suspension, oral: Sulfamethoxazole 200 mg and trimethoprim 40 mg per 5 mL (20 mL, 100 mL, 150 mL, 200 mL, 480 mL)

Tablet: Sulfamethoxazole 400 mg and trimethoprim 80 mg

Tablet, double strength: Sulfamethoxazole 800 mg and trimethoprim 160 mg

References

Naber K, Vergin H, and Weigand W, "Pharmacokinetics of Co-trimoxazole and Co-tetroxazine in Geriatric Patients." *Infection*, 1981, 9(5):239-43.

Varoquaux O, Lajoie D, Gobert C, et al, "Pharmacokinetics of the Trimethoprim-Sulfamethoxazole Combination in the Elderly," *Br J Clin Pharmacol*, 1985, 20:575-81.

Coumadin® see Warfarin Sodium *on page 739*

CPM see Cyclophosphamide *on page 196*

Cremacoat®2 [OTC] see Guaifenesin *on page 331*

Cromoglycic Acid see Cromolyn Sodium *on this page*

Cromolyn Sodium (kroe' moe lin)

Brand Names Gastrocrom®; Intal®; Nasalcrom®; Opticrom®

Synonyms Cromoglycic Acid; Disodium Cromoglycate; DSCG

Therapeutic Class Antihistamine, Inhalation; Inhalation, Miscellaneous

Use Adjunct in the prophylaxis of allergic disorders, including rhinitis, giant papillary conjunctivitis, and asthma; inhalation product may be used for relief and prevention of exercise-induced bronchospasm; systemic mastocytosis, food allergy, and treatment of inflammatory bowel disease; **cromolyn is a prophylactic drug with no benefit for acute situations**

Contraindications Hypersensitivity to cromolyn or any component; acute asthma attacks

Warnings Aerosol inhalant should not be used in patients with cardiac arrhythmias

Precautions Caution should be used when withdrawing the drug or tapering the dose as symptoms may reoccur; use with caution in patients with a history of cardiac arrhythmia; use with caution in patients with renal and hepatic impairment

Adverse Reactions
Central nervous system: Dizziness, headache
Dermatologic: Rash, urticaria
Gastrointestinal: Nausea, vomiting, diarrhea
Local: Nasal burning
Neuromuscular & skeletal: Joint pain
Ocular: Ocular stinging, lacrimation
Respiratory: Coughing, wheezing, throat irritation, eosinophilic pneumonia, pulmonary infiltrates, hoarseness

Overdosage Symptoms of overdose include bronchospasm, laryngeal edema, dysuria

Stability Compatible with metaproterenol sulfate, isoproterenol hydrochloride, 0.25% isoetharine hydrochloride, epinephrine hydrochloride, terbutaline sulfate, and 20% acetylcysteine solution for at least 1 hour after their admixture

Mechanism of Action Prevents the mast cell release of histamine, leukotrienes, and slow-reacting substance of anaphylaxis by inhibiting degranulation after contact with antigens

Pharmacokinetics
Absorption:
Inhalation: ~8% of dose reaches the lungs upon inhalation of the powder and is well absorbed
Oral: Only 0.5% to 2%
Half-life: 80-90 minutes
Time to peak: Inhalation: Peak serum levels occur within 15 minutes
Elimination: Absorbed cromolyn is equally excreted unchanged in urine and feces (via bile); small amounts are exhaled

Usual Dosage Geriatrics and Adults:
Inhalation: 20 mg 4 times/day (Spinhaler®) or nebulization solution, 2 inhalations 4 times/day by metered spray
For prevention of exercise-induced bronchospasm: Single dose of 2 inhalations (aerosol) or 20 mg (powder inhalation) just prior to exercise (no more than 1 hour)
Nasal: 1 spray in each nostril 3-4 times/day
Ophthalmic: Instill 1-2 drops 4-6 times/day

Systemic mastocytosis: Oral: 200 mg 4 times/day

Food allergy and inflammatory bowel disease: Oral: 200 mg 4 times/day 15-20 minutes before meal, up to 400 mg 4 times/day (investigational)

Monitoring Parameters Pulmonary function tests, spirometry

Patient Information Do not discontinue abruptly; not effective for acute relief of symptoms; must be taken on a regularly scheduled basis; unless instructed otherwise, capsules are for inhalation, not oral ingestion; store nebulizer solution away from light; follow instructions that come with the product

Nursing Implications Advise patient to clear as much mucus as possible before inhalation treatments

Additional Information Oral administration is strictly investigational; cromolyn is a prophylactic drug with no benefit for acute situations

Special Geriatric Considerations Assess the patient's ability to empty the capsules via the Spinhaler®. Older persons often have difficulty with inhaled dosage forms.

Dosage Forms
Capsule:
Oral: 100 mg
Powder for inhalation: 20 mg
Inhalation, oral: 800 mcg/spray 8.1 g inhaler
Solution:
Nasal: 40 mg/mL (13 mL)
Nebulizer: 10 mg/mL (2 mL)
Ophthalmic: 4% (10 mL)

Crotamiton (kroe tam' i tonn)
Brand Names Eurax®
Generic Available No
Therapeutic Class Antipruritic, Topical; Scabicidal Agent
(Continued)

Crotamiton *(Continued)*

Use Treatment of scabies and symptomatic treatment of pruritus

Contraindications Hypersensitivity to crotamiton or other components; patients who manifest a primary irritation response to topical medications

Precautions Avoid contact with face, eyes, mucous membranes, and urethral meatus; do not apply to acutely inflamed or raw skin

Adverse Reactions
Dermatologic: Pruritus, contact dermatitis
Local: Irritation, warm sensation

Overdosage Burning or irritation in the oral cavity may signify oral ingestion, burning of the esophagus and gastric mucosa, nausea, vomiting; no specific treatment

Usual Dosage Topical: Scabicide: Geriatrics and Adults: Wash thoroughly and scrub away loose scales, then towel dry; apply a thin layer and massage drug onto skin of the entire body from the neck to the toes (with special attention to skin folds, creases, and interdigital spaces). Repeat application in 24 hours; take a cleansing bath 48 hours after the final application.

Administration Lotion: Shake well before using; avoid contact with face, eyes, mucous membranes, and urethral meatus

Patient Information For topical use only; keep away from eyes and mucosa membranes, all contaminated clothing and bed linen should be washed to avoid reinfestation; shake lotion well

Nursing Implications See Administration

Additional Information Treatment may be repeated after 7-10 days if live mites are still present

Special Geriatric Considerations If cure is not achieved after 2 doses, use alternative therapy

Dosage Forms
Cream: 10%: 60 g
Lotion: 10%: 60 mL, 454 mL

Crystalline Penicillin *see* Penicillin G, Parenteral *on page 540*

Crystamine® *see* Cyanocobalamin *on this page*

Crysticillin® A.S. *see* Penicillin G Procaine, Aqueous *on page 541*

Crystodigin® *see* Digitoxin *on page 220*

C-Solve-2® *see* Erythromycin, Topical *on page 266*

C-Span® [OTC] *see* Ascorbic Acid *on page 57*

CTX *see* Cyclophosphamide *on page 196*

Cuprimine® *see* Penicillamine *on page 537*

Curretab® *see* Medroxyprogesterone Acetate *on page 437*

Cutivate™ Topical *see* Fluticasone Propionate *on page 309*

CyA *see* Cyclosporine *on page 199*

Cyanocobalamin *(sye an oh koe bal' a min)*

Brand Names Berubigen®; Betalin®l Cryste-12®; Cobex®; Crystamine®; Cyanoject®; Cyomin®l Rubisol-1000®; Redisol®; Rubramin-PC®; Sytobex®

Synonyms Vitamin B_{12}

Generic Available Yes

Therapeutic Class Vitamin, Water Soluble

Use Pernicious anemia; vitamin B_{12} deficiency; thyrotoxicosis, hemorrhage, malignancy, liver or kidney disease; hydroxocobalamin has been used to treat cyanide toxicity associated with nitroprusside

Contraindications Hypersensitivity to cyanocobalamin or any component, cobalt; patients with hereditary optic nerve atrophy

Warnings I.M. route used to treat pernicious anemia; vitamin B_{12} deficiency for >3 months results in irreversible degenerative CNS lesions; treatment of vitamin B_{12} megaloblastic anemia may result in severe hypokalemia, sometimes, fatal, when anemia corrects due to cellular potassium requirements

Precautions Folate doses exceeding 10 mcg/day may produce hematologic response in patients with folate deficiency. Indiscriminate folate use may mask the true diagnosis of pernicious anemia. Single deficiency is rare (except multiple deficiencies). Doses of folate >0.1 mg/day may reverse vitamin B_{12} hematologic abnormalities; however, the neurologic manifestations will not be treated or prevented, and irreversible neurologic damage will ensue; B_{12} deficiency masks signs of polycythemia vera; vegetarian diets may result in B_{12} deficiency; pernicious anemia occurs more often in gastric carcinoma than in general population

Adverse Reactions
Cardiovascular: Peripheral vascular thrombosis
Dermatologic: Itching, urticaria
Gastrointestinal: Diarrhea
Miscellaneous: Anaphylaxis

Toxicology Excess vitamin B_{12} is excreted in urine; toxic doses not known

Drug Interactions
Aminosalicylic acid may reduce therapeutic action of vitamin B_{12}
Chloramphenicol may decrease the hematologic effect of vitamin B_{12} in patients with pernicious anemia
Colchicine and prolonged alcohol (>2 weeks) use may decrease absorption of vitamin B_{12}

Stability Clear pink to red solutions are stable at room temperature; protect from light; incompatible with chlorpromazine, phytonadione, prochlorperazine, warfarin, ascorbic acid, dextrose, heavy metals, oxidizing or reducing agents; avoid freezing

Mechanism of Action Coenzyme for various metabolic functions, including fat and carbohydrate metabolism and protein synthesis, used in cell replication, hematopoiesis, and myelin synthesis

Pharmacokinetics
Absorption: From the terminal ileum in the presence of calcium; for absorption to occur, gastric "intrinsic factor" must be present to transfer the compound across the intestinal mucosa
Protein binding: Following absorption, bound to transcobalamin II (the major transport protein) and converted in the tissues to active coenzymes methylcobalamin and deoxyadenosylcobalamin; principally stored in the liver, also stored in the kidneys and adrenals. Hydroxocobalamin (vitamin B_{12a}) is bound highly to protein and is retained in the body longer than cyanocobalamin, but offers no clinical advantage.

Usual Dosage Geriatrics and Adults:
Pernicious anemia: I.M.: 100 mcg/day for at least 2 weeks; maintenance: 100 mcg/month; administer folic acid 1 mg/day for 1 month concomitantly

Vitamin B_{12} deficiency: I.M., S.C.: 100 mcg/day for 6-7 days followed by 100 μ/month for life; maximal oral absorption: 2-3 mcg/day
Oral: RDA: 2 mcg
Nutritional deficiency: 25-250 mcg/day (oral not recommended for pernicious anemia due to lack of absorption)

Reference Range Normal range of serum B_{12} is 150-750 pg/mL; this represents 0.1% of total body content. Metabolic requirements are 2-5 μg/day; years of deficiency required before hematologic and neurologic signs and symptoms are seen. Most commercial methods have in the past undergone modification. The lower limit of normal (critical to the diagnosis of B_{12} deficiency/pernicious anemia) has not been firmly established. Clinical correlation and multiple test documentation of the etiology of macrocytic anemia is advised. Occasional patients with significant neuropsychiatric abnormalities may have no hematologic abnormalities and normal serum cobalamin levels, 200 pg/mL (SI: >150 pmol/L), or more commonly between 100-200 pg/mL (SI: 75-150 pmol/L).

Test Interactions Methotrexate, pyrimethamine and most antibiotics interfere with microbiologic assays

Patient Information Patients with pernicious anemia will require monthly injections for life

Nursing Implications I.M. or deep S.C. are preferred routes of administration; oral therapy is markedly inferior to parenteral therapy; monitor potassium concentrations during early therapy; folate therapy may be necessary in first month B_{12} replacement

Additional Information Water-soluble vitamin with a wide margin of safety; oral therapy with hog mucosa intrinsic factor will not effectively or adequately treat pernicious anemia

Special Geriatric Considerations There exists evidence that people, particularly elderly whose serum cobalamin concentrations <300 pg/mL, should receive replacement parenteral therapy; this recommendation is based upon neuropsychiatric disorders and cardiovascular disorders associated with lower sodium cobalamin concentrations

Dosage Forms
Injection: 30 mcg/mL (30 mL); 100 mcg/mL (1 mL, 10 mL, 30 mL); 1000 mcg/mL (1 mL, 10 mL, 30 mL)
Tablet: 25 mcg, 50 mcg, 100 mcg, 250 mcg, 500 mcg, 1000 mcg

References
Lindenbaum J, Healton EB, Savage DG, et al, "Neuropsychiatric Disorders Caused by Cobalamin Deficiency in the Absence of Anemia or Macrocytosis," *N Engl J Med*, 1988, 318(26):1720-8.
Olszewski AJ, Szostak WB, Bialkowska M, et al, "Reduction of Plasma Lipid and Homocysteine Levels by Pyridoxine, Folate, Cobalamin, Choline, Riboflavin, and Troxerutin in Atherosclerosis," *Atherosclerosis*, 1989, 75(1):1-6.
Regland B, Gottfries CG, and Lindstedt G, "Dementia Patients With Low Serum Cobalamin Concentration: Relationship to Atrophic Gastritis," *Aging Milano*, 1992, 4(1):35-41.

Cyanoject® see Cyanocobalamin *on previous page*

Cyclandelate (sye klan' de late)
Brand Names Cyclospasmol®
Generic Available Yes
Therapeutic Class Vasodilator, Peripheral

(Continued)

Cyclandelate *(Continued)*

Use Considered as "possibly effective" for adjunctive therapy in peripheral vascular disease and possibly senility due to cerebrovascular disease or multi-infarct dementia; migraine prophylaxis, vertigo, tinnitus, and visual disturbances secondary to cerebrovascular insufficiency and diabetic peripheral polyneuropathy

Contraindications Hypersensitivity to cyclandelate or any component

Warnings Use caution when using in patients with active bleeding or hemorrhage potential; use extreme caution in patients with obliterative cerebral vascular or coronary artery disease as these areas may have their perfusion altered by peripheral vasodilatation

Precautions Use caution in patients with glaucoma, use with caution in elderly

Adverse Reactions
Cardiovascular: Mild flushing, tachycardia, hypotension, syncope
Central nervous system: Headache, pain
Gastrointestinal: Heartburn, abdominal pain, eructation
Neuromuscular & skeletal: Weakness

Overdosage Symptoms of overdose include drowsiness, weakness, respiratory depression, hypotension

Toxicology Treatment following decontamination is supportive; fluids followed by vasopressors are most helpful

Drug Interactions May enhance action of drugs causing vasodilation/hypotension

Mechanism of Action Cyclandelate, 3,3,5-trimethylcyclohexyl mandelate is a vasodilator that exerts a direct, papaverine-like action on smooth muscles, particularly that found within the blood vessels. Animal data indicate that cyclandelate also has antispasmodic properties; exhibits no adrenergic stimulation or blocking action; action exceeds that of papaverine; mild calcium channel blocking agent, may benefit in mild hypercalcemia; calcium channel blocking activity may explain some of its pharmacologic effects (enhanced blood flow) and inhibition of platelet aggregation

Usual Dosage Geriatrics and Adults: Initial dose: 1200-1600 mg/day in 3-4 doses until response noted; start with lowest dose in elderly due to hypotensive potential; decrease dose by 200 mg decrements to achieve minimal maintenance dose; usual maintenance: 400-800 mg/day in divided doses; may not be possible to decrease dose when treating dementia states; improvement may usually be seen over weeks of therapy and prolonged use; short courses of therapy usually ineffective and not recommended; use in dementia states questionable; see Special Geriatric Considerations

Monitoring Parameters Monitor for hypotension; worsening of cerebral or coronary artery disease

Patient Information Take medication with meals or antacids to decrease gastrointestinal side effects. Note: Use of antacids not recommended with reduced renal function (Cl_{cr} <30 mL/minute) or where antacids affect bowel function in elderly

Nursing Implications Administer with meals; observe for orthostatic hypotension

Special Geriatric Considerations Vasodilators have been used to treat dementia upon the premise that dementia is secondary to a cerebral blood flow insufficiency. The hypothesis is that if blood flow could be increased, cognitive function would be increased. This hypothesis is no longer valid. The use of vasodilators for cognitive dysfunction is not recommended or proven by appropriate scientific study.

Dosage Forms
Capsule: 200 mg, 400 mg
Tablet: 200 mg, 400 mg

References
Erwin WG, "Senile Dementia of the Alzheimer Type," *Clin Pharm*, 1984, 3:497-504.
Higbee MD, "Noncholinergic Approaches to Treating Senile Dementia of the Alzheimer's Type," *Consult Pharm*, 1992, 7(6):635-41.
Waters C, "Cognitive Enhancing Agents: Current Status in the Treatment of Alzheimer's Disease," *Can J Neurol Sci*, 1988, 15:249-56.
Yesavage JA, Tinklenberg JR, Hollister LE, et al, "Vasodilators in Senile Dementias: A Review of the Literature," *Arch Gen Psychiatry*, 1979, 36:220-3.

Cyclizine *(sye' kli zeen)*

Brand Names Marezine® [OTC]

Generic Available No

Therapeutic Class Antiemetic; Antihistamine

Use Prevention and treatment of nausea, vomiting and vertigo associated with motion sickness; control of postoperative nausea and vomiting

Contraindications Hypersensitivity to meclizine, cyclizine, or any component

Precautions Use with caution in patients with angle-closure glaucoma or prostatic hypertrophy; elderly may be at risk for anticholinergic side effects such as glaucoma, prostate hypertrophy, constipation, gastrointestinal obstructive disease

Adverse Reactions
Cardiovascular: Palpitations, tachycardia, hypotension
Central nervous system: Drowsiness, fatigue, restlessness, excitation, insomnia, confusion, euphoria, vertigo

Dermatologic: Rash, urticaria
Gastrointestinal: Dry mouth, anorexia, nausea, vomiting, diarrhea, constipation
Genitourinary: Urinary frequency, urinary retention, difficult urination
Hepatic: Cholestatic jaundice
Ocular: Blurred vision, diplopia, visual hallucinations
Otic: Tinnitus, auditory hallucinations
Miscellaneous: Dry nose

Overdosage Excitation alternating with drowsiness, respiratory depression, hallucinations

Toxicology There is no specific treatment for an antihistamine overdose, however, most of its clinical toxicity is due to anticholinergic effects. Anticholinesterase inhibitors may be useful by reducing acetylcholinesterase. Anticholinesterase inhibitors include physostigmine, neostigmine, pyridostigmine and edrophonium. For anticholinergic overdose with severe life-threatening symptoms, physostigmine 1-2 mg I.V., slowly may be given to reverse these effects.

Drug Interactions See Adverse Reactions; may enhance actions of drugs with similar adverse reactions and pharmacologic actions

Mechanism of Action Has antiemetic, anticholinergic, and antihistaminic activity; has central anticholinergic action by blocking chemoreceptor trigger zone; decreases excitability of the middle ear labyrinth and blocks conduction in the middle ear vestibular-cerebellar pathways

Pharmacodynamics
Onset of action: Oral: Within 30-60 minutes
Duration: 4-6 hours

Pharmacokinetics
Metabolism: Reportedly in the liver
Half-life: 6 hours
Elimination: As metabolites in urine and as unchanged drug in feces

Usual Dosage Geriatrics and Adults:
Oral: 25-50 mg taken 30 minutes before departure, may repeat in 4-6 hours if needed, up to 200 mg/day
I.M.: 25-50 mg every 4-6 hours as needed

Monitoring Parameters Monitor for CNS side effects in elderly

Patient Information May impair ability to perform hazardous tasks; may cause drowsiness; may cause dry mouth, constipation, difficulty urinating, confusion

Nursing Implications See Precautions and Special Geriatric Considerations

Special Geriatric Considerations Due to anticholinergic action, use lowest dose in divided doses to avoid side effects and their inconvenience; limit use if possible; may cause confusion or aggravate symptoms of confusion in those with dementia

Dosage Forms
Injection: 50 mg/mL (1 mL)
Tablet: 50 mg

Cyclobenzaprine Hydrochloride (sye kloe ben' za preen)

Brand Names Flexeril®
Generic Available Yes
Therapeutic Class Skeletal Muscle Relaxant
Use Treatment of muscle spasm associated with acute painful musculoskeletal conditions

Contraindications Hypersensitivity to cyclobenzaprine or any component; do not use concomitantly or within 14 days of MAO inhibitors; acute recovery phase of myocardial infarction, arrhythmias, heart block, conduction disturbances, congestive heart failure or hyperthyroidism

Warnings Use only for short periods of time (2-3 weeks); cyclobenzaprine shares the toxic potentials of the tricyclic antidepressants; the usual precautions of tricyclic antidepressant therapy should be observed

Precautions Because it has anticholinergic effects, use with caution in patients with urinary hesitancy or angle-closure glaucoma

Adverse Reactions
Cardiovascular: Tachycardia, hypotension, arrhythmias
Central nervous system: Drowsiness, headache, dizziness, fatigue, asthenia, nervousness, convulsions, confusion
Dermatologic: Rash
Gastrointestinal: Dyspepsia, nausea, constipation, dry mouth, vomiting, diarrhea, unpleasant taste
Genitourinary: Urinary frequency or retention
Hepatic: Abnormal liver function
Ocular: Blurred vision

Overdosage Symptoms of overdose include drowsiness, hypothermia, tachycardia, arrhythmias, dilated pupils, convulsions, severe hypotension, stupor, and coma

Toxicology Following initiation of essential overdose management, toxic symptoms should be treated. Ventricular arrhythmias often respond to systemic alkalinization

(Continued)

195

Cyclobenzaprine Hydrochloride *(Continued)*

(sodium bicarbonate 0.5-2 mEq/kg I.V.) and/or phenytoin 15-20 mg/kg. Arrhythmias unresponsive to this therapy may respond to lidocaine 1 mg/kg I.V. followed by a titrated infusion. Physostigmine 1-2 mg I.V. slowly may be indicated in reversing cardiac arrhythmias that are life-threatening. Seizures usually respond to 5-10 mg diazepam I.V. boluses. If seizures are unresponsive or recur, phenytoin or phenobarbital may be required.

Drug Interactions Do not use concomitantly or within 14 days after MAO inhibitors
Increased effect/toxicity with alcohol, barbiturates, CNS depressants
Increased toxicity with MAO inhibitors, TCAs, anticholinergics

Mechanism of Action Reduces tonic somatic motor activity influencing both alpha and gamma motor neurons

Pharmacodynamics
Onset of action: Commonly occurs within 1 hour
Duration: 12-24 hours

Pharmacokinetics
Absorption: Oral: Completely
Protein binding: 93%
Metabolism: Hepatic; may undergo enterohepatic recycling; metabolized to glucuronide-like conjugate
Half-life: 1-3 days
Time to peak serum concentration: Within 3-8 hours
Elimination: Renally as inactive metabolites and in feces (via bile) as unchanged drug

Usual Dosage Oral: **Note:** Do not use longer than 2-3 weeks
Geriatrics: See Special Geriatric Considerations
Adults: Initial: 10 mg 3 times/day; range: 20-40 mg/day in divided doses; maximum dose: 60 mg/day

Monitoring Parameters Relief of pain and muscle spasm, liver function tests, mental status

Patient Information May cause drowsiness, dizziness, or blurred vision; use caution performing activities requiring alertness; avoid alcohol and CNS depressants; may cause dry mouth

Nursing Implications Raise bed rails, institute safety measures, assist with ambulation

Special Geriatric Considerations High doses in the elderly caused drowsiness and dizziness; therefore, use the lowest dose possible. Because cyclobenzaprine causes anticholinergic effects, it may not be the skeletal muscle relaxant of choice in the elderly.

Dosage Forms Tablet: 10 mg

Cyclophosphamide (sye kloe foss' fa mide)
Brand Names Cytoxan®; Neosar®
Synonyms CPM; CTX; CYT
Generic Available No
Therapeutic Class Antineoplastic Agent, Alkylating Agent (Nitrogen Mustard)
Use Management of Hodgkin's disease, malignant lymphomas, multiple myeloma, leukemias, small cell carcinoma of the lungs, mycosis fungoides, neuroblastoma, ovarian carcinoma, breast carcinoma, a variety of other tumors; nephrotic syndrome, lupus erythematosus, severe rheumatoid arthritis, rheumatoid vasculitis, multiple sclerosis, polyarteritis nodosa, and polymyositis
Contraindications Hypersensitivity to cyclophosphamide or any component, severely depressed bone marrow function
Warnings The U.S. Food and Drug Administration (FDA) currently recommends that procedures for proper handling and disposal of antineoplastic agents be considered.

Cardiac toxicity with necrosis: Reported with high doses (120-170 mg/kg given over a few days); no residual cardiac effects seen with EKG or echocardiogram

Genitourinary: Hemorrhagic cystitis occurs in 7% to 12% of patients; higher percentages have been reported. This sterile hemorrhagic cystitis is related to the concentration of metabolites in bladder (acrolein); may result in bladder telangiectasis fibrosis and bladder cancer

Pulmonary: Pulmonary fibrosis has been reported

Skin: May interfere with normal wound healing

Hypersensitivity: Type I reactions have occurred; anaphylaxis is rare

Renal: Use cautiously in renal impairment since alterations in renal function may result in altered pharmacokinetics. No evidence for a need to alter dose for renal function; long-term free water clearance may be impaired

Carcinogenesis: Long-term follow up indicates an increased incidence of leukemia (myeloproliferative and lymphoproliferative malignancies); these secondary malignancies have occurred most frequently in patients with primary myeloproliferative/lymphoproliferative diseases; most frequent malignancies occur in the bladder;

some cases of secondary malignancies have occurred years after discontinuation of cyclophosphamide

Precautions Use with caution in patients with bone marrow depression and impaired renal or hepatic function

Adverse Reactions
Cardiovascular: Cardiotoxicity with high dose therapy
Dermatologic: Alopecia
Endocrine & metabolic: Hypokalemia, amenorrhea, SIADH, hyperuricemia
Gastrointestinal: Nausea, vomiting, taste distortion
Genitourinary: Oligospermia
Hematologic: Leukopenia nadir at 8-15 days, hemolytic anemia, myelosuppression, positive Coombs' test
Renal: Hemorrhagic cystitis
Respiratory: Interstitial pulmonary fibrosis, nasal stuffiness

Overdosage Symptoms of overdose include myelosuppression, alopecia, nausea, vomiting, cystitis

Toxicology Institute general supportive care; cyclophosphamide and its metabolites are dialyzable; no specific antidote is known

Drug Interactions
Cardiotoxic drugs (eg, doxorubicin); drugs that affect hepatic microsomal enzymes (eg, phenobarbital, phenytoin, chloramphenicol); barbiturates, allopurinol, imipramine, phenothiazines, succinylcholine
Digoxin serum concentrations may decrease
Thiazide diuretics enhance leukopenia

Stability Reconstituted solution is stable for 24 hours at room temperature and 6 days when refrigerated; if powder for injection is not reconstituted with bacteriostatic water for injection, USP, use within 6 hours; does not contain antimicrobial agent; assure sterile preparation

Mechanism of Action Cyclophosphamide is converted through hepatic metabolism to active metabolites: non-nitrogen mustard and phosphoramide mustard. Acrolein is a significant metabolite thought to cause bladder toxicity. The active metabolites interfere with the normal function of DNA by alkylation and cross-linking the strands of DNA, and by possible protein modification.

Pharmacokinetics
Absorption: Completely from GI tract
Metabolism: In the liver to active metabolite
Half-life: 3-12 hours
Time to peak: Oral: Peak serum levels occur within 1 hour
Elimination: In urine as unchanged drug (<30%) and as metabolites (85% to 90%)
Alkylating activity is lost 10 hours after oral administration

Usual Dosage
Geriatrics (refer to individual protocols): Initial and maintenance: 1-2 mg/kg/day; adjust for renal clearance

Adults with no hematologic problems:
Induction:
Oral: 1-5 mg/kg/day
I.V.: 40-50 mg/kg (1.5-1.8 g/m^2) in divided doses over 2-5 days
Maintenance:
Oral: 1-5 mg/kg/day
I.V.: 10-15 mg/kg (350-550 mg/m^2) every 7-10 days or 3-5 mg/kg (110-185 mg/m^2) twice weekly

Dosing adjustment in renal impairment:
Cl_{cr} 25-50 mL/minute: Decrease dose by 50%
Cl_{cr} <25 mL/minute: Avoid use
Moderately dialyzable (20% to 50%)

Adults:
SLE: I.V.: 500-750 mg/m^2 every month; maximum: 1 g/m^2
BMT-conditioning regimen: I.V.: 50 mg/kg/day once daily for 3-4 days
Nephrotic syndrome: Oral: 2-3 mg/kg/day every day for up to 12 weeks when corticosteroids are unsuccessful

Monitoring Parameters Monitor WBC and platelets; observe for signs of infection, bleeding, and bladder irritation; monitor urinalysis for blood; see Additional Information

Test Interactions Increased prothrombin time (S), potassium (S)

Patient Information Drink plenty of fluids before and after doses; report any blood in the urine. May cause nausea, vomiting, and diarrhea. If these side effects persist, call physician; report any bruising, bleeding, chills, cough, shortness of breath, unusual lumps, seizures, sores in mouth, flank or joint pain

Nursing Implications Encourage adequate hydration and frequent voiding to help prevent hemorrhagic cystitis; see Monitoring Parameters and Patient Information

Additional Information Myelosuppressive effects:
WBC: Moderate

(Continued)

Cyclophosphamide *(Continued)*

Platelets: Moderate
Onset (days): 7
Nadir (days): 10-14
Recovery (days): 21

Special Geriatric Considerations Toxicity to immunosuppressives is increased in elderly. Start with lowest recommended adult doses. Signs of infection, such as fever and WBC rise, may not occur. Lethargy and confusion may be more prominent signs of infection; adjust dose for renal function in elderly

Dosage Forms
Injection: 100 mg, 200 mg, 500 mg, 1 g, 2 g
Tablet: 25 mg, 50 mg

References
Bostrom BC, Weisdorf DJ, Kim TH, et al, "Bone Marrow Transplantation for Advanced Acute Leukemia: A Pilot Study of High-Energy Total Body Irradiation, Cyclophosphamide and Continuous Infusion Etoposide," *Bone Marrow Transplant*, 1990, 5(2):83-9.
Hutchins LF and Lipschitz DA, "Cancer, Clinical Pharmacology, and Aging," *Clin Geriatr Med*, 1987, 3(3):483-503.
Kaplan HG, "Use of Cancer Chemotherapy in the Elderly," *Drug Treatment in the Elderly*, Vestal RE, ed, Boston, MA: ADIS Health Science Press, 1984, 338-49.
McCune WJ, Golbus J, Zeldes W, et al, "Clinical and Immunologic Effects of Monthly Administration of Intravenous Cyclophosphamide in Severe Systemic Lupus Erythematosus," *N Engl J Med*, 1988, 318(22):1423-31.

Cycloserine *(sye kloe ser' een)*

Brand Names Seromycin® Pulvules®

Therapeutic Class Antibiotic, Miscellaneous; Antitubercular Agent

Use Adjunctive treatment in pulmonary or extrapulmonary tuberculosis; treatment of acute urinary tract infections caused by *E. coli* or *Enterobacter* sp when less toxic conventional therapy has failed or is contraindicated

Contraindications Known hypersensitivity to cycloserine; epilepsy, depression, severe anxiety or psychosis, severe renal insufficiency, chronic alcoholism

Precautions Adjust dosage with renal impairment

Adverse Reactions
Cardiovascular: Cardiac arrhythmias
Central nervous system: Drowsiness, headache, dizziness, vertigo, seizures, confusion, psychosis, coma, paresis
Dermatologic: Rash
Hepatic: Elevated liver enzymes
Neuromuscular & skeletal: Tremors
Miscellaneous: Vitamin B_{12} deficiency, folate deficiency

Overdosage Symptoms of overdose include confusion, CNS depression, psychosis, coma,

Toxicology Seizures; decontaminate with activated charcoal; can be hemodialyzed; management is supportive; administer 100-300 mg/day of pyridoxine to reduce neurotoxic effects; acute toxicity can occur with ingestions of >1 g

Drug Interactions Alcohol increases risk of seizures, isoniazid may increase cycloserine CNS side effects

Mechanism of Action Inhibits bacterial cell wall synthesis by competing with amino acid (D-alanine) for incorporation into the bacterial cell wall

Pharmacokinetics
Absorption: Oral: ~70% to 90% from GI tract
Half-life: Normal renal function: 10 hours
Time to peak: Oral: Peak serum levels occur within 3-4 hours
Elimination: 60% to 70% of oral dose excreted unchanged in urine by glomerular filtration within 72 hours, small amounts excreted in feces, remainder is metabolized

Usual Dosage Oral:
Tuberculosis: Geriatrics and Adults: Initial: 250 mg every 12 hours for 14 days, then give 500 mg to 1 g/day in 2 divided doses for 18-24 months (maximum daily dose: 1 g)

Urinary tract infection: Adults: 250 mg every 12 hours for 14 days; patients with impaired renal function should have their dose adjusted based upon blood levels; see Monitoring Parameters and Reference Range

Dosing interval in renal impairment:
Cl_{cr} 10-50 mL/minute: Administer every 12-24 hours
Cl_{cr} <10 mL/minute: Administer every 24 hours

Monitoring Parameters Check blood levels weekly for patients with decreased renal function, receiving >500 mg/day, or when toxicity is suspected

Reference Range Adequate CSF penetration; toxicity is greatly increased at levels >30 µg/mL

Patient Information May cause drowsiness; notify physician if skin rash, mental confusion, dizziness, headache, or tremors occur

Nursing Implications Some of the neurotoxic effects may be relieved or prevented by the concomitant administration of pyridoxine

Additional Information Administer 100-300 mg/day of pyridoxine to relieve neurotoxic effects

Special Geriatric Considerations See Usual Dosage; adjust dose for renal function

Dosage Forms Capsule: 250 mg

Cyclospasmol® *see* Cyclandelate *on page 193*

Cyclosporin A *see* Cyclosporine *on this page*

Cyclosporine (sye' kloe spor een)
Related Information
Drug Levels Commonly Monitored Guidelines *on page 771-772*

Brand Names Sandimmune®

Synonyms CyA; Cyclosporin A

Generic Available No

Therapeutic Class Immunosuppressant Agent

Use Immunosuppressant used with corticosteroids to prevent graft versus host disease in patients with kidney, liver, heart, and bone marrow transplants.

Unlabeled use: Rheumatoid arthritis

Contraindications Hypersensitivity to cyclosporine or polyoxyethylated castor oil

Warnings Administer with adrenal corticosteroids; infection and possible development of lymphoma may result; make dose adjustments (to avoid toxicity or possible organ rejection) via cyclosporine blood levels because absorption is erratic

Precautions Dosage needs to be adjusted in patients with hepatic and renal dysfunction

Adverse Reactions
Cardiovascular: Hypertension, hypotension, tachycardia, warmth, flushing
Central nervous system: Seizure, paresthesias, headache
Dermatologic: Hirsutism
Endocrine & metabolic: Hyperkalemia, hypomagnesemia, hyperuricemia
Gastrointestinal: Abdominal discomfort, gingival hyperplasia
Hepatic: Hepatotoxicity
Neuromuscular & skeletal: Myositis, tremors
Renal: Nephrotoxicity, renal dysfunction
Respiratory: Respiratory distress
Miscellaneous: Increased susceptibility to infection, and sensitivity to temperature extremes

Toxicology Minimal experience with overdosage; may see transient hepatotoxicity and nephrotoxicity; not dialyzable, not cleared well by charcoal hemoperfusion

Drug Interactions
Decreased levels: Carbamazepine, barbiturates, phenytoin, rifampin
Increased levels: Diltiazem, erythromycin, fluconazole, ketoconazole, nicardipine, imipenem-cilastatin, metoclopramide
Increased toxicity: Aminoglycosides, amphotericin B, NSAIDs, co-trimoxazole, digoxin (increased digoxin levels)
Increased risk of gingival hyperplasia when given with nifedipine

Stability Stability of injection of parenteral admixture at room temperature (25°C): 6 hours in PVC, 12 hours in glass; do not refrigerate; protect I.V. ampuls from light; use contents of oral solution within 2 months after opening

Mechanism of Action Inhibition of production and release of interleukin II and inhibits interleukin II-induced activation of resting T lymphocytes

Pharmacokinetics
Absorption: Oral: Incomplete and erratic
Protein binding: 90% of dose binds to blood proteins
Metabolism: By mixed function oxidase enzymes in the liver
Bioavailability: Gut dysfunction, commonly seen in BMT recipients reduces oral bioavailability further
Half-life: Adults: 19-40 hours
Time to peak serum concentration: 3-4 hours
Elimination: Primarily in bile, clearance is decreased in patients with liver disease

Usual Dosage Geriatrics and Adults:
Oral: Initial: 14-18 mg/kg/dose daily, beginning 4-12 hours prior to organ transplantation; maintenance: 5-10 mg/kg/day
I.V.: Initial: 5-6 mg/kg/day in divided doses every 12-24 hours; patients should be switched to oral cyclosporine as soon as possible

Rheumatoid arthritis: Oral: 5-10 mg/kg/day

Administration For I.V. use, dilute to a concentration of 50 mg per 20-100 mL; infuse over 2-6 hours; do not administer liquid from plastic or styrofoam cup; mixing with milk, chocolate milk, or orange juice preferably at room temperature, improves palatability; stir well and drink at once; do not allow to stand before drinking; rinse with more diluent to ensure that the total dose is taken; after use, dry outside of pipette; do not rinse with water or other cleaning agents

(Continued)

Cyclosporine *(Continued)*

Monitoring Parameters Cyclosporine levels, serum electrolytes, renal function, hepatic function, blood pressure, pulse

Reference Range Reference ranges are **method dependent and specimen dependent**. Trough levels should be obtained 12-18 hours after oral dose (chronic usage), 12 hours after I.V. dose, or immediately prior to next dose.

Therapeutic: Not well defined, dependent on organ transplanted, time after transplant, organ function and CSA toxicity

Toxic: Not well defined, nephrotoxicity usually occurs at level above 400 ng/mL, but may occur at any level

Test Interactions Specific whole blood, HPLC assay for cyclosporine may be falsely elevated if sample is drawn from the same line through which dose was administered (even if flush has been administered and/or dose was given hours before)

Patient Information Use glass droppers or glass to hold dose; may mix with milk or juice for flavor; rinse container to get full dose

Nursing Implications May cause inflamed gums; see Administration

Additional Information Should be mixed in glass containers

Special Geriatric Considerations Cyclosporine has not been specifically studied in the elderly

Dosage Forms
Injection: 50 mg/mL (5 mL)
Solution, oral: 100 mg/mL (50 mL)

References
Burckart GJ, Canafax DM, and Yee GC, "Cyclosporine Monitoring," *Drug Intell Clin Pharm*, 1986, 20(9):649-52.

Cycrin® *see* Medroxyprogesterone Acetate *on page 437*

Cyomin®I Rubisol-1000® *see* Cyanocobalamin *on page 192*

Cyproheptadine Hydrochloride (si proe hep' ta deen)

Brand Names Periactin®

Generic Available Yes

Therapeutic Class Antihistamine

Use Perennial and seasonal allergic rhinitis and other allergic symptoms including cold urticaria

Unlabeled use: Appetite stimulant, vascular cluster headaches, migraine headache prophylaxis

Contraindications Hypersensitivity to cyproheptadine or any component; narrow-angle glaucoma, bladder neck obstruction, asthmatic attack, stenosing peptic ulcer, GI tract obstruction, those on MAO inhibitors

Warnings Antihistamines are more likely to cause dizziness, excessive sedation, syncope, toxic confusional states, and hypotension in the elderly.

Precautions Use with caution in patients with heart disease, hypertension, thyroid disease, and asthma

Adverse Reactions
Cardiovascular: Tachycardia
Central nervous system: Sedation, CNS stimulation, seizures
Gastrointestinal: Appetite stimulation, weight gain
Hematologic: Hemolytic anemia, leukopenia, thrombocytopenia
Miscellaneous: Allergic reactions

Overdosage Symptoms of overdose include CNS depression or stimulation, dry mouth, flushed skin, fixed and dilated pupils, apnea

Toxicology There is no specific treatment for an antihistamine overdose, however, most of its clinical toxicity is due to anticholinergic effects. Anticholinesterase inhibitors may be useful by reducing acetylcholinesterase. Anticholinesterase inhibitors include physostigmine, neostigmine, pyridostigmine and edrophonium. For anticholinergic overdose with severe life-threatening symptoms, physostigmine 1-2 mg I.V. slowly may be given to reverse these effects.

Drug Interactions Increased toxicity: MAO inhibitors, CNS depressants, alcohol

Mechanism of Action Competes with histamine for H_1-receptor sites on effector cells in the gastrointestinal tract, blood vessels, and respiratory tract; also has antiserotonin effects

Pharmacokinetics
Metabolism: Almost completely
Elimination: >50% excreted in urine (primarily as metabolites) and ~25% excreted in feces

Usual Dosage Oral:
Geriatrics: Initial: 4 mg twice daily
Adults: Initial: 4 mg 3 times/day; maximum: do not to exceed 0.5 mg/kg/day
Appetite stimulant: 4 mg 3-4 times/day

Dosing adjustment in hepatic impairment: Dosage should be reduced in patients with significant hepatic dysfunction

Monitoring Parameters Relief of symptoms, weight

Test Interactions Diagnostic antigen skin tests

Patient Information May cause drowsiness; avoid CNS depressants and alcohol

Nursing Implications Monitor relief of symptoms, weight, eating habits

Additional Information May stimulate appetite

Special Geriatric Considerations In case reports, cyproheptadine has promoted weight gain in anorexic adults, though it has not been specifically studied in the elderly. All cases of weight loss or decreased appetite should be adequately assessed. Cyproheptadine may cause less sedation than diphenhydramine or hydroxyzine and, therefore, may be useful for pruritus in the elderly; elderly may not tolerate anticholinergic effects.

Dosage Forms
Syrup: 2 mg/5 mL with alcohol 5% (473 mL)
Tablet: 4 mg

Cystospaz® see Hyoscyamine Sulfate on page 359

Cystospaz-M® see Hyoscyamine Sulfate on page 359

CYT see Cyclophosphamide on page 196

Cytomel® see Liothyronine Sodium on page 408

Cytotec® see Misoprostol on page 475

Cytovene® see Ganciclovir on page 318

Cytoxan® see Cyclophosphamide on page 196

D₃ see Cholecalciferol on page 161

D-3-Mercaptovaline see Penicillamine on page 537

Dacodyl® [OTC] see Bisacodyl on page 87

Dalalone L.A.® see Dexamethasone on page 207

Dalcaine® see Lidocaine Hydrochloride on page 406

Dalmane® see Flurazepam Hydrochloride on page 305

Dantrium® see Dantrolene Sodium on this page

Dantrolene Sodium (dan' troe leen)

Brand Names Dantrium®

Generic Available No

Therapeutic Class Antidote, Malignant Hyperthermia; Hyperthermia, Treatment; Skeletal Muscle Relaxant

Use Treatment of spasticity associated with spinal cord injury, stroke, cerebral palsy, or multiple sclerosis; also used as treatment of malignant hyperthermia

Unlabeled use: Neuroleptic malignant syndrome, heat stroke

Contraindications Active hepatic disease; should not be used where spasticity is used to maintain posture or balance

Warnings Has potential for hepatotoxicity; overt hepatitis has been most frequently observed between the third and twelfth month of therapy; hepatic injury appears to be greater in females and in patients >35 years of age

Precautions Use with caution in patients with impaired cardiac function or impaired pulmonary function

Adverse Reactions
Cardiovascular: Pleural effusion with pericarditis
Central nervous system: Seizures, drowsiness, dizziness, lightheadedness, confusion, headache
Dermatologic: Rash
Gastrointestinal: Diarrhea, nausea, vomiting
Hepatic: Hepatitis
Neuromuscular & skeletal: Muscle weakness

Overdosage Symptoms of overdose include CNS depression, nausea, vomiting; employ supportive measures, gastric lavage

Drug Interactions
Decreased protein binding: Warfarin, clofibrate

Definite drug interaction with estrogen has not been established, but increased hepatotoxicity is seen in women >35 years of age using both drugs
Increased hyperkalemia and cardiac depression with verapamil

Stability Add 60 mL of sterile water for injection USP (not **bacteriostatic water for injection**); protect from light; use within 6 hours

Mechanism of Action Acts directly on skeletal muscle by interfering with release of calcium ion from the sarcoplasmic reticulum; prevents or reduces the increase in myoplasmic calcium ion concentration that activates the acute catabolic processes associated with malignant hyperthermia

(Continued)

Dantrolene Sodium *(Continued)*

Pharmacokinetics
Absorption: Slow and incomplete from GI tract
Metabolism: Slowly in the liver
Half-life: 8.7 hours
Elimination: 25% in urine as metabolites and unchanged drug, and 45% to 50% in feces via bile

Usual Dosage Geriatrics and Adults:
Spasticity: Oral: 25 mg/day to start, increase frequency to 3-4 times/day, then increase dose by 25 mg every 4-7 days to a maximum of 100 mg 2-4 times/day or 400 mg/day

Hyperthermia:
Oral: 4-8 mg/kg/day in 4 divided doses
I.V.: 1 mg/kg; may repeat dose up to cumulative dose of 10 mg/kg (mean effective dose is 2.5 mg/kg), then switch to oral dosage

Monitoring Parameters Blood pressure, pulse, temperature, liver function tests, motor performance

Test Interactions Increased serum AST (SGOT), ALT (SGPT), alkaline phosphatase, LDH, BUN, and total serum bilirubin

Patient Information Avoid unnecessary exposure to sunlight (or use sunscreen, protective clothing); avoid alcohol and other CNS depressants; patients should use caution while driving or performing other tasks requiring alertness

Nursing Implications 36 vials needed for adequate hyperthermia therapy; exercise caution at meals on the day of administration because difficulty swallowing and choking has been reported

Additional Information Avoid glass bottles for I.V. infusion

Special Geriatric Considerations There is little experience with this drug in the elderly; see Warnings and Monitoring Parameters

Dosage Forms
Capsule: 25 mg, 50 mg, 100 mg
Injection: 20 mg

Extemporaneous Preparation(s) A suspension can be prepared by mixing 500 mg (from capsules) with 150 mg citric acid, 10 mL distilled water, and sufficient simple syrup to bring the total volume to 100 mL (final concentration 5 mg/mL)

Dapa® [OTC] *see* Acetaminophen *on page 13*

Dapiprazole Hydrochloride *(da' pi pray zole)*

Brand Names Rēv-Eyes™
Generic Available No
Therapeutic Class Alpha-Adrenergic Blocking Agent, Ophthalmic
Use Reverse dilation due to drugs (adrenergic or parasympathomimetic) after eye exams
Contraindications In the presence of conditions where miosis is unacceptable, such as acute iritis and in patients with a history of hypersensitivity to any component of the formulation
Warnings For ophthalmic use only
Adverse Reactions
Central nervous system: Headache
Local: Burning sensation in the eyes, lid edema, ptosis, lid erythema, chemosis, itching, punctate keratitis, corneal edema
Ocular: Photophobia
Stability After reconstitution, drops are stable at room temperature for 21 days
Mechanism of Action Dapiprazole is a selective alpha-adrenergic blocking agent, exerting effects primarily on alpha$_1$-adrenoceptors. It induces miosis via relaxation of the smooth dilator (radial) muscle of the iris, which causes pupillary constriction. It is devoid of cholinergic effects. Dapiprazole also partially reverses the cycloplegia induced with parasympatholytic agents such as tropicamide. Although the drug has no significant effect on the ciliary muscle per se, it may increase accommodative amplitude therefore relieving the symptoms of paralysis of accommodation. Does not significantly alter intraocular pressure in eyes that are normotensive or with increased intraocular pressure.
Usual Dosage Geriatrics and Adults: Administer 2 drops followed 5 minutes later by an additional 2 drops applied to the conjunctiva of each eye; should not be used more frequently than once a week in the same patient
Administration Finger pressure should be applied to lacrimal sac for 1-2 minutes after instillation to decrease risk of absorption and systemic reactions; do not touch eye with dropper
Patient Information May still be sensitive to sunlight and sensitivity may return in 2 or more hours; store at room temperature
Special Geriatric Considerations No specific data in the elderly; see Usual Dosage
Dosage Forms Powder, lyophilized: 25 mg [0.5% solution when mixed with supplied diluent]

Darvocet-N® *see* Propoxyphene and Acetaminophen *on page 604*

Darvon® *see* Propoxyphene *on page 603*

Darvon-N® *see* Propoxyphene *on page 603*

Datril® [OTC] *see* Acetaminophen *on page 13*

Daypro™ *see* Oxaprozin *on page 522*

Dazamide® *see* Acetazolamide *on page 15*

DDAVP® *see* Desmopressin Acetate *on page 206*

DDI *see* Didanosine *on page 216*

1-Deamino-8-D-Arginine Vasopressin *see* Desmopressin Acetate *on page 206*

Debrisan® [OTC] *see* Dextranomer *on page 209*

Debrox® Otic [OTC] *see* Carbamide Peroxide *on page 119*

Decaderm® *see* Dexamethasone *on page 207*

Decadron® *see* Dexamethasone *on page 207*

Decadron®-LA *see* Dexamethasone *on page 207*

Decadron® Turbinaire® *see* Dexamethasone *on page 207*

Decaject-L.A.® *see* Dexamethasone *on page 207*

Decaspray® *see* Dexamethasone *on page 207*

Declomycin® *see* Demeclocycline Hydrochloride *on this page*

Decofed® Syrup [OTC] *see* Pseudoephedrine *on page 609*

Deficol® [OTC] *see* Bisacodyl *on page 87*

Degest® 2 [OTC] *see* Naphazoline Hydrochloride *on page 492*

Dehist® *see* Brompheniramine Maleate *on page 95*

Dekasol-L.A.® *see* Dexamethasone *on page 207*

Delaxin® *see* Methocarbamol *on page 454*

Delestrogen® *see* Estradiol *on page 269*

Delsym® [OTC] *see* Dextromethorphan *on page 209*

Delta-Cortef® *see* Prednisolone *on page 584*

Deltacortisone *see* Prednisone *on page 586*

Delta-D® *see* Cholecalciferol *on page 161*

Deltadehydrocortisone *see* Prednisone *on page 586*

Deltahydrocortisone *see* Prednisolone *on page 584*

Deltasone® *see* Prednisone *on page 586*

Demadex® *see* Torsemide *on page 706*

Demeclocycline Hydrochloride (dem e kloe sye' kleen)

Brand Names Declomycin®

Synonyms Demethylchlortetracycline

Therapeutic Class Antibiotic, Tetracycline Derivative

Use Treatment of susceptible bacterial infections (acne, gonorrhea, pertussis and urinary tract infections) caused by both gram-negative and gram-positive organisms; used when penicillin is contraindicated; the treatment of chronic syndrome of inappropriate secretion of antidiuretic hormone (SIADH)

Contraindications Hypersensitivity to demeclocycline, tetracyclines, or any component

Warnings Photosensitivity reactions occur frequently with this drug, avoid prolonged exposure to sunlight, do not use tanning equipment

Adverse Reactions
Cardiovascular: Pericarditis
Central nervous system: Paresthesia, increased intracranial pressure
Dermatologic: Pruritus, pigmentation of nails, exfoliative dermatitis, photosensitivity
Endocrine & metabolic: Diabetes insipidus syndrome
Gastrointestinal: Nausea, vomiting, diarrhea, esophagitis, anorexia, abdominal cramps
Genitourinary: Azotemia
Renal: Acute renal failure
Miscellaneous: Superinfections, anaphylaxis

Overdosage Symptoms of overdose include photosensitivity, diabetes insipidus, nausea, anorexia, diarrhea

Drug Interactions
Do not administer with antacids, milk or dairy products, zinc, and iron preparations which may decrease absorption

(Continued)

Demeclocycline Hydrochloride *(Continued)*

Carbamazepine, barbiturates, hydantoins may decrease effect
Increased effect of warfarin

Stability Tetracyclines form toxic products when outdated or when exposed to light, heat, or humidity (Fanconi-like syndrome)

Mechanism of Action Inhibits protein synthesis by binding with the 30S and possibly the 50S ribosomal subunit(s) of susceptible bacteria; may also cause alterations in the cytoplasmic membrane

Pharmacodynamics Onset of action for diuresis in SIADH: Several days

Pharmacokinetics

Absorption: ~50% to 80% from GI tract (food and dairy products reduce absorption)

Protein binding: 41% to 50%

Metabolism: Small amounts metabolized in the liver to inactive metabolites; enterohepatically recycled

Half-life: 10-17 hours (prolonged with reduced renal function)

Time to peak: Oral: Peak serum levels occur within 3-6 hours

Elimination: As unchanged drug (42% to 50%) in urine

Usual Dosage Geriatrics and Adults: 150 mg 4 times/day or 300 mg twice daily

Uncomplicated gonorrhea (penicillin-sensitive): 600 mg stat, 300 mg every 12 hours for 4 days (3 g total)

SIADH: 900-1200 mg/day or 13-15 mg/kg/day divided every 6-8 hours initially, then decrease to 0.6-0.9 g/day

Administration Administer 1 hour before or 2 hours after food or milk with plenty of fluid

Monitoring Parameters CBC, renal and hepatic function; PT or INR in patients on anticoagulants

Test Interactions May interfere with tests for urinary glucose (false-negative urine glucose using Clinistix®, Tes-Tape®); may suppress bacterial growth in blood and urine for several days after discontinuance

Patient Information Avoid prolonged exposure to sunlight or sunlamps; avoid taking antacids before tetracyclines

Nursing Implications See Administration

Special Geriatric Considerations Has not been studied exclusively in the elderly, see Usual Dosage

Dosage Forms

Capsule: 150 mg

Tablet: 150 mg, 300 mg

References

Troyer AD, "Demeclocycline. Treatment for Syndrome of Inappropriate Antidiuretic Hormone Secretion," *JAMA*, 1977, 237(25):2723-6.

Demerol® *see* Meperidine Hydrochloride *on page 441*

Demethylchlortetracycline *see* Demeclocycline Hydrochloride *on previous page*

Depakene® *see* Valproic Acid and Derivatives *on page 728*

Depakote® *see* Valproic Acid and Derivatives *on page 728*

Depen® *see* Penicillamine *on page 537*

depGynogen® *see* Estradiol *on page 269*

depMedalone® *see* Methylprednisolone *on page 461*

Depo®-Estradiol *see* Estradiol *on page 269*

Depogen® *see* Estradiol *on page 269*

Depoject® *see* Methylprednisolone *on page 461*

Depo-Medrol® *see* Methylprednisolone *on page 461*

Deponit® *see* Nitroglycerin *on page 505*

Depopred® *see* Methylprednisolone *on page 461*

Depo-Provera® *see* Medroxyprogesterone Acetate *on page 437*

Deprenyl *see* Selegiline Hydrochloride *on page 640*

Dermabet® *see* Betamethasone *on page 82*

Dermacomb® Topical *see* Nystatin and Triamcinolone *on page 514*

Dermatop® *see* Prednicarbate *on page 583*

DermiCort® [OTC] *see* Hydrocortisone *on page 351*

Dermolate® [OTC] *see* Hydrocortisone *on page 351*

DES *see* Diethylstilbestrol *on page 217*

Desenex® [OTC] *see* Tolnaftate *on page 705*

Desiccated Thyroid *see* Thyroid *on page 691*

Desipramine Hydrochloride (dess ip' ra meen)

Related Information

Antidepressant Agents Comparison *on page 800*

Drug Levels Commonly Monitored Guidelines *on page 771-772*

Brand Names Norpramin®; Pertofrane®

Synonyms Desmethylimipramine HCl

Generic Available Yes: Tablet

Therapeutic Class Antidepressant, Tricyclic

Use Treatment of various forms of depression, often in conjunction with psychotherapy; as an analgesic in chronic pain, peripheral neuropathies

Contraindications Hypersensitivity to desipramine (cross-sensitivity with other tricyclic antidepressants may occur); patients receiving MAO inhibitors within past 14 days; narrow-angle glaucoma

Warnings Some formulations contain tartrazine which may cause allergic reaction; do not discontinue abruptly in patients receiving long-term high dose therapy

Precautions Use with caution in patients with cardiovascular disease, conduction disturbances, urinary retention; seizure disorders, bipolar illness, renal or hepatic impairment, hyperthyroidism or those receiving thyroid replacement; an EKG prior to the start of therapy is advised

Adverse Reactions Less sedation and anticholinergic adverse effects than amitriptyline or imipramine

Cardiovascular: Arrhythmias, hypotension

Central nervous system: Sedation, confusion, delirium, dizziness, excitation, headache, seizures

Dermatologic: Photosensitivity

Endocrine & metabolic: SIADH

Gastrointestinal: Dry mouth, constipation, nausea, vomiting, increased appetite, weight gain, craving sweets, GE reflux, unpleasant taste

Genitourinary: Urinary retention

Hematologic: Blood dyscrasias

Hepatic: Hepatitis, cholestatic jaundice, increased liver enzymes

Ocular: Increased intraocular pressure, blurred vision

Otic: Tinnitus

Miscellaneous: Hypersensitivity reactions, associated with falls, excessive sweating

Overdosage Symptoms of overdose include agitation, confusion, hallucinations, hyperthermia, urinary retention, CNS depression, cyanosis, dry mucous membranes

Toxicology Following initiation of essential overdose management, toxic symptoms should be treated. Ventricular arrhythmias often respond to phenytoin 15-20 mg/kg with concurrent systemic alkalinization (sodium bicarbonate 0.5-2 mEq/kg I.V.). Arrhythmias unresponsive to this therapy may respond to lidocaine 1 mg/kg I.V. followed by a titrated infusion. Physostigmine (1-2 mg I.V. slowly) may be indicated in reversing cardiac arrhythmias that are due to vagal blockade or for anticholinergic effects. Seizures usually respond to diazepam I.V. boluses (5-10 mg, up to 30 mg). If seizures are unresponsive or recur, phenytoin or phenobarbital may be required.

Drug Interactions

May decrease effects of guanethidine and clonidine resulting in hypertensive crisis

May increase effects of CNS depressants, adrenergic agents, dicumarol, anticholinergic agents

With MAO inhibitors, hyperpyrexia, tachycardia, hypertension, seizures, and death may occur; interactions similar to other tricyclics may occur

Cimetidine, fluoxetine, methylphenidate, and haloperidol may decrease the metabolism and/or increase TCA levels

Phenobarbital may increase TCA metabolism

Mechanism of Action Traditionally believed to increase the synaptic concentration of norepinephrine in the central nervous system by inhibition of its reuptake by the presynaptic neuronal membrane. However, additional receptor effects have been found including desensitization of adenyl cyclase, down regulation of beta-adrenergic receptors, and down regulation of serotonin receptors.

Pharmacodynamics Onset of action: 1-3 weeks; norepinephrine only

Pharmacokinetics

Absorption: Well absorbed from GI tract

Protein binding: 90%

Metabolism: In the liver

Half-life: 12-57 hours

Plasma concentration and half-life have been found to positively correlate with age; mean half-life: >75 hours, twice that of young patients

Elimination: 70% excreted in urine

Usual Dosage Oral:

Geriatrics: Initial dose: 10-25 mg/day; increase by 10-25 mg every 3 days for inpatients and every week for outpatients if tolerated; usual maintenance dose: 75-100 mg/day, but doses up to 300 mg may be necessary

(Continued)

Desipramine Hydrochloride *(Continued)*

Adults: Initial: 75 mg/day in divided doses; increase gradually to 150-200 mg/day in divided or single dose; maximum: 300 mg/day

Monitoring Parameters Improvement in depressive symptoms; blood pressure, pulse

Reference Range
Therapeutic: 125-160 ng/mL
Possible toxicity: >300 ng/mL (SI: 1070 nmol/L)
Toxic: >1000 ng/mL (SI: >3750 nmol/L)
In geriatric patients the response rate is greatest with steady-state plasma concentrations >115 ng/mL

Test Interactions Increased glucose

Patient Information Avoid alcohol ingestion; do not discontinue medication abruptly; may cause urine to turn blue-green; may cause drowsiness, dry mouth, blurred vision or dizziness; rise slowly to prevent dizziness

Nursing Implications Monitor blood pressure and pulse rate prior to and during initial therapy; evaluate mental status; monitor weight, may increase appetite

Additional Information Avoid unnecessary exposure to sunlight

Special Geriatric Considerations Preferred agent because of its milder side effect profile; patients may experience excitation or stimulation; in such cases give as a single morning dose or divided dose

Dosage Forms
Capsule: 25 mg, 50 mg
Tablet: 10 mg, 25 mg, 50 mg, 75 mg, 100 mg, 150 mg

References
Nelson JC, Jatlow PI, and Mazure C, "Desipramine Plasma Levels and Response in Elderly Melancholic Patients," *J Clin Psychopharmacol*, 1985, 5(4):217-20.
Nies A, Robinson DS, Friedman MS, et al, "Relationship Between Age and Tricyclic Antidepressant Plasma Levels," *Am J Psychiatry*, 1977, 134:790-3.

Desmethylimipramine HCl *see Desipramine Hydrochloride on previous page*

Desmopressin Acetate *(des moe press' in)*

Brand Names DDAVP®; Stimate™

Synonyms 1-Deamino-8-D-Arginine Vasopressin

Therapeutic Class Antihemophilic Agent; Hemostatic Agent; Vasopressin Analog, Synthetic

Use Treatment of diabetes insipidus; control bleeding in certain types of hemophilia; primary nocturnal enuresis (intranasal)

Contraindications Hypersensitivity to desmopressin or any component; avoid using in patients with type IIB or platelet-type von Willebrand's disease; or patients with <5% factor VIII activity level

Precautions Avoid overhydration especially when drug is used for its hemostatic effect; use with caution in patients with serious cardiovascular disease

Adverse Reactions
Cardiovascular: Facial flushing, increase in blood pressure, arrhythmias, decreased cardiac output
Central nervous system: Headache, dizziness
Endocrine & metabolic: Hyponatremia, water intoxication
Gastrointestinal: Nausea, abdominal cramps
Genitourinary: Vulval pain
Local: Pain at the injection site
Respiratory: Nasal congestion

Overdosage Symptoms of overdose include drowsiness, headache, confusion, anuria, water intoxication

Drug Interactions
Decreased effect: Demeclocycline, lithium → ↓ ADH effect
Increased effect: Chlorpropamide, fludrocortisone → ↑ ADH response

Stability Keep in refrigerator, avoid freezing; discard discolored solutions

Mechanism of Action Enhances reabsorption of water in the kidneys by increasing cellular permeability of the collecting ducts; possibly causes smooth muscle constriction with resultant vasoconstriction

Pharmacodynamics
Intranasal administration:
Onset of ADH effects: Within 1 hour
Peak effect: Within 1-5 hours
Duration: 5-21 hours
I.V. infusion:
Onset of increased factor VIII activity: Within 15-30 minutes
Peak effect: 0.75-3 hours

Pharmacokinetics
Absorption: Nasal: Slow, 10% to 20%

ALPHABETICAL LISTING OF DRUGS

Metabolism: Unknown
Half-life: Terminal elimination: 75 minutes

Usual Dosage Geriatrics and Adults:
Diabetes insipidus:
Intranasal: 5-40 mcg/day 1-3 times/day
I.V., S.C.: 2-4 mcg/day in 2 divided doses or $^1/_{10}$ of the maintenance intranasal dose

Hemophilia:
Intranasal: 2-4 mcg/kg/dose
I.V.: 0.3 mcg/kg by slow infusion

Administration Infuse over 15-30 minutes; dilute in 10-50 mL 0.9% sodium chloride

Monitoring Parameters Blood pressure and pulse should be monitored during I.V. infusion
Diabetes insipidus: Fluid intake, urine volume, specific gravity, plasma and urine osmolality, serum electrolytes
Hemophilia: Factor VIII antigen levels, APTT

Test Interactions Decreased sodium (S)

Patient Information Avoid overhydration; notify physician if headache, shortness of breath, heartburn, nausea, abdominal cramps or vulval pain occurs; follow administration guidelines for intranasal products

Nursing Implications See Administration

Additional Information Manufacturer supplies a flexible tubing for administering the nasal solution

Special Geriatric Considerations Elderly patients should be cautioned not to increase their fluid intake beyond that sufficient to satisfy their thirst in order to avoid water intoxication and hyponatremia. Under experimental conditions, the elderly have been shown to have a decreased responsiveness to vasopressin with respect to its effects on water homeostasis.

Dosage Forms
Injection: 4 mcg/mL (1 mL)
Solution, nasal: 0.1 mg/mL (2.5 mL, 5 mL)

References
Asplund R and Aberg H, "Desmopressin in Elderly Subjects With Increased Nocturnal Diuresis: A Two-Month Treatment Study," *Scand J Urol Nephrol*, 1993, 27(1):77-82.
Lindeman RD, Lee TD Jr, Yiengst MJ, et al, "Influence of Age, Renal Disease, Hypertension, Diuretics, and Calcium on the Antidiuretic Responses to Suboptimal Infusions of Vasopressin," *J Lab Clin Med*, 1966, 68(2):206-23.
Miller JH and Shock NW, "Age Differences in the Renal Tubular Response to Antidiuretic Hormone," *J Gerontol*, 1953, 8:446-50.

Desoxyphenobarbital *see* Primidone *on page 587*

Desyrel® *see* Trazodone *on page 709*

Devrom® [OTC] *see* Bismuth *on page 88*

Dexacidin® Ophthalmic *see* Neomycin, Polymyxin B, and Dexamethasone *on page 495*

Dex-A-Diet® [OTC] *see* Phenylpropanolamine Hydrochloride *on page 559*

Dexair® *see* Dexamethasone *on this page*

Dexamethasone (dex a meth' a sone)
Related Information
Antacid Drug Interactions *on page 764*
Corticosteroids Comparison, Systemic *on page 808*
Corticosteroids Comparison, Topical *on page 809*

Brand Names Aeroseb-Dex®; AK-Dex®; Alba-Dex®; Baldex®; Dalalone L.A.®; Decaderm®; Decadron®; Decadron®-LA; Decadron® Turbinaire®; Decaject-L.A.®; Decaspray®; Dekasol-L.A.®; Dexair®; Dexasone L.A.®; Dexone®; Hexadrol®; I-Methasone®; Maxidex®; Ocu-Dex®; Solurex L.A.®

Generic Available Yes

Therapeutic Class Antiemetic; Anti-inflammatory Agent; Anti-inflammatory Agent, Ophthalmic; Corticosteroid, Inhalant; Corticosteroid, Ophthalmic; Corticosteroid, Systemic; Corticosteroid, Topical (Low Potency)

Use Systemically and locally for chronic inflammation, allergic, hematologic, neoplastic, and autoimmune diseases; may be used in management of cerebral edema, septic shock, and as a diagnostic agent

Contraindications Active untreated infections; viral, fungal, or tuberculous diseases of the eye

Warnings Fatalities have occurred due to adrenal insufficiency in asthmatic patients during and after transfer from systemic corticosteroids to aerosol steroids; during this period, aerosol steroids do **not** provide the systemic steroid needed to treat patients having trauma, surgery or infections

Precautions Use with caution in patients with hypothyroidism, cirrhosis, hypertension, congestive heart failure, nonspecific ulcerative colitis, thromboembolic disorders and

(Continued)

Dexamethasone (Continued)

in patients with increased risk for peptic ulcer disease; gradually taper dose to withdraw therapy

Adverse Reactions

Cardiovascular: Hypertension, edema, accelerated atherogenesis

Central nervous system: Euphoria, mental changes, headache, vertigo, seizures, psychoses, pseudotumor cerebri

Dermatologic: Folliculitis, hypertrichosis, acneiform eruption, dermatitis, maceration, skin atrophy, acne, impaired wound healing, hirsutism

Endocrine & metabolic: Growth suppression, Cushing's syndrome, pituitary-adrenal axis suppression, alkalosis, glucose intolerance, hypokalemia, postmenopausal bleeding, hot flashes

Gastrointestinal: Peptic ulcer, nausea, vomiting, pancreatitis

Local: Burning, irritation

Neuromuscular & skeletal: Muscle weakness, osteoporosis, fractures, aseptic necrosis of femoral and humeral heads, steroid myopathy

Ocular: Cataracts, glaucoma

Miscellaneous: Increased susceptibility to infection

Toxicology When consumed in excessive quantities for prolonged periods, systemic hypercorticism and adrenal suppression may occur; in those cases, discontinuation and withdrawal of the corticosteroid should be done judiciously

Drug Interactions

Steroids decrease the effect of anticholinesterases, isoniazid, salicylates, insulin, oral hypoglycemics

Decreased effect: Barbiturates, phenytoin, rifampin

Increased effect (hypokalemia) of potassium-depleting diuretics

Increased risk of digoxin toxicity (due to hypokalemia)

Increased effect: Estrogens, ketoconazole

Stability

Stability of injection of parenteral admixture at room temperature (25°C): 24 hours

Stability of injection of parenteral admixture at refrigeration temperature (4°C): 2 days; protect from light and freezing

Mechanism of Action Decreases inflammation by suppression of migration of polymorphonuclear leukocytes and reversal of increased capillary permeability; suppresses normal immune response

Pharmacodynamics Duration of metabolic effects: Can last for 72 hours

Pharmacokinetics

Metabolism: In the liver

Half-life: 1.8-3.5 hours; biologic half-life: 36-54 hours

Time to peak serum concentration:

Oral: Within 1-2 hours

I.M.: Within 8 hours

Elimination: In urine and bile

Usual Dosage

Geriatrics: Use lowest effective dose

Adults:

Anti-inflammatory: Oral, I.M., I.V.: 0.75-9 mg/day in divided doses every 6-12 hours

Cerebral edema: I.V.: 10 mg stat, 4 mg I.M./I.V. every 6 hours until response is maximized, then switch to oral regimen, then taper off if appropriate

Inoperable brain tumor: Oral: 2 mg 2-4 times/day

Diagnosis for Cushing's syndrome: Oral: 1 mg at 11 PM, draw blood at 8 AM

Ophthalmic:

Suspension: Instill 1 drop 3-4 times/day

Ointment: Apply a thin layer 3-4 times/day, gradually taper dose

Inhalation: 3 inhalations 3-4 times/day; maximum: 12 inhalations/day

Nasal: 2 sprays in each nostril 2-3 times/day; maximum: 12 sprays/day

Topical: Apply 2-4 times/day

Monitoring Parameters Blood pressure, blood glucose, electrolytes, symptoms of fluid retention

Reference Range Dexamethasone suppression test, overnight: 8 AM cortisol <6 μg/100 mL (dexamethasone 1 mg)

Test Interactions Increased amylase (S), cholesterol (S), glucose, protein, sodium (S); decreased calcium (S), chloride (S), potassium (S), thyroxine (S)

Patient Information Notify physician of any signs of infection or injuries during therapy; inform physician or dentist before surgery if you are taking a corticosteroid; may cause GI upset; take with food or milk; do not stop abruptly; for topical products, use a thin layer; do not overuse; follow instructions with inhaled products

Nursing Implications Give with meals to decrease GI upset; do not use topical products on open wounds; acetate injection is not for I.V. use

Special Geriatric Considerations Because of the risk of adverse effects, systemic corticosteroids should be used cautiously in the elderly in the smallest possible dose, and for the shortest possible time.

Dosage Forms
  Aerosol:
    Nasal, as sodium phosphate: 0.1 mg/spray (15 mg/12.6 g, 12.6 g)
    Oral, as sodium phosphate: 0.01% (58 g); 0.04% (25 g)
    Topical: 0.075 mg/spray (25 g)
  Cream, as sodium phosphate: 0.1% (15 g)
  Elixir: 0.5 mg/5 mL (100 mL, 273 mL)
  Gel: 0.01% (30 g)
  Injection, as acetate: 8 mg/mL (1 mL, 5 mL); 16 mg/mL (1 mL, 5 mL)
  Injection, as sodium phosphate: 4 mg/mL (1 mL, 5 mL, 10 mL, 25 mL, 30 mL); 10 mg/mL (1 mL, 10 mL); 20 mg/mL (5 mL)
  Ointment, ophthalmic, as sodium phosphate: 0.05% (3.5 g)
  Solution:
    Concentrate: 0.5 mg/0.5 mL (30 mL)
    Oral: 0.5 mg/5 mL (5 mL, 20 mL, 500 mL)
  Suspension, ophthalmic, as sodium phosphate: 0.1% with methylcellulose 0.5% (15 mL)
  Tablet: 0.25 mg, 0.5 mg, 0.75 mg, 1 mg, 1.5 mg, 2 mg, 4 mg, 6 mg

Dexasone L.A.® *see* Dexamethasone *on page 207*

Dexasporin® Ophthalmic *see* Neomycin, Polymyxin B, and Dexamethasone *on page 495*

Dexatrim® [OTC] *see* Phenylpropanolamine Hydrochloride *on page 559*

Dexone L.A.® *see* Dexamethasone *on page 207*

Dextranomer (dex tran' oh mer)
Brand Names Debrisan® [OTC]
Generic Available No
Therapeutic Class Topical Skin Product
Use Clean exudative ulcers and wounds such as venous stasis ulcers, decubitus ulcers, and infected traumatic and surgical wounds; no controlled studies have found dextranomer to be more effective than conventional therapy
Contraindications Deep fistulas, sinus tracts, hypersensitivity to any component
Precautions Do not use in deep fistulas or any area where complete removal is not assured; do not use on dry wounds (ineffective); avoid contact with eyes
Adverse Reactions
  Dermatologic: Maceration may occur
  Local: Transitory pain, bleeding, blistering, erythema
Mechanism of Action Dextranomer is a network of dextran-sucrose beads possessing a great many exposed hydroxy groups; when this network is applied to an exudative wound surface, the exudate is drawn by capillary forces generated by the swelling of the beads, with vacuum forces producing an upward flow of exudate into the network
Usual Dosage Geriatrics and Adults: Apply to affected area once or twice daily in a ¼" layer; apply a dressing and seal on all four sides
Administration Sprinkle beads into ulcer (or apply paste) to ¼" thickness; change dressings 1-4 times/day depending on drainage; change dressing before it is completely dry to facilitate removal. Remove beads or paste when they become saturated. Occasionally vigorous irrigation, soaking, or whirlpool may be needed to remove the product. Each container should only be used for one patient to avoid cross-contamination.
Patient Information Avoid contact with eyes; for external use only
Nursing Implications Discontinue treatment when the area is free of exudate and edema or when healthy granulation tissue is present
Special Geriatric Considerations Preventive skin care should be instituted in all older patients at high risk for decubitus ulcers. Debrisan® is indicated in stage 3 and 4 decubitus ulcers.
Dosage Forms
  Beads: 4 g, 25 g, 60 g, 120 g
  Paste, premixed and sterile: 10 g foil packets
References
Chamberlain TM, Cali TJ, Cuzzell J, et al, "Assessment and Management of Pressure Sores in Long-Term Care Facilities," *Consult Pharm*, 1992, 7(12):1328-40.

Dextromethorphan (dex troe meth or' fan)
Brand Names Benylin® DM; Delsym® [OTC]; Vicks® Formula 44®
Generic Available Yes
Therapeutic Class Antitussive
Use Symptomatic relief of coughs caused by minor viral upper respiratory tract infections or inhaled irritants; most effective for a chronic nonproductive cough
(Continued)

Dextromethorphan *(Continued)*

Contraindications Hypersensitivity to dextromethorphan or any component

Warnings Should not be used for chronic productive coughs

Adverse Reactions
Central nervous system: Drowsiness, dizziness, coma
Gastrointestinal: Nausea, constipation
Respiratory: Respiratory depression

Overdosage Symptoms of overdose include nausea, vomiting, drowsiness, blurred vision, nystagmus, urinary retention, stupor, hallucinations

Toxicology Naloxone 2 mg I.V. with repeat administration as necessary up to a total of 10 mg

Drug Interactions
Decreased metabolism: Quinidine, amiodarone
Increased toxicity: MAO inhibitors, selegiline, alcohol, CNS depressants

Mechanism of Action Chemical relative of morphine lacking narcotic properties; controls cough by depressing the medullary cough center

Pharmacodynamics
Onset of antitussive action: Within 15-30 minutes
Duration: Up to 6 hours; higher doses may have longer duration

Pharmacokinetics
Metabolism: In the liver
Elimination: Principally in urine

Usual Dosage Geriatrics and Adults: Oral: 10-20 mg every 4 hours or 30 mg every 6-8 hours; extended release: 60 mg twice daily; maximum: 120 mg/day

Monitoring Parameters Cough, mental status

Patient Information May cause drowsiness. Avoid CNS depressants and alcohol; do not use for persistent or chronic cough

Nursing Implications See Monitoring Parameters

Additional Information Dextromethorphan is considered approximately half as potent as codeine as an antitussive; dextromethorphan is a component in many cough and cold preparations

Special Geriatric Considerations See Warnings

Dosage Forms
Capsule (Drixoral® Cough Liquid Caps): 30 mg
Liquid:
Pertussin® CS: 3.5 mg/5 mL (120 mL)
Pertussin® ES, Vicks Formula 44®: 15 mg/5 mL (120 mL, 240 mL)
Liquid, sustained release, as polistirex (Delsym®): 30 mg/5 mL (89 mL)
Lozenges:
Scot-Tussin® DM Cough Chasers: 2.5 mg
Hold® DM, Robitussin® Cough Calmers, Sucrets® Cough Calmers: 5 mg
Suppress®, Trocal®: 7.5 mg
Syrup: Benylin® DM, Silphen DM®: 10 mg/5 mL (120 mL, 3780 mL)

Dextromethorphan and Guaifenesin *see* Guaifenesin and Dextromethorphan *on page 332*

Dextropropoxyphene *see* Propoxyphene *on page 603*

Dey-Dose® Isoproterenol *see* Isoproterenol *on page 380*

Dey-Dose® Metaproterenol *see* Metaproterenol Sulfate *on page 449*

Dey-Lube® *see* Ocular Lubricant *on page 515*

Dey-Lute® Isoetharine *see* Isoetharine *on page 378*

Dezone® *see* Dexamethasone *on page 207*

DHPG Sodium *see* Ganciclovir *on page 318*

DHT™ *see* Dihydrotachysterol *on page 224*

Diaβeta® *see* Glyburide *on page 324*

Diabinese® *see* Chlorpropamide *on page 156*

Dialose® [OTC] *see* Docusate *on page 236*

Dialume® [OTC] *see* Aluminum Hydroxide *on page 28*

Diamine T.D.® [OTC] *see* Brompheniramine Maleate *on page 95*

Diamox® *see* Acetazolamide *on page 15*

Diaqua® *see* Hydrochlorothiazide *on page 347*

Diar-Aid® [OTC] *see* Attapulgite *on page 66*

Diasorb® [OTC] *see* Attapulgite *on page 66*

Diazepam (dye az' e pam)

Related Information
Antacid Drug Interactions *on page 764*
Anxiolytic/Hypnotic Use in Long-Term Care Facilities *on page 755-756*
Benzodiazepines Comparison *on page 802-803*

Brand Names Valium®; Valrelease®; Zetran®

Generic Available Yes

Therapeutic Class Antianxiety Agent; Anticonvulsant, Benzodiazepine; Benzodiazepine; Sedative

Use Management of general anxiety disorders, panic disorders, and to provide preoperative sedation, light anesthesia, and amnesia; treatment of status epilepticus, alcohol withdrawal symptoms; used as a skeletal muscle relaxant

Restrictions C-IV

Contraindications Hypersensitivity to diazepam or any component; there may be a cross-sensitivity with other benzodiazepines; do not use in a comatose patient, in those with pre-existing CNS depression, respiratory depression, narrow-angle glaucoma, or severe uncontrolled pain

Precautions Use with caution in patients receiving other CNS depressants, patients with low albumin, hepatic dysfunction, in patients with a history of drug dependence, and in the elderly

Adverse Reactions
Cardiovascular: Cardiac arrest, hypotension, bradycardia, cardiovascular collapse
Central nervous system: Drowsiness, confusion, dizziness, ataxia, amnesia, slurred speech, paradoxical excitement or rage
Local: Phlebitis, pain with injection
Neuromuscular & skeletal: Impaired coordination
Ocular: Blurred vision, diplopia
Respiratory: Decrease in respiratory rate, apnea, laryngospasm
Miscellaneous: Physical and psychological dependence with prolonged use

Overdosage Symptoms of overdose include somnolence, confusion, coma, hypoactive reflexes, dyspnea, hypotension, slurred speech, impaired coordination

Toxicology Treatment for benzodiazepine overdose is supportive. Rarely is mechanical ventilation required. Flumazenil has been shown to selectively block the binding of benzodiazepines to CNS receptors, resulting in a reversal of benzodiazepine-induced CNS depression, but not respiratory depression.

Drug Interactions Benzodiazepines may increase digoxin concentrations and may decrease the effect of levodopa; probenecid may increase onset of action and prolong the effect of benzodiazepine
Decreased metabolism: Cimetidine, fluoxetine
Increased metabolism: Rifampin
Increased toxicity: CNS depressants, alcohol

Stability Protect parenteral dosage form from light; potency is retained for up to 3 months when kept at room temperature; most stable at pH 4-8, hydrolysis occurs at pH <3; do not mix I.V. product with other medications

Mechanism of Action Benzodiazepines appear to potentiate the effects of GABA and other inhibitory neurotransmitters by binding to specific benzodiazepine-receptor sites in various areas of the CNS

Pharmacodynamics
Onset of action: Almost immediate with short duration of action (20-30 minutes) when given I.V. for status epilepticus.
Studies have shown that the elderly are more sensitive to the effects of benzodiazepines as compared to younger adults.

Pharmacokinetics
Absorption: Oral: 85% to 100%
Distribution: V_d: Increased in elderly
Protein binding: 98%
Metabolism: In liver; active major metabolite is desmethyldiazepam
Half-life: 20-50 hours, increased half-life in elderly (~90 hours) and those with severe hepatic disorders; desmethyldiazepam has a half-life of 50-100 hours and can be prolonged in the elderly; accumulation of diazepam is extensive

Usual Dosage
Geriatrics:
Anxiety: Oral: Initial: 1-2 mg 1-2 times/day; increase gradually as needed, rarely need to use >10 mg/day
Skeletal muscle relaxation: 2-5 mg 2-4 times/day

Adults:
Anxiety:
Oral: 2-10 mg 2-4 times/day
I.M., I.V.: 2-10 mg, may repeat in 3-4 hours if needed
Skeletal muscle relaxation:
Oral: 2-10 mg 2-4 times/day
I.M., I.V.: 5-10 mg, may repeat in 2-4 hours

(Continued)

Diazepam *(Continued)*

Status epilepticus: I.V.: 5-10 mg every 10-20 minutes up to 30 mg in an 8-hour period; may repeat in 2-4 hours

Reference Range Therapeutic: Diazepam: 0.2-1.5 μg/mL (SI: 0.7-5.3 μmol/L); N-desmethyldiazepam (nordiazepam): 0.1-0.5 μg/mL (SI: 0.35-1.8 μmol/L)

Test Interactions False-negative urinary glucose determinations when using Clinistix® or Diastix®

Patient Information Avoid alcohol and other CNS depressants; may cause drowsiness; avoid activities needing good psychomotor coordination until CNS effects are known; may cause physical or psychological dependence; avoid abrupt discontinuation after prolonged use

Nursing Implications Do not exceed 5 mg/minute IVP; provide safety measures (ie, side rails, night light, and call button); remove smoking materials from area; supervise ambulation

Additional Information Oral absorption more reliable than I.M.

Special Geriatric Considerations See Pharmacodynamics and Pharmacokinetics; due to its long-acting metabolite, diazepam is not considered a drug of choice in the elderly; long-acting benzodiazepines have been associated with falls in the elderly; interpretive guidelines from the Health Care Financing Administration (HCFA) discourage the use of this agent in residents of long-term care facilities

Dosage Forms

Capsule, sustained release: 15 mg
Injection: 5 mg/mL (1 mL, 2 mL, 5 mL, 10 mL)
Solution:
Oral: 5 mg/5 mL (5 mL, 10 mL, 500 mL)
Oral, concentrate: 5 mg/mL (30 mL)
Tablet: 2 mg, 5 mg, 10 mg

References

Klotz U, Avant GR, Hoyumpa A, et al, "The Effects of Age and Liver Disease on the Disposition and Elimination of Diazepam in Adult Man," *J Clin Invest*, 1975, 55(2):347-59.

Pomara N, Stanley B, Block R, et al, "Increased Sensitivity of the Elderly to the Central Depressant Effects of Diazepam," *J Clin Psychiatry*, 1985, 46(5):185-7.

Reidenberg MM, Levy M, Warner H, et al, "Relationship Between Diazepam Dose, Plasma Level, Age, and Central Nervous System Depression," *Clin Pharmacol Ther*, 1978, 23(4):371-4.

Dibent® *see* Dicyclomine Hydrochloride *on page 215*

Dibenzyline® *see* Phenoxybenzamine Hydrochloride *on page 556*

Dicarbosil® [OTC] *see* Calcium Salts (Oral) *on page 111*

Dichysterol *see* Dihydrotachysterol *on page 224*

Diclofenac Sodium *(dye kloe' fen ak)*

Brand Names Cataflam®; Voltaren®; Voltaren® Ophthalmic Solution

Generic Available No

Therapeutic Class Analgesic, Non-narcotic; Anti-inflammatory Agent; Anti-inflammatory Agent, Ophthalmic; Nonsteroidal Anti-Inflammatory Agent (NSAID), Ophthalmic; Nonsteroidal Anti-inflammatory Agent (NSAID), Oral

Use Acute and chronic treatment of rheumatoid arthritis, ankylosing spondylitis, and osteoarthritis; also used for gout, mild to moderate pain relief, acute painful shoulder, sunburn; ophthalmic used for treatment of postoperative inflammation following cataract removal

Contraindications Known hypersensitivity to diclofenac, any component, aspirin or other nonsteroidal anti-inflammatory drugs (NSAIDs); porphyria

Warnings Hypersensitivity to diclofenac or any component of product used; GI toxicity (bleeding, ulceration, perforation); systemic effects from ocular absorption may occur (ie, bleeding); CNS effects may occur (headaches, confusion, depression); hypersensitivity, anaphylactoid reactions (intermittent tolmetin use more often); cross-sensitivity with aspirin and other NSAIDs exists; renal function decline, acute renal insufficiency, interstitial nephritis, dysuria, cystitis, hematuria, nephrotic syndrome, hyperkalemia in acute renal insufficiency, hyponatremia, papillary necrosis, hepatic function impairment; elderly have increased risk for adverse reactions to NSAIDs. **Note:** Use caution with ophthalmic solutions if patient wears soft contact lenses; eye irritation, burning, and redness reported; see Special Geriatric Considerations

Precautions Use with caution in patients with congestive heart failure, hypertension, decreased renal or hepatic function, history of GI disease (bleeding or ulcers), or those receiving anticoagulants; perform ophthalmologic evaluation for those who develop eye complaints during therapy (blurred vision, diminished vision, changes in color vision, retinal changes); NSAIDs may mask signs/symptoms of infections; photosensitivity reported

Adverse Reactions

Cardiovascular: Congestive heart failure, angina, hypertension, hypotension, fluid retention, arrhythmias, edema

Central nervous system: Headache, drowsiness, vertigo, dizziness, fatigue, hallucinations, confusion, depression, emotional lability, psychotic behavior, asthenia, pyrexia

Dermatologic: Rash, urticaria, angioedema, Stevens-Johnson syndrome, exfoliative dermatitis, ecchymosis, petechiae, purpura, bruising

Endocrine & metabolic: Hyperglycemia, hypoglycemia, hyperkalemia, gynecomastia, hyponatremia

Gastrointestinal: Dyspepsia, heartburn, nausea, diarrhea, constipation, flatulence, stomatitis, vomiting, abdominal pain, peptic ulcer, GI bleeding, GI perforation, gingival ulcers, pancreatitis, proctitis, paralytic ulcers, colitis, anorexia, weight loss

Genitourinary: Azotemia, impotence

Hematologic: Neutropenia, anemia, agranulocytosis, bone marrow suppression, hemolytic anemia, hemorrhage, inhibition of platelet aggregation

Hepatic: Hepatitis, elevated LFTs, cholestatic jaundice

Neuromuscular & skeletal: Involuntary muscle movements, muscle weakness, tremors

Ocular: Vision changes, burning, redness, irritation, keratitis, elevated IOP, anterior chamber reaction, ocular allergy

Otic: Tinnitus

Renal: Dysuria, polyuria, pyuria, oliguria, anuria, acute renal failure

Respiratory: Exacerbation of asthma, dyspnea

Miscellaneous: Dry mucous membranes, thirst, sweating

Overdosage Acute renal failure (2.5 g); symptoms include drowsiness, lethargy, disorientation, confusion, dizziness, numbness, paresthesia, nausea, vomiting, gastric irritation, abdominal pain, headache, tinnitus, sweating, blurred vision, muscle twitching, seizures, coma, acute renal failure, increased BUN and serum creatinine, hypotension, tachycardia, and metabolic acidosis

Toxicology Management of a nonsteroidal anti-inflammatory agent (NSAID) intoxication is primarily supportive and symptomatic. Fluid therapy is commonly effective in managing the hypotension that may occur following an acute NSAID overdose, except when this is due to an acute blood loss. Seizures tend to be very short-lived and often do not require drug treatment although recurrent seizures should be treated with I.V. diazepam. Since many of the NSAIDs undergo enterohepatic cycling, multiple doses of charcoal may be needed to reduce the potential for delayed toxicities. NSAIDs are highly bound to plasma proteins, therefore hemodialysis and peritoneal dialysis are not useful.

Drug Interactions

May increase nephrotoxicity of cyclosporin

Diclofenac + K⁺ sparing diuretics → ↑ serum K⁺

Concomitant insulin or oral hypoglycemic agents → ↑ or ↓ serum glucose

May increase digoxin, methotrexate, and lithium serum concentrations

Aspirin or other salicylates may decrease NSAID serum concentrations

Other NSAIDs may increase adverse GI effects; increased prothrombin time with anticoagulants

Decreased antihypertensive effects of ACE inhibitors, beta-blockers, and thiazide diuretics

Increased response to sympathomimetics

Probenecid may increase toxicity of NSAIDs by increase in serum concentrations

Effects of loop diuretics may decrease

Concomitant use with loop diuretics may enhance azotemia in elderly

Mechanism of Action Inhibits prostaglandin synthesis, acts on the hypothalamus heat-regulating center to reduce fever, blocks prostaglandin synthetase action which prevents formation of the platelet-aggregating substance thromboxane A_2; decreases pain receptor sensitivity. Other proposed mechanisms of action are lysosomal stabilization, kinin and leukotriene production, alteration of chemotactic factors, and inhibition of neutrophil activation. This latter mechanism may be the most significant pharmacologic action to reduce inflammation.

Pharmacokinetics

Absorption: Completely

Protein binding: 99%

Metabolism: In the liver to inactive metabolites

Half-life: 1-2 hours

Time to peak: Peak serum levels occur within 2-3 hours

Elimination: Primarily in urine

Usual Dosage Geriatrics and Adults:

Oral (maximum daily dose: 200 mg):

Rheumatoid arthritis: 150-200 mg/day in 2-4 divided doses (do not exceed 200 mg/day)

Osteoarthritis: 100-150 mg/day in 2-3 divided doses

Ankylosing spondylitis: 100-125 mg/day in 4-5 divided doses

Mild to moderate pain: 25 mg 3-4 times/day

Ophthalmic: Instill 1 drop to affected eye 4 times/day starting 24 hours after cataract surgery and continue for 2 weeks of postoperative care

Monitoring Parameters Monitor response (pain, range of motion, grip strength, mobility, ADL function), inflammation; observe for weight gain, edema; monitor renal function; observe for bleeding, bruising; evaluate gastrointestinal effects (abdominal

(Continued)

Diclofenac Sodium *(Continued)*

pain, bleeding, dyspepsia); mental confusion, disorientation, CBC, serum, creatinine, BUN, liver function tests

Patient Information Do not crush delayed release (enteric coated) tablets. Serious gastrointestinal bleeding can occur as well as ulceration and perforation. Pain may or may not be present. Avoid aspirin and aspirin-containing products while taking this medication. If gastric upset occurs, take with food, milk, or antacid. If gastric adverse effects persist, contact physician. May cause drowsiness, dizziness, blurred vision, and confusion. Use caution when performing tasks which require alertness (eg, driving). Do not take for more than 3 days for fever or 10 days for pain without physician advice.

Nursing Implications Do not crush enteric coated tablets; see Monitoring Parameters, Overdosage, Patient Information, and Special Geriatric Considerations

Additional Information There are no clinical guidelines to predict which NSAID will give response in a particular patient. Trials with each must be initiated until response determined. Consider dose, patient convenience, and cost.

Special Geriatric Considerations Elderly are a high-risk population for adverse effects from nonsteroidal anti-inflammatory agents. As much as 60% of elderly can develop peptic ulceration and/or hemorrhage asymptomatically. The concomitant use of H_2 blockers, omeprazole, and sucralfate is not effective as prophylaxis. Misoprostol is the only prophylactic agent proven effective. Also, concomitant disease and drug use contribute to the risk for GI adverse effects. Use lowest effective dose for shortest period possible. Consider renal function decline with age. Use of NSAIDs can compromise existing renal function especially when Cl_{cr} is $\leq$30 mL/minute. Tinnitus may be a difficult and unreliable indication of toxicity due to age-related hearing loss or eighth cranial nerve damage. CNS adverse effects such as confusion, agitation, and hallucination are generally seen in overdose or high dose situations, but elderly may demonstrate these adverse effects at lower doses than younger adults.

Dosage Forms

Solution, ophthalmic: 0.1% (2.5 mL, 5 mL)

Tablet: 50 mg

Tablet, enteric coated (Voltaren®): 25 mg, 50 mg, 75 mg

References

Brooks PM, Day RO, "Nonsteroidal Anti-inflammatory Drugs – Differences and Similarities," *N Engl J Med*, 1991, 324(24):1716-25.

Clinch D, Banerjee AK, Ostick G, "Absence of Abdominal Pain in Elderly Patients With Peptic Ulcer," *Age Ageing*, 1984, 13:120-3.

Clive DM, Stoff JS, "Renal Syndromes Associated With Nonsteroidal Anti-inflammatory Drugs," *N Engl J Med*, 1984, 310(9):563-72.

Graham DY, "Prevention of Gastroduodenal Injury Induced by Chronic Nonsteroidal Anti-inflammatory Drug Therapy," *Gastroenterology*, 1989, 96(2 Pt 2 Suppl):675-81.

Gurwitz JH, Avarn J, Ross-Degan D, et al, "Nonsteroidal Anti-Inflammatory Drug-Associated Azotemia in the Very Old," *JAMA*, 1990, 264(4):471-5.

Knodel LC, "Preventing NSAID-Induced Ulcers: The Role of Misoprostol," *Consult Pharm*, 1989, 4:37-41.

Pounder R, "Silent Peptic Ulceration: Deadly Silence or Golden Silence?" *Gastroenterology*, 1989, 96(2 Pt 2 Suppl):626-31.

Dicloxacillin Sodium *(dye klox a sill' in)*

Brand Names Dycill®; Dynapen®; Pathocil®

Generic Available Yes

Therapeutic Class Antibiotic, Penicillin

Use Treatment of systemic infections such as pneumonia, skin and soft tissue infections and osteomyelitis caused by penicillinase-producing staphylococci

Contraindications Known hypersensitivity to dicloxacillin, penicillin, or any components

Precautions Use with caution in patients with cephalosporin allergy

Adverse Reactions

Central nervous system: Fever

Dermatologic: Rash

Gastrointestinal: Nausea, vomiting, diarrhea

Hematologic: Eosinophilia, neutropenia, leukopenia, thrombocytopenia

Hepatic: Elevation in liver enzymes

Miscellaneous: Serum sickness-like reaction

Overdosage Symptoms of overdose include neuromuscular hypersensitivity, convulsions

Toxicology Many beta-lactam-containing antibiotics have the potential to cause neuromuscular hyperirritability or convulsive seizures. Hemodialysis may be helpful to aid in the removal of the drug from the blood, otherwise most treatment is supportive or symptom directed.

Drug Interactions

Decreased effect of warfarin

Increased effect with probenecid

Food/Drug Interactions Food decreases rate and extent of absorption

Stability Refrigerate suspension after reconstitution; discard after 14 days if refrigerated or 7 days if kept at room temperature

Mechanism of Action Interferes with bacterial cell synthesis during active multiplication causing cell death and resultant bactericidal activity against susceptible bacteria

Pharmacokinetics
Absorption: 35% to 76% from GI tract
Half-life: 0.6-0.8 hours, half-life is slightly prolonged in patients with renal impairment
Protein binding: 96%
Time to peak: Peak serum levels occur within 0.5-2 hours
Elimination: Partially by the liver and excreted in bile, 56% to 70% is eliminated in urine as unchanged drug
The percent unbound has been reported to be increased in the elderly compared to young healthy volunteers (8.8% vs 7.3%), but this is not felt to be clinically significant

Usual Dosage Geriatrics and Adults: Oral: 125-500 mg every 6 hours
Not dialyzable (0% to 5%)

Administration Give 1 hour before or 2 hours after meals; give around-the-clock rather than 4 times/day, 3 times/day, etc (ie, 12-6-12-6, not 9-1-5-9) to promote less variation in peak and trough serum levels

Monitoring Parameters Signs and symptoms of infection; mental status; monitor PT or INR if patient concurrently on warfarin

Reference Range
Level guidelines: 10-25 μg/mL
Panic value: >100 μg/mL
Time to draw levels: 2 hours after dose

Test Interactions Increased protein

Patient Information Complete full course of therapy; report diarrhea or if symptoms not improving to physician or pharmacist

Nursing Implications See Administration

Additional Information
Sodium content of 250 mg capsule: 13 mg (0.6 mEq)
Sodium content of suspension 65 mg/5 mL: 27 mg (1.2 mEq)

Special Geriatric Considerations See Pharmacokinetics; no dosage adjustment for renal function is necessary

Dosage Forms
Capsule: 125 mg, 250 mg, 500 mg
Suspension, oral: 62.5 mg/5 mL (80 mL, 100 mL, 200 mL)

References
Pacifici GM, Viani A, Taddeucci-Brunelli G, et al, "Plasma Protein Binding of Dicloxacillin: Effects of Age and Diseases," *Int J Clin Pharmacol Ther Toxicol*, 1987, 25(11):622-6.

Dicyclomine Hydrochloride (dye sye' kloe meen)

Brand Names Antispas®; Bemote®; Bentyl® Hydrochloride; Byclomine®; Dibent®; Dilomine®; Di-Spaz®; Neoquess® Injection; Or-tyl®

Synonyms Dicycloverine Hydrochloride

Generic Available Yes

Therapeutic Class Antispasmodic Agent, Gastrointestinal

Use Treatment of functional disturbances of GI motility such as irritable bowel syndrome

Unlabeled use: Urinary incontinence

Contraindications Hypersensitivity to any anticholinergic drug; narrow-angle glaucoma, tachycardia, GI obstruction, obstruction of the urinary tract, myasthenia gravis

Precautions Use with caution in patients with hepatic or renal disease, ulcerative colitis, hyperthyroidism, cardiovascular disease, hypertension

Adverse Reactions
Cardiovascular: Tachycardia, palpitations
Central nervous system: Seizures, coma, nervousness, excitement, confusion, insomnia, headache **(the elderly may be at increased risk for confusion and hallucinations)**
Gastrointestinal: Nausea, vomiting, constipation, dry mouth
Genitourinary: Urinary retention
Neuromuscular & skeletal: Muscular hypotonia
Ocular: Blurred vision
Respiratory: Respiratory distress, asphyxia

Overdosage Symptoms of overdose include CNS stimulation followed by depression, confusion, delusions, nonreactive pupils, tachycardia, hypertension

Toxicology Anticholinergic toxicity is caused by strong binding of the drug to cholinergic receptors. Anticholinesterase inhibitors reduce acetylcholinesterase, the enzyme that breaks down acetylcholine and thereby allows acetylcholine to accumulate and compete for receptor binding with the offending anticholinergic. For anticholinergic overdose with severe life-threatening symptoms, physostigmine 1-2 mg S.C. or I.V., slowly may be given to reverse these effects.

(Continued)
215

Dicyclomine Hydrochloride *(Continued)*

Drug Interactions

Decreased effect of phenothiazines, anti-Parkinson's drugs, haloperidol, tacrine, sustained release dosage forms; decreased effect with antacids

Increased effect/toxicity with anticholinergics, amantadine, narcotic analgesics, type I antiarrhythmics, antihistamines, phenothiazines, tricyclic antidepressants

Mechanism of Action Blocks the action of acetylcholine at parasympathetic sites in smooth muscle, secretory glands and the CNS

Pharmacodynamics

Onset of action: 1-2 hours

Duration: Up to 4 hours

Pharmacokinetics

Absorption: Oral: Well absorbed

Metabolism: Extensive

Elimination: In urine with only a small amount excreted as unchanged drug

Usual Dosage

Geriatrics: 10-20 mg 4 times/day; increasing as necessary to 160 mg/day

Adults:

Oral: Begin with 80 mg/day in 4 equally divided doses, then increase up to 160 mg/day; if no effects after 2 weeks, discontinue the medication

I.M. (**should not be used I.V.**): 80 mg/day in 4 divided doses (20 mg/dose); do not use for longer than 1-2 days

Monitoring Parameters Pulse, anticholinergic effects, urinary output, GI symptoms

Patient Information Take 30-60 minutes before a meal; may cause drowsiness, dizziness, or blurred vision; may cause dry mouth, difficult urination, or constipation

Nursing Implications Do not administer I.V.

Special Geriatric Considerations Long-term use of antispasmodics should be avoided in the elderly. The potential for a toxic reaction is greater than the potential benefit. In addition, the anticholinergic effects of dicyclomine are not well tolerated in the elderly; see Adverse Reactions.

Dosage Forms

Capsule: 10 mg, 20 mg

Injection: 10 mg/mL (2 mL, 10 mL)

Syrup: 10 mg/5 mL (118 mL, 473 mL, 946 mL)

Tablet: 20 mg

References

Beers MH, Ouslander JG, Rollingher I, et al, "Explicit Criteria for Determining Inappropriate Medication Use in Nursing Home Residents," *Arch Intern Med*, 1991, 151(9):1825-32.

Dicycloverine Hydrochloride *see* Dicyclomine Hydrochloride
on previous page

Didanosine *(dye dan' oh seen)*

Brand Names Videx®

Synonyms DDI

Generic Available No

Therapeutic Class Antiviral Agent, Oral

Use Treatment of advanced HIV infection in patients who are intolerant of zidovudine therapy or who have demonstrated significant clinical or immunologic deterioration during zidovudine therapy

Contraindications Hypersensitivity to any component

Warnings Didanosine is indicated for treatment of HIV infection only in patients intolerant of zidovudine or who have failed zidovudine. Patients receiving didanosine may still develop opportunistic infections. Peripheral neuropathy occurs in ~35% of patients receiving the drug; pancreatitis, which in some cases can be fatal, occurs in ~17% of patients receiving didanosine; patients should undergo retinal examination every 6 months to 1 year. Use with caution in patients with decreased renal or hepatic function; in high concentrations, didanosine is mutagenic; use with caution in patients with edema or congestive heart failure; use with caution in patients with hyperuricemia.

Adverse Reactions

Central nervous system: Anxiety, headache (32% to 36%), irritability, insomnia, restlessness, seizures

Gastrointestinal: Abdominal pain, nausea, diarrhea (18%), pancreatitis (9%)

Hematologic: Anemia, granulocytopenia, leukopenia, thrombocytopenia

Hepatic: Elevated liver enzymes, hepatic failure

Neuromuscular & skeletal: Peripheral neuropathy

Ocular: Retinal depigmentation

Miscellaneous: Hypersensitivity

Overdosage Chronic overdose may cause pancreatitis, peripheral neuropathy, diarrhea, hyperuricemia, and hepatic impairment

Toxicology There is no known antidote for didanosine overdose

Drug Interactions
Decreased absorption of tetracyclines and quinolones if given together; administer drugs whose absorption is pH dependent at least 2 hours prior to dosing
H_2 antagonists and antacids may increase absorption

Food/Drug Interactions Food decreases extent of absorption and peak concentration by 50%

Mechanism of Action Didanosine, a purine nucleoside analogue and the deamination product of dideoxyadenosine (ddA), inhibits HIV replication *in vitro* in both T cells and monocytes. Didanosine is converted within the cell to the monophosphates, diphosphates, and triphosphates of ddA. These ddA-triphosphates act as substrate and inhibitor of HIV reverse transcriptase substrate and inhibitor of HIV reverse transcriptase thereby blocking viral DNA synthesis and suppressing HIV replication.

Pharmacokinetics
Absorption: 20% to 25% more bioavailable from the tablet than the powder form; absolute: 30% to 33%
Distribution: V_d: 22-103 L; CSF levels equal 21% of serum levels
Half-life:
Serum: 0.8 hours
Intracellular: Much longer

Usual Dosage Geriatrics and Adults: Oral (administer on an empty stomach), dosing is based on patient weight:
35-49 kg: 125 mg tablets twice daily or 167 mg buffered powder twice daily
50-74 kg: 200 mg tablets twice daily or 250 mg buffered powder twice daily
≥75 kg: 300 mg tablets twice daily or 375 mg buffered powder twice daily

Note: Adults should receive 2 tablets per dose for adequate buffering and absorption; tablets should be chewed

Dosing adjustment in renal impairment: Should be considered in patients with Cl_{cr} <60 mL/minute

Dosing adjustment in hepatic impairment: Should be considered

Administration Give on an empty stomach; administer liquified powder immediately after dissolving

Monitoring Parameters Serum potassium, uric acid, creatinine, hemoglobin, CBC with neutrophil and platelet count, CD_4 cells, liver function tests, amylase, weight gain; perform dilated retinal exam every 6 months

Patient Information Thoroughly chew tablets or manually crush or disperse 2 tablets in 1 oz of water prior to taking; for powder, open packet and pour contents into 4 oz of liquid; do not mix with fruit juice or other acid-containing liquid; stir until dissolved, drink immediately; do not take with meals

Nursing Implications Avoid creating dust if powder spilled, use wet mop or damp sponge; see Administration

Additional Information Sodium content of buffered tablets: 264.5 mg (11.5 mEq)

Special Geriatric Considerations Since the elderly often have a creatinine clearance <60 mL/minute, monitor closely for adverse reactions; see Adverse Reactions and Monitoring Parameters; adjust dose accordingly to maintain efficacy (CD_4 counts)

Dosage Forms
Powder for oral solution: Buffered (single dose packet): 100 mg, 167 mg, 250 mg, 375 mg
Tablet, buffered, chewable (mint flavor): 25 mg, 50 mg, 100 mg, 150 mg

Didronel® *see* Etidronate Disodium *on page 276*

Diethylstilbestrol (dye eth il stil bess' trole)

Brand Names Diethylstilbestrol Enseals®; Stilphostrol®

Synonyms DES; Stilbestrol

Generic Available Yes

Therapeutic Class Estrogen Derivative

Use Management of severe vasomotor symptoms of menopause, for estrogen replacement, and for palliative treatment of inoperable metastatic prostatic carcinoma

Contraindications Undiagnosed vaginal bleeding, during pregnancy; breast cancer except in select patients with metastatic disease

Warnings Estrogens have been reported to increase the risk of endometrial carcinoma; this risk can be reduced by cycling with a progestin (ie, medroxyprogesterone) for the last 10-13 days of each month

Precautions Use with caution in patients with a history of breast cancer, thromboembolism, stroke, myocardial infarction (especially >40 years of age who smoke), liver tumor, hypertension, cardiac, renal or hepatic insufficiency

Adverse Reactions
Cardiovascular: Hypertension, thromboembolism, stroke, myocardial infarction, edema

(Continued)

217

Diethylstilbestrol *(Continued)*

Central nervous system: Migraine, dizziness, anxiety, depression, headache

Dermatologic: Chloasma, melasma, rash

Endocrine & metabolic: Decreased glucose tolerance, alterations in frequency and flow of menses, breast tenderness or enlargement, breast tumors

Gastrointestinal: Nausea, GI distress, anorexia, vomiting, diarrhea

Genitourinary: Increased libido (female), decreased libido (male)

Hepatic: Increased triglycerides and LDL, cholestatic jaundice

Miscellaneous: Increased susceptibility to *Candida* infection, intolerance to contact lenses

Overdosage Symptoms of overdose include nausea

Drug Interactions

Estrogens may reduce the effects of anticoagulants, alter the effects of antidepressants; estrogen effects may be reduced by barbiturates, rifampin, and other agents that induce hepatic microsomal enzymes

Corticosteroids may decrease the clearance and increase the half-life of estrogens

Mechanism of Action Competes with estrogenic and androgenic compounds for binding onto tumor cells and thereby inhibits their effects on tumor growth

Pharmacokinetics

Metabolism: In the liver

Elimination: In urine and feces

Usual Dosage Geriatrics and Adults:

Menopausal symptoms: Oral: 0.1-2 mg/day for 3 weeks and then off 1 week

Postmenopausal breast carcinoma: Oral: 15 mg/day

Prostate carcinoma: Oral: 1-3 mg/day

Prostatic cancer: I.V.: 0.5 g to start, then 1 g every 2-5 days followed by 0.25-0.5 g 1-2 times/week as maintenance

Diphosphate:

Oral: 50 mg 3 times/day; increase up to 200 mg or more 3 times/day

I.V.: Give 0.5 g, dissolved in 250 mL of saline or D_5W, administer slowly the first 10-15 minutes then adjust rate so that the entire amount is given in 1 hour

Monitoring Parameters Mammography should be performed in all women prior to starting estrogen therapy and then annually; blood pressure, PAP smear annually

Test Interactions

Increased prothrombin and factors VII, VIII, IX, X

Decreased antithrombin III

Increased platelet aggregability

Increased thyroid binding globulin

Increased total thyroid hormone (T_4)

Decreased serum folate concentration

Increased serum triglycerides/phospholipids

Patient Information Patients should inform their physicians if signs or symptoms of any of the following occur: thromboembolic or thrombotic disorders including sudden severe headache or vomiting, disturbance of vision or speech, loss of vision, numbness or weakness in an extremity, sharp or crushing chest pain, calf pain, shortness of breath, severe abdominal pain or mass, mental depression or unusual bleeding. Women should perform regular self-exams on breasts.

Nursing Implications Give 0.5 g I.V., dissolved in 250 mL of saline or D_5W, administer slowly the first 10-15 minutes then adjust rate so that the entire amount is given in 1 hour

Special Geriatric Considerations The benefits of postmenopausal estrogen therapy may be substantial for some women. Diethylstilbestrol is not the drug of choice for vasomotor symptoms, to prevent bone loss, or to treat vaginal atrophy or urinary incontinence secondary to estrogen deficiency. Diethylstilbestrol does have a role in the treatment of inoperable, progressive prostatic carcinoma and inoperable, progressive breast cancer in select men and women.

Dosage Forms

Injection: 50 mg/mL (5 mL)

Injection, as diphosphate sodium (Stilphostrol®): 0.25 g (5 mL)

Tablet: 0.25 mg, 0.5 mg, 1 mg, 5 mg

Tablet, enteric coated: 0.1 mg, 0.25 mg, 0.5 mg, 1 mg, 5 mg

Tablet (Stilphostrol®): 50 mg

Diethylstilbestrol Enseals® *see Diethylstilbestrol on previous page*

Diflucan® *see Fluconazole on page 295*

Diflunisal *(dye floo' ni sal)*

Related Information

Antacid Drug Interactions *on page 764*

Brand Names Dolobid®

Generic Available No

Therapeutic Class Analgesic, Non-narcotic; Anti-inflammatory Agent; Nonsteroidal Anti-inflammatory Agent (NSAID), Oral

Use Management of inflammatory disorders usually including rheumatoid arthritis and osteoarthritis; can be used as an analgesic for treatment of mild to moderate pain

Contraindications Hypersensitivity to diflunisal or any component, may be a cross-sensitivity with other nonsteroidal anti-inflammatory agents including aspirin; should not be used in patients with active GI bleeding; factor VII or IX deficiencies; may cause reaction in patients with tartrazine dye sensitivity

Warnings Tinnitus or impaired hearing may indicate toxicity; discontinue use 1 week prior to surgical procedures

Precautions Ophthalmologic effects; impaired renal function, use lower dosage; peripheral edema; elevation in liver tests; use with caution in patients with platelet and bleeding disorders, renal dysfunction, hepatic disease, history of salicylate-induced gastric irritation, peptic ulcer disease, erosive gastritis, bleeding disorders, hypoprothrombinemia, and vitamin K deficiency; use cautiously in asthmatics, especially those with aspirin intolerance and nasal polyps

Adverse Reactions
Cardiovascular: Palpitations, chest pain, syncope
Central nervous system: Headache, dizziness, somnolence, nervousness, hallucinations, confusion, depression, insomnia, vertigo, fatigue, asthenia
Dermatologic: Rash, pruritus, dry mucous membranes, TEN, Stevens-Johnson syndrome, photosensitivity
Gastrointestinal: Nausea, dyspepsia, GI pain, diarrhea, vomiting, constipation, flatulence, urticaria, GI bleeding/perforation
Hematologic: Agranulocytosis (rare)
Neuromuscular & skeletal: Muscle cramps
Ocular: Blurred vision
Otic: Tinnitus
Renal: Dysuria, interstitial nephritis, proteinuria, hematuria
Respiratory: Dyspnea
Miscellaneous: Sweating

Overdosage 10-30 g; symptoms of overdose include tinnitus, headache, dizziness, confusion, metabolic acidosis, hyperpyrexia, hyperpnea, tachypnea, nausea, vomiting, irritability, disorientation, hallucinations, lethargy, stupor, dehydration, hyperventilation, hyperthermia, hyperactivity, depression leading to coma, respiratory failure, and collapse; laboratory abnormalities include hypokalemia, hypoglycemia or hyperglycemia with alterations in pH

Toxicology Lowest fatal dose: 15 g. The "Done" nomogram is very helpful for estimating the severity of aspirin poisoning and directing treatment using serum salicylate levels. Treatment can also be based upon symptomatology. See table.

Aspirin or Other Salicylate Toxicity

Toxic Symptoms	Treatment
Overdose	Induce emesis with ipecac, and/or lavage with saline, followed with activated charcoal
Dehydration	I.V. fluids with KCl (no D_5W only)
Metabolic acidosis (must be treated)	Sodium bicarbonate
Hyperthermia	Cooling blankets or sponge baths
Coagulopathy/hemorrhage	Vitamin K I.V.
Hypoglycemia (with coma, seizures or change in mental status)	Dextrose 25 g I.V.
Seizures	Diazepam 5–10 mg I.V.

Drug Interactions
Diflunisal – digoxin → increased digoxin plasma concentration
Diflunisal – methotrexate → increased methotrexate plasma concentrations
Diflunisal – anticoagulants → increased prothrombin time
Hydantoins, sulfonamides, and sulfonylureas may be displayed → increase activity
Lithium – diflunisal → increase lithium level
Diflunisal – anticoagulants and thrombolytics increased bleeding without increased PT or PTT but with increased bleeding time
Increased acetaminophen levels, hydrochlorothiazide levels, indomethacin levels
Decreased hyperuricemic effects of hydrochlorothiazide
Decreased levels of sulindac
Aspirin or other salicylates may decrease serum concentrations of NSAIDs
Effects of loop diuretics may be decreased; may increase azotemia when used with loop diuretics

(Continued)

Diflunisal *(Continued)*

Mechanism of Action Unknown; proposed that is inhibits prostaglandin synthesis by decreasing the activity of the enzyme, cyclo-oxygenase, which results in decreased formation of prostaglandin precursors; see Additional Information

Pharmacodynamics
Onset of analgesia: Within 60 minutes
Duration of action: 8-12 hours

Pharmacokinetics
Absorption: Well absorbed from GI tract
Plasma protein binding: >90% bound
Metabolism: Extensive in the liver
Half-life: 8-12 hours, prolonged with renal impairment
Time to peak: Oral: Peak serum levels occur within 2-3 hours
Elimination: In urine within 72-96 hours, ~3% as unchanged drug and 90% as glucuronide conjugates

Usual Dosage Geriatrics and Adults: Oral (see Additional Information):
Pain: Initial: 500-1000 mg followed by 250-500 mg every 8-12 hours

Osteoarthritis: 500-750 mg/day in divided doses

Inflammatory condition: 500-1000 mg/day in 2 divided doses; do not exceed doses of 1.5 g/day

Monitoring Parameters Fecal blood loss, renal function; hearing changes or tinnitus; monitor for response (ie, pain, inflammation, range of motion, grip strength); observe for abnormal bleeding, bruising, weight gain

Test Interactions Increased chloride (S), glucose, ketone (U), uric acid (S), sodium (S); decreased uric acid (S), catecholamines (U), glucose, potassium (S), prothrombin time (S), uric acid (S)

Patient Information May cause GI upset, take with water, milk, or meals; do not take aspirin with diflunisal, swallow tablets whole, do not crush or chew

Nursing Implications See Monitoring Parameters, Patient Information, Additional Information, and Special Geriatric Considerations

Additional Information Diflunisal is a salicylic acid derivative which is chemically different than aspirin and is not metabolized to salicylic acid. Diflunisal 500 mg is equal in analgesic efficacy to aspirin 650 mg, acetaminophen 650 mg, and acetaminophen 650 mg/propoxyphene napsylate 100 mg, but has a longer duration of effect (8-12 hours). Not recommended as an antipyretic. Not found to be clinically useful to treat fever; at doses of ≥2 g/day, platelets are reversibly inhibited in function. Diflunisal is uricosuric at 500-750 mg/day; causes less GI and renal toxicity than aspirin and other NSAIDs; fecal blood loss is $\frac{1}{2}$ that of aspirin at 2.6 g/day

Special Geriatric Considerations Elderly are a high-risk population for adverse effects from nonsteroidal anti-inflammatory agents. As much as 60% of elderly can develop peptic ulceration and/or hemorrhage asymptomatically. The concomitant use of H_2 blockers, omeprazole, and sucralfate is not effective as prophylaxis. Misoprostol is the only prophylactic agent proven effective. Also, concomitant disease and drug use contribute to the risk for GI adverse effects. Use lowest effective dose for shortest period possible. Consider renal function decline with age. Use of NSAIDs can compromise existing renal function especially when Cl_{cr} is ≤30 mL/minute. Tinnitus may be a difficult and unreliable indication of toxicity due to age-related hearing loss or eighth cranial nerve damage. CNS adverse effects such as confusion, agitation, and hallucination are generally seen in overdose or high dose situations, but elderly may demonstrate these adverse effects at lower doses than younger adults.

Dosage Forms Tablet: 250 mg, 500 mg

References
Gurwitz JH, Avarn J, Ross-Degan D, et al, "Nonsteroidal Anti-Inflammatory Drug-Associated Azotemia in the Very Old," *JAMA*, 1990, 264(4):471-5.

Di-Gel® [OTC] *see* Aluminum Hydroxide, Magnesium Hydroxide and Simethicone *on page 31*

Digitoxin (di ji tox' in)

Brand Names Crystodigin®

Generic Available Yes

Therapeutic Class Antiarrhythmic Agent, Miscellaneous; Cardiac Glycoside

Use Treatment of congestive heart failure; slows the ventricular rate in tachyarrhythmias; atrial fibrillation; atrial flutter; paroxysmal atrial tachycardia; and cardiogenic shock

Contraindications Hypersensitivity to digitoxin or any component (rare); digitalis toxicity, beriberi heart disease, A-V block, idiopathic hypertrophic subaortic stenosis, constrictive pericarditis, ventricular fibrillation, or tachycardia

Warnings Use with caution in patients with hypoxia, hypothyroidism, acute myocarditis, suspected digitalis toxicity must be ruled out; do not use to treat obesity; patients with incomplete A-V block (Stokes-Adams attack) may progress to complete block with digitalis drug administration; use with caution in patients with acute myocardial infarction, severe pulmonary disease, advanced heart failure, idiopathic hypertrophic subaortic stenosis, Wolff-Parkinson-White syndrome, sick sinus syndrome (bradyarrhythmias), amyloid heart disease, and constrictive cardiomyopathies; adjust dose with renal impairment and aged patients; elderly may develop exaggerated serum/tissue concentrations due to decreased lean body mass, total body water, and age-related reduction in renal function; hepatic disease or failure requires dose reduction

Precautions When changing from oral (tablets or liquid) or I.M. to I.V. therapy, dosage should be reduced by 20% to 25%; use with caution in patients with hypoxia, myxedema, hypokalemia, hypomagnesemia, hypercalcemia, hypothyroidism, acute myocarditis

Adverse Reactions
Cardiovascular: Sinus bradycardia, A-V block, S-A block, atrial or nodal ectopic beats, ventricular arrhythmias, bigeminy, trigeminy, atrial tachycardia with A-V block
Central nervous system: Drowsiness, fatigue, headache, lethargy, vertigo, disorientation, restlessness, delirium, hallucinations, psychosis, apathy, depression, confusion, seizures, neuralgia
Endocrine & metabolic: Hyperkalemia with acute toxicity
Gastrointestinal: Vomiting, nausea, anorexia, abdominal pain, diarrhea
Neuromuscular & skeletal: Weakness
Ocular: Blurred vision, halos, yellow or green vision, diplopia, photophobia, flashing lights

Overdosage Symptoms of overdose include anorexia, nausea, vomiting, diarrhea, abdominal discomfort, headache, weakness, drowsiness, visual disturbances, mental depression, confusion, restlessness, disorientation, seizures, hallucinations; cardiac abnormalities include ventricular tachycardia, unifocal or multifocal PVCs (bigeminal, trigeminal); paroxysmal nodal rhythms, A-V dissociation; excessive slowing of the pulse, A-V block of varying degree; P-R prolongation, S-T depression; occasional atrial fibrillation; ventricular fibrillation is common cause of death (alterations in cardiac rate an rhythm can result in any type or known arrhythmia)

Toxicology Antidote: Life-threatening digitoxin toxicity is treated with Digibind®; discontinue digitalis preparation; administer potassium 40-80 mEq in divided doses in D_5W at 20 mEq/hour I.V.; do not give potassium with complete heart block secondary to digitalis product or in cases of renal failure; digitalis-induced arrhythmias not responsive to potassium may be treated with phenytoin (0.5 mg/kg I.V. at 50 mg/minute), lidocaine (1 mg/kg over 5 minutes); cholestyramine, colestipol, activated charcoal may decrease absorption; other agents to consider, based on EKG and clinical assessment are atropine, quinidine, procainamide, and propranolol. Note: Other antiarrhythmics appear more dangerous to use in toxicity.

Drug Interactions
Aminosalicylic acid, antacids, cholestyramine; colestipol, kaolin and pectin, metoclopramide, sulfasalazine, and some combinations of antineoplastic agents decrease gastrointestinal absorption
Aminoglutethimide, rifampin, phenylbutazone, barbiturates, and hydantoins increase metabolism of digitoxin
Nondepolarizing muscle relaxants, succinylcholine have increased toxic effect
Potassium-sparing diuretics increase toxic effects
Diuretics enhance toxicity due to potassium decrease
Thyroid replacement may decrease effect of digitoxin

Mechanism of Action Digitalis binds to and inhibits magnesium and adenosine triphosphate dependent sodium and potassium ATPase thereby increasing the influx of calcium ions, from extracellular to intracellular cytoplasm due to the inhibition of sodium and potassium ion movement across the myocardial membranes; this increase in calcium ions results in a potentiation of the activity of the contractile heart muscle fibers and an increase in the force of myocardial contraction (positive inotropic effect); digitalis may also increase intracellular entry or calcium via slow calcium channel influx; stimulates release and blocks re-uptake of norepinephrine; decreases conduction through the S-A and A-V nodes

Pharmacodynamics Onset: 1-4 hours

Pharmacokinetics
Absorption: 90% to 100%
Protein binding: 90% to 97%
Half-life: 7-8 days
Time to peak serum concentration: 8-12 hours
Elimination:
Hepatic: 50% to 70%
Renal: Metabolites (digoxin)

Usual Dosage Geriatrics and Adults: Oral:
Rapid loading dose: Initial: 0.6 mg followed by 0.4 mg and then 0.2 mg at intervals of 4-6 hours

Slow loading dose: 0.2 mg twice daily for a period of 4 days followed by a maintenance dose

Maintenance: 0.05-0.3 mg/day
Most common dose: 0.15 mg/day

Not dialyzable (0% to 5%)

(Continued)

221

ALPHABETICAL LISTING OF DRUGS

Digitoxin *(Continued)*

Monitoring Parameters Monitor apical pulse, peripheral pulse, serum concentrations, EKG in critical cases of toxicity or arrhythmias

Reference Range Therapeutic: 20-35 ng/mL; Toxic: >45 ng/mL

Test Interactions Will give confusing and misleading results if a digoxin level is measured; **must** measure digitoxin level

Patient Information Do not discontinue medication without physician's advice; instruct patients to notify physician if they suffer loss of appetite, visual changes, nausea, vomiting, weakness, drowsiness, headache, confusion, or depression

Nursing Implications Check apical pulse before giving; monitor blood pressure and EKG closely

Special Geriatric Considerations Digitalis preparations (primarily digoxin) are frequently used to treat common cardiac diseases in elderly (congestive heart failure, atrial fibrillation). Elderly are at risk for toxicity due to age-related changes; volume of distribution is diminished significantly; half-life is increased as a result of decreased total body clearance. Additionally, elderly frequently have concomitant diseases which affect the pharmacokinetics in digitalis glycosides; hypo- and hyperthyroidism and renal function decline will affect clearance of digoxin. Must be observant for noncardiac signs of toxicity in elderly such as anorexia, vision changes (blurred), confusion, and depression.

Dosage Forms
Injection: 0.2 mg/mL
Tablet: 0.05 mg, 0.1 mg, 0.15 mg, 0.2 mg

References
Nolan PE and Mooradian AD, "Digoxin," Bressler R and Katz MD eds, *Geriatric Pharmacology*, New York, NY: McGraw-Hill, 1993, 7:151-63.

Digoxin *(di jox' in)*

Related Information
Antacid Drug Interactions *on page 764*
Drug Levels Commonly Monitored Guidelines *on page 771-772*

Brand Names Lanoxicaps®; Lanoxin®

Generic Available Yes: Tablet

Therapeutic Class Antiarrhythmic Agent, Miscellaneous; Cardiac Glycoside

Use Treatment of congestive heart failure; slows the ventricular rate in tachyarrhythmias such as atrial fibrillation, atrial flutter, supraventricular tachycardia (paroxysmal atrial tachycardia), cardiogenic shock

Contraindications Hypersensitivity to digoxin or any component (rare); digitalis toxicity, beriberi, heart disease, A-V block, idiopathic hypertrophic subaortic stenosis, constrictive pericarditis, ventricular fibrillation, or tachycardia

Warnings Use with caution in patients with hypoxia, hypothyroidism, acute myocarditis, suspected digitalis toxicity must be ruled out; do not use to treat obesity; patients with incomplete A-V block (Stokes-Adams attack) may progress to complete block with digitalis drug administration; use with caution in patients with acute myocardial infarction, severe pulmonary disease, advanced heart failure, idiopathic hypertrophic subaortic stenosis, Wolff-Parkinson-White syndrome, sick sinus syndrome (bradyarrhythmias), amyloid heart disease, and constrictive cardiomyopathies; adjust dose with renal impairment and aged patients; elderly may develop exaggerated serum/tissue concentrations due to decreased lean body mass, total body water, and age-related reduction in renal function

Precautions When changing from oral (tablets or liquid) or I.M. to I.V. therapy, dosage should be reduced by 20% to 25%

Adverse Reactions
Cardiovascular: Sinus bradycardia, A-V block, S-A block, atrial or nodal ectopic beats, ventricular arrhythmias, bigeminy, trigeminy, atrial tachycardia with A-V block
Central nervous system: Drowsiness, fatigue, headache, lethargy, vertigo, disorientation, restlessness, delirium, hallucinations, psychosis, apathy, depression, confusion, seizures, neuralgia
Endocrine & metabolic: Hyperkalemia with acute toxicity
Gastrointestinal: Vomiting, nausea, anorexia, abdominal pain, diarrhea
Neuromuscular & skeletal: Weakness
Ocular: Blurred vision, halos, yellow or green vision, diplopia, photophobia, flashing lights

Overdosage Symptoms of overdose include anorexia, nausea, vomiting, diarrhea, abdominal discomfort, headache, weakness, drowsiness, visual disturbances, mental depression, confusion, restlessness, disorientation, seizures, hallucinations; cardiac abnormalities include ventricular tachycardia, unifocal or multifocal PVCs (bigeminal, trigeminal); paroxysmal nodal rhythms, A-V dissociation; excessive slowing of the pulse, A-V block of varying degree; P-R prolongation, S-T depression; occasional arterial fibrillation; ventricular fibrillation is common cause of death (alterations in cardiac rate an rhythm can result in any type or known arrhythmia)

Toxicology Antidote: Life-threatening digoxin toxicity is treated with Digibind®; discontinue digitalis preparation; administer potassium 40-80 mEq in divided doses in D_5W

at 20 mEq/hour I.V.; do not give potassium with complete heart block secondary to digitalis product or in cases of renal failure; digitalis-induced arrhythmias not responsive to potassium may be treated with phenytoin (0.5 mg/kg I.V. at 50 mg/minute), lidocaine (1 mg/kg over 5 minutes); cholestyramine, colestipol, activated charcoal may decrease absorption; other agents to consider, based on EKG and clinical assessment are atropine, quinidine, procainamide, and propranolol. Note: Other antiarrhythmics appear more dangerous to use in toxicity.

Drug Interactions

Antacids, psyllium, kaolin-pectin, aminosalicylic acid, colestipol, sulfasalazine, antineoplastics, cholestyramine, and metoclopramide may decrease absorption of digoxin

Quinidine, indomethacin, verapamil (20% to 30% decrease in clearance of digoxin), nifedipine, diltiazem, esmolol, flecainide, hydroxychloroquine, ibuprofen, quinine, tolbutamide, amiodarone, erythromycin, tetracycline, and spironolactone (25% decrease in digoxin clearance) may increase digoxin serum concentration; penicillamine may decrease digoxin's pharmacologic effects

Captopril, diltiazem decreased renal clearance

Anticholinergics increased absorption

Disopyramide, nondepolarizing muscle relaxants, succinylcholine, potassium-sparing diuretics

Amiloride may decrease inotropic effects

Triamterene may increase pharmacologic effects

Diuretics decrease potassium

Thyroid replacement and penicillamine may decrease therapeutic effects

Stability Protect elixir and injection from light; solution compatibility: D_5W, $D_{10}W$, NS, sterile water for injection (when diluted fourfold or greater)

Mechanism of Action Digitalis binds to and inhibits magnesium and adenosine triphosphate dependent sodium and potassium ATPase thereby increasing the influx of calcium ions, from extracellular to intracellular cytoplasm due to the inhibition of sodium and potassium ion movement across the myocardial membranes; this increase in calcium ions results in a potentiation of the activity of the contractile heart muscle fibers and an increase in the force of myocardial contraction (positive inotropic effect); digitalis may also increase intracellular entry or calcium via slow calcium channel influx; stimulates release and blocks re-uptake of norepinephrine; decreases conduction through the S-A and A-V nodes

Pharmacodynamics

Onset of effects:
I.V.: 5-30 minutes
Oral: 1-2 hours
Peak effect:
I.V.: 1-4 hours
Oral: 2-8 hours
Duration: 3-4 days

Pharmacokinetics

Distribution: V_d: Geriatrics: 194 L (range: 129-314 L)
Protein binding: 25%
Bioavailability: Dependent upon formulation:
Elixir: 70% to 85%
Tablets: 60% to 80% (76% in elderly)
Capsules: 90% to 100%
Half-life:
Geriatrics: 69 hours (average)
Adults: 38-48 hours
Anephric Adults: >4.5 days
Time to peak serum concentration:
Oral: 2-6 hours
I.V.: 1-5 hours
Elimination: Renal

Usual Dosage Geriatrics and Adults (based on lean body weight and normal renal function for age. Decrease dose in patients with decreased renal function)

Total digitalizing dose: Give $\frac{1}{2}$ as initial dose, then give $\frac{1}{4}$ of the total digitalizing dose (TDD) in each of 2 subsequent doses at 8- to 12-hour intervals. Obtain EKG 6 hours after each dose to assess potential toxicity.
Oral: 0.75-1.5 mg
I.M., I.V.: 0.5-1 mg

Daily maintenance dose:
Oral: 0.125-0.5 mg
I.M., I.V.: 0.1-0.4 mg

Monitoring Parameters Monitor apical pulse, peripheral pulse, serum concentrations, EKG in critical cases of toxicity or arrhythmias

Reference Range Therapeutic: 1-2 ng/mL (SI: 1.3-2.6 nmol/L); <0.5 ng/mL (SI: <0.6 nmol/L) probably indicates underdigitalization unless there are special circumstances; Toxic: >2 ng/mL (SI: >2.6 nmol/L)

(Continued)

Digoxin (Continued)

Test Interactions Endogenous digoxin-like immunoreactive substances (DLISs) and metabolites of digoxin may accumulate to cross-react with the antibodies used in immunoassays. This occurs in renal impairment, uremic states, and hepatic disease; need to communicate with laboratory to use another more specific assay (ie, monoclonal antibody assay as a radioimmunoassay with a double antibody system to eliminate cross-reactivity problems).

Patient Information Do not discontinue medication without physician's advice; instruct patients to notify physician if they suffer loss of appetite, visual changes, nausea, vomiting, weakness, drowsiness, headache, confusion, or depression

Nursing Implications Check apical pulse before giving; monitor blood pressure and EKG closely

Special Geriatric Considerations Digitalis preparations (primarily digoxin) are frequently used to treat common cardiac diseases in elderly (congestive heart failure, atrial fibrillation). Elderly are at risk for toxicity due to age-related changes; volume of distribution is diminished significantly; half-life is increased as a result of decreased total body clearance. Additionally, elderly frequently have concomitant diseases which affect the pharmacokinetics in digitalis glycosides; hypo- and hyperthyroidism and renal function decline will affect clearance of digoxin. Exercise in elderly will reduce serum concentrations of digoxin due to increased skeletal muscle uptake. Therefore, a knowledge of the physical activity of the elderly helps interpret serum assays. Must be observant for noncardiac signs of toxicity in elderly such as anorexia, vision changes (blurred), confusion, and depression. Changes in dose may be necessary with declining renal function with age; monitor closely.

Dosage Forms
Capsule: 0.05 mg, 0.1 mg, 0.2 mg
Injection: 0.25 mg/mL (1 mL, 2 mL)
Tablet: 0.125 mg, 0.25 mg, 0.5 mg

References
Nolan PE and Mooradian AD, "Digoxin," Bressler R and Katz MD eds, *Geriatric Pharmacology*, New York, NY: McGraw-Hill, 1993, 7:151-63.

Dihydrohydroxycodeinone *see* Oxycodone Hydrochloride *on page 529*

Dihydromorphinone *see* Hydromorphone Hydrochloride *on page 352*

Dihydrotachysterol (dye hye droe tak iss' ter ole)
Brand Names DHT™; Hytakerol®
Synonyms Dichysterol
Generic Available Yes
Therapeutic Class Vitamin D Analog
Use Treatment of hypocalcemia associated with hypoparathyroidism; prophylaxis of hypocalcemic tetany following thyroid surgery
Contraindications Hypercalcemia, known hypersensitivity to dihydrotachysterol, vitamin D toxicity, malabsorption syndrome, decreased renal function
Warnings Must give concomitant calcium supplementation; maintain adequate fluid intake; calcium-phosphate product (serum calcium and phosphorus) must not exceed 70; avoid hypercalcemia; renal function impairment with secondary hyperparathyroidism
Precautions Use with caution in coronary artery disease, decreased renal function, renal stones, and elderly
Adverse Reactions
Cardiovascular: Cardiac arrhythmias
Central nervous system: Somnolence
Endocrine & metabolic: Hypercalcemia
Gastrointestinal: Nausea, vomiting, anorexia, weight loss, convulsions, constipation, metallic taste, dry mouth
Hematologic: Anemia
Hepatic: Elevated AST/ALT
Neuromuscular & skeletal: Metastatic calcification, muscle pain, bone pain, weakness
Ocular: Photophobia
Renal: Renal damage, polyuria, polydipsia
Overdosage Symptoms of overdose include hypercalcemia, anorexia, nausea, weakness, constipation, diarrhea, vague aches, mental confusion, tinnitus, ataxia, depression, hallucinations, syncope, coma; polyuria, polydipsia, nocturia, hypercalciuria, irreversible renal insufficiency or proteinuria, azotemia; will spread tissue calcifications, hypertension
Toxicology Following withdrawal of the drug, treatment consists of bed rest, liberal intake of fluids, reduced calcium intake, and cathartic administration. Severe hypercalcemia requires I.V. hydration and forced diuresis with I.V. furosemide (20-40 mg I.V. every 4-6 hours). Urine output should be monitored and maintained at >3 mL/kg/hour. I.V. saline can quickly and significantly increase excretion of calcium into the urine.

Calcitonin, cholestyramine, prednisone, sodium EDTA, and mithramycin have all been used successfully to treat the more resistant cases of vitamin D-induced hypercalcemia.

Drug Interactions

Vitamin D may increase absorption of magnesium from magnesium compounds; hypercalcemia may be precipitated by vitamin D and, therefore, may increase cardiac arrhythmias in patients taking digitalis glycosides and verapamil; hypoparathyroid patients may develop hypercalcemia when using thiazide diuretics

Phenytoin and barbiturates decrease half-life of vitamin D; mineral oil with prolonged use decreases vitamin D absorption; cholestyramine reduces absorption of vitamin D

Stability Protect from light

Mechanism of Action Stimulates calcium and phosphate absorption from the small intestine, promotes secretion of calcium from bone to blood (calcium hemostasis); promotes renal tubule resorption or phosphate

Pharmacodynamics

Onset of action: Maximum hypercalcemic effects occur within 2-4 weeks

Duration: Can be as long as 9 weeks

Pharmacokinetics

Absorption: Well from GI tract

Elimination: In bile and feces; stored in liver, fat, skin, muscle, and bone

Usual Dosage Geriatrics and Adults: Oral:

Hypoparathyroidism: 0.5-1 mg/day

Nutritional rickets: 0.5 mg as a single dose or 13-50 mcg/day until healing occurs

Renal osteodystrophy: 0.6-6 mg/24 hours; maintenance: 0.25-0.6 mg/24 hours adjusted as necessary to achieve normal serum calcium levels and promote bone healing. 1 mg is equal to 3 mg vitamin D_2 (120,000 IU) not recommended for daily supplementation due to dosage form strengths; not easily divided to deliver 800 IU

Monitoring Parameters Monitor renal function, serum calcium and phosphate concentrations; if hypercalcemia is encountered, discontinue agent until serum calcium returns to normal

Reference Range Calcium (serum) 9-10 mg/dL (4.5-5 mEq/L); phosphate 2.5-5 mg/dL

Test Interactions Increased calcium (S), cholesterol (S)

Patient Information Do not take more than the recommended amount. While taking this medication, your physician may want you to follow a special diet or take a calcium supplement. Follow this diet closely. Avoid taking magnesium supplements or magnesium containing antacids. Early symptoms of hypercalcemia include weakness, fatigue, somnolence, headache, anorexia, dry mouth, metallic taste, nausea, vomiting, cramps, diarrhea, muscle pain, bone pain, and irritability.

Nursing Implications Monitor calcium and phosphate levels closely; monitor symptoms of hypercalcemia; see Adverse Reactions

Additional Information Synthetic analog of vitamin D with a faster onset of action; dose adjustment should be based on serum calcium level

Special Geriatric Considerations Recommended daily allowances (RDA) have not been developed for persons >65 years of age; vitamin D, folate, and B_{12} (cyanocobalamin) have decreased absorption with age, but the clinical significance is yet unknown. Calorie requirements decrease with age and therefore, nutrient density must be increased to ensure adequate nutrient intake, including vitamins and minerals. Therefore, the use of a daily supplement with a multiple vitamin with minerals is recommended. Elderly consume less vitamin D, absorption may be decreased, and many elderly have decreased sun exposure; therefore, elderly should receive supplementation with 800 units of vitamin D (20 mcg)/day. This is a recommendation of particular need to those with high risk for osteoporosis.

Dosage Forms

Capsule: 0.125 mg

Solution: 0.25 mg/mL in oil (15 mL); 0.2 mg/5 mL (500 mL)

Solution, concentrate: 0.2 mg/mL (30 mL)

Tablet: 0.125 mg, 0.2 mg, 0.4 mg

References

Letsou AP and Price LS, "Health Aging and Nutrition: An Overview," *Clin Geriatr Med*, 1987, 3(2):253-60.

Myrianthopoulos M, "Dietary Treatment of Hyperlipidemia in the Elderly," *Clin Geriatr Med*, 1987, 3(2):343-59.

Riggs BL and Melton LJ, "The Prevention and Treatment of Osteoporosis," *N Engl J Med*, 1992, 327(9):620-7.

1,25 dihydroxycholecalciferol *see Calcitriol on page 105*

Dihydroxypropyl Theophylline *see Dyphylline on page 247*

Diiodohydroxyquin *see Iodoquinol on page 375*

Dilacor™ XR *see Diltiazem on next page*

Dilantin® *see Phenytoin on page 559*

Dilatair® Ophthalmic Solution *see* Phenylephrine Hydrochloride *on page 557*

Dilaudid® *see* Hydromorphone Hydrochloride *on page 352*

Dilaudid® Cough Syrup *see* Hydromorphone Hydrochloride *on page 352*

Dilitrate®-SR *see* Isosorbide Dinitrate *on page 382*

Dilocaine® *see* Lidocaine Hydrochloride *on page 406*

Dilomine® *see* Dicyclomine Hydrochloride *on page 215*

Dilor® *see* Dyphylline *on page 247*

Diltiazem (dil tye' a zem)

Related Information
Calcium Channel Blocking Agents Comparison *on page 806-807*

Brand Names Cardizem®; Cardizem® CD; Cardizem® SR; Dilacor™ XR

Generic Available No

Therapeutic Class Antianginal Agent; Calcium Channel Blocker

Use Management of angina pectoris due to coronary insufficiency (chronic, stable, and vasospastic), hypertension, Raynaud's syndrome

Unlabeled use: Prevent non-Q-wave myocardial infarction, tardive dyskinesia; diastolic dysfunction

Contraindications Severe hypotension or second and third degree heart block; hypersensitivity to other calcium channel blockers, adenosine; atrial and ventricular arrhythmias; acute myocardial infarction, and pulmonary congestion

Warnings Monitor EKG and blood pressure closely in patients receiving I.V. therapy; hypotension, congestive heart failure; cardiac conduction defects, PVCs, idiopathic hypertrophic subaortic stenosis; may cause platelet intubation; do not abruptly withdraw (chest pain); hepatic dysfunction, renal function impairment, increased angina, increased intracranial pressure with cranial tumors; elderly may have greater hypotensive effect

Precautions Sick sinus syndrome, severe left ventricular dysfunction, congestive heart failure, hepatic or renal impairment, hypertrophic cardiomyopathy (especially obstructive), concomitant therapy with beta-blockers or digoxin, edema

Adverse Reactions
Cardiovascular: Tachycardia, hypotension, bradycardia, first, second, or third degree A-V block, worsening heart failure, palpitations, congestive heart failure, myocardial infarction, angina, bundle-branch block

Central nervous system: Amnesia, dizziness, headache, fatigue, seizures (occasionally with I.V. use), lightheadedness, psychotic symptoms, paresthesia, asthenia, insomnia

Gastrointestinal: Thirst, constipation (more of a problem in elderly), nausea, abdominal discomfort, diarrhea, gingival hyperplasia, dry mouth

Hepatic: Increase in hepatic enzymes

Neuromuscular & skeletal: Gait abnormality

Ocular: Amblyopia, eye irritation, blurred vision

Respiratory: May precipitate insufficiency of respiratory muscle function in Duchenne muscular dystrophy

Miscellaneous: Peripheral edema

Overdosage Symptoms of overdose include heartblock, hypotension, asystole

Toxicology Ipecac-induced emesis can hypothetically worsen calcium antagonist toxicity, since it can produce vagal stimulation. The potential for seizures precipitously following acute ingestion of large doses of a calcium antagonist may also contraindicate the use of ipecac. Supportive and symptomatic treatment, including I.V. fluids and Trendelenburg positioning, should be initiated as intoxication may cause hypotension. Although calcium (calcium chloride I.V. 1-2 g) has been used as an "antidote" for acute intoxications, there is limited experience to support its routine use, and should be reserved for those cases where definite signs of myocardial depression are evident. Heart block may respond to isoproterenol, glucagon, atropine and/or calcium, although a temporary pacemaker may be required.

Drug Interactions
Calcium channel blockers (CCB) and H_2 blockers → ↑ bioavailability CCB
CCB and beta-blockers → ↑ cardiac depressant effects on A-V conduction
CCB and carbamazepine → ↑ carbamazepine levels (nifedipine does not appear to interact with carbamazepine)
CCB and cyclosporine → ↑ cyclosporine levels
CCB and digitalis → ↑ digitalis levels
CCB and theophylline → ↑ pharmacologic actions of theophylline

Stability Store injections in refrigerator at 2°C to 8°C (36°F to 46°F); stable for 24 hours

Mechanism of Action Inhibits calcium ion from entering the "slow channels" or select voltage-sensitive areas of vascular smooth muscle and myocardium during depolarization, producing a relaxation of coronary vascular smooth muscle and coronary vasodilation; increases myocardial oxygen delivery in patients with vasospastic angina

Pharmacodynamics
Onset of action: 30-60 minutes after oral administration (including sustained release)
Peak effects: 2-3 hours for plain tablets, 6-11 hours for sustained release

Pharmacokinetics
Absorption: 80% to 90%
Distribution: V_d: 1.7 L/kg
Protein binding: 77% to 85%
Metabolism: Extensive in the liver
Bioavailability: Around 40% to 65% due to a significant first-pass effect following oral administration
Half-life: 4-6 hours (may increase with renal impairment), 5-7 hours for sustained release
Time to peak: Peak serum levels occur within 2-3 hours
Elimination: In urine and in bile mostly as metabolites

Usual Dosage Geriatrics and Adults:
Oral: Initial dose: 30 mg 3-4 times/day, then 30-120 mg 3-4 times/day; dosage should be increased gradually, at 1- to 2-day intervals until optimum response is obtained; not to exceed 360 mg/day
Sustained-release capsules: Initial dose: 60-120 mg twice daily; increase dose at 14-day intervals
Cardizem® CD and Dilacor™ XR: 180-240 mg once daily; increase dose at 14-day intervals
Parenteral: Initial dose: 0.25 mg/kg as a bolus over 2 minutes (20 mg is an average dose); second bolus: 0.35 mg/kg over 2 minutes (25 mg is an average dose)
Continuous I.V.: After bolus, 5-10 mg/hour; see Additional Information

Dosing adjustment in renal impairment: None

Monitoring Parameters Heart rate, blood pressure, signs and symptoms of congestive heart failure

Reference Range Therapeutic: 50-200 ng/mL

Patient Information Sustained release products should be taken with food and not crushed; limit caffeine intake; avoid alcohol; notify physician if angina pain is not reduced when taking this drug, irregular heartbeat, shortness of breath, swelling, dizziness, constipation, nausea, or hypotension occur; do not stop therapy without advice of physician

Nursing Implications Do not crush sustained release capsules; see Warnings, Precautions, Monitoring Parameters, and Special Geriatric Considerations

Additional Information Mix injection for continuous infusion in D_5W, NS, $D_5\frac{1}{2}NS$

Special Geriatric Considerations Elderly may experience a greater hypotensive response; constipation may be more of a problem in elderly; calcium channel blockers are no more effective in elderly than other therapies; however, they do not cause significant CNS effects which is an advantage over some antihypertensive agents.

Dosage Forms
Capsule, sustained release: 60 mg, 90 mg, 120 mg, 180 mg, 240 mg, 300 mg
Injection: 25 mg/5 mL (5 mL); 50 mg/5 mL (10 mL)
Tablet: 30 mg, 60 mg, 90 mg, 120 mg

Dimaphen® [OTC] see Brompheniramine and Phenylpropanolamine on page 94

Dimenhydrinate (dye men hye' dri nate)
Brand Names Calm-X® [OTC]; Dimetabs®; Dinate®; Dommanate®; Dramamine® [OTC]; Dramilin®; Dramocen®; Dramoject®; Dymenate®; Hydrate®; Marmine® [OTC]; Tega-Cert® [OTC]; TripTone® Caplets® [OTC]; Wehamine®

Generic Available Yes

Therapeutic Class Antiemetic; Antihistamine

Use Treatment and prevention of nausea, vertigo, and vomiting associated with motion sickness

Contraindications Hypersensitivity to dimenhydrinate or any component; chlorotheophylline and theophylline

Warnings Use with caution when giving with antibiotics which may cause ototoxicity since dimenhydrinate may mask signs of ototoxicity (vestibular toxicity)

Precautions Use with caution with prostatic hypertrophy, peptic ulcer, pyloroduodenal obstruction, bladder neck obstruction, narrow-angle glaucoma, bronchial asthma, and cardiac arrhythmias

Adverse Reactions
Cardiovascular: Hypotension
Central nervous system: Drowsiness, headache, paradoxical CNS stimulation, dizziness, confusion, nervousness, restlessness, insomnia, vertigo, lassitude
Gastrointestinal: Anorexia
Genitourinary: Urinary frequency
Local: Pain at the injection site
Neuromuscular & skeletal: Heaviness and weakness of hands

(Continued)
227

Dimenhydrinate *(Continued)*

Ocular: Blurred vision, diplopia
Otic: Tinnitus
Respiratory: Chest tightness, wheezing, thickening of bronchial secretions
Miscellaneous: Dry mucous membranes

Overdosage Toxicity may resemble atropine overdosage; CNS depression or stimulation; convulsions, coma, respiratory depression with massive overdosage

Toxicology There is no specific treatment for an antihistamine overdose, however, most of its clinical toxicity is due to anticholinergic effects. Anticholinesterase inhibitors may be useful by reducing acetylcholinesterase. Anticholinesterase inhibitors include physostigmine, neostigmine, pyridostigmine, and edrophonium. For anticholinergic overdose with severe life-threatening symptoms, physostigmine 1-2 mg I.V., slowly may be given to reverse these effects; treat convulsions with diazepam.

Drug Interactions CNS depressants, drugs with anticholinergic effects, ototoxic drugs, alcohol

Mechanism of Action Competes with histamine for H_1-receptor sites on effector cells in the gastrointestinal tract, blood vessels, and respiratory tract; blocks chemoreceptor trigger zone, diminishes vestibular stimulation and depresses labyrinthine function through its central anticholinergic activity

Pharmacodynamics

Onset of action: Oral: Within 15-30 minutes following administration
Duration: ~4-6 hours

Pharmacokinetics

Absorption: Well absorbed from GI tract
Metabolism: Extensive in the liver

Usual Dosage Geriatrics and Adults: Oral, I.M., I.V.: 50-100 mg every 4-6 hours, not to exceed 400 mg/day; start elderly at lowest dose recommended; do not inject intra-arterially; see Nursing Implications

Monitoring Parameters Monitor for anticholinergic side effects; emetic episodes and nausea

Patient Information May cause drowsiness

Nursing Implications I.V. injection must be diluted to 10 mL with NS and given at 25 mg/minute over at least 2 minutes

Special Geriatric Considerations Monitor for anticholinergic side effects (confusion, constipation, etc); limit use if possible to short-term therapy

Dosage Forms

Capsule: 50 mg
Injection: 50 mg/mL (1 mL, 5 mL, 10 mL)
Liquid: 12.5 mg/4 mL; 15.62 mg/5 mL
Tablet: 50 mg
Tablet, chewable: 50 mg

Dimetabs® *see* Dimenhydrinate *on previous page*

Dimetane® [OTC] *see* Brompheniramine Maleate *on page 95*

Dimetapp® [OTC] *see* Brompheniramine and Phenylpropanolamine *on page 94*

Dimethoxyphenyl Penicillin Sodium *see* Methicillin Sodium *on page 453*

β,β-Dimethylcysteine *see* Penicillamine *on page 537*

Dinate® *see* Dimenhydrinate *on previous page*

Diocto-C® [OTC] *see* Docusate and Casanthranol *on page 237*

Diocto® [OTC] *see* Docusate *on page 236*

Dioctyl Calcium Sulfosuccinate *see* Docusate *on page 236*

Dioctyl Sodium Sulfosuccinate *see* Docusate *on page 236*

Dioeze® [OTC] *see* Docusate *on page 236*

Dionex® [OTC] *see* Docusate *on page 236*

Diosuccin® [OTC] *see* Docusate *on page 236*

Diothron® [OTC] *see* Docusate and Casanthranol *on page 237*

Dioval® *see* Estradiol *on page 269*

Dipentum® *see* Olsalazine Sodium *on page 516*

Diphenhydramine Hydrochloride *(dye fen hye' dra meen)*

Related Information

Anxiolytic/Hypnotic Use in Long-Term Care Facilities *on page 755-756*

Brand Names AllerMax® [OTC]; Banophen® [OTC]; Beldin® [OTC]; Belix® [OTC]; Benadryl® [OTC]; Benylin® Cough Syrup [OTC]; Compoz® [OTC]; Diphen® Cough [OTC]; Genahist®; Nidryl® [OTC]; Nordryl®; Nytol® [OTC]; Sleep-eze 3® [OTC]; Sominex® [OTC]; Tusstat®; Twilite® [OTC]; Valdrene®

Generic Available Yes

Therapeutic Class Antidote, Hypersensitivity Reactions; Antihistamine; Sedative

Use Symptomatic relief of allergic symptoms caused by histamine release which include nasal allergies and allergic dermatosis; mild nighttime sedation, prevention of motion sickness, as an antitussive

Unlabeled use: Parkinson's disease (anticholinergic effects)

Contraindications Hypersensitivity to diphenhydramine or any component; should not be used in acute attacks of asthma

Warnings Antihistamines are more likely to cause dizziness, excessive sedation, syncope, toxic confusional states, and hypotension in the elderly

Precautions Use with caution in patients with angle-closure glaucoma, peptic ulcer, urinary tract obstruction, hyperthyroidism; some preparations contain sodium bisulfite; syrup contains alcohol

Adverse Reactions

Cardiovascular: Hypotension, palpitations

Central nervous system: Sedation, dizziness, paradoxical excitement, fatigue, insomnia

Gastrointestinal: Nausea, vomiting

Genitourinary: Urinary retention

Neuromuscular & skeletal: Tremors

Ocular: Blurred vision

Miscellaneous: Dry mucous membranes

Overdosage Symptoms of overdose include CNS depression or stimulation, dry mouth, flushed skin, fixed and dilated pupils, apnea

Toxicology There is no specific treatment for an antihistamine overdose, however, most of its clinical toxicity is due to anticholinergic effects. Anticholinesterase inhibitors may be useful by reducing acetylcholinesterase. Anticholinesterase inhibitors include physostigmine, neostigmine, pyridostigmine and edrophonium. For anticholinergic overdose with severe life-threatening symptoms, physostigmine 1-2 mg I.V., slowly may be given to reverse these effects.

Drug Interactions Increased effect/toxicity: CNS depressants, alcohol, tricyclic antidepressants, monoamine oxidase inhibitors; elixir should not be given to patients taking drugs that can cause disulfiram reactions (ie, metronidazole, chlorpropamide) due to alcohol content

Stability Protect from light

Mechanism of Action Competes with histamine for H_1-receptor sites on effector cells in the gastrointestinal tract, blood vessels, and respiratory tract

Pharmacodynamics Duration of action: 4-7 hours

Pharmacokinetics

Absorption: Oral: ~65%

Metabolism: Extensive in the liver, and to smaller degrees in the lung and kidneys

Half-life:

Elderly: 13.5 hours

Adults: 2-8 hours

Time to peak serum concentration: 2-4 hours; one study showed significant increase in peak concentration in elderly

Elimination: Total body clearance is decreased in elderly

Usual Dosage

Geriatrics: Initial: 25 mg 2-3 times/day increasing as needed

Dosing interval in renal impairment:

Cl_{cr} 10-50 mL/minute: Increase dosing interval to 6-12 hours

Cl_{cr} <10 mL/minute: Increase dosing interval to 12-18 hours

Adults:

Oral:

Antihistamine: 25-50 mg every 4-6 hours

Antitussive: 25 mg every 4 hours

Antiemetic: 25-50 mg 3-4 times/day

Parkinson's disease: 25-50 mg 3-4 times/day

Sleep aid: 50 mg at bedtime (maximum)

I.M., I.V.: 10-50 mg in a single dose every 2-4 hours, not to exceed 400 mg/day

Topical: Apply to affected area for not longer than 7 days

Monitoring Parameters Relief of symptoms, mental alertness

Reference Range Therapeutic: Not established; Toxic: >0.1 μg/mL

Test Interactions May suppress the wheal and flare reactions to skin test antigens

Patient Information May cause drowsiness. Avoid CNS depressants and alcohol.

Nursing Implications I.V. must be given slowly; monitor patient for sedation

Additional Information Has antinauseant and topical anesthetic properties

Special Geriatric Considerations Diphenhydramine has high sedative and anticholinergic properties, so it may not be considered the antihistamine of choice for prolonged use in the elderly. Its use as a sleep aid is discouraged due to its anticholinergic effects; interpretive guidelines issued by the Health Care Financing Administration (HCFA) discourage the use of diphenhydramine as a sedative or anxiolytic in long-term care facilities; see Pharmacokinetics

(Continued)

Diphenhydramine Hydrochloride (Continued)

Dosage Forms
Capsule: 25 mg, 50 mg
Cream: 2% (30 g, 60 g)
Elixir: 12.5 mg/5 mL (4 mL, 120 mL, 240 mL)
Injection: 10 mg/mL (10 mL, 30 mL); 50 mg/mL (1 mL, 10 mL)
Lotion: 1% (75 mL)
Solution, spray: 1% (60 mL)
Syrup: 12.5 mg/5 mL (120 mL, 240 mL, 473 mL, 4000 mL); 13.3 mg/5 mL (473 mL, 946 mL)
Tablet: 25 mg, 50 mg

References
Simons KJ, Watson WT, Martin TJ, et al, "Diphenhydramine: Pharmacokinetics and Pharmacodynamics in Elderly Adults, Young Adults, and Children," *J Clin Pharmacol*, 1990, 30(7):665-71.

Diphenoxylate and Atropine (dye fen ox' i late)

Brand Names Lofene®; Logen®; Lomenate®; Lomodix®; Lomotil®; Lonox®; Lo-Trol®; Low-Quel®; Nor-Mil®

Synonyms Atropine and Diphenoxylate

Generic Available Yes

Therapeutic Class Antidiarrheal

Use Adjunctive treatment of diarrhea

Restrictions C-V

Contraindications Hypersensitivity to diphenoxylate, atropine or any component; severe liver disease, jaundice, dehydrated patient, and narrow-angle glaucoma, diarrhea due to pseudomembranous enterocolitis or enterotoxin-producing bacteria

Warnings Reduction of intestinal motility may be deleterious in diarrhea resulting from *Shigella*, *Salmonella*, toxigenic strains of *E. coli* and from pseudomembranous enterocolitis associated with broad spectrum antibiotics; diphenoxylate may induce toxic megacolon in patients with ulcerative colitis; discontinue use if abdominal distention occurs; hepatic coma may be precipitated when used in patients with significant or severe hepatic disease

Precautions High doses may cause addiction; use with caution in patients with ulcerative colitis, dehydration, and hepatic dysfunction; use with caution in patients performing hazardous tasks (driving, etc)

Adverse Reactions
Cardiovascular: Tachycardia
Central nervous system: Sedation, dizziness, euphoria, headache, anaphylaxis, headache, confusion, delirium, sedation, malaise, lethargy, restlessness, hyperthermia
Dermatologic: Pruritus, urticaria, dry skin, angionecrotic edema
Gastrointestinal: Nausea, vomiting, abdominal discomfort, paralytic ileus, pancreatitis, dry mouth, toxic megacolon
Genitourinary: Urinary retention
Neuromuscular & skeletal: Weakness
Ocular: Blurred vision
Respiratory: Respiratory depression
Miscellaneous: Swelling

Overdosage Symptoms of overdose include drowsiness, hypotension, blurred vision (mydriasis), flushing, dry mouth, miosis, dry mucous membranes, restlessness, hyperthermia, tachycardia, lethargy; and then coma, hypotonic reflexes, nystagmus, respiratory depression; respiratory depression may occur 12-30 hours after ingestion

Toxicology Naloxone 2 mg I.V. with repeat administration as necessary to maintain respiration, up to a total of 10 mg. Duration of diphenoxylate is longer than naloxone. Repeated doses necessary. Monitor closely for 48 hours. For the anticholinergic overdose with severe life-threatening symptoms, physostigmine 1-2 mg S.C. or I.V., slowly may be given to reverse these effects. Administration of activated charcoal will reduce bioavailability of diphenoxylate. Gastric lavage can be used in place of activated charcoal therapy.

Drug Interactions Diphenoxylate may precipitate hypertensive crises with monoamine oxidase inhibitors; diphenoxylate may increase CNS depressant effects of barbiturates, alcohol, major and minor tranquilizers

Stability Protect liquid from light

Mechanism of Action Diphenoxylate inhibits excessive GI motility and GI propulsion; this is both a peripheral and central mechanism of action; commercial preparations contain a subtherapeutic amount of atropine to discourage abuse; diphenoxylate is a congener of meperidine but lacks analgesic activity; high doses (40-60 mg) exhibit opioid activity

Pharmacodynamics
Onset of action: Within 45-60 minutes
Duration: 3-4 hours

Pharmacokinetics
Absorption: Oral: Well absorbed

Metabolism: Diphenoxylate is extensively metabolized in the liver to diphenoxylic acid (active)

Half-life:

Diphenoxylate: 2.5 hours

Diphenoxylic acid (difenoxine): 12-14 hours

Time to peak: Plasma concentrations occur at 2 hours

Elimination: Primarily in feces (via bile) and ~14% excreted in urine; <1% excreted unchanged in urine

Usual Dosage Geriatrics and Adults: Oral (as diphenoxylate): 15-20 mg/day in 3-4 divided doses initially; reduce dosage as soon as symptoms are controlled; maintenance dose is $\frac{1}{4}$ of initial dose; see Additional Information

Monitoring Parameters Monitor number and consistency of stools; observe for signs of toxicity, fluid and electrolyte loss, hypotension, and respiratory depression

Patient Information Drowsiness, dizziness, dry mouth; use caution while driving or performing hazardous tasks; avoid alcohol or other CNS depressants; do not exceed prescribed dose; report persistent diarrhea, fever, or palpitations to physician

Nursing Implications Watch for signs of atropinism (dryness of skin and mucous membranes, tachycardia, thirst, flushing), hypotension, respiratory depression, confusion; see Monitoring Parameters

Additional Information If there is no response within 48 hours, the drug is unlikely to be effective and should be discontinued. If chronic diarrhea is not improved symptomatically within 10 days at maximum dosage of 20 mg/day, control is unlikely with further use. Diarrhea should also be treated with dietary measures (ie, clear liquids), and avoid milk products and high sodium foods such as bouillon and soups.

Special Geriatric Considerations Elderly are particularly sensitive to fluid and electrolyte loss. This generally results in lethargy, weakness, and confusion. Repletion and maintenance of electrolytes and water are essential in the treatment of diarrhea. Drug therapy must be limited in order to avoid toxicity with this agent.

Dosage Forms

Solution, oral: Diphenoxylate hydrochloride 2.5 mg and atropine sulfate 0.025 mg per 5 mL (60 mL)

Tablet: Diphenoxylate hydrochloride 2.5 mg and atropine sulfate 0.025 mg

Diphen® Cough [OTC] *see* Diphenhydramine Hydrochloride
on page 228

Diphenylan Sodium® *see* Phenytoin *on page 559*

Diphenylhydantoin *see* Phenytoin *on page 559*

Diphtheria and Tetanus Toxoid (dif theer' ee a)

Related Information

Immunization Guidelines *on page 759-762*

Synonyms DT; Tetanus and Diphtheria Toxoid

Therapeutic Class Toxoid

Use Active immunity against diphtheria and tetanus

Contraindications Patients receiving immunosuppressive agents, prior anaphylactic, allergic, or systemic reactions, hypersensitivity to diphtheria and tetanus toxoid or any component

Warnings Do not use to treat active tetanus or diphtheria infections

Precautions Hypersensitivity may occur; primary immunization should be postponed until the second year of life due to possibility of CNS damage or convulsion

Adverse Reactions

Cardiovascular: Flushing, tachycardia, hypotension, especially those who have received many booster injections

Central nervous system: Drowsiness, malaise, neurologic symptoms are uncommon (ie, radial nerve paralysis, swallowing difficulties, etc), severe fever, convulsions rarely

Dermatologic: Urticaria, rash, pruritus, redness

Gastrointestinal: Anorexia, vomiting

Local: Pain, tenderness, palpable nodules and sterile abscesses may occur at injection site

Neuromuscular & skeletal: Generalized aches and pains

Miscellaneous: Arthus-type hypersensitivity reactions, swelling

Drug Interactions Immunosuppressive agents

Stability Refrigerate

Usual Dosage Geriatrics and Adults: I.M.: Two primary doses of 0.5 mL each, given at an interval of 4-6 weeks; third (reinforcing) dose of 0.5 mL 6-12 months later; boosters every 10 years

Patient Information A nodule may be palpable at the injection site for a few weeks

Nursing Implications Shake well before giving, advise patient of adverse reactions; must be given I.M.; do not inject the same site more than once; federal law requires that the date of administration, the vaccine manufacturer, lot number of vaccine, and the administering person's name, title, and address be entered into the patient's permanent medical record

(Continued)

Diphtheria and Tetanus Toxoid *(Continued)*

Special Geriatric Considerations Tetanus is a rare disease in U.S. with <100 cases annually; 66% of cases occur in persons >50 years of age; protective tetanus and diphtheria antibodies decline with age; it is estimated that <50% of elderly are protected.

Elderly are at risk because:
Many lack proper immunization maintenance
Higher case fatality ratio
Immunizations are not available from childhood

Indications for vaccination:
Primary series with combined tetanus-diphtheria (Td) should be given to all elderly lacking a clear history of vaccination
Boosters should be given at 10-year intervals; earlier for wounds
Elderly are more likely to require tetanus immune globulin with infection of tetanus due to lower antibody titer

Dosage Forms See table.

Diphtheria and Tetanus Toxoid

Manufacturer	Diphtheria in Lf units per 0.5 mL	Tetanus in Lf units per 0.5 mL
Connaught Td	2	5
Lederle Td	2	5
Sclavo Td	2	10
Wyeth Td	1.5	5

Td — adult use

References
Bentley DW, "Vaccinations," *Clin Geriatr Med*, 1992, 8(4):745-60.
Gardner P and Schaffner W, "Immunization of Adults," *N Engl J Med*, 1993, 328(17):1242-8.

Dipivalyl Epinephrine *see* Dipivefrin *on this page*

Dipivefrin (dye piʹ ve frin)

Related Information
Glaucoma Drug Therapy Comparison *on page 810*
Brand Names Propine®
Synonyms Dipivalyl Epinephrine; DPE
Generic Available No
Therapeutic Class Adrenergic Agonist Agent, Ophthalmic; Ophthalmic Agent, Vasoconstrictor
Use Reduce elevated intraocular pressure in chronic open-angle glaucoma; also used to treat ocular hypertension, low tension, and secondary glaucomas
Contraindications Hypersensitivity to dipivefrin, ingredients in the formulation, or epinephrine; contraindicated in patients with angle-closure glaucoma
Warnings Contains sulfites which cause allergic-type reactions in susceptible persons
Precautions Use with caution in patients with vascular hypertension or cardiac disorders and in aphakic patients
Adverse Reactions
Cardiovascular: Tachycardia, arrhythmia, hypertension
Central nervous system: Headache
Local: Burning, stinging
Ocular: Ocular congestion, photophobia, mydriasis, blurred vision, ocular pain, bulbar conjunctival follicles, blepharoconjunctivitis, cystoid macular edema
Drug Interactions Effects when used with other agents to lower intraocular pressure may be additive or synergistic; cyclopropane and halothane (general anesthetics) sensitize the heart to sympathomimetics; chymotrypsin is inactivated by epinephrine, exaggerated adrenergic pressor effects with monoamine oxidase inhibitors and tricyclic antidepressants
Stability Avoid exposure to light and air, discolored or darkened solutions indicate loss of potency
Mechanism of Action Dipivefrin is a prodrug of epinephrine which is the active agent that stimulates alpha- and/or beta-adrenergic receptors increasing aqueous humor outflow
Pharmacodynamics
Ocular pressure effects: Within 30 minutes

Duration: 12 hours or longer; mydriasis may occur within 30 minutes and last for several hours

Pharmacokinetics Absorption: Rapid into the aqueous humor; converted to epinephrine

Usual Dosage Geriatrics and Adults: Ophthalmic: Initial: Instill 1 drop every 12 hours

Monitoring Parameters Intraocular pressure; heart rate and blood pressure

Patient Information Discolored solutions should be discarded; do not touch dropper to eye; slight amount of discomfort may follow instillation; headache or browache may occur at start of therapy; report any change in vision to physician immediately

Nursing Implications Instruct on how to give eye drops

Additional Information Contains sodium metabisulfite

Special Geriatric Considerations Use with caution in patients with heart disease. Assess patient's ability to self-administer drops.

Dosage Forms Solution, ophthalmic: 0.1% (5 mL, 10 mL, 15 mL)

Diprolene® see Betamethasone on page 82

Diprolene® AF see Betamethasone on page 82

Dipropylacetic Acid see Valproic Acid and Derivatives on page 728

Diprosone® see Betamethasone on page 82

Dipyridamole (dye peer id' a mole)
Brand Names Persantine®
Generic Available Yes
Therapeutic Class Antiplatelet Agent; Vasodilator, Coronary
Use Maintain patency after surgical grafting procedures including coronary artery bypass; with warfarin to decrease thrombosis in patients after artificial heart valve replacement; for chronic management of angina pectoris; with aspirin to prevent coronary artery thrombosis; in combination with aspirin or warfarin to prevent other thromboembolic disorders
Contraindications Hypersensitivity to dipyridamole or any component
Warnings Use with caution in patients with hypotension
Precautions May further decrease blood pressure in patients with hypotension due to peripheral vasodilation
Adverse Reactions
  Cardiovascular: Vasodilatation, flushing, syncope
  Central nervous system: Dizziness, headache
  Dermatologic: Rash, pruritus, bruising
  Gastrointestinal: Abdominal distress
  Hematologic: Bleeding
  Neuromuscular & skeletal: Weakness
Overdosage Symptoms of overdose include hypotension, peripheral vasodilation
Drug Interactions Heparin, aspirin, adenosine
Mechanism of Action Inhibits the activity of adenosine deaminase and phosphodiesterase, which causes an accumulation of adenosine, adenine nucleotides, and cyclic AMP; these mediators then inhibit platelet aggregation and may cause vasodilation; may also stimulate release of prostacyclin or PGD$_2$
Pharmacokinetics
  Absorption: Readily from GI tract
  Distribution: V_d: Adults: 2-3 L/kg
  Protein binding: 91% to 99%
  Metabolism: Concentrated and metabolized in the liver
  Bioavailability: Ranges from 37% to 66%
  Half-life (terminal): 10-12 hours
  Time to peak: Peak serum levels occur within 2-2.5 hours
  Elimination: In feces via bile as glucuronide conjugates and unchanged drug
Usual Dosage Geriatrics and Adults: Oral: 75-400 mg/day in 3-4 divided doses before meals; see Additional Information
Additional Information Dipyridamole may also be given 2 days prior to open heart surgery to prevent platelet activation by extracorporeal bypass pump; differences in bioavailability between products observed; evidence exists that doses of 400-600 mg/day have been shown to have **no effect** on platelet aggregation; this casts doubt on clinical usefulness as an antiplatelet agent
Special Geriatric Considerations Since evidence suggests that clinically used doses are ineffective for prevention of platelet aggregation, consideration for low dose aspirin (81-325 mg/day) alone may be necessary; this will decrease cost as well as inconvenience
Dosage Forms Tablet: 25 mg, 50 mg, 75 mg
References
Fitzgerald GA, "Dipyridamole," N Engl J Med, 1987, 316(20):1247-57.

Disalcid® see Salsalate on page 637

ALPHABETICAL LISTING OF DRUGS

Disalicylic Acid *see* Salsalate *on page 637*

Disanthrol® [OTC] *see* Docusate and Casanthranol *on page 237*

Disodium Cromoglycate *see* Cromolyn Sodium *on page 190*

d-Isoephedrine Hydrochloride *see* Pseudoephedrine *on page 609*

Disolan® Capsules [OTC] *see* Docusate and Phenolphthalein *on page 238*

Disopyramide Phosphate (dye soe peer' a mide)

Brand Names Norpace®; Norpace® CR

Generic Available Yes

Therapeutic Class Antiarrhythmic Agent, Class IA

Use Suppression and prevention of unifocal and multifocal premature ventricular complexes, coupled ventricular tachycardia considered to be life threatening; also effective in the conversion of atrial fibrillation, atrial flutter, and paroxysmal atrial tachycardia to normal sinus rhythm and prevention of the reoccurrence of these arrhythmias after conversion by other methods

Contraindications Pre-existing second or third degree A-V block; cardiogenic shock or known hypersensitivity to the drug

Warnings Demonstrates proarrhythmic effect to the extent it is not recommended for arrhythmias capable of being treated with less toxic, more traditional therapy, has not been shown to increase survival; negative inotropic action may result in congestive heart failure or hypotension; QRS widening, QT_c prolongation; atrial arrhythmias; use with caution in sick sinus syndrome, Wolff-Parkinson-White syndrome, and patients with heart block; hypoglycemia reported; disopyramide has strong anticholinergic activity; use with caution and reduce dosage in renal ($Cl_{cr} \leq 40$ mL/minute) and hepatic impairment

Precautions Pre-existing urinary retention, family history or existing angle-closure glaucoma, myasthenia gravis, hypotension during initiation of therapy, congestive heart failure unless caused by an arrhythmias, widening of QRS complex during therapy or Q-T interval (>25% to 50% of baseline QRS complex or Q-T interval), sick sinus syndrome or WPW, renal or hepatic impairment require decrease in dosage; disopyramide ineffective in hypokalemia and potentially toxic with hyperkalemia

Adverse Reactions

Cardiovascular: Hypotension, congestive heart failure, edema, chest pain, syncope, conduction disturbances including A-V block, widening QRS complex and lengthening of Q-T interval

Central nervous system: Nervousness, acute psychosis, depression, dizziness, fatigue, headache, malaise, pain

Dermatologic: Generalized rashes

Endocrine & metabolic: Hypoglycemia, increased cholesterol and triglycerides; hyperkalemia may enhance toxicities

Gastrointestinal: Constipation, dry mouth, weight gain, nausea, vomiting, diarrhea, gas, anorexia

Genitourinary: Urinary retention, urinary hesitancy

Neuromuscular & skeletal: Weakness

Ocular: Blurred vision

Respiratory: Dyspnea

Miscellaneous: Dry nose, eyes, and throat

Overdosage Symptoms of overdose include anticholinergic effects, hypotension, loss of consciousness, respiratory arrest, cardiac conduction disturbances, arrhythmias, widening of the QRS complex and Q-T interval, bradycardia, congestive heart failure, asystole and seizures

Toxicology General supportive care: Induce emesis or perform gastric lavage followed by cathartic or activated charcoal; use of pressor agents (isoproterenol, dopamine), diuretics, cardiac glycosides, intra-aortic balloon counterpulsation, mechanical ventilation may be necessary as indicated; hemodialysis and charcoal hemoperfusion are effective to help eliminate disopyramide

Drug Interactions

Hepatic microsomal enzyme inducing agents (ie, phenytoin, phenobarbital, rifampin) may increase metabolism of disopyramide

Erythromycin may increase disopyramide serum concentrations

Anticoagulants may have decreased PTs after discontinuation of disopyramide

Digoxin and quinidine serum concentrations may be increased, and drugs with anticholinergic effects will be augmented

Mechanism of Action Class IA antiarrhythmic: Decreases myocardial excitability and conduction velocity; reduces disparity in refractory between normal and infarcted myocardium; possesses anticholinergic, peripheral vasoconstrictive and negative inotropic effects

Pharmacodynamics

Onset of action: 0.5-3.5 hours

Duration of effect: 1.5-8.5 hours

Pharmacokinetics
Protein binding: Concentration-dependent ranging from 20% to 60%
Metabolism: In the liver to inactive metabolites
Bioavailability: 60% to 83%
Half-life: 4-10 hours with Cl_{cr} <40 mL/minute; half-life: 8-18 hours; increased half-life with hepatic or renal disease
Time to peak: Peak levels occur in 1-2 hours
Elimination: 40% to 60% unchanged in urine and 10% to 15% in feces
Total body clearance of unbound disopyramide averages 3.2-5.4 mL/minute/kg; total disopyramide clearance range: 0.7-1.2 mL/minute/kg; the total body clearance (bound and unbound) is decreased in elderly

Usual Dosage Oral (initiate therapy in hospital):
Geriatrics and Adults:
Initial loading: 300 mg (<50 kg: 200 mg); follow with 200 mg every 6 hours (if no toxicity or response after 6 hours); if no response in 48 hours, increase carefully to 250 mg every 6 hours or stop drug
<50 kg: 100 mg every 6 hours or 200 mg every 12 hours (controlled release)
>50 kg: 150 mg every 6 hours or 300 mg every 12 hours (controlled release); if no response, may increase to 200 mg every 6 hours; most adults respond to 600 mg/day; maximum dose required for patients with severe refractory ventricular tachycardia may be 400 mg every 6 hours. When switching from immediate release to controlled release dosage form, initiate controlled release dose 6 hours following last dose of immediate release preparation.

Dosing adjustment in renal impairment: Adults: 100 mg (nonsustained release) given at the following intervals; see table.

Cl_{cr} (mL/min)	Dosage Interval
30–40	q8h
15–30	q12h
<15	q24h

Monitoring Parameters Congestive heart failure, hypotension and urinary retention; monitor EKG, blood pressure, pulse, and serum levels

Reference Range
Therapeutic:
Atrial arrhythmias: 2.8-3.2 µg/mL (SI: 8.3-9.4 µmol/L)
Ventricular arrhythmias: 3.3-7.5 µg/mL (SI: 9.7-22 µmol/L)
Toxic: >7 µg/mL (SI: >20.7 µmol/L)

Test Interactions Decreased glucose

Patient Information May cause dry mouth, difficulty with urination, dizziness, dyspnea, blurred vision, and constipation; do not break or chew sustained release capsules

Nursing Implications Give around-the-clock rather than 4 times/day, 3 times/day, etc (ie, 12-6-12-6, not 9-1-5-9) to promote less variation in peak and trough serum levels; do not crush controlled release capsules

Special Geriatric Considerations Due to changes in total clearance (decreased) in elderly, monitor closely; the anticholinergic action may be intolerable and require discontinuation; monitor for CNS anticholinergic effects (confusion, agitation, hallucinations, etc). **Note:** Dose needs to be altered with Cl_{cr} <40 mL/minute which may be found frequently in elderly

Dosage Forms
Capsule: 100 mg, 150 mg
Capsule, sustained action: 100 mg, 150 mg

References
Fenster PE and Nolan PE, "Antiarrhythmic Drugs," *Geriatric Pharmacology*, Bressler R and Katz MD, eds, New York, NY: McGraw-Hill, 1993, 6:105-49.

Di-Sosul® [OTC] *see* Docusate *on next page*

Di-Spaz® *see* Dicyclomine Hydrochloride *on page 215*

Dispos-a-Med® Isoproterenol *see* Isoproterenol *on page 380*

Ditropan® *see* Oxybutynin Chloride *on page 527*

Diuril® *see* Chlorothiazide *on page 151*

Divalproex Sodium *see* Valproic Acid and Derivatives *on page 728*

Dizmiss® [OTC] *see* Meclizine Hydrochloride *on page 434*

dl-Norephedrine Hydrochloride *see* Phenylpropanolamine Hydrochloride *on page 559*

Dobutamine Hydrochloride (doe byoo' ta meen)

Brand Names Dobutrex®

Generic Available No

Therapeutic Class Adrenergic Agonist Agent

Use Short-term management of patients with cardiac decompensation due to depressed contractility

Contraindications Hypersensitivity to sulfites (commercial preparation contains sodium bisulfite); patients with idiopathic hypertrophic subaortic stenosis (IHSS)

Warnings Potent drug, must be diluted prior to use; patient's hemodynamic status should be monitored

Precautions Continuously monitor EKG and blood pressure; hypovolemia should be corrected prior to use; infiltration causes local inflammatory changes, extravasation may cause dermal necrosis; use with extreme caution following myocardial infarction

Adverse Reactions

Cardiovascular: Ectopic heartbeats, increased heart rate, chest pain, angina, palpitations, elevation in blood pressure; in higher doses ventricular tachycardia or arrhythmias may be seen. **Patients with atrial fibrillation or flutter are at risk of developing a rapid ventricular response.**

Central nervous system: Tingling sensation, paresthesia, headache

Gastrointestinal: Nausea, vomiting

Neuromuscular & skeletal: Mild leg cramps

Respiratory: Dyspnea

Overdosage Symptoms of overdose include fatigue, nervousness, tachycardia, hypertension, arrhythmias

Toxicology Reduce rate of administration or discontinue infusion until condition stabilizes

Drug Interactions

General anesthetics (ie, halothane or cyclopropane) and usual doses of dobutamine have resulted in ventricular arrhythmias in animals. In animals, the cardiac effects of dobutamine are antagonized by beta-adrenergic blockers, resulting in predominance of alpha-adrenergic effects and increased peripheral resistance.

Bretylium and tricyclic antidepressants may potentiate dobutamine's effects

Stability Incompatible with alkaline solutions (sodium bicarbonate); store reconstituted solution under refrigeration for 48 hours or 6 hours at room temperature; after dilution, the solution is stable for 24 hours at room temperature; pink discoloration of solution indicates slight oxidation but **no** significant loss of potency.

Mechanism of Action Stimulates beta$_1$-adrenergic receptors, causing increased cardiac output, with little effect on beta$_2$- or alpha-receptors; heart rate is not usually increased; dobutamine does not cause the release of norepinephrine

Pharmacodynamics

Onset of action: I.V.: 1-10 minutes following administration

Peak effect: Within 10-20 minutes

Pharmacokinetics

Metabolism: In tissues and liver to inactive metabolites

Half-life: 2 minutes

Elimination: In urine

Usual Dosage Geriatrics and Adults: I.V. infusion: 2.5-15 mcg/kg minute; maximum: 40 mcg/kg/minute, titrate to desired response; administer with an infusion device to control the flow rate

Administration Do not give through same I.V. line as heparin, hydrocortisone sodium succinate, cefazolin, or penicillin; administer into large vein; use infusion device to control rate of flow

Monitoring Parameters EKG, blood pressure, pulse, hemodynamic status

Nursing Implications See Administration

Additional Information Most clinical experience with dobutamine is short-term (several hours)

Standard diluent: 250 mg/500 mL D$_5$W

Minimum volume: 500 mg/250 mL D$_5$W

Special Geriatric Considerations A recent study demonstrated beneficial hemodynamic effects in elderly patients; monitor closely; see Adverse Reactions - Cardiovascular

Dosage Forms Injection: 250 mg (20 mL)

References

Rich MN, Woods WL, Davila-Roman VG, et al, "A Randomized Comparison of Intravenous Amrinone Versus Dobutamine in Older Patients With Decompensated Congestive Heart Failure," *J Am Geriatr Soc*, 1995, 43(3):271-4.

Dobutrex® see Dobutamine Hydrochloride *on this page*

Docusate (dok' yoo sate)

Brand Names Colace® [OTC]; Dialose® [OTC]; Diocto® [OTC]; Dioeze® [OTC]; Dionex® [OTC]; Diosuccin® [OTC]; Di-Sosul® [OTC]; Duosol® [OTC]; Surfak® [OTC]

Synonyms Dioctyl Calcium Sulfosuccinate; Dioctyl Sodium Sulfosuccinate; DOSS; DSS

Generic Available Yes

Therapeutic Class Laxative, Surfactant; Stool Softener

Use Stool softener in patients who should avoid straining during defecation and constipation associated with hard, dry stools; prophylaxis for straining (Valsalva) following myocardial infarction

Contraindications Concomitant use of mineral oil; intestinal obstruction, acute abdominal pain, nausea, vomiting; hypersensitivity to docusate or any component

Warnings Excessive use may lead to fluid and electrolyte balance

Adverse Reactions
Dermatologic: Rash
Gastrointestinal: Diarrhea, abdominal cramping
Miscellaneous: Throat irritation

Drug Interactions Mineral oil

Mechanism of Action Reduces surface tension of the oil-water interface of the stool resulting in enhanced incorporation of water and fat allowing for stool softening in small and large intestine; may also cause increased intestinal secretion

Pharmacodynamics Onset of action: 12-72 hours

Usual Dosage Geriatrics and Adults:
Oral: 100-400 mg/day in 1-4 divided doses
Rectal: Add 50-100 mg of docusate liquid to enema fluid (saline or water); give as retention or flushing enema

Patient Information Patients should assure proper dietary fiber and fluid intake with adequate exercise if medically appropriate; do not use if abdominal pain, nausea, or vomiting are present; laxative use should be used for a short period of time (<1 week); prolonged use may result in abuse, dependence, as well as fluid and electrolyte loss; notify physician if bleeding occurs or if constipation is not relieved

Nursing Implications Docusate liquid can be given with milk or fruit juice to mask the bitter taste

Additional Information Docusate salts are interchangeable; the amount of sodium, calcium, or potassium per dosage unit is clinically insignificant; should institute nonpharmacologic therapy (ie, fluid, fiber, exercise)

Special Geriatric Considerations A safe agent to be used in elderly; some evidence that doses <200 mg are ineffective; stool softeners are unnecessary if stool is well hydrated or "mushy" and soft; shown to be ineffective used long-term

Dosage Forms
Capsule: 50 mg, 60 mg, 100 mg, 240 mg, 250 mg, 300 mg
Solution: 10 mg/mL (30 mL, 480 mL); 50 mg/mL (60 mL, 4000 mL)
Syrup: 16.7 mg/5 mL (30 mL); 20 mg/5 mL (15 mL, 30 mL, 60 mL, 240 mL, 473 mL)
Tablet: 50 mg, 100 mg

Docusate and Casanthranol (dok' yoo sate & ka san' thra nole)

Related Information
Docusate *on previous page*

Brand Names Diocto-C® [OTC]; Diothron® [OTC]; Disanthrol® [OTC]; Peri-Colace® [OTC]; Peri-DOS® [OTC]

Synonyms Casanthranol and Docusate; DSS With Casanthranol

Generic Available Yes

Therapeutic Class Laxative, Surfactant; Stool Softener

Use Treatment of constipation generally associated with dry, hard stools and decreased intestinal motility

Contraindications Concomitant use of mineral oil; intestinal obstruction; acute abdominal pain; nausea, vomiting, appendicitis, acute surgical abdomen; hypersensitivity to docusate or casanthranol

Warnings Do not use when abdominal pain, nausea, or vomiting are present; excessive use may lead to fluid and electrolyte balance

Precautions Drug is habit-forming and may result in laxative dependence and loss of normal bowel function with prolonged use; rectal bleeding and failure to respond to therapy may require further evaluation; discoloration of urine may occur

Adverse Reactions
Gastrointestinal: Diarrhea, abdominal cramping, griping, nausea, vomiting, bloating, flatulence
Miscellaneous: Throat irritation, sweating

Overdosage Symptoms of overdose include fluid/electrolyte loss, hypotension, fatigue, lethargy, diarrhea, abdominal pain, nausea, vomiting

Drug Interactions Mineral oil

Stability Store in tight, light-resistant containers

Mechanism of Action Casanthranol has direct action on intestinal mucosa (colon) which stimulates the myenteric plexus, increases water and electrolyte secretion into intestine

Pharmacodynamics Onset of action: 6-12 hours after administration but may require up to 24 hours

Usual Dosage Adults: Oral: 1-2 capsules or 15-30 mL syrup at bedtime, may be increased to 2 capsules or 30 mL twice daily or 3 capsules at bedtime

(Continued)

Docusate and Casanthranol *(Continued)*

Monitoring Parameters Monitor stools daily or weekly; fluid/electrolyte status

Patient Information Patients should assure proper dietary fiber and fluid intake with adequate exercise if medically appropriate; do not use if abdominal pain, nausea, or vomiting are present; laxative use should be used for a short period of time (<1 week); prolonged use may result in abuse, dependence, as well as fluid and electrolyte loss; notify physician if bleeding occurs or if constipation is not relieved

Nursing Implications See Contraindications and Special Geriatric Considerations

Special Geriatric Considerations The chronic use of stimulant cathartics is inappropriate and should be avoided; although constipation is a common complaint from elderly, such complaints require evaluation; short term use of stimulants is best; if prophylaxis is desired, this can be accomplished with bulk agents (psyllium), stool softeners, and hyperosmotic agents (sorbitol 70%); stool softeners are unnecessary if stools are well hydrated, soft, or "mushy"

Dosage Forms

Capsule: Docusate sodium 100 mg and casanthranol 30 mg

Syrup: Docusate sodium 20 mg and casanthranol 10 mg per 5 mL (240 mL, 480 mL, 4000 mL)

Docusate and Phenolphthalein (dok' yoo sate & fee noe thay' leen)

Related Information

Docusate *on page 236*

Phenolphthalein *on page 556*

Brand Names Colax® [OTC]; Correctol® [OTC]; Disolan® Capsules [OTC]; Doxidan® [OTC]; Extra Gentle Ex-Lax® [OTC]; Feen-A-Mint® Pills [OTC]; FemiLax® [OTC]; Modane® Plus [OTC]; Phillips® LaxCaps® [OTC]; Unilax® [OTC]

Therapeutic Class Laxative, Stimulant; Laxative, Surfactant; Stool Softener

Use Management of chronic functional constipation

Contraindications Concomitant use of mineral oil; intestinal obstruction; acute abdominal pain; nausea, vomiting, appendicitis, acute surgical abdomen; hypersensitivity to docusate or phenolphthalein

Warnings Do not use when abdominal pain, nausea, or vomiting are present; excessive use may lead to fluid and electrolyte balance

Precautions Drug is habit-forming and may result in laxative dependence and loss of normal bowel function with prolonged use; rectal bleeding and failure to respond to therapy may require further evaluation; discoloration of urine may occur

Adverse Reactions

Gastrointestinal: Diarrhea, abdominal cramping, griping, nausea, vomiting, bloating, flatulence

Miscellaneous: Sweating, throat irritation, may discolor urine pink-red, red-violet, or red-brown

Overdosage Symptoms of overdose include fluid/electrolyte loss, hypotension, fatigue, lethargy

Drug Interactions Mineral oil

Mechanism of Action Has direct action on intestinal mucosa (colon) which stimulates the myenteric plexus, increases water and electrolyte secretion into intestine

Pharmacodynamics Onset of action: 6-12 hours after administration but may require up to 24 hours

Usual Dosage Geriatrics and Adults: Oral: 1-2 capsules/day given at bedtime for 2-3 nights until bowel movements are normal; use for <7 days is preferable

Monitoring Parameters Monitor stools daily or weekly; fluid/electrolyte status

Patient Information Patients should assure proper dietary fiber and fluid intake with adequate exercise if medically appropriate; do not use if abdominal pain, nausea, or vomiting are present; laxative use should be used for a short period of time (<1 week); prolonged use may result in abuse, dependence, as well as fluid and electrolyte loss; notify physician if bleeding occurs or if constipation is not relieved

Nursing Implications See Contraindications and Special Geriatric Considerations

Special Geriatric Considerations The chronic use of stimulant cathartics is inappropriate and should be avoided; although constipation is a common complaint from elderly, such complaints require evaluation; short term use of stimulants is best; if prophylaxis is desired, this can be accomplished with bulk agents (psyllium), stool softeners, and hyperosmotic agents (sorbitol 70%); stool softeners are unnecessary if stools are well hydrated, soft, or "mushy"

Dosage Forms

Capsule (Doxidan®): Docusate potassium 60 mg and phenolphthalein 65 mg

Tablet (Correctol®): Docusate sodium 100 mg and phenolphthalein 65 mg

Doktors® Nasal Solution [OTC] *see* Phenylephrine Hydrochloride *on page 557*

Dolacet® *see* Hydrocodone and Acetaminophen *on page 350*

Dolene® AP-65 *see* Propoxyphene and Acetaminophen *on page 604*

Dolobid® *see* Diflunisal *on page 218*

Dolophine® *see* Methadone Hydrochloride *on page 450*

Dommanate® *see* Dimenhydrinate *on page 227*

Donnapectolin®-PG *see* Hyoscyamine, Atropine, Scopolamine, Kaolin, Pectin and Opium *on page 358*

Donnatal® *see* Hyoscyamine, Atropine, Scopolamine and Phenobarbital *on page 357*

Dopamine Hydrochloride (doe' pa meen)

Brand Names Dopastat®; Intropin®

Generic Available Yes

Therapeutic Class Adrenergic Agonist Agent

Use Adjunct in the treatment of shock which persists after adequate fluid volume replacement; dose related inotropic and vasopressor effects; stimulates dopaminergic, beta- and alpha-receptors

Contraindications Hypersensitivity to sulfites (commercial preparation contains sodium bisulfite); pheochromocytoma, ventricular fibrillation, or uncorrected tachyarrhythmias

Warnings Potent drug; must be diluted prior to use. Patient's hemodynamic status should be monitored.

Precautions Hypovolemia should be corrected by appropriate plasma volume expanders before administration; closely monitor patients with a history of occlusive vascular disease; extravasation may cause tissue necrosis

Adverse Reactions
Cardiovascular: Ectopic heartbeats, tachycardia, vasoconstriction, hypotension, cardiac conduction abnormalities, widened QRS complex, bradycardia, hypertension, ventricular arrhythmias, gangrene of the extremities
Central nervous system: Anxiety, headache, piloerection
Gastrointestinal: Nausea, vomiting
Genitourinary: Decreased urine output, azotemia
Respiratory: Dyspnea

Overdosage Symptoms of overdose include severe hypertension, cardiac arrhythmias, acute renal failure

Toxicology Reduce rate of administration or discontinue infusion until condition stabilizes

Drug Interactions
Decreased effect: Tricyclic antidepressants
Increased effect/toxicity: MAO inhibitors, alpha- and beta-adrenergic blockers, general anesthetics, phenytoin

Stability Do not mix with alkaline solutions (bicarbonate); protect from light; do **not** use if solution is discolored
Stability of parenteral admixture at room temperature (25°C): 2 days (prepared); manufacturer's expiration date (premixed)
Stability of parenteral admixture at refrigeration temperature (4°C): 7 days (prepared)

Mechanism of Action Stimulates both adrenergic and dopaminergic receptors, lower doses are mainly dopaminergic stimulating and produces renal and mesenteric vasodilation, higher doses stimulate both dopaminergic and beta$_1$-adrenergic and produces cardiac stimulation and renal vasodilation, large doses stimulate alpha-adrenergic receptors

Pharmacodynamics
Onset of action: 5 minutes upon administration
Duration of action: <10 minutes

Pharmacokinetics
Metabolism: In plasma, kidneys, and liver 75% to inactive metabolites by monoamine oxidase and 25% to norepinephrine (active)
Half-life: 2 minutes
Elimination: In urine; clearance is more prolonged with combined hepatic and renal dysfunction

Usual Dosage I.V. infusion:
Geriatrics and Adults: 1 mcg/kg/minute up to 50 mcg/kg/minute, titrate to desired response; administer with an infusion device to control flow rate

If dosages >20-30 mcg/kg/minute are needed, a more direct-acting pressor may be more beneficial (ie, epinephrine, norepinephrine)

The hemodynamic effects of dopamine are dose-dependent:
Low dose: 1-5 mcg/kg/minute, increased renal blood flow and urine output
Intermediate dose: 5-15 mcg/kg/minute, increased renal blood flow, heart rate, cardiac contractility, and cardiac output

(Continued)

Dopamine Hydrochloride *(Continued)*

High dose: > 15 mcg/kg/minute, alpha-adrenergic effects begin to predominate, vasoconstriction, increased blood pressure

Administration Administer into large vein to prevent the possibility of extravasation; monitor continuously for free flow; use infusion device to control rate of flow; add 200-400 mg to 250-500 mL of D$_5$W, NS, D$_5$NS, D$_5$^{1}/$_2$NS, D$_5$LR, LR, or Normosol® to dilute

Monitoring Parameters Urine output, cardiac hemodynamic status, blood pressure, EKG, pulse

Nursing Implications When discontinuing the infusion, gradually decrease the dose of dopamine

Additional Information Important: Antidote for peripheral ischemia: To prevent sloughing and necrosis in ischemic areas, the area should be infiltrated as soon as possible with 10-15 mL of saline solution containing from 5-10 mg of Regitine® (brand of phentolamine), an adrenergic blocking agent. A syringe with a fine hypodermic needle should be used, and the solution liberally infiltrated throughout the ischemic area. Sympathetic blockade with phentolamine causes immediate and conspicuous local hyperemic changes if the area is infiltrated within 12 hours. Therefore, phentolamine should be given as soon as possible after the extravasation is noted.

Special Geriatric Considerations Has not been specifically studied in the elderly; monitor closely, especially due to increase in cardiovascular disease with age

Dosage Forms

Infusion: 0.8 mg/mL in D$_5$W (250 mL, 500 mL); 1.6 mg/mL in D$_5$W (250 mL, 500 mL); 3.2 mg/mL in D$_5$W (250 mL, 500 mL)

Injection: 40 mg/mL (5 mL, 10 mL, 20 mL); 80 mg/mL (5 mL, 20 mL); 160 mg/mL (5 mL)

Dopar® *see* Levodopa *on page 402*

Dopastat® *see* Dopamine Hydrochloride *on previous page*

Dopram® *see* Doxapram Hydrochloride *on this page*

Doral® *see* Quazepam *on page 614*

Dorcol® [OTC] *see* Acetaminophen *on page 13*

Doryx® *see* Doxycycline *on page 243*

DOSS *see* Docusate *on page 236*

Dovonex® *see* Calcipotriene *on page 104*

Doxapram Hydrochloride (dox' a pram)

Brand Names Dopram®

Therapeutic Class Central Nervous System Stimulant, Nonamphetamine; Respiratory Stimulant

Use Respiratory and CNS stimulant; stimulate respiration in patients with drug-induced CNS depression or postanesthesia respiratory depression; in hospitalized patients with COPD associated with acute hypercapnia

Contraindications Hypersensitivity to doxapram or any component; epilepsy, cerebral edema, head injury, severe pulmonary disease, pheochromocytoma, cardiovascular disease, hypertension, hyperthyroidism

Warnings Assure an adequate airway and oxygenation; may only serve as an adjunct therapy in persons with severe respiratory depression

Precautions May cause severe CNS toxicity, seizures

Adverse Reactions

Cardiovascular: Hypertension (dose related), tachycardia, ectopic beats, arrhythmias, hypotension, flushing, feeling of warmth, vasoconstriction

Central nervous system: CNS stimulation, restlessness, lightheadedness, jitters, hallucinations, irritability, seizures, headache, hyperpyrexia

Gastrointestinal: Abdominal distension, nausea, vomiting, retching

Genitourinary: Urinary retention

Hematologic: Hemolysis

Local: Phlebitis

Neuromuscular & skeletal: Hyperreflexia, bilateral Babinski, tremors

Ocular: Lacrimation, mydriasis

Respiratory: Coughing, laryngospasm, dyspnea

Miscellaneous: Sweating

Overdosage Symptoms of overdose include tachycardia, dyspnea, hypertension

Toxicology Supportive care is the preferred treatment; seizures are unlikely and can be treated with benzodiazepines

Drug Interactions Sympathomimetic drugs and MAO inhibitors may cause significant elevation in blood pressure; doxapram may mask effects of muscle relaxants; halothane, cyclopropane, and enflurane may sensitize the myocardium to catecholamine and epinephrine which is released at the initiation of doxapram, hence, separate discontinuation of anesthetics and start of doxapram by at least 10 minutes

Stability Incompatible with aminophylline, thiopental, or sodium bicarbonate (alkali drugs)

Mechanism of Action Stimulates respiration through action on peripheral carotid chemoreceptors and at higher doses on respiratory center in medulla

Pharmacodynamics
Onset of respiratory stimulation: I.V.: 20-40 seconds
Peak effect: Within 1-2 minutes
Duration: 5-12 minutes

Pharmacokinetics
Metabolism: In the liver
Half-life: Mean: 3.4 hours
Elimination: In urine as metabolites within 24-48 hours

Usual Dosage Geriatrics and Adults: I.V.:
Respiratory depression following anesthesia:
Initial: 0.5-1 mg/kg; may repeat at 5-minute intervals; maximum total dose: 2 mg/kg
I.V. infusion: Initial: 5 mg/minute until adequate response or adverse effects seen; decrease to 1-3 mg/minute; usual total dose: 0.5-4 mg/kg; maximum: 300 mg
Drug-induced CNS depression: Priming dose of 2 mg/kg and repeat in 5 minutes; repeat every 1-2 hours until patient wakes up; if patient relapses, then resume injections every 1-2 hours until patient awakens or maximum daily dose of 3 g is given
COPD with acute hypercapnia: Start an infusion of 1-2 mg/minute and increase to a maximum of 3 mg/minute

Administration Dilute to 1 mg/mL in D_5W or NS for continuous infusion; rotate infusion site on a regular basis to prevent phlebitis

Monitoring Parameters Blood pressure and deep tendon reflexes; arterial blood gas, respiratory rate

Nursing Implications See Administration

Special Geriatric Considerations Has not been studied in the elderly; see Adverse Reactions and Warnings

Dosage Forms Injection: 20 mg/mL (20 mL)

Doxazosin (dox ay' zoe sin)
Brand Names Cardura®
Generic Available No
Therapeutic Class Alpha-Adrenergic Blocking Agent, Oral
Use Alpha-blocking agent for treatment of hypertension

Unlabeled use: Symptoms of benign prostatic hypertrophy

Contraindications Hypersensitivity to doxazosin or any component

Warnings Can cause marked hypotension and syncope with sudden loss of consciousness with the first few doses. Anticipate a similar effect if therapy is interrupted for a few days, if dosage is increased rapidly, or if another antihypertensive drug is introduced.

Precautions Use with caution in patients with renal impairment, patients receiving first dose, or dosage increase of doxazosin

Adverse Reactions
Cardiovascular: Syncope, palpitations, edema, tachycardia
Central nervous system: Dizziness, lightheadedness, drowsiness, headache
Dermatologic: Rash
Gastrointestinal: Nausea, dry mouth
Genitourinary: Urinary frequency or incontinence
Neuromuscular & skeletal: Weakness

Overdosage Symptoms of overdose include severe hypotension, drowsiness, tachycardia

Toxicology Hypotension usually responds to I.V. fluids or Trendelenburg positioning. If unresponsive to these measures, the use of a parenteral vasoconstrictor may be required (eg, norepinephrine 0.1-0.2 mcg/kg/minute titrated to response). Treatment is primarily supportive and symptomatic.

Drug Interactions Increased effect with other antihypertensive agents

Mechanism of Action Competitively inhibits postsynaptic alpha-adrenergic receptors which results in vasodilation of veins and arterioles and a decrease in total peripheral resistance and blood pressure

Pharmacodynamics
Peak effect: Occurs 2-6 hours after a dose
Duration of effect: 24 hours

Pharmacokinetics Increased age does not significantly affect pharmacokinetics of doxazosin
Protein binding: 98%
Metabolism: Extensive in the liver
Half-life: 22 hours
Time to peak serum concentration: 2-3 hours

Usual Dosage Oral:
Geriatrics: Initial: 0.5 mg once daily
Adults: 1 mg once daily, may be increased to 2 mg once daily thereafter up to 16 mg if needed

(Continued)

241

Doxazosin *(Continued)*

Monitoring Parameters Blood pressure, standing and sitting/supine

Patient Information Rise from sitting/lying carefully; may cause dizziness; take the first dose at bedtime

Nursing Implications Syncope may occur, usually within 90 minutes of the initial dose

Additional Information First-dose hypotension occurs less frequently with doxazosin as compared to prazosin; this may be due to its slower onset of action

Special Geriatric Considerations Adverse reactions such as dry mouth and urinary problems can be particularly bothersome in the elderly; see Warnings

Dosage Forms Tablet: 1 mg, 2 mg, 4 mg, 8 mg

Doxepin Hydrochloride (dox' e pin)

Related Information

Antidepressant Agents Comparison *on page 800*

Brand Names Adapin®; Sinequan®

Generic Available Yes

Therapeutic Class Antianxiety Agent; Antidepressant, Tricyclic

Use Treatment of various forms of depression, usually in conjunction with psychotherapy; treatment of anxiety disorders; analgesic for certain chronic and neuropathic pain

Contraindications Hypersensitivity to doxepin or any component (cross-sensitivity with other tricyclic antidepressants may occur); narrow-angle glaucoma

Warnings Do not discontinue abruptly in patients receiving chronic high dose therapy

Precautions Use with caution in patients with cardiovascular disease, conduction disturbances, seizure disorders, urinary retention, hyperthyroidism or those receiving thyroid replacement; an EKG prior to the start of therapy is advised

Adverse Reactions Pronounced sedation and anticholinergic adverse effects may occur

Cardiovascular: Hypotension, arrhythmias

Central nervous system: Sedation, confusion, dizziness, delirium

Dermatologic: Photosensitivity

Endocrine & metabolic: SIADH

Gastrointestinal: Constipation, nausea, vomiting, dry mouth, weight gain

Genitourinary: Urinary retention

Hematologic: Blood dyscrasias

Hepatic: Hepatitis

Neuromuscular & skeletal: Associated with falls

Ocular: Blurred vision, increased intraocular pressure

Otic: Tinnitus

Miscellaneous: Hypersensitivity

Overdosage Symptoms of overdose include confusion, hallucinations, seizure, urinary retention, hypothermia, hypotension, tachycardia, cyanosis

Toxicology Following initiation of essential overdose management, toxic symptoms should be treated. Ventricular arrhythmias often respond to phenytoin 15-20 mg/kg with concurrent systemic alkalinization (sodium bicarbonate 0.5-2 mEq/kg I.V.). Arrhythmias unresponsive to this therapy may respond to lidocaine 1 mg/kg I.V. followed by a titrated infusion. Physostigmine (1-2 mg I.V. slowly) may be indicated in reversing cardiac arrhythmias that are due to vagal blockade or for anticholinergic effects. Seizures usually respond to diazepam I.V. boluses (5-10 mg, up to 30 mg). If seizures are unresponsive or recur, phenytoin or phenobarbital may be required.

Drug Interactions

Decreased effect of bretylium, guanethidine, clonidine, levodopa; decreased effect with ascorbic acid, cholestyramine

Increased effect/toxicity of carbamazepine, amphetamines, thyroid preparations, sympathomimetics

Increased toxicity with fluoxetine (seizures), thyroid preparations, MAO inhibitors, albuterol, CNS depressants (ie, benzodiazepines, opiate analgesics, phenothiazines, alcohol), anticholinergics, cimetidine

Stability Protect from light

Mechanism of Action Traditionally believed to increase the synaptic concentration of serotonin and/or norepinephrine in the central nervous system by inhibition of their reuptake by the presynaptic neuronal membrane. However, additional receptor effects have been found including desensitization of adenyl cyclase, down regulation of beta-adrenergic receptors, and down regulation of serotonin receptors

Pharmacodynamics Maximum antidepressant effects usually occur after more than 2 weeks; anxiolytic effects may occur sooner; 5-HT >NE

Pharmacokinetics

Protein binding: 80% to 85%

Metabolism: Hepatically to metabolites, including desmethyldoxepin (active)

Half-life: 6-8 hours

Elimination: Renal

Usual Dosage Oral:

Geriatrics: Initial: 10-25 mg at bedtime; increase by 10-25 mg every 3 days for inpatients and weekly for outpatients if tolerated; rarely does the maximum dose required exceed 75 mg/day; a single bedtime dose is recommended

Adults: Initial: 30-150 mg/day at bedtime or in 2-3 divided doses; may increase up to 300 mg/day; single dose should not exceed 150 mg; select patients may respond to 25-50 mg/day

Reference Range Therapeutic: >110 ng/mL for sum of doxepin and desmethyl-doxepin; Toxic: >500 ng/mL

Test Interactions Elevated glucose

Patient Information Avoid unnecessary exposure to sunlight; avoid alcohol ingestion; do not discontinue medication abruptly; may cause urine to turn blue-green; may cause drowsiness, dry mouth, sedation, urinary retention, blurred vision; rise slowly to prevent dizziness

Nursing Implications Monitor sitting and standing blood pressure and pulse rate prior to and during initial therapy; evaluate mental status; monitor weight, may increase appetite

Additional Information Entire daily dose may be given at bedtime; avoid unnecessary exposure to sunlight

Special Geriatric Considerations Preferred agent when sedation is a desired property; less anticholinergic than amitriptyline and less orthostatic hypotension than imipramine. The pharmacokinetics of doxepin have not been studied in older patients.

Dosage Forms
Capsule: 10 mg, 25 mg, 50 mg, 75 mg, 100 mg, 150 mg
Concentrate, oral: 10 mg/mL (120 mL)

References
Lakshmanan M, Mion LC, and Frengley JD, "Effective Low Dose Tricyclic Antidepressant Treatment for Depressed Geriatric Rehabilitation Patients. A Double-Blind Study," *J Am Geriatr Soc*, 1986, 34(6):421-6.

Doxidan® [OTC] *see* Docusate and Phenolphthalein *on page 238*

Doxy-200® *see* Doxycycline *on this page*

Doxy-Caps® *see* Doxycycline *on this page*

Doxychel® *see* Doxycycline *on this page*

Doxycycline (dox i sye' kleen)

Brand Names Doryx®; Doxy-200®; Doxy-Caps®; Doxychel®; Doxy-Tabs®; Vibramycin®; Vibra-Tabs®

Synonyms Doxycycline Hyclate; Doxycycline Monohydrate

Generic Available Yes

Therapeutic Class Antibiotic, Tetracycline Derivative

Use Principally in the treatment of infections caused by susceptible *Rickettsia*, *Chlamydia*, and *Mycoplasma* along with uncommon susceptible gram-negative and gram-positive organisms; unapproved use as treatment for syphilis in penicillin allergic patients or traveler's diarrhea

Contraindications Hypersensitivity to doxycycline, tetracycline or any component; severe hepatic dysfunction

Warnings Photosensitivity reaction may occur with this drug; avoid prolonged exposure to sunlight or tanning equipment

Precautions Prolonged use may result in superinfection

Adverse Reactions
Central nervous system: Increased intracranial pressure
Dermatologic: Rash, photosensitivity
Gastrointestinal: Nausea, diarrhea, esophagitis
Hematologic: Neutropenia, eosinophilia
Hepatic: Hepatotoxicity
Local: Phlebitis

Overdosage Symptoms of overdose include photosensitivity, nausea, anorexia, diarrhea

Toxicology Following GI decontamination, supportive care only; fluid support may be required for hypotension

Drug Interactions
Antacids containing aluminum, calcium or magnesium, iron and bismuth subsalicylate may decrease doxycycline bioavailability
Barbiturates, phenytoin, and carbamazepine decrease doxycycline's half-life
Effects of warfarin may be increased

Stability Tetracyclines form toxic products when outdated or when exposed to light, heat, or humidity; reconstituted solution is stable for 72 hours (refrigerated); for I.V. infusion in NS or D_5W solution, complete infusion should be completed within 12 hours; discard remaining solution

Mechanism of Action Inhibits protein synthesis by binding with the 30S and possibly the 50S ribosomal subunits of susceptible bacteria; may also cause alterations in the cytoplasmic membrane

(Continued)

Doxycycline *(Continued)*

Pharmacokinetics

Absorption: Almost completely from GI tract; can be reduced by food or milk by 20%

Protein binding: 90%

Metabolism: Not metabolized in the liver, instead partially inactivated in GI tract by chelate formation

Half-life: 12-15 hours (usually increases to 22-24 hours with multiple dosing); may be slightly increased and serum and tissue concentrations have been reported to be higher in the elderly

Time to peak: Peak serum levels occur within 1.5-4 hours

Elimination: Urine (23%), feces (30%)

Usual Dosage Geriatrics and Adults: Oral, I.V.: 100-200 mg/day in 1-2 divided doses

Sclerosing agent for pleural effusion injection: 500 mg as a single dose in 30-50 mL of NS or SWI

Not dialyzable (0% to 5%)

Administration Infuse I.V. doxycycline over 1 hour; do not give with antacids, iron products, or dairy products

Monitoring Parameters Signs and symptoms of infection including mental status

Test Interactions False-negative urine glucose using Clinistix®, Tes-Tape®

Patient Information Avoid unnecessary exposure to sunlight; do not take with antacids, iron products, or dairy products; complete full course of therapy

Nursing Implications See Administration

Additional Information

Doxycycline hyclate: Oral suspension

Doxycycline monohydrate: Capsule, tablet, and injection

Special Geriatric Considerations See Pharmacokinetics; dose adjustment for renal function is not necessary

Dosage Forms

Capsule, as hyclate: 50 mg, 100 mg

Capsule, coated pellets, as hyclate: 100 mg

Injection, as hyclate: 100 mg, 200 mg

Suspension, as monohydrate: 25 mg/5 mL (60 mL)

Syrup, as calcium: 50 mg/5 mL (30 mL, 473 mL)

Tablet, as hyclate: 50 mg, 100 mg

References

Böcker R, Mühlberg W, Platt D, et al, "Serum Level, Half-Life and Apparent Volume of Distribution of Doxycycline in Geriatric Patients," *Eur J Clin Pharmacol*, 1986, 30(1):105-8.

Ljungberg B and Nilsson-Ehle I, "Pharmacokinetics of Antimicrobial Agents in the Elderly," *Rev Infect Dis*, 1987, 9(2):250-64.

Doxycycline Hyclate *see Doxycycline on previous page*

Doxycycline Monohydrate *see Doxycycline on previous page*

Doxy-Tabs® *see Doxycycline on previous page*

DPA *see Valproic Acid and Derivatives on page 728*

DPE *see Dipivefrin on page 232*

D-Penicillamine *see Penicillamine on page 537*

DPH *see Phenytoin on page 559*

Dramamine® [OTC] *see Dimenhydrinate on page 227*

Dramilin® *see Dimenhydrinate on page 227*

Dramocen® *see Dimenhydrinate on page 227*

Dramoject® *see Dimenhydrinate on page 227*

Dr Caldwell Senna Laxative® [OTC] *see Senna on page 641*

Drisdol® *see Ergocalciferol on page 259*

Dristan® Long Lasting Nasal Solution [OTC] *see Oxymetazoline Hydrochloride on page 530*

Droperidol *(droe per' i dole)*

Related Information

Antipsychotic Medication Guidelines *on page 754*

Brand Names Inapsine®

Generic Available Yes

Therapeutic Class Antiemetic; Antipsychotic Agent

Use Tranquilizer and antiemetic in surgical and diagnostic procedures; antiemetic for cancer chemotherapy; preoperative medication

Contraindications Hypersensitivity to droperidol or any component of droperidol; since this is a butyrophenone derivative, caution should be used in patients with a hypersensitivity to haloperidol

Warnings

Tardive dyskinesia: Prevalence rate may be 40% in elderly; elderly women especially at risk; embarrassment from dyskinesias may lead to greater social isolation; development of the syndrome and the irreversible nature are proportional to duration and total cumulative dose over time. May be reversible if diagnosed early in therapy; intermittent use of antipsychotics (not proven use) helps decrease total cumulative dose.

EPS: Extrapyramidal reactions are more common in elderly with up to 50% developing these reactions after age 60. These reactions may be more common in dementia patients. Drug-induced **Parkinson's syndrome** occurs often. Discontinuation usually resolves symptoms but may take weeks to months (12+) to clear. **Akathisia** is the most common EPS reaction in elderly. The symptoms of motor restlessness are difficult to diagnose in demented elderly; increased nervousness, assertiveness, restlessness with constant movement may indicate this adverse event. Consider decreasing dose if antipsychotic to treat as well as diagnose problem; usually see this reaction within 2-3 months of initiating antipsychotic drug.

Anticholinergic effects: These side effects most common with low potency antipsychotics (eg, thioridazine, chlorpromazine). CNS toxicity occurs more frequently and severely in elderly; increased confusion, memory loss, psychotic behavior, and agitation frequently occur as a consequence of anticholinergic effects to antipsychotic agents. Peripheral anticholinergic action troublesome to elderly; most peripheral anticholinergic effects last only 2-3 weeks; see Adverse Reactions.

Orthostatic hypotension: More common with low potency agents (eg, thioridazine, chlorpromazine, and clozapine) but of concern with all antipsychotic agents; orthostasis due to alpha-receptor blockade by antipsychotic agents. Elderly present many risk factors for orthostatic hypotension: blunted baroreceptor reflexes, decreased vascular tone, decreased vascular volume, and possible presence of cardiac diseases which result in decreased cardiac output.

Sedation: Common side effect with antipsychotic therapy; should not be used as a hypnotic unless insomnia is associated with target behavior symptoms treated with antipsychotic medications; see Special Geriatric Considerations. Anecdotal reports suggesting antipsychotic sedation in nonpsychotic patients is extremely unpleasant due to feelings of depersonalization, derealization, and dysphoria. Due to the long duration of action with antipsychotic drugs, these reactions may last up to 24 hours and result in decreased daytime function.

Cardiac toxicity: Life-threatening arrhythmias have occurred at therapeutic doses of antipsychotics. Thioridazine more commonly demonstrates EKG changes than other antipsychotics; suggested to use high potency antipsychotic agents (ie, haloperidol) in patients with cardiac conduction defects.

Precautions May cause severe hypotension; use with caution in patients with hepatic or renal insufficiency; watch for hypotension when administering I.M. or I.V.; use with caution in patients with cardiovascular disease, seizures, and Parkinson's disease; benefits of therapy must be weighed against risks of therapy

Adverse Reactions

Cardiovascular: Hypotension, tachycardia

Central nervous system: Dystonic reactions, akathisia, anxiety, hyperactivity, drowsiness, dizziness, hallucinations, chills

Ocular: Oculogyric crisis

Respiratory: Laryngospasm, bronchospasm, respiratory depression

Overdosage Symptoms of overdose include hypotension, tachycardia, hallucinations, extrapyramidal symptoms; administer O_2 if hypoventilation or apnea present; assist respiratory function as needed; maintain fluid intake; maintain body warmth; observe for 24 hours; see Toxicology

Toxicology Following initiation of essential overdose management, toxic symptom treatment and supportive treatment should be initiated. Hypotension usually responds to I.V. fluids or Trendelenburg positioning. If unresponsive to these measures the use of a parenteral inotrope may be required (eg, norepinephrine 0.1-0.2 mcg/kg/minute titrated to response). Do not use epinephrine. Seizures commonly respond to diazepam (I.V. 5-10 mg bolus every 15 minutes if needed up to a total of 30 mg) or to phenytoin or phenobarbital. Also critical cardiac arrhythmias often respond to I.V. phenytoin (15 mg/kg up to 1 g), while other antiarrhythmics can be used. Neuroleptics often cause extrapyramidal symptoms (eg, dystonic reactions) requiring management with diphenhydramine 1-2 mg/kg up to a maximum of 50 mg I.M. or I.V. slow push followed by a maintenance dose for 48-72 hours. When these reactions are unresponsive to diphenhydramine, benztropine mesylate I.V. 1-2 mg may be effective. These agents are generally effective within 2-5 minutes.

Drug Interactions

Other CNS depressants → additive effects (CNS, respiratory depression, etc)

Droperidol plus fentanyl or other other analgesics → ↑ blood pressure

Induction anesthesia may increase hypotension; droperidol plus epinephrine → ↓ blood pressure due to alpha-adrenergic blockade effects of droperidol

(Continued)

Droperidol *(Continued)*

Stability Stable in D_5W for injection; 0.9% sodium chloride for injection and lactated Ringer's for injection for 7-10 days in glass bottles and 7 days for plastic bags

Mechanism of Action Alters the action of dopamine in the CNS, at subcortical levels, to produce sedation; produces mild alpha-adrenergic blockade resulting in decreased peripheral blood pressure and possibly pulmonary artery pressure; may reduce epinephrine-induced arrhythmias

Pharmacodynamics

Onset of action: I.M., I.V.: 3-10 minutes

Peak effect: Parenteral: Within 30 minutes

Duration: 2-4 hours (may extend to 12 hours)

Pharmacokinetics

Metabolism: In the liver

Half-life: 2.3 hours

Elimination: In urine (75%) and feces (22%); ~1% excreted in urine unchanged

Usual Dosage

Geriatrics: Elderly patients should be started on lowest dose recommendations for adults; titrate carefully to desired effect

Adults:

Premedication: I.M.: 2.5-10 mg 30 minutes to 1 hour preoperatively

Adjunct to general anesthesia: I.V. induction: 0.22-0.275 mg/kg; maintenance: 1.25-2.5 mg/dose

Alone in diagnostic procedures: I.M.: Initial: 2.5-10 mg 30 minutes to 1 hour before; then 1.25-2.5 mg if needed

Nausea and vomiting: I.M., I.V.: 2.5-5 mg/dose every 3-4 hours as needed

Monitoring Parameters Monitor blood pressure, respiratory rate; observe for dystonias, extrapyramidal side effects, and temperature changes

Nursing Implications Administration recommendations for all doses: I.V.: Over 2-5 minutes; see Monitoring Parameters

Additional Information Has good antiemetic effect as well as sedative and antianxiety effects

Special Geriatric Considerations See Warnings

Many elderly patients receive antipsychotic medications for inappropriate nonpsychotic behavior. Before initiating antipsychotic medication, the clinician should investigate any possible reversible cause; any stress or stress from any disease can cause acute "confusion" or worsening of baseline nonpsychotic behavior. Most commonly acute changes in behavior are due to increases in drug dose or addition of new drug to regimen; fluid electrolyte loss; infections; and changes in environment.

Any changes in disease status in any organ system can result in behavior changes.

Dosage Forms Injection: 2.5 mg/mL (1 mL, 2 mL, 5 mL, 10 mL)

Drug Levels Commonly Monitored Guidelines *see page 771*

DSCG *see* Cromolyn Sodium *on page 190*

DSS *see* Docusate *on page 236*

DSS With Casanthranol *see* Docusate and Casanthranol *on page 237*

DT *see* Diphtheria and Tetanus Toxoid *on page 231*

Dulcolax® [OTC] *see* Bisacodyl *on page 87*

DuoCet™ *see* Hydrocodone and Acetaminophen *on page 350*

Duolube® [OTC] *see* Ocular Lubricant *on page 515*

Duosol® [OTC] *see* Docusate *on page 236*

Duo-Trach® *see* Lidocaine Hydrochloride *on page 406*

Duotrate® *see* Pentaerythritol Tetranitrate *on page 543*

Duotrate® 45 *see* Pentaerythritol Tetranitrate *on page 543*

Duphalac® *see* Lactulose *on page 397*

Duracillin® A.S. *see* Penicillin G Procaine, Aqueous *on page 541*

Dura-Estrin® *see* Estradiol *on page 269*

Duragen® *see* Estradiol *on page 269*

Duragesic™ *see* Fentanyl *on page 284*

Duralone® *see* Methylprednisolone *on page 461*

Duramorph® *see* Morphine Sulfate *on page 481*

Duraphyl™ *see* Theophylline *on page 681*

Duraquin® *see* Quinidine *on page 618*

Duratears® [OTC] *see* Ocular Lubricant *on page 515*

Duration® Nasal Solution [OTC] *see* Oxymetazoline Hydrochloride
on page 530

Duricef® *see* Cefadroxil Monohydrate *on page 125*

Duvoid® *see* Bethanechol Chloride *on page 85*

Dyazide® *see* Hydrochlorothiazide and Triamterene *on page 349*

Dycill® *see* Dicloxacillin Sodium *on page 214*

Dymelor® *see* Acetohexamide *on page 17*

Dymenate® *see* Dimenhydrinate *on page 227*

DynaCirc® *see* Isradipine *on page 385*

Dynapen® *see* Dicloxacillin Sodium *on page 214*

Dyphylline (dye' fi lin)

Brand Names Dilor®; Lufyllin®; Neothylline®

Synonyms Dihydroxypropyl Theophylline

Generic Available Yes

Therapeutic Class Bronchodilator; Theophylline Derivative

Use Bronchodilator in reversible airway obstruction due to asthma or COPD

Contraindications Hypersensitivity to xanthines; peptic ulcer, uncontrolled seizure disorders, uncontrolled arrhythmias, hyperthyroidism

Warnings May precipitate or worsen existing arrhythmias

Precautions Use with caution in patients with peptic ulcer, hyperthyroidism, hypertension, and patients with compromised cardiac function; hepatic function, esophageal reflux disease, alcoholism, and elderly

Adverse Reactions

Cardiovascular: Palpitations, sinus tachycardia, extrasystoles, hypotension, ventricular arrhythmias, flushing

Central nervous system: Irritability, restlessness, fever, headache, insomnia, seizures

Endocrine & metabolic: Hyperglycemia

Gastrointestinal: Nausea, vomiting, esophageal reflux, diarrhea, hematemesis, rectal bleeding, epigastric pain

Neuromuscular & skeletal: Muscle twitching, tremors

Renal: Proteinuria, diuresis

Respiratory: Tachypnea, respiratory arrest

Adverse reactions are uncommon at serum theophylline concentrations <20 mcg/mL

Overdosage Symptoms of overdose include tachycardia, extrasystoles, nausea, vomiting, anorexia, tonic-clonic seizures, insomnia, circulatory failure; agitation, irritability, headache

Toxicology If seizures have not occurred, induce vomiting; ipecac syrup is preferred. Do not induce emesis in the presence of impaired consciousness. Repeated doses of charcoal have been shown to be effective in enhancing the total body clearance of theophylline. Do not repeat charcoal doses if an ileus is present. Charcoal hemoperfusion may be considered if the serum theophylline level exceed 40 mcg/mL, the patient is unable to tolerate repeated oral charcoal administrations, or if severe toxic symptoms are present. Clearance with hemoperfusion is better than clearance from hemodialysis. Administer a cathartic, especially if sustained release agents were used. Phenobarbital administered prophylactically may prevent seizures.

Drug Interactions

Theophylline may decrease the effects of phenytoin, lithium, and neuromuscular blocking agents; theophylline may have synergistic toxicity with sympathomimetics

Cimetidine, ranitidine, allopurinol, beta-blockers (nonspecific), erythromycin, influenza virus vaccine, corticosteroids, ephedrine, quinolones, thyroid hormones, oral contraceptives, amiodarone, troleandomycin, clindamycin, carbamazepine, isoniazid, loop diuretics, and lincomycin may increase theophylline concentrations

Cigarette and marijuana smoking, rifampin, barbiturates, hydantoins, ketoconazole, sulfinpyrazone, sympathomimetics, isoniazid, loop diuretics, carbamazepine, and aminoglutethimide may decrease theophylline concentrations

Tetracyclines enhance toxicity and benzodiazepine's action may be antagonized

Mechanism of Action Causes bronchodilatation, diuresis, CNS and cardiac stimulation, and gastric acid secretion by blocking phosphodiesterase which increases tissue concentrations of cyclic adenine monophosphate (cAMP) which in turn promotes catecholamine stimulation of lipolysis, glycogenolysis, and gluconeogenesis and induces release of epinephrine from adrenal medulla cells. Other proposed mechanisms include inhibition of extracellular adenosine, stimulation of endogenous catecholamines, antagonism of PGE_2 and $PGE_{2\alpha}$, mobilization of intracellular calcium, and increased sensitivity of beta-adrenergic receptors in reactive airways.

Pharmacodynamics Dyphylline use may result in fewer adverse drug reactions than theophylline salts; however, blood levels and drug response are lower

Pharmacokinetics Dyphylline is a derivative of theophylline and is not a salt of theophylline. Dyphylline is **not** metabolized to theophylline *in vivo*. Dyphylline is 70% by

(Continued)

247

Dyphylline *(Continued)*

weight theophylline, however, the amount for equivalency is not known. Specific dyphylline serum concentrations must be used to monitor therapy since serum theophylline concentration analysis will **not** measure dyphylline. The minimal effective serum concentration is 12 mcg/mL.

Usual Dosage Geriatrics and Adults:
Oral: Up to 15 mg/kg 4 times/day, individualize dosage
I.M.: 250-500 mg, do not exceed total dosage of 15 mg/kg every 6 hours

Monitoring Parameters Heart rate, CNS effects (insomnia, irritability); respiratory rate (COPD patients often have resting controlled respiratory rates in low 20's)

Reference Range Minimum effective level: 12 μg/mL

Patient Information Oral preparations should be taken with a full glass of water; avoid drinking or eating large quantities of caffeine-containing beverages or food; take at regular intervals; take with food if GI upset occurs; notify physician if nausea, vomiting, insomnia, nervousness, irritability, palpitations, seizures occur; do not change from one brand to another without consulting physician and pharmacist; do not change doses without consulting your physician

Nursing Implications Not for I.V. administration, inject slowly; give oral administration around-the-clock rather than 4 times/day, 3 times/day, etc (ie, 12-6-12-6, not 9-1-5-9) to promote less variation in peak and trough serum levels; monitor vital signs, serum concentrations, and CNS effects (insomnia, irritability); encourage patient to drink adequate fluids (2 L/day) to decrease mucous viscosity in airways

Additional Information This drug is rarely used today. Requires a special laboratory measuring procedure rather than the standard theophylline assay. Saliva levels are approximately equal to 60% of plasma levels; charcoal-broiled foods may increase elimination, reducing half-life by 50%; cigarette smoking may require an increase of dosage by 50% to 100%. Because different salts of theophylline have different theophylline content, various salts are not equivalent.

The following are percent content of theophylline for various salts:
Theophylline anhydrous: 100%
Theophylline monohydrate: 91%
Aminophylline anhydrous: 86%
Oxtriphylline: 64%

Special Geriatric Considerations Although there is a great intersubject variability for half-lives of methylxanthines (2-10 hours), the elderly as a group have slower hepatic clearance. Therefore, use lower initial doses and monitor closely for response and adverse reactions. Additionally, elderly are at greater risk for toxicity due to concomitant disease (eg, congestive heart failure, arrhythmias), and drug use (eg, cimetidine, ciprofloxacin, etc); see Precautions and Drug Interactions

Dosage Forms
Elixir: 100 mg/15 mL, 160 mg/15 mL
Injection, I.M. only: 250 mg/mL (10 mL)
Tablet: 200 mg, 400 mg

Dyrenium® *see* Triamterene *on page 712*

Easprin® *see* Aspirin *on page 58*

Echothiophate Iodide *(ek oh thye' oh fate)*
Related Information
Glaucoma Drug Therapy Comparison *on page 810*
Brand Names Phospholine Iodide®
Synonyms Ecostigmine Iodide
Therapeutic Class Ophthalmic Agent, Miotic
Use Reverse toxic CNS effects caused by anticholinergic drugs; used as miotic in treatment of open-angle glaucoma; may be useful in specific case of narrow-angle glaucoma; accommodative esotropia

Contraindications Hypersensitivity to echothiophate or any component; most cases of angle-closure glaucoma; active uveal inflammation or any inflammatory disease of the iris or ciliary body, glaucoma associated with iridocyclitis; GI or GU obstruction, asthma, diabetes, gangrene

Warnings Tolerance may develop after prolonged use; a rest period restores response to the drug

Adverse Reactions
Dermatologic: Eczematoid dermatitis
Local: Stinging, burning
Ocular: Lacrimation, activation of latent iritis or uveitis may occur, lens opacities, paradoxical increase in intraocular pressure, retinal detachment, vitreous hemorrhage, conjunctival thickening, iris cysts may form, myopia, follicular conjunctivitis

Overdosage Symptoms of overdose include excessive salivation, urinary incontinence, dyspnea, diarrhea, profuse sweating

Toxicology If systemic effects occur, give parenteral atropine; for severe muscle weakness, pralidoxime may be used in addition to atropine

Drug Interactions Increased toxicity: Carbamate or organophosphate insecticides and pesticides; succinylcholine; systemic acetylcholinesterases may increase neuromuscular effects

Stability Reconstituted solutions remain stable for 30 days at room temperature or 6 months when refrigerated

Mechanism of Action Produces miosis and changes in accommodation by inhibiting cholinesterase, thereby preventing the breakdown of acetylcholine; acetylcholine is therefore allowed to continuously stimulate the iris and ciliary muscles of the eye

Pharmacodynamics
Onset of action: Following ophthalmic instillation, miosis occurs within 10-30 minutes and a decrease in intraocular pressure (IOP) occurs within 4-8 hours
Duration: Miosis and IOP reduction can persist for 1-4 weeks

Usual Dosage Geriatrics and Adults: Ophthalmic:
Glaucoma: Instill 1 drop in affected eye(s) 1-2 times/day; some patients may have an adequate response with every other day dosing

Accommodative esotropia:
Diagnosis: Instill 1 drop of 0.125% once daily into both eyes at bedtime for 2-3 weeks
Treatment: Use lowest concentration and frequency which gives satisfactory response, with a maximum dose of 0.125% once daily, although more intensive therapy may be used for short periods of time

Monitoring Parameters Intraocular pressure

Patient Information Be sure of solution expiration date; local irritation and headache may occur; notify physician if abdominal cramps, diarrhea, or salivation occurs; use caution if driving at night or performing hazardous tasks; do not touch dropper to eye; report any change in vision to physician

Nursing Implications Instruct patient on how to administer drops

Special Geriatric Considerations Assess patient's ability to self-administer eye drops

Dosage Forms Solution, ophthalmic: 0.03% = 1.5 mg/5 mL (5 mL) ; 0.06% = 3 mg/5 mL (5 mL); 0.125% = 6.25 mg/5 mL (5 mL); 0.25% = 12.5 mg/5 mL (5 mL)

Econochlor® see Chloramphenicol on page 148

Econopred® see Prednisolone on page 584

Econopred® Plus see Prednisolone on page 584

Ecostigmine Iodide see Echothiophate Iodide on previous page

Ecotrin® [OTC] see Aspirin on page 58

Ectasule® see Ephedrine Sulfate on page 255

E-Cypionate® see Estradiol on page 269

Edecrin® see Ethacrynic Acid on page 272

E.E.S.® see Erythromycin on page 263

E.E.S. 400® see Erythromycin on page 263

E.E.S.® Chewable see Erythromycin on page 263

E.E.S.® Granules see Erythromycin on page 263

Efedron® see Ephedrine Sulfate on page 255

Effer-Syllium® [OTC] see Psyllium on page 610

Effexor® see Venlafaxine on page 733

EHDP see Etidronate Disodium on page 276

Elavil® see Amitriptyline Hydrochloride on page 43

Eldepryl® see Selegiline Hydrochloride on page 640

Elimite™ see Permethrin on page 548

Elixicon® see Theophylline on page 681

Elixophyllin® see Theophylline on page 681

Elixophyllin® SR see Theophylline on page 681

Elocon® Topical see Mometasone Furoate on page 479

Emete-Con® see Benzquinamide Hydrochloride on page 79

Empirin® [OTC] see Aspirin on page 58

Empirin® With Codeine see Aspirin and Codeine on page 61

Emulsoil® [OTC] see Castor Oil on page 124

E-Mycin® see Erythromycin on page 263

E-Mycin-E® see Erythromycin on page 263

Enalapril (e nal' a pril)

Brand Names Vasotec®

Synonyms Enalaprilat

Generic Available No

Therapeutic Class Angiotensin-Converting Enzyme (ACE) Inhibitors

Use Management of hypertension, treatment of congestive heart failure, and asymptomatic left ventricular dysfunction; increase circulation in Raynaud's phenomenon; idiopathic edema; diabetic nephropathy

Unlabeled use: Hypertensive crisis, diabetic nephropathy, rheumatoid arthritis, diagnosis of anatomic renal artery stenosis, hypertension secondary to scleroderma renal crisis, diagnosis of aldosteronism, idiopathic edema, Bartter's syndrome, postmyocardial infarction for prevention of ventricular failure

Contraindications Hypersensitivity to enalapril, enalaprilat or any component or any ACE inhibitor

Warnings Neutropenia, agranulocytosis, angioedema, decreased renal function (hypertension, renal artery stenosis, congestive heart failure), hepatic dysfunction (elimination, activation), proteinuria, first-dose hypotension (hypovolemia, congestive heart failure, dehydrated patients at risk, eg, diuretic use, elderly), elderly (due to renal function changes)

Precautions Use with caution and modify dosage in patients with renal impairment (especially renal artery stenosis), hyponatremia, hypovolemia, severe congestive heart failure or with coadministered diuretic therapy; valvular stenosis, hyperkalemia (>5.7 mEq/L), anesthesia

Adverse Reactions

Cardiovascular: Hypotension, syncope, orthostatic hypotension, arrhythmias, tachycardia, atrial fibrillation, bradycardia, cardiac arrest, CVA, myocardial infarction, chest pain, palpitations, angina, vasculitis

Central nervous system: Fatigue, vertigo, insomnia, dizziness, asthenia, headache, paresthesias, somnolence, ataxia, confusion, depression, nervousness

Dermatologic: Rash, alopecia, urticaria, pemphigus, erythema multiforme, exfoliative dermatitis, flushing, Stevens-Johnson syndrome, photosensitivity, angioedema

Endocrine & metabolic: Hypoglycemia, hyperkalemia

Gastrointestinal: Nausea, ileus, diarrhea, dry mouth, dyspepsia, glossitis, abdominal pain, vomiting, dysgeusia, anorexia, constipation, pancreatitis

Genitourinary: Impotence

Hematologic: Agranulocytosis, neutropenia, anemia, eosinophilia, thrombocytopenia

Hepatic: Hepatitis, cholestatic jaundice

Neuromuscular & skeletal: Muscle cramps, myalgia, arthralgia, arthritis

Ocular: Blurred vision

Otic: Tinnitus

Renal: Deterioration in renal function (20%), especially with renal artery stenosis, oliguria

Respiratory: Chronic cough (nonproductive, persistent; more often in women and seen in 15% to 30% of patients), asthma, bronchitis, bronchospasm, dyspnea, pulmonary embolism

Miscellaneous: Loss of taste perception, fever, sweating

Overdosage Symptoms of overdose include severe hypotension

Toxicology Following initiation of essential overdose management, toxic symptom treatment and supportive treatment should be initiated. Hypotension usually responds to I.V. fluids or Trendelenburg positioning. If unresponsive to these measures, the use of a parenteral inotrope may be required (eg, norepinephrine 0.1-0.2 mcg/kg/minute titrated to response). Seizures commonly respond to diazepam (I.V. 5-10 mg bolus in adults every 15 minutes if needed up to a total of 30 mg) or to phenytoin or phenobarbital.

Drug Interactions

Hypotensive agent or diuretics → ↑ hypotensive effect

Enalapril and potassium-sparing diuretics → additive hyperkalemic effect

Enalapril and indomethacin or nonsteroidal anti-inflammatory agents → reduced antihypertensive response to enalapril

Allopurinol and enalapril → neutropenia

Antacids and ACE inhibitors → ↓ absorption of ACE inhibitors

Phenothiazines and ACE inhibitors → ↑ ACE inhibitor effect

Probenecid and ACE inhibitors (enalapril) → ↑ ACE inhibitors (enalapril) levels

Rifampin and ACE inhibitors (enalapril) → ↓ ACE inhibitor effect

Digoxin and ACE inhibitors → ↑ serum digoxin levels

Lithium and ACE inhibitors → ↑ lithium serum levels

Tetracycline and ACE inhibitors (enalapril) → ↓ tetracycline absorption (up to 37%)

Food decreases enalapril absorption, see Additional Information

Stability Solutions for I.V. infusion mixed in NS, D_5NS, D_5LR, or D_5W and Isolyte® E are stable for 24 hours at room temperature

Mechanism of Action Competitive inhibitor of angiotensin-converting enzyme (ACE); prevents conversion of angiotensin I to angiotensin II, a potent vasoconstrictor; results in lower levels of angiotensin II which causes an increase in plasma renin activity and a reduction in aldosterone secretion; a CNS mechanism may also be involved in hypotensive effect as angiotensin II increases adrenergic outflow from CNS; vasoactive kallikreins may be decreased in conversion to active hormones by ACE inhibitors, thus reducing blood pressure

Pharmacodynamics
Onset of action: Oral: ~1 hour following administration
Peak effect: 4-8 hours
Duration: 12-24 hours

Pharmacokinetics
Absorption: Oral: 55% to 75% (enalapril)
Protein binding: 50% to 60%
Enalapril is a prodrug and undergoes biotransformation to enalaprilat in the liver
Half-life:
Enalapril: 1-2 hours
Enalapril half-life (CHF): 3.4-5.8 hours
Enalaprilat half-life: 11 hours
Time to peak: Peak serum levels occur within 0.5-1.5 hours, while peak serum levels of enalaprilat (active) occur within 3-4.5 hours
Elimination: Principally in urine (60% to 80%) with some fecal excretion

Usual Dosage Use lower listed initial dose in patients with hyponatremia, hypovolemia, severe congestive heart failure, decreased renal function, or in those receiving diuretics

Geriatrics and Adults:
Oral: **Enalapril:** 2.5-5 mg/day then increase as required in 2.5-5 mg increments at 1- to 2-week intervals; daily dose range is usually 10-40 mg/day in 1-2 divided doses
I.V.: **Enalaprilat:** 0.625-1.25 mg/dose, given over 5 minutes every 6 hours; for conversion from I.V. to oral, administer 2.5 mg orally once daily for those who responded to 0.625 mg I.V. every 6 hours

Asymptomatic left ventricular dysfunction: 2.5 mg twice daily; titrate carefully as tolerated to a recommended 20 mg/day in divided doses

Dosing interval in renal impairment:
Cl_{cr} 10-50 mL/minute: Administer 75% to 100% of the usual dose
Cl_{cr} <10 mL/minute: Administer 50% of the usual dose
Enalaprilat is dialyzable (62 mL/minute)

Monitoring Parameters Serum potassium levels, BUN, serum creatinine, renal function, and WBC

Test Interactions Increased potassium (S); increased serum creatinine/BUN

Patient Information Do not stop therapy except under prescriber advice; notify physician if you develop sore throat, fever, swelling of hands, feet, face, eyes, lips, and tongue; difficult breathing, irregular heartbeats, chest pains, or cough. May cause dizziness, fainting, and lightheadedness, especially in first week of therapy, sit and stand up slowly; may cause changes in taste or rash; do not add a salt substitute (potassium) without advice of physician.

Nursing Implications May cause depression in some patients; discontinue if angioedema of the face, extremities, lips, tongue, or glottis occurs; watch for hypotensive effect within 1-3 hours of first dose or new higher dose; see Precautions, Warnings, Monitoring Parameters, and Special Geriatric Considerations

Additional Information Severe hypotension may occur in patients who are sodium and/or volume depleted; initiate lower doses and monitor closely when starting therapy in these patients

Special Geriatric Considerations Due to frequent decreases in glomerular filtration (also creatinine clearance) with aging, elderly patients may have exaggerated responses to ACE inhibitors; differences in clinical response due to hepatic changes are not observed. ACE inhibitors may be preferred agents in elderly patients with congestive heart failure and diabetes mellitus. Diabetic proteinuria is reduced and insulin sensitivity is enhanced. In general, the side effect profile is favorable in elderly and causes little or no CNS confusion; use lowest dose recommendations initially; adjust dose for renal function in elderly.

Dosage Forms
Injection, as enalaprilat: 1.25 mg/mL (2 mL)
Tablet: 2.5 mg, 5 mg, 10 mg, 20 mg

References
McAreavey D and Robertson JIS, "Angiotensin Converting Enzyme Inhibitors and Moderate Hypertension," *Drugs*, 1990, 40(3):326-45.

Enalaprilat see Enalapril *on previous page*

Encainide Hydrochloride (en kay' nide)
Brand Names Enkaid®
Generic Available No
Therapeutic Class Antiarrhythmic Agent, Class IC

(Continued)

Encainide Hydrochloride *(Continued)*

Use Life-threatening ventricular arrhythmias; supraventricular arrhythmias. **Note:** Manufacturer has withdrawn from market due to implications of CAST study; however, the drug is available for those who responded to it and physician does not believe a substitution should occur (contact Bristol-Myers-Squibb)

Contraindications Hypersensitivity to encainide or any component, second or third degree A-V block, premature ventricular complexes, nonsustained ventricular arrhythmias, cardiogenic shock

Warnings Can cause new or worsened arrhythmias; such proarrhythmic effects range from an increase in frequency of PVCs to the development of more severe ventricular tachycardia (eg, tachycardia that is more sustained or more resistant to conversion to sinus rhythm, with potentially fatal consequences); aggravate or cause congestive heart failure; electrolyte abnormalities alter drug response; therefore, correct any prior to therapy, use with caution in patients with sick sinus syndrome, and renal and hepatic dysfunction (caution when Cl_{cr} <20 mL/minute)

Precautions Use with caution in patients with a history of congestive heart failure or myocardial dysfunction; use is recommended only in patients with life-threatening arrhythmias

Adverse Reactions
  Cardiovascular: Arrhythmogenic effects range from an increased frequency of ventricular premature complexes (VPCs) to the development of new and/or more severe and potentially fatal ventricular tachyarrhythmias; bradycardia, first degree A-V block; negative inotropic effect, chest pain, congestive heart failure, palpitations
  Central nervous system: Dizziness, headache, insomnia, nervousness, somnolence
  Dermatologic: Rash
  Gastrointestinal: Abdominal pain, constipation, nausea, vomiting, diarrhea, dry mouth, dyspepsia, anorexia
  Neuromuscular & skeletal: Generalized pain, tremors
  Ocular: Visual disturbances
  Respiratory: Cough, dyspnea
  Miscellaneous: Peripheral edema

Overdosage Symptoms of overdose include second or third degree A-V block, sinus arrest, hypotension, convulsions, widening of QRS complex

Toxicology Cardiac dysrhythmias and hypotension often respond to bolus I.V. injections of hypertonic sodium bicarbonate 1-2 mEq/kg, while conventional type IA antiarrhythmics tend to worsen conduction defects, especially ventricular arrhythmias. In those patients displaying seizures along with conduction defects, phenytoin may be most effective in reducing these symptoms.

Drug Interactions Beta-blockers (possible negative inotropic effects); diuretics, cimetidine, other cardiac medications that affect conduction or inotropic function

Mechanism of Action Encainide is a class IC agent that blocks the sodium channel of the Purkinje fibers; it slows conduction, reduces membrane responsiveness, increases the effective refractory period to the action potential, and inhibits automaticity.

Pharmacokinetics
  Absorption: Well absorbed
  Metabolism: Extensive in the liver to two active metabolites; o-dimethyl encainide (ODE) and 3-methoxy-o-dimethyl encainide (MODE)
  Bioavailability: Wide intrapatient differences
  Half-life: 1-2.7 hours
  Half-life: Active metabolites:
    ODE half-life: 3-4 hours
    MODE half-life: 6-12 hours
  Elimination: In urine and bile

Usual Dosage Geriatrics and Adults: Oral (hospitalization is necessary to initiate therapy): 25 mg every 8 hours; may increase to 35 mg every 8 hours after 3-5 days if needed; increase to 50 mg every 8 hours in another 3-5 days if response is not achieved

Monitoring Parameters EKG, heart rate, blood pressure

Reference Range Therapeutic: 50-85 μg/L (SI: 130-220 nmol/L)
  ODE: 180-220 μg/L (SI: 460-565 nmol/L)
  MODE: 140-185 μg/L (SI: 360-475 nmol/L) (normal phenotype)

Patient Information Take as directed; do not change dose except from advice of your physician; report any chest pain and irregular heartbeats

Nursing Implications Give around-the-clock rather than 4 times/day, 3 times/day, etc (ie, 12-6-12-6, not 9-1-5-9) to promote less variation in peak and trough serum levels

Additional Information Based on adverse outcomes noted with encainide in the CAST trial, the FDA recommends that use of encainide be limited to patients with life-threatening ventricular arrhythmias

Special Geriatric Considerations Prolonged half-life of the two active metabolites ODE and MODE; consider age changes in renal and hepatic function since this may alter clearance, see Warnings; there are no guidelines, therefore, monitor closely

Dosage Forms Capsule: 25 mg, 35 mg, 50 mg

References

Fenster PE and Nolan PE, "Antiarrhythmic Drugs," *Geriatric Pharmacology*, Bressler R and Katz MD, eds, New York, NY: McGraw-Hill, 1993, 6:105-49.

Endep® *see* Amitriptyline Hydrochloride *on page 43*

Engerix-B® *see* Hepatitis B Vaccine *on page 342*

Enkaid® *see* Encainide Hydrochloride *on page 251*

Enovil® *see* Amitriptyline Hydrochloride *on page 43*

Enoxacin

Brand Names Penetrex™

Generic Available No

Therapeutic Class Antibiotic, Quinolone

Use Complicated and uncomplicated urinary tract infections caused by susceptible gram-negative and gram-positive bacteria; uncomplicated urethral or cervical gonorrhea

Contraindications Hypersensitivity to enoxacin, the fluoroquinolones, or the quinolone group

Warnings Prolonged use may result in superinfection, including pseudomembranous colitis; use with caution in patients with seizure disorders or renal impairment; not effective for syphilis, may mask signs or symptoms and patients treated for gonorrhea should have serologic testing in 3 months

Precautions Modify dosage in patients with renal insufficiency; CNS stimulation may occur and manifest as tremor, restlessness, confusion, and very rarely seizures. Use with caution in patients with known or suspected CNS disorders; phototoxicity (patients may need sunglasses)

Adverse Reactions

Central nervous system: Restlessness, dizziness, confusion, seizures, headache, confusion, depersonalization, hypertonia, seizures

Dermatologic: Rash, photosensitivity

Gastrointestinal: Nausea, diarrhea, vomiting, GI bleeding, anorexia, pseudomembranous colitis

Genitourinary: Vaginitis

Hematologic: Anemia

Hepatic: Increased liver enzymes

Neuromuscular & skeletal: Arthralgia, myalgia, tremors

Renal: Acute renal failure

Overdosage Symptoms of overdose include acute renal failure, seizures

Toxicology GI decontamination and supportive care; for acute overdose, empty stomach contents by inducing vomiting or gastric lavage; observe and treat the patient symptomatically; maintain fluid status; diazepam for seizures; not removed by peritoneal or hemodialysis

Drug Interactions

Antacids, iron salts, sucralfate, and zinc salts may reduce absorption if given at the same time

Antineoplastic agents may decrease fluoroquinolone serum concentrations

Bismuth subsalicylate decreased enoxacin's bioavailability

Cimetidine decreased elimination

Probenecid decreased clearance

Caffeine's clearance is reduced

Digoxin serum levels may be increased

Anticoagulant effects may be increased

Cyclosporine may increase nephrotoxic effects when used with a quinolone

Decreased theophylline clearance and increased serum concentrations

Mechanism of Action Exerts a broad spectrum antimicrobial effect. The primary target of the fluoroquinolones is DNA gyrase (topoisomerase II) an essential bacterial enzyme that maintains the superhelical structure of DNA. DNA gyrase is required for DNA replication and transcription, DNA repair, recombination, and transposition.

Pharmacodynamics Bactericidal

Pharmacokinetics

Absorption: Peak plasma concentration in 1-3 hours; 98%

Distribution: Concentrations in the cervix, fallopian tube, and myometrium 1-2 times greater than plasma; renal and prostate concentration 2-4 times greater than plasma

Metabolism: 15% to 20% of dose metabolized to 1 of 5 metabolites; inhibits selected cytochrome P-450 isoenzymes resulting in the decreased metabolism of certain drugs; see Drug Interactions

Elimination: Renal, clearance: 2.28 mL/minute/kg in young adults

Half-life: 7.34 hours

In the elderly, mean peak serum concentrations were 50% greater than younger adults, statistically, a nonsignificant finding. One study found a significantly re-

(Continued)

Enoxacin *(Continued)*

duced renal clearance in the elderly, compared to younger adults (1.39 vs 2.28 mL/minute/kg); the mean half-life in older subjects has been reported to be 6.11-7.3 hours which is similar to younger adults. A dosage adjustment is recommended if the patient's estimated Cl_{cr} ≤30 mL/minute/1.73 m²; see Usual Dosage.

Usual Dosage Oral:

Geriatrics: Normal adult dose adjusted for renal function

Adults:
Uncomplicated urinary tract infection: 200 mg every 12 hours for 7 days
Complicated urinary tract infection: 400 mg every 12 hours for 14 days
Uncomplicated gonorrhea: 400 mg as a single dose

Dosing adjustment in renal impairment: Cl_{cr} ≤30 mL/minute/1.73 m²: For all indications, give normal initial dose, then ½ the recommended dose every 12 hours for the prescribed duration

Monitoring Parameters Signs and symptoms of infection (temperature, WBC, mental status, appetite); urinalysis; appropriate cultures and sensitivity; patients receiving concurrent theophylline should have their serum concentrations monitored; patients receiving concurrent warfarin therapy should have their prothrombin time or INR monitored; patients receiving cyclosporine should be monitored for nephrotoxicity

Patient Information Complete full course of therapy; take on empty stomach (1 hour before or 2 hours after meals); drink fluids liberally; warn of potential phototoxicity and sensitivity

Nursing Implications Hold antacids for 3-4 hours before or after giving; give on an empty stomach; encourage fluids

Special Geriatric Considerations See Pharmacokinetics and Usual Dosage; adjust dose for renal function

Dosage Forms Tablet: 400 mg

References

Dobbs BR, Gazeley LR, Campbell AJ, et al, "The Effect of Age on the Pharmacokinetics of Enoxacin," *Eur J Clin Pharmacol*, 1987, 33(1):101-4.

Wise R, Baker SL, Misra M, et al, "The Pharmacokinetics of Enoxacin in Elderly Patients," *J Antimicrob Chemother*, 1987, 19(3):343-50.

Enoxaparin Sodium *(e nox ah pair' in)*

Brand Names Lovenox®

Therapeutic Class Anticoagulant

Use Prevention of deep vein thrombosis following hip replacement surgery

Contraindications Active major bleeding or hemophilia; hypersensitivity to heparin or pork products; drug-induced thrombocytopenia

Warnings Heparin-induced thrombocytopenia, bacterial endocarditis, congenital or acquired bleeding disorders, active ulceration and angiodysplastic gastrointestinal disease, hemorrhagic stroke, status post brain, spinal, or ophthalmological surgery, uncontrolled arterial hypertension, recent CNS surgery, elderly, and lactation. Never give by intramuscular injection. Conventional heparin has possibly been associated with an increased risk of bleeding in females >60 years of age; it is unknown whether low molecular weight heparins pose the same risk; these agents should be used with caution in this population.

Adverse Reactions

Cardiovascular: Edema
Central nervous system: Confusion
Dermatologic: Ecchymosis, erythema
Hematologic: Hemorrhage, thrombocytopenia, hematoma, hypochromic anemia
Gastrointestinal: Nausea
Hepatic: Asymptomatic increases in liver transaminases (AST, ALT)
Miscellaneous: Local irritation, pain, fever

Overdosage Symptoms of overdose include hemorrhage

Toxicology Protamine zinc has been used to reverse effects

Drug Interactions Increased toxicity with oral anticoagulants, platelet inhibitors

Pharmacodynamics

Peak effect: 3 hours
Duration: 275 minutes

Pharmacokinetics

Half-life: 275 minutes
Elimination: In the kidney

Usual Dosage Geriatrics and Adults: S.C.: 30 mg within 24 hours of surgery, then twice daily for 7-10 days; 14 days maximum; a single daily dose of 40 mg has also been shown to be safe and effective in prevention of thromboembolism in patients undergoing orthopedic or gynecologic surgical procedures

Administration S.C. only; do not give I.M. injection

Monitoring Parameters Periodic CBC including platelets, occult blood, and anti-Xa activity, if available

Nursing Implications See Administration

Special Geriatric Considerations No specific recommendations; see Usual Dosage

Dosage Forms Injection, preservative free: 30 mg/0.3 mL

Entacef® *see* Cephalexin Monohydrate *on page 142*
Enulose® *see* Lactulose *on page 397*

Ephedrine Sulfate (e fed' rin)
Brand Names Ectasule®; Efedron®; Ephedsol®; Vicks Vatronol®
Generic Available Yes
Therapeutic Class Adrenergic Agonist Agent
Use Bronchial asthma; nasal congestion; acute bronchospasm

Unlabeled use: Urinary incontinence, stress type; carotid sinus syncope; malignant vasovagal syndrome

Contraindications Hypersensitivity to ephedrine or any component, cardiac arrhythmias, angle-closure glaucoma, patients on other sympathomimetic agents

Warnings Use caution in patients with unstable vasomotor symptoms, diabetes, hyperthyroidism, prostatic hypertrophy, or a history of seizures; also use caution in the elderly and those patients with cardiovascular disorders such as coronary artery disease, arrhythmias, and hypertension. Ephedrine may cause hypertension resulting in intracranial hemorrhage. Long-term use may cause anxiety and symptoms of paranoid schizophrenia.

Adverse Reactions
Cardiovascular: Tachycardia, palpitations, elevation or depression of blood pressure
Central nervous system: CNS-stimulating effects, nervousness, anxiety, apprehension, fear, tension, agitation, excitation, restlessness, irritability, insomnia, hyperactivity
Gastrointestinal: Nausea, anorexia, GI upset
Genitourinary: Difficult painful urination; urinary retention may occur in men with enlarged prostates
Neuromuscular & skeletal: Tremors (more common in the elderly), weakness

Overdosage Symptoms of overdose include dysrhythmias, CNS excitation, respiratory depression, vomiting, convulsions

Toxicology There is no specific antidote for ephedrine intoxication and the bulk of the treatment is supportive. Hyperactivity and agitation usually respond to reduced sensory input, however with extreme agitation, haloperidol may be required. Hyperthermia is best treated with external cooling measures, or when severe or unresponsive, muscle paralysis with pancuronium may be needed. Hypertension is usually transient and generally does not require treatment unless severe. For diastolic blood pressures >110 mm Hg, a nitroprusside infusion should be initiated. Seizures usually respond to diazepam I.V. and/or phenytoin maintenance regimens.

Drug Interactions
Decreased effect of guanethidine; decreased effect with alpha-blockers, beta-blockers, methyldopa, reserpine
Increased effect/toxicity with acetazolamide, sympathomimetics, theophylline, MAO inhibitors (increased blood pressure), atropine (increased blood pressure), digoxin, general anesthetics, albuterol, sodium bicarbonate

Stability Protect all dosage forms from light

Mechanism of Action Releases tissue stores of epinephrine and thereby produces an alpha- and beta-adrenergic stimulation. It is longer acting but less potent than epinephrine. In urinary incontinence, the alpha-adrenergic activity of ephedrine stimulates contraction of the internal urethral sphincter.

Pharmacodynamics
Onset of bronchodilation: Oral: 15-60 minutes
Duration: 3-6 hours

Pharmacokinetics
Metabolism: Little hepatic metabolism
Half-life: 3-6 hours
Elimination: 60% to 77% of dose excreted as unchanged drug in urine within 24 hours; renal excretion is dependent on urine pH; decreased excretion with alkaline urine

Usual Dosage
Geriatrics: Urinary incontinence: 25-50 mg every 6 hours

Adults:
Nasal congestion:
Oral: 25-50 mg every 3-4 hours as needed
I.M., S.C.: 25-50 mg
I.V.: 10-25 mg slow I.V. push; repeat every 5-10 minutes, not to exceed 150 mg/24 hours

Monitoring Parameters Blood pressure, pulse, urinary output, mental status
Patient Information May cause wakefulness or nervousness; available over-the-counter, but elderly patients should consult physician before using
Nursing Implications Protect from light; do not administer unless solution is clear; monitor urinary output, mental status, vital signs
Additional Information Ephedrine is generally not used as a bronchodilator since newer beta$_2$-specific agents are less toxic

(Continued)
255

Ephedrine Sulfate *(Continued)*

Special Geriatric Considerations Avoid as a bronchodilator. Most often used for stress incontinence in the elderly to increase internal sphincter tone. Use caution since it crosses the blood-brain barrier and may cause confusion; see Warnings, Adverse Reactions

Dosage Forms
Capsule: 25 mg, 50 mg
Injection: 25 mg/mL (1 mL); 50 mg/mL (1 mL)
Syrup: 20 mg/5 mL

Ephedsol® *see Ephedrine Sulfate on previous page*

Epifrin® *see Epinephrine on this page*

Epinal® *see Epinephrine on this page*

Epinephrine *(ep i nef' rin)*

Related Information
Glaucoma Drug Therapy Comparison *on page 810*

Brand Names Adrenalin®; AsthmaHaler®; AsthmaNefrin® [OTC]; Breatheasy®; Bronitin®; Bronkaid® Mist [OTC]; Epifrin®; Epinal®; EpiPen®; EpiPen® Jr; Epitrate®; Glaucon® Eppy/N®; Medihaler-Epi®; microNefrin®; Primatene® Mist [OTC]; Sus-Phrine®; Vaponefrin®

Synonyms Adrenaline; Epinephrine Bitartrate; Epinephrine Hydrochloride; Racemic Epinephrine

Generic Available Yes

Therapeutic Class Adrenergic Agonist Agent; Antidote, Hypersensitivity Reactions; Bronchodilator

Use Bronchospasm; anaphylactic reactions; cardiac arrest; management of open-angle (chronic simple) glaucoma

Contraindications Hypersensitivity to epinephrine or any component; cardiac arrhythmias, angle-closure glaucoma

Precautions Use with caution in geriatric patients, patients with diabetes mellitus or cardiovascular diseases, thyroid disease or cerebral arteriosclerosis

Adverse Reactions
Cardiovascular: Pallor, tachycardia, hypertension, increased myocardial oxygen consumption, cardiac arrhythmias, sudden death
Central nervous system: Anxiety, headache, insomnia, dizziness
Gastrointestinal: Nausea, vomiting
Neuromuscular & skeletal: Weakness, tremors
Ocular: Precipitation of or exacerbation of narrow-angle glaucoma
Renal: Decreased renal and splanchnic blood flow, acute urinary retention in patients with bladder outflow obstruction
Miscellaneous: Increased sweating
Rapid I.V. infusion may cause death from cerebrovascular hemorrhage or cardiac arrhythmias

Overdosage Symptoms of overdose include hypertension which may result in subarachnoid hemorrhage and hemiplegia; arrhythmias, unusually large pupils, pulmonary edema, renal failure, metabolic acidosis

Toxicology There is no specific antidote for epinephrine intoxication and the bulk of the treatment is supportive. Hyperactivity and agitation usually respond to reduced sensory input, however, with extreme agitation haloperidol may be required. Hyperthermia is best treated with external cooling measures, or when severe or unresponsive, muscle paralysis with pancuronium may be needed. Hypertension is usually transient and generally does not require treatment unless severe. For diastolic blood pressures >110 mm Hg, a nitroprusside infusion should be initiated. Seizures usually respond to diazepam I.V. and/or phenytoin maintenance regimens.

Drug Interactions
Hypertension may occur if administered with beta-blockers, guanethidine, tricyclic antidepressants
Arrhythmias may occur if administered with bretylium, halogenated hydrocarbon anesthetics
Epinephrine decreases the effect of hypoglycemic agents

Stability Protect from light, oxidation turns drug pink, then a brown color; solutions should not be used if they are discolored or contain a precipitate; stability of injection of parenteral admixture at room temperature and refrigeration: 24 hours; do not use D_5W as a diluent; D_5W is incompatible with epinephrine

Mechanism of Action Stimulates alpha-, beta₁- and beta₂-adrenergic receptors; small doses can cause vasodilation via beta₂ vascular receptors; decreases production of aqueous humor and increases aqueous outflow; dilates the pupil by contracting the dilator muscle

Pharmacodynamics
Onset of action:
S.C.: Bronchodilation occurs within 3-5 minutes following administration

Inhalation: Within 1 minute

Following conjunctival instillation, intraocular pressures fall within 1 hour with a maximal response occurring within 4-8 hours

Duration: Ocular effects persist for 12-24 hours; decreased beta-receptor responsiveness has been seen in the elderly

Pharmacokinetics

Absorption: Oral: Degraded in the GI tract and, therefore, is not useful

Metabolism: Following administration, drug is taken up into the adrenergic neuron and metabolized by monoamine oxidase and catechol-o-methyltransferase, circulating drug is metabolized in the liver

Elimination: Inactive metabolites (metanephrine and the sulfate and hydroxy derivatives of mandelic acid) and a small amount of unchanged drug is excreted in urine

Usual Dosage Geriatrics and Adults:

Bronchodilator: I.M., S.C.: 0.1-0.5 mg every 10-15 minutes; I.V.: 0.1-0.25 mg (single dose maximum: 1 mg)

Nebulizer: Instill 8-15 drops into nebulizer reservoir; administer 1-3 inhalations 4-6 times/day

Cardiac arrest: I.V., intracardiac: 0.1-1 mg every 5 minutes as needed; intratracheal: 1 mg

Hypersensitivity reaction: I.M., S.C.: 0.2-0.5 mg every 20 minutes to 4 hours (single dose maximum: 1 mg)

Ophthalmic: Instill 1-2 drops in eye(s) once or twice daily

Monitoring Parameters Pulmonary function, blood pressure, pulse, intraocular pressure

Reference Range Therapeutic: 31-95 pg/mL (SI: 170-520 pmol/L)

Test Interactions Increased bilirubin (S), catecholamines (U), glucose, uric acid (S)

Patient Information Instruct patient on proper instillation of ophthalmic preparation; after instilling, apply pressure on the side of the nose near the eye to minimize systemic absorption; stinging may occur upon instillation; headache or aching in the brow area may occur

Nursing Implications Protect from light; oxidation turns dark pink, then brown – solutions should not be used if they are discolored or contain a precipitate; epinephrine is unstable in alkaline solution

Additional Information Oral inhalation of epinephrine is **not** the preferred route of administration. Patients should be cautioned to avoid the use of over-the-counter epinephrine inhalation products. Beta$_2$-adrenergic agents for inhalation are preferred.

Epinephrine: Primatene® Mist, Bronkaid® Mist, Sus-Phrine®

Epinephrine bitartrate: AsthmaHaler®, Bronitin®, Epitrate®, Medihaler-Epi®; Primatene® Mist

Epinephrine hydrochloride: Adrenalin®, Epifrin®, EpiPen®, EpiPen® Jr.

Racemic epinephrine: AsthmaHaler®, Breatheasy®, microNefrin®, Vaponefrin®

Epinephryl borate: Epinal®

Special Geriatric Considerations The use of epinephrine in the treatment of acute exacerbations of asthma was studied in older adults. A dose of 0.3 mg S.C. every 20 minutes for three doses was well tolerated in older patients with no history of angina or recent myocardial infarction. There was no significant difference in the incidence of ventricular arrhythmias in older adults versus younger adults; see Pharmacodynamics and Additional Information.

Dosage Forms

Aerosol, as bitartrate: 0.16 mg/inhalation (10 mL, 15 mL)

Inhalation, as hydrochloride: 1% (15 mL)

Solution for nebulization, as hydrochloride: Racemic epinephrine is equivalent to 2.25% epinephrine base (7.5 mL, 15 mL, 30 mL)

Solution:

Injection: 1 mg/mL = 1:1000 (1 mL, 2 mL, 30 mL); 0.1 mg/mL = 1:10,000 (3 mL, 10 mL); 0.01 mg/mL (5 mL)

Nasal: 1 mg/mL = 1:1000 (30 mL)

Ophthalmic, as bitartrate: 1% (7.5 mL)

Ophthalmic, as borate: 0.5% (7.5 mL); 1% (7.5 mL); 2% (7.5 mL)

Ophthalmic, as hydrochloride: 0.1% (1 mL, 30 mL); 0.25% (15 mL); 0.5% (15 mL); 1% (1 mL, 10 mL, 15 mL); 2% (10 mL, 15 mL)

Topical: 0.1% (30 mL)

Suspension, injection: 1.5 mg/0.3 mL = 1:200 (0.3 mL)

References

Cydulka R, Davison R, Grammer L, et al, "The Use of Epinephrine in the Treatment of Older Adult Asthmatics," *Ann Emerg Med,* 1988, 17(4):322-6.

Epinephrine Bitartrate *see* Epinephrine *on previous page*

Epinephrine Hydrochloride *see* Epinephrine *on previous page*

EpiPen® *see* Epinephrine *on previous page*

EpiPen® Jr *see* Epinephrine *on page 256*

Epitol® *see* Carbamazepine *on page 117*

Epitrate® *see* Epinephrine *on page 256*

EPO *see* Epoetin Alfa *on this page*

Epoetin Alfa (e poe' e tin)

Brand Names Epogen®; Procrit®

Synonyms EPO; Erythropoietin; HuEPO

Therapeutic Class Recombinant Human Erythropoietin

Use

Anemia associated with end stage renal disease (FDA-approved indication)

Anemia related to therapy with AZT-treated HIV-infected patients (FDA-approved indication)

Endogenous serum erythropoietin (EPO) level which are inappropriately low for hemoglobin level (anemia of neoplasia) (FDA approved indication)

Patients undergoing autologous blood donation prior to surgery – EPO may accelerate recovery of hemoglobin level and, in some cases, permit more units of blood to be donated

rHuEPO-α is not beneficial in the acute treatment of anemia (onset of reticulocyte response does not appear until 7-10 days and hemoglobin rise appears over 2-6 weeks after starting therapy). Therefore, emergency/stat orders for the drug are not appropriate.

Contraindications Known hypersensitivity to human albumin; uncontrolled hypertension

Warnings Use with caution in patients with porphyria, hypertension, or a history of seizures; prior to and during therapy, iron stores must be evaluated

Adverse Reactions

Cardiovascular: Hypertension, edema, chest pain, myocardial infarction

Central nervous system: Fatigue, dizziness, headache, seizure, CVA/TIA

Dermatologic: Rash

Gastrointestinal: Nausea

Hematologic: Clotted access

Neuromuscular & skeletal: Arthralgias

Miscellaneous: Hypersensitivity reactions

Overdosage Symptoms of overdose include polycythemia

Toxicology Adequate airway and other supportive measures and agents for treating anaphylaxis should be present when I.V. drug is given

Stability Do not shake; refrigerate; vials are stable 2 weeks at room temperature

Mechanism of Action Induces erythropoiesis by stimulating the division and differentiation of committed erythroid progenitor cells; induces the release of reticulocytes from the bone marrow into the bloodstream, where they mature to erythrocytes

Pharmacodynamics

Onset on action: Increase in reticulocyte count in 10 days, with an increase in RBC count, hemoglobin, and hematocrit within 2-6 weeks

Peak effect: 2-3 weeks

Pharmacokinetics

Distribution: V_d: 9 L; rapid in the plasma compartment; majority of drug is taken up by the liver, kidneys, and bone marrow

Metabolism: Some metabolic degradation does occur

Bioavailability: S.C.: ~21% to 31%; intraperitoneal epoetin in a few patients demonstrated a bioavailability of only 3%

Half-life: Circulating: 4-13 hours in patients with chronic renal failure; 20% shorter in patients with normal renal function

Time to peak serum concentrations: S.C.: 2-8 hours after administration

Elimination: Small amounts recovered in the urine; majority hepatically eliminated; 10% excreted unchanged in the urine of normal volunteers

Epoetin Alfa: General Therapeutic Guidelines

Starting dose	50 to 100 U/kg 3 times weekly I.V.: Dialysis patients I.V. or SC: nondialysis CRF patients
Reduce dose when	1. Target range is reached, or 2. Hematocrit increases >4 points in any 2–week period
Increase dose if	Hematocrit does not increase by 5 to 6 points after 8 weeks of therapy, and hematocrit is below target range
Maintenance dose	Individualize. General dosage range: 25 units/kg (3 times weekly)
Target hematocrit range	30–33% (maximum 36%)

Usual Dosage Geriatrics and Adults:

In patients on dialysis epoetin alfa usually has been administered as an I.V. bolus 3 times/week. While the administration is independent of the dialysis procedure, it may be administered into the venous line at the end of the dialysis procedure to obviate the need for additional venous access; in patients with CRF not on dialysis, epoetin alfa may be given either as an I.V. or S.C. injection. See table on previous page.

AZT-treated HIV-infected patients: I.V., S.C.: Initial: 100 units/kg/dose 3 times/week for 8 weeks; after 8 weeks of therapy the dose can be adjusted by 50-100 units/kg increments 3 times/week to a maximum dose of 300 units/kg 3 times/week; if the hematocrit exceeds 40%, the dose should be discontinued until the hematocrit drops to 36%

Monitoring Parameters

Careful monitoring of blood pressure is indicated; problems with hypertension have been noted in renal failure patients treated with rHuEPO-α. Other patients are less likely to develop this complication.

Follow serum ferritin and serum transferrin saturation monthly

Hematocrit should be determined twice weekly until stabilization within the target range (30% to 33%), and twice weekly at least 2 to 6 weeks after a dose increase

Baseline and follow-up of blood urea nitrogen (BUN), uric acid, serum creatinine, phosphorous, and potassium

Reference Range Hematocrit: 30% to 33%

Patient Information Frequent blood tests are needed to determine the correct dose; notify physician if any severe headache develops

Nursing Implications Monitor for access clotting, blood pressure; see Stability

Additional Information Epogen® reimbursement hotline number for information regarding coverage of epoetin alfa is 1-800-2-PAY-EPO. ProCrit™ reimbursement hotline is 1-800-441-1366.

Special Geriatric Considerations There is limited information about the use of epoetin alfa in the elderly. Endogenous erythropoietin secretion has been reported to be decreased in older adults with normocytic or iron deficiency anemias or those with a serum hemoglobin level <12 g/dL; one study did not find such a relationship in elderly with chronic anemia. A blunted erythropoietin response to anemia has been reported in patients with cancer, rheumatoid arthritis, and AIDS.

Dosage Forms Injection, preservative free: 2000 units (1 mL); 3000 units (1 mL); 4000 units (1 mL); 10,000 units (1 mL)

References

Carpenter MA, Kendall RG, O'Brien AE, et al, "Reduced Erythropoietin Response to Anaemia in Elderly Patients With Normocytic Anaemia," Eur J Haematol, 1992, 49(3):119-21.

Erslev AJ, "Erythropoietin," N Engl J Med, 1991, 324(19):1339-44.

Joosten E, Van Hove L, Lesaffre E, et al, "Serum Erythropoietin Levels in Elderly Inpatients With Anemia of Chronic Disorders and Iron Deficiency Anemia," J Am Geriatr Soc, 1993, 41(12):1301-4.

Kario K, Matsuo T, and Nakao K, "Serum Erythropoietin Levels in the Elderly," Gerontology, 1991, 37(6):345-8.

Nafziger J, Pailla K, Luciani L, et al, "Decreased Erythropoietin Responsiveness to Iron Deficiency Anemia in the Elderly," Am J Hematol, 1993, 43(3):172-6.

Powers JS, Krantz SB, Collins JC, et al, "Erythropoietin Response to Anemia as a Function of Age," J Am Geriatr Soc, 1991, 39(1):30-2.

Epogen® see Epoetin Alfa on previous page

Epsom Salt [OTC] see Magnesium Salts (Various Salts) on page 430

Epsom Salts see Magnesium Salts (Various Salts) on page 430

Equalactin® Chewable Tablet [OTC] see Calcium Polycarbophil on page 110

Equanil® see Meprobamate on page 443

Equilet® [OTC] see Calcium Salts (Oral) on page 111

Ercaf® see Ergotamine on page 261

Ergocalciferol (er goe kal sif' e role)

Brand Names Calciferol™; Drisdol®

Synonyms Activated Ergosterol; Viosterol; Vitamin D₂

Generic Available Yes

Therapeutic Class Vitamin D Analog

Use Refractory rickets; hypophosphatemia; hypoparathyroidism

Contraindications Hypercalcemia, hypersensitivity to ergocalciferol or any component; malabsorption syndrome; evidence of vitamin D toxicity, decreased renal function

Warnings Administer with extreme caution in patients with impaired renal function, heart disease, renal stones, or arteriosclerosis; must give concomitant calcium supplementation for adequate response to vitamin D; maintain adequate fluid intake; calcium-phosphate product (serum calcium and phosphorus) must not exceed 70; avoid hypercalcemia; renal function impairment with secondary hyperparathyroidism

(Continued)

Ergocalciferol *(Continued)*

Adverse Reactions
Cardiovascular: Hypertension, arrhythmias

Central nervous system: Drowsiness, irritability, headache, convulsions, somnolence

Endocrine & metabolic: Acidosis, polydipsia

Gastrointestinal: Nausea, vomiting, anorexia, dry mouth, constipation, weight loss, metallic taste

Genitourinary: Reversible azotemia

Hematologic: Anemia

Hepatic: Elevated AST/ALT

Neuromuscular & skeletal: Weakness, muscle and bone pain, metastatic calcification

Ocular: Photophobia

Renal: Polyuria, nephrocalcinosis, renal damage

Miscellaneous: Ectopic calcifications

Overdosage
Symptoms of overdose include hypercalcemia, hypercalciuria, hyperphosphatemia

Toxicology
Following withdrawal of the drug, treatment consists of bed rest, liberal intake of fluids, reduced calcium intake, and cathartic administration. Severe hypercalcemia requires I.V. hydration and forced diuresis with I.V. furosemide (20-40 mg I.V. every 4-6 hours). Urine output should be monitored and maintained at >3 mL/kg/hour. I.V. saline can quickly and significantly increase excretion of calcium into the urine. Calcitonin, cholestyramine, prednisone, sodium EDTA, and mithramycin have all been used successfully to treat the more resistant cases of vitamin D-induced hypercalcemia.

Drug Interactions
Vitamin D may increase absorption of magnesium from magnesium compounds; hypercalcemia may be precipitated by vitamin D and, therefore, may increase cardiac arrhythmias in patients taking digitalis glycosides and verapamil; hypoparathyroid patients may develop hypercalcemia when using thiazide diuretics

Phenytoin and barbiturates decrease half-life of vitamin D; mineral oil with prolonged use decreases vitamin D absorption; cholestyramine reduces absorption of vitamin D

Stability
Protect from light

Mechanism of Action
Stimulates calcium and phosphate absorption from the small intestine, promotes secretion of calcium from bone to blood (calcium homeostasis); promotes renal tubule phosphate resorption

Pharmacodynamics
Peak effect: Within a month following daily doses

Pharmacokinetics
Absorption: Readily from GI tract; absorption requires intestinal levels of bile

Inactive until hydroxylated in the liver and the kidney to calcifediol and then to calcitriol (most active form)

Usual Dosage
Geriatrics and Adults (see Additional Information):

RDA: 400 IU/day; many elderly require 800 IU/day; see Special Geriatric Considerations

Renal failure: Oral: 0.5 mg/day (20,000 units)

Hypoparathyroidism: Oral: 625 mcg to 5 mg/day (25,000-200,000 units) and calcium supplements (500 mg elemental calcium 6 times/day)

Vitamin D-dependent rickets: Oral: 250 mcg to 1.5 mg/day (10,000-60,000 units)

Nutritional rickets and osteomalacia: Oral: Adults (with normal absorption): 25 mcg/day (1000 units)

Familial phosphatemia: 10,000-80,000 IU/day and phosphorus 1-2 g/day

I.M. therapy may be required with liver, gastrointestinal, or biliary disease

Monitoring Parameters
Measure serum calcium, BUN, and phosphorus every 1-2 weeks

Reference Range
Serum calcium times phosphorus should not exceed 70 mg/dL to avoid ectopic calcification; serum calcium should be maintained between 9-10 mg/dL; phosphorus 2.5-5 mg/dL

Test Interactions
Increased calcium (S), cholesterol (S); false increased serum cholesterol levels with the Zlavkis-Zak reaction

Patient Information
Early symptoms of hypercalcemia include weakness, fatigue, somnolence, headache, anorexia, dry mouth, metallic taste, nausea, vomiting, cramps, diarrhea, muscle pain, bone pain and irritability; do not take more than the recommended amount. While taking this medication, your physician may want you to follow a special diet or take a calcium supplement. Follow this diet closely. Avoid taking magnesium supplements or magnesium containing antacids.

Nursing Implications
Parenteral injection for I.M. use only; monitor serum calcium, phosphorus and BUN every 2 weeks; administer with extreme caution in patients with impaired renal function, heart disease, renal stones, or arteriosclerosis; see Warnings and Reference Range

Additional Information
1.25 mg ergocalciferol provides 50,000 units of vitamin D activity

Special Geriatric Considerations Recommended daily allowances (RDA) have not been developed for persons >65 years of age; vitamin D, folate, and B_{12} (cyanocobalamin) have decreased absorption with age, but the clinical significance is yet unknown. Calorie requirements decrease with age and therefore, nutrient density must be increased to ensure adequate nutrient intake, including vitamins and minerals. Therefore, the use of a daily supplement with a multiple vitamin with minerals is recommended. Elderly consume less vitamin D, absorption may be decreased and many elderly have decreased sun exposure; therefore, elderly should receive supplementation with 800 units (20 mcg)/day. This is a recommendation of particular need to those with high risk for osteoporosis.

Dosage Forms
Capsule: 50,000 units = 1.25 mg
Injection: 500,000 units/mL = 12.5 mg/mL
Solution: 8000 units/mL = 200 mcg/mL
Tablet: 50,000 units = 1.25 mg

References
Letsou AP and Price LS, "Health Aging and Nutrition: An Overview," *Clin Geriatr Med*, 1987, 3(2):253-60.

Myrianthopoulos M, "Dietary Treatment of Hyperlipidemia in the Elderly," *Clin Geriatr Med*, 1987, 3(2):343-59.

Riggs BL and Melton LJ, "The Prevention and Treatment of Osteoporosis," *N Engl J Med*, 1992, 327(9):620-7.

Ergotamine (er got' a meen)

Brand Names Cafergot®; Ercaf®; Ergomar®; Ergostat®; Lanatrate®; Medihaler Ergotamine®; Migergot®; Wigraine®

Generic Available Yes

Therapeutic Class Adrenergic Blocking Agent; Ergot Alkaloid

Use Vascular headache, such as migraine or cluster

Contraindications Hypersensitivity to ergotamine, caffeine or any component; peripheral vascular disease, hepatic or renal disease, hypertension, peptic ulcer disease, sepsis, coronary artery disease

Precautions Avoid prolonged administration or excessive dosage because of the danger of ergotism and gangrene; patients who take ergotamine for extended periods of time may become dependent on it

Adverse Reactions
Cardiovascular: Tachycardia, bradycardia, arterial spasm, claudication and vasoconstriction
Central nervous system: Paresthesia
Dermatologic: Pruritus
Gastrointestinal: Nausea, vomiting, diarrhea
Neuromuscular & skeletal: Weakness in the legs, abdominal, or muscle pain
Miscellaneous: Rebound headache may occur with sudden withdrawal of the drug in patients on prolonged therapy, vasospasm, local edema

Overdosage Symptoms include vasospastic effects, nausea, vomiting, lassitude, impaired mental function, hypotension, hypertension, unconsciousness, seizures, shock and death.

Toxicology Treatment includes general supportive therapy, gastric lavage, or induction of emesis, activated charcoal, saline cathartic; keep extremities warm. Activated charcoal is effective at binding certain chemicals, and this is especially true for ergot alkaloids; treatment is symptomatic with heparin, vasodilators (nitroprusside); vasodilators should be used with caution to avoid exaggerating any pre-existing hypotension.

Drug Interactions
Decreased antianginal effect with nitrates
Increased toxicity: Beta-blockers, macrolide antibiotics
Increased pressor effects with vasodilators

Mechanism of Action Ergot alkaloid alpha-adrenergic blockade directly stimulates vascular smooth muscle to vasoconstrict peripheral and cerebral vessels; may also have antagonist effects on serotonin; may inhibit receptor reuptake of norepinephrine

Pharmacokinetics
Absorption:
Oral, rectal: Erratic; enhanced by caffeine coadministration
Inhalation: Rapid and complete
Metabolism: Extensive in the liver
Bioavailability: Poor overall (<5%)
Time to peak serum concentration: Within 0.5-3 hours following administration
Elimination: In bile as metabolites (90%)

Usual Dosage Geriatrics and Adults:
Oral:
Cafergot®: 2 tablets at onset of attack; then 1 tablet every 30 minutes as needed; maximum: 6 tablets per attack; do not exceed 10 tablets/week

(Continued)

Ergotamine *(Continued)*

Ergostat®: 1 tablet under tongue at first sign, then 1 tablet every 30 minutes if necessary; maximum: 3 tablets/24 hours; do not exceed 5 tablets/week

Inhalation: 1 inhalation at start of attack; repeat every 5 minutes if necessary; maximum: 6 inhalations/24 hours; do not exceed 15 inhalations/week

Rectal (Cafergot® suppositories, Wigraine® suppositories, Cafergot® P-B suppositories): 1 at first sign of an attack; follow with second dose after 1 hour, if needed; maximum: 2 per attack; do not exceed 5/week

Monitoring Parameters Relief of symptoms, blood pressure, pulse, peripheral circulation

Patient Information Any symptoms such as nausea, vomiting, numbness or tingling, and chest, muscle, or abdominal pain should be reported to the physician. Initiate therapy at first sign of attack. Do **not** exceed recommended dosage.

Nursing Implications Do not crush sublingual drug product

Additional Information
Ergotamine tartrate: Ergostat®
Ergotamine tartrate and caffeine: Cafergot®
Ergotamine, caffeine, belladonna alkaloids and pentobarbital: Cafergot® P-B

Special Geriatric Considerations May be harmful due to reduction in cerebral blood flow; may precipitate angina, myocardial infarction, or aggravate intermittent claudication; therefore, not considered a drug of choice in the elderly; see Contraindications and Precautions

Dosage Forms
Aerosol: 360 mcg/metered spray
Suppository, rectal: Ergotamine tartrate 2 mg and caffeine 100 mg (12/box)
Tablet: Ergotamine tartrate 1 mg and caffeine 100 mg
Tablet, sublingual: 2 mg

Eryc® *see* Erythromycin *on next page*

Erycette® *see* Erythromycin, Topical *on page 266*

EryDerm® *see* Erythromycin, Topical *on page 266*

Erymax® *see* Erythromycin, Topical *on page 266*

Erypar® *see* Erythromycin *on next page*

Ery-Tab® *see* Erythromycin *on next page*

Erythrityl Tetranitrate *(e ri' thri till)*

Brand Names Cardilate®

Generic Available Yes

Therapeutic Class Antianginal Agent; Nitrate; Vasodilator, Coronary

Use Prophylaxis and long-term treatment of frequent or recurrent anginal pain and reduced exercise tolerance associated with angina pectoris

Unlabeled use: Reduce cardiac workload in CHF or following a myocardial infarction; adjunct in treatment of Raynaud's disease

Contraindications Severe anemia, closed-angle glaucoma, postural hypotension, cerebral hemorrhage, head trauma, hypersensitivity to erythrityl tetranitrate or any component

Warnings Do not crush or chew sublingual dosage form; do not crush chewable tablets before administration; use with caution in patients with hypovolemia, glaucoma, increased intracranial pressure, hypotension

Precautions Increased intracranial pressure; do not stop use abruptly to avoid withdrawal reactions (angina); must gradually reduce daily doses to withdraw; tolerance to vascular effects of nitrates has been demonstrated; see Usual Dosage for recommendation to minimize development of tolerance

Adverse Reactions
Cardiovascular: Tachycardia, flushing, postural hypotension
Central nervous system: Restlessness, dizziness, headache, vertigo
Dermatologic: Rash
Gastrointestinal: Nausea, vomiting, diarrhea, GI upset
Hematologic: Methemoglobinemia
Neuromuscular & skeletal: Weakness

Overdosage Symptoms of overdose include hypotension, throbbing headache, palpitations, visual disturbances, flushing, perspiring skin, vertigo, diaphoresis, dizziness, syncope, nausea, vomiting, anorexia, dyspnea, heart block, confusion, fever, paralysis

Toxicology Formation of methemoglobinemia is dose-related and unusual in normal doses; high levels can cause signs and symptoms of hypoxemia; treatment consists of placing patient in recumbent position and administer fluids; alpha-adrenergic vasopressors may be required; treat methemoglobinemia with oxygen and methylene blue at a dose of 1-2 mg/kg I.V. slowly

Drug Interactions
May antagonize the anticoagulant effect of heparin; alcohol (increased hypotension) Aspirin (increases serum nitrate concentration); calcium channel blockers (increases hypotension)

Mechanism of Action Erythrityl tetranitrate, like other organic nitrates, induces vasodilation by dephosphorylation of the myosin light chain in smooth muscles. This is accomplished by activation of guanylate cyclase, which eventually stimulates a cyclic GMP-dependent protein kinase that alters the phosphorylation of the myosin. Venodilation causes peripheral blood pooling, which decreases venous return to the heart, central venous pressure, and pulmonary capillary wedge pressure. A reduction in pulmonary vascular resistance occurs secondary to pulmonary arteriolar dilation and afterload may be decreased by a lowering of systemic arterial pressure.

Pharmacodynamics
Onset of action:
Oral: 15-30 minutes
Tablets, sublingual/chewable: 5 minutes
Duration:
Oral: 6 hours
Tablets, sublingual/chewable: 3 hours

Pharmacokinetics
Absorption: Oral, sublingual: Well absorbed
Metabolism: Hepatic biotransformation through reductive hydrolysis catalyzed by glutathione-organic nitrate reductase

Usual Dosage Geriatrics and Adults: 5 mg sublingual or placed in the buccal pouch 3 times/day or 10 mg orally before meals or food, 3 times/day, increasing in 2-3 days if needed by adding doses in the midmorning and midafternoon to control symptoms; some patients may need bedtime doses if they experience nocturnal symptoms

Monitoring Parameters Monitor anginal episodes, orthostatic blood pressures; a decrease of 15 mm Hg pressure systolic and/or 10 mm Hg diastolic or an increase in heart rate of 10 beats/minute from baseline (no drug) indicates approximate maximal cardiodynamic effects to nitrates and end point for dosing

Test Interactions Decreased cholesterol (S)

Patient Information Dispense drug in easy-to-open container; do not chew or crush sublingual tablet; not for acute use; do not change brands without consulting your pharmacist or physician; patient should be instructed to take sublingual and chewable tablets while sitting down; any angina that persists for more than 20 minutes should be evaluated by a physician immediately

Nursing Implications Do not crush sublingual drug product; monitor blood pressure reduction for maximal effect and orthostatic hypotension

Additional Information Doses up to 100 mg are generally well tolerated; headache may occur when increasing doses; should headache occur, reduce dose for 2-3 days; may use analgesics to treat headache

Special Geriatric Considerations The first dose of nitrates should be taken in a physician's office to observe for maximal cardiovascular dynamic effects (see Monitoring Parameters) and adverse effects (orthostatic blood pressure drop, headache). The use of nitrates for angina may occasionally promote reflux esophagitis. This may require dose adjustments or changing therapeutic agents to correct this adverse effect. This agent offers no benefit over other nitrate products.

Dosage Forms Tablet, oral or sublingual (scored): 10 mg

Erythrocin® *see* Erythromycin *on this page*

Erythromycin (er ith roe mye' sin)
Brand Names E.E.S.®; E.E.S. 400®; E.E.S.® Chewable; E.E.S.® Granules; E-Mycin®; E-Mycin-E®; Eryc®; Erypar®; Ery-Tab®; Erythrocin®; Ilosone®; Ilosone® Pulvules®; Ilotycin® Gluceptate; PCE®; Wyamycin®

Synonyms Erythromycin Base; Erythromycin Estolate; Erythromycin Ethylsuccinate; Erythromycin Gluceptate; Erythromycin Lactobionate; Erythromycin Stearate

Generic Available Yes

Therapeutic Class Antibiotic, Macrolide; Antibiotic, Ophthalmic

Use Treatment of susceptible bacterial infections including *M. pneumoniae*, *Legionella* pneumonia, diphtheria, pertussis, chancroid, *Chlamydia*, and *Campylobacter* gastroenteritis; used in conjunction with neomycin for decontaminating the bowel

Unlabeled use: Gastroparesis

Contraindications Hepatic impairment, known hypersensitivity to erythromycin or its any components

Warnings Hepatic impairment with or without jaundice has occurred, it may be accompanied by malaise, nausea, vomiting, abdominal colic, and fever; discontinue use if these occur

Precautions Use with caution in patients with hepatic dysfunction

Adverse Reactions
Cardiovascular: Thrombophlebitis, ventricular arrhythmias

(Continued)

Erythromycin *(Continued)*

Central nervous system: Fever

Dermatologic: Skin rash

Gastrointestinal: Abdominal pain, cramping, nausea, vomiting, diarrhea, hypertrophic pyloric stenosis

Hematologic: Eosinophilia

Hepatic: Cholestatic hepatitis

Otic: Ototoxicity

Miscellaneous: Allergic reactions

Overdosage Symptoms of overdose include nausea, vomiting, diarrhea, prostration, reversible pancreatitis, hearing loss with or without tinnitus or vertigo

Toxicology General and supportive care only

Drug Interactions

Erythromycin decreased clearance of carbamazepine, cyclosporine, terfenadine, and triazolam

Increased effects of anticoagulants, increased bromocriptine, cyclosporine, disopyramide, digoxin, methylprednisolone, and ergot alkaloid serum concentrations have been reported; erythromycin may decrease theophylline clearance and increased theophylline's half-life by up to 60% (patients on high dose theophylline and erythromycin or who have received erythromycin for >5 days may be at higher risk)

Stability Erythromycin lactobionate should be reconstituted with sterile water for injection without preservatives to avoid gel formation; the reconstituted solution is stable for 2 weeks when refrigerated or 24 hours at room temperature. Erythromycin I.V. infusion solution is stable at pH 6-8. Do not use D_5W as a diluent unless sodium bicarbonate is added to solution.

Mechanism of Action Inhibits RNA-dependent protein synthesis at the chain elongation step; binds to the 50S ribosomal subunit resulting in blockage of transpeptidation

Pharmacokinetics

Absorption: Variable but better with salt forms than with base form; 18% to 45% absorbed orally

Protein binding: 75% to 90%

Metabolism: In the liver by demethylation

Half-life: 1.5-2 hours, prolonged with reduced renal function

Time to peak: Peak levels occur at 4 hours for the base, 3 hours for the stearate, 0.5-2.5 hours for the ethylsuccinate, 2-4 hours for the estolate; after oral administration peak serum levels occur within 4 hours (delayed in the presence of food except when using the estolate)

Elimination: 2% to 15% excreted as unchanged drug in urine and major excretion in feces (via bile)

Usual Dosage Geriatrics and Adults:

Ophthalmic: Instill 1 or more times/day depending on the severity of the infection

Oral:

Base: 333 mg every 8 hours

Estolate, stearate or base: 250-500 mg every 6-12 hours

Ethylsuccinate: 400-800 mg every 6-12 hours

Pre-op bowel preparation: 1 g erythromycin base at 1, 2, and 11 PM on the day before surgery combined with mechanical cleansing of the large intestine and oral neomycin

I.V.: 2-4 g/day divided every 6 hours

Bacterial endocarditis prophylaxis: Oral: 1 g 2 hours before procedure, then 500 mg 6 hours after initial dose

Administration Can give with food to decrease GI upset; tablets should be swallowed whole, do not crush or chew; burning at I.V. site and phlebitis, change I.V. site frequently; see Stability

Monitoring Parameters Signs and symptoms of infection

Test Interactions False-positive urinary catecholamines

Patient Information Complete full course of therapy, do not skip doses; refrigerate after reconstitution; chewable tablets should not be swallowed whole; notify physician or pharmacist if GI side effects are intolerable, diarrhea develops, or symptoms are not improving

Nursing Implications GI upset, including diarrhea, is common

Additional Information

Erythromycin base: E-Mycin®, Eryc®, Ery-Tab®, PCE®, Ilotycin®, Robimycin®

Erythromycin estolate: Ilosone®

Erythromycin ethylsuccinate: E.E.S.®, E-Mycin® E, EryPed®, Wyamycin® E

Erythromycin gluceptate: Ilotycin® Gluceptate

Erythromycin lactobionate: Erythrocin® Lactobionate-IV

Erythromycin stearate: Eramycin®, Erypar®, Erythrocin®, Ethril®, Wintrocin®, Wyamycin® S

Due to differences in absorption, 200 mg erythromycin ethylsuccinate produces the same serum levels as erythromycin base or estolate; do not use D_5W as a diluent unless sodium bicarbonate is added to solution; infuse over 30 minutes

Sodium content of oral suspension (ethyl succinate) 200 mg/5 mL: 29 mg (1.3 mEq)
Sodium content of base Filmtab® 250 mg: 70 mg (3 mEq)

Special Geriatric Considerations Dose of erythromycin does not need to be adjusted in the elderly unless there is severe renal impairment or hepatic dysfunction; has not been studied in the elderly

Dosage Forms
Capsule, as estolate: 125 mg, 250 mg
Capsule, delayed release: 250 mg
Ointment, ophthalmic: 5 mg/g (3.5 g)
Suspension, as estolate: 125 mg/5 mL (480 mL); 250 mg/5 mL (480 mL)
Suspension, as ethylsuccinate: 200 mg/5 mL (480 mL); 400 mg/5 mL (480 mL)
Tablet:
Chewable, as estolate: 125 mg, 250 mg
Chewable, as ethylsuccinate: 200 mg
Delayed release, as base: 250 mg, 333 mg, 500 mg
Film coated: 250 mg, 500 mg
Film coated, as ethylsuccinate: 400 mg
Polymer coated particles, as base: 333 mg
Tablet, as estolate: 500 mg

References
Yoshikawa TT, "Antimicrobial Therapy for the Elderly Patient," *J Am Geriatr Soc*, 1990, 38(12):1353-72.

Erythromycin and Sulfisoxazole (er ith roe mye' sin & sul fi sox' a zole)

Related Information
Erythromycin *on page 263*
Sulfisoxazole *on page 662*
Brand Names Eryzole®; E.S.P.®; Sulfimycin®
Synonyms Sulfisoxazole and Erythromycin
Generic Available Yes
Therapeutic Class Antibiotic, Macrolide; Antibiotic, Sulfonamide Derivative
Use Treatment of susceptible bacterial infections of the upper and lower respiratory tract; and other infections in patients allergic to penicillin
Contraindications Hepatic dysfunction, known hypersensitivity to erythromycin or sulfonamides; patients with porphyria
Precautions Use with caution in patients with impaired renal or hepatic function, G-6-PD deficiency (hemolysis may occur)
Adverse Reactions
Central nervous system: Headache
Dermatologic: Rash, Stevens-Johnson syndrome, toxic epidermal necrolysis
Gastrointestinal: Abdominal cramping, nausea, vomiting, diarrhea
Hematologic: Agranulocytosis, aplastic anemia
Hepatic: Hepatic necrosis
Renal: Toxic nephrosis, crystalluria
Overdosage Symptoms of overdose include nausea, vomiting, diarrhea, prostration, reversible pancreatitis, hearing loss with or without tinnitus or vertigo
Toxicology General and supportive care only; keep patient well hydrated
Drug Interactions
Erythromycin may decrease theophylline clearance and increase theophylline's half-life by up to 60% (patients on high doses of theophylline and erythromycin or on >5 days of erythromycin may be at higher risk)
Increased effect/toxicity/levels of alfentanil, anticoagulants, astemizole, terfenadine, loratadine, bromocriptine, carbamazepine, cyclosporine, digoxin, disopyramide, triazolam, and warfarin
Stability Reconstituted suspension is stable for 14 days when refrigerated
Mechanism of Action Erythromycin inhibits bacterial protein synthesis; sulfisoxazole competitively inhibits bacterial synthesis of folic acid from para-aminobenzoic acid
Pharmacokinetics
Erythromycin ethylsuccinate:
Absorption: Well from the GI tract
Protein binding: 75% to 90%
Metabolism: In the liver
Half-life: 1-1.5 hours
Elimination: Unchanged drug excreted and concentrated in bile
Sulfisoxazole acetyl:
Hydrolyzed in GI tract to sulfisoxazole which is readily absorbed
Protein binding: 85%
Half-life: 6 hours, prolonged in renal impairment
Elimination: 50% excreted in urine as unchanged drug
Usual Dosage Geriatrics and Adults: Oral (dosage recommendation is based on the product's erythromycin content): 400 mg erythromycin and 1200 mg sulfisoxazole every 6 hours

(Continued)

Erythromycin and Sulfisoxazole *(Continued)*

Dosing adjustment in renal impairment (sulfisoxazole must be adjusted in renal impairment):

Cl_{cr} 10-50 mL/minute: Administer every 8-12 hours

Cl_{cr} <10 mL/minute: Administer every 12-24 hours

Monitoring Parameters CBC and periodic liver function test

Test Interactions False-positive urinary protein

Patient Information Maintain adequate fluid intake; avoid prolonged exposure to sunlight; discontinue if rash appears

Special Geriatric Considerations See individual agents; not recommended for use in the elderly, see Usual Dosage; adjust dose for renal function

Dosage Forms Suspension, oral: Erythromycin ethylsuccinate 200 mg and sulfisoxazole acetyl 600 mg per 5 mL (100 mL, 150 mL, 200 mL)

Erythromycin Base *see* Erythromycin *on page 263*

Erythromycin Estolate *see* Erythromycin *on page 263*

Erythromycin Ethylsuccinate *see* Erythromycin *on page 263*

Erythromycin Gluceptate *see* Erythromycin *on page 263*

Erythromycin Lactobionate *see* Erythromycin *on page 263*

Erythromycin Stearate *see* Erythromycin *on page 263*

Erythromycin, Topical (er ith roe mye' sin)

Brand Names Akne-Mycin®; A/T/S®; C-Solve-2®; Erycette®; EryDerm®; Erymax®; E-Solve-2®; ETS-2%®; Staticin®; T-Stat®

Therapeutic Class Acne Products; Antibiotic, Topical

Use Topical treatment of acne vulgaris

Contraindications Known hypersensitivity to erythromycin

Precautions External use only

Adverse Reactions Dermatologic: Erythema, desquamation, dryness, pruritus

Drug Interactions Antagonism with clindamycin, inactivated by acids; sodium alginate, pectin, bentonite, calamine, silicate, and polysorbate 80 all decrease activity

Mechanism of Action Erythromycin works by binding to the bacterial 50S ribosomal subunit, apparently interfering with the translocation reaction in which the growing peptide chain is moved from the receptor to the donor site; this causes disruption of protein synthesis

Usual Dosage Geriatrics and Adults: Apply twice daily

Patient Information Contains benzoyl peroxide which may stain or bleach clothing

Special Geriatric Considerations Not for infected wounds or pressure sores

Dosage Forms

Gel: 2% (30 g, 60 g)

Gel (A/T/S®, Emgel™, Erygel®): 2% (27 g, 30 g, 60 g)

Ointment:

Ophthalmic (Ilotycin®, AK-Mycin®): 0.5% (1 g, 3.5 g, 3.75 g)

Topical (Akne-Mycin®): 2% (25 g)

Pad (T-Stat®): 2% (60s)

Solution, topical:

Staticin®: 1.5% (60 mL)

Akne-Mycin®, A/T/S®, Del-Mycin®, Eryderm™, Ery-sol®, ETS-2%®, Romycin®, Theramycin Z®, T-Stat®: 2% (60 mL, 66 mL, 120 mL)

Swab (Erycette®): 2% (60s)

Erythropoietin *see* Epoetin Alfa *on page 258*

Eryzole® *see* Erythromycin and Sulfisoxazole *on previous page*

Eserine Salicylate *see* Physostigmine *on page 562*

Esidrix® *see* Hydrochlorothiazide *on page 347*

Eskalith® *see* Lithium *on page 413*

Esmolol Hydrochloride (ess' moe lol)

Related Information

Beta-Blockers Comparison *on page 804-805*

Brand Names Brevibloc®

Therapeutic Class Antiarrhythmic Agent, Class II; Beta-Adrenergic Blocker

Use Supraventricular tachycardia (primarily to control ventricular rate) and sinus tachycardia

Contraindications Sinus bradycardia or heart block, uncompensated congestive heart failure, cardiogenic shock, hypersensitivity to esmolol, any component, or other beta-blockers

Warnings Caution should be exercised when discontinuing esmolol infusions to avoid withdrawal effects; although esmolol primarily blocks beta₁-receptors, high doses can result in beta$_2$-receptor blockade. Abrupt withdrawal of beta-blockers may result in an exaggerated cardiac beta-adrenergic responsiveness in coronary artery disease, however, this has not been reported with esmolol. Symptomatology has included reports of tachycardia, hypertension, ischemia, angina, myocardial infarction, and sudden death.

Precautions Use with extreme caution in patients with hyper-reactive airway disease; use lowest dose possible and discontinue infusion if bronchospasm occurs; use with caution in diabetes mellitus, hypoglycemia, renal failure; avoid extravasation, if extravasation occurs, use another I.V. site. Avoid use of butterfly needles.

Adverse Reactions

Cardiovascular: Hypotension (especially with higher doses), bradycardia, Raynaud's phenomena

Central nervous system: Dizziness, somnolence, confusion, lethargy, depression, headache

Gastrointestinal: Nausea, vomiting

Local: Skin necrosis after extravasation, phlebitis

Respiratory: Bronchoconstriction (less than propranolol, but more likely with higher doses)

Miscellaneous: Cold extremities, diaphoresis

Overdosage Symptoms of overdose include hypotension

Toxicology Sympathomimetics (eg, epinephrine or dopamine), glucagon or a pacemaker can be used to treat the toxic bradycardia, asystole, and/or hypotension. Initially, fluids may be the best treatment for toxic hypotension. Patients should remain supine; serum glucose and potassium should be measured. Use supportive measures: lavage, syrup of ipecac; atenolol may be removed by hemodialysis. I.V. glucose should be administered for hypoglycemia; seizures may be treated with phenytoin or diazepam intravenously; continuous monitoring of blood pressure and EKG is necessary. If PVCs occur, treat with lidocaine or phenytoin; avoid quinidine, procainamide, and disopyramide since these agents further depress myocardial function. Bronchospasm can be treated with theophylline or beta$_2$ agonists (epinephrine).

Drug Interactions

Pharmacologic action of beta-antagonists may be decreased by aluminum compounds, calcium salts, barbiturates, cholestyramine, colestipol, NSAIDs, penicillins (ampicillin), rifampin, salicylates, sulfinpyrazone, thyroid hormones; hypoglycemic effect of sulfonylureas may be blunted

Pharmacologic effect of beta-antagonists may be enhanced with concomitant use of calcium channel blockers, oral contraceptives, flecainide (bioavailability and effect of flecainide also enhanced), haloperidol (hypotensive effects of both drugs), H$_2$ antagonists (decreased metabolism), hydralazine (both drugs hypotensive effects increased), loop diuretics (increased serum levels of beta-blockers except atenolol), MAO inhibitors, phenothiazines, propafenone, quinidine, quinolones, thioamines

Beta-blockers may decrease clearance of acetaminophen; beta-blockers may increase anticoagulant effects of warfarin (propranolol)

Benzodiazepine effects enhanced by the lipophilic beta-blockers (atenolol does not interact)

Significant and fatal increases in blood pressure have occurred after decrease in dose or discontinuation of clonidine in patients receiving both clonidine and beta-blockers together (reduce doses of each cautiously with small decreases)

Peripheral ischemia of ergot alkaloids enhanced by beta-blockers

Beta-blockers increase serum concentration of lidocaine; beta-blockers increase hypotensive effect of prazosin

Stability Diluted I.V. infusion solution is stable for 24 hours at room temperature; compatible with the following I.V. solutions: 5% dextrose injection, 5% dextrose in lactated Ringer's injection, 5% dextrose in Ringer's injection, 5% dextrose and 0.9% **or** 0.45% sodium chloride injection, lactated Ringer's injection, potassium chloride (40 mEq/L) in 5% dextrose injection, and 0.9% or 0.45% sodium chloride injection. Esmolol is **not** compatible with 5% sodium bicarbonate injection.

Mechanism of Action Class II antiarrhythmic: Competitively blocks response to beta$_1$-adrenergic receptors, with little or no effect on beta$_2$-receptors except at high doses

Pharmacodynamics

Onset of action: Beta blockade occurs within 2-10 minutes following initiation of I.V. administration (onset of effects is quickest when loading doses are administered)

Duration: Short (10-30 minutes)

Pharmacokinetics

Protein binding: 55%

Metabolism: By esterase in cytosol or red blood cells

Half-life: 9 minutes

Elimination: ~69% of dose excreted in urine as metabolites and 2% as unchanged drug

Usual Dosage Must be adjusted to individual response and tolerance

Geriatrics and Adults: I.V.: Loading dose: 500 mcg/kg over 1 minute; follow with a 50 mcg/kg/minute infusion for 4 minutes; if response is inadequate, rebolus with anoth-

(Continued)

Esmolol Hydrochloride *(Continued)*

er 500 mcg/kg loading dose over 1 minute, and increase the maintenance infusion to 100 mcg/kg/minute. Repeat this process until a therapeutic effect has been achieved or to a maximum recommended maintenance dose of 200 mcg/kg/minute. Usual dosage range: 50-200 mcg/kg/minute with average dose = 100 mcg/kg/minute.

Monitoring Parameters Blood pressure, apical and peripheral pulse, EKG

Test Interactions Increased cholesterol (S), glucose

Nursing Implications The 250 mg/mL ampul is **not** for direct I.V. injection, but rather must first be diluted to a final concentration of 10 mg/mL (ie, 2.5 g in 250 mL or 5 g in 500 mL)

Special Geriatric Considerations Due to alterations in the beta-adrenergic autonomic nervous system, beta-adrenergic blockade may result in less hemodynamic response than seen in younger adults. Studies indicate that despite decreased sensitivity to the chronotropic effects of beta blockade with age, there appears to be an increased myocardial sensitivity to the negative inotropic effect during stress (ie, exercise). Controlled trials have shown the overall response rate for propranolol to be only 20% to 50% in elderly populations. Therefore, all beta-adrenergic blocking drugs may result in a decreased response as compared to younger adults.

Dosage Forms Injection: 10 mg/mL (10 mL); 250 mg/mL (10 mL)

References

Vincent RN, Click LA, Williams HM, et al, "Esmolol As an Adjunct in the Treatment of Systemic Hypertension After Operative Repair of Coarctation of the Aorta," *Am J Cardiol*, 1990, 65(13):941-3.

E-Solve-2® *see* Erythromycin, Topical *on page 266*

E.S.P.® *see* Erythromycin and Sulfisoxazole *on page 265*

Estazolam *(eh sta' zo lam)*

Related Information

Antacid Drug Interactions *on page 764*

Anxiolytic/Hypnotic Use in Long-Term Care Facilities *on page 755-756*

Benzodiazepines Comparison *on page 802-803*

Brand Names ProSom™

Generic Available No

Therapeutic Class Benzodiazepine; Hypnotic; Sedative

Use Short-term management of insomnia

Restrictions C-IV

Contraindications Hypersensitivity to estazolam, cross-sensitivity with other benzodiazepines may occur, severe uncontrolled pain, pre-existing CNS depression, narrow-angle glaucoma, sleep apnea

Warnings Abrupt discontinuance may precipitate withdrawal or rebound insomnia

Precautions Potential for drug dependence and abuse; use with caution in patients with the potential for drug dependence

Adverse Reactions

Central nervous system: Drowsiness, amnesia, confusion, dizziness, headache, ataxia, impaired coordination

Gastrointestinal: Nausea, vomiting, dry mouth

Hepatic: Cholestatic jaundice

Miscellaneous: Physical and psychological dependence may occur with prolonged use

Overdosage Symptoms of overdose include somnolence, confusion, coma, and diminished reflexes

Toxicology Treatment for benzodiazepine overdose is supportive; rarely is mechanical ventilation required; flumazenil has been shown to selectively block the binding of benzodiazepines to CNS receptors, resulting in a reversal of benzodiazepine-induced sedation; however, its use may not alter the course of overdose

Drug Interactions Increased toxicity: CNS depressants, alcohol

Mechanism of Action Benzodiazepines appear to potentiate the effects of GABA and other inhibitory neurotransmitters by binding to specific benzodiazepine-receptor sites in various areas of the CNS

Pharmacodynamics Studies have shown that the elderly are more sensitive to the effects of benzodiazepines as compared to younger adults

Pharmacokinetics

Metabolism: Rapid and extensive in the liver to inactive metabolites

Half-life: 10-24 hours (no significant changes in the elderly)

Time to peak serum concentration: 0.5-1.6 hours

Elimination: <5% excreted unchanged in urine

Usual Dosage Oral:

Geriatrics: Initial: 0.5-1 mg at bedtime

Adults: 1-2 mg at bedtime

Monitoring Parameters Respiratory, cardiovascular, and mental status

Patient Information Avoid alcohol and other CNS depressants; may cause drowsi-

ness; avoid activities needing good psychomotor coordination until CNS effects are
known; may cause physical or psychological dependence; avoid abrupt discontinuation after prolonged use

Nursing Implications Provide safety measures (ie, side rails, night light, and call button); remove smoking materials from area; supervise ambulation

Special Geriatric Considerations There has been little experience with this drug in
the elderly, but because of its lack of active metabolites, estazolam would be a rea-
sonable choice when a benzodiazepine hypnotic is indicated; see Pharmacodynamics

Dosage Forms Tablet: 1 mg, 2 mg

Estivin® II [OTC] *see* Naphazoline Hydrochloride *on page 492*

Estrace® *see* Estradiol *on this page*

Estraderm® *see* Estradiol *on this page*

Estradiol (ess tra dye' ole)

Brand Names Delestrogen®; depGynogen®; Depo®-Estradiol; Depogen®; Dioval®;
Dura-Estrin®; Duragen®; E-Cypionate®; Estrace®; Estraderm®; Estro-Cyp®; Es-
trofem®; Estroject-L.A.®; Estronol-LA®; Ru-Est-Span®; Valergen®

Synonyms Estradiol Cypionate; Estradiol Valerate

Generic Available Yes

Therapeutic Class Estrogen Derivative

Use Treatment of atrophic vaginitis, urinary incontinence secondary to estrogen deficiency, atrophic dystrophy of vulva, menopausal symptoms, female hypogonadism,
oophorectomy, ovariectomy, primary ovarian failure, inoperable breast cancer, inoperable prostatic cancer, mild to severe vasomotor symptoms associated with menopause, prevention of osteoporosis

Contraindications Undiagnosed genital bleeding, diplopia, active liver disease; carcinoma of the breast (with certain exceptions), estrogen-dependent tumor, present or
past thromboembolic disease, cerebrovascular disease

Warnings Estrogens have been reported to increase the risk of endometrial carcinoma; this risk can be reduced by cycling with a progestin (ie, medroxyprogesterone)
for the last 10-13 days of estrogen therapy each month or administering daily throughout the month

Precautions Use with caution in patients with renal or hepatic insufficiency; in patients
with a history of thromboembolism, stroke, liver tumor, hypertension

Adverse Reactions
Cardiovascular: Increase in blood pressure, edema, thromboembolic disorders
Central nervous system: Depression, headache
Dermatologic: Chloasma, melasma, scalp hair loss
Endocrine & metabolic: Hypercalcemia, folate deficiency, breakthrough bleeding,
spotting, endometrial carcinoma
Gastrointestinal: Nausea, vomiting, bloating
Genitourinary: Increased libido (female), decreased libido (male)
Hepatic: Cholestatic jaundice, increased LDL and triglycerides
Local: Pain at injection site, enlargement of breasts (female and male), breast tender-
ness

Overdosage Symptoms of overdose include fluid retention, jaundice, thrombophlebitis

Toxicology Toxicity is unlikely following single exposures of excessive doses, any
treatment following emesis and charcoal administration should be supportive and
symptomatic

Drug Interactions
Rifampin, barbiturates, cigarette smoking, and other agents that induce hepatic metabolism can increase estrogen clearance and decrease serum concentrations
Increased toxicity (potential) with anticoagulants, tricyclic antidepressants, corticosteroids

Mechanism of Action Increases the synthesis of DNA, RNA, and various proteins in
target tissues; reduces the release of gonadotropin-releasing hormone from the hypothalamus; reduces FSH and LH release from the pituitary

Pharmacokinetics
Absorption: Readily through skin and GI tract
Protein binding: 80%
Half-life: 50-60 minutes
Elimination: Principally degraded in the liver and excreted in urine as conjugates;
small amounts excreted in feces via bile, reabsorbed from the GI tract and entero-
hepatically recycled

Usual Dosage Geriatrics and Adults (all doses need to be adjusted based upon the
patient's response):

Male:
Prostate cancer: Valerate: I.M.: ≥30 mg or more every 1-2 weeks
Prostate cancer (androgen-dependent, inoperable, progressing): Oral: 10 mg 3
times/day for at least 3 months

(Continued)

269

Estradiol (Continued)

Female:
Hypogonadism:
Oral: 1-2 mg/day
I.M.: Valerate: 10-20 mg/month
Transdermal: 0.05 mg patch initially (titrate dosage to response) applied twice weekly
Osteoporosis prevention: Oral: 0.5 mg/day
Breast cancer (inoperable, progressing): Oral: 10 mg 3 times/day for at least 3 months
Atrophic vaginitis, kraurosis vulvae: Vaginal: Insert 2-4 g/day for 2 weeks then gradually reduce to $\frac{1}{2}$ the initial dose for 2 weeks followed by a maintenance dose of 1 g 1-3 times/week
Moderate to severe vasomotor symptoms: I.M.:
Cypionate: 1-5 mg every 3-4 months
Valerate: 10-20 mg every 4 weeks

Monitoring Parameters Mammography should be performed in all women prior to starting estrogen therapy and then every 18-24 months; blood pressure; PAP smear at baseline and then every 2 years; clinical breast exam annually

Reference Range Male: 10-50 pg/mL (SI: 37-184 pmol/L); postmenopausal female: 0-30 pg/mL (SI: 0-110 pmol/L)

Test Interactions Increased chloride (S), glucose, iron (B), sodium (S), thyroxine (S); decreased protein, prothrombin time (S)

Patient Information Women should inform their physicians if signs or symptoms of any of the following occur: thromboembolic or thrombotic disorders including sudden severe headache or vomiting, disturbance of vision or speech, loss of vision, numbness or weakness in an extremity, sharp or crushing chest pain, calf pain, shortness of breath, severe abdominal pain or mass, mental depression or unusual bleeding. Women should perform regular self exams on breasts. Notify physician if area under dermal patch becomes irritated or a rash develops.

Nursing Implications For intramuscular use only

Special Geriatric Considerations Before prescribing estrogen therapy to postmenopausal women, the risks and benefits must be weighed for each patient. Women should be informed of these risks and benefits, as well as possible side effects and the return of menstrual bleeding (when cycled with a progestin), and be involved in the decision to prescribe. Oral therapy may be more convenient for vaginal atrophy and urinary incontinence.

Dosage Forms

Cream, vaginal (Estrace®): 0.1 mg/g (42.5 g)
Injection, as cypionate (depGynogen®, Depo®-Estradiol, Depogen®, Dura-Estrin®, Estra-D®, Estro-Cyp®, Estroject-L.A.®): 5 mg/mL (5 mL, 10 mL)
Injection, as valerate:
Delestrogen®, Valergen®: 10 mg/mL (5 mL, 10 mL); 20 mg/mL (1 mL, 5 mL, 10 mL); 40 mg/mL (5 mL, 10 mL)
Dioval®, Duragen®, Estra-L®, Gynogen L.A.®: 20 mg/mL (10 mL); 40 mg/mL (10 mL)
Tablet, micronized (Estrace®): 1 mg, 2 mg
Transdermal system (Estraderm®):
0.05 mg/24 hours [10 cm²], total estradiol 4 mg
0.1 mg/24 hours [20 cm²], total estradiol 8 mg

References

American College of Physicians, "Guidelines for Counseling Postmenopausal Women About Preventive Hormone Therapy," *Ann Intern Med*, 1992, 117(12):1038-41.
Belchetz PE, "Hormone Treatment for Postmenopausal Women," *N Engl J Med*, 1994, 330(15):1062-71.

Estradiol Cypionate see Estradiol on previous page

Estradiol Valerate see Estradiol on previous page

Estro-Cyp® see Estradiol on previous page

Estrofem® see Estradiol on previous page

Estrogenic Substances, Conjugated see Estrogens, Conjugated on this page

Estrogens, Conjugated (ess' troe jenz)

Brand Names Premarin®
Synonyms C.E.S.; Estrogenic Substances, Conjugated
Generic Available Yes: Tablet
Therapeutic Class Estrogen Derivative
Use Atrophic vaginitis; atrophic dystrophy of vulva, urinary incontinence secondary to estrogen deficiency; hypogonadism; primary ovarian failure; vasomotor symptoms of menopause; prostatic carcinoma; prevention of osteoporosis, inoperable breast cancer

Contraindications Undiagnosed vaginal bleeding; hypersensitivity to estrogens or any component; thrombophlebitis, liver disease, breast cancer (with certain exceptions)

Warnings Estrogens have been reported to increase the risk of endometrial carcinoma; this risk can be reduced by cycling with a progestin (ie, medroxyprogesterone) for the last 10-13 days of estrogen therapy each month

Precautions Use with caution in patients with asthma, epilepsy, migraine, diabetes, cardiac or renal dysfunction

Adverse Reactions
Cardiovascular: Increase in blood pressure, edema, thromboembolic disorder
Central nervous system: Depression, headache
Dermatologic: Chloasma, melasma, scalp hair loss
Endocrine & metabolic: Breast tenderness, hypercalcemia, breakthrough bleeding, spotting, endometrial carcinoma
Gastrointestinal: Nausea, vomiting
Hepatic: Cholestatic jaundice
Local: Pain at injection site

Overdosage Symptoms of overdose include fluid retention, jaundice, thrombophlebitis

Toxicology Toxicity is unlikely following single exposures of excessive doses, any treatment following emesis and charcoal administration should be supportive and symptomatic

Drug Interactions
Rifampin, barbiturates, cigarette smoking, and other agents that induce hepatic metabolism can increase estrogen clearance and decrease serum concentrations
Increased toxicity (potential) with anticoagulants, tricyclic antidepressants, corticosteroids

Stability Refrigerate injection

Mechanism of Action Increases the synthesis of DNA, RNA, and various proteins in target tissues; reduces the release of gonadotropin-releasing hormone from the hypothalamus; reduces FSH and LH release from the pituitary

Pharmacokinetics
Absorption: Readily from GI tract
Metabolism: To inactive compounds occurs in the liver
Elimination: In bile and urine

Usual Dosage Geriatrics and Adults:
Abnormal uterine bleeding:
Oral: 2.5-5 mg/day for 7-10 days; then decrease to 1.25 mg/day for 2 weeks
I.V.: 25 mg every 6-12 hours until bleeding stops

Osteoporosis: Oral: 0.625 mg/day chronically

Vasomotor symptoms: 0.3-1.25 mg/day; recommended duration: 5 years

Vaginal atrophy/urinary continence:
Oral: 0.3-0.625 mg/day; treat for 3 months and repeat as necessary
Cream: 2-4 g/day ($\frac{1}{2}$ to 1 applicatorful)

Monitoring Parameters Mammography should be performed in all women prior to starting estrogen therapy and then annually; blood pressure; PAP smear annually

Reference Range Male: 15-40 μg/24 hours (SI: 52-139 μmol/day); Female, postmenopausal: <20 μg/24 hours (SI: 69 μmol/day) (values at Mayo Medical Laboratories)

Test Interactions Increased chloride (S), glucose (S), iron (B), sodium (S), thyroxine (S); decreased protein, prothrombin time (S); endocrine function test may be altered

Patient Information Women should inform their physicians if signs or symptoms of any of the following occur: thromboembolic or thrombotic disorders including sudden severe headache or vomiting, disturbance of vision or speech, loss of vision, numbness or weakness in an extremity, sharp or crushing chest pain, calf pain, shortness of breath, severe abdominal pain or mass, mental depression or unusual bleeding; women should perform regular self-exams on breasts

Nursing Implications May also be administered intramuscularly; give at bedtime to minimize occurrence of adverse effects; when administered I.V. drug should be administered slowly to avoid the occurrence of a flushing reaction

Special Geriatric Considerations Before prescribing estrogen therapy to postmenopausal women, the risks and benefits must be weighed for each patient; women should be informed of these risks and benefits, as well as possible side effects and the return of menstrual bleeding (when cycled with a progestin), and be involved in the decision to prescribe. Oral therapy may be more convenient for vaginal atrophy and urinary incontinence.

Dosage Forms
Cream, vaginal: 0.625 mg/g (42.5 g)
Injection: 25 mg (5 mL)
Tablet: 0.3 mg, 0.625 mg, 0.9 mg, 1.25 mg, 2.5 mg

References

American College of Physicians, "Guidelines for Counseling Postmenopausal Women About Preventive Hormone Therapy," Ann Intern Med, 1992, 117(12):1038-41.
Belchetz PE, "Hormonal Treatment of Postmenopausal Women," N Engl J Med, 1994, 330 (15): 1062-71.

ALPHABETICAL LISTING OF DRUGS

Estroject-L.A.® *see* Estradiol *on page 269*

Estronol-LA® *see* Estradiol *on page 269*

Ethacrynic Acid (eth a krin' ik)

Brand Names Edecrin®

Generic Available No

Therapeutic Class Diuretic, Loop

Use Management of edema associated with congestive heart failure; hepatic cirrhosis or renal disease; short-term management of ascites due to malignancy, idiopathic edema, and lymphedema

Contraindications Hypersensitivity to ethacrynic acid or any component; anuria, hypotension, dehydration with low serum sodium concentrations; metabolic alkalosis with hypokalemia, or history of severe, watery diarrhea from ethacrynic acid

Warnings Loop diuretics are potent diuretics; excess amount can lead to profound diuresis with fluid and electrolyte loss; close medical supervision and dose evaluation is required, particularly in the elderly

Precautions Use with caution in patients with advanced hepatic cirrhosis or diabetes mellitus

Adverse Reactions
Cardiovascular: Hypotension
Central nervous system: Headache
Dermatologic: Rash
Endocrine & metabolic: Fluid and electrolyte imbalances (fluid depletion, hypokalemia, hyponatremia), hyperuricemia
Gastrointestinal: GI irritation, diarrhea
Hematologic: Thrombocytopenia, neutropenia, agranulocytosis
Hepatic: Abnormal liver function tests
Ocular: Blurred vision
Otic: Ototoxicity
Renal: Renal injury

Overdosage Symptoms of overdose include electrolyte depletion, volume depletion, dehydration, circulatory collapse

Toxicology Following GI decontamination, treatment is supportive; hypotension responds to fluids and Trendelenburg position

Drug Interactions
Decreased effect: Indomethacin, other NSAIDs
Increased hypotensive effect: Other antihypertensives
Increased level of lithium
Increased risk of ototoxicity: Aminoglycosides, other loop diuretics, vancomycin
Increased effect/toxicity of warfarin, lithium
When given with digoxin, diuretic-induced hypokalemia increases the risk of digoxin toxicity

Mechanism of Action Inhibits reabsorption of sodium and chloride in the ascending loop of Henle and distal renal tubule, interfering with the chloride-binding cotransport system, thus causing increased excretion of water, sodium, chloride, magnesium, and calcium

Pharmacodynamics
Onset of action:
Oral: Following administration diuretic effects occur within 30 minutes and peak in 2 hours
I.V.: Diuresis occurs in 5 minutes and peaks in 30 minutes
Duration of action:
Oral: 12 hours
I.V.: 2 hours

Pharmacokinetics
Absorption: Oral: Rapid
Metabolism: In the liver to active cysteine conjugate
Elimination: In bile and urine

Usual Dosage
Geriatrics: Oral: Initial: 25-50 mg/day
Adults:
Oral: Initial: 50-200 mg/day in 1-2 divided doses; increase by 25-50 mg/day to desired response
I.V.: 0.5-1 mg/kg/dose (maximum: 50 mg/dose); repeat doses not recommended

Administration Injection should **not** be given S.C. or I.M. due to local pain and irritation; single I.V. doses should not exceed 100 mg; use a new injection site if a second dose is needed, to avoid possible thrombophlebitis

Monitoring Parameters Blood pressure (both standing and sitting/supine), serum electrolytes, renal function, auditory function, weight, I & O

Test Interactions Increased ammonia (B), amylase (S), glucose, uric acid (S); decreased calcium (S); chloride (S), magnesium, sodium (S)

Patient Information May be taken with food or milk; get up slowly from a lying or sitting position to minimize dizziness, lightheadedness, or fainting; also use extra care when exercising, standing for long periods of time and during hot weather; take in the morning; take the last dose of multiple doses before 6 PM unless instructed otherwise

Nursing Implications See Monitoring Parameters and Administration

Additional Information Injection form may be given orally while hospitalized; ethacrynic acid should be saved for patients who are either allergic or resistant to furosemide or bumetanide

Special Geriatric Considerations Ethacrynic acid is rarely used because of its increased incidence of ototoxicity as compared to the other loop diuretics; see Additional Information

Dosage Forms
Injection, as ethacrynate sodium: 1 mg/mL (50 mL)
Tablet: 25 mg, 50 mg

Ethambutol Hydrochloride (e tham' byoo tole)

Brand Names Myambutol®

Therapeutic Class Antitubercular Agent

Use Treatment of tuberculosis and other mycobacterial diseases in conjunction with other antituberculosis agents

Contraindications Hypersensitivity to ethambutol or any component; optic neuritis

Precautions Dosage modification required in patients with renal insufficiency

Adverse Reactions
Central nervous system: Malaise, peripheral neuritis, mental confusion, fever, headache
Dermatologic: Rash, pruritus
Endocrine & metabolic: Elevated uric acid levels
Gastrointestinal: Nausea, vomiting, abdominal pain, anorexia
Hepatic: Abnormal liver function tests
Ocular: Optic neuritis
Miscellaneous: Anaphylaxis, acute gout

Overdosage Symptoms of overdose include decrease in visual acuity, anorexia, joint pain, numbness of the extremities, toxic epidermal necrolysis

Toxicology Following GI decontamination, treatment is supportive

Drug Interactions Aluminum salts may delay absorption; take separately

Mechanism of Action Suppresses mycobacteria multiplication by interfering with RNA synthesis

Pharmacokinetics
Absorption: Oral: ~80%
Distribution: Well throughout the body with high concentrations in kidneys, lungs, saliva and red blood cells
Protein binding: 20% to 30%
Metabolism: 20% by the liver to inactive metabolite
Half-life: 2.5-3.6 hours (up to 7 hours or longer with renal impairment)
Time to peak: Peak serum levels occur in 2-4 hours
Elimination: ~50% in urine and 20% excreted in feces as unchanged drug

Usual Dosage Geriatrics and Adults: Oral: 15-25 mg/kg/day once daily, not to exceed 2.5 g/day

Dosing interval in renal impairment:
Cl_{cr} 10-50 mL/minute: Administer every 24-36 hours
Cl_{cr} <10 mL/minute: Administer every 48 hours and/or reduce daily dose

Monitoring Parameters Periodic visual testing in patients receiving more than 15 mg/kg/day; periodic renal, hepatic, and hematopoietic tests

Test Interactions Increased uric acid (S)

Patient Information Report any visual changes to physician; may cause stomach upset, take with food

Nursing Implications Reinforce compliance

Special Geriatric Considerations Since most elderly patients acquired their tuberculosis before current antituberculin regimens were available, ethambutol is only indicated when patients are from areas where drug resistant M. tuberculosis is endemic, in HIV-infected elderly patients, and when drug resistant M. tuberculosis is suspected; see dose adjustments for renal impairment

Dosage Forms Tablet: 100 mg, 400 mg

References
Yoshikawa TT, "Tuberculosis in Aging Adults," *J Am Geriatr Soc*, 1992, 40(2):178-87.

Ethionamide (e thye on am' ide)

Brand Names Trecator®-SC

Therapeutic Class Antitubercular Agent

Use In conjunction with other antituberculosis agents in the treatment of tuberculosis and other mycobacterial diseases

Contraindications Contraindicated in patients with severe hepatic impairment or in patients who are hypersensitive to the drug

(Continued)

Ethionamide *(Continued)*

Precautions Use with caution in diabetic patients and patients receiving cycloserine or isoniazid

Adverse Reactions
Cardiovascular: Postural hypotension
Central nervous system: Drowsiness, dizziness, optic neuritis, peripheral neuritis, seizures, headache
Dermatologic: Rash, stomatitis
Endocrine & metabolic: Hypoglycemia, goiter, gynecomastia
Gastrointestinal: Nausea, vomiting, abdominal pain, diarrhea, anorexia, metallic taste
Hematologic: Thrombocytopenia
Hepatic: Hepatitis

Overdosage Symptoms of overdose include peripheral neuropathy, anorexia, joint pain

Toxicology Following GI decontamination, treatment is supportive; pyridoxine may be given to prevent peripheral neuropathy

Mechanism of Action Inhibits peptide synthesis

Pharmacokinetics
Protein binding: 10%
Bioavailability: 80%
Half-life: 2-3 hours
Time to peak: Oral: Peak serum levels occur within 3 hours
Elimination: Metabolized and excreted as metabolites (active and inactive) and parent drug in urine

Usual Dosage Geriatrics and Adults: Oral: 500-1000 mg/day in 1-3 divided doses

Monitoring Parameters Initial and periodic serum AST and ALT

Test Interactions Decreased thyroxine (S)

Patient Information Take with meals, may cause upset stomach and loss of appetite, metallic taste or salivation

Nursing Implications Neurotoxic effects may be relieved by the administration of pyridoxine

Special Geriatric Considerations See Usual Dosage and Overdosage

Dosage Forms Tablet: 250 mg

Ethmozine® *see* Moricizine Hydrochloride *on page 479*

Ethopropazine Hydrochloride *(eth oh proe' pa zeen)*

Related Information
Antacid Drug Interactions *on page 764*

Brand Names Parsidol®

Generic Available No

Therapeutic Class Anti-Parkinson's Agent

Use Treatment of parkinsonism, drug-induced extrapyramidal reactions

Contraindications Patients with narrow-angle glaucoma; hypersensitivity to any component; pyloric or duodenal obstruction, stenosing peptic ulcers; bladder neck obstructions; achalasia; myasthenia gravis

Precautions Use with caution in hot weather or during exercise. Elderly patients frequently develop increased sensitivity and require strict dosage regulation – side effects may be more severe in elderly patients with atherosclerotic changes. Use with caution in patients with tachycardia, cardiac arrhythmias, hypertension, hypotension, prostatic hypertrophy (especially in the elderly) or any tendency toward urinary retention, liver or kidney disorders and obstructive disease of the GI or GU tract. May exacerbate mental symptoms and precipitate a toxic psychosis when used to treat extrapyramidal reactions resulting from phenothiazines. When given in large doses or to susceptible patients, may cause weakness and inability to move particular muscle groups. Anticholinergic agents can aggravate tardive dyskinesia caused by neuroleptic agents.

Adverse Reactions
Cardiovascular: Tachycardia
Central nervous system: Coma, nervousness, drowsiness, seizures, memory loss (**the elderly may be at increased risk for confusion and hallucinations**)
Dermatologic: Pigmentation of the skin
Gastrointestinal: Nausea, vomiting, constipation, dry mouth
Genitourinary: Urinary retention
Hepatic: Jaundice
Ocular: Blurred vision, mydriasis, pigmentation of the cornea, lens, retina
Miscellaneous: Heat intolerance

Overdosage Symptoms of overdose include CNS depression, confusion, nervousness, hallucinations, dizziness, blurred vision, nausea, vomiting, hyperthermia

Toxicology Anticholinergic toxicity is caused by strong binding of the drug to cholinergic receptors. Anticholinesterase inhibitors reduce acetylcholinesterase, the enzyme that breaks down acetylcholine and thereby allows acetylcholine to accumulate and compete for receptor binding with the offending anticholinergic. For anticholinergic overdose with severe life-threatening symptoms, physostigmine 1-2 mg S.C. or I.V., slowly may be given to reverse these effects.

Drug Interactions
Decreased effect of levodopa (decreased absorption); decreased effect with tacrine Increased toxicity (central anticholinergic syndrome): Narcotic analgesics, phenothiazines, and other antipsychotics, tricyclic antidepressants, some antihistamines, quinidine, disopyramide

Mechanism of Action Phenothiazine-derivative with strong atropine-like blocking effects on parasympathetic-innervated peripheral structures; also exhibits antihistamine activity

Pharmacokinetics No data available

Usual Dosage Geriatrics and Adults: Oral: Initial: 50 mg once or twice daily, increasing gradually; severe cases may need up to 600 mg/day

Monitoring Parameters Symptoms of EPS or Parkinson's, pulse, anticholinergic effects (ie, CNS, bowel and bladder function)

Patient Information Take after meals or with food if GI upset occurs; do not discontinue drug abruptly; notify physician if adverse GI effects, rapid or pounding heartbeat, confusion, eye pain, rash, fever or heat intolerance occurs. Observe caution when performing hazardous tasks or those that require alertness such as driving, as may cause drowsiness. Avoid alcohol and other CNS depressants. May cause dry mouth – adequate fluid intake or hard sugar-free candy may relieve. Difficult urination or constipation may occur – notify physician if effects persist; may increase susceptibility to heat stroke.

Nursing Implications Do not discontinue drug abruptly

Additional Information Ethopropazine is a phenothiazine with prominent anticholinergic effects. It is less effective than the synthetic anticholinergic agents. High doses of ethopropazine are relatively well tolerated in adults.

Special Geriatric Considerations Anticholinergic agents are generally not well tolerated in the elderly and their use should be avoided when possible; see Precautions and Adverse Reactions. In the elderly, anticholinergic agents should not be used as prophylaxis against extrapyramidal symptoms.

Dosage Forms Tablet: 10 mg, 50 mg

References
Feinberg M, "The Problems of Anticholinergic Adverse Effects in Older Patients," *Drugs Aging*, 1993, 3(4):335-48.

Ethosuximide (eth oh sux' i mide)

Brand Names Zarontin®

Generic Available No

Therapeutic Class Anticonvulsant, Succinimide

Use Management of absence (petit mal) seizures, myoclonic seizures, and akinetic epilepsy; considered to be drug of choice for simple absence seizures

Contraindications Known hypersensitivity to ethosuximide or any succinimide

Warnings Use with caution in patients with hepatic or renal disease; abrupt withdrawal of the drug may precipitate absence status; ethosuximide may increase tonic-clonic seizures in patients with mixed seizure disorders; ethosuximide must be used in combination with other anticonvulsants in patients with both absence and tonic-clonic seizures

Precautions Proceed slowly when increasing or decreasing dose of ethosuximide; use caution and monitor closely when adding or eliminating other medications

Adverse Reactions
Central nervous system: Sedation, fatigue, dizziness, lethargy, euphoria, ataxia, irritability, nervousness, hallucinations, insomnia, agitation, behavioral changes, headache, sleep disturbances, loss of concentration, confusion, depression, aggressiveness

Dermatologic: Rashes, urticaria, Stevens-Johnson syndrome, erythema multiforme, alopecia

Gastrointestinal: Nausea, vomiting, anorexia, abdominal pain, cramps, diarrhea, constipation

Genitourinary: Vaginal bleeding, urinary frequency, hematuria (also microscopic hematuria)

Hematologic: Rarely: Leukopenia, aplastic anemia, thrombocytopenia, eosinophilia, granulocytopenia, monocytosis, pancytopenia

Ocular: Blurred vision, periorbital edema

Miscellaneous: Rarely SLE, swelling of tongue, gingival hypertrophy, hiccups

Overdosage Acute overdosage can cause CNS depression, ataxia, stupor, coma, hypotension; chronic overdose can cause skin rash, confusion, ataxia, proteinuria, hepatic dysfunction, hematuria

Toxicology Treatment is supportive; hemoperfusion and hemodialysis may be useful

Drug Interactions
May increase serum concentrations of hydantoins (phenytoin)

(Continued)

Ethosuximide *(Continued)*

Decreases serum concentrations of phenobarbital and primidone
Serum concentrations of valproic acid may increase or decrease

Mechanism of Action Increases the seizure threshold and suppresses paroxysmal spike-and-wave pattern in absence seizures; depresses nerve transmission in the motor cortex

Pharmacokinetics
Absorption: Well absorbed from GI tract
Distribution: Adults: V_d: 0.62-0.72 L/kg
Metabolism: ~80% in the liver to three inactive metabolites
Half-life: 50-60 hours
Time to peak serum concentration:
Capsule: Within 3-7 hours
Syrup: <2-4 hours
Elimination: Slowly excreted in urine as metabolites (50%) and as unchanged drug (10% to 20%); small amounts excreted in feces

Usual Dosage Geriatrics and Adults: Oral: Initial: 250 mg twice daily; increase by 250 mg as needed every 4-7 days up to 1.5 g/day in 2 divided doses

Monitoring Parameters CBC, platelets, liver enzymes, trough ethosuximide serum concentration

Reference Range Therapeutic: 40-100 μg/mL (SI: 280-710 μmol/L); Toxic: >150 μg/mL (SI: >1062 μmol/L)

Test Interactions Increased alkaline phosphatase (S); positive Coombs' [direct]; decreased calcium (S)

Patient Information Take with food; do not discontinue abruptly; may cause drowsiness and impair judgment; patient should have a "Medic Alert" identification; call physician if experiencing rash, fever, sore throat, bleeding, dizziness, blurred vision

Nursing Implications Observe patient for excess sedation; maintain serum levels; monitor for bruising and bleeding

Additional Information Considered to be drug of choice for simple absence seizures

Special Geriatric Considerations No specific studies with the use of this medication in elderly; consider renal function and proceed slowly with dosing increases; monitor closely

Dosage Forms
Capsule: 250 mg
Syrup (raspberry flavor): 250 mg/5 mL (473 mL)

Ethoxynaphthamido Penicillin Sodium *see* Nacfillin Sodium
on page 487

Etidronate Disodium (e ti droe' nate)

Brand Names Didronel®

Synonyms EHDP; Sodium Etidronate

Therapeutic Class Antidote, Hypercalcemia; Biphosphonate Derivative

Use Symptomatic treatment of Paget's disease and heterotopic ossification due to spinal cord injury or after total hip replacement, hypercalcemia associated with malignancy

Unlabeled use: Postmenopausal osteoporosis

Contraindications Hypersensitivity to biphosphonates; patients with serum creatinine >5 mg/dL

Warnings Response may be slow; therefore, do not increase therapy prematurely or resume therapy before there is evidence of reactivation of disease process; renal dysfunction in hypercalcemic treatment (reversible)

Precautions Use with caution in patients with restricted calcium and vitamin D intake; dosage modification required in renal impairment; must maintain adequate calcium and vitamin D intake; do not administer during bouts of enterocolitis since it may aggravate or induce diarrhea; osteoid formation may delay mineralization, therefore, withhold therapy in patients with fractured bone until callus is evident; Paget's disease may fracture if doses are >20 mg/kg/day or are continuous for >6 months; hypocalcemia may occur during therapy; proximal renal tubular damage

Adverse Reactions
Central nervous system: Fever, seizures
Dermatologic: Angioedema, urticaria, rash, pruritus
Endocrine & metabolic: Hyperphosphatemia, hypocalcemia hypophosphatemia, hypomagnesemia
Gastrointestinal: Diarrhea, nausea, vomiting constipation, ulcerative stomatitis
Hepatic: Elevated hepatic enzymes
Neuromuscular & skeletal: Pain, increased risk of fractures
Renal: Nephrotoxicity fluid overload, elevated serum creatinine and BUN
Respiratory: Dyspnea
Miscellaneous: Altered taste, occult blood in stools, hypersensitivity reactions

Overdosage Symptoms of overdose include diarrhea, nausea, hypocalcemia; parenteral: EKG changes, bleeding, paresthesia, carpopedal spasm; renal insufficiency

Toxicology Gastric lavage, treat hypocalcemia (I.V. calcium); general supportive care, hypotension, and fever may be treated with corticosteroids

Drug Interactions Oral: Calcium, food decrease absorption

Stability Avoid heat >104°F (40°C)

Mechanism of Action Decreases bone resorption by inhibiting osteocystic osteolysis; decreases mineral release and matrix or collagen breakdown in bone

Pharmacodynamics
Onset of action: Within 1-3 months of therapy
Duration: 12 months without continuous therapy

Pharmacokinetics
Absorption: Oral: Dependent upon dose (1% at 5 mg/kg/day to 6% at 20 mg/kg/day) administered
Half-life:
Serum: 5-7 hours
Bone: >90 days
Metabolism: Not metabolized
Elimination: Excreted as unchanged drug primarily in urine with unabsorbed oral drug being eliminated in feces

Usual Dosage Geriatrics and Adults: Oral:

Paget's disease: Initial: 5 mg/kg/day given every day for no more than 6 months; may give 10-20 mg/kg/day for up to 3 months. Daily dose may be divided if adverse GI effects occur; do not exceed 20 mg/kg/day

Heterotropic ossification complications following total hip replacement: 20 mg/kg/day for 1 month preoperatively, followed by 20mg/kg/day for 3 months postoperatively

Heterotropic ossification with spinal cord injury: 20 mg/kg/day for 2 weeks, then 10 mg/kg/day for 10 weeks

Hypercalcemia associated with malignancy: I.V.: 7.5 mg/kg/day for 3 days; repeat treatment must be given at 7 days between treatments; oral therapy may be started following parenteral treatment, 20 mg/kg/day for 1 month; use for >90 days is recommended

Postmenopausal osteoporosis (investigational): 400 mg/day for 2 weeks followed by a 13-week period with no etidronate, then repeat cycle; maintain adequate calcium and vitamin D intake during entire 15-week treatment cycle

Monitoring Parameters Serum calcium, phosphorous, potassium

Reference Range Calcium (total): Adults: 9.0-11.0 mg/dL (2.05-2.54 mmol/L), may slightly decrease with aging; phosphorus: 2.5-4.5 mg/dL (0.81-1.45 mmol/L)

Patient Information Maintain adequate intake of calcium and vitamin D; take medicine on an empty stomach

Nursing Implications Dilute I.V. dose in at least 250 mL NS, ensure adequate hydration; dosage modification required in renal insufficiency

Special Geriatric Considerations Monitor serum electrolytes periodically since elderly are often receiving diuretics which can result in decreases in serum calcium, potassium, and magnesium

Dosage Forms
Injection: 50 mg/mL (6 mL)
Tablet: 200 mg, 400 mg

References
Storm T, Thamsborg G, Steiniche T, et al, "Effect of Intermittent Cyclical Etidronate Therapy on Bone Mass and Fracture Rate in Women With Postmenopausal Osteoporosis," *N Engl J Med*, 1990, 322(18):1265-71.
Watts NB, Harris ST, Genant HK, et al, "Intermittent Cyclical Etidronate Treatment of Postmenopausal Osteoporosis," *N Engl J Med*, 1990, 323(2):73-9.

Etodolac (ee toe doe' lak)

Brand Names Lodine®

Generic Available No

Therapeutic Class Analgesic, Non-narcotic; Anti-inflammatory Agent; Nonsteroidal Anti-inflammatory Agent (NSAID), Oral

Use Acute and long-term use in the management of signs and symptoms of osteoarthritis and management of pain

Unlabeled use: Rheumatoid arthritis, ankylosing spondylitis, tendonitis, bursitis, acute painful shoulder, acute gout

Contraindications Hypersensitivity to etodolac, aspirin or other NSAIDs

Warnings GI toxicity (bleeding, ulceration, perforation); CNS effects may occur (headaches, confusion, depression); hypersensitivity, anaphylactoid reactions (intermittent tolmetin use more often); renal function decline, acute renal insufficiency, interstitial nephritis, dysuria, cystitis, hematuria, nephrotic syndrome, hyperkalemia in acute renal insufficiency, hyponatremia, papillary necrosis, hepatic function impairment; elderly have increased risk for adverse reactions to NSAIDs; see Special Geriatric Considerations

Precautions Use with caution in patients with congestive heart failure, hypertension, decreased renal or hepatic function, history of GI disease (bleeding or ulcers), or

(Continued)

Etodolac (Continued)

those receiving anticoagulants; perform ophthalmologic evaluation for those who develop eye complaints during therapy (blurred vision, diminished vision, changes in color vision, retinal changes); NSAIDs may mask signs/symptoms of infections; photosensitivity reported

Adverse Reactions

Cardiovascular: Congestive heart failure, angina, hypertension, hypotension, fluid retention, arrhythmias, edema

Central nervous system: Headache, drowsiness, vertigo, dizziness, fatigue, hallucinations, confusion, depression, emotional lability, psychotic behavior, asthenia

Dermatologic: Rash, urticaria, angioedema, Stevens-Johnson syndrome, exfoliative dermatitis, ecchymosis, petechiae, purpura, bruising

Endocrine & metabolic: Hyperglycemia, hypoglycemia, hyperkalemia, gynecomastia, hyponatremia

Gastrointestinal: Dyspepsia, heartburn, nausea, diarrhea, constipation, flatulence, stomatitis, vomiting, abdominal pain, peptic ulcer, GI bleeding, GI perforation, gingival ulcers, pancreatitis, proctitis, paralytic ulcers, colitis, anorexia, weight loss

Genitourinary: Impotence, azotemia

Hematologic: Neutropenia, anemia, agranulocytosis, bone marrow suppression, hemolytic anemia, hemorrhage, inhibition of platelet aggregation

Hepatic: Hepatitis, elevated LFTs, cholestatic jaundice

Neuromuscular & skeletal: Involuntary muscle movements, muscle weakness, tremors

Ocular: Vision changes

Otic: Tinnitus

Renal: Dysuria, polyuria, pyuria, oliguria, anuria, acute renal failure

Respiratory: Exacerbation of asthma, dyspnea

Miscellaneous: Dry mucous membranes, thirst, pyrexia, sweating

Overdosage Symptoms include drowsiness, lethargy, disorientation, confusion, dizziness, numbness, paresthesia, nausea, vomiting, gastric irritation, abdominal pain, headache, tinnitus, sweating, blurred vision, muscle twitching, seizures, coma, acute renal failure, increased BUN and serum creatinine, hypotension, tachycardia, and metabolic acidosis

Toxicology Management of a nonsteroidal anti-inflammatory drug (NSAID) intoxication is primarily supportive and symptomatic. Fluid therapy is commonly effective in managing the hypotension that may occur following an acute NSAID overdose, except when this is due to an acute blood loss. Seizures tend to be very short-lived and often do not require drug treatment although recurrent seizures should be treated with I.V. diazepam. Since many of the NSAIDs undergo enterohepatic cycling, multiple doses of charcoal may be needed to reduce the potential for delayed toxicities. NSAIDs are highly bound to plasma proteins, therefore hemodialysis and peritoneal dialysis are not useful.

Drug Interactions

NSAIDs may decrease effect of loop diuretics

Cyclosporine may increase nephrotoxicity of both agents; may increase digoxin, methotrexate, and lithium serum concentrations

Aspirin or other salicylates may decrease NSAID serum concentrations

Other NSAIDs may increase adverse GI effects

Increased prothrombin time with anticoagulants

Decreased antihypertensive effects of ACE inhibitors, beta-blockers, and thiazide diuretics

Increased response to sympathomimetics

Probenecid may increase toxicity of NSAIDs by increase in serum concentrations

Concomitant use with loop diuretics may enhance azotemia in elderly

Stability Protect from moisture

Mechanism of Action Inhibits prostaglandin synthesis, acts on the hypothalamus heat-regulating center to reduce fever, blocks prostaglandin synthetase action which prevents formation of the platelet-aggregating substance thromboxane A_2; decreases pain receptor sensitivity. Other proposed mechanisms of action for salicylate anti-inflammatory action are lysosomal stabilization, kinin and leukotrienes production, alteration of chemotactic factors, and inhibition of neutrophil activation. This latter mechanism may be the most significant pharmacologic action to reduce inflammation.

Pharmacodynamics

Onset of analgesic action: Within 30 minutes to 1 hour

Duration: 4-12 hours

Pharmacokinetics

Absorption: Oral: Well absorbed

Distribution: V_d: 0.4 L/kg

Protein binding: Highly protein-bound

Half-life: 7 hours

Time to peak serum concentration: Within 1-2 hours

Usual Dosage Geriatrics and Adults: Oral:

Acute pain: 200-400 mg every 6-8 hours, as needed, not to exceed total daily doses of 1200 mg

Osteoarthritis: Initial: 800-1200 mg/day given in divided doses: 400 mg 2 or 3 times/day; 300 mg 2, 3 or 4 times/day; 200 mg 3 or 4 times/day; total daily dose should not exceed 1200 mg; for patients weighing <60 kg, total daily dose should not exceed 20 mg/kg

Monitoring Parameters Monitor CBC, liver enzymes; monitor BUN/serum creatinine in patients receiving diuretics; monitor response (pain, range of motion, grip strength, mobility, ADL function), inflammation; observe for weight gain, edema; monitor renal function; observe for bleeding, bruising; evaluate gastrointestinal effects (abdominal pain, bleeding, dyspepsia); mental confusion, disorientation

Test Interactions False-positive for urinary bilirubin and ketone

Patient Information Take with food, milk, or water; report any signs of blood in stool; serious gastrointestinal bleeding can occur as well as ulceration and perforation. Pain may or may not be present. Avoid aspirin and aspirin-containing products while taking this medication. If gastric upset occurs, take with food, milk, or antacid. If gastric adverse effects persist, contact physician. May cause drowsiness, dizziness, blurred vision, and confusion. Use caution when performing tasks which require alertness (eg, driving). Do not take for more than 3 days for fever or 10 days for pain without physician's advice.

Nursing Implications See Overdosage, Monitoring Parameters, Patient Information, and Special Geriatric Considerations

Additional Information Single dose of 76-100 mg is comparable to the analgesic effect of aspirin 650 mg; there are no clinical guidelines to predict which NSAID will give response in a particular patient. Trials with each must be initiated until response determined. Consider dose, patient convenience, and cost.

Special Geriatric Considerations Elderly are a high-risk population for adverse effects from nonsteroidal anti-inflammatory agents. As much as 60% of elderly who experience GI side effects can develop peptic ulceration and/or hemorrhage asymptomatically. The concomitant use of H_2 blockers, omeprazole, and sucralfate is not effective as prophylaxis. Misoprostol is the only prophylactic agent proven effective. Also, concomitant disease and drug use contribute to the risk for GI adverse effects. Use lowest effective dose for shortest period possible. Consider renal function decline with age. Use of NSAIDs can compromise existing renal function especially when Cl_{cr} is ≤30 mL/minute. Tinnitus may be a difficult and unreliable indication of toxicity due to age-related hearing loss or eighth cranial nerve damage. CNS adverse effects such as confusion, agitation, and hallucination are generally seen in overdose or high dose situations, but elderly may demonstrate these adverse effects at lower doses than younger adults. In patients ≥65 years, no substantial differences in the pharmacokinetics or side-effects profile were seen compared with the general population.

Dosage Forms Capsule: 200 mg, 300 mg

References

Brooks PM, Day RO, "Nonsteroidal Anti-inflammatory Drugs – Differences and Similarities," N Engl J Med, 1991, 324(24):1716-25.

Clinch D, Banerjee AK, Ostick G, "Absence of Abdominal Pain in Elderly Patients With Peptic Ulcer," Age Ageing, 1984, 13:120-3.

Clive DM, Stoff JS, "Renal Syndromes Associated With Nonsteroidal Anti-inflammatory Drugs," N Engl J Med, 1984, 310(9):563-72.

Graham DY, "Prevention of Gastroduodenal Injury Induced by Chronic Nonsteroidal Anti-inflammatory Drug Therapy," Gastroenterology, 1989, 96(2 Pt 2 Suppl):675-81.

Gurwitz JH, Avarn J, Ross-Degan D, et al, "Nonsteroidal Anti-Inflammatory Drug-Associated Azotemia in the Very Old," JAMA, 1990, 264(4):471-5.

Knodel LC, "Preventing NSAID-Induced Ulcers: The Role of Misoprostol," Consult Pharm, 1989, 4:37-41.

Pounder R, "Silent Peptic Ulceration: Deadly Silence or Golden Silence?" Gastroenterology, 1989, 96(2 Pt 2 Suppl):626-31.

Etrafon® see Amitriptyline and Perphenazine on page 43

ETS-2%® see Erythromycin, Topical on page 266

Eulexin® see Flutamide on page 308

Eurax® see Crotamiton on page 191

Euthroid® see Liotrix on page 410

Evac-U-Gen® [OTC] see Phenolphthalein on page 556

Evac-U-Lax® [OTC] see Phenolphthalein on page 556

E-Vista® see Hydroxyzine on page 356

Excedrin IB® [OTC] see Ibuprofen on page 360

Ex-Lax® [OTC] see Phenolphthalein on page 556

Ex-Lax® Gentle Nature® [OTC] see Senna on page 641

Extra Gentle Ex-Lax® [OTC] see Docusate and Phenolphthalein on page 238

ALPHABETICAL LISTING OF DRUGS

Extra Strength Doan's® [OTC] *see* Salicylates (Various Salts)
on page 633

Eye-Sed® [OTC] *see* Zinc Sulfate *on page 742*

Eye-Zine® [OTC] *see* Tetrahydrozoline Hydrochloride *on page 680*

F₃T *see* Trifluridine *on page 717*

Famotidine (fa moe' ti deen)
Brand Names Pepcid®
Generic Available No
Therapeutic Class Histamine-2 Antagonist
Use Therapy and treatment of duodenal ulcer, gastric ulcer, gastroesophageal reflux, pathological hypersecretory conditions, control gastric pH in critically ill patients

Unlabeled use: Prevent upper GI bleeding, prevent aspiration pneumonitis, symptomatic relief in gastritis, and active benign ulcer

Contraindications Hypersensitivity to famotidine or other H₂ antagonist
Warnings Adjust dosages in renal/hepatic impairment; elderly due to renal decline with age
Precautions Gastric malignancy may be masked, gynecomastia; cardiac arrhythmias and hypotension (I.V.); CNS side effects (confusion, depression, psychosis, hallucinations, anxiety)
Adverse Reactions
Cardiovascular: Flushing, palpitation, hypertension
Central nervous system: Headache, dizziness, fever, fatigue, paresthesia, hallucinations, anxiety, seizure, insomnia, drowsiness, depression
Dermatologic: Rash, acne, pruritus, urticaria, dry skin
Gastrointestinal: Constipation, anorexia, dry mouth, diarrhea, nausea, pancreatitis, abdominal discomfort, flatulence, belching
Genitourinary: Impotence, loss of libido
Hematologic: Thrombocytopenia
Neuromuscular & skeletal: Pain, weakness
Ocular: Orbital edema, conjunctival injection
Renal: Proteinuria, increases in BUN and creatinine
Respiratory: Bronchospasm
Overdosage No experience with intentional overdose; reported ingestions of 20 g have had transient side effects seen with recommended doses; animal data have shown respiratory failure, tachycardia, muscle tremors, vomiting, restlessness, hypotension, salivation, emesis, and diarrhea
Toxicology Treatment is primarily symptomatic and supportive; food may increase absorption
Drug Interactions
Binds weakly to cytochrome P-450 and, therefore, does not cause significant inhibition of drug metabolism
Antacids may decrease absorption; decreased absorption of diazepam may occur (ranitidine)
Increased serum levels of procainamide (ranitidine)
Increased hypoglycemic effects observed with sulfonylureas; serum concentrations may be increased (case reports with ranitidine)
May decrease warfarin clearance and increase anticoagulant effect (ranitidine) but data are conflicting
Stability Reconstituted I.V. solution is stable for 48 hours at room temperature; I.V. infusion in NS or D₅W solution is stable for 48 hours at room temperature; reconstituted oral solution is stable for 30 days at room temperature. Do not store powder in temperatures >40°C (104°F); after reconstitution, store in refrigerator <30°C (86°F); do not freeze; discard unused suspension in 30 days; store I.V. at 2°C to 8°C (36°F to 46°F).
Mechanism of Action Competitive inhibition of histamine at H₂ receptors of the gastric parietal cells, which inhibits gastric acid secretion; gastric volume and hydrogen ion concentration reduced
Pharmacodynamics
Onset of action: Oral: Gastrointestinal effects can be observed within 60 minutes following administration
Peak effects: Oral: Within 1-3 hours after doses
Duration: 10-12 hours
Duodenal ulcer healing rates at 40 mg/day: 4 weeks: 67% to 77%: 8 weeks: 82% to 95% in young adults
Pharmacokinetics
Protein binding: 15% to 20%
Metabolism: 30% to 35%
Bioavailability: Oral: 40% to 50%
Half-life: 2.5-3.5 hours (increases with renal impairment; oliguric half-life: 20 hours)
Elimination: Excreted unchanged drug in urine 25% to 30% oral and 65% to 70% I.V.; excreted in bile and feces

Usual Dosage Geriatrics and Adults: Oral:

Duodenal ulcer and gastric ulcer: 40 mg/day at bedtime for 4-8 weeks for adults, 12 weeks for elderly; prophylaxis: 20 mg at bedtime

Pathological hypersecretory conditions: 20 mg every 6 hours, higher doses may be needed; 160 mg every 6 hours have been used for Zollinger-Ellison syndrome

GERD: 20 mg every 6 hours for 6 weeks

Erosive esophagitis: 20-40 mg twice daily for 12 weeks

Dosing interval in renal impairment: Cl_{cr} <10 mL/minute: Dose may have to be reduced to 20 mg at bedtime

Monitoring Parameters Signs and symptoms of peptic ulcer disease, occult blood with GI bleeding, gastric pH where necessary; monitor renal function to correct dose; monitor for side effects

Patient Information Take with or immediately after meals; inform pharmacist and physician (nurse, practitioner) of any concomitant drug therapy; stagger doses with antacids

Nursing Implications Injection must be diluted prior to administration to a concentration of 20 mg/mL; reduce dosage in decreased renal function

Additional Information The expensive parenteral route should only be used when a patient is unable to take oral medication

Special Geriatric Considerations H_2 blockers are the preferred drugs for treating PUD in elderly due to cost and ease of administration. These agents are no less or more effective than any other therapy. The preferred agents (due to side effects, drug interaction profile, and pharmacokinetics) are ranitidine, famotidine, and nizatidine. Treatment for PUD in elderly is recommended for 12 weeks since their lesions are larger; therefore, take longer to heal. Always adjust dose based upon creatinine clearance.

Dosage Forms

Injection: 10 mg/mL (2 mL)

Tablet: 20 mg, 40 mg

References

Fennerty MD and Higbee M, "Drug Therapy of Gastrointestinal Disease," *Geriatric Pharmacology*, Bressler R and Katz MD, eds, New York, NY: McGraw-Hill, 1993, 585-608.

5-FC *see* Flucytosine *on page 296*

Feen-A-Mint® Pills [OTC] *see* Docusate and Phenolphthalein *on page 238*

Feen-A-Mint® [OTC] *see* Phenolphthalein *on page 556*

Feldene® *see* Piroxicam *on page 571*

Felodipine (fe loe' di peen)

Related Information

Calcium Channel Blocking Agents Comparison *on page 806-807*

Brand Names Plendil®

Generic Available No

Therapeutic Class Calcium Channel Blocker

Use Hypertension

Contraindications Hypersensitivity to felodipine or any component or other calcium channel blocker; severe hypotension or second and third degree heart block

Warnings Use with caution in titrating dosages for impaired hepatic function patients; use with caution in patients with congestive heart failure; may increase frequency, severity, duration of angina during initiation of therapy, increased intracranial pressure, idiopathic hypertrophic subaortic stenosis; do not abruptly withdraw therapy; use with caution in elderly due to greater propensity to hypotension

Precautions Sick sinus syndrome, severe left ventricular dysfunction, congestive heart failure, hepatic or renal impairment, hypertrophic cardiomyopathy (especially obstructive), concomitant therapy with beta-blockers or digoxin, edema

Adverse Reactions

Cardiovascular: Arrhythmia, bradycardia, hypotension, palpitations, tachycardia, congestive heart failure, myocardial infarction

Central nervous system: Dizziness, headache, fatigue, insomnia

Dermatologic: Rash

Gastrointestinal: Nausea, diarrhea, constipation, dry mouth

Hepatic: Mild to marked elevations in liver function tests

Ocular: Blurred vision

Respiratory: Shortness of breath

Miscellaneous: Peripheral edema

Overdosage Symptoms of overdose include hypotension

Toxicology Ipecac-induced emesis can hypothetically worsen calcium antagonist toxicity since it can produce vagal stimulation. The potential for seizures precipitously following acute ingestion of large doses of a calcium antagonist may also contraindicate the use of ipecac. Supportive and symptomatic treatment, including I.V. fluids

(Continued)

281

Felodipine (Continued)

and Trendelenburg positioning, should be initiated as intoxication may cause hypotension. Although calcium (calcium chloride I.V. 1-2 g with repeats as needed) has been used as an "antidote" for acute intoxications, there is limited experience to support its routine use and should be reserved for those cases where definite signs of myocardial depression are evident. Heart block may respond to isoproterenol, glucagon, atropine and/or calcium although a temporary pacemaker may be required.

Drug Interactions
Beta-blockers (increased cardiac and A-V conduction depression); fentanyl (increased volume requirements and hypotension); although this drug is new, other drug interactions not reported to the same degree as older agents; however, should be suspect of any drug interaction reported with other calcium channel blockers
Cimetidine, ranitidine may increase bioavailability
Digoxin levels may increase
Erythromycin may increase pharmacologic and toxic effects

Mechanism of Action Inhibits calcium ion from entering the "slow channels" or select voltage-sensitive areas of vascular smooth muscle and myocardium during depolarization, producing a relaxation of coronary vascular smooth muscle and coronary vasodilation; increases myocardial oxygen delivery in patients with vasospastic angina

Pharmacodynamics Onset of action: 2-5 hours

Pharmacokinetics
Absorption: 98% to 100%
Protein bound: 99%
Bioavailability: Due to first-pass elimination, absolute bioavailability is ~20%
Time to peak: Oral: Peak levels attained in 2-5 hours

Usual Dosage Oral:
Geriatrics: Initial dose: 5 mg/day; increase by 5 mg/day at 2-week intervals; monitor closely

Adults: 5-10 mg once daily; increase by 5 mg at 2-week intervals to a maximum of 20 mg/day

Dosing adjustment in hepatic impairment: Do not use doses >10 mg/day

Monitoring Parameters Heart rate, blood pressure

Reference Range None described

Patient Information Do not crush or chew tablets; do not discontinue abruptly; report any dizziness, shortness of breath, palpitations or edema occurs

Nursing Implications Do not crush sustained release capsules; see Warnings, Precautions, Monitoring Parameters, and Special Geriatric Considerations

Special Geriatric Considerations Elderly may experience a greater hypotensive response; constipation may be more of a problem in elderly; calcium channel blockers are no more effective in elderly than other therapies; however, they do not cause significant CNS effects which is an advantage over some antihypertensive agents.

Dosage Forms Tablet, extended release: 5 mg, 10 mg

FemiLax® [OTC] see Docusate and Phenolphthalein on page 238

Femiron® [OTC] see Ferrous Fumarate on page 286

Fenamates see Meclofenamate Sodium on page 435

Fenesin™ see Guaifenesin on page 331

Fenoprofen Calcium (fen oh proe' fen)

Brand Names Nalfon®

Generic Available Yes

Therapeutic Class Analgesic, Non-narcotic; Anti-inflammatory Agent; Nonsteroidal Anti-inflammatory Agent (NSAID), Oral

Use Symptomatic treatment of acute and chronic rheumatoid arthritis and osteoarthritis; relief of mild to moderate pain, sunburn, migraine headache prophylaxis

Contraindications Renal impairment, known hypersensitivity to fenoprofen or other NSAIDs including aspirin and other salicylates

Warnings GI toxicity (bleeding, ulceration, perforation); CNS effects may occur (headaches, confusion, depression); hypersensitivity, anaphylactoid reactions (intermittent tolmetin use more often); renal function decline, acute renal insufficiency, interstitial nephritis, dysuria, cystitis, hematuria, nephrotic syndrome, hyperkalemia in acute renal insufficiency, hyponatremia, papillary necrosis, hepatic function impairment; elderly have increased risk for adverse reactions to NSAIDs; see Special Geriatric Considerations

Precautions Use with caution in patients with congestive heart failure, hypertension, decreased renal or hepatic function, history of GI disease (bleeding or ulcers), or those receiving anticoagulants; perform ophthalmologic evaluation for those who develop eye complaints during therapy (blurred vision, diminished vision, changes in color vision, retinal changes); NSAIDs may mask signs/symptoms of infections; photosensitivity reported

Adverse Reactions

Cardiovascular: Congestive heart failure, angina, hypertension, hypotension, fluid retention, arrhythmias, edema

Central nervous system: Headache, drowsiness, vertigo, dizziness, fatigue, hallucinations, confusion, depression, emotional lability, psychotic behavior, asthenia

Dermatologic: Rash, urticaria, angioedema, Stevens-Johnson syndrome, exfoliative dermatitis, ecchymosis, petechiae, purpura, bruising

Endocrine & metabolic: Hyperglycemia, hypoglycemia, hyperkalemia, gynecomastia, hyponatremia

Gastrointestinal: Dyspepsia, heartburn, nausea, diarrhea, constipation, flatulence, anorexia, stomatitis, vomiting, abdominal pain, peptic ulcer, GI bleeding, GI perforation, gingival ulcers, pancreatitis, proctitis, paralytic ulcers, colitis, weight loss

Genitourinary: Impotence, azotemia

Hematologic: Neutropenia, anemia, agranulocytosis, bone marrow suppression, hemolytic anemia, hemorrhage, inhibition of platelet aggregation

Hepatic: Hepatitis, elevated LFTs, cholestatic jaundice

Neuromuscular & skeletal: Involuntary muscle movements, muscle weakness, tremors

Ocular: Vision changes

Otic: Tinnitus

Renal: Dysuria, polyuria, pyuria, oliguria, anuria, acute renal failure

Respiratory: Exacerbation of asthma, dyspnea

Miscellaneous: Dry mucous membranes, thirst, pyrexia, sweating

Overdosage Symptoms include drowsiness, lethargy, disorientation, confusion, dizziness, numbness, paresthesia, nausea, vomiting, gastric irritation, abdominal pain, headache, tinnitus, sweating, blurred vision, muscle twitching, seizures, coma, acute renal failure, increased BUN and serum creatinine, hypotension, tachycardia, and metabolic acidosis

Toxicology Management of a nonsteroidal anti-inflammatory agent (NSAID) intoxication is primarily supportive and symptomatic. Fluid therapy is commonly effective in managing the hypotension that may occur following an acute NSAID overdose, except when this is due to an acute blood loss. Seizures tend to be very short-lived and often do not require drug treatment although recurrent seizures should be treated with I.V. diazepam. Since many of the NSAIDs undergo enterohepatic cycling, multiple doses of charcoal may be needed to reduce the potential for delayed toxicities.

Drug Interactions

Cyclosporine may increase nephrotoxicity of both agents; may increase digoxin, methotrexate, and lithium serum concentrations

Aspirin and other salicylates may decrease NSAID serum concentrations

Other NSAIDs may increase adverse GI effects

Increased prothrombin time with anticoagulants

Decreased antihypertensive effects of ACE inhibitors, beta-blockers, and thiazide diuretics

Increased response to sympathomimetics

Probenecid may increase toxicity of NSAIDs by increase in serum concentrations

NSAIDs may decrease effects of loop diuretics

May enhance azotemia in elderly receiving loop diuretics

Mechanism of Action Inhibits prostaglandin synthesis, acts on the hypothalamus heat-regulating center to reduce fever, blocks prostaglandin synthetase action which prevents formation of the platelet-aggregating substance thromboxane A_2; decreases pain receptor sensitivity. Other proposed mechanisms of action for salicylate anti-inflammatory action are lysosomal stabilization, kinin and leukotriene production, alteration of chemotactic factors, and inhibition of neutrophil activation. This latter mechanism may be the most significant pharmacologic action to reduce inflammation.

Pharmacodynamics

Onset of anti-inflammatory action: 2 days

Maximum response: 2-3 weeks

Pharmacokinetics

Absorption: Rapid (to 80%) from upper GI tract

Protein binding: 99%

Metabolism: Extensive in the liver

Half-life: 2.5-3 hours

Time to peak serum concentration: Within 1-2 hours

Elimination: In urine 2% to 5% as unchanged drug; small amounts appear in feces

Usual Dosage Geriatrics and Adults: Oral:

Arthritis: 300-600 mg 3-4 times/day up to 3.2 g/day; maximum response may take 2-3 weeks

Pain: 200 mg every 4-6 hours as needed; do not exceed 3.2 g/day

Monitoring Parameters Monitor response (pain, range of motion, grip strength, mobility, ADL function), inflammation; observe for weight gain, edema; monitor renal function; observe for bleeding, bruising; evaluate gastrointestinal effects (abdominal pain, bleeding, dyspepsia); mental confusion, disorientation, CBC, serum, creatinine, BUN, liver function tests

(Continued)

283

Fenoprofen Calcium *(Continued)*

Reference Range Therapeutic: 20-65 µg/mL (SI: 82-268 µmol/L)

Test Interactions Increased chloride (S), increased sodium (S)

Patient Information Serious gastrointestinal bleeding can occur as well as ulceration and perforation. Pain may or may not be present. Avoid aspirin and aspirin-containing products while taking this medication. If gastric upset occurs, take with food, milk, or antacid. If gastric adverse effects persist, contact physician. May cause drowsiness, dizziness, blurred vision, and confusion. Use caution when performing tasks which require alertness (eg, driving). Do not take for more than 3 days for fever or 10 days for pain without physician advice.

Nursing Implications See Monitoring Parameters, Overdosage, Patient Information, and Special Geriatric Considerations

Additional Information There are no clinical guidelines to predict which NSAID will give response in a particular patient. Trials with each must be initiated until response determined. Consider dose, patient convenience, and cost.

Special Geriatric Considerations Elderly are a high-risk population for adverse effects from nonsteroidal anti-inflammatory agents. As much as 60% of elderly can develop peptic ulceration and/or hemorrhage asymptomatically. The concomitant use of H_2 blockers, omeprazole, and sucralfate is not effective as prophylaxis. Misoprostol is the only prophylactic agent proven effective. Also, concomitant disease and drug use contribute to the risk for GI adverse effects. Use lowest effective dose for shortest period possible. Consider renal function decline with age. Use of NSAIDs can compromise existing renal function especially when Cl_{cr} is ≤30 mL/minute. Tinnitus may be a difficult and unreliable indication of toxicity due to age-related hearing loss or eighth cranial nerve damage. CNS adverse effects such as confusion, agitation, and hallucination are generally seen in overdose or high-dose situations, but elderly may demonstrate these adverse effects at lower doses than younger adults.

Dosage Forms

Capsule: 200 mg, 300 mg

Tablet: 600 mg

References
Brooks PM, Day RO, "Nonsteroidal Anti-inflammatory Drugs – Differences and Similarities," *N Engl J Med*, 1991, 324(24):1716-25.

Clinch D, Banerjee AK, Ostick G, "Absence of Abdominal Pain in Elderly Patients With Peptic Ulcer," *Age Ageing*, 1984, 13:120-3.

Clive DM, Stoff JS, "Renal Syndromes Associated With Nonsteroidal Anti-inflammatory Drugs," *N Engl J Med*, 1984, 310(9):563-72.

Graham DY, "Prevention of Gastroduodenal Injury Induced by Chronic Nonsteroidal Anti-inflammatory Drug Therapy," *Gastroenterology*, 1989, 96(2 Pt 2 Suppl):675-81.

Gurwitz JH, Avarn J, Ross-Degan D, et al, "Nonsteroidal Anti-Inflammatory Drug-Associated Azotemia in the Very Old," *JAMA*, 1990, 264(4):471-5.

Knodel LC, "Preventing NSAID-Induced Ulcers: The Role of Misoprostol," *Consult Pharm*, 1989, 4:37-41.

Pounder R, "Silent Peptic Ulceration: Deadly Silence or Golden Silence?" *Gastroenterology*, 1989, 96(2 Pt 2 Suppl):626-31.

Fentanyl *(fen' ta nil)*

Related Information

Narcotic Agonist Comparative Pharmacology *on page 811*

Pharmacokinetics of Narcotic Agonist Analgesics *on page 812*

Brand Names Duragesic™; Sublimaze®

Generic Available Yes: Injection

Therapeutic Class Analgesic, Narcotic; General Anesthetic

Use Sedation; relief of pain; preoperative medication; adjunct to general or regional anesthesia; management of chronic pain (transdermal product)

Restrictions C-II

Contraindications Hypersensitivity to fentanyl or any component; increased intracranial pressure; severe respiratory depression; severe liver or renal insufficiency;

Transmucosal is contraindicated in unmonitored settings where a risk of unrecognized hypoventilation exists or in treating acute or chronic pain

Warnings Rapid I.V. infusion may result in skeletal muscle and chest wall rigidity which leads to impaired ventilation causing respiratory distress including apnea, bronchoconstriction, laryngospasm; inject slowly over 3-5 minutes; nondepolarizing skeletal muscle relaxant may be required. Transdermal product: Patients who experience adverse reactions should be monitored for at least 12 hours after the removal of the product. Transmucosal product is not recommended for use in those who have received MAO inhibitors within 14 days.

Precautions Fentanyl shares the toxic potentials of opiate agonists, and precautions of opiate agonist therapy should be observed; use with caution in patients with bradycardia

Adverse Reactions

Cardiovascular: Hypotension, bradycardia

Central nervous system: CNS depression, drowsiness, dizziness, sedation

Dermatologic: Erythema, pruritus

Endocrine & metabolic: ADH release

Gastrointestinal: Nausea, vomiting, constipation

Local: Edema (transdermal system)

Neuromuscular & skeletal: Skeletal and thoracic muscle rigidity especially following rapid I.V. administration

Ocular: Miosis

Respiratory: Respiratory depression

Miscellaneous: Physical and psychological dependence with prolonged use, biliary or urinary tract spasm

Overdosage Symptoms of overdose include CNS depression, respiratory depression, miosis

Toxicology Treatment of an overdose includes support of the patient's airway, establishment of an I.V. line and administration of naloxone 2 mg I.V. with repeat administration as necessary up to a total of 10 mg.

Drug Interactions Increased toxicity: CNS depressants, phenothiazines, tricyclic antidepressants

Stability Protect from light

Mechanism of Action Binds with stereospecific receptors at many sites within the CNS, increases pain threshold, alters pain reception, inhibits ascending pain pathways

Pharmacodynamics

Onset of analgesia:

I.M.: 7-15 minutes

I.V.: Almost immediate

Duration:

I.M.: 1-2 hours

I.V.: 30-60 minutes; respiratory depressant effect may last longer than analgesic effect; duration of action may be increased in the elderly; enhanced analgesia has been seen in elderly patients on therapeutic doses of narcotics

Transmucosal:

Onset of effect: 5-15 minutes with a maximum reduction in activity/apprehension

Peak analgesia: Within 20-30 minutes

Duration: Related to blood level of the drug

Pharmacokinetics

Absorption: Transmucosal: Rapid, ~25% from the buccal mucosa; 75% swallowed with saliva and slowly absorbed from gastrointestinal tract

Metabolism: In the liver

Half-life: 2-4 hours; transmucosal: 6.6 hours (range: 5-15 hours)

Elimination: In urine primarily as metabolites and 10% as unchanged drug

In the elderly, the clearance of fentanyl is decreased and the half-life increased; it is unknown how this affects the kinetics of the transdermal system

Transdermal: Serum concentrations increase gradually, leveling off between 12-24 hours with peak levels occurring 24-72 hours after application; after 72-hour application, steady-state fentanyl concentration is reached

Usual Dosage A wide range of doses may be used; when choosing a dose, take into consideration the following patient factors; age, weight, physical status, underlying disease states, other drugs used, type of anesthesia used, and the surgical procedure to be performed.

Geriatrics and Adults:

Preoperative sedation, adjunct to regional anesthesia, postoperative pain: I.M., I.V.: 50-100 mcg/dose

Adjunct to general anesthesia: I.M., I.V.: 2-50 mcg/kg depending on the procedure to be performed

General anesthesia without additional anesthetic agents: I.V. 50-100 mcg/kg with O_2 and skeletal muscle relaxant

Transdermal: Initial: 25 mcg/hour system applied every 72 hours (3 days); maximum dose: 300 mcg/hour, increase if necessary after 3 days; may take 6 days to reach equilibrium on new dose; if currently receiving opiates, calculate the 24-hour analgesia requirements and convert it to the equianalgesic oral morphine dose; use the table on the following page to choose the appropriate Duragesic™ dose.

Transmucosal:

Geriatrics: 2.5-5 mcg/kg; suck on lozenge vigorously approximately 20-40 minutes before the start of procedure

Adults; 5 mcg/kg; suck on lozenge as above

Administration Transmucosal product should begin 20-40 minutes prior to the anticipated start of surgery, diagnostic, or therapeutic procedure; foil overwrap should be removed just prior to administration; once removed, patient should place the unit in mouth and suck (not chew) it; unit should be removed after it is consumed or if patient has achieved an adequate sedation and anxiolytic level, and/or shows signs of respiratory depression

Monitoring Parameters Respiratory, cardiovascular status, mental status

(Continued)

Fentanyl *(Continued)*

Duragesic® Dose Prescription Based Upon Daily Morphine Equivalence Dose

Oral 24–hour Morphine (mg/day)	I.M. 24–hour Morphine (mg/day)	Duragesic® Dose (mcg/h)
45–134	8–22	25
135–224	23–37	50
225–314	38–52	75
315–404	53–67	100
405–494	68–82	125
495–584	83–97	150
585–674	98–112	175
675–764	113–127	200
765–854	128–142	225
855–944	143–157	250
945–1034	158–172	275
1035–1124	173–187	300

Patient Information Transdermal system: Apply to intact skin on the upper torso; clip hair at application site (do not shave) before applying system. If cleansing skin before application, use clear water and allow skin to dry completely before applying system; leave system in place for 72 hours; dispose of system by folding it (medication side in) and flushing down the toilet; may cause dizziness or drowsiness, avoid alcohol, and CNS depressants.

Nursing Implications May cause rebound respiratory depression postoperatively
Transdermal system: See Patient Information for instructions on applying the transdermal system. If gel from the patch contacts the health worker's skin, wash the area with water; do not use soap or solvents as this will enhance the drug's ability to penetrate the skin; during initiation of therapy, short-acting analgesics may be needed until the full effects of the system are obtained; monitor patients for at least 12 hours after the removal of the patch
Transmucosal: See Administration

Special Geriatric Considerations See Pharmacodynamics, Pharmacokinetics, and Usual Dosage. The elderly may be particularly susceptible to the CNS depressant and constipating effects of narcotics.

Dosage Forms
Injection, as citrate: 0.05 mg/mL (2 mL, 5 mL, 10 mL, 20 mL, 50 mL)
Lozenge, oral transmucosal (raspberry flavored): 200 mcg, 300 mcg, 400 mcg
Transdermal system: 25 mcg/hour [10 cm^2]; 50 mcg/hour [20 cm^2]; 75 mcg/hour [30 cm^2]; 100 mcg/hour [40 cm^2] (all available in 5s)

Feosol® [OTC] *see* Ferrous Sulfate *on page 289*

Feosol® Spansules® [OTC] *see* Ferrous Sulfate *on page 289*

Fergon® *see* Ferrous Gluconate *on page 288*

Fer-In-Sol® [OTC] *see* Ferrous Sulfate *on page 289*

Fero-Gradumet® [OTC] *see* Ferrous Sulfate *on page 289*

Feronim® *see* Iron Dextran Complex *on page 377*

Ferospace® [OTC] *see* Ferrous Sulfate *on page 289*

Ferralet® [OTC] *see* Ferrous Gluconate *on page 288*

Ferro-Sequels® [OTC] *see* Ferrous Fumarate *on this page*

Ferrous Fumarate *(fyoo' ma rate)*
Brand Names Femiron® [OTC]; Ferro-Sequels® [OTC]
Therapeutic Class Iron Salt
Use Prevention and treatment of iron deficiency anemias
Contraindications Hemochromatosis, hemolytic anemia, known hypersensitivity to iron salts
Precautions Avoid using for longer than 6 months except in patients with conditions that require prolonged therapy; avoid in patients with peptic ulcer, enteritis, or ulcerative colitis
Adverse Reactions
Gastrointestinal: GI irritation, epigastric pain, nausea, diarrhea, dark stool, vomiting

ALPHABETICAL LISTING OF DRUGS

Miscellaneous: Liquid preparations may temporarily stain the teeth, discolored urine

Overdosage Symptoms of overdose include lethargy, tarry stools, hypotension, acidosis, pulmonary edema, hyperthermia, convulsions

Toxicology Following treatment for fluid losses, metabolic acidosis, and shock, a severe iron overdose (when the serum iron concentration exceeds the total iron-binding capacity) may be treated with deferoxamine. Deferoxamine may be administered I.V. (80 mg/kg over 24 hours) or I.M. (40-90 mg/kg every 8 hours)

Drug Interactions

Absorption of oral preparation of iron and tetracyclines are decreased when both of these drugs are given together; concurrent administration of antacids or H_2 antagonists may decrease iron absorption; iron may decrease absorption of levodopa, methyldopa, quinolones, and penicillamine when given at the same time

Iron absorption may be increased in patients receiving chloramphenicol; concurrent administration ≥200 mg vitamin C per 30 mg elemental iron increases absorption of oral iron

Food/Drug Interactions Milk and eggs may decrease absorption of iron

Mechanism of Action Replaces iron found in hemoglobin, myoglobin, and other enzymes; allows the transportation of oxygen via hemoglobin

Pharmacodynamics

Onset of action: Hematologic response to oral iron in red blood cells form and color changes occur within 3-10 days

Peak action: Within 5-10 days, and hemoglobin values increase within 2-4 weeks

Pharmacokinetics

Absorption: Iron is absorbed in the duodenum and upper jejunum; in persons with normal iron stores 10% of an oral dose is absorbed, this is increased to 20% to 30% in persons with inadequate iron stores. Food and achlorhydria will decrease absorption; aging has not been shown to affect absorption, but the percent uptake by red cells decreases from 91.2% in healthy young adults to 60% in healthy older adults

Elimination: Iron is largely bound to serum transferrin and excreted in the urine, sweat, sloughing of intestinal mucosa, and by menstrual bleeding.

Usual Dosage Oral (to avoid GI upset, start with a single daily dose and increase by 1 tablet/day each week or as tolerated until desired daily dose is achieved):

Geriatrics and Adults: 200 mg 3-4 times/day

Administration Administer 2 hours prior to or 4 hours after antacids

Monitoring Parameters Hemoglobin, hematocrit, ferritin, reticulocyte count

Reference Range Therapeutic: Male: 75-175 µg/dL (SI: 13.4-31.3 µmol/L); Female: 65-165 µg/dL (SI: 11.6-29.5µmol/L); ranges may vary by laboratory

Test Interactions Increased serum iron

Patient Information May color stool black, take between meals for maximum absorption; may take with food if GI upset occurs, do not take with milk or antacids

Nursing Implications See Administration

Additional Information The elemental iron content in ferrous fumarate is 33% (ie, 200 mg ferrous fumarate is equivalent to 66 mg ferrous iron). Administration of iron for longer than 6 months should be avoided except in patients with continuous bleeding or menorrhagia.

Special Geriatric Considerations Anemia in the elderly is most often caused by "anemia of chronic disease" or associated with inflammation rather than blood loss. Iron stores are usually normal or increased, with a serum ferritin >50 ng/mL and a decreased total iron binding capacity. Hence, the anemia is not secondary to iron deficiency but the inability of the reticuloendothelial system to use available iron stores. Timed release iron preparations should be avoided due to their erratic absorption. Products combined with a laxative or stool softener should not be used unless the need for the combination is demonstrated.

Dosage Forms

Drops: 45 mg/0.6 mL

Tablet: 200 mg, 325 mg

Tablet, timed release (Ferro-Sequels®): Ferrous fumarate 150 mg and docusate sodium 100 mg

See table.

Elemental Iron Content of Iron Salts

Iron Salt	% Iron
Ferrous sulfate	20
Ferrous sulfate, exsiccated	~30
Ferrous gluconate	11.6
Ferrous fumarate	33

References
References

References

Lipschitz DA, "The Anemia of Chronic Disease," *J Am Geriatr Soc*, 1990, 38(11):1258-64.

(Continued)

Ferrous Fumarate *(Continued)*

Marx JJM, "Normal Iron Absorption and Decreased Red Cell Iron Uptake in the Aged," *Blood*, 1979, 53:204-11.

Ferrous Gluconate (gloo' koe nate)

Brand Names Fergon®; Ferralet® [OTC]

Therapeutic Class Iron Salt

Use Prevention and treatment of iron deficiency anemias

Contraindications Hemochromatosis, hemolytic anemia; known hypersensitivity to iron salts

Precautions Avoid using for longer than 6 months, except in patients with conditions that require prolonged therapy

Adverse Reactions

Gastrointestinal: GI irritation, epigastric pain, nausea, diarrhea, dark stool

Miscellaneous: Liquid preparations may temporarily stain the teeth

Overdosage Symptoms of overdose include lethargy, tarry stools, hypotension, acidosis, pulmonary edema, hyperthermia, convulsions

Toxicology Following treatment for fluid losses, metabolic acidosis, and shock, a severe iron overdose (when the serum iron concentration exceeds the total iron-binding capacity) may be treated with deferoxamine. Deferoxamine may be administered I.V. (80 mg/kg over 24 hours) or I.M. (40-90 mg/kg every 8 hours)

Drug Interactions

Absorption of oral preparation of iron and tetracyclines are decreased when both of these drugs are given together; concurrent administration of antacids or H_2 antagonists may decrease iron absorption; iron may decrease absorption of levodopa, methyldopa, quinolones, and penicillamine when given at the same time

Iron absorption may be increased in patients receiving chloramphenicol; concurrent administration ≥200 mg vitamin C per 30 mg elemental iron increases absorption of oral iron

Food/Drug Interactions Milk and eggs may decrease absorption of iron

Mechanism of Action Replaces iron, found in hemoglobin, myoglobin, and enzymes; allows the transportation of oxygen via hemoglobin

Pharmacodynamics

Onset of action: Hematologic response to either oral or parenteral iron salts is essentially the same; red blood cell form and color changes within 3-10 days

Peak effect: Within 5-10 days, and hemoglobin values increase within 2-4 weeks

Pharmacokinetics

Absorption: Iron is absorbed in the duodenum and upper jejunum; in persons with normal iron stores 10% of an oral dose is absorbed, this is increased to 20% to 30% in persons with inadequate iron stores. Food and achlorhydria will decrease absorption; aging has not been shown to affect absorption, but the percent uptake by red cells decreases from 91.2% in healthy young adults to 60% in healthy older adults

Elimination: Iron is largely bound to serum transferrin and excreted in the urine, sweat, sloughing of intestinal mucosa, and by menstrual bleeding

Usual Dosage Oral (to avoid GI upset, start with a single daily dose and increase by 1 tablet/day each week or as tolerated until desired daily dose is achieved):

Dose expressed in terms of elemental iron (see Additional Information):

Geriatrics and Adults:

Iron deficiency: 60 mg iron twice daily up to 60 mg iron 4 times/day

Prophylaxis: 60 mg iron/day

Administration Administer 2 hours before or 4 hours after antacids

Monitoring Parameters Hemoglobin, hematocrit, ferritin, reticulocyte count

Reference Range Therapeutic: Male: 75-175 µg/dL (SI: 13.4-31.3 µmol/L); Female: 65-165 µg/dL (SI: 11.6-29.5µmol/L); ranges may vary by laboratory

Test Interactions Increased serum iron

Patient Information May color the stool black; take between meals for maximum absorption; may take with food if GI upset occurs; do **not** take with milk or antacid

Nursing Implications See Administration

Additional Information Gluconate contains 12% elemental iron (ie, 300 mg ferrous gluconate is equivalent to 34 mg ferrous iron); administration of iron for longer than 6 months should be avoided except in patients with continued bleeding or menorrhagia

Special Geriatric Considerations Anemia in the elderly is most often caused by "anemia of chronic disease" or associated with inflammation rather than blood loss. Iron stores are usually normal or increased, with a serum ferritin >50 ng/mL and a decreased total iron binding capacity. Hence, the anemia is not secondary to iron deficiency but the inability of the reticuloendothelial system to use available iron stores. Timed release iron preparations should be avoided due to their erratic absorption. Products combined with a laxative or stool softener should not be used unless the need for the combination is demonstrated.

Dosage Forms

Capsule: 86 mg, 325 mg, 435 mg

Elixir: 300 mg/5 mL (473 mL)
Tablet: 300 mg, 320 mg, 325 mg

References

Lipschitz DA, "The Anemia of Chronic Disease," *J Am Geriatr Soc*, 1990, 38(11):1258-64.
Marx JJM, "Normal Iron Absorption and Decreased Red Cell Iron Uptake in the Aged," *Blood*, 1979, 53:204-11.

Ferrous Sulfate (fer' us)

Brand Names Feosol® [OTC]; Feosol® Spansules® [OTC]; Fer-In-Sol® [OTC]; Fero-Gradumet® [OTC]; Ferospace® [OTC]; Ferr-TD® [OTC]; Mol-Iron® [OTC]

Synonyms FeSO₄

Generic Available Yes

Therapeutic Class Iron Salt

Use Prevention and treatment of iron deficiency anemias

Contraindications Hemochromatosis, hemolytic anemia; known hypersensitivity to iron salts

Precautions Avoid using for longer than 6 months, except in patients with conditions that require prolonged therapy

Adverse Reactions

Gastrointestinal: GI irritation, epigastric pain, nausea, diarrhea, dark stool
Miscellaneous: Liquid preparations may temporarily stain the teeth

Overdosage Symptoms of overdose include acute GI irritation; erosion of GI mucosa, hepatic and renal impairment, coma, hematemesis, lethargy, acidosis

Toxicology Following treatment for fluid losses, metabolic acidosis, and shock, a severe iron overdose (when the serum iron concentration exceeds the total iron-binding capacity) may be treated with deferoxamine. Deferoxamine may be administered I.V. (80 mg/kg over 24 hours) or I.M. (40-90 mg/kg every 8 hours). Lethal dose of elemental iron is 180-300 mg/kg.

Drug Interactions

Absorption of oral preparation of iron and tetracyclines are decreased when both of these drugs are given together; concurrent administration of antacids or H₂ antagonists may decrease iron absorption; iron may decrease absorption of levodopa, methyldopa, quinolones, and penicillamine when given at the same time

Iron absorption may be increased in patients receiving chloramphenicol; concurrent administration ≥200 mg vitamin C per 30 mg elemental iron increases absorption of oral iron

Food/Drug Interactions Milk and eggs may decrease absorption of iron

Mechanism of Action Replaces iron, found in hemoglobin, myoglobin, and other enzymes; allows the transportation of oxygen via hemoglobin

Pharmacodynamics

Onset of action: Hematologic response to either oral or parenteral iron salts is essentially the same; red blood cell form and color changes within 3-10 days

Peak effect: Reticulocytosis occurs in 5-10 days, and hemoglobin values increase within 2-4 weeks

Pharmacokinetics

Absorption: Iron is absorbed in the duodenum and upper jejunum; in persons with normal serum iron stores, 10% of an oral dose is absorbed; this is increased to 20% to 30% in persons with inadequate iron stores. Food and achlorhydria will decrease absorption; aging has not been shown to affect absorption, but the percent uptake by red cells decreases from 91.2% in healthy young adults to 60% in healthy older adults.

Elimination: Iron is largely bound to serum transferrin and excreted in the urine, sweat, sloughing of the intestinal mucosa, and by menstrual bleeding

Usual Dosage Oral (to avoid GI upset, start with a single daily dose and increase by 1 tablet/day each week or as tolerated until desired daily dose is achieved):

Dose expressed in terms of elemental iron (see Additional Information):
Geriatrics and Adults:
Iron deficiency: 60 mg iron twice daily up to 60 mg iron 4 times/day or 50 mg iron (extended release) 1-2 times/day
Prophylaxis: 60 mg iron/day

Administration Administer 2 hours prior to or 4 hours after antacids

Monitoring Parameters Hemoglobin, hematocrit, ferritin, reticulocyte count

Reference Range Therapeutic: Male: 75-175 µg/dL (SI: 13.4-31.3 µmol/L); Female: 65-165 µg/dL (SI: 11.6-29.5 µmol/L); values may vary by laboratory

Test Interactions Increased serum iron

Patient Information May color stool black, take between meals for maximum absorption; may take with food if GI upset occurs, do not take with milk or antacids

Nursing Implications See Administration

Additional Information The elemental iron content of ferrous sulfate is 20% (ie, 300 mg ferrous sulfate is equivalent to 60 mg ferrous iron). Administration of iron for longer than 6 months should be avoided except in patients with continued bleeding, or menorrhagia.

(Continued)

Ferrous Sulfate *(Continued)*

Special Geriatric Considerations Anemia in the elderly is most often caused by "anemia of chronic disease" or associated with inflammation rather than blood loss. Iron stores are usually normal or increased, with a serum ferritin >50 ng/mL and a decreased total iron binding capacity. Hence, the anemia is not secondary to iron deficiency but the inability of the reticuloendothelial system to use available iron stores. Timed release iron preparations should be avoided due to their erratic absorption. Products combined with a laxative or stool softener should not be used unless the need for the combination is demonstrated.

Dosage Forms
Capsule, timed release: 150 mg, 250 mg, 390 mg
Drops: 75 mg/0.6 mL (50 mL); 125 mg/mL (50 mL)
Elixir: 220 mg/5 mL (473 mL, 4000 mL)
Liquid: 300 mg/5 mL unit dose
Syrup: 90 mg/5 mL; 300 mg/5 mL (480 mL)
Tablet: 325 mg
Tablet, timed release: 525 mg

References
Lipschitz DA, "The Anemia of Chronic Disease," *J Am Geriatr Soc*, 1990, 38(11):1258-64.
Marx JJM, "Normal Iron Absorption and Decreased Red Cell Iron Uptake in the Aged," *Blood*, 1979, 53:204-11.

Ferr-TD® [OTC] *see* Ferrous Sulfate *on previous page*

FeSO₄ *see* Ferrous Sulfate *on previous page*

Feverall™ [OTC] *see* Acetaminophen *on page 13*

Fiberall® Chewable Tablet [OTC] *see* Calcium Polycarbophil *on page 110*

Fiberall® [OTC] *see* Psyllium *on page 610*

FiberCon® Tablet [OTC] *see* Calcium Polycarbophil *on page 110*

Fiber-Lax® Tablet [OTC] *see* Calcium Polycarbophil *on page 110*

FiberNorm® [OTC] *see* Calcium Polycarbophil *on page 110*

Filgrastim *(fil gra' stim)*

Brand Names Neupogen® Injection
Synonyms G-CSF; Granulocyte Colony Stimulating Factor
Generic Available No
Therapeutic Class Colony Stimulating Factor
Use Decreases the period of neutropenia and the associated risk of infection in patients with nonmyeloid malignancies receiving myelosuppressive chemotherapeutic regimens associated with a significant incidence of severe neutropenia with fever; it has also been used in AIDS patients on zidovudine and in patients with noncancer chemotherapy-induced neutropenia
Contraindications Hypersensitivity to *E. coli* derived proteins or G-CSF
Warnings Complete blood count and platelet count should be obtained prior to chemotherapy. Do not use G-CSF in the period 24 hours before to 24 hours after administration of cytotoxic chemotherapy because of the potential sensitivity of rapidly dividing myeloid cells to cytotoxic chemotherapy. Precaution should be exercised in the usage of G-CSF in any malignancy with myeloid characteristics. G-CSF can potentially act as a growth factor for any tumor type, particularly myeloid malignancies. Tumors of nonhematopoietic origin may have surface receptors for G-CSF.
Adverse Reactions
Cardiovascular: Transient decrease in blood pressure, vasculitis
Central nervous system: Fever
Dermatologic: Exacerbation of pre-existing skin disorders
Endocrine & metabolic: Reversible increase in uric acid, lactate dehydrogenase, alkaline phosphatase
Gastrointestinal: Splenomegaly, nausea
Hematologic: Thrombocytopenia
Neuromuscular & skeletal: Medullary bone pain (24% incidence) is generally dose related, localized to the lower back, posterior iliac crests, and sternum, osteoporosis
Renal: Hematuria, proteinuria
Toxicology Leukocytosis which was not associated with any clinical adverse effects; after discontinuing the drug there is a 50% decrease in circulating levels of neutrophils within 1-2 days, return to pretreatment levels within 1-7 days. No clinical adverse effects seen with high-dose producing ANC >10,000/mm³
Stability Store at 2°C to 8°C (36°F to 46°F); do not expose to freezing or dry ice. Prior to administration, filgrastim may be allowed to be at room temperature for a maximum of 24 hours. It may be diluted in dextrose 5% in water to a concentration of ≥15 mcg/mL for I.V. infusion administration. Minimum concentration is 15 mcg/mL; concentrations <15 mcg/mL require addition of albumin (1 mL of 5%) to the bag to prevent ab-

sorption. This diluted solution is stable for 7 days under refrigeration or at room temperature. **Filgrastim is incompatible with 0.9% sodium chloride (normal saline)**. Standard diluent: $\geq$375 mcg/25 mL D_5W

Mechanism of Action Stimulates the production, maturation, and activation of neutrophils, G-CSF activates neutrophils to increase both their migration and cytotoxicity. Natural proteins which stimulate hematopoietic stem cells to proliferate, prolong cell survival, stimulate cell differentiation, and stimulate functional activity of mature cells. CSFs are produced by a wide variety of cell types. Specific mechanisms of action are not yet fully understood, but possibly work by a second-messenger pathway with resultant protein production. See table.

Proliferation/Differentiation	G-CSF (Filgrastim)	GM-CSF (Sargramostim)
Neutrophils	Yes	Yes
Eosinophils	No	Yes
Macrophages	No	Yes
Neutrophil migration	Enhanced	Inhibited

Pharmacodynamics
  Onset of action: Rapid elevation in neutrophil counts within the first 24 hours, reaching a plateau in 3-5 days
  Duration: ANC decreases by 50% within 2 days after discontinuing G-CSF white counts return to the normal range in 4-7 days
Pharmacokinetics
  Absorption: S.C.: 100%; peak plasma levels can be maintained for up to 12 hours
  Distribution: V_d: 150 mL/kg; no evidence of drug accumulation over a 11- to 20-day period
  Metabolism: Systemic
  Bioavailability: Oral: Not bioavailable
  Half-life: 1.8-3.5 hours
  Time to peak serum concentration: S.C.: Within 2-6 hours
Usual Dosage Geriatrics and Adults:
  Initial dosing recommendations: 5 mcg/kg/day administered S.C. or I.V. as a single daily infusion over 20-30 minutes

  Doses may be increased in increments of 5 mcg/kg for each chemotherapy cycle, according to the duration and severity of the absolute neutrophil count (ANC) nadir. In phase III trials, efficacy was observed at doses of 4-6 mcg/kg/day. Discontinue therapy if the ANC count is > 10,000/mm^3 after the ANC nadir has occurred.

  Length of therapy:
    Bone marrow transplant patients: G-CSF should be administered daily for up to 30 days, until the ANC has reached 1000/mm^3 for 3 consecutive days following the expected chemotherapy-induced neutrophil nadir.
    Chemotherapy-treated patients: G-CSF may be administered daily for up to 2 weeks until the ANC has reached 10,000/mm^3 following the expected chemotherapy-induced neutrophil nadir. Duration of therapy needed to attenuate chemotherapy-induced neutropenia may be dependent on the myelosuppressive potential of the chemotherapy regimen employed. Duration of therapy in clinical studies has ranged from 2 weeks to 3 years. Safety and efficacy of chronic administration have not been established.

  Premature discontinuation of G-CSF therapy prior to the time of recovery from the expected neutrophil is generally not recommended; a transient increase in neutrophil counts is typically seen 1-2 days after initiation of therapy
Administration Infuse I.V. dose over 20-30 minutes
Monitoring Parameters Complete blood cell count and platelet count should be obtained twice weekly. Leukocytosis (white blood cell counts of $\geq$100,000/mm^3) has been observed in ~2% of patients receiving G-CSF at doses above 5 mcg/kg/day. Monitor platelets and hematocrit regularly. Monitor patients with pre-existing cardiac conditions closely as cardiac events (myocardial infarctions, arrhythmias) have been reported in premarketing clinical studies.
Reference Range No clinical benefit seen with ANC > 10,000/mm^3
Patient Information Possible bone pain
Nursing Implications Do not mix with sodium chloride solutions; see Administration
Additional Information Reimbursement hotline: 1-800-28-AMGEN
Special Geriatric Considerations No specific data available for the elderly; see Usual Dosage and Monitoring Parameters
Dosage Forms Injection, preservative free: 300 mcg/mL (1 mL, 1.6 mL)

ALPHABETICAL LISTING OF DRUGS

Finasteride

Brand Names Proscar®

Therapeutic Class Antiandrogen; Urinary Tract Product

Use Early data indicate that finasteride is useful in the treatment of symptomatic benign prostatic hyperplasia (BPH)

Unlabeled use: Adjuvant monotherapy after radical prostatectomy in the treatment of prostatic cancer

Contraindications History of hypersensitivity to drug

Warnings Women who are pregnant or who may become pregnant should not handle crushed finasteride tablets because of potential effects on a male fetus; pregnant women should also avoid exposure to the semen of a patient on finasteride

Precautions Use with caution in patients with impaired hepatic function; patients should be evaluated for prostate cancer before initiating therapy with finasteride

Adverse Reactions Genitourinary: <4% incidence of impotence, decreased libido, decreased volume of ejaculate

Drug Interactions Finasteride decreased theophylline half-life by 10%, but this was not clinically significant

Mechanism of Action

Finasteride is a 4-azo analog of testosterone and is a competitive inhibitor of both tissue and hepatic 5-alpha reductase. This results in inhibition of the conversion of testosterone to dihydrotestosterone and markedly suppresses serum dihydrotestosterone levels; depending on dose and duration, serum testosterone concentrations may or may not increase. Testosterone-dependent processes such as fertility, muscle strength, potency, and libido are not affected by finasteride.

Pharmacodynamics

Onset of clinical effect: Within 12 weeks to 6 months of ongoing therapy

Duration of action:

After a single oral dose as small as 0.5 mg: 65% depression of plasma dihydrotestosterone levels persists 5-7 days

After 6 months of treatment with 5 mg/day: Circulating dihydrotestosterone levels are reduced to castrate levels without significant effects on circulating testosterone; levels return to normal within 14 days of discontinuation of treatment

Pharmacokinetics

Absorption: Oral: Extent of absorption may be reduced if administered with food

Bioavailability: Mean: 63%

Half-life:

Elderly: 8 hours

Adults: 6 hours (3-16)

Protein binding: 90%

Elimination: Excreted as metabolites in urine and feces; elimination rate is decreased in the elderly, but no dosage adjustment is needed

Usual Dosage Geriatrics and Adults: Oral: 5 mg/day as a single dose; clinical response occurs within 12 weeks to 6 months of initiation of therapy; long-term administration is recommended for maximal response

Monitoring Parameters Objective and subjective signs of relief of benign prostatic hyperplasia, including improvement in urinary flow, reduction in symptoms of urgency, and relief of difficulty in micturition

Test Interactions Finasteride does not influence plasma FSH, LH, cortisol, or estradiol levels; plasma dihydrotestosterone and prostate specific antigen levels are suppressed; plasma testosterone levels are usually increased; no clinically significant effects on serum lipids

Patient Information See Warnings; explain that it may take 6-12 months to see a response; in patients who respond, treatment is for life

Nursing Implications See Warnings

Additional Information Finasteride may be useful in men with moderately symptomatic BPH who either refuse prostatectomy or are poor surgical candidates. Risk:benefit ratio and cost must be explained to the patient. Currently, there is no way to predict which men will respond to finasteride.

Special Geriatric Considerations Clearance of finasteride is decreased in the elderly, but no dosage reductions are necessary; see Precautions

Dosage Forms Tablet: 5 mg

Fisalamine *see* Mesalamine *on page 445*

Flagyl® *see* Metronidazole *on page 467*

Flavorcee® [OTC] *see* Ascorbic Acid *on page 57*

Flavoxate (fla vox' ate)

Brand Names Urispas®

Generic Available No

Therapeutic Class Antispasmodic Agent, Urinary

Use Antispasmodic to provide symptomatic relief of dysuria, nocturia, suprapubic pain, urgency, and incontinence due to detrusor instability and hyper-reflexia in elderly with cystitis, urethritis, urethrocystitis, urethrotrigonitis, and prostatitis

292

Contraindications Pyloric or duodenal obstruction, GI hemorrhage, GI obstruction; ileus; achalasia; obstructive uropathies of lower urinary tract (BPH)

Warnings Glaucoma

Precautions May cause drowsiness, vertigo, and ocular disturbances; give cautiously in patients with suspected glaucoma

Adverse Reactions
Cardiovascular: Tachycardia, palpitation
Central nervous system: Nervousness, fatigue, mental confusion (especially in geriatrics), vertigo, headache, drowsiness (>10%), hyperpyrexia
Dermatologic: Urticaria, other dermatoses
Gastrointestinal: Constipation, nausea, vomiting, dry mouth (>10%)
Hematologic: Eosinophilia; one case of reversible leukopenia has been reported
Ocular: Blurred vision, increased ocular tension (<1%)
Renal: Dysuria
Miscellaneous: Dry throat (>10%)

Overdosage Symptoms of overdose include clumsiness, dizziness, drowsiness, flushing, hallucinations, irritability

Toxicology Treatment is general supportive care

Drug Interactions See Adverse Reactions; may enhance the anticholinergic effects of drugs exhibiting anticholinergic pharmacologic action

Mechanism of Action Synthetic antispasmotic with similar actions to that of propantheline; it exerts a direct relaxant effect on smooth muscles via phosphodiesterase inhibition, providing relief to a variety of smooth muscle spasms; it is especially useful for the treatment of bladder spasticity, whereby it produces an increase in urinary capacity

Pharmacodynamics Onset of action: 55-60 minutes

Pharmacokinetics
Metabolism: To methyl; flavone carboxylic acid active
Elimination: 10% to 30% in urine within 6 hours

Usual Dosage Geriatrics and Adults: Oral: 100-200 mg 3-4 times/day; reduction of dose may be possible with symptomatic improvement

Monitoring Parameters Monitor incontinence episodes; postvoid residual (PVR); monitor for anticholinergic side effects

Patient Information May cause drowsiness, dizziness, or visual disturbances; use with caution if performing tasks requiring coordination or mental alertness; avoid other substances that may cause similar effects (eg, alcohol)

Nursing Implications Monitor incontinence and PVR; see Adverse Reactions, Overdosage

Special Geriatric Considerations Caution should be used in elderly due to anticholinergic activity (eg, confusion, constipation, blurred vision, and tachycardia)

Dosage Forms Tablet: 100 mg

Flecainide Acetate (fle kay' nide)

Brand Names Tambocor®
Generic Available No
Therapeutic Class Antiarrhythmic Agent, Class IC
Use Prevention and suppression of documented life-threatening ventricular arrhythmias (ie, sustained ventricular tachycardia); controlling symptomatic, disabling supraventricular tachycardias in patients without structural heart disease
Contraindications Pre-existing second or third degree A-V block; right bundle-branch block associated with left hemiblock (bifascicular block) or trifascicular block; cardiogenic shock, myocardial depression; known hypersensitivity to the drug
Warnings Due to the results of the CAST study, the manufacturer and FDA recommend that this drug be reserved for life-threatening ventricular arrhythmias unresponsive to conventional therapy. Its use for symptomatic nonsustained ventricular tachycardia, frequent premature ventricular complexes (PVCs), uniform and multiform PVCs and/or coupled PVCs is no longer recommended. Flecainide can worsen or cause arrhythmias with an associated risk of death. Proarrhythmic effects range from an increased number of PVCs to more severe ventricular tachycardias (eg, tachycardias that are more sustained or more resistant to conversion to sinus rhythm). Electrolyte abnormalities alter effects of drug; correct abnormalities prior to treatment, see Adverse Reactions.
Precautions Pre-existing sinus node dysfunction, sick sinus syndrome, history of congestive heart failure or myocardial dysfunction; increases in P-R interval ≥300 MS, QRS ≥180 MS, Q-T$_c$ interval increases and/or new bundle-branch block; patients with pacemakers, renal impairment and/or hepatic impairment
Adverse Reactions
Cardiovascular: Bradycardia, heart block, increased P-R, QRS duration; worsening ventricular arrhythmias, congestive heart failure, palpitations, chest pain, edema, syncope
Central nervous system: Dizziness, fatigue, nervousness, headache, lightheadedness, hypoesthesia, paresthesia

(Continued)
293

ALPHABETICAL LISTING OF DRUGS
Flecainide Acetate *(Continued)*

Dermatologic: Rashes
Gastrointestinal: Nausea, constipation, abdominal pain, diarrhea, anorexia, dyspepsia, flatulence, dysgeusia, dry mouth
Hematologic: Blood dyscrasias
Hepatic: Possible hepatic dysfunction
Neuromuscular & skeletal: Tremors
Ocular: Blurred vision
Respiratory: Dyspnea

Overdosage Increases in PR, QRS, Q-T intervals and amplitude of the T wave, reduced heart rate and myocardial contractility, conduction disturbances, hypotension and death

Toxicology Supportive monitoring, charcoal hemoperfusion; may be useful as well as acidification of the urine; flecainide-induced ventricular tachycardia should be treated with ventricular pacing, antiarrhythmic drugs and/or cardioversion, however it is commonly refractory to these measures

Drug Interactions
Digoxin (increased plasma digoxin concentrations), beta-blockers (possible additive negative inotropic effects)
Alkalinizing agents (high-dose antacids, carbonic anhydrase inhibitors or sodium bicarbonate) may decrease flecainide's clearance

Mechanism of Action Class IC antiarrhythmic; slows conduction in cardiac tissue by altering transport of ions across cell membranes; causes slight prolongation of refractory periods; decreases the rate of rise of the action potential without affecting its duration; increases electrical stimulation threshold of ventricle, HIS-Purkinje system; possesses local anesthetic and moderate negative inotropic effects

Pharmacokinetics
Absorption: Oral: Rapid
Distribution: V_d: Adults: 5-13.4 L/kg
Protein binding: 40% to 50% (alpha$_1$ glycoprotein)
Metabolism: In the liver
Bioavailability: 85% to 90%
Half-life: Adults: 7-22 hours (average: 14 hours); increased half-life with congestive heart failure or renal dysfunction
Time to peak serum levels: Within 1.5-3 hours
Elimination: 80% to 90% in urine as unchanged drug and metabolites (10% to 50%)

Usual Dosage Geriatrics and Adults: Oral:
Ventricular arrhythmias: Initial: 100 mg every 12 hours, increase by 50 mg/day (given in 2 doses/day) every 4 days to maximum of 400 mg/day; for patients receiving 400 mg/day who are not controlled and have trough concentrations <0.6 µg/mL, dosage may be increased to 600 mg/day

Supraventricular arrhythmias: 50 mg every 12 hours; increase by 50 mg twice daily at 4-day intervals; maximum daily dose: 300 mg

Dosing interval in severe renal impairment: Cl_{cr} <35 mL/minute/1.73 m^2: Decrease the usual dose by 25% to 50%

When transferring from another antiarrhythmic agent, allow for 2-4 half-lives of the agent to pass before initiating flecainide therapy

Monitoring Parameters EKG, blood pressure, pulse, periodic serum concentrations, especially in patients with renal or hepatic impairment

Reference Range Therapeutic: 0.2-1 µg/mL (SI: 0.4-2 µmol/L)

Patient Information Take as directed; do not change dose except from advice of your physician; report any chest pain or irregular heartbeats

Nursing Implications Give around-the-clock rather than 4 times/day, 3 times/day, etc (ie, 12-6-12-6, not 9-1-5-9) to promote less variation in peak and trough serum levels

Special Geriatric Considerations Decreased clearance and, therefore, prolonged half-life is possible; however, studies have shown no difference in response to usual doses in elderly despite slight decrease in clearance; calculate or measure Cl_{cr} since many elderly have Cl_{cr} <35 mL/minute; see Usual Dosage

Dosage Forms Tablet: 50 mg, 100 mg, 150 mg

References
Fenster PE and Nolan PE, "Antiarrhythmic Drugs," *Geriatric Pharmacology*, Bressler R and Katz MD, eds, New York, NY: McGraw-Hill, 1993, 6:105-49.

Fleet® Laxative [OTC] *see* Bisacodyl *on page 87*

Fleet® Flavored Castor Oil [OTC] *see* Castor Oil *on page 124*

Fleet® Babylax® [OTC] *see* Glycerin *on page 325*

Fleet® Mineral Oil Enema [OTC] *see* Mineral Oil *on page 473*

Fletcher's Castoria® [OTC] *see* Senna *on page 641*

Flexeril® *see* Cyclobenzaprine Hydrochloride *on page 195*

Flint SSD® *see* Silver Sulfadiazine *on page 644*

Flonase® Intranasal Spray *see* Fluticasone Propionate *on page 309*

Florical® [OTC] *see* Calcium Salts (Oral) *on page 111*

Florinef® Acetate *see* Fludrocortisone Acetate *on page 297*

Floxin® *see* Ofloxacin *on page 515*

Flubenisolone *see* Betamethasone *on page 82*

Fluconazole (floo koe' na zole)

Brand Names Diflucan®

Generic Available No

Therapeutic Class Antifungal Agent, Systemic

Use Treatment of susceptible fungal infections including oropharyngeal and esophageal candidiasis; treatment of systemic candidal infections including urinary tract infection, peritonitis, and pneumonia; treatment of cryptococcal meningitis

Contraindications Known hypersensitivity to fluconazole or other azoles

Warnings Patients who develop abnormal liver function tests during fluconazole therapy should be monitored closely for the development of more severe hepatic injury; if clinical signs and symptoms consistent with liver disease develop that may be attributable to fluconazole, fluconazole should be discontinued

Precautions Should be used with caution in patients with renal and hepatic dysfunction or previous hepatotoxicity from other azole derivatives.

Adverse Reactions

Cardiovascular: Pallor

Central nervous system: Dizziness, headache

Dermatologic: Skin rash, exfoliative skin disorders

Endocrine & metabolic: Hypokalemia

Gastrointestinal: Nausea, abdominal pain, vomiting, diarrhea

Hepatic: Elevated AST, ALT, or alkaline phosphatase

Overdosage Symptoms of overdose include decreased lacrimation, salivation, respiration, and GI motility; urinary incontinence, cyanosis

Toxicology Hemodialysis for 3 hours reduces plasma levels by ~50%

Drug Interactions

May increase cyclosporine levels when high doses used, may increase phenytoin serum concentration; fluconazole may also inhibit warfarin's metabolism

Rifampin decreased concentrations of fluconazole

Cimetidine has been reported to decrease fluconazole's absorption

Hydrochlorothiazide has been reported to increase fluconazole's absorption

Fluconazole may increase ethinyl estradiol absorption; fluconazole given concurrently with tolbutamide, glyburide, and glipizide has resulted in increased maximum concentrations and AUC of the oral hypoglycemics with hypoglycemia

Stability Do not add other medications to I.V. unit

Mechanism of Action Interferes with cytochrome P-450 activity, decreasing ergosterol synthesis (principal sterol in fungal cell membrane) and inhibiting cell membrane formation

Pharmacokinetics

Protein binding, plasma: 11% to 12%

Bioavailability: Oral: >90%

Half-life: Normal renal function: 25-30 hours

Time to peak: Oral: Peak concentrations achieved within 2-4 hours

Elimination: 80% of dose excreted unchanged in urine

Usual Dosage The daily dose of fluconazole is the same for oral and I.V. administration Geriatrics and Adults: Oral, I.V.: For once daily dosing, see table.

Indication	Day 1	Daily Therapy	Minimum Duration of Therapy
Oropharyngeal candidiasis	200 mg	100 mg	14 d
Esophageal candidiasis	200 mg	100 mg	21 d
Systemic candidiasis	400 mg	200 mg	28 d
Cryptococcal meningitis acute	400 mg	200 mg	10–12 wk after CSF culture becomes negative
relapse	200 mg	200 mg	

Vaginal candidiasis: 150 mg as a single dose

Dosing adjustment in renal impairment: Cl$_{cr}$ 11-50 mL/minute: Administer 50% of recommended dose

Administration Parenteral fluconazole must be administered by I.V. infusion over ~1-2 hours; do not exceed 200 mg/hour when giving I.V. infusion

(Continued)

Fluconazole *(Continued)*

Monitoring Parameters AST, ALT, and alkaline phosphatase, potassium

Patient Information Complete full course of therapy; contact physician or pharmacist if side effects develop

Nursing Implications Monitor renal function as dosage adjustments are required with significant changes in renal function; do not unwrap unit until ready for use; do not use if cloudy or precipitated; see Administration and Stability

Additional Information An expensive oral alternative to I.V. amphotericin B infusions; in some clinical studies it has been as effective as amphotericin B, but is less likely to cause serious adverse reactions

Special Geriatric Considerations See Usual Dosage and dosing in renal impairment; has not been specifically studied in the elderly

Dosage Forms
Injection: 2 mg/mL (100 mL, 200 mL)
Powder, for oral suspension: 10 mg/mL, 40 mg/mL when reconstituted
Tablet: 50 mg, 100 mg, 150 mg, 200 mg

References
Grant SM and Clissold SP, "Fluconazole: A Review of Its Pharmacodynamic and Pharmacokinetic Properties and Therapeutic Potential in Superficial and Systemic Mycoses," *Drugs*, 1990, 39(6):877-916.

Flucytosine (floo sye' toe seen)

Brand Names Ancobon®

Synonyms 5-FC; 5-Flurocytosine

Therapeutic Class Antifungal Agent, Systemic

Use Treatment of susceptible fungal infections, usually strains of *Candida* or *Cryptococcus*

Unlabeled use: Treatment of chromomycosis

Contraindications Hypersensitivity to flucytosine or any component

Warnings Use with extreme caution in patients with renal impairment, bone marrow depression; patients with AIDS

Precautions Dosage modification required in patients with impaired renal function

Adverse Reactions
Cardiovascular: Cardiac arrest
Central nervous system: Confusion, sedation, paresthesia, parkinsonism, hallucinations, psychosis, headache, ataxia
Dermatologic: Rash, photosensitivity
Endocrine & metabolic: Hypoglycemia, hypokalemia
Gastrointestinal: Nausea, vomiting, diarrhea, abdominal pain, loss of appetite
Hematologic: Bone marrow depression, anemia, leukopenia, thrombocytopenia
Hepatic: Elevated liver enzymes, jaundice
Otic: Hearing loss
Respiratory: Respiratory arrest

Overdosage Symptoms of overdose include nausea, vomiting, diarrhea

Toxicology Treatment is supportive

Drug Interactions Amphotericin dose must be reduced when used at the same time; cytosine may inactivate flucytosine

Stability Protect from light

Mechanism of Action Penetrates fungal cells and is converted to fluorouracil which competes with uracil interfering with fungal RNA and protein synthesis

Pharmacokinetics
Absorption: Oral: 75% to 90%
Protein binding: 2% to 4%
Metabolism: Minimal
Half-life: 3-8 hours (may be as long as 200 hours in anuria)
Time to peak: Peak serum levels occur within 2-6 hours
Elimination: 75% to 90% excreted unchanged in urine by glomerular filtration

Usual Dosage Geriatrics and Adults: Oral: 50-150 mg/kg/day in divided doses every 6 hours

Dosing interval in renal impairment:
Cl_{cr} <50 mL/minute: Administer every 12 hours
Cl_{cr} <10 mL/minute: Administer every 24 hours
Dialyzable (50% to 100%)

Monitoring Parameters Serum creatinine, BUN, alkaline phosphatase, AST, ALT, CBC; serum flucytosine concentrations

Reference Range Therapeutic: 50-100 μg/mL (SI: 390-775 μmol/L)

Test Interactions Flucytosine causes markedly false elevations in serum creatinine values when the Ektachem® analyzer is used

Patient Information Take capsules a few at a time with food over a 15-minute period

Nursing Implications Give around-the-clock rather than 4 times/day, 3 times/day, etc (ie, 12-6-12-6, not 9-1-5-9) to promote less variation in peak and trough serum levels; perform hematologic, renal and hepatic function tests

Special Geriatric Considerations See Usual Dosage; adjust for renal function
Dosage Forms Capsule: 250 mg, 500 mg

Fludrocortisone Acetate (floo droe kor' ti sone)

Related Information
Corticosteroids Comparison, Systemic *on page 808*
Brand Names Florinef® Acetate
Synonyms Fluohydrisone Acetate; Fluohydrocortisone Acetate; 9α-Fluorohydrocortisone Acetate
Generic Available No
Therapeutic Class Mineralocorticoid
Use Addison's disease; partial replacement therapy for adrenal insufficiency and for treatment of salt-losing forms of congenital adrenogenital syndrome

Unlabeled use: Severe orthostatic hypotension; Shy-Drager syndrome
Contraindications Known hypersensitivity to fludrocortisone; congestive heart failure, systemic fungal infections
Precautions Addison's disease, sodium retention and potassium loss, infection
Adverse Reactions
Cardiovascular: Hypertension, edema, congestive heart failure
Central nervous system: Convulsions, headache
Dermatologic: Acne, rash, bruising
Endocrine & metabolic: Hypokalemic alkalosis, suppression of growth, hyperglycemia, HPA suppression
Gastrointestinal: Peptic ulcer
Neuromuscular & skeletal: Muscle weakness, steroid myopathy
Ocular: Cataracts, glaucoma
Overdosage Symptoms of overdose include hypertension, edema, hypokalemia, and weight gain; muscle weakness may develop due to hypokalemia
Toxicology Treat by discontinuing medication; administer potassium supplement, if necessary
Drug Interactions
Steroids decrease the effect of anticholinesterases, isoniazid, salicylates, insulin, oral hypoglycemics
Decreased effect: Barbiturates, phenytoin, rifampin
Increased effect (hypokalemia) of potassium-depleting diuretics
Increased risk of digoxin toxicity (due to hypokalemia)
Increased effect: Estrogens, ketoconazole
Mechanism of Action Promotes increased reabsorption of sodium and loss of potassium from distal tubules
Pharmacodynamics Duration of action: 1-2 days
Pharmacokinetics
Absorption: Rapid and completely from GI tract
Protein binding: 42%
Metabolism: In the liver
Half-life: 30-35 minutes; biological: 18-36 hours
Time to peak serum concentration: 1-7 hours
Usual Dosage Geriatrics and Adults: Oral: 0.05-0.2 mg/day
Orthostatic hypotension: 0.1 mg 2-3 times/day
Monitoring Parameters Blood pressure, standing and sitting/lying down, signs of edema, electrolytes
Test Interactions Increased amylase (S), chloride (S), increased cholesterol (S), increased glucose, increased protein, increased sodium (S); decreased calcium (S), decreased chloride (S), decreased potassium (S), decreased thyroxine (S)
Patient Information Notify physician if dizziness, severe or continuing headaches, swelling of feet or lower legs or unusual weight gain occur
Nursing Implications See Monitoring Parameters
Additional Information Very potent mineralocorticoid with high glucocorticoid activity
Special Geriatric Considerations The most common use of fludrocortisone in the elderly is orthostatic hypotension that is unresponsive to more conservative measures; attempt nonpharmacologic measures before starting drug therapy
Dosage Forms Tablet: 0.1 mg

Flu-Imune® *see* Influenza Virus Vaccine *on page 371*
Flumadine® Oral *see* Rimantadine Hydrochloride *on page 629*

Flunisolide (floo niss' oh lide)
Brand Names AeroBid®; Nasalide®
Generic Available No
Therapeutic Class Anti-inflammatory Agent; Corticosteroid, Inhalant
(Continued)

Flunisolide *(Continued)*

Use Steroid-dependent asthma; nasal solution is used for seasonal or perennial rhinitis

Contraindications Known hypersensitivity to flunisolide, acute status asthmaticus; viral, tuberculosis, fungal or bacterial respiratory infections

Warnings Fatalities have occurred due to adrenal insufficiency in asthmatic patients during and after transfer from systemic corticosteroids to aerosol steroids; several months may be required for recovery of this syndrome; during this period, aerosol steroids do **not** provide the systemic steroid needed to treat patients having trauma, surgery or infections

Precautions Use with caution in patients with hypothyroidism, cirrhosis, hypertension, congestive heart failure, ulcerative colitis, thromboembolic disorders; do not stop medication abruptly if on prolonged therapy

Adverse Reactions
Central nervous system: Dizziness, headache
Endocrine & metabolic: Adrenal suppression
Local: Nasal burning, nasal congestion, nasal dryness, sore throat, bitter taste
Respiratory: Sneezing, atrophic rhinitis, *Candida* infections of the nose or pharynx

Toxicology When consumed in excessive quantities for prolonged periods, systemic hypercorticism and adrenal suppression may occur; in those cases, discontinuation and withdrawal of the corticosteroid should be done judiciously

Drug Interactions Although there have been no reported drug interactions to date, one would expect flunisolide could potentially interact with drugs known to interact with other corticosteroids

Mechanism of Action Decreases inflammation by suppression of migration of polymorphonuclear leukocytes and reversal of increased capillary permeability; does not depress hypothalamus; in asthma, flunisolide may enhance effectiveness of beta-adrenergic drugs, inhibit bronchoconstrictor mechanisms, or produce direct smooth muscle relaxation

Pharmacokinetics
Absorption: Nasal inhalation: ~50%
Metabolism: Rapid in the liver to active metabolites
Half-life: 1.8 hours
Elimination: Equally excreted in urine and feces

Usual Dosage Geriatrics and Adults:
Oral inhalation: 2 inhalations twice daily up to 8 inhalations/day
Nasal: 2 sprays in each nostril twice daily; maximum: 8 sprays/day in each nostril; after desired effect is obtained, decrease dose to the smallest one possible; some patients may be maintained on 1 spray per nostril per day

Monitoring Parameters Relief of symptoms

Patient Information Follow instructions that accompany the product; do not exceed recommended dosage

Nursing Implications Shake well before giving; do not use Nasalide® orally; dispose of product after it has been opened for 3 months; allow at least 1 minute between inhalations

Additional Information Does not contain fluorocarbons; contains polyethylene glycol vehicle

Special Geriatric Considerations Many elderly patients have difficulty using metered dose inhalers, which can limit their effectiveness. Assess technique in all older patients. A spacer device may be useful for the oral inhaler.

Dosage Forms Inhalant:
Nasal (Nasalide®): 25 µg/actuation [200 sprays] (25 mL)
Oral:
AeroBid®: 250 µg/actuation [100 metered doses] (7 g)
AeroBid-M® (menthol flavor): 250 µg/actuation [100 metered doses] (7 g)

Fluocet® *see Fluocinolone Acetonide on this page*

Fluocinolone Acetonide *(floo oh sin' oh lone)*
Related Information
Corticosteroids Comparison, Topical *on page 809*

Brand Names Fluocet®; Fluonid®; Flurosyn®; Synalar®; Synemol®

Generic Available Yes

Therapeutic Class Corticosteroid, Topical (Medium Potency)

Use Relief of susceptible inflammatory and pruritic dermatosis

Contraindications Fungal infection, hypersensitivity to fluocinolone or any component, TB of skin, herpes (including varicella)

Precautions Systemic absorption of topical corticosteroids has produced reversible HPA axis suppression. This is more likely to occur when the preparation is used on large surface or denuded areas for prolonged periods of time or with an occlusive dressing.

Adverse Reactions
Dermatologic: Acne, hypopigmentation, allergic dermatitis, maceration of the skin, skin atrophy

Endocrine & metabolic: HPA suppression, Cushing's syndrome, growth retardation

Local: Burning, itching, irritation, dryness, folliculitis, hypertrichosis

Miscellaneous: Secondary infection

Mechanism of Action Topical corticosteroids have anti-inflammatory, antipruritic, vasoconstrictive, and antiproliferative actions

Usual Dosage Topical: Apply thin layer to affected areas 2-4 times/day

Monitoring Parameters Relief of symptoms

Patient Information Use only as prescribed and for no longer than the period prescribed; apply sparingly in a thin film and rub in lightly; avoid contact with eyes; notify physician if condition persists or worsens

Nursing Implications Use sparingly

Additional Information Considered a moderate-potency steroid; avoid prolonged use on the face, may cause atrophic changes

Special Geriatric Considerations See Precautions; due to age-related changes in skin, limit use of topical glucocorticosteroids

Dosage Forms

Cream: 0.01% (15 g, 30 g, 60 g, 425 g); 0.025% (15 g, 60 g, 425 g); 0.2% (12 g)

Ointment: 0.025% (15 g, 30 g, 60 g, 425 g)

Solution, topical: 0.01% (20 mL, 60 mL)

Fluocinonide (floo oh sin' oh nide)

Related Information

Corticosteroids Comparison, Topical *on page 809*

Brand Names Lidex®; Lidex® E; Vasoderm®; Vasoderm-D®

Generic Available Yes

Therapeutic Class Corticosteroid, Topical (High Potency)

Use Anti-inflammatory, antipruritic, relief of inflammatory and pruritic manifestations

Contraindications Viral, fungal, or tubercular skin lesions, herpes simplex, known hypersensitivity to fluocinonide

Precautions Systemic absorption of topical corticosteroids has produced reversible HPA axis suppression. This is more likely to occur when the preparation is used on large surface or denuded areas for prolonged periods of time or with an occlusive dressing.

Adverse Reactions

Dermatologic: Acne, hypopigmentation, allergic dermatitis, maceration of the skin, skin atrophy

Endocrine & metabolic: HPA suppression, Cushing's syndrome, growth retardation

Local: Burning, itching, irritation, dryness, folliculitis, hypertrichosis

Miscellaneous: Secondary infection

Mechanism of Action Topical corticosteroids have anti-inflammatory, antipruritic, vasoconstrictive, and antiproliferative actions

Usual Dosage Topical: Apply thin layer to affected area 2-4 times/day depending on the severity of the condition

Monitoring Parameters Relief of symptoms

Patient Information Use only as prescribed and for no longer than the period prescribed; apply sparingly in a thin film and rub in lightly; avoid contact with eyes; notify physician if condition persists or worsens

Nursing Implications Use sparingly

Additional Information Considered a high potency steroid; avoid prolonged use on the face; may cause atrophic changes

Special Geriatric Considerations See Precautions; due to age-related changes in skin, limit use of topical glucocorticosteroids

Dosage Forms

Cream: 0.05% (15 g, 30 g, 60 g, 120 g)

Gel, topical: 0.05% (15 g, 30 g, 60 g, 120 g)

Ointment, topical: 0.05% (15 g, 30 g, 60 g, 120 g)

Solution, topical: 0.05% (20 mL, 60 mL)

Fluogen® *see Influenza Virus Vaccine on page 371*

Fluohydrisone Acetate *see Fludrocortisone Acetate on page 297*

Fluohydrocortisone Acetate *see Fludrocortisone Acetate on page 297*

Fluonid® *see Fluocinolone Acetonide on previous page*

Fluoride

Brand Names ACT® [OTC]; Fluorigard®; Fluorineed®; Fluoritab®; Fluorode®; Flura®; Gel-Kam®; Gel-Tin®; Karidium®; Karigel®; Luride®; Luride®-SF F. Lozi-Tabs®; Phos-Flur®; Prevident®; Thera-Flur® Gel

Synonyms Acidulated Phosphate Fluoride; Sodium Fluoride; Stannous Fluoride

Generic Available Yes

Therapeutic Class Mineral, Oral; Mineral, Oral Topical

Use Prevention of dental caries

(Continued)

Fluoride *(Continued)*

Unlabeled use: Treatment of osteoporosis

Contraindications Hypersensitivity to fluoride or any component; when fluoride content of drinking water exceeds 0.7 ppm

Precautions Prolonged ingestion with excessive doses may result in dental fluorosis and osseous changes; do **not** exceed recommended dosage

Adverse Reactions

Dermatologic: Rash

Gastrointestinal: GI upset, nausea, vomiting, especially with large doses for treatment of bone diseases

Neuromuscular & skeletal: Pain in lower extremities

Respiratory: Ulceration of mucous membranes

Miscellaneous: Stannous fluoride may stain the teeth

Overdosage

Hypersalivation, salty or soapy taste, epigastric pain, nausea, vomiting, diarrhea, rash, muscle weakness, tremor, seizure, cardiac failure, respiratory arrest, shock, death

Treatment of overdose: Gastric lavage with calcium chloride or $Ca(OH)_2$ solution; give large quantity of milk at frequent intervals; $Al(OH)_3$ may also bind the fluoride ion

Toxicology Fatal dose not known; adults: 7-140 mg/kg

Drug Interactions Magnesium-, aluminum-, and calcium-containing products (including foods) may decrease absorption of fluoride

Stability Store in tight plastic containers (not glass)

Mechanism of Action Reduces acid production by dental bacteria; increases tooth resistance to acid dissolution by formation of fluorohydroxyapatite; direct stimulation of osteoblasts

Pharmacokinetics

Absorption: In the GI tract, lungs and skin; 50% of fluoride is deposited in teeth and bone after ingestion; topical application works superficially on enamel and plaque

Elimination: In urine and feces

Usual Dosage Recommended daily fluoride supplement: Not recommended for persons >14 years of age

Geriatrics and Adults: Oral:

Dental rinse or gel: 10 mL rinse or apply to teeth and spit daily after brushing

Treatment of osteoporosis: 50-75 mg/day in divided doses

Patient Information Take with food (but not milk) to eliminate GI upset; with dental rinse or dental gel do **not** eat or drink for 30 minutes after use; notify physician of GI or lower extremity complaints

Nursing Implications Avoid giving with milk or dairy products, antacids

Additional Information 2.2 mg of sodium fluoride is equivalent to 1 mg of fluoride ion

Special Geriatric Considerations Postmenopausal women taking high doses of sodium fluoride have increased their bone density in the lumbar spine by 35% with a smaller increase in the femoral neck. In spite of these increases, the overall rate of vertebral fracture did not decline significantly while the rate of hip fracture increased. At the present time, fluoride treatment for osteoporosis cannot be considered safe or effective and should be restricted to investigational protocols.

Dosage Forms

Gel, as sodium: 1.1% (24 g, 125 g)

Gel, oral topical, as stannous: 0.4%

Gel, oral topical, acidulated phosphate: 1.1% (480 mL)

Paste, as sodium: 33.3%

Solution:

Oral, as acidulated phosphate: 0.044% (250 mL, 500 mL)

Oral, as sodium: 1.1 mg/mL (50 mL); 4.4 mg/mL (30 mL); 4.97 mg/mL (50 mL); 12.3 mg/mL (24 mL); 13 mg/mL (19 mL)

Rinsing: 0.02%, 0.05%, 0.2%

Tablet, as sodium: 2.2 mg

Tablet, chewable, as sodium: 0.55 mg, 1.1 mg, 2.2 mg

References

Riggs BL, Hodgson SF, O'Fallon WM, et al, "Effect of Fluoride Treatment on the Fracture Rate in Postmenopausal Women With Osteoporosis," *N Engl J Med*, 1990, 322(12):802-9.

Fluorigard® *see Fluoride on previous page*

Fluorineed® *see Fluoride on previous page*

Fluoritab® *see Fluoride on previous page*

Fluorode® *see Fluoride on previous page*

9α-Fluorohydrocortisone Acetate *see Fludrocortisone Acetate on page 297*

Fluoxetine Hydrochloride (floo ox' e teen)

- **Related Information**
    Antidepressant Agents Comparison *on page 800*
- **Brand Names** Prozac®
- **Generic Available** No
- **Therapeutic Class** Antidepressant; Serotonin Antagonist
- **Use** Treatment of major depression
- **Contraindications** Hypersensitivity to fluoxetine; patients receiving MAO inhibitors currently or in past 2 weeks
- **Precautions** Due to limited experience, use with caution in patients with renal or hepatic impairment, seizure disorders, diabetes mellitus; use with caution in patients at high risk for suicide
- **Adverse Reactions**
    Cardiovascular: Chest pain
    Central nervous system: Headache, nervousness, insomnia, abnormal dreams, drowsiness, anxiety, dizziness, fatigue, sedation, seizures, extrapyramidal reactions (rare)
    Dermatologic: Rash, pruritus
    Endocrine & metabolic: Hypoglycemia, hyponatremia (elderly or volume-depleted patients), SIADH
    Gastrointestinal: Nausea, diarrhea, dry mouth, anorexia, dyspepsia, constipation, vomiting, weight loss
    Genitourinary: Frequent urination, ejaculation problems
    Neuromuscular & skeletal: Tremors, muscle pain, weakness
    Ocular: Visual disturbances
    Respiratory: Nasal congestion
    Miscellaneous: Swollen glands, excessive sweating
- **Overdosage** Symptoms of overdose include nausea, vomiting, agitation, hypomania, seizures
- **Toxicology** Following initiation of essential overdose management (emesis, lavage, activated charcoal), toxic symptoms should be treated. Seizures usually respond to diazepam I.V. boluses (5-10 mg, up to 30 mg). If seizures are unresponsive or recur, phenytoin or phenobarbital may be required.
- **Drug Interactions**
    Increased effect with tricyclics (2 times increased plasma level)
    Increased/decreased effect of lithium (both increased and decreased level has been reported)
    Increased toxicity of diazepam, trazodone via decreased clearance; increased toxicity with MAO inhibitors (hyperpyrexia, tremors, seizures, delirium, coma)
    Displace protein bound drugs
    Cyproheptadine may decrease or reverse effect of fluoxetine
    Carbamazepine and hydantoin levels may be increased, increasing pharmacologic effects
- **Mechanism of Action** Inhibits CNS neuron serotonin uptake; minimal or no effect on reuptake of norepinephrine or dopamine; does not significantly bind to alpha-adrenergic, histamine or cholinergic receptors; may therefore be useful in patients at risk from sedation, hypotension and anticholinergic effects of tricyclic antidepressants
- **Pharmacodynamics** Peak antidepressant effects: Usually occur after more than 4 weeks; due to long half-life, resolution of adverse reactions after discontinuation may be slow
- **Pharmacokinetics**
    Absorption: Oral: Well absorbed
    Metabolism: To norfluoxetine (active)
    Half-life (adults): 2-3 days
    Time to peak: Peak serum levels occurring within 4-8 hours
    Elimination: In urine as fluoxetine (2.5% to 5%) and norfluoxetine (10%)
    Geriatrics: Similar to younger patients after a single dose; has not been evaluated under steady-state conditions
- **Usual Dosage** Oral:
    Geriatrics: Some patients may require an initial dose of 10 mg/day with dosage increases of 10 and 20 mg every several weeks as tolerated; should not be taken at night unless patient experiences sedation

    Adults: 20 mg/day in the morning; may increase after several weeks by 20 mg/day increments; maximum: 80 mg/day; doses >20 mg should be divided into morning and noon doses. **Note:** Lower doses of 5 mg/day have been used for initial treatment

    Dosing adjustment in hepatic impairment:
    Cirrhosis patients: Administer a lower dose or less frequent dosing interval
    Compensated cirrhosis without ascites: Administer 50% of normal dose
- **Monitoring Parameters** Signs and symptoms of depression, anxiety, sleep, appetite, and weight
- **Reference Range** Therapeutic: Fluoxetine 100-800 ng/mL (SI: 289-2314 nmol/L); norfluoxetine 100-600 ng/mL (SI: 289-1735 nmol/L); not well correlated

(Continued)

Fluoxetine Hydrochloride *(Continued)*

Test Interactions Increased albumin in urine

Patient Information Use sugarless hard candy for dry mouth; avoid alcoholic beverages, may cause drowsiness or insomnia, improvement may take several weeks; rise slowly to prevent dizziness

Nursing Implications Offer patient sugarless hard candy for dry mouth

Special Geriatric Considerations Fluoxetine's favorable side effect profile makes it a useful alternative to the traditional tricyclic antidepressants; its potential stimulating and anorexic effects may be bothersome to some patients; has not been shown to be superior in efficacy to the traditional tricyclic antidepressants or other SSRIs; the long half-life in the elderly makes it less attractive compared to other SSRIs

Dosage Forms
Capsule: 10 mg, 20 mg
Solution: 20 mg/5 mL

Extemporaneous Preparation(s) A 20 mg capsule may be mixed with 4 oz of water, apple juice, or Gatorade to provide a solution that is stable for 14 days under refrigeration

References

Beasley CM, Bosomworth JC, and Wernicke JF, "Fluoxetine: Relationships Among Dose, Response, Adverse Events, and Plasma Concentrations in the Treatment of Depression," *Psychopharmacol Bull*, 1990, 26(1):18-24.

Feighner JP and Cohn JB, "Double-blind Comparative Trials of Fluoxetine and Doxepin in Geriatric Patients With Major Depressive Disorder," *J Clin Psychiatry*, 1985, 46(3 Pt 2):20-5.

Lemberger L, Bergstrom RF, Wolen RL, et al, "Fluoxetine: Clinical Pharmacology and Physiologic Disposition," *J Clin Psychiatry*, 1985, 46(3 Pt 2):14-9.

Schone W and Ludwig M, "A Double-Blind Study of Paroxetine Compared With Fluoxetine in Geriatric Patients With Major Depression," *J Clin Psychopharmacol*, 1993, 13(6 Suppl 2):34S-9S.

Fluphenazine *(floo fen' a zeen)*

Related Information
Antacid Drug Interactions *on page 764*
Antipsychotic Agents Comparison *on page 801*
Antipsychotic Medication Guidelines *on page 754*

Brand Names Prolixin®; Prolixin Decanoate®; Prolixin Enanthate®

Synonyms Fluphenazine Decanoate; Fluphenazine Enanthate; Fluphenazine Hydrochloride

Generic Available Yes

Therapeutic Class Antipsychotic Agent; Phenothiazine Derivative

Use Management of manifestations of psychotic disorders; depressive neurosis; alcohol withdrawal; nausea and vomiting; nonpsychotic symptoms associated with dementia in elderly; Tourette's syndrome; Huntington's chorea; spiromatic torticollis and Reye's syndrome; see Special Geriatric Considerations

Contraindications Hypersensitivity to fluphenazine or any component, cross-sensitivity with other phenothiazines may exist; avoid use in patients with narrow-angle glaucoma, bone marrow depression, severe liver or cardiac disease; subcortical brain damage; circulatory collapse, severe hypotension or hypertension

Warnings

Tardive dyskinesia: Prevalence rate may be 40% in elderly; elderly women especially at risk; embarrassment from dyskinesias may lead to greater social isolation; development of the syndrome and the irreversible nature are proportional to duration and total cumulative dose over time. May be reversible if diagnosed early in therapy; intermittent use of antipsychotics (not proven use) helps decrease total cumulative dose.

EPS: Extrapyramidal reactions are more common in elderly with up to 50% developing these reactions after age 60. These reactions may be more common in dementia patients. Drug-induced **Parkinson's syndrome** occurs often. Discontinuation usually resolves symptoms but may take weeks to months (12+) to clear. **Akathisia** is the most common EPS reaction in elderly. The symptoms of motor restlessness are difficult to diagnose in demented elderly; increased nervousness, assertiveness, restlessness with constant movement may indicate this adverse event. Consider decreasing dose if antipsychotic to treat as well as diagnose problem; usually see this reaction within 2-3 months of initiating antipsychotic drug.

Anticholinergic effects: These side effects most common with low potency antipsychotics (eg, thioridazine, chlorpromazine). CNS toxicity occurs more frequently and severely in elderly; increased confusion, memory loss, psychotic behavior, and agitation frequently occur as a consequence of anticholinergic effects to antipsychotic agents. Peripheral anticholinergic action troublesome to elderly; most peripheral anticholinergic effects last only 2-3 weeks; see Adverse Reactions.

Orthostatic hypotension: More common with low potency agents (eg, thioridazine, chlorpromazine, and clozapine) but of concern with all antipsychotic agents; orthostasis due to alpha-receptor blockade by antipsychotic agents. Elderly present many risk factors for orthostatic hypotension: blunted baroreceptor reflexes, decreased vascular tone, decreased vascular volume, and possible presence of cardiac diseases which result in decreased cardiac output.

Sedation: Common side effect with antipsychotic therapy; should not be used as a hypnotic unless insomnia is associated with target behavior symptoms treated with antipsychotic medications; see Special Geriatric Considerations. Anecdotal reports suggesting antipsychotic sedation in nonpsychotic patients is extremely unpleasant due to feelings of depersonalization, derealization, and dysphoria. Due to the long duration of action with antipsychotic drugs, these reactions may last up to 24 hours and result in decreased daytime function.

Cardiac toxicity: Life-threatening arrhythmias have occurred at therapeutic doses of antipsychotics. Thioridazine more commonly demonstrates EKG changes than other antipsychotics; suggested to use high potency antipsychotic agents (ie, haloperidol) in patients with cardiac conduction defects.

Precautions Use with caution in patients with cardiovascular disease, seizures, and Parkinson's disease; benefits of therapy must be weighed against risks of therapy; adverse effects may be of longer duration with Depot® form

Adverse Reactions

Cardiovascular: EKG changes, orthostatic hypotension, tachycardia, arrhythmias, abnormal T waves with prolonged ventricular repolarization

Central nervous system: Sedation, drowsiness, restlessness, anxiety, extrapyramidal reactions, pseudoparkinsonian signs and symptoms, tardive dyskinesia, neuroleptic malignant syndrome, seizures, altered central temperature regulation

Dermatologic: Hyperpigmentation, pruritus, rash, photosensitivity (rare)

Endocrine & metabolic: Amenorrhea, galactorrhea, gynecomastia

Gastrointestinal: GI upset, dry mouth (problem for denture users), constipation, adynamic ileus, weight gain

Genitourinary: Urinary retention, overflow incontinence, priapism, impotence, sexual dysfunction (up to 60%)

Hematologic: Agranulocytosis, leukopenia (usually in patients with large doses for prolonged periods), thrombocytopenia, hemolytic anemia, eosinophilia

Hepatic: Cholestatic jaundice (rare)

Ocular: Retinal pigmentation (more common than with chlorpromazine), blurred vision, decreased visual acuity (may be irreversible)

Miscellaneous: Anaphylactoid reactions

Overdosage Symptoms of overdose include deep sleep, coma, extrapyramidal symptoms, abnormal involuntary muscle movements, hypotension or hypertension; agitation, restlessness, fever, hypothermia or hyperthermia, seizures, cardiac arrhythmias, EKG changes

Toxicology Following initiation of essential overdose management, toxic symptom treatment and supportive treatment should be initiated. Hypotension usually responds to I.V. fluids or Trendelenburg positioning. If unresponsive to these measures the use of a parenteral inotrope may be required (eg, norepinephrine 0.1-0.2 mcg/kg/minute titrated to response). Do not use epinephrine. Seizures commonly respond to diazepam (I.V. 5-10 mg bolus in adults every 15 minutes if needed up to a total of 30 mg) or to phenytoin or phenobarbital. Also critical cardiac arrhythmias often respond to I.V. phenytoin (15 mg/kg up to 1 g), while other antiarrhythmics can be used. Neuroleptics often cause extrapyramidal symptoms (eg, dystonic reactions) requiring management with diphenhydramine 1-2 mg/kg up to a maximum of 50 mg I.M. or I.V. slow push followed by a maintenance dose for 48-72 hours. When these reactions are unresponsive to diphenhydramine, benztropine mesylate I.V. 1-2 mg may be effective. These agents are generally effective within 2-5 minutes.

Drug Interactions

Alcohol may increase CNS sedation

Anticholinergic agents may decrease pharmacologic effects; increase anticholinergic side effects; may enhance tardive dyskinesia

Aluminum salts may decrease absorption of phenothiazines

Barbiturates may decrease phenothiazine serum concentrations

Bromocriptine may have decreased efficacy when administered with phenothiazines

Guanethidine's hypotensive effect is decreased by phenothiazines

Lithium administration with phenothiazines may increase disorientation

Meperidine and phenothiazine coadministration increases sedation and hypotension

Methyldopa administration with phenothiazine (trifluoperazine) may significantly increase blood pressure

Norepinephrine, epinephrine have decreased pressor effect when administered with chlorpromazine; therefore, be aware of possible decreased effectiveness or when any phenothiazine is used

Phenytoin serum concentrations may increase or decrease with phenothiazines; tricyclic antidepressants may have increased serum concentrations with concomitant administration with phenothiazines

Propranolol administered with phenothiazines may increase serum concentrations of both drugs

Valproic acid may have increased half-life when administered with phenothiazines (chlorpromazine)

(Continued)

303

Fluphenazine *(Continued)*

Stability Avoid freezing; protect all dosage forms from light, clear or slightly yellow solutions may be used; should be dispensed in amber or opaque vials/bottles. Solutions may be diluted or mixed with fruit juices or other liquids but must be administered immediately after mixing; do not prepare bulk dilutions or store bulk dilutions.

Mechanism of Action Blocks postsynaptic mesolimbic dopaminergic D_1 and D_2 receptors in the brain; exhibits a strong alpha-adrenergic blocking and anticholinergic effect, depresses the release of hypothalamic and hypophyseal hormones; believed to depress the reticular activating system thus affecting basal metabolism, body temperature, wakefulness, vasomotor tone, and emesis

Pharmacodynamics

Onset of action: I.M., S.C.: 24-72 hours

Peak effects: 48-96 hours; derivative dependent; the hydrochloride salt acts quickly and persists briefly, while the decanoate lasts the longest and requires more time for onset

Following hydrochloride derivative administration, the onset of activity occurs within 1 hour yet persists for only 6-8 hours

Pharmacokinetics

Absorption: Oral: May be affected by the inherent anticholinergic action on the gastrointestinal tissue causing variable absorption. Absorption from tablets is erratic with less variation seen with solutions. These agents are widely distributed in tissues with CNS concentrations exceeding that of plasma due to their lipophilic characteristics.

Protein binding: Antipsychotic agents are bound 90% to 99% to plasma or proteins; highly bound to brain and lung tissue and other tissues with a high blood perfusion

Half-life (derivative dependent):
Enanthate: 84-96 hours
Hydrochloride: 33 hours
Decanoate: 163-232 hours

Time to peak: Peak concentrations occur between 2-4 hours

Elimination: Excretion occurs through hepatic metabolism (oxidation) where numerous active metabolites are produced; active metabolites excreted in urine; elimination half-lives of antipsychotics ranges from 20-40 hours which may be extended in elderly due to decline in oxidative hepatic reactions (phase I) with age.

The biologic effect of a single dose persists for 24 hours. When the patient has accommodated to initial side effects (sedation), once daily dosing is possible due to the long half-life of antipsychotics.

Steady-state plasma levels are achieved in 4-7 days; therefore, if possible, do not make dose adjustments more than once in a 7-day period.

Due to the long half-lives of antipsychotics, as needed (PRN) use is ineffective since repeated doses are necessary to achieve therapeutic tissue concentrations in the CNS

Usual Dosage

Geriatrics: Initial (nonpsychotic patient; dementia behavior): 1-2.5 mg/day; increase dose at 4- to 7-day intervals by 1-2.5 mg/day; increase dosing intervals (bid, tid) as necessary to control response or side effects. Maximum daily dose: 20 mg; gradual increases (titration) may prevent some side effects or decrease their severity.

Adults:
Oral: 0.5-10 mg/day; dose is 2-3 times the parenteral dose
I.M.: 2.5-10 mg/day
I.M., S.C. (Decanoate®): 12.5 mg every 3 weeks
I.M., S.C. (Enanthate®): 12.5-25 mg every 3 weeks

Conversion ratio from hydrochloride salt to decanoate salt is ~0.5 mL (12.5 mg) decanoate every 3 weeks for every 10 mg of hydrochloride salt daily.

Not dialyzable (0% to 5%)

Monitoring Parameters Orthostatic blood pressures; tremors; gait changes, abnormal movement in trunk, neck, buccal area or extremities; monitor target behaviors for which the agent is given

Reference Range Therapeutic: 0.13-2.8 ng/mL; correlation of serum concentrations and efficacy is controversial; most often dosed to best response

Test Interactions Increased cholesterol (S), increased glucose; decreased uric acid (S)

Patient Information Oral concentrate must be diluted in 2-4 oz of liquid (water, fruit juice, carbonated drinks, milk, or pudding); do not take antacid within 1 hour of taking drug; avoid alcohol; avoid excess sun exposure (use sun block); may cause drowsiness, rise slowly from recumbent position; use of supportive stockings may help prevent orthostatic hypotension

Nursing Implications Watch for hypotension when administering I.M. or I.V.; Dilute the oral concentrate with water or juice before administration; avoid skin contact with oral suspension or solution; may cause contact dermatitis; monitor orthostatic blood pressures 3-5 days after initiation of therapy or a dose increase; observe for tremor and abnormal movement or posturing (extrapyramidal symptoms)

Additional Information Oral liquid to be diluted in the following **only**: water, saline, 7-UP, homogenized milk, carbonated orange beverages, pineapple, apricot, prune, orange, V-8 juice, tomato, and grapefruit juices; do not mix with beverages containing caffeine, tannins, or pectin (ie, coffee, tea, apple juice)

Special Geriatric Considerations See Warnings

Many elderly patients receive antipsychotic medications for inappropriate nonpsychotic behavior. Before initiating antipsychotic medication, the clinician should investigate any possible reversible cause; any stress or stress from any disease can cause acute "confusion" or worsening of baseline nonpsychotic behavior. Most commonly acute changes in behavior are due to increases in drug dose or addition of new drug to regimen; fluid electrolyte loss; infections; and changes in environment.

Any changes in disease status in any organ system can result in behavior changes.

Dosage Forms

Concentrate, as hydrochloride: 5 mg/mL with alcohol 14% (120 mL)

Elixir, as hydrochloride: 2.5 mg/5 mL with alcohol 14% (60 mL)

Injection, as decanoate ester: 25 mg/mL (1 mL, 5 mL)

Injection, as enanthate: 25 mg/mL (5 mL)

Injection, as hydrochloride: 2.5 mg/mL (10 mL)

Tablet, as hydrochloride: 1 mg, 2.5 mg, 5 mg, 10 mg

Fluphenazine Decanoate see Fluphenazine on page 302

Fluphenazine Enanthate see Fluphenazine on page 302

Fluphenazine Hydrochloride see Fluphenazine on page 302

Flura® see Fluoride on page 299

Flurazepam Hydrochloride (flure az' e pam)

Related Information

Antacid Drug Interactions on page 764

Anxiolytic/Hypnotic Use in Long-Term Care Facilities on page 755-756

Benzodiazepines Comparison on page 802-803

Brand Names Dalmane®

Generic Available Yes

Therapeutic Class Benzodiazepine; Hypnotic; Sedative

Use Short-term treatment of insomnia

Restrictions C-IV

Contraindications Hypersensitivity to flurazepam or any component; there may be cross-sensitivity with other benzodiazepines; pre-existing CNS depression, respiratory depression, narrow-angle glaucoma

Precautions Use with caution in patients receiving other CNS depressants, patients with low albumin, and hepatic dysfunction, or a history of drug dependence

Adverse Reactions

Cardiovascular: Hypotension

Central nervous system: Drowsiness, dizziness, confusion, residual daytime sedation, paradoxical reactions, hyperactivity and excitement (rare), ataxia, hallucinations

Respiratory: Decrease in respiratory rate, apnea, laryngospasm

Miscellaneous: Physical and psychological dependence with prolonged use, falls in the elderly

Toxicology Treatment for benzodiazepine overdose is supportive. Rarely is mechanical ventilation required. Flumazenil has been shown to selectively block the binding of benzodiazepines to CNS receptors, resulting in a reversal of benzodiazepine-induced CNS depression, but not respiratory depression.

Drug Interactions Benzodiazepines may increase digoxin concentrations and may decrease the effect of levodopa

Decreased metabolism: Cimetidine, fluoxetine

Increased metabolism: Rifampin

Increased toxicity: CNS depressants, alcohol

Stability Store in light-resistant containers

Mechanism of Action Benzodiazepines appear to potentiate the effects of GABA and other inhibitory neurotransmitters by binding to specific benzodiazepine-receptor sites in various areas of the CNS

Pharmacodynamics Because of a long-acting metabolite, residual, daytime sedation or "hangover effect" may occur, particularly in the elderly. Studies have shown that the elderly are more sensitive to the effects of benzodiazepines as compared to younger adults.

Hypnotic effects:

Onset of action: 15-20 minutes

Peak effect: 3-6 hours

Duration of action: 7-8 hours

Pharmacokinetics

Metabolism: In liver to N-desalkylflurazepam (active)

(Continued)

Flurazepam Hydrochloride *(Continued)*

Half-life (active metabolite): Adults: 40-114 hours
Elimination: Prolonged in elderly; accumulation of the parent drug and its metabolite occurs

Usual Dosage Oral:
Geriatrics: 15 mg at bedtime
Adults: 15-30 mg at bedtime

Monitoring Parameters Respiratory, cardiovascular, and mental status

Reference Range Therapeutic: 0-4 ng/mL (SI: 0-9 nmol/L); metabolite N-desalkylflurazepam: 20-110 ng/mL (SI: 43-240 nmol/L); Toxic: >0.12 µg/mL

Patient Information Avoid alcohol and other CNS depressants, may cause drowsiness or "hangover" effect; avoid activities needing good psychomotor coordination until CNS effects are known; may cause physical or psychological dependence; avoid abrupt discontinuation after prolonged use

Nursing Implications Provide safety measures (ie, side rails, night light, and call button); remove smoking materials from area; supervise ambulation; avoid abrupt discontinuance in patients with prolonged therapy or seizure disorders; observe for orthostasis

Special Geriatric Considerations See Pharmacodynamics and Pharmacokinetics; due to its long-acting metabolite, flurazepam is not considered a drug of choice in the elderly; long-acting benzodiazepines have been associated with falls in the elderly; interpretive guidelines from the Health Care Financing Administration (HCFA) discourage the use of this agent in residents of long-term care facilities

Dosage Forms Capsule: 15 mg, 30 mg

References

Maletta G, Mattox KM, and Dysken M, "Guidelines for Prescribing Psychoactive Drugs in the Elderly: Part 1," *Geriatrics*, 1991, 46(9):40-7.

Reidenberg MM, Levy M, Warner H, et al, "Relationship Between Diazepam Dose, Plasma Level, Age, and Central Nervous System Depression," *Clin Pharmacol Ther*, 1978, 23(4):371-4.

Flurbiprofen Sodium (flure bi' proe fen)

Brand Names Ansaid®; Ocufen®

Generic Available Tablet: Yes

Therapeutic Class Analgesic, Non-narcotic; Anti-inflammatory Agent; Anti-inflammatory Agent, Ophthalmic; Nonsteroidal Anti-Inflammatory Agent (NSAID), Ophthalmic

Use Acute or long-term treatment of signs and symptoms of rheumatoid arthritis and osteoarthritis; inhibition of intraoperative miosis; topical treatment of cystoid macular edema; postcataract surgery inflammation and uveitis syndromes

Unlabeled use: Ankylosing spondylitis, mild to moderate pain, tendonitis, bursitis, acute painful shoulder, acute gout, sunburn, for aborting acute migraine headache attacks; ophthalmic: prevention and management of postoperative ocular inflammation and postoperative cystoid macular edema

Contraindications Hypersensitivity to flurbiprofen or any component; hypersensitivity to aspirin or other NSAIDs; dendritic keratitis

Warnings Potential cross-sensitivity to aspirin and other NSAIDs exists; systemic effects from ocular absorption may occur (ie, bleeding): GI toxicity (bleeding, ulceration, perforation); CNS effects may occur (headaches, confusion, depression); hypersensitivity, anaphylactoid reactions (intermittent tolmetin use more often); renal function decline, acute renal insufficiency, interstitial nephritis, dysuria, cystitis, hematuria, nephrotic syndrome, hyperkalemia in acute renal insufficiency, hyponatremia, papillary necrosis, hepatic function impairment; should be used with caution in patients with a history of herpes simplex, keratitis, and patients who might be affected by inhibition of platelet aggregation; patients in whom asthma, rhinitis, or urticaria is precipitated by aspirin or other NSAIDs; systemic absorption occurs with ocular application; elderly have increased risk for adverse reactions to NSAIDs; see Special Geriatric Considerations

Precautions Use with caution in patients with congestive heart failure, hypertension, decreased renal or hepatic function, history of GI disease (bleeding or ulcers), or those receiving anticoagulants; perform ophthalmologic evaluation for those who develop eye complaints during therapy (blurred vision, diminished vision, changes in color vision, retinal changes); should be used with caution in patients with a history of herpes simplex, keratitis, and patients who might be affected by inhibition of platelet aggregation; slowing of corneal wound healing; NSAIDs may mask signs/symptoms of infections; photosensitivity reported

Adverse Reactions
Cardiovascular: Congestive heart failure, angina, hypertension, hypotension, fluid retention, arrhythmias, edema
Central nervous system: Headache, drowsiness, vertigo, dizziness, fatigue, hallucinations, confusion, depression, emotional lability, psychotic behavior, asthenia
Dermatologic: Rash, urticaria, angioedema, Stevens-Johnson syndrome, exfoliative dermatitis, ecchymosis, petechiae, purpura, slowing of corneal wound healing, bruising

Endocrine & metabolic: Hyperglycemia, hypoglycemia, hyperkalemia, gynecomastia, hyponatremia

Gastrointestinal: Dyspepsia, heartburn, nausea, diarrhea, constipation, flatulence, anorexia, stomatitis, vomiting, abdominal pain, peptic ulcer, GI bleeding, GI perforation, gingival ulcers, pancreatitis, proctitis, paralytic ulcers, colitis, weight loss

Genitourinary: Impotence, azotemia

Hematologic: Neutropenia, anemia, agranulocytosis, bone marrow suppression, hemolytic anemia, hemorrhage, inhibition of platelet aggregation

Hepatic: Hepatitis, elevated LFTs, cholestatic jaundice

Neuromuscular & skeletal: Tremors

Ocular: Vision changes, transient stinging, burning, ocular irritation

Otic: Tinnitus

Renal: Dysuria, polyuria, pyuria, oliguria, anuria, acute renal failure

Respiratory: Exacerbation of asthma, dyspnea

Miscellaneous: Dry mucous membranes, thirst, pyrexia, sweating

Overdosage Symptoms include drowsiness, lethargy, disorientation, confusion, dizziness, numbness, paresthesia, nausea, vomiting, gastric irritation, abdominal pain, headache, tinnitus, sweating, blurred vision, muscle twitching, seizures, coma, acute renal failure, increased BUN and serum creatinine, hypotension, tachycardia, and metabolic acidosis

Toxicology Management of a nonsteroidal anti-inflammatory drug (NSAID) intoxication is primarily supportive and symptomatic. Fluid therapy is commonly effective in managing the hypotension that may occur following an acute NSAID overdose, except when this is due to an acute blood loss. Seizures tend to be very short-lived and often do not require drug treatment although recurrent seizures should be treated with I.V. diazepam. Since many of the NSAIDs undergo enterohepatic cycling, multiple doses of charcoal may be needed to reduce the potential for delayed toxicities. NSAIDs are highly bound to plasma proteins; therefore, hemodialysis and peritoneal dialysis are not useful.

Drug Interactions

May increase digoxin, methotrexate, and lithium serum concentrations

Aspirin or other salicylates may decrease NSAID serum concentrations

Other NSAIDs may increase adverse GI effect

Increased prothrombin time with anticoagulants; decreased antihypertensive effects of ACE inhibitors, beta-blockers, and thiazide diuretics; increased response to sympathomimetics

Probenecid may increase toxicity of NSAIDs by increase in serum concentrations

Effects of loop diuretics may be decreased

When used concurrently with flurbiprofen, acetylcholine chloride and carbachol may be ineffective

Mechanism of Action Inhibits prostaglandin synthesis by decreasing the activity of the enzyme, cyclo-oxygenase, which results in decreased formation of prostaglandin precursors; acts on the hypothalamus heat-regulating center to reduce fever, blocks prostaglandin synthetase action which prevents formation of the platelet-aggregating substance, thromboxane A_2; decreases pain receptor sensitivity. Other proposed mechanisms of action for salicylate anti-inflammatory action are lysosomal stabilization, kinin and leukotrienes production, alteration of chemotactic factors, and inhibition of neutrophil activation. This latter mechanism may be the most significant pharmacologic action to reduce inflammation; prostaglandins are believed to play a role in constricting the iris sphincter during ocular surgery.

Pharmacodynamics Onset of action: Within 1-2 hours

Pharmacokinetics

Absorption: Oral: Rapid

Protein binding: 99%

Metabolism: Metabolized in the liver

Half-life: 5-6 hours

Time to peak serum concentration: Within 1-2 hours

Elimination: Excreted by kidneys primarily as glucuronides and sulfates

Usual Dosage Geriatrics and Adults:

Oral: Rheumatoid arthritis and osteoarthritis: Initial: 50 mg 4 times/day to 100 mg 3 times/day; do not give more than 100 mg for any single dose; maximum dose: 300 mg/day

Ophthalmic: Instill 1 drop every 30 minutes, 2 hours prior to surgery (total of 4 drops to each affected eye)

Monitoring Parameters Monitor response (pain, range of motion, grip strength, mobility, ADL function), inflammation; observe for weight gain, edema; monitor renal function; observe for bleeding, bruising; evaluate gastrointestinal effects (abdominal pain, bleeding, dyspepsia); mental confusion, disorientation, CBC, serum creatinine, BUN, liver function tests

Test Interactions Increased chloride (S), increased sodium (S)

Patient Information Serious gastrointestinal bleeding can occur as well as ulceration and perforation. Pain may or may not be present. Avoid aspirin and aspirin-containing products while taking this medication. If gastric upset occurs, take with food, milk, or

(Continued)

Flurbiprofen Sodium *(Continued)*

antacid. If gastric adverse effects persist, contact physician. May cause drowsiness, dizziness, blurred vision, and confusion. Use caution when performing tasks which require alertness (eg, driving). Do not take for more than 3 days for fever and 10 days for pain without physician's advice.

Ophthalmic: May sting on instillation; do not touch dropper to eye; visual acuity may be decreased after administration; assess patient's or caregiver's ability to administer

Nursing Implications See Monitoring Parameters, Overdosage, Patient Information, and Special Geriatric Considerations

Additional Information There are no clinical guidelines to predict which NSAID will give response in a particular patient. Trials with each must be initiated until response is determined. Consider dose, patient convenience, and cost.

Special Geriatric Considerations Elderly are a high-risk population for adverse effects from nonsteroidal anti-inflammatory agents. As much as 60% of elderly can develop peptic ulceration and/or hemorrhage asymptomatically. The concomitant use of H_2 blockers, omeprazole, and sucralfate is not effective as prophylaxis. Misoprostol is the only prophylactic agent proven effective. Also, concomitant disease and drug use contribute to the risk for GI adverse effects. Use lowest effective dose for shortest period possible. Consider renal function decline with age. Use of NSAIDs can compromise existing renal function especially when Cl_{cr} is ≤30 mL/minute. Tinnitus may be a difficult and unreliable indication of toxicity due to age-related hearing loss or eighth cranial nerve damage. CNS adverse effects such as confusion, agitation, and hallucination are generally seen in overdose or high-dose situations, but elderly may demonstrate these adverse effects at lower doses than younger adults.

Dosage Forms

Solution, ophthalmic: 0.03% (2.5 mL, 5 mL, 10 mL)

Tablet: 50 mg, 100 mg

References

Brooks PM, Day RO, "Nonsteroidal Anti-inflammatory Drugs – Differences and Similarities," *N Engl J Med*, 1991, 324(24):1716-25.

Clinch D, Banerjee AK, Ostick G, "Absence of Abdominal Pain in Elderly Patients With Peptic Ulcer," *Age Ageing*, 1984, 13:120-3.

Clive DM, Stoff JS, "Renal Syndromes Associated With Nonsteroidal Anti-inflammatory Drugs," *N Engl J Med*, 1984, 310(9):563-72.

Graham DY, "Prevention of Gastroduodenal Injury Induced by Chronic Nonsteroidal Anti-inflammatory Drug Therapy," *Gastroenterology*, 1989, 96(2 Pt 2 Suppl):675-81.

Knodel LC, "Preventing NSAID-Induced Ulcers: The Role of Misoprostol," *Consult Pharm*, 1989, 4:37-41.

Pounder R, "Silent Peptic Ulceration: Deadly Silence or Golden Silence?" *Gastroenterology*, 1989, 96(2 Pt 2 Suppl):626-31.

5-Flurocytosine *see* Flucytosine *on page 296*

Flurosyn® *see* Fluocinolone Acetonide *on page 298*

Flutamide *(floo' ta mide)*

Brand Names Eulexin®

Generic Available No

Therapeutic Class Antiandrogen

Use In combination therapy with LHRH agonistic (leuprolide) in treatment of metastatic prostatic carcinoma; see Additional Information

Contraindications Known hypersensitivity to flutamide or any component

Warnings Animal data (based on using doses higher than recommended for humans) produced testicular interstitial cell adenoma

Precautions Do not discontinue therapy without physician's advice

Adverse Reactions

Cardiovascular: Edema, hypertension

Central nervous system: Drowsiness, nervousness, depression, anxiety, confusion

Endocrine & metabolic: Gynecomastia, hot flashes

Gastrointestinal: Diarrhea, nausea, anorexia

Genitourinary: Impotence, loss of libido

Hepatic: Elevated LFTs (usually transient)

Overdosage Symptoms of overdose include hypoactivity, ataxia, anorexia, vomiting, piloerection, decreased respiration, tranquilization, lacrimation

Toxicology Induce vomiting; general supportive care; dialysis not effective

Mechanism of Action Inhibiting androgen uptake or inhibits binding of androgen in target tissues

Pharmacokinetics

Absorption: Oral: Rapid and complete

Metabolism: Extensive to more than 10 metabolites

Half-life: 5-6 hours

Elimination: All excreted primarily in urine

Usual Dosage Geriatrics and Adults: Oral: 2 capsules (250 mg) every 8 hours

Monitoring Parameters LFTs, tumor reduction, testosterone/estrogen, and phosphatase serum levels

Patient Information Do not discontinue therapy without physician's advice

Nursing Implications See Monitoring Parameters

Additional Information To achieve benefit to combination therapy, both drugs need to be started simultaneously; most common side effect with this dual therapy is diarrhea

Special Geriatric Considerations A study has shown that the addition of flutamide to leuprolide therapy in patients with advanced prostatic cancer increased median actuarial survival time to 34.9 months versus 27.9 months with leuprolide alone. No specific dose alterations are necessary in elderly.

Dosage Forms Capsule: 125 mg

References
Crawford ED, Eisenberger MA, McLeod DG, et al, "A Controlled Trial of Leuprolide With and Without Flutamide in Prostatic Carcinoma," *N Engl J Med* , 1989, 321(7):419-24.

Flutex® *see* Triamcinolone *on page 710*

Fluticasone Propionate (floo tik' a sone)
Related Information
Corticosteroids Comparison, Topical *on page 809*

Brand Names Cutivate™ Topical; Flonase® Intranasal Spray

Generic Available No

Therapeutic Class Corticosteroid, Topical (Medium Potency)

Use
Intranasal: Management of seasonal and perennial allergic rhinitis
Topical: Relief of inflammation and pruritus associated with corticosteroid-responsive dermatoses

Contraindications Hypersensitivity to any component, bacterial infections, ophthalmic use

Warnings Adverse systemic effects may occur when used on large areas of the body, denuded areas, for prolonged periods of time, and/or with an occlusive dressing

Adverse Reactions
Dermatologic: Acne, hypopigmentation, allergic dermatitis, maceration of the skin, skin atrophy
Endocrine & metabolic: HPA suppression, Cushing's syndrome, growth retardation
Local: Burning, itching, irritation, dryness, folliculitis, hypertrichosis
Miscellaneous: Secondary infection

Toxicology
Signs and symptoms: When consumed in excessive quantities, systemic hypercorticism and adrenal suppression may occur
Treatment: Discontinuation and withdrawal of the corticosteroid should be done judiciously

Mechanism of Action Fluticasone belongs to a new group of corticosteroids which utilizes a fluorocarbothioate ester linkage at the 17 carbon position; extremely potent vasoconstrictive and anti-inflammatory activity; has a weak hypothalamic-pituitary-adrenocortical axis (HPA) inhibitory potency when applied topically, which gives the drug a high therapeutic index. Although HPA suppression does occur after I.V. administration, fluticasone is inactive when administered orally due to first-pass hydrolysis of the carbothioate ester to the corresponding carboxylic acid, which is inactive.

Usual Dosage Geriatrics and Adults:
Intranasal: 2 sprays (50 mcg each) per nostril once daily or 1 spray per nostril twice daily; do not exceed a total daily dosage of 200 mcg; after a few days of use, the dosage may be decreased to 1 spray per nostril once daily
Topical: Apply sparingly in a thin film twice daily

Monitoring Parameters Relief of symptoms

Patient Information A thin film of cream or ointment is effective; do not overuse; use only as prescribed, and for no longer than the period prescribed; apply topical product sparingly in light film, rub in lightly, avoid contact with eyes; notify physician if condition being treated persists or worsens; for intranasal product, follow the instructions accompanying the medication

Nursing Implications Use sparingly; spray is for intranasal use only

Dosage Forms
Cream: 0.05% (15 g, 30 g, 60 g)
Ointment, topical: 0.005% (15 g, 60 g)
Spray (intranasal): 9 g (60 activations) and 16 g (120 actuations)

Fluvastatin
Brand Names Lescol®

Therapeutic Class Antilipemic Agent; HMG-CoA Reductase Inhibitor

Use Adjunct to dietary therapy to decrease elevated serum total and LDL cholesterol concentrations in primary hypercholesterolemia

(Continued)

Fluvastatin *(Continued)*

Contraindications Active liver disease or unexplained persistent elevations of LFTs, hypersensitivity to fluvastatin or other HMG-CoA reductase inhibitors

Warnings Musculoskeletal effects include myopathy (myalgia and/or muscle weakness accompanied by markedly elevated CR concentrations), rash and/or pruritus

Precautions May elevate aminotransferases; LFTs should be performed before and every 4- 6 weeks during the first 12-15 months of therapy and periodically thereafter; serum cholesterol and triglyceride concentrations should be determined prior to and regularly during therapy; use with caution in patients who consume large quantities of alcohol

Adverse Reactions

Central nervous system: Headache, dizziness, insomnia, fatigue

Dermatologic: Rash, pruritus

Gastrointestinal: Nausea, vomiting, diarrhea, abdominal cramps, constipation, flatulence, dyspepsia

Neuromuscular & skeletal: Muscle cramps, back pain, arthropathy

Respiratory: Upper respiratory infection, rhinitis, cough, pharyngitis, sinusitis, bronchitis

Miscellaneous: Influenza, allergy

Overdosage Few cases have been reported; no patients were symptomatic and all recovered without adverse effects

Drug Interactions Increased anticoagulant effect of warfarin; concurrent use of niacin, gemfibrozil, erythromycin, and cyclosporine increases the risk of rhabdomyolysis or myopathy

Mechanism of Action Acts by competitively inhibiting 3-hydroxy-3-methylglutaryl-coenzyme A (HMG-CoA) reductase, the enzyme that catalyzes the rate-limiting step in cholesterol biosynthesis

Usual Dosage Geriatrics and Adults: Oral: 20 mg at bedtime; maximum: 40 mg/day

No dose adjustment needed in mild to moderate renal impairment

Administration May be taken without regard to meals; if concomitant therapy with a bile acid resin, take at least 2 hours later

Monitoring Parameters Serum cholesterol (total and fractionated); reduce dose if indicated

Patient Information Promptly report any unexplained muscle pain, tenderness or weakness, especially if accompanied by malaise or fever; follow prescribed diet; take with meals

Special Geriatric Considerations The definition of and, therefore, when to treat hyperlipidemia in the elderly is a controversial issue. The National Cholesterol Education Program recommends that all adults 20 years of age and older maintain a plasma cholesterol of <200 mg/dL. By this definition, 60% of all elderly would be considered to have a borderline high (200-239 mg/dL) or high blood (≥240 mg/dL) elevated cholesterol. However, plasma cholesterol has been shown to be a less reliable predictor of coronary heart disease in the elderly. Therefore, it is the authors' belief that pharmacologic treatment be reserved for those who are unable to obtain a desirable plasma cholesterol level by diet alone and for whom the benefits of treatment are believed to outweigh the potential adverse effects, drug interactions, and cost of treatment.

Dosage Forms Capsule: 20 mg, 40 mg

References

"Summary of the Second Report of the National Cholesterol Education Program (NCEP) Expert Panel on Detection, Evaluation, and Treatment of High Blood Cholesterol in Adults (Adult Treatment Panel II)," *JAMA*, 1993, 269(23):3015-23.

Fluzone® *see Influenza Virus Vaccine on page 371*

Folacin *see Folic Acid on this page*

Folate *see Folic Acid on this page*

Folex® *see Methotrexate on page 455*

Folex® PFS *see Methotrexate on page 455*

Folic Acid *(foe' lik)*

Brand Names Folvite®

Synonyms Folacin; Folate; Pteroylglutamic Acid

Generic Available Yes

Therapeutic Class Vitamin, Water Soluble

Use Treatment of megaloblastic and macrocytic anemias due to folate deficiency

Contraindications Pernicious, aplastic, or normocytic anemias

Warnings Large doses may mask the hematologic effects of B_{12} deficiency, thus obscuring the diagnosis of pernicious anemia while allowing the neurologic complications due to B_{12} deficiency to progress; injection contains benzyl alcohol (1.5%) as preservative

Precautions Doses above 0.1 mg/day may obscure pernicious anemia; patients with pernicious anemia may show hematologic improvement with doses as low as 0.25

mg/day with continuing irreversible nerve damage progression. Resistance to treatment may occur with depressed hematopoiesis, alcoholism, deficiencies of other vitamins; should rule out pernicious anemia with Schilling Test and serum vitamin concentration

Adverse Reactions
Dermatologic: Pruritus
Miscellaneous: Allergic reaction

Overdosage Not described; see Additional Information

Toxicology Not described; see Additional Information

Drug Interactions In folate-deficient patients, folic acid therapy may increase phenytoin metabolism resulting in decreased phenytoin serum concentrations. Phenytoin, primidone, para-aminosalicylic acid, and sulfasalazine have been reported to decrease serum folate concentrations and may cause deficiency. Concurrent administration of chloramphenicol and folic acid in these patients may result in antagonism of the hematopoietic response to folic acid.

Stability Incompatible with oxidizing and reducing agents and heavy metal ions

Mechanism of Action Folic acid is necessary for formation of a number of coenzymes in many metabolic systems, particularly for purine and pyrimidine synthesis; required for nucleoprotein synthesis and maintenance in erythropoiesis; stimulates WBC and platelet production in folate deficiency anemia

Pharmacodynamics Peak effects: Oral: Within 30-60 minutes

Pharmacokinetics Absorption: In the proximal part of the small intestine

Usual Dosage Geriatrics and Adults: RDA: 0.4 mg
Folic acid deficiency: Oral, I.M., I.V., S.C.: Initial: 1 mg/day; replacement requires only 2-3 weeks; maintenance dose: 0.5 mg/day; 1 mg/day may be needed for patients taking anticonvulsant therapy

Monitoring Parameters Reticulocyte count within 5-10 days of initiation of therapy; hematocrit, hemoglobin, RBC count at monthly intervals; diarrheal episodes should stop in 2-3 days of therapy; monitor seizure activity, serum phenytoin concentration should be monitored more often

Reference Range Therapeutic: 0.005-0.015 μg/mL

Test Interactions Falsely low serum concentrations may occur with the *Lactobacillus casei* assay method in patients on anti-infectives (eg, tetracycline)

Patient Information Take folic acid replacement only under recommendation of physician

Nursing Implications Oral, but may also be administered by deep I.M., S.C., or I.V. injection; a diluted solution for oral or for parenteral administration may be prepared by diluting 1 mL of folic acid injection (5 mg/mL), with 49 mL sterile water for injection; resulting solution is 0.1 mg folic acid per 1 mL; see Monitoring Parameters

Additional Information Water-soluble vitamin with a wide margin of safety

Special Geriatric Considerations Elderly frequently have combined nutritional deficiencies; must rule out vitamin B_{12} deficiency before initiating folate therapy; elderly RDA requirements from 1989 RDA are 200 mcg minimum (0.2 mg). Elderly, due to decreased nutrient intake, may benefit from daily intake of a multiple vitamin with minerals.

Dosage Forms
Injection, as sodium folate: 5 mg/mL (10 mL); 10 mg/mL (10 mL)
Tablet: 0.1 mg, 0.4 mg, 0.8 mg, 1 mg

References
Olszewski AJ, Szostak WB, Bialkowska M, et al, "Reduction of Plasma Lipid and Hymocysteine Levels by Pyridoxine, Folate, Cobalamin, Choline, Riboflavin, and Troxerutin in Atherosclerosis," *Atherosclerosis*, 1989, 75(1):1-6.

Folvite® *see* Folic Acid *on previous page*

Fortaz® *see* Ceftazidime *on page 137*

Foscarnet

Brand Names Foscavir®

Generic Available No

Therapeutic Class Antiviral Agent, Parenteral

Use Alternative to ganciclovir for treatment of CMV retinitis and other CMV infections; alternative to acyclovir for treatment of acyclovir-resistant HSV infections

Contraindications Hypersensitivity to foscarnet; a Cl_{cr} <0.4 mL/minute/kg during therapy

Warnings Impairment of renal function is the major toxicity and is experienced to some extent in most patients, thus renal function should be closely monitored; see Monitoring Parameters. Imbalance of serum electrolytes or minerals occurs in 6% to 18% of patients (hypocalcemia, low ionized calcium, hypo- or hyperphosphatemia, hypomagnesemia or hypokalemia). Patients with a low ionized calcium may experience perioral tingling, numbness, paresthesias, tetany, and seizures. Seizures have been experienced by up to 10% of AIDS patients. Risk factors for seizures include a low baseline absolute neutrophil count (ANC), impaired baseline renal function and low

(Continued)

Foscarnet *(Continued)*

total serum calcium. Some patients who have experienced seizures have died, while others have been able to continue or resume foscarnet treatment after their mineral or electrolyte abnormality has been corrected, their underlying disease state treated or their dose decreased. Foscarnet has been shown to be mutagenic *in vitro* and in mice at very high doses.

Precautions Diagnosis of CMV retinitis should be made by an ophthalmologist familiar with the presentation and differentiation of CMV from other ophthalmic conditions with similar presentations (ie, candidiasis, toxoplasmosis, etc); local irritation at the infusion site and penile and vulvovaginal ulcerations have been reported. The risk of these irritations may be minimized by infusion into a large enough vein for quick dilution and maintaining adequate hydration, respectively.

Adverse Reactions
Central nervous system: Headache, seizures, fever, dizziness, anxiety, hypothermia, confusion, fatigue
Endocrine & metabolic: Electrolyte imbalance
Gastrointestinal: Diarrhea, nausea, vomiting
Neuromuscular & skeletal: Rigors
Renal: Renal impairment

Overdosage Symptoms of overdose include seizures, coma, renal impairment, paresthesias, hypocalcemia and hypo- or hyperphosphatemia

Toxicology No specific antidote is available; in overdose situations, maintain hydration and monitor renal function and electrolytes; hydration and hemodialysis may be useful but have not been well studied.

Drug Interactions
Concurrent treatment with aminoglycosides, amphotericin B, or I.V. pentamidine or other potential nephrotoxic drugs; foscarnet's elimination may be decreased by drugs that block renal tubular secretion (ie, probenecid)
I.V. pentamidine (hypocalcemia); zidovudine (anemia); any drug that may influence serum calcium levels (ie, furosemide) may increase risk for hypocalcemia or lower serum ionized calcium levels

Stability Give in normal saline or 5% dextrose solution; administer no other drug or supplement concurrently via the same catheter. Incompatible with 30% dextrose, amphotericin B, and calcium-containing solutions such as Ringer's lactate and TPN. See package insert for a complete list of incompatibilities.

Mechanism of Action Pyrophosphate analogue which acts as a noncompetitive inhibitor of many viral RNA and DNA polymerases as well as HIV reverse transcriptase. Inhibitory effects occur at concentrations which do not affect host cellular DNA polymerases; however, some human cell growth suppression has been observed with high *in vitro* concentrations. Similar to ganciclovir, foscarnet is a virostatic agent; foscarnet does not require activation by thymidine kinase.

Pharmacokinetics
Absorption: Oral: Poor; I.V. therapy is needed for the treatment of viral infections in AIDS patients
Distribution: Up to 28% of cumulative I.V. dose may be deposited in bone
Metabolism: Biotransformation does not occur
Half-life: ~3 hours
Elimination: Up to 28% excreted unchanged in urine

Usual Dosage I.V.:
Geriatrics: Adjust dose based upon estimated renal function

Adults:
Induction treatment: 60 mg/kg at a constant rate of infusion over at least 1 hour every 8 hours for 2-3 weeks
Maintenance treatment: 90-120 mg/kg/day at a constant rate of infusion over 2 hours
Dosing adjustment in renal impairment: See table.

Administration Do not give by rapid or bolus I.V. injection; an infusion pump must be used to avoid overdose. Administer diluted to 12 mg/mL through a peripheral line; may be administered undiluted through a central line; see Stability and Usual Dosage

Monitoring Parameters Measure serum electrolytes, minerals, creatinine and estimated creatinine clearance at baseline, 2-3 times/week during induction therapy, and at least once every 1-2 weeks during maintenance therapy. More frequent monitoring and dosage adjustments may be necessary in patients with fluctuating renal function. A 24-hour creatinine clearance in selected patients; serum electrolytes and minerals should be monitored at the time (or as close as possible) that a patient experiences symptoms of electrolyte abnormalities

Patient Information Close monitoring is important and any symptom of electrolyte abnormalities should be reported immediately; maintain adequate fluid intake and hydration; regular ophthalmic examinations are necessary. Foscarnet is not a cure for CMV retinitis; progression may occur during or following treatment.

Nursing Implications See Administration, Monitoring Parameters, and Stability

Special Geriatric Considerations Information on the use of foscarnet is lacking in the elderly; dose adjustments and proper monitoring must be performed because of the decreased renal function common in older patients; see Warnings and Usual Dosage

Dosage Forms Injection: 24 mg/mL (250 mL, 500 mL)

Dose Adjustment for Renal Impairment

The induction dose of foscarnet should be adjusted according to creatinine clearance as follows:

Creatinine Clearance (mL/min/kg)	Foscarnet Induction Dose (mg/kg q8h)
1.6	60
1.5	57
1.4	53
1.3	49
1.2	46
1.1	42
1	39
0.9	35
0.8	32
0.7	28
0.6	25
0.5	21
0.4	18

The maintenance dose of foscarnet should be adjusted according to creatinine clearance as follows:

Creatinine Clearance (mL/min/kg)	Foscarnet Maintenance Dose (mg/kg/day)
1.4	90–120
1.2–1.4	78–104
1–1.2	75–100
0.8–1	71–94
0.6–0.8	63–84
0.4–0.6	57–75

Foscavir® *see* Foscarnet *on page 311*

Fosinopril (foe sin' oh pril)
Brand Names Monopril®
Generic Available No
Therapeutic Class Angiotensin-Converting Enzyme (ACE) Inhibitors
Use Treatment of hypertension, either alone or in combination with other antihypertensive agents
Contraindications Renal impairment, collagen vascular disease, hypersensitivity to fosinopril, any component, or other angiotensin-converting enzyme inhibitors
Warnings Use with caution and modify dosage in patients with renal impairment (decrease dosage) (especially renal artery stenosis), severe congestive heart failure or with coadministered diuretic therapy. Severe hypotension may occur in patients who are sodium and/or volume depleted, initiate lower doses and monitor closely when starting therapy in these patients; observe for hyperkalemia (>5.7 mEq/L) first-dose hypotension, proteinuria, neutropenia, agranulocytosis, and angioedema.

Adverse Reactions
Cardiovascular: Hypotension, tachycardia, arrhythmias, orthostatic blood pressure changes, angina, palpitations, chest pain, CVA, myocardial infarction, syncope, flushing, hypertensive crisis, claudication
Central nervous system: Nervousness, depression, confusion, somnolence, fatigue, dizziness, headache, paresthesias, insomnia, vertigo

(Continued)

313

Fosinopril *(Continued)*

Dermatologic: Rash, urticaria, photosensitivity, pruritus, angioedema

Endocrine & metabolic: Hyperkalemia, hypoglycemia

Gastrointestinal: Pancreatitis, constipation, anorexia, nausea, heartburn, flatulence, vomiting, diarrhea, abdominal pain, dry mouth, dysphagia, abdominal distention

Genitourinary: Azotemia, impotence, decreased libido

Hematologic: Anemia, neutropenia, leukopenia, eosinophilia, agranulocytosis

Hepatic: Hepatitis

Neuromuscular & skeletal: Myalgia, arthralgia, muscle cramps

Ocular: Blurred vision

Otic: Tinnitus

Renal: Proteinuria, oliguria, deterioration in renal function, increased BUN and serum creatinine

Respiratory: Cough, dyspnea, asthma, bronchospasm, sinusitis

Miscellaneous: Loss of taste perception, sweating

Overdosage Symptoms of overdose include severe hypotension

Toxicology Following initiation of essential overdose management, toxic symptom treatment and supportive treatment should be initiated. Hypotension usually responds to I.V. fluids or Trendelenburg positioning. If unresponsive to these measures, the use of a parenteral inotrope may be required (eg, norepinephrine 0.1-0.2 mcg/kg/minute titrated to response). Seizures commonly respond to diazepam (I.V. 5-10 mg bolus in adults every 15 minutes if needed up to a total of 30 mg) or to phenytoin or phenobarbital.

Drug Interactions

Fosinopril and potassium-sparing diuretics → additive hyperkalemic effect

Fosinopril and indomethacin or nonsteroidal anti-inflammatory agents → reduced antihypertensive response to fosinopril

Allopurinol and fosinopril → neutropenia

Antacids and ACE inhibitors → ↓ absorption of ACE inhibitors

Phenothiazines and ACE inhibitors → ↑ ACE inhibitor effect

Probenecid and ACE inhibitors (fosinopril) → ↑ ACE inhibitors (fosinopril) levels

Rifampin and ACE inhibitors (enalapril) → ↓ ACE inhibitor effect

Digoxin and ACE inhibitors → ↑ serum digoxin levels

Lithium and ACE inhibitors → ↑ lithium serum levels

Tetracycline and ACE inhibitors (quinapril) → ↓ tetracycline absorption (up to 37%)

Food decreases fosinopril absorption, see Additional Information

Mechanism of Action Competitive inhibitor of angiotensin-converting enzyme (ACE); prevents conversion of angiotensin I to angiotensin II, a potent vasoconstrictor; results in lower levels of angiotensin II which causes an increase in plasma renin activity and a reduction in aldosterone secretion; a CNS mechanism may also be involved in hypotensive effect as angiotensin II increases adrenergic outflow from CNS; vasoactive kallikreins may be decreased in conversion to active hormones by ACE inhibitors, thus reducing blood pressure

Pharmacodynamics Duration of effect: ~12-24 hours

Pharmacokinetics

Absorbed: 36%

Metabolism: Fosinopril is a prodrug and is hydrolyzed to its active metabolite fosinoprilat by intestinal wall and hepatic esterases

Half-life, serum (fosinoprilat): 12 hours

Time to peak serum concentration: ~3 hours

Elimination: In the urine and bile as fosinoprilat and it conjugates in roughly equal proportions (45% to 50%)

Usual Dosage Geriatrics and Adults: Oral: Initial: 10 mg/day and increase to a maximum dose of 40 mg/day; most patients are maintained on 20-40 mg/day; see Additional Information

Moderately dialyzable (20% to 50%)

Monitoring Parameters Serum potassium levels, BUN, serum creatinine, renal function, WBC

Test Interactions Increases BUN, creatinine, potassium, positive Coombs' [direct]; decreases cholesterol (S); may cause false-positive results in urine acetone determinations using sodium nitroprusside reagent

Patient Information Notify physician if vomiting, diarrhea, excessive perspiration, or dehydration should occur; also if swelling of face, lips, tongue, or difficulty in breathing occurs or if persistent cough develops; may be taken with meals; do not stop therapy or add a potassium salt replacement without physician's advice

Nursing Implications May cause depression in some patients; discontinue if angioedema of the face, extremities, lips, tongue, or glottis occurs; watch for hypotensive effects within 1-3 hours of first dose or new higher dose; see Precautions and Special Geriatric Considerations

Additional Information Some patients may have a decreased hypotensive effect between 12-16 hours; consider dividing total daily dose into 2 doses 12 hours apart; if patient is receiving a diuretic, a potential for first-dose hypotension is increased; to decrease this potential, stop diuretic for 2-3 days prior to initiating fosinopril if possible; continue diuretic if needed to control blood pressure

Special Geriatric Considerations Due to frequent decreases in glomerular filtration (also creatinine clearance) with aging, elderly patients may have exaggerated responses to ACE inhibitors; differences in clinical response due to hepatic changes are not observed. ACE inhibitors may be preferred agents in elderly patients with congestive heart failure and diabetes mellitus. Diabetic proteinuria is reduced and insulin sensitivity is enhanced. In general, the side effect profile is favorable in elderly and causes little or no CNS confusion; use lowest dose recommendations initially.

Dosage Forms Tablet: 10 mg, 20 mg

References
McAreavey D and Robertson JIS, "Angiotensin Converting Enzyme Inhibitors and Moderate Hypertension," *Drugs*, 1990, 40(3):326-45.

Frusemide see Furosemide *on this page*

Fulvicin® P/G see Griseofulvin *on page 330*

Fulvicin-U/F® see Griseofulvin *on page 330*

Fungizone® see Amphotericin B *on page 50*

Furadantin® see Nitrofurantoin *on page 504*

Furalan® see Nitrofurantoin *on page 504*

Furan® see Nitrofurantoin *on page 504*

Furanite® see Nitrofurantoin *on page 504*

Furazolidone (fur a zoe' li done)
Brand Names Furoxone®

Therapeutic Class Antibiotic, Miscellaneous; Antidiarrheal; Antiprotozoal

Use Treatment of bacterial or protozoal diarrhea and enteritis caused by susceptible organisms: *Giardia lamblia* and *Vibrio cholerae*

Contraindications Known hypersensitivity to furazolidone; concurrent use of alcohol; MAO inhibitors, tyramine-containing foods

Precautions Use caution in patients with G-6-PD deficiency

Adverse Reactions
Cardiovascular: Orthostatic hypotension
Central nervous system: Dizziness, drowsiness, malaise, fever, headache
Dermatologic: Rash
Endocrine & metabolic: Hypoglycemia, disulfiram-like reaction after alcohol ingestion
Gastrointestinal: Nausea, vomiting
Hematologic: Agranulocytosis, hemolysis in patients with G-6-PD deficiency

Overdosage Hypertensive crisis after doses greater than recommended or if taken for more than 5 days

Drug Interactions Alcohol, MAO inhibitors, indirect-acting sympathomimetic amines, tyramine-containing food, levodopa, guanethidine, tricyclic antidepressant, meperidine, sedatives, antihistamines, narcotics, insulin and sulfonylureas

Mechanism of Action Inhibits several vital enzymatic reactions causing antibacterial and antiprotozoal action

Pharmacokinetics
Absorption: Oral: Poor
Elimination: 33% of oral dose excreted in urine as active drug and metabolites

Usual Dosage Geriatrics and Adults: Oral: 100 mg 4 times/day; not more than 8.8 mg/kg/day; treatment duration: 7 days

Test Interactions False-positive results for urine glucose with Clinitest®

Patient Information May discolor urine to a brown tint; avoid drinking alcohol or eating tyramine-containing foods; if result not achieved at the end of treatment contact physician

Special Geriatric Considerations See Adverse Reactions and Usual Dosage

Dosage Forms
Liquid: 50 mg/15 mL (60 mL, 473 mL)
Tablet: 100 mg

Furazosin see Prazosin Hydrochloride *on page 582*

Furomide® see Furosemide *on this page*

Furosemide (fur oh' se mide)
Brand Names Furomide®; Lasix®; Lo-Aqua®

Synonyms Frusemide

Generic Available Yes

Therapeutic Class Diuretic, Loop

Use Management of edema associated with congestive heart failure and hepatic or renal disease; used alone or in combination with antihypertensives in treatment of hypertension

(Continued)

Furosemide (Continued)

Contraindications Hypersensitivity to furosemide or any component; allergy to sulfonamides may result in cross-sensitivity to furosemide

Warnings Loop diuretics are potent diuretics; excess amounts can lead to profound diuresis with fluid and electrolyte loss; close medical supervision and dose evaluation is required, particularly in the elderly

Adverse Reactions
Cardiovascular: Hypotension
Central nervous system: Dizziness
Dermatologic: Urticaria, rash, photosensitivity
Endocrine & metabolic: Hypokalemia, hyponatremia, hypochloremia, alkalosis, dehydration, hypercalciuria, hyperuricemia
Gastrointestinal: Pancreatitis, nausea, diarrhea
Genitourinary: Prerenal azotemia
Hematologic: Agranulocytosis, anemia, thrombocytopenia
Otic: Potential ototoxicity
Renal: Nephrocalcinosis, interstitial nephritis

Overdosage Symptoms of overdose include electrolyte depletion, volume depletion, hypotension, dehydration, circulatory collapse

Toxicology Following GI decontamination, treatment is supportive; hypotension responds to fluids and Trendelenburg position; replace electrolytes as necessary

Drug Interactions
Decreased effect: Indomethacin, other NSAIDs
Increased hypotensive effect: Other antihypertensives
Increased level of lithium
Increased risk of ototoxicity: Aminoglycosides, other loop diuretics, vancomycin
When given with digoxin, diuretic-induced hypokalemia increases the risk of digoxin toxicity

Stability Protect from light; do not dispense discolored tablets or injection; I.V. infusion solution mixed in NS or D_5W solution is stable for 24 hours at room temperature

Mechanism of Action Inhibits reabsorption of sodium and chloride in the ascending loop of Henle and distal renal tubule, interfering with the chloride-binding cotransport system, thus causing increased excretion of water, sodium, chloride, magnesium, and calcium

Pharmacodynamics
Oral:
Onset of action: Diuresis begins within 30-60 minutes
Peak effect: Within 1-2 hours
Duration: 6-8 hours
I.V.:
Onset of action: Diuresis starts in 5 minutes
Peak effect: Reduced and delayed in the elderly as compared to younger adults
Duration: 2 hours

Pharmacokinetics
Absorption: Oral: 60% to 67%
Protein binding: >90%
Elimination: In the elderly, total clearance is decreased and dependent on renal function

Usual Dosage Oral, I.M., I.V.:
Geriatrics: Initial: 20 mg/day, increase slowly to desired response
Adults: 20-80 mg/day in divided doses every 6-12 hours up to 600 mg/day

Acute renal failure: Up to 100 mg/day may be necessary to initiate desired response

Dosing adjustment/comments in hepatic disease: Diminished natriuretic effect with increased sensitivity to hypokalemia and volume depletion in cirrhosis; monitor effects, particularly with high doses

Administration Maximum rate of administration is 4 mg/minute

Monitoring Parameters Blood pressure both standing and sitting/supine, serum electrolytes, renal function, I & O, weight; in high doses monitor auditory function

Reference Range Therapeutic: 1-2 µg/mL (SI: 3-6 µmol/L)

Test Interactions Increased ammonia (B), increased amylase (S), increased glucose, increased uric acid (S); decreased calcium (S), decreased chloride (S), decreased magnesium, decreased sodium (S)

Patient Information May be taken with food or milk; get up slowly from a lying or sitting position to minimize dizziness, lightheadedness or fainting; also use extra care when exercising, standing for long periods of time and during hot weather; take in the morning; may cause increased sensitivity to sunlight

Nursing Implications I.V. injections should be given slowly over 1-2 minutes; replace parenteral therapy with oral therapy as soon as possible; for continuous infusion furosemide in patients with severely impaired renal function, do not exceed 4 mg/minute; be alert to complaints about hearing difficulty; check the patient for orthostasis; see Monitoring Parameters

Additional Information Injection contains 0.162 mEq of sodium per mL; do not use solutions that are yellow in color

Standard diluent: Dose/50 mL D$_5$W
Minimum volume: 50 mL D$_5$W

Special Geriatric Considerations Severe loss of sodium and/or increases in BUN can cause confusion. For any change in mental status in patients on furosemide, monitor electrolytes and renal function; see Pharmacodynamics and Pharmacokinetics.

Dosage Forms
Injection: 10 mg/mL (2 mL, 4 mL, 5 mL, 6 mL, 8 mL, 10 mL, 12 mL)
Solution, oral: 10 mg/mL (60 mL, 120 mL); 40 mg/5 mL (5 mL, 10 mL, 500 mL)
Tablet: 20 mg, 40 mg, 80 mg

References
Chaudhry AY, Bing RF, Castleden CM, et al, "The Effect of Aging on the Response to Frusemide in Normal Subjects," *Eur J Clin Pharmacol*, 1984, 27(3):303-6.
Mühlberg W, "Pharmacokinetics of Diuretics in Geriatric Patients," *Arch Gerontol Geriatr*, 1989, 9(3):283-90.

Furoxone® *see* Furazolidone *on page 315*

Gabapentin

Brand Names Neurontin®
Generic Available No
Therapeutic Class Anticonvulsant, Miscellaneous
Use Adjunct for treatment of drug-refractory partial and secondarily generalized seizures
Contraindications Hypersensitivity to the drug or any component or preparation
Warnings Gabapentin may be associated with a slight incidence (0.6%) of status epilepticus and sudden deaths (0.0038 deaths/patient year); rat studies demonstrated an association with pancreatic adenocarcinoma in male rats; clinical implication unknown
Precautions See Reference Range; routine monitoring not needed
Adverse Reactions
Cardiovascular: Syncope
Central nervous system: Somnolence, dizziness, ataxia, fatigue, nervousness, dysarthria, amnesia, depression, anxiety, hallucinations, psychosis, paranoia, paresthesias, hyperkinesia
Dermatologic: Pruritus
Gastrointestinal: Dyspepsia, dryness of mouth/throat, constipation
Genitourinary: Impotence
Hematologic: Leukopenia
Neuromuscular & skeletal: Back pain, myalgia
Ocular: Diplopia, amblyopia, nystagmus
Respiratory: Rhinitis, bronchospasm
Miscellaneous: Hiccups, peripheral edema
Overdosage Symptoms of overdose include ataxia, ptosis, sedation, excitation, dyspnea, diplopia, lethargy, diarrhea, slurred speech
Toxicology Treatment: Hemodialysis can be performed since it is dialyzable; give general supportive care
Drug Interactions
Antacids reduce the bioavailability of gabapentin by 20%
Cimetidine may decrease clearance of gabapentin
Mechanism of Action Exact mechanism of action is not known, but does have properties in common with other anticonvulsants; although structurally related to GABA, it does not interact with GABA receptors
Pharmacokinetics
Absorption: ~60%
Half-life: 5-7 hours in normal renal function; increases with decreasing creatinine clearance; must have dose adjusted (see Usual Dosage)
Usual Dosage Geriatric and Adults: Oral: 900-1800 mg/day administered in 3 divided doses; therapy is initiated with a rapid titration, beginning with 300 mg on day 1, 300 mg twice daily on day 2, and 300 mg 3 times/day on day 3; dose is then titrated as needed up to 1800 mg/day; doses up to 2400-3600 mg/day have been used safely

Dosing adjustment in renal impairment:
Cl$_{cr}$ >60 mL/minute: Administer 1200 mg/day
Cl$_{cr}$ 30-60 mL/minute: Administer 600 mg/day
Cl$_{cr}$ 15-30 mL/minute: Administer 300 mg/day
Cl$_{cr}$ <15 mL/minute: Administer 150 mg/day
Hemodialysis: 200-300 mg after each 4-hour dialysis following a loading dose of 300-400 mg
Reference Range Minimum effective serum concentration may be 2 µg/mL; **routine monitoring of drug levels is not required even with concomitant drug therapy**
Patient Information Take only as prescribed; may cause dizziness, somnolence, and other symptoms and signs of CNS depression; do not operate machinery or drive a car until you have experience with the drug; may be administered without regard to meals
(Continued)

Gabapentin *(Continued)*

Nursing Implications See Adverse Reactions and Overdosage; note dosage must be adjusted for renal function and elderly often have reduced renal function

Special Geriatric Considerations No clinical studies to specifically evaluate this drug in elderly have been performed; however, in premarketing studies, patients >65 years of age did not demonstrate any difference in side effect profiles from younger adults; since gabapentin is eliminated renally, dose **must** be adjusted for creatinine clearance in the elderly patient

Dosage Forms Capsule: 100 mg, 300 mg, 400 mg

Gamastan® *see* Immune Globulin *on page 366*

Gamimune® N *see* Immune Globulin *on page 366*

Gamma Benzene Hexachloride *see* Lindane *on page 407*

Gammagard® *see* Immune Globulin *on page 366*

Gamma Globulin *see* Immune Globulin *on page 366*

Gammar® *see* Immune Globulin *on page 366*

Gammar®-IV *see* Immune Globulin *on page 366*

Ganciclovir *(gan sye' kloe vir)*

Brand Names Cytovene®

Synonyms DHPG Sodium; GCV Sodium; Nordeoxyguanosine

Generic Available No

Therapeutic Class Antiviral Agent, Parenteral

Use CMV retinitis treatment of immunocompromised individuals, including patients with acquired immunodeficiency syndrome; treatment of CMV pneumonia in marrow transplant recipients, promising results have been achieved in AIDS patients and organ transplant recipients with CMV colitis, pneumonitis, and multiorgan involvement; attenuation of CMV infection in transplant patients

Contraindications Absolute neutrophil count <500/mm^3; platelet count <25,000/mm^3; known hypersensitivity to ganciclovir or acyclovir

Warnings Dosage adjustment or interruption of ganciclovir therapy may be necessary in patients with neutropenia and/or thrombocytopenia and patients with impaired renal function. Ganciclovir may adversely affect spermatogenesis and fertility; due to its mutagenic potential, contraceptive precautions for female and male patients need to be followed during and for at least 90 days after therapy with the drug; take care to administer only into veins with good blood flow.

Adverse Reactions

Cardiovascular: Edema, arrhythmias, hypertension

Central nervous system: Headache, seizure, confusion, nervousness, dizziness, hallucinations, coma, fever, encephalopathy, malaise

Dermatologic: Rash, urticaria

Gastrointestinal: Nausea, vomiting, diarrhea

Hematologic: Neutropenia, thrombocytopenia, leukopenia, anemia, eosinophilia

Hepatic: Elevation in liver function tests

Local: Phlebitis

Ocular: Retinal detachment

Renal: Hematuria, increased BUN and serum creatinine

Respiratory: Dyspnea

Overdosage Symptoms of overdose include neutropenia, vomiting, hypersalivation, bloody diarrhea, cytopenia, testicular atrophy

Toxicology Hemodialysis removes 50% of drug; hydration may be of some benefit

Drug Interactions

Increased effect/toxicity with probenecid, imipenem/cilastatin

Increased toxicity in rapidly dividing cells with cytotoxic drugs; increased hematologic toxicity with zidovudine

Stability Reconstituted solution is stable for 12 hours at room temperature; **do not refrigerate**; reconstitute with sterile water **not** bacteriostatic water because parabens may cause precipitation

Mechanism of Action Ganciclovir is phosphorylated to a substrate which competitively inhibits the binding of deoxyguanosine triphosphate to DNA polymerase resulting in inhibition of viral DNA synthesis

Pharmacokinetics

Protein binding: 1% to 2%

Half-life: 1.7-5.8 hours; increases with impaired renal function

Elimination: Majority (94% to 99%) is excreted as unchanged drug in urine

Usual Dosage Slow I.V. infusion (dosing is based on total body weight):

Geriatrics and Adults:

Induction therapy: 5 mg/kg/dose every 12 hours for 14-21 days followed by maintenance therapy

Maintenance therapy: 5 mg/kg/day as a single daily dose for 7 days/week or 6 mg/kg/day for 5 days/week

Dosing interval in renal impairment:
Cl_{cr} 50-79 mL/minute per 1.73 m^2: Administer 2.5 mg/kg/dose every 12 hours
Cl_{cr} 25-49 mL/minute per 1.73 m^2: Administer 2.5 mg/kg/dose every 24 hours
Cl_{cr} <25 mL/minute per 1.73 m^2: Administer 1.25 mg/kg/dose every 24 hours
40% to 50% removed by a 4-hour hemodialysis

Monitoring Parameters CBC with differential and platelet count, serum creatinine, ophthalmologic exams

Patient Information Ganciclovir is not a cure for CMV retinitis; regular ophthalmologic examinations should be done; close monitoring of blood counts should be done while on therapy and dosage adjustments may need to be made

Nursing Implications Must be prepared in vertical flow hood; use chemotherapy precautions during administration; discard appropriately

Additional Information Sodium content of 500 mg vial: 46 mg

Special Geriatric Considerations Adjust dose based upon renal function; see Usual Dosage

Dosage Forms Powder for injection, lyophilized: 500 mg (10 mL)

Gantanol® *see Sulfamethoxazole on page 660*

Gantrisin® *see Sulfisoxazole on page 662*

Garamycin® *see Gentamicin Sulfate on next page*

Gastrocrom® *see Cromolyn Sodium on page 190*

Gastrosed™ *see Hyoscyamine Sulfate on page 359*

Gas-X® [OTC] *see Simethicone on page 645*

Gaviscon-2® [OTC] *see Aluminum Hydroxide, Magnesium Trisilicate, Sodium Bicarbonate and Alginic Acid on page 32*

Gaviscon® [OTC] *see Aluminum Hydroxide, Magnesium Trisilicate, Sodium Bicarbonate and Alginic Acid on page 32*

Gaviscon® Extra Strength Relief Formula [OTC] *see Aluminum Hydroxide, Magnesium Trisilicate, Sodium Bicarbonate and Alginic Acid on page 32*

G-CSF *see Filgrastim on page 290*

GCV Sodium *see Ganciclovir on previous page*

Gel-Kam® *see Fluoride on page 299*

Gel-Tin® *see Fluoride on page 299*

Gelusil® [OTC] *see Aluminum Hydroxide, Magnesium Hydroxide and Simethicone on page 31*

Gemfibrozil (jem fi' broe zil)

Brand Names Lopid®

Synonyms CI-719

Generic Available No

Therapeutic Class Antilipemic Agent

Use Hypertriglyceridemia in types IV and V hyperlipidemia for patients who are at greater risk for pancreatitis and who have not responded to dietary intervention; reduction of coronary heart disease in type IIb patients who have low HDL cholesterol, increased LDL cholesterol, and decreased triglycerides

Contraindications Renal or hepatic dysfunction, primary biliary cirrhosis, gallbladder disease, hypersensitivity to gemfibrozil or any component

Precautions Estrogen therapy may increase triglycerides, consider this if appropriate before prescribing

Adverse Reactions
Central nervous system: Headache, dizziness, drowsiness, somnolence, paresthesia, fatigue, mental depression
Dermatologic: Eczema and rash, alopecia, angioedema
Gastrointestinal: Abdominal pain, weight loss, cholelithiasis have been reported, nausea, vomiting, diarrhea, constipation, dyspepsia, alteration in taste, and flatulence occur less frequently
Genitourinary: Impotence and decreased male fertility
Hematologic: Anemia, leukopenia, thrombocytopenia
Ocular: Blurred vision
Miscellaneous: Lupus-like syndrome

Drug Interactions May potentiate the effects of warfarin; concomitant use with lovastatin or other HMG-CoA reductase inhibitors may lead to rhabdomyolysis

Mechanism of Action The exact mechanism of action of gemfibrozil is unknown, however, several theories exist regarding the VLDL effect; it can inhibit lipolysis and decrease subsequent hepatic fatty acid uptake as well as inhibit hepatic secretion of VLDL; together these actions decrease serum VLDL levels; increases HDL cholesterol; the mechanism behind HDL elevation is currently unknown

(Continued)

319

Gemfibrozil *(Continued)*

Pharmacokinetics

Absorption: Oral: Well absorbed

Protein binding: 99%; a portion of the drug undergoes enterohepatic recycling

Metabolism: In the liver by oxidation to 2 inactive metabolites

Half-life: 1.4 hours

Time to peak: Peak serum levels occur within 1-2 hours

Elimination: In urine (70%) primarily as glucuronide conjugate; some enterohepatic recycling

Usual Dosage Geriatrics and Adults: Oral: 1200 mg/day in 2 divided doses, 30 minutes before breakfast and supper

Monitoring Parameters Fractionated cholesterol and triglycerides; CBC; liver function tests; blood glucose, especially in diabetics

Test Interactions Decreased glucose, increased LFTs, decreased hemoglobin or hematocrit, WBC, platelets; positive ANA

Patient Information May cause dizziness or blurred vision, medication may cause abdominal or epigastric pain, diarrhea, nausea, or vomiting; notify physician if these become pronounced; take before meals

Nursing Implications See Monitoring Parameters

Additional Information If no appreciable triglyceride or cholesterol lowering effect occurs after 3 months, the drug should be discontinued

Special Geriatric Considerations Gemfibrozil is the drug of choice for the treatment of hypertriglyceridemia and hypoalphaproteinemia in the elderly; it is usually well tolerated; myositis may be more common in patients with poor renal function

Dosage Forms Capsule: 300 mg, 600 mg

Genabid® *see* Papaverine Hydrochloride *on page 533*

Genac® [OTC] *see* Triprolidine and Pseudoephedrine *on page 723*

Genagesic® *see* Propoxyphene and Acetaminophen *on page 604*

Genahist® *see* Diphenhydramine Hydrochloride *on page 228*

Genapap® [OTC] *see* Acetaminophen *on page 13*

Genasal® Nasal Solution [OTC] *see* Oxymetazoline Hydrochloride *on page 530*

Genaspor® [OTC] *see* Tolnaftate *on page 705*

Genatuss® [OTC] *see* Guaifenesin *on page 331*

Gencalc® 600 [OTC] *see* Calcium Salts (Oral) *on page 111*

Generlac® *see* Lactulose *on page 397*

Gen-K® *see* Potassium Chloride *on page 576*

Genoptic® *see* Gentamicin Sulfate *on this page*

Genpril® [OTC] *see* Ibuprofen *on page 360*

Gentacidin® *see* Gentamicin Sulfate *on this page*

Gentafair® *see* Gentamicin Sulfate *on this page*

Gentak® *see* Gentamicin Sulfate *on this page*

Gentamicin and Prednisolone *see* Prednisolone and Gentamicin *on page 585*

Gentamicin Sulfate *(jen ta mye' sin)*

Related Information

Aminoglycoside Dosing Guidelines *on page 753*

Drug Levels Commonly Monitored Guidelines *on page 771-772*

Prednisolone *on page 584*

Brand Names Garamycin®; Genoptic®; Gentacidin®; Gentafair®; Gentak®; Gentrasul®; I-Gent®; Jenamicin®; Ocumycin®

Therapeutic Class Antibiotic, Aminoglycoside; Antibiotic, Ophthalmic; Antibiotic, Topical

Use Treatment of susceptible bacterial infections, normally gram-negative organisms including *Pseudomonas, Proteus, Serratia*, treatment of bone infections, CNS infections, respiratory tract infections, skin and soft tissue infections, as well as abdominal and urinary tract infections, endocarditis, and septicemia

Contraindications Hypersensitivity to gentamicin or other aminoglycosides

Warnings

Not intended for long-term therapy due to toxic hazards associated with extended administration; pre-existing renal insufficiency, vestibular or cochlear impairment, myasthenia gravis, hypocalcemia, conditions which depress neuromuscular transmission

Parenteral aminoglycosides are associated with significant nephrotoxicity or ototoxicity; the ototoxicity is directly proportional to the amount of drug given and the duration of treatment; tinnitus or vertigo are indications of vestibular injury and impending irreversible bilateral deafness; nephrotoxicity is associated with trough concentrations >2 µg/mL and is usually reversible

Precautions Use with caution in patients with renal impairment; pre-existing auditory or vestibular impairment; and in patients with neuromuscular disorders; dosage modification required in patients with impaired renal function

Adverse Reactions
Dermatologic: Rash, skin itching, photosensitivity
Gastrointestinal: Diarrhea, pseudomembranous colitis
Neuromuscular & skeletal: Neuromuscular blockade
Ocular: Lacrimation, itching, edema of the eyelids, keratitis
Otic: Ototoxicity
Renal: Nephrotoxicity (high trough levels)

Overdosage Symptoms of overdose include ototoxicity, nephrotoxicity, and neuromuscular toxicity

Toxicology The treatment of choice following a single acute overdose appears to be the maintenance of good urine output of at least 3 mL/kg/hour. Dialysis is of questionable value in the enhancement of aminoglycoside elimination. If required, hemodialysis is preferred over peritoneal dialysis in patients with normal renal function. Careful hydration may be all that is required to promote diuresis and therefore the enhancement of the drug's elimination. Chelation with penicillins is experimental.

Drug Interactions Penicillins, cephalosporins, amphotericin B, loop diuretics → ↑ nephrotoxic potential; neuromuscular blocking agents → ↑ neuromuscular blockade

Stability I.V. infusion solutions mixed in NS or D$_5$W solution are stable for 24 hours at room temperature; incompatible with penicillins

Mechanism of Action Interferes with bacterial protein synthesis by binding to 30S and 50S ribosomal subunits resulting in a defective bacterial cell membrane

Pharmacokinetics
Distribution: V$_d$: Increased by edema, ascites, fluid overload; decreased in patients with dehydration
Adults: 0.2-0.3 L/kg
Protein binding: <30%
Half-life: Adults: 1.5-3 hours; with anuria: 36-70 hours
Time to peak serum concentration:
I.M.: Within 30-90 minutes
I.V.: 30 minutes after a 30-minute I.V. infusion
Elimination: Clearance is directly related to renal function, eliminated almost completely by glomerular filtration of unchanged drug with excretion into the urine
The pharmacokinetics of the aminoglycosides are heterogeneous in the elderly; it is best to assume that clearance is reduced and half-life prolonged in the elderly, while volume of distribution is usually unchanged. The establishment of each patient's pharmacokinetic parameters is important for proper dosing in order to achieve optimal therapeutic benefit and minimize the risk of toxicity.

Usual Dosage
Individualization is critical because of the low therapeutic index. Use of ideal body weight (IBW) for determining the mg/kg/dose appears to be more accurate than dosing on the basis of total body weight (TBW). In morbid obesity, dosage requirement may best be estimated using a dosing weight of IBW + 0.4 (TBW - IBW). Initial and periodic peak and trough plasma drug levels should be determined, particularly in critically ill patients with serious infections or in disease states known to significantly alter aminoglycoside pharmacokinetics (eg, cystic fibrosis, burns, or major surgery).

Dosage should be based on an estimate of ideal body weight. All patients receiving I.M. or I.V. dosing should receive 1.5-2 mg/kg based on ideal body weight as a loading dose regardless of renal function, then give 3-5 mg/kg in 3 divided doses or as indicated by adjustment for renal function
Geriatrics and Adults:
Intrathecal: 4-8 mg/day
I.M., I.V.: 1-5 mg/kg/day in 1-2 divided doses

Dosing adjustment in renal impairment: 2 mg/kg (2-3 serum level measurements should be obtained after the initial dose to measure the half-life in order to determine the frequency of subsequent doses)
Dialyzable (50% to 100%)
   * Some patients may require larger or more frequent doses (eg, every 6 hours) if serum levels document the need (ie, cystic fibrosis or febrile granulocytopenic patients)
   ** 2-3 serum level measurements should be obtained after the initial dose to measure the half-life in order to determine the frequency of subsequent doses

Topical: Apply 1-4 times/day to affected area
Ophthalmic:
Solution: Instill 1-2 drops every 2-4 hours
Ointment: Instill ½" (1.25 cm) 2-3 times/day to every 3-4 hours

(Continued)

Gentamicin Sulfate *(Continued)*

Dosing adjustment/comments in hepatic disease: Monitor plasma concentrations

Monitoring Parameters Urinalysis, urine output, BUN, serum creatinine; hearing should be tested before, during, and after treatment; particularly in those at risk for ototoxicity or who will be receiving prolonged therapy (>2 weeks). Obtain peak levels 30 minutes after the end of a 30-minute infusion; trough levels are drawn within 30 minutes before the next dose.

Reference Range

Therapeutic:
Peak: 4-8 μg/mL (SI: 8-17 μmol/L)
Trough: <2 μg/mL (SI: 4 μmol/L) (peak depends in part on the minimal inhibitory concentration of drug against organism being treated)

Toxic:
Peak: >12 μg/mL (SI: >21 μmol/L)
Trough: >2 μg/mL (SI: >8.4 μmol/L)

Test Interactions Increased protein; decreased magnesium; increased BUN, AST, GPT, alk phos, serum creatinine; decreased potassium, sodium, calcium

Patient Information Report any dizziness or sensations of ringing or fullness in ears; do not touch ophthalmics to eye; use no other eye drops within 5-10 minutes of instilling ophthalmic

Nursing Implications When injected into the muscles of paralyzed patients the results are different than in normal patients, slower absorption and lower peak concentrations probably due to poor circulation in the atrophic muscles, suggest I.V. route; aminoglycoside levels measured in blood taken from Silastic® central catheters can sometime give falsely high readings. Give other antibiotic drugs at least 1 hour before or after gentamicin. Hearing should be tested before, during, and after treatment.

Special Geriatric Considerations The aminoglycosides are important therapeutic interventions for infections due to susceptible organisms and as empiric therapy in seriously ill patients. Their use is not without risk of toxicity, however, these risks can be minimized if initial dosing is adjusted for estimated renal function and appropriate monitoring performed.

Dosage Forms

Cream, topical: 0.1% (15 g)
Injection: 40 mg/mL (1 mL, 2 mL, 10 mL, 20 mL)
Intrathecal: 2 mg/mL (2 mL)
Ointment:
Ophthalmic: 0.3% (3.5 g)
Topical: 0.1% (15 g)
Solution, ophthalmic: 0.3% (1 mL, 5 mL, 15 mL)

References

Matzke GR, Jameson JJ, and Halstenson CE, "Gentamicin Disposition in Young and Elderly Patients With Various Degrees of Renal Function," *J Clin Pharmacol*, 1987, 27(3):216-20.
Zaske DE, Irvine P, Strand LM, et al, "Wide Interpatient Variations in Gentamicin Dose Requirements for Geriatric Patients," *JAMA*, 1982, 248(23):3122-6.

Gentlax® [OTC] *see* Senna *on page 641*

Gentle Nature® [OTC] *see* Senna *on page 641*

Gentrasul® *see* Gentamicin Sulfate *on page 320*

Gen-XENE® *see* Clorazepate Dipotassium *on page 178*

Geocillin® *see* Carbenicillin *on page 120*

Geopen® *see* Carbenicillin *on page 120*

Geridium® *see* Phenazopyridine Hydrochloride *on page 552*

German Measles Vaccine *see* Rubella Virus Vaccine, Live *on page 632*

Gesterol® *see* Progesterone *on page 596*

GG *see* Guaifenesin *on page 331*

GG-Cen® [OTC] *see* Guaifenesin *on page 331*

Glaucoma Drug Therapy Comparison *see page 810*

Glaucon® Eppy/N® *see* Epinephrine *on page 256*

Glibenclamide *see* Glyburide *on page 324*

Glipizide *(glip' i zide)*

Brand Names Glucotrol®
Synonyms Glydiazinamide
Generic Available No
Therapeutic Class Antidiabetic Agent; Hypoglycemic Agent, Oral; Sulfonylurea Agent
Use Management of noninsulin-dependent diabetes mellitus (type II)
Contraindications Hypersensitivity to glipizide or any component, other sulfonamides, type I diabetes mellitus

Warnings Use with caution in patients with severe hepatic disease

Precautions Avoid alcohol and alcohol-containing products

Adverse Reactions
Cardiovascular: Edema
Central nervous system: Headache, dizziness
Dermatologic: Rash, hives, photosensitivity
Endocrine & metabolic: Hypoglycemia, hyponatremia
Gastrointestinal: Anorexia, nausea, vomiting, diarrhea, heartburn
Hematologic: Blood dyscrasias
Hepatic: Jaundice
Renal: Diuretic effect

Overdosage Symptoms of overdose include low blood sugar, tingling of lips and tongue, nausea, yawning, confusion, agitation, tachycardia, sweating, convulsions, stupor, and coma

Toxicology Intoxications with sulfonylureas can cause hypoglycemia and are best managed with glucose administration (oral for milder hypoglycemia or by injection in more severe forms)

Drug Interactions
Increased effect: H_2 antagonists, anticoagulants, androgens, fluconazole, salicylates, gemfibrozil, sulfonamides, tricyclic antidepressants, probenecid, MAO inhibitors, methyldopa, digitalis glycosides, urinary acidifiers
Decreased effect: Beta-blockers, cholestyramines, hydantoins, rifampin, thiazide diuretics, urinary alkalines, charcoal

Mechanism of Action Stimulates insulin release from the pancreatic beta cells; reduces glucose output from the liver; insulin sensitivity is increased at peripheral target sites

Pharmacodynamics
Onset of action: Oral: Maximal blood glucose reductions occur within 1.5-2 hours
Duration of action: 12-24 hours

Pharmacokinetics
Protein binding: 92% to 99% nonionic; has been reported to be as low as 64% in elderly diabetics
Metabolism: In the liver with metabolites (91% to 97%)
Half-life: 2-4 hours
Elimination: In urine (60% to 80%) and feces (11%)

Usual Dosage Oral:
Geriatrics: Initial: 2.5-5 mg/day; increase by 2.5-5 mg/day every 1-2 weeks

Adults: 2.5-40 mg/day; doses > 15-20 mg/day should be divided and given twice daily

Monitoring Parameters Fasting blood glucose, hemoglobin A_{1c}, fructosamine

Reference Range Glucose: Geriatrics: 100-150 mg/dL; Adults: 80-140 mg/dL

Test Interactions Decreased prothrombin time (S), decreased sodium (S)

Patient Information Patients must be counseled by someone experienced in diabetes education, signs and symptoms of hyper- and hypoglycemia, exercise and diet, blood glucose monitoring, and other related topics; eat regularly, do not skip meals; carry quick source of sugar; medical alert bracelet

Nursing Implications Monitor for signs and symptoms of hypoglycemia; give 30 minutes before meals to avoid erratic absorption

Special Geriatric Considerations A useful agent since few drug to drug interactions and not dependent upon renal elimination of active drug. How "tightly" a geriatric patient's blood glucose should be controlled is controversial; however, a fasting blood sugar of <150 mg/dL is now an acceptable end point. Such a decision should be based on the patient's functional and cognitive status, how well they recognize hypoglycemic or hyperglycemic symptoms, and how to respond to them and their other disease states.

Dosage Forms Tablet: 5 mg, 10 mg

References
Brodows RG, "Benefits and Risks With Glyburide and Glipizide in Elderly NIDDM Patients," *Diabetes Care*, 1992, 15(1):75-80.
Kradjan WA, Kobayashi KA, Bauer LA, et al, "Glipizide Pharmacokinetics: Effects of Age, Diabetes, and Multiple Dosing," *J Clin Pharmacol*, 1989, 29(12):1121-7.
Rosenstock J, Corrao PJ, Goldberg RB, et al, "Diabetes Control in the Elderly: A Randomized, Comparative Study of Glyburide Versus Glipizide in Noninsulin Dependent Diabetes Mellitus," *Clin Ther*, 1993, 15(6):1031-40.

Glucagon (gloo' ka gon)

Generic Available No

Therapeutic Class Antihypoglycemic Agent

Use Hypoglycemia; diagnostic aid in the radiologic examination of GI tract when a hypotonic state is needed; used with some success as a cardiac stimulant in management of severe cases of beta-adrenergic blocking agent overdosage

Contraindications Hypersensitivity to glucagon or any component

Warnings Use with caution in patients with a history of insulinoma and/or pheochromocytoma

(Continued)

ALPHABETICAL LISTING OF DRUGS

Glucagon *(Continued)*

Adverse Reactions
Gastrointestinal: Nausea, vomiting
Miscellaneous: Hypersensitivity reactions

Overdosage Symptoms of overdose include hypokalemia, nausea, vomiting

Drug Interactions Increased toxicity: Oral anticoagulant – hypoprothrombinemic effects may be increased possibly with bleeding

Stability After reconstitution, use immediately; may be kept at 5°C for up to 48 hours if necessary

Mechanism of Action Stimulates adenylate cyclase to produce increased cyclic AMP, which promotes hepatic glycogenolysis and gluconeogenesis, causing a raise in blood glucose levels

Pharmacokinetics
Peak effect on blood glucose levels: Parenteral: Within 5-20 minutes
Duration of action: 1-1.5 hours
Metabolism: In the liver with some inactivation occurring in the kidneys and plasma
Half-life, plasma: 3-10 minutes

Usual Dosage Geriatrics and Adults:
Hypoglycemia or insulin shock therapy: I.M., I.V., S.C.: 0.5-1 mg, may repeat in 20 minutes as needed

Diagnostic aid: I.M., I.V.: 0.25-2 mg 10 minutes prior to procedure

Administration Reconstitute powder for injection by adding 1 or 10 mL of sterile diluent to a vial containing 1 or 10 units of the drug, respectively, to provide solutions containing 1 mg of glucagon/mL; if dose to be administered is <2 mg of the drug → use only the diluent provided by the manufacturer; if >2 mg → use sterile water for injection; use immediately after reconstitution

Monitoring Parameters Blood pressure, blood glucose

Patient Information Instruct a close associate on how to prepare and administer as a treatment for insulin shock

Additional Information 1 unit = 1 mg

Special Geriatric Considerations No specific recommendations needed; use as indicated in Usual Dosage

Dosage Forms Powder for injection, lyophilized: 1 mg [1 unit]; 10 mg [10 units]

Glucotrol® *see* Glipizide *on page 322*

Glu-K® *see* Potassium Gluconate *on page 578*

Glyate® [OTC] *see* Guaifenesin *on page 331*

Glyburide *(glye' byoor ide)*
Brand Names Diaβeta®; Micronase®
Synonyms Glibenclamide
Generic Available No
Therapeutic Class Antidiabetic Agent; Hypoglycemic Agent, Oral; Sulfonylurea Agent
Use Management of noninsulin-dependent diabetes mellitus (type II)
Contraindications Hypersensitivity to glyburide or any component, or other sulfonamides; type I diabetes mellitus
Precautions Use with caution in patients with renal and hepatic impairment
Adverse Reactions
Central nervous system: Paresthesia
Dermatologic: Pruritus, rash, photosensitivity
Endocrine & metabolic: Hypoglycemia
Gastrointestinal: Nausea, epigastric fullness, heartburn, constipation, diarrhea, anorexia
Genitourinary: Nocturia
Hematologic: Leukopenia, thrombocytopenia, hemolytic anemia
Hepatic: Cholestatic jaundice
Neuromuscular & skeletal: Joint pain
Renal: Diuretic effect

Overdosage Symptoms of overdose include low blood sugar, tingling of lips and tongue, nausea, yawning, confusion, agitation, tachycardia, sweating, convulsions, stupor, and coma

Toxicology Intoxications with sulfonylureas can cause hypoglycemia and are best managed with glucose administration (oral for milder hypoglycemia or by injection in more severe forms)

Drug Interactions
Decreased effect: Thiazides and beta-blockers → ↓ effectiveness of glyburide
Increased effect: Increased hypoglycemia with phenylbutazone, oral anticoagulants, hydantoins, salicylates, NSAIDs, MAO inhibitors
Increased toxicity: Increased disulfiram reactions with alcohol

Mechanism of Action Stimulates insulin release from the pancreatic beta cells; reduces glucose output from the liver; insulin sensitivity is increased at peripheral target sites

Pharmacodynamics
Insulin levels in the serum begin to increase within 15-60 minutes after a single oral dose and persist for up to 24 hours
Duration of action: 18 hours

Pharmacokinetics
Protein binding: 99% ionic/nonionic
Metabolism: To one moderately active and several inactive metabolites
Half-life: 5-16 hours, may be prolonged with renal insufficiency
Time to peak: Oral: Peak serum levels occur within 2-4 hours

Usual Dosage Oral: Doses >10 mg/day should be divided
Geriatrics: Initial: 1.25-2.5 mg/day, increase by 1.25-2.5 mg/day every 1-3 weeks; maximum daily dose: 20 mg/day

Adults: 1.25-5 mg to start then 1.25-20 mg maintenance dose/day divided in 1-2 doses

Monitoring Parameters Fasting blood glucose, hemoglobin A_{1c}, fructosamine

Reference Range Fasting blood glucose: Geriatrics: 100-150 mg/dL; Adults: 80-140 mg/dL

Test Interactions Decreased prothrombin time (S), decreased sodium (S)

Patient Information Patients must be counseled by someone experienced in diabetes education, signs and symptoms of hyper- and hypoglycemia, exercise and diet, blood glucose monitoring, and other related topics; eat regularly, do not skip meals; carry quick source of sugar; medical alert bracelet

Nursing Implications Monitor for signs and symptoms of hypoglycemia; patients who are anorexic or NPO may need to have their dose held to avoid hypoglycemia

Special Geriatric Considerations Rapid and prolonged hypoglycemia (>12 hours) despite hypertonic glucose injections have been reported; age, hepatic, and renal impairment are independent risk factors for hypoglycemia; dosage titration should be made at weekly intervals. How "tightly" a geriatric patient's blood glucose should be controlled is controversial; however, a fasting blood sugar of <150 mg/dL is now an acceptable end point. Such a decision should be based on the patient's functional and cognitive status, how well they recognize hypoglycemic or hyperglycemic symptoms, and how to respond to them and their other disease states. Use with caution in elderly with renal insufficiency.

Dosage Forms Tablet: 1.25 mg, 2.5 mg, 5 mg

References
Brodowa RG, "Benefits and Risks With Glyburide and Glipizide in Elderly NIDDM Patients," *Diabetes Care*, 1992, 15(1):75-80.
Rosenstock J, Corrao PJ, Goldberg RB, et al, "Diabetes Control in the Elderly: A Randomized, Comparative Study of Glyburide Versus Glipizide in Noninsulin-Dependent Diabetes Mellitus," *Clin Ther*, 1993, 15(6):1031-40.
Sonnenblick M and Shilo S, "Glibenclamide Induced Prolonged Hypoglycaemia," *Age Ageing*, 1986, 15:185-9.

Glycerin (glis' er in)

Brand Names Fleet® Babylax® [OTC]; Glyrol®; Ophthalgan®; Osmoglyn®; Sani-Supp® [OTC]

Synonyms Glycerol

Generic Available Yes

Use Constipation; reduction of intraocular pressure; reduction of corneal edema; glycerin has been administered orally to reduce intracranial pressure acutely

Therapeutic Class Laxative, Hyperosmolar

Contraindications Known hypersensitivity to glycerin, anuria, acute pulmonary edema, severe dehydration

Warnings Use oral glycerin with caution in patients with cardiac, renal or hepatic disease and in diabetics

Adverse Reactions
Central nervous system: Dizziness, headache
Endocrine & metabolic: Hyperglycemia
Gastrointestinal: Diarrhea, nausea, tenesmus, vomiting
Local: Pain, rectal irritation, cramping pain
Miscellaneous: Thirst

Stability Protect from heat; freezing should be avoided

Mechanism of Action Osmotic dehydrating agent which increases osmotic pressure; draws fluid into colon and thus stimulates evacuation

Pharmacodynamics
Onset of action:
For glycerin suppository: 15-30 minutes
In decreasing IOP: Within 10-30 minutes
Peak effects: Following oral absorption, within 60-90 minutes
Duration of action: 4-8 hours; increased intracranial pressure decreases within 10-60 minutes following an oral dose with a duration of action around 2-3 hours

(Continued)

325

Glycerin *(Continued)*

Pharmacokinetics

Absorbed:

Oral: Well absorbed

Rectal: Poor

Metabolism: Primarily in the liver with 20% metabolized in the kidney

Half-life: 30-45 minutes

Elimination: Only a small percentage of drug is excreted unchanged in urine

Usual Dosage Geriatrics and Adults:

Constipation: Rectal: 1 suppository as needed

Reduction of intraocular pressure: Oral: 1-1.8 g/kg 1 to 1$\frac{1}{2}$ hours preoperatively; additional doses may be administered at 5-hour intervals

Reduction of corneal edema: Instill 1-2 drops in eye(s) every 3-4 hours

Reduction of intracranial pressure: Oral: 1.5 g/kg/day divided every 4 hours; dose of 1 g/kg/dose every 6 hours has also been used

Administration Apply topical anesthetic before instilling ophthalmic drops

Patient Information Do not use if experiencing abdominal pain, nausea, or vomiting

Nursing Implications See Administration

Additional Information Suppository needs to melt to provide laxative effect

Special Geriatric Considerations The primary use of glycerin in the elderly is as a laxative, although it is not recommended as a first-line treatment

Dosage Forms

Liquid: 4 mL/applicator (220 mL); 75% (120 mL)

Solution:

Oral: 50%

Sterile: With chlorobutanol 0.55% (7.5 mL)

Suppositories: Glycerin and sodium stearate

References

Heinemeyer G, "Clinical Pharmacokinetic Considerations in the Treatment of Increased Intracranial Pressure," *Clin Pharmacokinet*, 1987, 13(1):1-25.

Rottenberg DA, Hurwitz BJ, and Posner JB, "The Effect of Oral Glycerol on Intraventricular Pressure in Man," *Neurology*, 1977, 27(7):600-8.

Glycerol *see* Glycerin *on previous page*

Glycerol Guaiacolate *see* Guaifenesin *on page 331*

Glyceryl Trinitrate *see* Nitroglycerin *on page 505*

Glycopyrrolate *(glye koe pye' roe late)*

Brand Names Robinul®

Synonyms Glycopyrronium Bromide

Generic Available Yes

Therapeutic Class Anticholinergic Agent; Antispasmodic Agent, Gastrointestinal

Use Adjunct in treatment of peptic ulcer disease; inhibit salivation and excessive secretions of the respiratory tract preoperatively; reversal of neuromuscular blockade; control of upper airway secretions

Contraindications Narrow-angle glaucoma, acute hemorrhage, tachycardia, hypersensitivity to glycopyrrolate or any component; ulcerative colitis, obstructive uropathy

Warnings Blondes and patients with Down's syndrome may be hypersensitive to antimuscarinic effects

Precautions Use with caution in the elderly, autonomic neuropathy, glaucoma, hepatic disease, ulcerative colitis, hiatal hernia with reflux esophagitis, renal disease, prostatic hypertrophy, congestive heart failure, coronary artery disease, arrhythmias, or hypertension

Adverse Reactions

Cardiovascular: Tachycardia, palpitations

Central nervous system: Fatigue, delirium, restlessness, headache (the elderly are at increased risk for confusion and hallucinations, ataxia)

Dermatologic: Dry hot skin

Gastrointestinal: Impaired GI motility, xerostomia

Genitourinary: Urinary hesitancy/retention

Neuromuscular & skeletal: Tremors

Ocular: Mydriasis, blurred vision

Overdosage Symptoms of overdose include blurred vision, urinary retention, tachycardia, absent bowel sounds

Toxicology Anticholinergic toxicity is caused by strong binding of the drug to cholinergic receptors. Anticholinesterase inhibitors reduce acetylcholinesterase, the enzyme that breaks down acetylcholine and thereby allows acetylcholine to accumulate and compete for receptor binding with the offending anticholinergic. For anticholinergic overdose with severe life-threatening symptoms, physostigmine 1-2 mg S.C. or I.V., slowly may be given to reverse these effects.

Drug Interactions

Decreased effect of levodopa (decreased absorption); decreased effect with tacrine

Increased toxicity (central anticholinergic syndrome): Narcotic analgesics, phenothiazines, and other antipsychotics, tricyclic antidepressants, some antihistamines, quinidine, disopyramide

Stability Unstable at pH >6

Mechanism of Action Blocks the action of acetylcholine at parasympathetic sites in smooth muscle, secretory glands and the CNS

Pharmacodynamics
Onset of action:
Oral: Within 50 minutes
I.M.: 20-40 minutes
I.V.: 10-15 minutes
Peak effect: Oral: Within 1 hour

Pharmacokinetics
Absorption: Oral: Poor and erratic
Bioavailability: ~10%

Usual Dosage Geriatrics and Adults:
Reverse neuromuscular blockade: I.V.: 0.2 mg for each 1 mg of neostigmine or 5 mg of pyridostigmine administered

Peptic ulcer:
Oral: 1-2 mg 2-3 times/day
I.M., I.V.: 0.1-0.2 mg 3-4 times/day

Preoperative: I.M.: 4 mcg/kg 30-60 minutes before procedure

Administration For I.V. administration, glycopyrrolate may also be administered via the tubing of a running I.V. infusion of a compatible solution

Monitoring Parameters Pulse, anticholinergic effects

Patient Information Maintain good oral hygiene habits, because lack of saliva may increase chance of cavities. Observe caution while driving or performing other tasks requiring alertness, as may cause drowsiness, dizziness, or blurred vision. Notify physician if skin rash, flushing or eye pain occurs; or if difficulty in urinating, constipation or sensitivity to light becomes severe or persists.

Nursing Implications Monitor for anticholinergic effects

Additional Information Because of its bothersome and potentially dangerous side effects, glycopyrrolate is rarely used for the treatment of peptic ulcer disease

Special Geriatric Considerations Anticholinergic agents are generally not well tolerated in the elderly and their use should be avoided when possible; see Precautions and Adverse Reactions

Dosage Forms
Injection: 0.2 mg/mL (1 mL, 2 mL, 5 mL, 20 mL)
Tablet: 1 mg, 2 mg

Glycopyrronium Bromide see Glycopyrrolate on previous page

Glycotuss® [OTC] see Guaifenesin on page 331

Glydiazinamide see Glipizide on page 322

Gly-Oxide® Oral [OTC] see Carbamide Peroxide on page 119

Glyrol® see Glycerin on page 325

Glytuss® [OTC] see Guaifenesin on page 331

Gold Sodium Thiomalate

Brand Names Myochrysine®

Therapeutic Class Gold Compound

Use Adjunctive treatment in adult active rheumatoid arthritis; alternative or adjunct in treatment of pemphigus; for psoriatic patients who do not respond to NSAIDs

Contraindications Severe hepatic or renal dysfunction; hypersensitivity to gold compounds or any component; systemic lupus erythematosus; history of blood dyscrasias; congestive heart failure, exfoliative dermatitis, colitis

Warnings Explain the possibility of adverse reactions before initiating therapy; signs of gold toxicity include: decrease in hemoglobin, leukopenia, granulocytes and platelets; proteinuria, hematuria, pruritus, stomatitis, persistent diarrhea, rash, metallic taste; diabetes mellitus and congestive heart failure should be in control before initiating therapy; use cautiously in patients with a history of blood dyscrasias, bone marrow depression, inflammatory bowel disease, allergic hemolytic anemias, drug allergy, or hypersensitivity, skin rash, history of renal or liver disease, uncontrolled hypertension, or compromised cerebral or cardiovascular circulation. Therapy should be discontinued if platelet count falls <100,000/mm³; <4000 WBC, <1500 granulocytes/mm³.

Precautions Frequent monitoring of patients for signs and symptoms of toxicity will prevent serious adverse reactions; must not be injected I.V.; use with caution in patients with impaired renal or hepatic function; NSAIDs and corticosteroids may be discontinued over time after initiating gold therapy; do not use with penicillamine, antimalarials, immunosuppressives, other than corticosteroids; for mild or minor adverse reactions, hold therapy until reaction resolves then may resume therapy of reduced doses; moderate to severe reaction require discontinuation of gold therapy

(Continued)

Gold Sodium Thiomalate *(Continued)*

Adverse Reactions
Cardiovascular: Flushing

Central nervous system: Dizziness, confusion, fever, hallucinations, seizures, fainting, headache

Dermatologic: Dermatitis, alopecia, pruritus, gray-to-blue pigmentation

Gastrointestinal: Stomatitis, metallic taste, nausea, vomiting, abdominal cramps, abdominal pain, constipation, flatulence, dyspepsia, melena, GI bleeding, mouth ulcers, dysgeusia, dysphagia

Genitourinary: Vaginitis

Hematologic: Leukopenia, thrombocytopenia, eosinophilia

Hepatic: Hepatitis, increased LFTs, jaundice

Neuromuscular & skeletal: Weakness

Ocular: Iritis, corneal ulcers, deposits of gold

Renal: Hematuria, proteinuria, nephrotic syndrome, glomerulitis

Respiratory: Bronchitis, interstitial pneumonitis, fibrosis

Miscellaneous: Sweating

Overdosage Symptoms of overdose include hematuria, proteinuria, fever, nausea, vomiting, diarrhea

Toxicology For mild gold poisoning, dimercaprol 2.5 mg/kg 4 times/day for 2 days or for more severe forms of gold intoxication, dimercaprol 3-5 mg/kg every 4 hours for 2 days, should be initiated. Then after 2 days, the initial dose should be repeated twice daily on the third day, and once daily thereafter for 10 days. Other chelating agents have been used with some success.

Drug Interactions Penicillamine, antimalarials, cytotoxic drugs, or immunosuppressive agents, phenylbutazone, oxyphenbutazone

Stability Should not be used if solution is darker than pale yellow

Mechanism of Action The exact mechanism of action of gold is unknown; gold is taken up by macrophages which result in inhibition of phagocytosis and lysosomal membrane stabilization; other actions observed are decreased serum rheumatoid factor and alterations in immunoglobulins. Additionally, complement activation is decreased, prostaglandin synthesis is inhibited and lysosomal enzyme activity is decreased.

Pharmacodynamics Gold injections may result in decreased morning stiffness in 1-2 months; significant benefit may not be noted for 3-6 months

Pharmacokinetics
Protein binding: 95% to 99%

Half-life: 3-27 days (single dose); 14-40 days (third dose); up to 168 days (11th dose)

Time to peak: I.M.: Peak serum levels occur within 2-6 hours

Elimination: Majority (60% to 90%) is excreted in urine with smaller amounts (10% to 40%) excreted in feces (via bile)

Usual Dosage Geriatrics and Adults: I.M. (gluteal muscle preferable): 10 mg first week; 25 mg second week; then 25-50 mg/week until 1 g cumulative dose has been given. If improvement occurs without adverse reactions, give 25-50 mg every week for 2-20 weeks; then every 3-4 weeks if patient is stable; may give maintenance 25-50 mg I.M. every 3-4 weeks indefinitely; if no response after cumulative dose of 1 g, discontinue therapy

Monitoring Parameters Each visit, the patient should have urinalysis, CBC with platelets initially; then every 6 months on maintenance therapy; monitor for other adverse reactions; see Adverse Reactions

Reference Range Gold: Normal: 0-0.1 µg/mL (SI: 0-0.0064 µmol/L); Therapeutic: 1-3 µg/mL (SI: 0.06-0.18 µmol/L); urine <0.1 µg/24 hours

Patient Information Minimize exposure to sunlight; report any signs of toxicity to physician (ie, pruritus, rash, sore mouth, indigestion, metallic taste); joint pain may take 1-2 months to start to subside

Nursing Implications Therapy should be discontinued if platelet count falls <100,000/mm^3; deep I.M. injection into the upper outer quadrant of the gluteal region; addition of 0.1 mL of 1% lidocaine to each injection may reduce the discomfort with injection; vial should be thoroughly shaken before withdrawing a dose; explain the possibility of adverse reactions before initiating therapy; advise patients to report any symptoms of toxicity; monitor serum levels, CBC, platelets, urine protein; see Adverse Reactions

Special Geriatric Considerations Tolerance to gold decreases with advanced age; use cautiously only after traditional therapy and other disease modifying antirheumatic drugs (DMARDs) have been attempted

Dosage Forms Injection: 25 mg/mL (1 mL); 50 mg/mL (1 mL, 10 mL); contains 50% gold

Granisetron *(gra ni' se tron)*

Brand Names Kytril®

Therapeutic Class Antiemetic

Use Prophylaxis and treatment of chemotherapy-related nausea and emesis; may be prescribed for patients who are refractory to or have severe adverse reactions to standard antiemetic therapy. Granisetron may be prescribed for young patients (ie, <45 years of age who are more likely to develop extrapyramidal reactions to high-dose metoclopramide) who are to receive highly emetogenic chemotherapeutic agents as listed:

Agents with high emetogenic potential (>90%) (dose/m^2):
  Carmustine ≥200 mg
  Cisplatin ≥75 mg
  Cyclophosphamide ≥1000 mg
  Cytarabine ≥1000 mg
  Dacarbazine ≥500 mg
  Ifosfamide ≥1000 mg
  Lomustine ≥60 mg
  Mechlorethamine
  Pentostatin
  Streptozocin

or two agents classified as having high or moderately high emetogenic potential as listed:

Agents with moderately high emetogenic potential (60% to 90%) (dose/m^2):
  Carmustine <200 mg
  Cisplatin <75 mg
  Cyclophosphamide 1000 mg
  Cytarabine 250-1000 mg
  Dacarbazine <500 mg
  Doxorubicin ≥75 mg
  Ifosfamide
  Lomustine <60 mg
  Methotrexate ≥250 mg
  Mitomycin
  Mitoxantrone
  Procarbazine

Granisetron should not be prescribed for chemotherapeutic agents with a low emetogenic potential (eg, bleomycin, busulfan, cyclophosphamide <1000 mg, etoposide, 5-fluorouracil, vinblastine, vincristine)

Contraindications Previous hypersensitivity to granisetron

Warnings Use with caution in patients with liver disease; hepatocellular carcinomas and adenomas were induced in rats at doses 400 times recommended for use in humans; see Special Geriatric Considerations

Adverse Reactions
  Cardiovascular: Transient blood pressure changes, sinus bradycardia, atrial fibrillation, A-V block, ventricular ectopy
  Central nervous system: Headache, somnolence, agitation, asthenia, fever, extrapyramidal effects
  Dermatologic: Rash
  Endocrine & metabolic: Hot flashes
  Gastrointestinal: Constipation, diarrhea, taste changes
  Hepatic: Increased LFTs (AST, ALT)
  Neuromuscular & skeletal: Weakness
  Miscellaneous: Anaphylactic reactions

Overdosage Doses up to 38.5 mg have been reported without symptoms or slight headache

Toxicology No specific antidote; give general supportive care

Drug Interactions Drugs which inhibit clearance by cytochrome P-450 system may change clearance of granisetron; induction may occur as well and decrease half-life of granisetron

Stability Stable when mixed in NS or D$_5$W for 24 hours at room temperature; protect from light; do not freeze vials

Mechanism of Action Selective 5-HT$_3$ receptor antagonist, blocking serotonin, both peripherally on vagal nerve terminals and centrally in the chemoreceptor trigger zone

Pharmacodynamics
  Onset of action: Commonly controls emesis within 1-3 minutes of administration
  Duration: Effects generally last no more than 24 hours maximum

Pharmacokinetics
  Distribution: V$_d$: 2-3 L/kg (range: 0.85-10 L/kg); widely distributed throughout the body
  Half-life:
    Cancer patients: 10-12 hours (range: 1-31 hours)
    Healthy volunteers: 3-4 hours
  Elimination: Primarily hepatic, 8% to 15% of a dose is excreted unchanged in urine within 48 hours

Usual Dosage Geriatrics and Adults:
  Oral: 1 mg twice daily on days receiving chemotherapy
  I.V.: 10 mcg/kg for 1-3 doses; doses should be administered as a single IVPB over 5 minutes to 1 hour, given just prior to chemotherapy (15-60 minutes before) and only on days when receiving chemotherapy

(Continued)

Granisetron *(Continued)*

As intervention therapy for breakthrough nausea and vomiting, during the first 24 hours following chemotherapy, 2 or 3 repeat infusions (same dose) have been administered, separated by at least 10 minutes

Dosing interval in renal impairment: Creatinine clearance values have no relationship to granisetron clearance

Administration As a general precaution, do not mix in solution with other medications

Monitoring Parameters Monitor for control of nausea and vomiting

Nursing Implications Doses should be given at least 15-60 minutes prior to initiation of chemotherapy

Special Geriatric Considerations Clinical trials with patients older than 65 years of age are limited; however, the data indicates that safety and efficacy are similar to that observed in younger adults; no adjustment in dose necessary for elderly

Dosage Forms
Injection, preservative free: 1 mg/mL (1 mL)
Tablet: 1 mg

Extemporaneous Preparation(s) Injection: 1 mg/mL as free base (1.12 mg/mL as HCl salt); 1 mL vial

Granulex *see* Trypsin, Balsam Peru, and Castor Oil *on page 724*

Granulocyte Colony Stimulating Factor *see* Filgrastim *on page 290*

Grifulvin® V *see* Griseofulvin *on this page*

Grisactin® *see* Griseofulvin *on this page*

Grisactin® Ultra *see* Griseofulvin *on this page*

Griseofulvin *(gri see oh ful' vin)*

Brand Names Fulvicin® P/G; Fulvicin-U/F®; Grifulvin® V; Grisactin®; Grisactin® Ultra; Gris-PEG®

Synonyms Griseofulvin Microsize; Griseofulvin Ultramicrosize

Generic Available No

Therapeutic Class Antifungal Agent, Systemic

Use Treatment of susceptible tinea infections of the skin, hair, and nails

Contraindications Hypersensitivity to griseofulvin or any component; severe liver disease, porphyria (interferes with porphyrin metabolism)

Warnings During long-term therapy, periodic assessment of hepatic, renal, and hematopoietic functions should be performed; avoid exposure to intense sunlight to prevent photosensitivity reactions; hypersensitivity cross-reaction between penicillins and griseofulvin is possible

Adverse Reactions
Central nervous system: Fatigue, confusion, impaired judgment, insomnia, paresthesia, headache, incoordination
Dermatologic: Rash, urticaria, photosensitivity
Gastrointestinal: Nausea, vomiting, diarrhea
Hematologic: Leukopenia, granulocytopenia
Hepatic: Hepatotoxicity
Renal: Proteinuria
Miscellaneous: Lupus-like syndrome

Overdosage Symptoms of overdose include lethargy, vertigo, blurred vision, nausea, vomiting, diarrhea

Toxicology Following GI decontamination, supportive care only

Drug Interactions
Decreased effect of anticoagulants, oral contraceptives; decreased effect/levels with barbiturates
Disulfiram-like reaction with alcohol

Mechanism of Action Inhibits fungal cell mitosis at metaphase; binds to human keratin making it resistant to fungal invasion

Pharmacokinetics
Absorption: Ultramicrosize griseofulvin is almost complete; absorption of microsize griseofulvin is variable (25% to 70% of an oral dose); absorption is enhanced by ingestion of a fatty meal
Distribution: Deposited in varying concentrations in the keratin layer of the skin, hair, and nails; only a very small fraction is distributed in the body fluids and tissues
Metabolism: Extensive in the liver
Half-life: 9-22 hours
Time to peak serum concentration: ~4 hours
Elimination: <1% excreted unchanged in urine; also excreted in feces and perspiration

Usual Dosage
Geriatrics and Adults: Oral:
Microsize: 500-1000 mg/day in single or divided doses

Ultramicrosize: 330-375 mg/day in single or divided doses; doses up to 750 mg/day have been used for infections more difficult to eradicate such as tinea unguium and tinea pedis

Duration of therapy depends on the site of infection:
Tinea corporis: 2-4 weeks
Tinea capitis: 4-6 weeks or longer
Tinea pedis: 4-8 weeks
Tinea unguium: 4-6 months

Monitoring Parameters Periodic renal, hepatic, and hematopoietic function tests

Test Interactions False-positive urinary VMA levels

Patient Information Avoid exposure to sunlight, take with fatty meal; if patient gets headache, it usually goes away with continued therapy; may cause dizziness, drowsiness, and impair judgment

Additional Information
Microsize: Fulvicin-U/F®, Grifulvin® V, Grisactin®
Ultramicrosize: Fulvicin® P/G, Grisactin® Ultra, Gris-PEG®; GI absorption of ultramicrosize is ~1.5 times that of microsize

Special Geriatric Considerations No specific changes in dosing are needed; see Usual Dosage

Dosage Forms
Microsize:
Capsule (Grisactin®): 125 mg, 250 mg
Suspension, oral (Grifulvin® V): 125 mg/5 mL with alcohol 0.2% (120 mL)
Tablet:
Fulvicin-U/F®, Grifulvin® V: 250 mg
Fulvicin-U/F®, Grifulvin® V, Grisactin-500®: 500 mg

Ultramicrosize:
Tablet:
Fulvicin® P/G: 165 mg, 330 mg
Fulvicin® P/G, Grisactin® Ultra, Gris-PEG®: 125 mg, 250 mg
Grisactin® Ultra: 330 mg

Griseofulvin Microsize *see* Griseofulvin *on previous page*

Griseofulvin Ultramicrosize *see* Griseofulvin *on previous page*

Gris-PEG® *see* Griseofulvin *on previous page*

Guaifenesin (gwye fen' e sin)

Brand Names Amonidrin® [OTC]; Anti-Tuss® [OTC]; Breonesin® [OTC]; Cremacoat®2 [OTC]; Fenesin™; Genatuss® [OTC]; GG-Cen® [OTC]; Glyate® [OTC]; Glycotuss® [OTC]; Glytuss® [OTC]; Guaituss® [OTC]; Halotussin® [OTC]; Humibid® L.A.; Humibid® Sprinkle; Hytuss-2X® [OTC]; Malotuss [OTC]; Medi-Tuss® [OTC]; Mytussin® [OTC]; Naldecon® Senior EX [OTC]; Nortussin® [OTC]; Robafen® [OTC]; Robitussin® [OTC]; Uni Tussin® [OTC]

Synonyms GG; Glycerol Guaiacolate

Generic Available Yes

Therapeutic Class Expectorant

Use Symptomatic relief of respiratory conditions characterized by a dry, nonproductive cough and in the presence of mucous in the respiratory tract

Contraindications Hypersensitivity to guaifenesin or any component

Warnings Should not be used for persistent or chronic coughs

Adverse Reactions
Central nervous system: Drowsiness, headache
Dermatologic: Rash
Gastrointestinal: Nausea, vomiting, stomach pain

Overdosage Symptoms of overdose include vomiting

Toxicology Treatment is supportive

Stability Protect from light

Mechanism of Action Thought to act as an expectorant by irritating the gastric mucosa and stimulating respiratory tract secretions, thereby increasing respiratory fluid volumes and decreasing phlegm viscosity

Pharmacokinetics
Absorption: Well absorbed from the GI tract
Metabolism: Undergoes hepatic metabolism (60%)
Elimination: Renal excretion of changed and unchanged drug

Usual Dosage Geriatrics and Adults: Oral: 100-400 mg (5-20 mL) every 4 hours to a maximum of 2.4 g/day (60 mL/day)

Monitoring Parameters Cough, sputum consistency and volume

Test Interactions Decreased uric acid (S)

Patient Information Take with a large quantity of fluid to ensure proper action; if cough persists for more than 1 week, is recumbent, or is accompanied by fever, rash or persistent headache, physician should be consulted

(Continued)

Guaifenesin *(Continued)*

Nursing Implications Give with large quantity of water to ensure proper action; some products contain alcohol

Additional Information Should not be used for persistent or chronic cough such as that occurring with smoking, asthma, chronic bronchitis, or emphysema or for cough associated with excessive phlegm. There is a lack of convincing studies to document the efficacy of guaifenesin. Guaifenesin is available in various combinations. These include phenylpropanolamine; pseudoephedrine; dextromethorphan; codeine; pseudoephedrine and codeine; phenylpropanolamine and dextromethorphan.

Special Geriatric Considerations See Additional Information

Dosage Forms

Capsule: 200 mg
Capsule, sustained release: 300 mg
Liquid: 200 mg/5 mL (118 mL)
Syrup: 100 mg/5 mL (120 mL, 240 mL, 473 mL, 946 mL)
Tablet: 100 mg, 200 mg
Tablet, sustained release: 600 mg

Guaifenesin and Codeine (gwye fen' e sin & koe' deen)

Related Information

Codeine *on page 183*
Guaifenesin *on previous page*

Brand Names Cheracol®; Guaituss AC®; Medi-Tuss® AC; Mytussin® AC; Robitussin® A-C; Tolu-Sed®

Synonyms Codeine and Guaifenesin

Generic Available Yes

Therapeutic Class Antitussive; Cough Preparation; Expectorant

Use Temporary control of cough due to minor throat and bronchial irritation

Restrictions C-V

Contraindications Hypersensitivity to guaifenesin, codeine or any component

Warnings Should not be used for chronic productive coughs

Precautions Use with caution in patients who have undergone thoracotomies or laparotomies

Adverse Reactions

Codeine:
Cardiovascular: Hypotension, palpitations, bradycardia, peripheral vasodilation, increased intracranial pressure
Central nervous system: CNS depression, dizziness, drowsiness, sedation
Endocrine & metabolic: Antidiuretic hormone release
Gastrointestinal: Nausea, vomiting, constipation
Ocular: Miosis
Respiratory: Respiratory depression
Miscellaneous: Physical and psychological dependence with prolonged use, biliary or urinary tract spasm, histamine release

Guaifenesin: Gastrointestinal: Nausea, vomiting

Overdosage Symptoms of overdose include lethargy, coma, respiratory depression

Toxicology Naloxone 2 mg I.V. with repeat administration as necessary up to a total of 10 mg

Drug Interactions Increased toxicity: Opiate agonists, general anesthetics, tranquilizers, sedatives, hypnotics, TCAs, MAO inhibitors, alcohol, CNS depressants

Usual Dosage Geriatrics and Adults: Oral: 10 mL every 6-8 hours

Monitoring Parameters Cough, sputum consistency and volume, mental status, respiratory status

Patient Information Take with a large quantity of fluid to ensure proper action. May cause drowsiness; avoid CNS depressants and alcohol; do not use for chronic or persistent coughs

Nursing Implications Give with a large quantity of fluid; see Monitoring Parameters

Special Geriatric Considerations The elderly may be more sensitive to the CNS depressant effects of codeine; monitor closely for excessive sedation

Dosage Forms Syrup: Guaifenesin 100 mg and codeine phosphate 10 mg per 5 mL (60 mL, 120 mL, 480 mL)

Guaifenesin and Dextromethorphan (dex troe meth or' fan)

Brand Names Guaituss DM® [OTC]; Halotussin® DM [OTC]; Mytussin® DM [OTC]; Queltuss® [OTC]; Robitussin-DM® [OTC]

Synonyms Dextromethorphan and Guaifenesin

Generic Available Yes

Therapeutic Class Antitussive; Cough Preparation; Expectorant

Use Temporary control of cough due to minor throat and bronchial irritation

Contraindications Hypersensitivity to guaifenesin, dextromethorphan or any component; patients receiving monoamine oxidase inhibitors

Warnings Should not be used for chronic or persistent coughs

Precautions Some products contain tartrazine dye (FD & C yellow No 5); others contain aspartame which breaks down to phenylalanine; labels should be checked carefully if these substances are to be avoided

Adverse Reactions
Central nervous system: Drowsiness, headache
Dermatologic: Rash
Gastrointestinal: Nausea, vomiting, constipation

Overdosage Symptoms of overdose include nausea, vomiting, drowsiness, dizziness, blurred vision, nystagmus, ataxia, shallow respiration, urinary retention, stupor, toxic psychosis, coma

Toxicology CNS depression in overdose may be reversed by naloxone

Drug Interactions
Monoamine oxidase inhibitors, selegiline; coadministration of MAO inhibitors and dextromethorphan has caused hypotension, hyperpyrexia, and coma
Increased toxicity: CNS depressants, alcohol

Stability Protect from light

Usual Dosage Geriatrics and Adults: Oral: 10 mL every 6-8 hours

Monitoring Parameters Cough, sputum consistency and volume, mental status

Patient Information Take with a large quantity of fluid to ensure proper action; if cough persists for more than 1 week, is recumbent, or is accompanied by fever, rash or persistent headache, physician should be consulted; may cause drowsiness; avoid CNS depressants and alcohol

Nursing Implications Give with a large quantity of fluid; see Monitoring Parameters

Additional Information Should not be used for persistent or chronic cough such as that occurring with smoking, asthma, chronic bronchitis, or emphysema or for cough associated with excessive phlegm

Special Geriatric Considerations See Warnings and Additional Information

Dosage Forms Syrup: Guaifenesin 100 mg and dextromethorphan hydrobromide 10 mg per 5 mL (120 mL, 240 mL); guaifenesin 100 mg and dextromethorphan hydrobromide 15 mg per 5 mL (120 mL, 240 mL)

Guaituss AC® *see* Guaifenesin and Codeine *on previous page*

Guaituss DM® [OTC] *see* Guaifenesin and Dextromethorphan *on previous page*

Guaituss® [OTC] *see* Guaifenesin *on page 331*

Guanabenz Acetate (gwahn' a benz)

Brand Names Wytensin®
Generic Available No
Therapeutic Class Alpha-Adrenergic Agonist
Use Management of hypertension
Contraindications Hypersensitivity to guanabenz or any component
Precautions Do not abruptly discontinue this medication; use with caution in patients with severe coronary insufficiency, recent myocardial infarction, severe renal or hepatic impairment

Adverse Reactions
Central nervous system: Drowsiness, dizziness, headache
Gastrointestinal: Dry mouth
Neuromuscular & skeletal: Weakness

Overdosage Symptoms of overdose include CNS depression, hypothermia, apnea, lethargy, diarrhea, hypotension, bradycardia

Toxicology Treatment is primarily supportive and symptomatic. Hypotension usually responds to I.V. fluids or Trendelenburg positioning. If unresponsive to these measures the use of a parenteral vasoconstrictor may be required (eg, norepinephrine 0.1-0.2 mcg/kg/minute titrated to response). Naloxone may be utilized in treating the hypotension, CNS depression and/or apnea and should be given I.V. 0.4-2 mg, with repeats as needed. Atropine 15 mcg/kg I.V. or I.M. may be needed for symptomatic bradycardia.

Drug Interactions
Decreased hypotensive effect of guanabenz with tricyclic antidepressants
Increased effect: Other hypotensive agents

Mechanism of Action Stimulates alpha$_2$-adrenoreceptors in the brain stem, thus activating an inhibitory neuron, resulting in reduced sympathetic outflow, producing a decrease in vasomotor tone and heart rate

Pharmacodynamics Onset of antihypertensive effect: Within 60 minutes

Pharmacokinetics
Absorption: Oral: ~75% administration
Metabolism: Extensive
Half-life: 7-10 hours
Elimination: <1% of dose excreted as unchanged drug in urine

(Continued)

Guanabenz Acetate *(Continued)*

Usual Dosage Oral:
Geriatrics: Initial: 4 mg once daily, increase every 1-2 weeks
Adults: Initial: 4 mg twice daily, increase by 4-8 mg/day every 1-2 weeks; usual dosage range: 4-32 mg twice daily

Monitoring Parameters Blood pressure, standing and sitting/supine

Test Interactions Increased sodium (S)

Patient Information May cause drowsiness; rise from sitting/lying position carefully, may cause dizziness; do not discontinue without notifying physician

Nursing Implications Monitor for orthostasis; do not abruptly discontinue

Additional Information Guanabenz is considered an alternate to clonidine; it causes less sodium retention than clonidine or methyldopa

Special Geriatric Considerations Because of its CNS adverse effects, guanabenz is not considered a drug of choice in the elderly.

Dosage Forms Tablet: 4 mg, 8 mg

Guanadrel Sulfate *(gwahn' a drel)*

Brand Names Hylorel®

Generic Available No

Therapeutic Class Alpha-Adrenergic Agonist

Use Management of hypertension usually combined with a diuretic

Contraindications Known hypersensitivity to guanadrel, pheochromocytoma, congestive heart failure, patients taking MAO inhibitors

Warnings Use cautiously in asthmatic patients; orthostatic hypotension occurs frequently

Precautions Salt and water retention may occur; use cautiously in patients with peptic ulcers

Adverse Reactions
Cardiovascular: Orthostatic hypotension, palpitations, chest pain
Central nervous system: Fatigue, dizziness, faintness, headache, drowsiness
Gastrointestinal: Diarrhea, increased bowel movements
Genitourinary: Ejaculation disturbances, nocturia
Neuromuscular & skeletal: Weakness
Ocular: Blurred vision
Respiratory: Shortness of breath on exertion
Miscellaneous: Peripheral edema

Overdosage Symptoms of overdose include hypotension, blurred vision, dizziness, syncope

Toxicology Treatment is primarily supportive and symptomatic. Hypotension usually responds to I.V. fluids or Trendelenburg positioning. If unresponsive to these measures the use of a parenteral vasoconstrictor may be required (eg, norepinephrine 0.1-0.2 mcg/kg/minute titrated to response).

Drug Interactions
Decreased effect with tricyclic antidepressants, indirect-acting amines (ephedrine, phenylpropanolamine), phenothiazines
Increased toxicity of direct-acting amines (epinephrine, norepinephrine)
Increased effect: Beta-blockers, vasodilators

Mechanism of Action Acts as a false neurotransmitter that blocks the adrenergic actions of norepinephrine; it displaces norepinephrine from its presynaptic storage granules and thus exposes it to degradation; it thereby produces a reduction in total peripheral resistance and therefore blood pressure

Pharmacodynamics
Peak effect: Within 4-6 hours
Duration of action: 4-14 hours

Pharmacokinetics
Absorption: Oral: Rapid
Distribution: Hydrophilic and, therefore, does not cross the blood-brain barrier
Protein binding: 20%
Half-life:
Initial: 1-4 hours
Terminal: 5-45 hours
Time to peak serum concentration: Within 1.5-2 hours
Elimination: Biphasic; excreted in urine 40% as unchanged drug

Usual Dosage
Geriatrics: Initial: 5 mg once daily
Adults: Initial: 10 mg/day (5 mg twice daily); adjust dosage until blood pressure is controlled, usual dosage: 20-75 mg/day, given twice daily
Dosing interval in renal impairment:
Cl_{cr} 10-50 mL/minute: Administer every 12-24 hours
Cl_{cr} <10 mL/minute: Administer every 24-48 hours

Monitoring Parameters Blood pressure, standing and sitting/supine

Test Interactions Increased sodium (S)

Patient Information Change positions slowly; do not take any over-the-counter or prescription cold medications without consulting your physician

ALPHABETICAL LISTING OF DRUGS

Nursing Implications Monitor for orthostasis
Additional Information Considered an alternative to guanethidine
Special Geriatric Considerations Because of its CNS adverse effects and high incidence of orthostasis, guanadrel is not considered a drug of choice in the elderly; if used, adjust dose for renal function in elderly
Dosage Forms Tablet: 10 mg, 25 mg

Guanethidine Sulfate (gwahn eth' i deen)
Brand Names Ismelin®
Generic Available Yes
Therapeutic Class Alpha-Adrenergic Agonist
Use Treatment of moderate to severe hypertension
Contraindications Pheochromocytoma, MAO inhibitors, hypersensitivity to guanethidine or any component
Warnings Should be withdrawn 2 weeks prior to surgery to decrease chance of vascular collapse and cardiac arrest during anesthesia
Precautions Orthostatic hypotension can occur frequently; avoid the use of guanethidine in the elderly; use with caution in patients with CHF, asthma, or peptic ulcer disease
Adverse Reactions
Cardiovascular: Orthostatic hypotension, edema, syncope
Central nervous system: Dizziness, headache
Gastrointestinal: Diarrhea, increased bowel movements, dry mouth
Genitourinary: Nocturia, ejaculation disturbances
Neuromuscular & skeletal: Weakness
Ocular: Blurred vision
Respiratory: Shortness of breath
Overdosage Symptoms of overdose include hypotension, blurred vision, dizziness, syncope
Toxicology Hypotension usually responds to I.V. fluids or Trendelenburg positioning. If unresponsive to these measures the use of a parenteral vasoconstrictor may be required (eg, norepinephrine 0.1-0.2 mcg/kg/minute titrated to response). Treatment is primarily supportive and symptomatic.
Drug Interactions
Decreased effect with tricyclic antidepressants, indirect-acting amines (ephedrine, phenylpropanolamine), phenothiazines, MAO inhibitors
Increased toxicity of direct-acting amines (epinephrine, norepinephrine)
Mechanism of Action Acts as a false neurotransmitter that blocks the adrenergic actions of norepinephrine; it displaces norepinephrine from its presynaptic storage granules and thus exposes it to degradation; it thereby produces a reduction in total peripheral resistance and therefore blood pressure
Pharmacodynamics
Onset of action: Within 0.5-2 hours
Peak antihypertensive effect: Within 6-8 hours
Duration: 24-48 hours
Pharmacokinetics
Absorption: Oral: Irregular (3% to 55)
Metabolism: Hepatic to inactive metabolites, followed by 25% to 60% of a dose
Half-life: 5-10 days
Elimination: Unchanged in urine, small amounts also appear in feces
Usual Dosage Oral:
Geriatrics: Initial: 5 mg once daily
Adults: Initial: 10 mg; increase by 10-25 mg every 5-7 days; usual dose: 25-50 mg once daily
Monitoring Parameters Blood pressure, standing and sitting/supine
Test Interactions Increased sodium (S); decreased catecholamines (U)
Patient Information May cause drowsiness; rise from sitting/lying carefully, may cause dizziness; do not take any OTC or prescription cough or cold medication without consulting physician
Nursing Implications Tablet may be crushed; monitor for orthostasis
Special Geriatric Considerations Because of its CNS adverse effects and high incidence of orthostatic hypotension, guanethidine is not considered a drug of choice in the elderly.
Dosage Forms Tablet: 10 mg, 25 mg

Guanfacine Hydrochloride (gwahn' fa seen)
Brand Names Tenex®
Generic Available No
Therapeutic Class Alpha-Adrenergic Agonist
Use Management of hypertension
Contraindications Hypersensitivity to guanfacine or any component
(Continued)

Guanfacine Hydrochloride *(Continued)*

Precautions Use with caution in patients with severe coronary insufficiency, recent myocardial infarction, severe renal or hepatic impairment

Adverse Reactions
Central nervous system: Drowsiness, dizziness, headache
Gastrointestinal: Nausea, dry mouth, constipation
Neuromuscular & skeletal: Leg cramps, weakness
Respiratory: Dyspnea

Overdosage Symptoms of overdose include CNS depression, hypothermia, apnea, lethargy, diarrhea, hypotension, bradycardia

Toxicology Treatment is primarily supportive and symptomatic. Hypotension usually responds to I.V. fluids or Trendelenburg positioning. If unresponsive to these measures the use of a parenteral vasoconstrictor may be required (eg, norepinephrine 0.1-0.2 mcg/kg/minute titrated to response). Naloxone may be utilized in treating the hypotension, CNS depression and/or apnea and should be given I.V. 0.4-2 mg, with repeats as needed. Atropine 15 mcg/kg I.V. or I.M. may be needed for symptomatic bradycardia.

Drug Interactions
Decreased hypotensive effect of guanfacine with tricyclic antidepressants
Increased effect: Other hypotensive agents

Mechanism of Action Acts as a false neurotransmitter that blocks the adrenergic actions of norepinephrine; it displaces norepinephrine form its presynaptic storage granules and thus exposes it to degradation; it thereby produces a reduction in total peripheral resistance and therefore blood pressure

Pharmacodynamics
Peak effect: Within 8-11 hours
Duration: 24 hours

Pharmacokinetics
Protein binding: 20% to 30%
Metabolism: In the liver to glucuronide and sulfate metabolites
Bioavailability: 80% to 100%
Half-life: 17 hours
Time to peak serum concentration: Oral: 1-4 hours
Elimination: Renal excretion of changed and unchanged drug (30%)

Usual Dosage Geriatrics and Adults: 1 mg usually at bedtime, may increase if needed; 1 mg/day is most common dose; adverse reactions increase with doses >3 mg/day

Monitoring Parameters Blood pressure, standing and sitting/supine

Patient Information May cause drowsiness, dizziness; do not discontinue this medication without consulting your physician; take at bedtime

Nursing Implications Administer dose at bedtime; observe for orthostasis

Additional Information Usually given with a thiazide diuretic

Special Geriatric Considerations Because of adverse effects such as CNS depression, dry mouth, and constipation, guanfacine may not be considered a drug of choice in the elderly.

Dosage Forms Tablet: 1 mg

Gyne-Lotrimin® [OTC] *see* Clotrimazole *on page 180*

Halazepam *(hal az' e pam)*

Related Information
Anxiolytic/Hypnotic Use in Long-Term Care Facilities *on page 755-756*
Benzodiazepines Comparison *on page 802-803*

Brand Names Paxipam®

Generic Available No

Therapeutic Class Benzodiazepine

Use Management of anxiety disorders; short-term relief of the symptoms of anxiety

Restrictions C-IV

Contraindications Hypersensitivity to halazepam or any component, cross-sensitivity with other benzodiazepines may exist; avoid using in patients with pre-existing CNS depression, severe uncontrolled pain, or narrow-angle glaucoma

Warnings May cause drug dependency; avoid abrupt discontinuance in patients with prolonged therapy or seizure disorders

Precautions Use with caution in patients with a history of drug dependence

Adverse Reactions
Central nervous system: Drowsiness, confusion, dizziness, ataxia, amnesia, slurred speech, paradoxical excitement or rage
Neuromuscular & skeletal: Impaired coordination
Ocular: Blurred vision, diplopia
Respiratory: Decrease in respiratory rate, apnea, laryngospasm
Miscellaneous: Physical and psychological dependence with prolonged use cardiac arrest

Overdosage Symptoms of overdose include somnolence, confusion, coma, and diminished reflexes

Toxicology Treatment for benzodiazepine overdose is supportive; rarely is mechanical ventilation required; flumazenil has been shown to selectively block the binding of benzodiazepines to CNS receptors, resulting in a reversal of benzodiazepine-induced sedation; however, its use may not alter the course of overdose

Drug Interactions Benzodiazepines may increase digoxin concentrations and may decrease the effect of levodopa

Decreased metabolism: Cimetidine, fluoxetine

Increased metabolism: Rifampin

Increased toxicity: CNS depressants, alcohol

Mechanism of Action Benzodiazepines appear to potentiate the effects of GABA and other inhibitory neurotransmitters by binding to specific benzodiazepine-receptor sites in various areas of the CNS

Pharmacodynamics

Onset of action: 2-3 hours

Studies have shown that the elderly are more sensitive to the effects of benzodiazepines as compared to younger adults

Pharmacokinetics

Half-life:

Parent: 14 hours

Active metabolite (desmethyldiazepam): 50-100 hours

Peak level: 1-3 hours

Elimination: <1% excreted unchanged in urine

Usual Dosage Oral:

Geriatrics: 20 mg 1-2 times/day

Adults: 20-40 mg 3 or 4 times/day

Monitoring Parameters Respiratory, cardiovascular and mental status, symptoms of anxiety

Patient Information Avoid alcohol and other CNS depressants; may cause drowsiness; avoid activities needing good psychomotor coordination until CNS effects are known; may cause physical or psychological dependence; avoid abrupt discontinuation after prolonged use

Nursing Implications Assist patient with ambulation, monitor for alertness

Additional Information Halazepam offers no significant advantage over other benzodiazepines

Special Geriatric Considerations Much of halazepam's pharmacologic activity can be attributed to its long-acting metabolite, desmethyldiazepam; therefore, it cannot be considered short-acting, even though the Health Care Financing Administration lists halazepam as a short acting agent (see Appendix). Long-acting benzodiazepines have been associated with falls in the elderly; therefore, halazepam is not considered a drug of choice; see Pharmacodynamics.

Dosage Forms Tablet: 20 mg, 40 mg

Halcion® *see* Triazolam *on page 713*

Haldol® *see* Haloperidol *on this page*

Haldol® Decanoate *see* Haloperidol *on this page*

Halenol® [OTC] *see* Acetaminophen *on page 13*

Haley's M-O® [OTC] *see* Magnesium Hydroxide and Mineral Oil Emulsion *on page 428*

Haloperidol (ha loe per' i dole)

Related Information

Antacid Drug Interactions *on page 764*

Antipsychotic Agents Comparison *on page 801*

Antipsychotic Medication Guidelines *on page 754*

Brand Names Haldol®; Haldol® Decanoate

Generic Available Yes

Therapeutic Class Antipsychotic Agent

Use Management of psychotic disorders; nonpsychotic symptoms associated with dementia in elderly, Tourette's syndrome, Huntington's chorea; see Special Geriatric Considerations

Contraindications Hypersensitivity to haloperidol or any component; narrow-angle glaucoma, bone marrow depression, CNS depression, severe liver or cardiac disease, subcortical brain damage; circulatory collapse; severe hypotension or hypertension

Warnings

Tardive dyskinesia: Prevalence rate may be 40% in elderly; elderly women especially at risk; embarrassment from dyskinesias may lead to greater social isolation; development of the syndrome and the irreversible nature are proportional to duration and total cumulative dose over time. May be reversible if diagnosed early in therapy; intermittent use of antipsychotics (not proven use) helps decrease total cumulative dose.

EPS: Extrapyramidal reactions are more common in elderly with up to 50% developing these reactions after age 60. These reactions may be more common in dementia

(Continued)

Haloperidol (Continued)

patients. Drug-induced **Parkinson's syndrome** occurs often. Discontinuation usually resolves symptoms but may take weeks to months (12+) to clear. **Akathisia** is the most common EPS reaction in elderly. The symptoms of motor restlessness are difficult to diagnose in demented elderly; increased nervousness, assertiveness, restlessness with constant movement may indicate this adverse event. Consider decreasing dose if antipsychotic to treat as well as diagnose problem; usually see this reaction within 2-3 months of initiating antipsychotic drug.

Anticholinergic effects: These side effects most common with low potency antipsychotics (eg, thioridazine, chlorpromazine). CNS toxicity occurs more frequently and severely in elderly; increased confusion, memory loss, psychotic behavior, and agitation frequently occur as a consequence of anticholinergic effects to antipsychotic agents. Peripheral anticholinergic action troublesome to elderly; most peripheral anticholinergic effects last only 2-3 weeks; see Adverse Reactions.

Orthostatic hypotension: More common with low potency agents (eg, thioridazine, chlorpromazine, and clozapine) but of concern with all antipsychotic agents; orthostasis due to alpha-receptor blockade by antipsychotic agents. Elderly present many risk factors for orthostatic hypotension: blunted baroreceptor reflexes, decreased vascular tone, decreased vascular volume, and possible presence of cardiac diseases which result in decreased cardiac output.

Sedation: Common side effect with antipsychotic therapy; should not be used as a hypnotic unless insomnia is associated with target behavior symptoms treated with antipsychotic medications; see Special Geriatric Considerations. Anecdotal reports suggesting antipsychotic sedation in nonpsychotic patients is extremely unpleasant due to feelings of depersonalization, derealization, and dysphoria. Due to the long duration of action with antipsychotic drugs, these reactions may last up to 24 hours and result in decreased daytime function.

Cardiac toxicity: Life-threatening arrhythmias have occurred at therapeutic doses of antipsychotics. Thioridazine more commonly demonstrates EKG changes than other antipsychotics; suggested to use high potency antipsychotic agents (ie, haloperidol) in patients with cardiac conduction defects.

Precautions Watch for hypotension when administering I.M. or I.V.; use with caution in patients with cardiovascular disease, seizures, and Parkinson's disease; benefits of therapy must be weighed against risks of therapy; decanoate form should never be given I.V.

Adverse Reactions

Anticholinergic: Dry mouth (problem for denture user), urinary retention, constipation, adynamic ileus, overflow incontinence, blurred vision

Cardiovascular: Hypotension (especially orthostatic), tachycardia, arrhythmias, abnormal T waves with prolonged ventricular repolarization, EKG changes

Central nervous system: Sedation, drowsiness, restlessness, anxiety, extrapyramidal reactions, dystonic reactions, pseudoparkinsonian signs and symptoms, tardive dyskinesia, neuroleptic malignant syndrome, seizures, altered central temperature regulation

Dermatologic: Photosensitivity (rare)

Endocrine & metabolic: Amenorrhea, galactorrhea, gynecomastia

Gastrointestinal: Constipation, adynamic ileus, GI upset, dry mouth (problem for denture user), weight gain

Genitourinary: Urinary retention, overflow incontinence, priapism, sexual dysfunction (up to 60%)

Hematologic: Agranulocytosis, leukopenia (usually in patients with large doses for prolonged periods)

Hepatic: Cholestatic jaundice

Ocular: Blurred vision, retinal pigmentation, decreased visual acuity (may be irreversible)

Overdosage Symptoms of overdose include deep sleep, coma, extrapyramidal symptoms, abnormal involuntary muscle movements, hypotension or hypertension; agitation, restlessness, fever, hypothermia or hyperthermia, seizures, cardiac arrhythmias, EKG changes

Toxicology Following initiation of essential overdose management, toxic symptom treatment and supportive treatment should be initiated. Hypotension usually responds to I.V. fluids or Trendelenburg positioning. If unresponsive to these measures the use of a parenteral inotrope may be required (eg, norepinephrine 0.1-0.2 mcg/kg/ minute titrated to response). Do not use epinephrine. Seizures commonly respond to diazepam (I.V. 5-10 mg bolus in adults every 15 minutes if needed up to a total of 30 mg) or to phenytoin or phenobarbital. Also critical cardiac arrhythmias often respond to I.V. phenytoin (15 mg/kg up to 1 g), while other antiarrhythmics can be used. Neuroleptics often cause extrapyramidal symptoms (eg, dystonic reactions) requiring management with diphenhydramine 1-2 mg/kg up to a maximum of 50 mg I.M. or I.V. slow push followed by a maintenance dose for 48-72 hours. When these reactions are unresponsive to diphenhydramine, benztropine mesylate I.V. 1-2 mg may be effective. These agents are generally effective within 2-5 minutes.

Drug Interactions

Concurrent use with lithium has occasionally caused acute encephalopathy-like syndrome

Carbamazepine, barbiturates, phenytoin may decrease serum concentration of haloperidol

Fluoxetine reported to have EPS when administered with haloperidol

Guanethidine's hypotensive effect is decreased with haloperidol

Lithium administration with haloperidol may increase disorientation

Methyldopa may increase antipsychotic effect or cause psychosis with haloperidol

Propranolol administered with haloperidol may increase hypotensive effect of propranolol

Tricyclic antidepressants may have serum concentrations increased with concomitant administration with haloperidol

Stability Protect oral dosage forms from light

Mechanism of Action Blocks postsynaptic mesolimbic dopaminergic D_1 and D_2 receptors in the brain; exhibits a strong alpha-adrenergic blocking and anticholinergic effect, depresses the release of hypothalamic and hypophyseal hormones; believed to depress the reticular activating system thus affecting basal metabolism, body temperature, wakefulness, vasomotor tone, and emesis

Pharmacodynamics

Onset of action: I.M.: Within 1 hour following administration

Peak levels: Oral: Occur in 2-4 hours

Decanoate form: Duration of action: ~3 weeks

Pharmacokinetics

Absorption: Oral: May be affected by the inherent anticholinergic action on the gastrointestinal tissue causing variable absorption. Absorption from tablets is erratic with less variation seen with solutions. These agents are widely distributed in tissues with CNS concentrations exceeding that of plasma due to their lipophilic characteristics.

Protein binding: 90%; antipsychotic agents are bound 90% to 99% to plasma proteins; highly bound to brain and lung tissue and other tissues with a high blood perfusion

Metabolism: Metabolized in the liver to inactive compounds

Half-life: 20 hours

Elimination half-life: Antipsychotic range: 20-40 hours which may be extended in elderly due to decline in oxidative hepatic reactions (phase I) with age

Elimination: 33% to 40% excreted in the urine within 5 days; an additional 15% is excreted in the feces; elimination occurs through hepatic metabolism (oxidation) where numerous active metabolites are produced; active metabolites excreted in urine

The biologic effect of a single dose persists for 24 hours. When the patient has accommodated to initial side effects (sedation), once daily dosing is possible due to the long half-life of antipsychotics.

Steady-state plasma levels are achieved in 4-7 days; therefore, if possible, do not make dose adjustments more than once in a 7-day period. Due to the long half-lives of antipsychotics, as needed (PRN) use is ineffective since repeated doses are necessary to achieve therapeutic tissue concentrations in the CNS

Usual Dosage

Geriatrics (nonpsychotic patient; dementia behavior): Initial: 0.25-0.5 mg 1-2 times/day; increase dose at 4- to 7-day intervals by 0.25-0.5 mg/day; increase dosing intervals (bid, tid, etc) as necessary to control response or side effects; maximum daily dose: 4 mg; gradual increases (titration) may prevent some side effects or decrease their severity

Adults (do not give I.V.):

Oral: 0.5-5 mg 2-3 times/day; usual maximum: 100 mg/day

I.M. (as lactate): 2-5 mg every 4-8 hours as needed

I.M. (as decanoate): Initial: 10-15 times the daily oral dose administered at 4-week intervals

Not dialyzable (0% to 5%)

Monitoring Parameters Orthostatic blood pressures; tremors, gait changes, abnormal movement in trunk, neck, buccal area or extremities; monitor target behaviors for which the agent is given

Reference Range Therapeutic: 5-20 ng/mL (SI: 10-30 nmol/L) (psychotic disorders – less for Tourette's and mania); Toxic: >42 μg/mL (SI: >84 nmol/L). Therapeutic levels are controversial; dosed by response most commonly.

Test Interactions Decreased cholesterol (S)

Patient Information Oral concentrate must be diluted in 2-4 oz of liquid (water, fruit juice, carbonated drinks, milk, or pudding); do not take antacid within 1 hour of taking drug; avoid alcohol; avoid excess sun exposure (use sun block); may cause drowsiness, rise slowly from recumbent position; use of supportive stockings may help prevent orthostatic hypotension

Nursing Implications Dilute oral concentrate with water or juice before administration; avoid skin contact with oral suspension or solution; may cause contact dermati-

(Continued)

Haloperidol *(Continued)*

tis; monitor orthostatic blood pressures 3-5 days after initiation of therapy or a dose increase; observe for tremor and abnormal movement or posturing (extrapyramidal symptoms)

Special Geriatric Considerations See Warnings

Many elderly patients receive antipsychotic medications for inappropriate nonpsychotic behavior. Before initiating antipsychotic medication, the clinician should investigate any possible reversible cause; any stress or stress from any disease can cause acute "confusion" or worsening of baseline nonpsychotic behavior. Most commonly acute changes in behavior are due to increases in drug dose or addition of new drug to regimen; fluid electrolyte loss; infections; and changes in environment.

Any changes in disease status in any organ system can result in behavior changes.

Dosage Forms

Concentrate, oral: 2 mg/mL (5 mL, 10 mL, 15 mL, 120 mL, 240 mL)

Injection, as decanoate: 50 mg/mL (1 mL, 5 mL); 100 mg/mL (1 mL, 5 mL)

Injection, as lactate: 5 mg/mL (1 mL, 2 mL, 2.5 mL, 10 mL)

Tablet: 0.5 mg, 1 mg, 2 mg, 5 mg, 10 mg, 20 mg

Halotussin® [OTC] *see* Guaifenesin *on page 331*

Halotussin® DM [OTC] *see* Guaifenesin and Dextromethorphan *on page 332*

Haltran® [OTC] *see* Ibuprofen *on page 360*

Haponal® *see* Hyoscyamine, Atropine, Scopolamine and Phenobarbital *on page 357*

HBIG *see* Hepatitis B Immune Globulin *on page 342*

H-BIG® *see* Hepatitis B Immune Globulin *on page 342*

25-HCC *see* Calcifediol *on page 102*

HCTZ *see* Hydrochlorothiazide *on page 347*

Heavy Mineral Oil *see* Mineral Oil *on page 473*

Heparin *(hep' a rin)*

Brand Names Calciparine®; HepFlush®; Hep-Lock®; Liquaemin®

Synonyms Heparin Calcium; Heparin Lock Flush; Heparin Sodium

Generic Available Yes

Therapeutic Class Anticoagulant

Use Prophylaxis and treatment of thromboembolic disorders

Contraindications Hypersensitivity to heparin or any component; severe thrombocytopenia, subacute bacterial endocarditis, suspected intracranial hemorrhage, shock, severe hypotension, uncontrollable bleeding (unless secondary to disseminated intravascular coagulation)

Warnings Some preparations contain sulfite which may cause allergic reactions.

Precautions Use with caution as hemorrhage may occur; risk factors for hemorrhage include I.M. injections, peptic ulcer disease, intermittent I.V. injections (vs continuous I.V. infusion), increased capillary permeability, severe renal, hepatic, or biliary disease, and indwelling catheters

Adverse Reactions

Central nervous system: Fever, headache, chills

Dermatologic: Urticaria

Gastrointestinal: Nausea, vomiting

Hematologic: Hemorrhage, thrombocytopenia

Hepatic: Elevation of liver enzymes

Local: Irritation, ulceration, cutaneous necrosis has been rarely reported with deep S.C. injections

Neuromuscular & skeletal: Osteoporosis

Overdosage Symptoms of overdose include hemorrhage, nose bleeds, hematuria, and melena are signs of overdose

Toxicology Antidote is protamine; 1 mg neutralized 90 units of heparin

Drug Interactions

Decreased effect with digoxin, TCN, nicotine, antihistamine, I.V. NTG

Increased toxicity with NSAIDs, ASA, dipyridamole, dextran, hydroxychloroquine

Stability Stable at room temperature; protect from freezing

Mechanism of Action Potentiates the action of antithrombin III and thereby inactivates thrombin (as well as activated coagulation factors IX, X, XI, XII, and plasmin) and prevents the conversion of fibrinogen to fibrin; heparin also stimulates release of lipoprotein lipase (lipoprotein lipase hydrolyzes triglycerides to glycerol and free fatty acids)

Pharmacodynamics

Onset of action:

S.C.: Anticoagulation occurs within 20-30 minutes

I.V.: Immediate

Duration of action: Dose-dependent

Pharmacokinetics
Absorption: Oral, rectal, S.L., I.M.: Erratic
Metabolism: Believed to be partially metabolized in the reticuloendothelial system
Half-life: Mean: 90 minutes with range: 30 minutes to 3 hours (half-life affected by obesity, renal function, hepatic function, malignancy, presence of pulmonary embolism, and infections), half-life is dose-dependent
Elimination: Hepatic metabolism is followed by renal excretion, small amount excreted unchanged in urine

Usual Dosage Note: For full-dose heparin (ie, non-low dose), the dose should be titrated according to PTT results. For anticoagulation, an APTT 1.5-2.5 times normal is usually desired. APTT is usually measured prior to heparin therapy, 6-8 hours after initiation of a continuous infusion (following a loading dose), and 6-8 hours after changes in the infusion rate; increase or decrease infusion by 2-4 units/kg/hour dependent on PTT. Continuous I.V. infusion is preferred vs I.V. intermittent injections. For intermittent I.V. injections, PTT is measured 3.5-4 hours after I.V. injection.

Geriatrics and Adults:
Prophylaxis (low-dose heparin): S.C.: 5000 units every 8-12 hours
Intermittent I.V.: Initial: 10,000 units, then 50-70 units/kg (5000-10,000 units) every 4-6 hours
I.V. infusion: Initial: 75-100 units/kg, then 15 units/kg/hour with dose adjusted according to PTT results; usual range: 10-30 units/kg/hour

Administration Do not administer I.M. due to pain, irritation, and hematoma formation

Monitoring Parameters PTT, platelets, hemoglobin, hematocrit, and signs of bleeding

Reference Range Therapeutic: 0.3-0.5 units/mL

Test Interactions Increased thyroxine (S) (competitive protein binding methods)

Nursing Implications See Administration

Additional Information Heparin does not possess fibrinolytic activity and, therefore, cannot lyse established thrombi; discontinue heparin if hemorrhage occurs; severe hemorrhage or overdosage may require protamine; monitor platelet counts, signs of bleeding, PTT.

When using daily flushes of heparin to maintain patency of single and double lumen central catheters. Capped PVC catheters and peripheral heparin locks require flushing more frequently (eg, every 6-8 hours). Volume of heparin flush is usually similar to volume of catheter (or slightly greater) or may be standardized according to specific hospital's policy (eg, 2-5 mL/flush). Dose of heparin flush used should not approach therapeutic per kg dose. Additional flushes should be given when stagnant blood is observed in catheter, after catheter is used for drug or blood administration, and after blood withdrawal from catheter.

Heparin 1 unit/mL (final concentration) may be added to TPN solutions, both central and peripheral. (Addition of heparin to peripheral TPN has been shown to increase duration of line patency.)

Arterial lines are heparinized with a final concentration of 1 unit/mL.

Heparin Sodium
(Porcine Intestinal Mucosa)

Strength (units/mL)	Availability			
	MDV (mL)	SDV (mL)	UD (mL)	Hep Lock (mL)
10				1, 2, 2.5, 3, 5, 10, 30
100				1, 2, 2.5, 3, 5, 10, 30
1000	5, 10, 30	1	1, 2	
2500			1	
5000	10	1	0.5, 1	
7500			1	
10,000	4, 5, 10	1	1	
15,000			1	
20,000	2, 5, 10	1	1	
40,000	5	1		

MDV = multiple dose vials.
SDV = single dose vials (ampuls).
UD = unit dose.
Hep lock = heparin lock flush solution.

(Continued)

Heparin (Continued)

Special Geriatric Considerations In the clinical setting, age has not been shown to be a reliable predictor of a patient's anticoagulant response to heparin. However, it is common for older patients to have a "standard" response for the first 24-48 hours after a loading dose (5000 units) and a maintenance infusion of 800-1000 units/hour. After this period, they then have an exaggerated response (ie, elevated PTT), requiring a lower infusion rate. Hence, monitor closely during this period of therapy. Older women are more likely to have bleeding complications and osteoporosis may be a problem when used >3 months or total daily dose exceeds 30,000 units.

Dosage Forms See table on previous page.

References

Bohannon AD and Lyles KW, "Drug-Induced Bone Disease," *Clin Geriatr Med*, 1994, 10(4):611-23.

Bull BS, Korpman RA, Huse WM, et al, "Heparin Therapy During Extracorporeal Circulation. I. Problems Inherent in Existing Heparin Protocols," *J Thorac Cardiovasc Surg*, 1975, 69(5):674-84.

Jick H, Slone D, Borda IT, et al, "Efficacy and Toxicity of Heparin in Relation to Age and Sex," *N Engl J Med*, 1968, 279(6):284-6.

Heparin Calcium *see Heparin on previous page*

Heparin Lock Flush *see Heparin on previous page*

Heparin Sodium *see Heparin on previous page*

Hepatitis B Immune Globulin

Related Information

Immunization Guidelines *on page 759-762*

Brand Names H-BIG®; Hep-B-Gammagee®; HyperHep®

Synonyms HBIG

Therapeutic Class Immune Globulin

Use Provide passive immunity to hepatitis B infection to those individuals exposed

Contraindications Hypersensitivity to hepatitis B immune globulin or any component; allergies to gamma globulin or anti-immunoglobulin antibodies; allergies to thimerosal; IgA deficiency; I.M. injections in patients with thrombocytopenia or coagulation disorders

Warnings Do not give I.V., hypersensitivity reaction; should have epinephrine 1:1000 available to treat anaphylactic reactions; anaphylactic reactions rarely occur

Precautions Skin testing should not be performed due to misinterpretation of positive reaction

Adverse Reactions

Central nervous system: Dizziness, malaise

Dermatologic: Urticaria, rash, angioedema

Local: Pain, tenderness, swelling, erythema

Neuromuscular & skeletal: Joint pains

Miscellaneous: Rarely anaphylaxis

Drug Interactions Live virus vaccines

Stability Refrigerate at 2°C to 8°C (36°F to 46°F); do not freeze

Mechanism of Action Solution of immunoglobulin containing high titer of antibody to hepatitis B surface antigen (HB$_s$Ag)

Usual Dosage Geriatrics and Adults: I.M.: 0.06 mL/kg; usual dose: 3-5 mL for postexposure prophylaxis

Patient Information Be aware of adverse effects

Nursing Implications I.M. injection only; to prevent injury from injection care should be taken when giving to patients with thrombocytopenia or bleeding disorders; do not administer I.V.

Additional Information Hepatitis B immune globulin is not indicated for treatment of active hepatitis B infections and is ineffective in the treatment of chronic active hepatitis B infection; administration of HBIG preceding or concomitantly with hepatitis B vaccine does not interfere with the immune response to vaccine; the two together provide more rapid protective antibodies to hepatitis B than when vaccine is used alone; rapid levels may be necessary in certain settings

Special Geriatric Considerations No data to suggest different dosing in elderly than in younger adults

Dosage Forms Injection: 0.5 mL, 1 mL, 4 mL, 5 mL

Hepatitis B Vaccine

Related Information

Immunization Guidelines *on page 759-762*

Brand Names Engerix-B®; Heptavax-B®; Recombivax HB®

Therapeutic Class Vaccine, Inactivated Virus

Use Immunization against infection caused by all known subtypes of hepatitis B virus in individuals considered at high risk of potential exposure to hepatitis B virus or HB$_s$Ag-positive materials

Contraindications Hypersensitivity to yeast, hepatitis B vaccine, or any component

Warnings Acute hypersensitivity reaction (have epinephrine 1:1000 available); immunosuppressed patients may require larger doses; vaccine will not prevent disease if infected at time of vaccination

Precautions Not recommended for patients on hemodialysis or hematology/oncology patients; caution in patients with thrombocytopenia or bleeding disorders; delay vaccination in patients with active, serious infections; use caution in patients with compromised cardiopulmonary disease

Adverse Reactions
Cardiovascular: Syncope, flushing, hypotension, tachycardia, palpitations
Central nervous system: Headache, fever, dizziness, vertigo, lightheadedness, paresthesia, somnolence, insomnia, irritability, agitation, fatigue, migraine headache, Bell's palsy, chills, malaise
Dermatologic: Rash, angioedema, hives, petechiae, purpura, pruritus
Gastrointestinal: Nausea, vomiting, abdominal cramps, dyspepsia, anorexia, diarrhea
Hematologic: Thrombocytopenia
Hepatic: Abnormal LFTs
Local: Soreness (erythema, swelling), induration, pain, tenderness
Neuromuscular & skeletal: Arthralgia, myalgia, neck and shoulder pain, neck stiffness, generalized aches, weakness
Ocular: Visual disturbances
Respiratory: Cough, bronchospasm, URI, pharyngitis, rhinitis
Miscellaneous: Herpes zoster

Drug Interactions Immunosuppressive agents

Stability Refrigerate, do not freeze

Usual Dosage Geriatrics and Adults: I.M., S.C.: 1 mL (20 mcg), repeat in 1 month and 6 months following initial injection; booster: 1 mL (20 mcg). **Note**: The second dose **must** be given at 1 month (± 1 day) exactly. This will decrease the chance of not developing a positive response (titer). The third dose is not as "time critical" for response.

Monitoring Parameters Measure serum antibody titers

Reference Range Maintain >10 mIU/mL

Patient Information Inform patient of adverse effects

Nursing Implications I.M. injection preferred; S.C. can be used if patient cannot be given I.M. injection

Additional Information Recombivax HB® is a recombinant vaccine derived from HB₅Ag produced in yeast cells

Special Geriatric Considerations Institutionalized elderly may be at risk for hepatitis B such as from human bites; in these cases, administer HBIG 0.06 mL/kg I.M. and give hepatitis B vaccine I.M. at a separate site within 7 days of exposure; give second and third dose at 1 and 6 months; no dose adjustments for age is necessary; some studies demonstrate a lower antibody titer in elderly as compared to young adults

Dosage Forms Injection:
Engerix-B®: Hepatitis B surface antigen 20 mcg/mL
Heptavax-B®: Hepatitis B surface antigen 20 mcg/mL (3 mL)
Recombivax HB®: Hepatitis B surface antigen 10 mcg/mL (3 mL)

References
Gardner P and Schaffner W, "Immunization of Adults," *N Engl J Med*, 1993, 328(17):1252-8.

Hep-B-Gammagee® *see* Hepatitis B Immune Globulin *on previous page*

HepFlush® *see* Heparin *on page 340*

Hep-Lock® *see* Heparin *on page 340*

Heptavax-B® *see* Hepatitis B Vaccine *on previous page*

Herplex® Ophthalmic *see* Idoxuridine *on page 362*

Hexachlorocyclohexane *see* Lindane *on page 407*

Hexadrol® *see* Dexamethasone *on page 207*

Hexamethylenetetramine *see* Methenamine *on page 452*

Hibiclens® [OTC] *see* Chlorhexidine Gluconate *on page 151*

Hiprex® *see* Methenamine *on page 452*

Hismanal® *see* Astemizole *on page 61*

Histaject® *see* Brompheniramine Maleate *on page 95*

Homatropine Hydrobromide (hoe ma' troe peen)

Brand Names AK-Homatropine®; I-Homatrine®; Isopto® Homatropine
Generic Available Yes
Therapeutic Class Anticholinergic Agent, Ophthalmic; Ophthalmic Agent, Mydriatic
Use Producing cycloplegia and mydriasis for refraction; treatment of acute inflammatory conditions of the uveal tract
Contraindications Narrow-angle glaucoma, acute hemorrhage or hypersensitivity to the drug or any component in the formulation

(Continued)

343

Homatropine Hydrobromide *(Continued)*

Precautions Use with caution in patients with hypertension, cardiac disease, or increased intraocular pressure

Adverse Reactions
Cardiovascular: Vascular congestion, edema (local)
Central nervous system: Drowsiness, delirium, cognitive impairment
Dermatologic: Exudate, eczematoid dermatitis
Local: Stinging
Ocular: Follicular conjunctivitis, blurred vision, increased intraocular pressure, photophobia

Overdosage Symptoms of overdose include blurred vision, urinary retention, tachycardia

Toxicology Anticholinergic toxicity is caused by strong binding of the drug to cholinergic receptors. Anticholinesterase inhibitors reduce acetylcholinesterase, the enzyme that breaks down acetylcholine and thereby allows acetylcholine to accumulate and compete for receptor binding with the offending anticholinergic. For anticholinergic overdose with severe life-threatening symptoms, physostigmine 1-2 mg S.C. or I.V., slowly may be given to reverse these effects.

Stability Protect from light

Mechanism of Action Blocks response of iris sphincter muscle and the accommodative muscle of the ciliary body to cholinergic stimulation resulting in dilation and loss of accommodation

Pharmacodynamics
Onset of action: Following ophthalmic instillation, accommodation and pupil effects occur within 30-90 minutes
Duration: Mydriasis persists for 6-24 hours or more and cycloplegia lasts for 10-48 hours

Usual Dosage Geriatrics and Adults:
Mydriasis and cycloplegia for refraction: Instill 1-2 drops of 2% solution or 1 drop of 5% solution before the procedure; repeat at 5- to 10-minute intervals as needed

Uveitis: Instill 1-2 drops 2-3 times/day up to every 3-4 hours as needed

Administration Finger pressure should be applied to lacrimal sac for 1-2 minutes after instillation to decrease risk of absorption and systemic reactions

Patient Information If irritation persists or increases, discontinue use; may cause blurred vision and sensitivity to bright light

Nursing Implications See Administration

Special Geriatric Considerations See Adverse Reactions

Dosage Forms Solution, ophthalmic: 2% (1 mL, 5 mL, 15 mL); 5% (1 mL, 2 mL, 5 mL, 15 mL)

References
Barker DB and Solomon DA, "The Potential for Mental Status Changes Associated With Systemic Absorption of Anticholinergic Ophthalmic Medications: Concerns in the Elderly," *DICP Ann Pharmacother*, 1990, 24(9):847-50.

HuEPO *see* Epoetin Alfa *on page 258*

Humibid® L.A. *see* Guaifenesin *on page 331*

Humibid® Sprinkle *see* Guaifenesin *on page 331*

HuMIST® [OTC] *see* Sodium Chloride *on page 648*

Humulin® L *see* Insulin Preparations *on page 372*

Humulin® N *see* Insulin Preparations *on page 372*

Humulin® R *see* Insulin Preparations *on page 372*

Humulin® U *see* Insulin Preparations *on page 372*

Hyaluronidase *(hye al yoor on' i dase)*

Brand Names Wydase®

Generic Available No

Therapeutic Class Antidote, Extravasation

Use Increase the dispersion and absorption of other drugs; increase rate of absorption of parenteral fluids given by hypodermoclysis; enhance diffusion of locally irritating or toxic drugs in the management of I.V. extravasation

Contraindications Hypersensitivity to hyaluronidase or any component; do not inject in or around infected, inflamed, or cancerous areas

Warnings Drug infiltrates in which hyaluronidase is contraindicated: dopamine, alpha agonists

Precautions An intradermal skin test for sensitivity should be performed before actual administration using 0.02 mL of hyaluronidase

Adverse Reactions Allergic reactions are rare, isolated cases of anaphylactic-like reactions have occurred

Overdosage Symptoms of overdose include urticaria, erythema, chills, nausea, vomiting, dizziness, tachycardia, hypotension

Toxicology Treatment is supportive

Drug Interactions Decreased effect: Salicylates, cortisone, ACTH, estrogens, antihistamines

Stability Reconstituted hyaluronidase solution remains stable for only 24 hours when stored in the refrigerator; do not use discolored solutions

Mechanism of Action Modifies the permeability of connective tissue through hydrolysis of hyaluronic acid, one of the chief ingredients of tissue cement which offers resistance to diffusion of liquids through tissues

Pharmacodynamics
Onset of action by S.C. or intradermal routes for the treatment of extravasation: Immediate
Duration: 24-48 hours

Usual Dosage Geriatrics and Adults:
Absorption and dispersion of drugs: 150 units is added to the vehicle containing the drug

Hypodermoclysis: 1 mL (150 units) is added to 1000 mL of infusion fluid and 0.5 mL (75 units) is injected into each clysis site at the initiation of the infusion

Monitoring Parameters Fluid status, electrolytes

Nursing Implications Administer hyaluronidase within the first few minutes to 1 hour after the extravasation is recognized; do not administer I.V.

Additional Information The USP hyaluronidase unit is equivalent to the turbidity-reducing (TR) unit and the International Unit; each unit is defined as being the activity contained in 100 mcg of the International Standard Preparation

Special Geriatric Considerations The most common use of hyaluronidase in the elderly is in hypodermoclysis. Hypodermoclysis is very useful in dehydrated patients in whom oral intake is minimal and I.V. access is a problem.

Dosage Forms Injection:
Lyophilized: 150 units/mL (1 mL, 10 mL)
Stabilized: 150 units/mL (1 mL, 10 mL)

References
Berger EY, "Nutrition by Hypodermoclysis," *J Am Geriatr Soc*, 1984, 32(3):199-203.
Lipschitz S, Campbell AJ, Roberts MS, et al, "Subcutaneous Fluid Administration in Elderly Subjects: Validation of an Underused Technique," *J Am Geriatr Soc*, 1991, 39(1):6-9.

Hydeltrasol® *see* Prednisolone *on page 584*

Hydeltra-T.B.A.® *see* Prednisolone *on page 584*

Hydextran® *see* Iron Dextran Complex *on page 377*

Hydralazine and Hydrochlorothiazide
(hye dral' azeen & hye droe klor oh thye' a zide)

Related Information
Hydralazine Hydrochloride *on this page*
Hydrochlorothiazide *on page 347*

Brand Names Apresazide®

Generic Available Yes

Therapeutic Class Antihypertensive, Combination

Special Geriatric Considerations Combination products are not recommended for first-line treatment and divided doses of diuretics may increase the incidence of nocturia in the elderly

Dosage Forms Tablet: Hydralazine hydrochloride 50 mg and hydrochlorothiazide 50 mg; hydralazine hydrochloride 100 mg and hydrochlorothiazide 50 mg; hydralazine hydrochloride 25 mg and hydrochlorothiazide 25 mg; hydralazine hydrochloride 25 mg and hydrochlorothiazide 15 mg

Hydralazine and Reserpine

Related Information
Hydralazine Hydrochloride *on this page*
Reserpine *on page 625*

Brand Names Serpasil®-Apresoline®

Generic Available No

Therapeutic Class Rauwolfia Alkaloid; Vasodilator

Special Geriatric Considerations Combination products are not recommended for first-line treatment

Dosage Forms Tablet: Hydralazine hydrochloride 25 mg and reserpine 0.1 mg; hydralazine hydrochloride 50 mg and reserpine 0.2 mg

Hydralazine Hydrochloride (hye dral' a zeen)

Brand Names Apresoline®

Generic Available Yes

Therapeutic Class Vasodilator

Use Management of moderate to severe hypertension, congestive heart failure

Contraindications Hypersensitivity to hydralazine or any component, dissecting aor-

(Continued)

345

Hydralazine Hydrochloride *(Continued)*

tic aneurysm, mitral valve rheumatic heart disease, known or suspected coronary artery disease

Warnings Monitor blood pressure closely with I.V. use; some formulations may contain tartrazines or sulfites

Precautions Discontinue hydralazine in patients who develop SLE-like syndrome or positive ANA. Use with caution in patients with severe renal disease or cerebral vascular accidents.

Adverse Reactions

Cardiovascular: Palpitations, flushing, tachycardia, dizziness, edema, rarely orthostatic hypotension

Central nervous system: Peripheral neuritis, headache

Gastrointestinal: Anorexia, nausea, vomiting, diarrhea

Neuromuscular & skeletal: Weakness

Miscellaneous: SLE-like syndrome (fever, rash, arthralgias, malaise, positive ANA, positive LE cells); this may occur in patients on high doses (>200 mg/day) and prolonged therapy

Note: Because of blunted baroreceptor response, the elderly are less likely to experience reflex tachycardia; this puts them at greater risk for orthostatic hypotension

Overdosage Symptoms of overdose include hypotension, tachycardia, shock

Toxicology Hypotension usually responds to I.V. fluids or Trendelenburg positioning. If unresponsive to these measures the use of a parenteral vasoconstrictor may be required (eg, norepinephrine 0.1-0.2 mcg/kg/minute titrated to response). Treatment is primarily supportive and symptomatic.

Drug Interactions

Decreased effect: Indomethacin

Increased effect: MAO inhibitors, other hypotensive agents

Stability Changes color after contact with a metal filter; do not store intact ampuls in refrigerator

Mechanism of Action Direct vasodilation of arterioles (with little effect on veins) with decreased systemic resistance

Pharmacodynamics

Onset of action:

Oral: 20-30 minutes

I.V.: 5-20 minutes

Duration:

Oral: 6-8 hours

I.V.: 2-4 hours

Pharmacokinetics

Metabolism: Oral: Large first-pass effect

Bioavailability: 30% to 50%; enhanced by the concurrent ingestion of food

Usual Dosage

Geriatrics: Oral: Initial: 10 mg 2-3 times/day, increase by 10-25 mg/day every 2-5 days

Adults:

Oral: Initial: 10 mg 4 times/day, increase by 10-25 mg/dose every 2-5 days to maximum of 300 mg/day

I.M., I.V.: Hypertensive initial: 10-20 mg/dose every 4-6 hours as needed, may increase to 40 mg/dose; change to oral therapy as soon as possible

Monitoring Parameters Blood pressure, standing and sitting/supine

Test Interactions Increased calcium (S)

Patient Information Report flu-like symptoms, rise from sitting/lying carefully, may cause dizziness; take with meals

Nursing Implications Monitor blood pressure closely with I.V. use

Additional Information Has also been used to treat primary pulmonary hypertension. Slow acetylators, patients with decreased renal function and patients receiving >200 mg/day (chronically) are at higher risk for SLE. Titrate dosage to patient's response. Usually administered with diuretic and a beta-blocker to counteract side effects of sodium and water retention and reflex tachycardia although the beta-blocker may not be necessary in the elderly.

Special Geriatric Considerations See Adverse Reactions and Usual Dosage

Dosage Forms

Injection: 20 mg/mL (1 mL)

Tablet: 10 mg, 25 mg, 50 mg, 100 mg

References

Feinberg LE, "Hypertension in the Aged," *Clinical Internal Medicine in the Aged*, Schrier RW, ed, Philadelphia, PA: WB Saunders, 1982, 66-86.

Hydralazine, Hydrochlorothiazide, and Reserpine

Related Information

Hydralazine Hydrochloride *on previous page*

Hydrochlorothiazide *on next page*

Reserpine *on page 625*
Brand Names Ser-Ap-Es®
Generic Available Yes
Therapeutic Class Antihypertensive, Combination
Special Geriatric Considerations Combination products are not recommended for first-line treatment and divided doses of diuretics may increase the incidence of nocturia in the elderly
Dosage Forms Tablet: Hydralazine 25 mg, hydrochlorothiazide 15 mg and reserpine 0.1 mg

Hydrate® *see* Dimenhydrinate *on page 227*

Hydrated Chloral *see* Chloral Hydrate *on page 146*

Hydrea® *see* Hydroxyurea *on page 355*

Hydrocet® *see* Hydrocodone and Acetaminophen *on page 350*

Hydrochlorothiazide (hye droe klor oh thye' a zide)
Brand Names Aquazide-H®; Diaqua®; Esidrix®; HydroDIURIL®; Hydro-T®; Micrin®; Oretic®; Thiuretic®
Synonyms HCTZ
Generic Available Yes: Tablet
Therapeutic Class Diuretic, Thiazide
Use Management of mild to moderate hypertension; treatment of edema in congestive heart failure and nephrotic syndrome
Contraindications Anuria, renal decompensation, hypersensitivity to hydrochlorothiazide or any component, cross-sensitivity with other thiazides and sulfonamide derivatives
Precautions Hypokalemia, renal disease, hepatic disease, gout, lupus erythematosus, diabetes mellitus; use with caution in severe renal diseases; ineffective in patients with Cl_{cr} <30 mL/minute
Adverse Reactions
Cardiovascular: Hypotension
Central nervous system: Drowsiness, paresthesia
Dermatologic: Rash, photosensitivity
Endocrine & metabolic: Hypokalemia, hyponatremia, hyperglycemia
Gastrointestinal: Nausea, vomiting, anorexia
Genitourinary: Prerenal azotemia
Hematologic: Aplastic anemia, hemolytic anemia, leukopenia, agranulocytosis, thrombocytopenia (all rare)
Hepatic: Hepatitis
Renal: Polyuria
Overdosage Symptoms of overdose include electrolyte depletion, volume depletion, hypotension, dehydration, circulatory collapse
Toxicology Following GI decontamination, treatment is supportive; hypotension responds to fluids and Trendelenburg position
Drug Interactions
Decreased effect of oral hypoglycemics; decreased absorption with cholestyramine and colestipol
Increased effect with loop diuretics and other antihypertensives
Increased toxicity/levels of lithium; when given with digoxin, diuretic-induced hypokalemia increases the risk of digoxin toxicity
Mechanism of Action Inhibits sodium reabsorption in the distal tubules causing increased excretion of sodium and water as well as potassium and hydrogen ions
Pharmacodynamics
Peak effects require 4 hours while diuresis can continue for 6-12 hours
Onset of diuretic action: Oral: Within 2 hours
Duration of action: 6-12 hours
Pharmacokinetics Absorption: Oral: ~60% to 80%
Usual Dosage Oral:
Geriatrics: Initial: 12.5-25 mg once daily; minimal increase in response and more electrolyte disturbances are seen with doses >50 mg/day

Adults: 25-100 mg/day in 1-2 doses; maximum: 200 mg/day
Monitoring Parameters Blood pressure (both standing and sitting/supine), serum electrolytes, renal function, weight, I & O
Test Interactions Increased ammonia (B), increased amylase (S), increased calcium (S), increased chloride (S), increased cholesterol (S), increased glucose, increased uric acid (S); decreased chloride (S), decreased magnesium, decreased potassium (S), decreased sodium (S). Tyramine and phentolamine tests, histamine tests for pheochromocytoma.
Patient Information May be taken with food or milk; take early in day to avoid nocturia; take the last dose of multiple doses no later than 6 PM unless instructed otherwise. A few people who take this medication become more sensitive to sunlight and
(Continued)

Hydrochlorothiazide *(Continued)*

may experience skin rash, redness, itching or severe sunburn, especially if sun block SPF ≥15 is not used on exposed skin areas.

Nursing Implications See Monitoring Parameters; check patient for orthostasis

Additional Information Effect of drug may be decreased when used every day

Special Geriatric Considerations Hydrochlorothiazide is not effective in patients with a Cl_{cr} <30 mL/minute, therefore, it may not be a useful agent in many elderly patients; see Usual Dosage

Dosage Forms
Solution:
Oral: 50 mg/5 mL (5 mL, 500 mL)
Oral, concentrate: 100 mg/mL (30 mL)
Tablet: 25 mg, 50 mg, 100 mg

Hydrochlorothiazide and Amiloride *see* Amiloride and Hydrochlorothiazide *on page 38*

Hydrochlorothiazide and Methyldopa *see* Methyldopa and Hydrochlorothiazide *on page 459*

Hydrochlorothiazide and Reserpine

Related Information
Hydrochlorothiazide *on previous page*
Reserpine *on page 625*

Brand Names Hydropres®

Synonyms Reserpine and Hydrochlorothiazide

Generic Available Yes

Therapeutic Class Antihypertensive, Combination

Special Geriatric Considerations Combination products are not recommended for first-line treatment and divided doses of diuretics may increase the incidence of nocturia in the elderly

Dosage Forms Tablet:
25 Hydrochlorothiazide 25 mg and reserpine 0.125 mg
50 Hydrochlorothiazide 50 mg and reserpine 0.125 mg

Hydrochlorothiazide and Spironolactone (speer on oh lak' tone)

Related Information
Hydrochlorothiazide *on previous page*
Spironolactone *on page 655*

Brand Names Aldactazide®

Synonyms Spironolactone and Hydrochlorothiazide

Generic Available Yes

Therapeutic Class Antihypertensive, Combination; Diuretic, Combination

Use Management of mild to moderate hypertension; treatment of edema in congestive heart failure and nephrotic syndrome; cirrhosis of the liver accompanied by edema or ascites

Contraindications Anuria, hyperkalemia, renal or hepatic failure, hypersensitivity to hydrochlorothiazide, spironolactone, or any component

Warnings This fixed combination is not indicated for initial therapy of hypertension; therapy requires titration to the individual patient, if dosage so determined represents this fixed combination, its use may be more convenient; has been shown to be tumorigenic in toxicity studies using rats at 25 to 250 times the usual human dose

Adverse Reactions
Cardiovascular: Hypotension
Central nervous system: Lethargy, headache
Dermatologic: Rash
Endocrine & metabolic: Hyperkalemia, gynecomastia, hyperchloremic metabolic acidosis, dehydration, hyponatremia
Gastrointestinal: Anorexia, nausea, vomiting, diarrhea

Overdosage Symptoms of overdose include drowsiness, confusion, clinical signs of dehydration and electrolyte imbalance

Toxicology Ingestion of large amounts of potassium-sparing diuretics may result in life-threatening hyperkalemia. This can be treated with I.V. glucose (dextrose 25% in water), with concurrent I.V. sodium bicarbonate (1 mEq/kg up to 44 mEq/dose), and 0.2-0.5 units of rapid-acting insulin per gram of glucose. If needed, Kayexalate® oral or rectal solutions in sorbitol may also be useful.

Drug Interactions
Increased risk of hyperkalemia if given with other potassium-sparing diuretics, potassium supplements, or ACE inhibitors
NSAIDs may reduce therapeutic effect

Usual Dosage Oral:
Geriatrics: Initial: 1 tablet/day, increase as necessary
Adults: 1-8 tablets of Aldactazide®-25 (1-4 tablets of Aldactazide®-50) in 1-2 divided doses

Monitoring Parameters Blood pressure, serum electrolytes, renal function, weight, I & O

Test Interactions Plasma and urinary cortisol levels

Patient Information Take in the morning; take the last dose of multiple doses before 6 PM unless instructed otherwise; may cause increased sensitivity to sunlight; avoid excessive ingestion of foods high in potassium or use of salt substitutes

Nursing Implications May interfere with digoxin serum assays; monitor for signs of hyperkalemia; see Monitoring Parameters

Additional Information See individual components for full prescribing information

Special Geriatric Considerations The efficacy of hydrochlorothiazide is limited in patients with a Cl_{cr} <30 mL/minute; monitor serum potassium; see Warnings

Dosage Forms Tablet:
25/25: Hydrochlorothiazide 25 mg and spironolactone 25 mg
50/50: Hydrochlorothiazide 50 mg and spironolactone 50 mg

Hydrochlorothiazide and Triamterene (trye am' ter een)

Related Information
Hydrochlorothiazide on page 347
Triamterene on page 712

Brand Names Dyazide®; Maxzide®; Maxzide®-25

Synonyms Triamterene and Hydrochlorothiazide

Generic Available Yes (Dyazide® strength only)

Therapeutic Class Diuretic, Combination

Use Management of mild to moderate hypertension; treatment of edema in congestive heart failure and nephrotic syndrome

Contraindications Anuria, hyperkalemia, renal, or hepatic failure, hypersensitivity to hydrochlorothiazide, triamterene or any component; concurrent use of potassium supplements

Warnings This fixed combination is not indicated for initial therapy of hypertension; therapy requires titration to the individual patient, if dosage so determined represents this fixed combination, its use may be more convenient

Adverse Reactions
Cardiovascular: Hypotension
Central nervous system: Dizziness, headache
Endocrine & metabolic: Electrolyte disturbances
Gastrointestinal: Nausea, vomiting

Overdosage Symptoms of overdose include drowsiness, confusion, clinical signs of dehydration and electrolyte imbalance

Toxicology Ingestion of large amounts of potassium-sparing diuretics may result in life-threatening hyperkalemia. This can be treated with I.V. glucose (dextrose 25% in water), with concurrent I.V. sodium bicarbonate (1 mEq/kg up to 44 mEq/dose), and 0.2-0.5 units of rapid-acting insulin per gram of glucose. If needed, Kayexalate® oral or rectal solutions in sorbitol may also be useful.

Drug Interactions
Increased risk of hyperkalemia if given with other potassium-sparing diuretics, potassium supplements, or ACE inhibitors
NSAIDs may reduce therapeutic effect

Food/Drug Interactions Avoid excessive ingestions of foods high in potassium or use of salt substitutes

Stability Protect from light

Usual Dosage
Geriatrics: Oral:
Dyazide®: Initial: 1 capsule/day or every other day
Maxzide®-25: Initial: 1 capsule/day or every other day

Adults:
Dyazide®, Maxzide®-25: 1-2 capsules twice daily after meals
Maxzide®: 1 capsule/day

Monitoring Parameters Blood pressure, serum electrolytes, renal function, weight, I & O

Test Interactions Serum creatinine and BUN, bentiromide test, fluorescent measurement of quinidine

Patient Information Take in the morning with meals or milk; may cause increased sensitivity to sunlight; avoid excessive ingestion of foods high in potassium or use of salt substitutes

Nursing Implications See Monitoring Parameters; monitor for signs of hyperkalemia

Additional Information Dyazide® and Maxzide® are not bioequivalent. *One product should not be substituted for the other.* Retitration and appropriate changes in dosage may be necessary if patients are to be transferred from one dosage form to the other. Serum potassium concentrations do not necessarily indicate the true body potassium concentration. A rise in plasma pH or an increase in the circulating levels of insulin or epinephrine may cause a decrease in plasma potassium concentration and an increase in the intracellular potassium concentration.

(Continued)

Hydrochlorothiazide and Triamterene *(Continued)*

Special Geriatric Considerations The efficacy of hydrochlorothiazide is limited in patients with Cl_{cr} <30 mL/minute; monitor serum potassium; see Warnings and Additional Information

Dosage Forms

Capsule (Dyazide®): Hydrochlorothiazide 25 mg and triamterene 37.5 mg

Tablet:

Maxzide®-25: Hydrochlorothiazide 25 mg and triamterene 37.5 mg

Maxzide®: Hydrochlorothiazide 50 mg and triamterene 75 mg

Hydrocil® [OTC] *see* Psyllium *on page 610*

Hydrocodone and Acetaminophen (hye droe koe' done)

Related Information

Narcotic Agonist Comparative Pharmacology *on page 811*

Pharmacokinetics of Narcotic Agonist Analgesics *on page 812*

Brand Names Anexia®; Bancap HC®; Co-Gesic®; Dolacet®; DuoCet™; Hydrocet®; Hydrogesic®; Hy-Phen®; Lortab®; Norcet®; T-Gesic®; Vicodin®; Zydone®

Synonyms Acetaminophen and Hydrocodone

Generic Available Yes

Therapeutic Class Analgesic, Narcotic

Use Relief of moderate to severe pain; antitussive (hydrocodone)

Restrictions C-III

Contraindications CNS depression, hypersensitivity to hydrocodone, acetaminophen or any component; severe respiratory depression

Warnings Some tablets contain sulfites which may cause allergic reactions

Precautions Contains sulfites which may cause allergic reactions; use with caution in patients with hypersensitivity reactions to other phenanthrene derivative opioid agonists (morphine, codeine, hydromorphone, oxycodone, oxymorphone, levorphanol)

Adverse Reactions

Cardiovascular: Hypotension, bradycardia, peripheral vasodilation

Central nervous system: CNS depression, drowsiness, dizziness, sedation, confusion, increased intracranial pressure

Endocrine & metabolic: Antidiuretic hormone release

Gastrointestinal: Nausea, vomiting, constipation

Ocular: Miosis

Respiratory: Respiratory depression

Miscellaneous: Physical and psychological dependence with prolonged use, biliary or urinary tract spasm, histamine release

Overdosage Symptoms of overdose include hepatic necrosis, blood dyscrasias, respiratory depression

Toxicology Treatment of an overdose includes support of the patient's airway, establishment of an I.V. line and administration of naloxone 2 mg I.V. with repeat administration as necessary. Mucomyst® (acetylcysteine) 140 mg/kg orally (loading) followed by 70 mg/kg (maintenance) every 4 hours for 17 doses. Therapy should be initiated based upon laboratory analysis suggesting high probability of hepatotoxic potential.

Drug Interactions

Decreased effect with phenothiazines

Increased effect with dextroamphetamine

Increased toxicity with CNS depressants, TCAs

Mechanism of Action

Hydrocodone: Binds to opiate receptors in the CNS, causing inhibition of ascending pain pathways, altering the perception of and response to pain; causes cough suppression by direct central action in the medulla; produces generalized CNS depression

Acetaminophen: See individual agent

Pharmacodynamics

Onset of action: Oral: Narcotic analgesia occurs within 10-20 minutes following administration

Duration: 3-6 hours; enhanced analgesia has been seen in elderly patients on therapeutic doses of narcotics; duration of action may be increased in the elderly

Pharmacokinetics

Metabolism: In the liver

Half-life: 3.8 hours

Elimination: In urine

Usual Dosage Doses should be titrated to appropriate analgesic effect

Geriatrics: 2.5-5 mg of the hydrocodone component every 4-6 hours; do not exceed 4 g/day of acetaminophen

Adults: 1-2 tablets or capsules every 4-6 hours

Monitoring Parameters Pain relief, respiratory and mental status, blood pressure

Patient Information May cause drowsiness; avoid alcoholic beverages; do not exceed recommended dose

Nursing Implications Observe patient for excessive sedation, respiratory depression

Special Geriatric Considerations See Adverse Reactions and Pharmacodynamics; the elderly may be particularly susceptible to the CNS depressant action (sedation, confusion) and constipating effects of narcotics; if one tablet/dose is used, it may be useful to add an additional 325 mg of acetaminophen to maximize analgesic effect

Dosage Forms

Capsule: Hydrocodone bitartrate 5 mg and acetaminophen 500 mg

Solution: Hydrocodone bitartrate 2.5 mg and acetaminophen 120 mg per 5 mL (480 mL)

Tablet: Hydrocodone bitartrate 2.5 mg and acetaminophen 500 mg; hydrocodone bitartrate 5 mg and acetaminophen 500 mg; hydrocodone bitartrate 7.5 mg and acetaminophen 500 mg

Hydrocortisone (hye droe kor' ti sone)

Related Information

Antacid Drug Interactions *on page 764*

Corticosteroids Comparison, Systemic *on page 808*

Corticosteroids Comparison, Topical *on page 809*

Brand Names Aeroseb-HC®; A-hydroCort®; CaldeCORT®; Cetacort®; Cortaid® [OTC]; Cort-Dome®; Cortef®; Cortifoam®; Cortril®; DermiCort® [OTC]; Dermolate® [OTC]; Hydrocortone®; Hydro-Tex®; Hytone®; Lexocort®; Locoid®; Nutracort®; Orabase® HCA; Penecort®; Proctocort™; Solu-Cortef®; Synacort®; U-Cort™; Westcort®

Synonyms Compound F; Cortisol; Hydrocortisone Acetate; Hydrocortisone Cypionate; Hydrocortisone Sodium Phosphate; Hydrocortisone Sodium Succinate

Generic Available Yes

Therapeutic Class Adrenal Corticosteroid; Anti-inflammatory Agent; Corticosteroid, Rectal; Corticosteroid, Systemic; Corticosteroid, Topical (Low Potency)

Use Management of adrenocortical insufficiency; relief of inflammation of corticosteroid-responsive dermatoses; adjunctive treatment of ulcerative colitis

Contraindications Serious infections, except septic shock or tuberculous meningitis; known hypersensitivity to hydrocortisone; viral, fungal, or tubercular skin lesions

Warnings Acute adrenal insufficiency may occur with abrupt withdrawal after long-term therapy or with stress

Precautions Use with caution in patients with hyperthyroidism, cirrhosis, nonspecific ulcerative colitis, hypertension, osteoporosis, thromboembolic tendencies, congestive heart failure, convulsive disorders, myasthenia gravis, thrombophlebitis, peptic ulcer, diabetes

Adverse Reactions

Cardiovascular: Hypertension, edema, accelerated atherogenesis

Central nervous system: Euphoria, insomnia, headache, vertigo, seizures, psychoses, pseudotumor cerebri

Dermatologic: Acne, dermatitis, skin atrophy, impaired wound healing, hirsutism

Endocrine & metabolic: Hypokalemia, hyperglycemia, Cushing's syndrome, alkalosis, pituitary-adrenal, hot flashes, postmenopausal bleeding, axis suppression, glucose intolerance

Gastrointestinal: Peptic ulcer, pancreatitis, nausea, vomiting

Neuromuscular & skeletal: Osteoporosis, fractures, aseptic necrosis of femoral and humeral heads, steroid myopathy

Ocular: Cataracts, glaucoma

Miscellaneous: Immunosuppression

Toxicology When consumed in excessive quantities for prolonged periods, systemic hypercorticism and adrenal suppression may occur; in those cases, discontinuation and withdrawal of the corticosteroid should be done judiciously

Drug Interactions

Steroids decrease the effect of anticholinesterases, isoniazid, salicylates, insulin, oral hypoglycemics

Decreased effect: Barbiturates, phenytoin, rifampin

Increased effect (hypokalemia) of potassium-depleting diuretics

Increased risk of digoxin toxicity (due to hypokalemia)

Increased effect: Estrogens, ketoconazole

Mechanism of Action Decreases inflammation by suppression of migration of polymorphonuclear leukocytes and reversal of increased capillary permeability

Pharmacokinetics

Absorption: Rapid by all routes, except rectally

Metabolism: In the liver and excreted renally, mainly as 17-hydroxysteroids and 17-ketosteroids

Half-life: Biologic: 8-12 hours

Usual Dosage

Acute adrenal insufficiency: Geriatrics and Adults: I.M., I.V., S.C.: 15-240 mg every 12 hours of hydrocortisone phosphate

Anti-inflammatory or immunosuppressive:

Geriatrics: Use lowest effective dose

(Continued)

Hydrocortisone *(Continued)*

Adults: Oral, I.M., S.C., I.V.: 15-240 mg every 12 hours

Shock: Geriatrics and Adults: I.M., I.V.: 500 mg to 2 g every 2-6 hours (succinate)

Geriatrics and Adults:
Rectal: Apply 1 application 1-2 times/day for 2-3 weeks
Topical: Apply to affected area 3-4 times/day

Monitoring Parameters Blood pressure, blood glucose, electrolytes, weight, symptoms of fluid retention

Reference Range Therapeutic: AM: 5-25 μg/dL (SI: 138-690 nmol/L); PM: 2-9 μg/dL (SI: 55-248 nmol/L) depending on test, assay

Test Interactions Increased amylase (S), chloride (S), increased cholesterol (S), increased glucose, increased protein, increased sodium (S); decreased calcium (S), decreased chloride (S), decreased potassium (S), decreased thyroxine (S)

Patient Information Notify surgeon or dentist before surgical repair; may cause GI upset; take with food or milk; notify physician if any sign of infection occurs; avoid abrupt withdrawal when on long-term oral therapy; do not use topical products on broken skin

Nursing Implications Give with meals to decrease GI upset; apply sparingly

Additional Information
Hydrocortisone: Cortone® tablet, Hydrocortone®
Hydrocortisone acetate: Hydrocortone® acetate injection
Hydrocortisone cipionate: Cortef® suspension
Hydrocortisone sodium phosphate: Hydrocortone® phosphate injection
Hydrocortisone sodium succinate: A-hydroCort® injection, Solu-Cortef® injection

Special Geriatric Considerations Because of the risk of adverse effects, systemic corticosteroids should be used cautiously in the elderly, in the smallest possible dose, and for the shortest possible time.

Dosage Forms
Aerosol, topical: 0.53 mg/1 sec spray (58 g)
Cream, as acetate: 0.5% (15 g, 30 g); 1% (30 g, 120 g)
Cream, as butyrate: 0.1% (15 g, 45 g, 60 g)
Cream:
Rectal: 1% (30 g with applicator)
Topical: 0.25% (30 g); 0.5% (15 g, 30 g, 120 g, 454 g); 1% (15 g, 20 g, 30 g, 120 g, 454 g); 2.5% (20 g, 30 g, 60 g, 454 g)
Topical, as valerate: 0.2% (15 g, 45 g, 60 g)
Enema: 100 mg/60 mL each unit (7 units/box)
Foam, rectal, as acetate: 10% (20 g)
Injection, as acetate: 25 mg/mL (3 mL, 10 mL); 50 mg/mL (5 mL, 10 mL)
Injection, as sodium phosphate: 50 mg/mL (2 mL, 10 mL)
Injection, as succinate: 100 mg, 250 mg, 500 mg
Injection, as sodium succinate: 100 mg, 250 mg, 500 mg, 1000 mg
Lotion: 0.25% (30 mL, 120 mL); 0.5% (30 mL, 60 mL, 120 mL); 1% (30 mL, 60 mL, 120 mL); 2.5% (60 mL, 120 mL)
Lotion, as acetate: 0.5% (30 mL)
Ointment, as acetate: 0.5% (15 g); 1% (30 g)
Ointment, as butyrate: 0.1% (15 g, 45 g)
Ointment:
Topical: 0.5% (30 g)
Topical, as valerate: 0.2% (15 g, 45 g, 60 g)
Paste, oral topical, as acetate: 0.5%
Suppository, as acetate: 25 mg
Suspension, as cipionate, oral: 10 mg/5 mL (120 mL)
Tablet: 5 mg, 10 mg, 20 mg

Hydrocortisone Acetate *see Hydrocortisone on previous page*

Hydrocortisone Cypionate *see Hydrocortisone on previous page*

Hydrocortisone Sodium Phosphate *see Hydrocortisone on previous page*

Hydrocortisone Sodium Succinate *see Hydrocortisone on previous page*

Hydrocortone® *see Hydrocortisone on previous page*

HydroDIURIL® *see Hydrochlorothiazide on page 347*

Hydrogesic® *see Hydrocodone and Acetaminophen on page 350*

Hydromagnesium aluminate *see Magaldrate on page 424*

Hydromorphone Hydrochloride *(hye droe mor' fone)*

Related Information
Narcotic Agonist Comparative Pharmacology *on page 811*
Pharmacokinetics of Narcotic Agonist Analgesics *on page 812*

Brand Names Dilaudid®; Dilaudid® Cough Syrup

Synonyms Dihydromorphinone

Generic Available Yes

Therapeutic Class Analgesic, Narcotic; Antitussive

Use Management of moderate to severe pain; antitussive at lower doses

Restrictions C-II

Contraindications Hypersensitivity to hydromorphone or any component

Warnings Injection contains benzyl alcohol

Precautions Tablet and cough syrup contain tartrazine which may cause allergic reactions; hydromorphone shares toxic potential of opiate agonists, and precaution of opiate agonist therapy should be observed; extreme caution should be taken to avoid confusing the highly concentrated injection with the less concentrated injectable product. Use caution in postoperative and pulmonary patients since hydromorphone can suppress the cough reflex. Use caution in impaired hepatic and/or renal function, and in patients allergic to other phenanthrene opiates

Adverse Reactions

Cardiovascular: Palpitations, hypotension, bradycardia, peripheral vasodilation

Central nervous system: CNS depression

Dermatologic: Pruritus

Endocrine & metabolic: Antidiuretic hormone release

Gastrointestinal: Nausea, vomiting, constipation

Ocular: Miosis

Respiratory: Respiratory depression

Miscellaneous: Increased intracranial pressure, physical and psychological dependence, histamine release, biliary or urinary tract spasm

Overdosage Symptoms of overdose include CNS depression, respiratory depression, miosis, apnea, pulmonary edema

Toxicology Maintain airway, establish I.V. line and give naloxone 2 mg I.V. with repeat administration as necessary up to a total of 10 mg

Drug Interactions Increased toxicity: CNS depressants, phenothiazines, tricyclic antidepressants

Stability Protect tablets from light; do not store intact ampuls in refrigerator; a slightly yellowish discoloration has not been associated with a loss of potency; not compatible with alkalies, bromides and iodides

Mechanism of Action Binds to opiate receptors in the CNS, causing inhibition of ascending pain pathways, altering the perception of and response to pain; causes cough supression by direct central action in the medulla; produces generalized CNS depression

Pharmacodynamics

Onset of action: Oral: Following administration, analgesic effects occur within 15-30 minutes

Peak effects: Within 30-90 minutes

Duration: 4-5 hours; enhanced analgesia has been seen in elderly patients on therapeutic doses of narcotics; duration of action may be increased in the elderly

Pharmacokinetics

Metabolism: Primarily in the liver

Bioavailability: 62%

Half-life: 1-3 hours

Elimination: In urine principally as glucuronide conjugates

Usual Dosage Doses should be titrated to appropriate analgesic effects; when changing routes of administration, note that oral doses are less than half as effective as parenteral doses (may be only 20% as effective)

Pain:

Geriatrics: Oral: 1-2 mg every 4-6 hours

Adults:

Oral, I.M., I.V., S.C.: 1-4 mg/dose every 4-6 hours as needed; usual adult dose: 2 mg/dose

Rectal: 3 mg every 6-8 hours

Antitussive: Geriatrics and Adults: Oral: 1 mg every 3-4 hours as needed

Monitoring Parameters Pain relief, respiratory and mental status, blood pressure

Test Interactions Increased aminotransferase [ALT (SGPT)/AST (SGOT)] (S)

Patient Information May cause drowsiness; avoid the use of alcohol and other CNS depressants

Nursing Implications Observe patient for oversedation, respiratory depression

Additional Information Equianalgesic doses: Morphine 10 mg I.M. = hydromorphone 1.5 mg I.M.

Special Geriatric Considerations The elderly may be particularly susceptible to the CNS depressant and constipating effects of the narcotics; see Pharmacodynamics

Dosage Forms

Injection: 1 mg/mL (1 mL); 2 mg/mL (1 mL, 20 mL); 3 mg/mL (1 mL); 4 mg/mL (1 mL); 10 mg/mL (1 mL, 2 mL, 5 mL)

Suppository, rectal: 3 mg

Syrup: Hydromorphone hydrochloride 1 mg and guaifenesin 100 mg/5 mL (450 mL)

(Continued)

Hydromorphone Hydrochloride *(Continued)*

Tablet: 1 mg, 2 mg, 3 mg, 4 mg

References

Ferrell BA, "Pain Management in Elderly People," *J Am Geriatr Soc*, 1991, 39(1):64-73.

Kaiko RF, Wallenstein SL, Rogers AG, et al, "Narcotics in the Elderly," *Med Clin North Am*, 1982, 66(5):1079-89.

Hydropres® *see* Hydrochlorothiazide and Reserpine *on page 348*

Hydro-T® *see* Hydrochlorothiazide *on page 347*

Hydro-Tex® *see* Hydrocortisone *on page 351*

Hydroxacen® *see* Hydroxyzine *on page 356*

Hydroxycarbamide *see* Hydroxyurea *on next page*

Hydroxychloroquine Sulfate (hye drox ee klor' oh kwin)

Brand Names Plaquenil®

Generic Available No

Therapeutic Class Antimalarial Agent

Use Suppresses and treats acute attacks of malaria; treatment of systemic lupus erythematosus and rheumatoid arthritis

Contraindications Retinal or visual field changes attributable to 4-aminoquinolines; hypersensitivity to hydroxychloroquine, 4-aminoquinoline derivatives, or any component

Warnings Use with caution in patients with hepatic disease, G-6-PD deficiency, psoriasis, and porphyria; perform baseline and periodic (6 months) ophthalmologic examinations; test periodically for muscle weakness

Adverse Reactions

Central nervous system: Insomnia, nervousness, nightmares, psychosis, ataxia, headache, confusion, agitation

Dermatologic: Lichenoid dermatitis, bleaching of the hair, pruritus

Gastrointestinal: GI irritation, anorexia, nausea, vomiting

Hematologic: Bone marrow depression

Neuromuscular & skeletal: Muscle weakness

Ocular: Visual field defects, blindness, retinitis

Overdosage Symptoms of overdose include headache, drowsiness, visual changes, cardiovascular collapse, and seizures followed by respiratory and cardiac arrest

Toxicology Treatment is symptomatic; activated charcoal will bind the drug following GI decontamination; urinary alkalinization will enhance renal elimination; seizures can be treated with diazepam 0.01 mg/kg; shock and hypotension should be treated with fluids and pressors if needed

Drug Interactions Increased digoxin serum levels

Mechanism of Action Interferes with digestive vacuole function within sensitive malarial parasites by increasing the pH and interfering with lysosomal degradation of hemoglobin; inhibits locomotion of neutrophils and chemotaxis of eosinophils; impairs complement-dependent antigen-antibody reactions

Pharmacokinetics

Absorption: Oral: Complete

Protein binding: 55%

Metabolism: In the liver

Elimination: Metabolites and unchanged drug slowly excreted in urine, may be enhanced by urinary acidification

Usual Dosage Geriatrics and Adults: Oral:

Chemoprophylaxis of malaria: 2 tablets weekly on same day each week; begin 2 weeks before exposure; continue for 4-6 weeks after leaving endemic area

Acute attack: 4 tablets first dose day 1; 2 tablets in 6 hours day 1; 2 tablets in 1 dose day 2; and 2 tablets in 1 dose on day 3

Rheumatoid arthritis: 2-3 tablets/day to start taken with food or milk; usually after 4-12 weeks dose should be reduced by $^1/_2$ and a maintenance dose of 1-2 tablets/day given

Lupus erythematosus: 2 tablets every day or twice daily for several weeks depending on response; 1-2 tablets/day for prolonged maintenance therapy

Monitoring Parameters Ophthalmologic exam, CBC

Patient Information Take with food or milk; complete full course of therapy; wear sunglasses in bright sunlight; notify physician if blurring or other vision changes, ringing in the ears, or hearing loss occurs

Nursing Implications Periodic blood counts and eye examinations are recommended when patient is on chronic therapy; give with food or milk

Special Geriatric Considerations No specific recommendations for dosing; see Monitoring Parameters and Adverse Reactions

Dosage Forms Tablet: 200 mg [base 155 mg]

Hydroxyurea (hye drox ee yoor ee' a)

Brand Names Hydrea®

Synonyms Hydroxycarbamide

Generic Available No

Therapeutic Class Antineoplastic Agent, Miscellaneous

Use CML in chronic phase; radiosensitizing agent in the treatment of primary brain tumors; head and neck tumors; uterine cervix and non-small cell lung cancer; psoriasis; sickle cell anemia and other hemoglobinopathies; hematologic conditions such as essential thrombocythemia, polycythemia vera, hypereosinophilia, and hyperleukocytosis due to acute leukemia. Has shown activity against renal cell cancer, malignant melanoma, ovarian cancer, head and neck cancer, and prostate cancer.

Contraindications Severe anemia, severe bone marrow depression; WBC <2500/mm^3 or platelet count <100,000/mm^3; hypersensitivity to hydroxyurea

Warnings The U.S. Food and Drug Administration (FDA) currently recommends that procedures for proper handling and disposal of antineoplastic agents be considered. Use with caution in patients with renal impairment, in patients who have received prior irradiation therapy, and in the elderly.

Precautions Patient who has received irradiation may experience postirradiation erythema; bone marrow suppression is a common side effect; self-limiting megaloblastic erythropoiesis seen commonly upon initiation of hydroxyurea; use with caution in renal impairment and in elderly

Adverse Reactions

Central nervous system: Dizziness, disorientation, hallucinations, seizures, headache

Dermatologic: Maculopapular rash, facial erythema

Endocrine & metabolic: Hyperuricemia

Gastrointestinal: Nausea, vomiting, diarrhea, constipation, anorexia, stomatitis

Hematologic: Myelosuppression, megaloblastic anemia, thrombocytopenia

Hepatic: Elevation of hepatic enzymes

Renal: Dysuria, transient renal tubule dysfunction with increased BUN, serum creatinine, and uric acid

Overdosage Symptoms of overdose include myelosuppression, facial swelling, hallucinations, disorientation

Toxicology General supportive care; discontinue drug; consider transfusion of specific blood components

Drug Interactions Increased toxicity: Fluorouracil: The potential for neurotoxicity may be increased with concomitant administration

Stability Store capsules at room temperature; capsules may be opened and emptied into water (will not dissolve completely)

Mechanism of Action Interferes with synthesis of DNA, during the S phase of cell division, without interfering with RNA synthesis; inhibits ribonucleoside diphosphate reductase, preventing conversion of ribonucleotides to deoxyribonucleotides; cell-cycle specific for the S phase and may hold other cells in the G_1 phase of the cell cycle.

Pharmacokinetics

Absorption: Readily from GI tract (≥80%)

Distribution: Readily crosses the blood-brain barrier; well distributed into intestine, brain, lung, and kidney tissues

Metabolism: In the liver

Half-life: 3-4 hours

Time to peak serum concentration: Within 2 hours

Elimination: Renal excretion of urea (metabolite) and respiratory excretion of CO_2 (metabolic end product); 50% of the drug is excreted unchanged in urine

Usual Dosage Oral (**refer to individual protocols**):

Geriatrics and Adults: Dose should always be titrated to patient response and WBC counts. Usual oral doses range from 10-30 mg/kg/day or 500-3000 mg/day; if WBC count falls <2500 cells/mm^3, or the platelet count <100,000/mm^3, therapy should be stopped for at least 3 days and resumed when values rise toward normal

Solid tumors: Intermittent therapy: 80 mg/kg as a single dose every third day; continuous therapy: 20-30 mg/kg/day given as a single dose/day

Concomitant therapy with irradiation: 80 mg/kg as a single dose every third day starting at least 7 days before initiation of irradiation

Resistant chronic myelocytic leukemia: 20-30 mg/kg/day as a single daily dose

Dosing adjustment in renal impairment:

Cl_{cr} 10-50 mL/minute: Administer 50% of normal dose

Cl_{cr} <10 mL/minute: Administer 20% of normal dose

Monitoring Parameters CBC with differential, platelets, hemoglobin, renal function and liver function tests, serum uric acid

Patient Information Contents of capsule may be emptied into a glass of water if taken immediately; inform the physician if you develop fever, sore throat, bruising, or bleeding; may cause drowsiness, constipation, and loss of hair

Nursing Implications See Monitoring Parameters

(Continued)

Hydroxyurea (Continued)

Additional Information
Myelosuppressive effects:
WBC: Moderate
Platelets: Moderate
Onset (days): 7
Nadir (days): 10
Recovery (days): 21

Special Geriatric Considerations Elderly may be more sensitive to the effects of this drug; advance dose slowly and adjust dose for renal function with careful monitoring

Dosage Forms Capsule: 500 mg

25-Hydroxyvitamin D_3 see Calcifediol on page 102

Hydroxyzine (hye drox' i zeen)

Related Information
Anxiolytic/Hypnotic Use in Long-Term Care Facilities on page 755-756

Brand Names Anxanil®; Atarax®; E-Vista®; Hydroxacen®; Hy-Pam®; Quiess®; Vistaril®; Vistazine®

Synonyms Hydroxyzine Hydrochloride; Hydroxyzine Pamoate

Generic Available Yes

Therapeutic Class Antianxiety Agent; Antiemetic; Antihistamine; Sedative

Use Treatment of anxiety, as a preoperative sedative, an antipruritic, an antiemetic, and in alcohol withdrawal symptoms

Contraindications Hypersensitivity to hydroxyzine or any component

Warnings Subcutaneous, intra-arterial and I.V. administration **not** recommended since thrombosis and digital gangrene can occur; extravasation can result in sterile abscess and marked tissue induration

Precautions Should be used with caution in patients with narrow-angle glaucoma, prostatic hypertrophy, and bladder neck obstruction; should also be used with caution in patients with asthma or COPD

Adverse Reactions
Cardiovascular: Hypotension
Central nervous system: Drowsiness, dizziness, headache, confusion (especially in the elderly), ataxia
Gastrointestinal: Dry mouth
Local: Pain at injection site
Neuromuscular & skeletal: Weakness
Miscellaneous: Anticholinergic effects (dry eyes, blurred vision, constipation, urinary retention)

Overdosage Symptoms of overdose include seizures, sedation, hypotension, confusion

Toxicology There is no specific treatment for an antihistamine overdose, however, most of its clinical toxicity is due to anticholinergic effects. Anticholinesterase inhibitors may be useful by reducing acetylcholinesterase. For anticholinergic overdose with severe life-threatening symptoms, physostigmine 1-2 mg I.V., slowly may be given to reverse these effects.

Drug Interactions
Decreased effect of epinephrine (decreased vasopressor effect)
Increased effect/toxicity: CNS depressants, anticholinergics

Stability Protect from light

Mechanism of Action Competes with histamine for H_1-receptor sites on effector cells in the gastrointestinal tract, blood vessels, and respiratory tract

Pharmacodynamics Onset of action: Within 15-30 minutes; one study found enhanced suppression of H_1-receptor activity in the elderly as compared to younger adults

Pharmacokinetics
Absorption: Oral: Rapid
Distribution: V_d: Increased in elderly
Metabolism: Exact metabolic fate is unknown
Half-life: 3-7 hours; increased in elderly
Time to peak serum concentration: Within 2 hours and lingers for 4-6 hours

Usual Dosage
Geriatrics: Management of pruritus: 10 mg 3-4 times/day; increase to 25 mg 3-4 times/day if necessary

Adults:
Antiemetic: I.M.: 25-100 mg/dose every 4-6 hours as needed
Anxiety: Oral: 25-100 mg 4 times/day; maximum: 600 mg/day
Preoperative sedation:
Oral: 50-100 mg
I.M.: 25-100 mg
Management of pruritus: Oral: 25 mg 3-4 times/day

Monitoring Parameters Relief of symptoms, mental status, blood pressure

Patient Information Will cause drowsiness, avoid alcohol and other CNS depressants, avoid driving and other hazardous tasks until the CNS effects are known

Nursing Implications S.C., intra-arterial, and I.V. administration **not** recommended since thrombosis and digital gangrene can occur; extravasation can result in sterile abscess and marked tissue induration; provide safety measures (ie, side rails, night light, and call button); remove smoking materials from area; supervise ambulation

Additional Information
Hydroxyzine hydrochloride: Anxanil®, Atarax®, E-Vista®, Hydroxacen®, Quiess®, Vistaril® injection, Vistazine®
Hydroxyzine pamoate: Hy-Pam®, Vistaril® capsule and suspension

Special Geriatric Considerations Anticholinergic effects are not well tolerated in the elderly. Hydroxyzine may be useful as a short-term antipruritic, but it is not recommended for use as a sedative or anxiolytic in the elderly. Interpretive guidelines issued by the Health Care Financing Administration (HCFA) discourage the use of hydroxyzine as a sedative or anxiolytic in long-term care facilities.

Dosage Forms
Capsule, as pamoate: 25 mg, 50 mg, 100 mg
Injection, as hydrochloride: 50 mg/mL (1 mL, 2 mL, 10 mL)
Suspension, as pamoate: 25 mg/5 mL (120 mL, 480 mL)
Syrup, as hydrochloride: 10 mg/5 mL (120 mL, 480 mL, 4000 mL)
Tablet, as hydrochloride: 10 mg, 25 mg, 50 mg, 100 mg

References
Simons KJ, Watson WT, Chen XY, et al, "Pharmacokinetic and Pharmacodynamic Studies of the H_1-Receptor Antagonist Hydroxyzine in the Elderly," *Clin Pharmacol Ther*, 1989, 45(1):9-14.

Hygroton® *see* Chlorthalidone *on page 159*

Hylorel® *see* Guanadrel Sulfate *on page 334*

Hyonatal® *see* Hyoscyamine, Atropine, Scopolamine and Phenobarbital *on this page*

Hyoscine *see* Scopolamine *on page 639*

Hyoscyamine, Atropine, Scopolamine and Phenobarbital

(hye oh sye' a meen, a' troe peen, skoe pol' a meen & fee noe bar' bi tal)

Brand Names Barophen®; Donnatal®; Haponal®; Hyonatal®; Hyosophen®; Kinesed®; Relaxadon®; Spasmolin; Spasquid®

Generic Available Yes

Therapeutic Class Anticholinergic Agent; Antispasmodic Agent, Gastrointestinal

Use Adjunct in the treatment of peptic ulcer disease, irritable bowel, spastic colitis, spastic bladder, and renal colic

Contraindications Hypersensitivity to hyoscyamine, atropine, scopolamine, phenobarbital, or any component; narrow-angle glaucoma, tachycardia, GI and GU obstruction, myasthenia gravis

Precautions Use with caution in patients with hepatic or renal disease, hyperthyroidism, cardiovascular disease, hypertension, prostatic hypertrophy, autonomic neuropathy

Adverse Reactions
Cardiovascular: Tachycardia, palpitations, hypotension
Central nervous system: Fatigue, delirium, restlessness, drowsiness, headache, ataxia, confusion, impairment of judgment and coordination
Dermatologic: Dry hot skin, skin rash
Gastrointestinal: Impaired GI motility, xerostomia
Genitourinary: Urinary hesitancy/retention
Neuromuscular & skeletal: Tremors
Ocular: Mydriasis, blurred vision, dry eyes
Respiratory: Respiratory depression

Overdosage Symptoms of overdose include unsteady gait, slurred speech, confusion, hypotension, respiratory collapse, dilated unreactive pupils, hot or flushed skin, diminished bowel sounds, urinary retention

Toxicology Anticholinergic toxicity is caused by strong binding of the drug to cholinergic receptors. Anticholinesterase inhibitors reduce acetylcholinesterase, the enzyme that breaks down acetylcholine and thereby allows acetylcholine to accumulate and compete for receptor binding with the offending anticholinergic. For anticholinergic overdose with severe life-threatening symptoms, physostigmine 1-2 mg S.C. or I.V., slowly may be given to reverse these effects.

Drug Interactions
Decreased effect with antacids; decreased effect of anticoagulants, tacrine
Increased effect/toxicity with CNS depressants, alcohol, amantadine, anticholinergics, narcotic analgesics, type I antiarrhythmics, antihistamines, phenothiazines, TCAs

Mechanism of Action Belladonna alkaloids inhibit muscarinic actions of acetylcholine at postganglionic receptor sites which decreases hypermotility and hypersecretory state of the gastrointestinal tract.

(Continued)

Hyoscyamine, Atropine, Scopolamine and Phenobarbital
(Continued)

Pharmacokinetics Absorption: Well absorbed from GI tract

Usual Dosage Geriatrics and Adults: Oral: 1-2 capsules or tablets 3-4 times/day; or 1 Donnatal® Extentab® in sustained release form every 12 hours; or 5-10 mL elixir 3-4 times/day or every 8 hours

Patient Information Maintain good oral hygiene habits, because lack of saliva may increase chance of cavities. Observe caution while driving or performing other tasks requiring alertness, as may cause drowsiness, dizziness, or blurred vision. Notify physician if skin rash, flushing or eye pain occurs; or if difficulty in urinating, constipation or sensitivity to light becomes severe or persists. Do not attempt tasks requiring mental alertness or physical coordination until you know the effects of the drug. Swallow extended release tablet whole, do not crush or chew.

Nursing Implications Do not crush extended release tablets

Special Geriatric Considerations Because of the anticholinergic effects of this product, it is not recommended for use in the elderly; see Contraindications, Precautions, Adverse Reactions

Dosage Forms

Elixir: Hyoscyamine sulfate 0.1037 mg, atropine sulfate 0.0194 mg, scopolamine hydrobromide 0.0065 mg and phenobarbital 16.2 mg per 5 mL (120 mL, 480 mL, 4000 mL)

Tablet: Hyoscyamine sulfate 0.1037 mg, atropine sulfate 0.0194 mg, scopolamine hydrobromide 0.0065 mg and phenobarbital 16.2 mg

Tablet:

Chewable: Hyoscyamine hydrobromide 0.12 mg, atropine sulfate 0.12 mg, scopolamine hydrobromide 0.12 mg and phenobarbital 16 mg

Long acting: Hyoscyamine sulfate 0.3111 mg, atropine sulfate 0.0582 mg, scopolamine hydrobromide 0.0195 mg and phenobarbital 48.6 mg

Hyoscyamine, Atropine, Scopolamine, Kaolin, Pectin and Opium (oh' pee um)

Brand Names Donnagel®-PG; Donnapectolin®-PG; Kapectolin® PG

Therapeutic Class Antidiarrheal

Use Treatment of diarrhea; also used in gastritis, enteritis, colitis, acute gastrointestinal upsets, and nausea which may accompany these conditions

Restrictions C-V

Contraindications Advanced renal or hepatic disease, narrow-angle glaucoma, known hypersensitivity to belladonna alkaloids, kaolin, pectin or opium, myocardial ischemia, tachycardia, gastrointestinal obstruction, paralytic ileus, intestinal atony (elderly), severe ulcerative colitis, toxic megacolon, obstructive uropathy, myasthenia gravis, asthma; pseudomembranous colitis (*Clostridium difficile* infections)

Warnings Drug dependence; incomplete intestinal obstruction (eg, ileostomy, colostomy) may present with diarrhea, thus needing evaluation before administering; sudden withdrawal of large doses of scopolamine in Parkinson's disease may precipitate malaise, vomiting, salivation, and sweating; heat prostration may occur in high environmental temperatures; gastric ulcer (delayed emptying time); anticholinergic psychosis; elderly may exhibit agitation, confusion, short-term memory loss, hallucinations, delirium with anticholinergic medications

Precautions Use with caution in geriatric patients, see Warnings; hazardous tasks (driving, etc); glaucoma (narrow-angle), ileus, hiatal hernia with reflux, prostatic hypertrophy, cardiac arrhythmias, congestive heart failure, hypertension, COPD, hyperthyroidism, and anatomic neuropathy

Adverse Reactions

Cardiovascular: Bradycardia (low-dose atropine), tachycardia (high dose), flushing, palpitations

Central nervous system: Confusion, insomnia, excitement, headache, drowsiness, hallucinations, delirium, nervousness

Gastrointestinal: Nausea, vomiting, heartburn, constipation, bloating, ileus, dry mouth, changes in taste perception

Genitourinary: Urinary retention, impotence

Ocular: Photophobia, dilated pupils, blurred vision, increased IOP

Overdosage Symptoms of overdose include dry mouth, thirst, vomiting, abdominal distention, difficulty swallowing, muscular weakness, CNS stimulation, delirium, drowsiness, anxiety, stupor, confusion, hallucinations, seizures, psychotic behavior, tachycardia, rapid respiration, hypertension or hypotension, respiratory depression, urinary urgency, blurred vision, dilated pupils, flushed hot dry skin

Toxicology Anticholinergic toxicity is caused by strong binding of the drug to cholinergic receptors. Anticholinesterase inhibitors reduce acetylcholinesterase, the enzyme that breaks down acetylcholine and thereby allows acetylcholine to accumulate and compete for receptor binding with the offending anticholinergic. For anticholinergic overdose with severe life-threatening symptoms, physostigmine 1-2 mg S.C. or I.V.

slowly may be given to reverse these effects. Induce emesis or perform gastric lavage and administer charcoal slurry; give supportive care. Diazepam, chloral hydrate are used to treat CNS stimulation.

Drug Interactions
Amantadine may enhance anticholinergic effects
Pharmacologic effects of atenolol may be increased; pharmacologic effects of digoxin may be enhanced
Phenothiazines may have decreased antipsychotic action but increased anticholinergic effects (additive)
Antidepressants (TCAs) may have increased anticholinergic effects (additive)
May increase anticholinergic effects of any drug with anticholinergic action

Mechanism of Action Belladonna alkaloids inhibit muscarinic actions of acetylcholine at postganglionic receptor sites which decreases hypermotility and hypersecretory state of the gastrointestinal tract. Opium delays transit of intraluminal contents, increases gut capacity, increases sphincter tone, stimulates fluid movement across gut mucosa, relieves tenesmus and pain.

Pharmacokinetics Atropine stimulates CNS; scopolamine is a CNS depressant
Absorption: Oral: Belladonna alkaloids are rapidly absorbed
Distribution: Readily crosses blood-brain barrier
Half-life: Atropine: 2.5 hours
Elimination: 94% of dose eliminated renally in 24 hours

Usual Dosage Geriatrics and Adults: Initial: 30 mL (1 fluid oz) followed by 15-30 mL after each loose stool (do not exceed 120 mL in 12 hours); use lower dose recommendations initially before increasing dose to 30 mL after each loose stool

Monitoring Parameters Monitor stool frequency, consistency; heart rate, signs of CNS toxicity; bladder dysfunction and respiratory rate with multiple doses, dehydration, fluid/electrolyte loss

Patient Information Shake well before using; do not exceed recommended doses; report failure to respond to physician

Nursing Implications See Warnings, Precautions, Monitoring Parameters, and Special Geriatric Considerations

Additional Information Hyoscyamine is dialyzable but is ineffective for atropine

Special Geriatric Considerations Elderly are particularly prone to CNS side effects to anticholinergics (ie, confusion, delirium, hallucinations). The use of this product is discouraged in elderly since systemic side effects often occur before clinical response obtained for GI problem.

Hyoscyamine Sulfate (hye oh sye' a meen)

Brand Names Anaspaz®; Cystospaz®; Cystospaz-M®; Gastrosed™; Levsin®; Levsinex®; Neoquess® Tablet
Synonyms l-Hyoscyamine Sulfate
Generic Available Yes
Therapeutic Class Anticholinergic Agent; Antispasmodic Agent, Gastrointestinal
Use GI tract disorders caused by spasm, adjunctive therapy for peptic ulcers, preoperative medication

Unlabeled use: Urinary incontinence
Contraindications Narrow-angle glaucoma, obstructive uropathy, obstructive GI tract disease, myasthenia gravis, known hypersensitivity to belladonna alkaloids
Precautions Use with caution in hot weather or during exercise. Elderly patients frequently develop increased sensitivity and require strict dosage regulation – side effects may be more severe in elderly patients with atherosclerotic changes. Use with caution in patients with tachycardia, cardiac arrhythmias, hypertension, hypotension, prostatic hypertrophy (especially in the elderly) or any tendency toward urinary retention, liver or kidney disorders and obstructive disease of the GI or GU tract. May exacerbate mental symptoms and precipitate a toxic psychosis when used to treat extrapyramidal reactions resulting from phenothiazines. When given in large doses or to susceptible patients, may cause weakness and inability to move particular muscle groups. Anticholinergic agents can aggravate tardive dyskinesia caused by neuroleptic agents.

Adverse Reactions
Cardiovascular: Tachycardia, palpitations
Central nervous system: Fatigue, delirium, restlessness, headache, ataxia, confusion (the elderly are at increased risk for confusion and hallucinations)
Dermatologic: Dry hot skin
Gastrointestinal: Impaired GI motility, constipation, dry mouth
Genitourinary: Urinary retention
Neuromuscular & skeletal: Tremors
Ocular: Mydriasis, blurred vision, dry eyes
Overdosage Symptoms of overdose include dilated, unreactive pupils; blurred vision; hot, dry flushed skin; dryness of mucous membranes; difficulty in swallowing, foul breath, diminished or absent bowel sounds, urinary retention, tachycardia, hyperthermia, hypertension, increased respiratory rate

(Continued)

Hyoscyamine Sulfate *(Continued)*

Toxicology Anticholinergic toxicity is caused by strong binding of the drug to cholinergic receptors. Anticholinesterase inhibitors reduce acetylcholinesterase, the enzyme that breaks down acetylcholine and thereby allows acetylcholine to accumulate and compete for receptor binding with the offending anticholinergic. For anticholinergic overdose with severe life-threatening symptoms, physostigmine 1-2 mg S.C. or I.V., slowly may be given to reverse these effects.

Drug Interactions
Decreased effect: Tacrine
Increased toxicity: Amantadine, phenothiazines, tricyclic antidepressants, other anticholinergic agents

Mechanism of Action Blocks the action of acetylcholine at parasympathetic sites in smooth muscle, secretory glands and the CNS; increases cardiac output, dries secretions, antagonizes histamine and serotonin

Pharmacodynamics
Onset of action: Within 2-3 minutes
Duration: 4-6 hours

Pharmacokinetics
Absorption: Oral: Absorbed well
Protein binding: 50%
Metabolism: In the liver
Half-life: 13% to 38%
Elimination: In urine

Usual Dosage Geriatrics and Adults:
Oral, S.L.: 0.125-0.25 mg 3-4 times/day before meals or food and at bedtime; 0.375-0.75 mg (timed release) every 12 hours
I.M., I.V., S.C.: 0.25-0.5 mg every 6 hours

Monitoring Parameters Pulse, anticholinergic effects, urine output, GI symptoms

Patient Information Take 30-60 minutes before a meal; maintain good oral hygiene habits, because lack of saliva may increase chance of cavities. Observe caution while driving or performing other tasks requiring alertness, as may cause drowsiness, dizziness, or blurred vision. Notify physician if skin rash, flushing or eye pain occurs; or if difficulty in urinating, constipation or sensitivity to light becomes severe or persists.

Nursing Implications Monitor patient for anticholinergic effects

Special Geriatric Considerations Avoid long-term use; the potential for toxic reactions is higher than the potential benefit, elderly are particularly prone to CNS side effects of anticholinergics (ie, confusion, delirium, hallucinations). Side effects often occur before clinical response is obtained; see Precautions.

Dosage Forms
Capsule, timed release: 0.375 mg
Elixir: 0.125 mg/5 mL alcohol 20%
Injection: 0.5 mg/mL (1 mL, 10 mL)
Solution: 0.125 mg/mL (15 mL)
Tablet: 0.125 mg, 0.15 mg

Hyosophen® *see* Hyoscyamine, Atropine, Scopolamine and Phenobarbital *on page 357*

Hy-Pam® *see* Hydroxyzine *on page 356*

HyperHep® *see* Hepatitis B Immune Globulin *on page 342*

Hyper-Tet® *see* Tetanus Immune Globulin, Human *on page 676*

Hy-Phen® *see* Hydrocodone and Acetaminophen *on page 350*

HypoTears® [OTC] *see* Ocular Lubricant *on page 515*

Hytakerol® *see* Dihydrotachysterol *on page 224*

Hytone® *see* Hydrocortisone *on page 351*

Hytrin® *see* Terazosin *on page 672*

Hytuss-2X® [OTC] *see* Guaifenesin *on page 331*

Ibidomide Hydrochloride *see* Labetalol Hydrochloride *on page 395*

Ibuprin® [OTC] *see* Ibuprofen *on this page*

Ibuprofen *(eye byoo proe' fen)*

Brand Names Advil® [OTC]; Excedrin IB® [OTC]; Genpril® [OTC]; Haltran® [OTC]; Ibuprin® [OTC]; Ibuprohm® [OTC]; Ibu-Tab®; Medipren® [OTC]; Menadol® [OTC]; Midol® 200 [OTC]; Motrin®; Motrin® IB [OTC]; Nuprin® [OTC]; Pamprin IB® [OTC]; Rufen®; Saleto-200® [OTC]; Saleto-400®; Trendar® [OTC]; Uni-Pro® [OTC]

Synonyms *p*-Isobutylhydratropic Acid

Generic Available Yes: Tablet

Therapeutic Class Analgesic, Non-narcotic; Anti-inflammatory Agent; Nonsteroidal Anti-inflammatory Agent (NSAID), Oral

Use Inflammatory diseases and rheumatoid disorders including rheumatoid arthritis; mild to moderate pain; fever; gout; osteoarthritis, sunburn, ankylosing spondylitis, acute migraine headache

Contraindications Hypersensitivity to ibuprofen, any component, aspirin or other non-steroidal anti-inflammatory drugs (NSAIDs)

Warnings GI toxicity (bleeding, ulceration, perforation); CNS effects may occur (headaches, confusion, depression); cross-sensitivity with aspirin and other NSAIDs exists; hypersensitivity, anaphylactoid reactions (intermittent tolmetin use more often); renal function decline, acute renal insufficiency, interstitial nephritis, dysuria, cystitis, hematuria, nephrotic syndrome, hyperkalemia in acute renal insufficiency, hyponatremia, papillary necrosis, hepatic function impairment; elderly have increased risk for adverse reactions to NSAIDs; see Special Geriatric Considerations

Precautions Use with caution in patients with congestive heart failure, hypertension, decreased renal or hepatic function, history of GI disease (bleeding or ulcers), or those receiving anticoagulants; perform ophthalmologic evaluation for those who develop eye complaints during therapy (blurred vision, diminished vision, changes in color vision, retinal changes); NSAIDs may mask signs/symptoms of infections; photosensitivity reported

Adverse Reactions

Cardiovascular: Congestive heart failure, angina, hypertension, hypotension, fluid retention, arrhythmias, edema

Central nervous system: Headache, drowsiness, vertigo, dizziness, fatigue, hallucinations, confusion, depression, emotional lability, psychotic behavior, asthenia

Dermatologic: Rash, urticaria, angioedema, Stevens-Johnson syndrome, exfoliative dermatitis, ecchymosis, petechiae, purpura, bruising

Endocrine & metabolic: Hyperglycemia, hypoglycemia, hyperkalemia, gynecomastia, hyponatremia

Gastrointestinal: Dyspepsia, heartburn, nausea, diarrhea, constipation, flatulence, stomatitis, vomiting, abdominal pain, peptic ulcer, GI bleeding, GI perforation, gingival ulcers, pancreatitis, proctitis, paralytic ulcers, colitis, anorexia, weight loss

Genitourinary: Impotence, azotemia

Hematologic: Neutropenia, anemia, agranulocytosis, bone marrow suppression, hemolytic anemia, hemorrhage, inhibition of platelet aggregation

Hepatic: Hepatitis, elevated LFTs, cholestatic jaundice

Neuromuscular & skeletal: Involuntary muscle movements, muscle weakness, tremors

Ocular: Vision changes

Otic: Tinnitus

Renal: Dysuria, polyuria, pyuria, oliguria, anuria, acute renal failure

Respiratory: Exacerbation of asthma, dyspnea

Miscellaneous: Dry mucous membranes, thirst, pyrexia, sweating

Overdosage Symptoms include drowsiness, lethargy, disorientation, confusion, dizziness, numbness, paresthesia, nausea, vomiting, gastric irritation, abdominal pain, headache, tinnitus, sweating, blurred vision, muscle twitching, seizures, coma, acute renal failure, increased BUN and serum creatinine, hypotension, tachycardia, and metabolic acidosis

Toxicology Management of a nonsteroidal anti-inflammatory agent (NSAID) intoxication is primarily supportive and symptomatic. Fluid therapy is commonly effective in managing the hypotension that may occur following an acute NSAID overdose, except when this is due to an acute blood loss. Seizures tend to be very short-lived and often do not require drug treatment although recurrent seizures should be treated with I.V. diazepam. Since many of the NSAIDs undergo enterohepatic cycling, multiple doses of charcoal may be needed to reduce the potential for delayed toxicities. NSAIDs are highly bound to plasma proteins, therefore hemodialysis and peritoneal dialysis are not useful.

Drug Interactions

May increase digoxin, methotrexate, and lithium serum concentrations

Aspirin and other salicylates may decrease NSAID serum concentrations

Other NSAIDs may increase adverse GI effects

Increased prothrombin time with anticoagulants

Decreased antihypertensive effects of ACE inhibitors, beta-blockers, and thiazide diuretics

Increased response to sympathomimetics

Probenecid may increase toxicity of NSAIDs by increase in serum concentrations

Effects of loop diuretics may be decreased

May enhance azotemia in elderly receiving loop diuretics; may increase risk for renal insufficiency when used with diuretics

Mechanism of Action Inhibits prostaglandin synthesis, acts on the hypothalamus heat-regulating center to reduce fever, blocks prostaglandin synthetase action which prevents formation of the platelet-aggregating substance thromboxane A_2; decreases pain receptor sensitivity. Other proposed mechanisms of action are lysosomal stabilization, kinin and leukotriene production, alteration of chemotactic factors, and inhibition of neutrophil activation. This latter mechanism may be the most significant pharmacologic action to reduce inflammation.

(Continued)

Ibuprofen (Continued)

Pharmacodynamics
Onset of analgesia: 30 minutes to 1 hour
Duration: 4-6 hours
Onset of anti-inflammatory: Up to 7 days
Peak action: 1-2 weeks

Pharmacokinetics
Absorption: Oral: Rapid, 85%
Protein binding: 90% to 99%
Metabolism: In the liver by oxidation
Half-life: 2-4 hours
Time to peak serum concentration: Within 1-2 hours
Elimination: In urine (1% as free drug); some biliary excretion occurs

Usual Dosage Geriatrics and Adults: Oral:
Inflammatory disease: 400-800 mg/dose 3-4 times/day; maximum dose: 3.2 g/day

Pain/fever: 200-400 mg/dose every 4-6 hours; maximum daily dose: 1.2 g

Monitoring Parameters Monitor response (pain, range of motion, grip strength, mobility, ADL function), inflammation; observe for weight gain, edema; monitor renal function; observe for bleeding, bruising; evaluate gastrointestinal effects (abdominal pain, bleeding, dyspepsia); mental confusion, disorientation, CBC, serum, creatinine, BUN, liver function tests

Reference Range Plasma concentrations >200 μg/mL may be associated with severe toxicity

Test Interactions Increased chloride (S), increased sodium (S)

Patient Information Serious gastrointestinal bleeding can occur as well as ulceration and perforation. Pain may or may not be present. Avoid aspirin and aspirin-containing products while taking this medication. If gastric upset occurs, take with food, milk, or antacid. If gastric adverse effects persist, contact physician. May cause drowsiness, dizziness, blurred vision, and confusion. Use caution when performing tasks which require alertness (eg, driving). Do not take for more than 3 days for fever or 10 days for pain without physician's advice.

Nursing Implications See Patient Information, Overdosage, Monitoring Parameters, and Special Geriatric Considerations

Additional Information There are no clinical guidelines to predict which NSAID will give response in a particular patient. Trials with each must be initiated until response determined. Consider dose, patient convenience, and cost.

Special Geriatric Considerations Elderly are a high-risk population for adverse effects from nonsteroidal anti-inflammatory agents. As much as 60% of elderly can develop peptic ulceration and/or hemorrhage asymptomatically. The concomitant use of H_2 blockers, omeprazole, and sucralfate is not effective as prophylaxis. Misoprostol is the only prophylactic agent proven effective. Also, concomitant disease and drug use contribute to the risk for GI adverse effects. Use lowest effective dose for shortest period possible. Consider renal function decline with age. Use of NSAIDs can compromise existing renal function especially when Cl_{cr} is ≤30 mL/minute. Tinnitus may be a difficult and unreliable indication of toxicity due to age-related hearing loss or eighth cranial nerve damage. CNS adverse effects such as confusion, agitation, and hallucination are generally seen in overdose or high dose situations, but elderly may demonstrate these adverse effects at lower doses than younger adults.

Dosage Forms
Suspension: 100 mg/5 mL (120 mL)
Tablet: 200 mg, 300 mg, 400 mg, 600 mg, 800 mg

References
Brooks PM, Day RO, "Nonsteroidal Anti-inflammatory Drugs – Differences and Similarities," N Engl J Med, 1991, 324(24):1716-25.

Clinch D, Banerjee AK, Ostick G, "Absence of Abdominal Pain in Elderly Patients With Peptic Ulcer," Age Ageing, 1984, 13(2):120-3.

Clive DM, Stoff JS, "Renal Syndromes Associated With Nonsteroidal Anti-inflammatory Drugs," N Engl J Med, 1984, 310(9):563-72.

Graham DY, "Prevention of Gastroduodenal Injury Induced by Chronic Nonsteroidal Anti-inflammatory Drug Therapy," Gastroenterology, 1989, 96(2 Pt 2 Suppl):675-81.

Gurwitz JH, Avarn J, Ross-Degan D, et al, "Nonsteroidal Anti-Inflammatory Drug-Associated Azotemia in the Very Old," JAMA, 1990, 264(4):471-5.

Knodel LC, "Preventing NSAID-Induced Ulcers: The Role of Misoprostol," Consult Pharm, 1989, 4:37-41.

Pounder R, "Silent Peptic Ulceration: Deadly Silence or Golden Silence?" Gastroenterology, 1989, 96:(2 Pt 2 Suppl)626-31.

Ibuprohm® [OTC] see Ibuprofen on page 360

Ibu-Tab® see Ibuprofen on page 360

I-Chlor® see Chloramphenicol on page 148

Idoxuridine (eye dox yoor' i deen)
Brand Names Herplex® Ophthalmic
Synonyms IDU; IUDR
Generic Available No

Therapeutic Class Antiviral Agent, Ophthalmic

Use Treatment of herpes simplex keratitis

Contraindications Hypersensitivity to idoxuridine or any component; concurrent use in patients receiving corticosteroids with superficial dendritic keratitis

Warnings Use with caution in patients with corneal ulceration or patients receiving corticosteroid applications; if no response in epithelial infections within 14 days, consider a second form of therapy

Adverse Reactions
Local: Irritation, pruritus, pain, inflammation
Ocular: Corneal clouding, photophobia, small punctate defects on the corneal epithelium, mild edema of the eyelids and cornea, follicular conjunctivitis; ointment may produce a temporary visual haze

Toxicology Due to frequent dosing, small defects on the epithelium may result. Mutagenic and cytotoxic and should be considered as being potentially carcinogenic; no treatment is indicated for accidental ingestion

Drug Interactions Increased toxicity (initiation): Do not coadminister with boric acid containing solutions

Stability Store in tight, light-resistant containers at 2 °C to 8°C until dispensed; do not mix with other medications; solution must be refrigerated

Mechanism of Action Incorporated into viral DNA in place of thymidine resulting in mutations and inhibition of viral replication

Pharmacokinetics
Absorption: Ophthalmic: Poor following instillation; tissue uptake is a function of cellular metabolism, which is inhibited by high concentrations of the drug (absorption decreases as the concentration of drug increases)
Metabolism: To iodouracil, uracil, and iodide
Elimination: Unchanged drug and metabolites excreted in urine

Usual Dosage Geriatrics and Adults: Ophthalmic:
Ointment: Instill 5 times/day (every 4 hours) in the conjunctival sac with last dose at bedtime; continue therapy for 5-7 days after healing appears complete
Solution: Instill 1 drop in eye(s) every hour during day and every 2 hours at night, continue until definite improvement is noted, then reduce daytime dose to 1 drop every 2 hours and every 4 hours at night; continue for 5-7 days after healing appears complete

Patient Information May cause sensitivity to bright light; minimize by wearing sunglasses; notify physician if improvement is not seen in 7-8 days, if condition worsens, or if pain, decreased vision, itching, or swelling of the eye occur; do not exceed recommended dose

Nursing Implications Idoxuridine solution should not be mixed with other medications

Special Geriatric Considerations Assess patient's ability to self-administer

Dosage Forms Ophthalmic:
Ointment: 0.5% (4 g)
Solution: 0.1% (15 mL)

IDU see Idoxuridine *on previous page*

IG see Immune Globulin *on page 366*

I-Gent® see Gentamicin Sulfate *on page 320*

IGIM see Immune Globulin *on page 366*

IGIV see Immune Globulin *on page 366*

I-Homatrine® see Homatropine Hydrobromide *on page 343*

Ilosone® see Erythromycin *on page 263*

Ilosone® Pulvules® see Erythromycin *on page 263*

Ilotycin® Gluceptate see Erythromycin *on page 263*

I-Methasone® see Dexamethasone *on page 207*

Imferon® see Iron Dextran Complex *on page 377*

Imipemide see Imipenem/Cilastatin *on this page*

Imipenem/Cilastatin (i mi pen' em)

Brand Names Primaxin®

Synonyms Imipemide

Generic Available No

Therapeutic Class Antibiotic, Miscellaneous

Use Treatment of documented multidrug resistant gram-negative infection due to organisms proven or suspected to be susceptible to imipenem/cilastatin; treatment of multiple organism infection in which other agents have an insufficient spectrum of activity or are contraindicated due to toxic potential

Contraindications Hypersensitivity to imipenem/cilastatin or any component

Warnings Prolonged use may result in superinfection; patients with CNS abnormalities at increased risk for seizures

(Continued)

Imipenem/Cilastatin *(Continued)*

Precautions Dosage adjustment required in patients with impaired renal function; use with caution in patients with penicillin or cephalosporin allergy

Adverse Reactions

Cardiovascular: Hypotension, palpitations

Central nervous system: Seizures

Dermatologic: Rash

Gastrointestinal: Nausea, vomiting, diarrhea, pseudomembranous colitis

Hematologic: Neutropenia, eosinophilia, positive Coombs' test

Local: Pain at injection site, phlebitis

Miscellaneous: Emergence of resistant strains of *P. aeruginosa*

Toxicology Discontinue the drug; many beta-lactam-containing antibiotics have the potential to cause neuromuscular hyperirritability or convulsive seizures; hemodialysis may be helpful to aid in the removal of the drug from the blood, otherwise most treatment is supportive or symptom directed. Diazepam 0.01 mg/kg can be used for seizures.

Drug Interactions Probenecid (minimal increase in imipenem plasma levels), ganciclovir (may increase risk for seizures)

Stability Stable for 10 hours at room temperature following reconstitution with 100 mL of 0.9% sodium chloride injection; up to 48 hours when refrigerated at 5°C. If reconstituted with 5% or 10% dextrose injection, 5% dextrose and sodium bicarbonate, 5% dextrose and 0.9% sodium chloride, is stable for 4 hours at room temperature and 24 hours when refrigerated.

Mechanism of Action Inhibits cell wall synthesis by binding to penicillin-binding proteins on the bacterial outer membrane; cilastatin prevents renal metabolism of imipenem by competitive inhibition of dehydropeptidase along the brush border of the proximal renal tubules

Pharmacokinetics

Protein binding: Cilastatin is 40% plasma protein bound

Metabolism:

Imipenem: Metabolized in the kidney by dehydropeptidase

Cilastatin: Partially metabolized in the kidneys

Half-life (both): 60 minutes, extended with renal insufficiency

Elimination: When imipenem is given with cilastatin, urinary excretion of unchanged imipenem increases to 70%

Cilastatin: 70% to 80% of a dose is excreted unchanged in the urine

Half-life and V_d (L/kg) have been reported to be increased and decreased, respectively, in the older adult compared to younger adults

Usual Dosage Geriatrics and Adults (dosage recommendation based on imipenem component. I.V. infusion):

Serious infection: 2-4 g/day in 3-4 divided doses

Mild to moderate infection: 1-2 g/day in 3-4 divided doses

Dosing adjustment in renal impairment:

Cl_{cr} <30-70 mL/minute/1.73m^2: Reduced dose

Moderately dialyzable (20% to 50%). See table.

Creatinine Clearance mL/min/1.73 m²	Frequency	% Decrease in Daily Maximum Dose
30–70	q6–8h	50
20–30	q8–12h	63
5–20	q12h	75

Administration Not for direct infusion; vial contents must be transferred to 100 mL of infusion solution; final concentration should not exceed 5 mg/mL; infuse over 30-60 minutes; watch for convulsions; I.M. preparation is for I.M. use only, I.V. preparation is for I.V. use only

Monitoring Parameters Signs and symptoms of infection; mental status, WBC, periodic renal, hepatic, and hematologic function tests

Test Interactions Interferes with urinary glucose determination using Clinitest®

Nursing Implications Do not mix with or physically add to other antibiotics; however, may administer concomitantly; see Administration

Additional Information Sodium content of 1 g: 3.2 mEq

Special Geriatric Considerations Imipenem/cilastatin's role is limited to the treatment of infections caused by susceptible multiresistant organism(s) and in patients whose bacterial infection(s) have failed to respond to other appropriate antimicrobials; many of the seizures attributed to imipenem/cilastatin were in elderly patients; dose must be adjusted for creatinine clearance

Dosage Forms Powder for injection: Imipenem 250 mg and cilastatin 250 mg (13 mL); imipenem 500 mg and cilastatin 500 mg (13 mL)

References

Finch RG, Craddock C, Kelly J, et al, "Pharmacokinetic Studies of Imipenem/Cilastatin in Elderly Patients," *J Antimicrob Chemother*, 1986, 18(Suppl E):103-7.

Toon S, Hopkins KJ, Garstang FM, et al, "Pharmacokinetics of Imipenem and Cilastatin After Their Simultaneous Administration to the Elderly," *Br J Clin Pharmacol*, 1987, 23(2):143-9.

Yoshikawa TT, "Antimicrobial Therapy for the Elderly Patient," *J Am Geriatr Soc*, 1990, 38(12):1353-72.

Imipramine (im ip' ra meen)

Related Information

Antidepressant Agents Comparison *on page 800*

Drug Levels Commonly Monitored Guidelines *on page 771-772*

Brand Names Janimine®; Tofranil®; Tofranil-PM®

Synonyms Imipramine Hydrochloride; Imipramine Pamoate

Generic Available Yes: Tablet

Therapeutic Class Antidepressant, Tricyclic

Use Treatment of various forms of depression, often in conjunction with psychotherapy

Unlabeled use: Neurogenic pain, urinary incontinence

Contraindications Hypersensitivity to imipramine (cross-sensitivity with other tricyclics may occur); patients receiving MAO inhibitors within past 14 days; narrow-angle glaucoma

Warnings To avoid cholinergic crisis do not discontinue abruptly in patients receiving long-term high dose therapy; some oral preparations contain tartrazine and injection contains sulfites both of which can cause allergic reactions

Precautions Use with caution in patients with cardiovascular disease, conduction disturbances, seizure disorders, urinary retention, bipolar illness, renal or hepatic impairment, hyperthyroidism or those receiving thyroid replacement; an EKG prior to the start of therapy is advised

Adverse Reactions

Cardiovascular: Arrhythmias, hypotension

Central nervous system: Drowsiness, sedation, confusion, delirium, dizziness, fatigue, anxiety, nervousness, sleep disorders, seizures

Dermatologic: Rash, photosensitivity

Gastrointestinal: Nausea, vomiting, constipation, dry mouth

Genitourinary: Urinary retention

Hematologic: Blood dyscrasias

Hepatic: Hepatitis, cholestatic jaundice

Neuromuscular & skeletal: Weakness

Ocular: Blurred vision, increased intraocular pressure

Miscellaneous: Has been associated with falls, hypersensitivity reactions

Less sedation and anticholinergic effects than amitriptyline

Overdosage Symptoms of overdose include confusion, hallucinations, seizure, constipation, cyanosis, tachycardia

Toxicology Following initiation of essential overdose management, toxic symptoms should be treated. Ventricular arrhythmias often respond to phenytoin 15-20 mg/kg with concurrent systemic alkalinization (sodium bicarbonate 0.5-2 mEq/kg I.V.). Arrhythmias unresponsive to this therapy may respond to lidocaine 1 mg/kg I.V. followed by a titrated infusion. Physostigmine (1-2 mg I.V. slowly) may be indicated in reversing cardiac arrhythmias that are due to vagal blockade or for anticholinergic effects. Seizures usually respond to diazepam I.V. boluses (5-10 mg, up to 30 mg). If seizures are unresponsive or recur, phenytoin or phenobarbital may be required.

Drug Interactions

May decrease or reverse effects of guanethidine and clonidine; may increase effects of CNS depressants, adrenergic agents, dicumarol, and anticholinergic agents

With MAO inhibitors, hyperpyrexia, tachycardia, hypertension, seizures and death may occur; similar interactions as with other tricyclics may occur

Cimetidine, fluoxetine, methylphenidate, and haloperidol may decrease the metabolism and/or increase TCA levels; phenobarbital may increase TCA metabolism

Stability Solutions stable at a pH of 4-5; turns yellowish or reddish on exposure to light. Slight discoloration does not affect potency; marked discoloration is associated with loss of potency. Capsules stable for 3 years following date of manufacture.

Mechanism of Action Traditionally believed to increase the synaptic concentration of serotonin and/or norepinephrine in the central nervous system by inhibition of their reuptake by the presynaptic neuronal membrane. However, additional receptor effects have been found including desensitization of adenyl cyclase, down regulation of beta-adrenergic receptors, and down regulation of serotonin receptors.

Pharmacodynamics Maximum antidepressant effects usually occur after ≥ 2 weeks; 5-HT >NE

Pharmacokinetics

Absorption: Oral: Well absorbed

(Continued)

Imipramine *(Continued)*

Metabolism: In the liver by microsomal enzymes to desipramine (active) and other metabolites; significant first-pass metabolism almost all compounds following metabolism; metabolism may be decreased in older patients

Half-life: 6-18 hours; mean half-life: ~24 hours

Elimination: In urine; utility of serum level monitoring controversial

Plasma levels and half-life are positively associated with age

Usual Dosage

Geriatrics: Initial: 10-25 mg at bedtime; increase by 10-25 mg every 3 days for inpatients and weekly for outpatients if tolerated; average daily dose to achieve a therapeutic concentration: 100 mg/day (range: 50-150 mg)

Adults:

Oral: Initial: 25 mg 3-4 times/day, increase dose gradually, total dose may be given at bedtime; maximum: 300 mg/day

I.M.: Initial: Up to 100 mg/day in divided doses; change to oral as soon as possible

Monitoring Parameters Improvement of depressive symptoms; blood pressure, pulse

Reference Range Therapeutic: Imipramine and desipramine 150-250 ng/mL (SI: 530-890 nmol/L); desipramine 150-300 ng/mL (SI: 560-1125 nmol/L); Toxic: >500 ng/mL (SI: 446-893 nmol/L)

Test Interactions Elevated glucose

Patient Information May require 2-4 weeks to achieve desired effect; avoid alcohol ingestion; do not discontinue medication abruptly; may cause urine to turn blue-green; may cause drowsiness, constipation, blurred vision; use water or hard candy for dry mouth; rise slowly to avoid dizziness

Nursing Implications Monitor blood pressure and pulse rate prior to and during initial therapy; evaluate mental status; monitor weight, may increase appetite; offer patient water or hard candy for dry mouth

Additional Information

Imipramine hydrochloride: Tofranil®, Janimine®

Imipramine pamoate: Tofranil-PM®

Special Geriatric Considerations Orthostatic hypotension is a concern with this agent, especially in patients taking other medications that may affect blood pressure; may precipitate arrhythmias in predisposed patients; may aggravate seizures; a less anticholinergic antidepressant may be a better choice

Dosage Forms

Capsule, as pamoate: 75 mg, 100 mg, 125 mg, 150 mg

Injection, as hydrochloride: 12.5 mg/mL (2 mL)

Tablet, as hydrochloride: 10 mg, 25 mg, 50 mg

References

Nies A, Robinson DS, Friedman MS, et al, "Relationship Between Age and Tricyclic Antidepressant Plasma Levels," *Am J Psychiatry*, 1977, 134:790-3.

Imipramine Hydrochloride *see* Imipramine *on previous page*

Imipramine Pamoate *see* Imipramine *on previous page*

Imitrex® *see* Sumatriptan Succinate *on page 666*

Immune Globulin

Related Information

Immunization Guidelines *on page 759-762*

Brand Names Gamastan®; Gamimune® N; Gammagard®; Gammar®; Gammar®-IV; Iveegam®; Sandoglobulin®; Venoglobulin®-I

Synonyms Gamma Globulin; IG; IGIM; IGIV; Immune Globulin Intramuscular; Immune Globulin Intravenous; Immune Serum Globulin; ISG

Therapeutic Class Immune Globulin

Use Immunodeficiency syndrome; idiopathic thrombocytopenia purpura; B-cell chronic lymphocytic leukemia; prophylaxis against hepatitis A, measles, varicella, and possibly rubella and immunoglobulin deficiency; Kawasaki syndrome

Contraindications Thrombocytopenia or coagulation disorder, hypersensitivity to immune globulin, thimerosal, IgA deficiency

Warnings Do not give I.V. except immune globulin I.V., hypersensitivity reactions should have epinephrine 1:1000 available for anaphylactic reactions; anaphylactic reaction more common with I.V. administration

Precautions Skin testing should not be performed; easy to misinterpret a positive reaction

Adverse Reactions

Cardiovascular: Chest tightness

Central nervous system: Lethargy, fever, chills

Dermatologic: Urticaria, angioedema

Gastrointestinal: Emesis, nausea

Local: Tenderness, induration, erythema

Neuromuscular & skeletal: Myalgia, muscle stiffness
Renal: Nephrotic syndrome
Miscellaneous: Rarely hypersensitivity reactions
Drug Interactions Live virus vaccines
Stability Keep in refrigerator; do not freeze
Mechanism of Action Provides passive immunity by increasing the antibody titer and antigen-antibody reaction potential
Pharmacodynamics Duration of immune effects: Usually 3-4 weeks
Pharmacokinetics
Half-life: 21-23 days
Time to peak:
I.M.: Peak antibody serum levels occur within 2-5 days
I.V. provides immediate antibody levels
Usual Dosage
I.M.:
Hepatitis A: 0.02 mL/kg
Travel into endemic areas:
1-3 months: 0.02 mL/kg
>3 months: 0.06 mL/kg; repeat every 4-6 months
IgG deficiency: 1.3 mL/kg then 0.66 mL/kg in 3-4 weeks
Measles: 0.25 mL/kg
Rubella: 0.55 mL/kg, within 72 hours of exposure
Varicella: 0.6-1.2 mL/kg
I.V.:
Immunodeficiency syndrome:
Sandoglobulin®: 200 mg/kg once monthly; may be increased to 300 mg/kg if prior dose insufficient; rate: 0.5-1 mL/minute for 15-30 minutes, increase to 1.5-2.5 mL/minute
Gammagard®: 200-400 mg/kg once monthly; rate: 0.5 mL/kg/hour
Gammar®-IV: 100-200 mg/kg every 3-4 weeks; rate: 0.01 mL/kg/minute; increase to 0.02 mL/kg/minute after 15-30 minutes, then, if tolerated 0.03-0.06 mL/kg/hour
Venoglobulin®-I: 200 mg/kg once monthly; increase to 300-400 mg/kg if response is insufficient; rate: 0.01-0.02 mL/kg/minute for 30 minutes; if tolerated, increase rate to 0.04 mL/kg/minute
Gamimune® N: 100-200 mg/kg once monthly; may increase to 400 mg/kg if insufficient response; rate: 0.01-0.02 mL/kg/minute for 30 minutes; if tolerated, increase to 0.08 mL/kg/minute
Iveegam®: 200 mg/kg once monthly; doses up to 800 mg/kg have been tolerated; rate: 1-2 mL/minute
Idiopathic thrombocytopenia purpura:
Sandoglobulin®: 400 mg/kg/day for 2-5 days
Gammagard®: 1000 mg/kg/day up to 3 doses on alternate days; monitor response by platelet counts
Venoglobulin®-I: 500 mg/kg/day for 2-7 days; maintenance (platelet counts <30,000/mm³): 500-2000 mg/kg as a single dose at 1- to 2-week intervals; monitor platelets
Gamimune® N: 400 mg/kg/day for 5 days
B-cell CLL: Gammagard®: 400 mg/kg as a single dose every 3-4 weeks
Monitoring Parameters I.V. may cause hypotension; monitor for anaphylaxis, platelet counts, serum IgG levels
Reference Range Serum IgG: 300 mg/dL
Test Interactions Skin tests should **not** be done
Nursing Implications Intramuscular injection only; do not mix with other medications; skin testing should not be performed as local irritation can occur and be misinterpreted as a positive reaction
Additional Information Epidemiologic and laboratory data indicate current IMIG products do not have a discernible risk of transmitting HIV
Special Geriatric Considerations No special recommendations are made for elderly, doses are same as recommended for younger adults
Dosage Forms Injection:
I.M.: 165 ± 15 mg (of protein)/mL (2 mL, 10 mL)
I.V.: 0.5 g, 1 g, 2.5 g, 3 g, 5 g, 6 g, 10 g; 5% (10 mL, 50 mL, 100 mL)

Immune Globulin Intramuscular *see* Immune Globulin *on previous page*
Immune Globulin Intravenous *see* Immune Globulin *on previous page*
Immune Serum Globulin *see* Immune Globulin *on previous page*
Immunization Guidelines *see page 759*
Imodium® *see* Loperamide Hydrochloride *on page 416*
Imodium® A-D Caplets [OTC] *see* Loperamide Hydrochloride *on page 416*

Imodium® A-D Liquid [OTC] *see* Loperamide Hydrochloride
on page 416

Imuran® *see* Azathioprine *on page 70*

I-Naphline® *see* Naphazoline Hydrochloride *on page 492*

Inapsine® *see* Droperidol *on page 244*

Indameth® *see* Indomethacin *on next page*

Indapamide (in dap' a mide)

Brand Names Lozol®

Generic Available No

Therapeutic Class Diuretic, Miscellaneous

Use Management of mild to moderate hypertension; treatment of edema in congestive heart failure and nephrotic syndrome

Contraindications Hypersensitivity to indapamide or any component

Adverse Reactions
Cardiovascular: Irregular heartbeats, weak pulse, hypotension
Central nervous system: Mood changes, numbness or tingling in hands, feet or lips
Dermatologic: Photosensitivity
Gastrointestinal: Dry mouth
Endocrine & metabolic: Hypokalemia, hyponatremia, hyperglycemia
Neuromuscular & skeletal: Muscle cramps or pain, unusual weakness
Respiratory: Shortness of breath
Miscellaneous: Increased thirst

Overdosage Symptoms of overdose include electrolyte depletion, volume depletion, hypotension, dehydration, circulatory collapse

Toxicology Following GI decontamination, treatment is supportive; hypotension responds to fluids and Trendelenburg position

Drug Interactions
Decreased effect of oral hypoglycemics; decreased absorption with cholestyramine and colestipol
Increased effect with loop diuretics and other antihypertensives
Increased toxicity/levels of lithium; when given with digoxin, diuretic-induced hypokalemia increases the risk of digoxin toxicity

Mechanism of Action Enhances sodium, chloride and water excretion by interfering with the transport of sodium ions across the renal tubular epithelium; diuretic effect is localized at the proximal segment of the distal tubule of the nephron; it does not appear to have significant effect on glomerular filtration rate nor renal blood flow; differs chemically from the thiazide

Pharmacokinetics
Absorption: Oral: Completely from GI tract
Protein binding: 71% to 79%
Metabolism: Extensive in the liver
Half-life: 14-18 hours
Time to peak serum concentration: 2-2.5 hours
Elimination: ~60% of dose excreted in urine within 48 hours, about 16% to 23% excreted via bile into feces

Usual Dosage Geriatrics and Adults: Oral:
Hypertension: 1.25 mg/day; if no response after 4 weeks, increase to 2.5 mg/day; maximum dose: 5 mg **Note:** There is little therapeutic benefit to increasing the dose above 5 mg/day; there is, however, an increased risk of electrolyte disturbances
Congestive heart failure: 2.5 mg/day; if no response after 1 week, increase to 5 mg

Monitoring Parameters Blood pressure (both standing and sitting/supine), serum electrolytes, renal function, weight, I & O

Test Interactions Increased ammonia (B), increased amylase (S), increased calcium (S), increased cholesterol (S), increased glucose, increased uric acid (S); decreased chloride (S), decreased magnesium, decreased potassium (S), decreased sodium (S)

Patient Information Take early in the day to avoid nocturia. May cause photosensitivity; use a sunblock with an SPF of 15 or more

Nursing Implications See Monitoring Parameters; check for orthostasis

Additional Information Indapamide offers no specific advantage over thiazides

Special Geriatric Considerations Thiazide diuretics lose efficacy when Cl_{cr} is <30-35 mL/minute; many elderly may have Cl_{cr} below this limit; calculate Cl_{cr} for elderly before initiating therapy; see Additional Information

Dosage Forms Tablet: 1.25 mg, 2.5 mg

Inderal® *see* Propranolol Hydrochloride *on page 605*

Inderal® LA *see* Propranolol Hydrochloride *on page 605*

Inderide® *see* Propranolol and Hydrochlorothiazide *on page 605*

Indocin® *see* Indomethacin *on next page*

Indocin® I.V. *see* Indomethacin *on this page*

Indocin® SR *see* Indomethacin *on this page*

Indo-Lemmon® *see* Indomethacin *on this page*

Indometacin *see* Indomethacin *on this page*

Indomethacin (in doe meth' a sin)

Brand Names Indameth®; Indocin®; Indocin® I.V.; Indocin® SR; Indo-Lemmon®

Synonyms Indometacin

Generic Available Yes

Therapeutic Class Analgesic, Non-narcotic; Anti-inflammatory Agent; Nonsteroidal Anti-inflammatory Agent (NSAID), Oral; Nonsteroidal Anti-Inflammatory Agent (NSAID), Parenteral

Use Management of inflammatory diseases and rheumatoid disorders; moderate pain; acute gouty arthritis; ankylosing spondylitis, osteoporosis, tendonitis, bursitis, acute painful shoulder, sunburn, migraine, headache prophylaxis, cluster headache

Contraindications Hypersensitivity to indomethacin, any component, aspirin, or other nonsteroidal anti-inflammatory drugs (NSAIDs); active GI bleeding, ulcer disease; impaired renal function, IVH, active bleeding, thrombocytopenia

Warnings GI toxicity (bleeding, ulceration, perforation); CNS effects may occur (headaches, confusion, depression); hypersensitivity, anaphylactoid reactions (intermittent tolmetin use more often); renal function decline, acute renal insufficiency, interstitial nephritis, dysuria, cystitis, hematuria, nephrotic syndrome, hyperkalemia in acute renal insufficiency, hyponatremia, papillary necrosis, hepatic function impairment; elderly have increased risk for adverse reactions to NSAIDs; see Special Geriatric Considerations

Precautions Use with caution in patients with congestive heart failure, hypertension, decreased renal or hepatic function, history of GI disease (bleeding or ulcers), or those receiving anticoagulants; perform ophthalmologic evaluation for those who develop eye complaints during therapy (blurred vision, diminished vision, changes in color vision, retinal changes); NSAIDs may mask signs/symptoms of infections; photosensitivity reported

Adverse Reactions

Cardiovascular: Headache, hypertension, edema

Central nervous system: Somnolence, vertigo, fatigue, depression, confusion, dizziness

Dermatologic: Rash

Endocrine & metabolic: Hyperkalemia, dilutional hyponatremia (I.V.), hypoglycemia (I.V.)

Gastrointestinal: Nausea, vomiting, diarrhea, constipation, flatulence, anorexia, epigastric pain, abdominal pain, anorexia, GI bleeding, ulcers, gingival ulcers, proctitis

Genitourinary: Cystitis

Hematologic: Hemolytic anemia, bone marrow depression, agranulocytosis, thrombocytopenia, inhibition of platelet aggregation

Hepatic: Hepatitis, cholestatic jaundice

Ocular: Papillary necrosis, perforation, corneal opacities

Otic: Tinnitus

Renal: Dysuria, hematuria, nephrotic syndrome, oliguria, renal failure

Miscellaneous: Hypersensitivity reactions

Elderly have high incidence of confusion and other adverse reactions; see Special Geriatric Considerations

Overdosage Symptoms include drowsiness, lethargy, disorientation, confusion, dizziness, numbness, paresthesia, nausea, vomiting, gastric irritation, abdominal pain, headache, tinnitus, sweating, blurred vision, muscle twitching, seizures, coma, acute renal failure, increased BUN and serum creatinine, hypotension, tachycardia, and metabolic acidosis

Toxicology Management of a nonsteroidal anti-inflammatory agent (NSAID) intoxication is primarily supportive and symptomatic. Fluid therapy is commonly effective in managing the hypotension that may occur following an acute NSAID overdose, except when this is due to an acute blood loss. Seizures tend to be very short-lived and often do not require drug treatment although recurrent seizures should be treated with I.V. diazepam. Since many of the NSAIDs undergo enterohepatic cycling, multiple doses of charcoal may be needed to reduce the potential for delayed toxicities.

Drug Interactions

Indomethacin may increase serum concentrations of digoxin, methotrexate, lithium, and aminoglycosides

May increase nephrotoxicity of cyclosporine

May decrease antihypertensive and diuretic effects of furosemide and thiazides

Effects of loop diuretics may decrease

May increase serum K^+ with potassium-sparing diuretics

May decrease antihypertensive effects of beta-blockers, hydralazine and captopril

Aspirin or other salicylates may decrease and probenecid may increase indomethacin serum concentrations

(Continued)

Indomethacin *(Continued)*

Concomitant administration with dipyridamole may cause enhance water retention
Indomethacin may increase bioavailability of penicillamine; coadministration with phe-
nylpropanolamine may increase blood pressure
Other NSAIDs may increase GI adverse effects
May increase or enhance azotemia in elderly receiving loop diuretics

Stability Protect from light; not stable in alkaline solution; reconstitute just prior to administration; discard any unused portion; do not use preservative containing diluents
for reconstitution

Mechanism of Action Inhibits prostaglandin synthesis, acts on the hypothalamus
heat-regulating center to reduce fever, blocks prostaglandin synthetase action which
prevents formation of the platelet-aggregating substance thromboxane A_2; decreases
pain receptor sensitivity. Other proposed mechanisms of action are lysosomal stabilization, kinin and leukotriene production, alteration of chemotactic factors, and inhibition of neutrophil activation. This latter mechanism may be the most significant pharmacologic action to reduce inflammation.

Pharmacodynamics

Onset of action: Within 30 minutes
Duration: 4-6 hours
Onset of anti-inflammatory action: Within 7 days
Peak effect: 1-2 weeks

Pharmacokinetics

Absorption: Promptly and extensively
Distribution: V_d: 0.34-1.57 L/kg
Protein binding: 90%
Metabolism: In the liver with significant enterohepatic recycling
Half-life: 4-6 hours
Time to peak serum concentration: Oral; Within 1-2 hours; sustained release: 2-4
hours
Elimination: In urine principally as glucuronide conjugates

Usual Dosage Geriatrics and Adults: 25-50 mg/dose 2-3 times/day; maximum dose:
200 mg/day; extended release capsule should be given on a 1-2 times/day schedule;
maximum dose for sustained release is 150 mg/day; best to start elderly on 25 mg
dose given 2-3 times/day

Monitoring Parameters Monitor response (pain, range of motion, grip strength, mobility, ADL function), inflammation; observe for weight gain, edema; monitor renal
function; observe for bleeding, bruising; evaluate gastrointestinal effects (abdominal
pain, bleeding, dyspepsia); mental confusion, disorientation, CBC, serum, creatinine,
BUN, liver function tests

Test Interactions Positive Coombs' [direct]

Patient Information Extended release capsules must be swallowed intact. Serious
gastrointestinal bleeding can occur as well as ulceration and perforation. Pain may or
may not be present. Avoid aspirin and aspirin-containing products while taking this
medication. If gastric upset occurs, take with food, milk, or antacid. If gastric adverse
effects persist, contact physician. May cause drowsiness, dizziness, blurred vision,
and confusion. Use caution when performing tasks which require alertness (eg, driving). Do not take for more than 3 days for fever or 10 days for pain without physician
advice.

Nursing Implications Extended release capsules must be swallowed intact; see
Overdosage, Monitoring Parameters, Patient Information, and Special Geriatric Considerations

Additional Information There are no clinical guidelines to predict which NSAID will
give response in a particular patient; trials with each must be initiated until response
determined; consider dose, patient convenience, and cost

Special Geriatric Considerations Elderly are a high-risk population for adverse effects from nonsteroidal anti-inflammatory agents. As much as 60% of elderly can develop peptic ulceration and/or hemorrhage asymptomatically. The concomitant use of
H_2 blockers, omeprazole, and sucralfate is not effective as prophylaxis. Misoprostol is
the only prophylactic agent proven effective. Also, concomitant disease and drug use
contribute to the risk for GI adverse effects. Use lowest effective dose for shortest period possible. Consider renal function decline with age. Use of NSAIDs can compromise existing renal function especially when Cl_{cr} is ≤ 30 mL/minute. Tinnitus may be
a difficult and unreliable indication of toxicity due to age-related hearing loss or eighth
cranial nerve damage. CNS adverse effects such as confusion, agitation, and hallucination are generally seen in overdose or high dose situations, but elderly may demonstrate these adverse effects at lower doses than younger adults.

Dosage Forms

Capsule: 25 mg, 50 mg
Capsule, sustained release: 75 mg
Suppository: 50 mg
Suspension, oral: 25 mg/5 mL (5 mL, 10 mL, 237 mL, 500 mL)

References

Brooks PM, Day RO, "Nonsteroidal Anti-inflammatory Drugs – Differences and Similarities," *N Engl
J Med*, 1991, 324(24):1716-25.

ALPHABETICAL LISTING OF DRUGS

Clinch D, Banerjee AK, Ostick G, "Absence of Abdominal Pain in Elderly Patients With Peptic Ulcer," *Age Ageing*, 1984, 13:120-3.

Clive DM, Stoff JS, "Renal Syndromes Associated With Nonsteroidal Anti-inflammatory Drugs," *N Engl J Med*, 1984, 310(9):563-72.

Graham DY, "Prevention of Gastroduodenal Injury Induced by Chronic Nonsteroidal Anti-inflammatory Drug Therapy," *Gastroenterology*, 1989, 96(2 Pt 2 Suppl):675-81.

Gurwitz JH, Avarn J, Ross-Degan D, et al, "Nonsteroidal Anti-Inflammatory Drug-Associated Azotemia in the Very Old," *JAMA*, 1990, 264(4):471-5.

Knodel LC, "Preventing NSAID-Induced Ulcers: The Role of Misoprostol," *Consult Pharm*, 1989, 4:37-41.

Pounder R, "Silent Peptic Ulceration: Deadly Silence or Golden Silence?" *Gastroenterology*, 1989, 96(2 Pt 2 Suppl):626-31.

I-N-Ethyl Sisomicin see Netilmicin Sulfate on page 496

Infectrol® Ophthalmic see Neomycin, Polymyxin B, and Dexamethasone on page 495

Inflamase® see Prednisolone on page 584

Inflamase® Mild see Prednisolone on page 584

Influenza Virus Vaccine (in floo en' za)
Related Information
Immunization Guidelines on page 759-762

Brand Names Flu-Imune®; Fluogen®; Fluzone®

Therapeutic Class Vaccine, Inactivated Virus

Use Provide active immunity to influenza virus strains contained in the vaccine; for high risk persons, previous year vaccines should not be to prevent present year influenza

Those at risk for influenza injection:

Persons ≥65 years of age

Institutionalized patients

Persons of any age with chronic disorders of pulmonary and/or cardiovascular system

Persons who have required medical follow-up following hospitalization for other chronic diseases such as diabetes, renal disease, immunodepressive disorders, etc

Travelers, especially those at risk (above)

Contraindications Persons with allergy history to eggs or egg products, chicken, chicken feathers or chicken dander, hypersensitivity to thimerosal, influenza virus vaccine or any component, presence of acute respiratory disease or other active infections or illnesses, delay immunization in a patient with an active neurological disorder

Warnings Hypersensitivity reaction (have epinephrine 1:1000 available); immunosuppressed patients may fail to develop protective antibody titers (amantadine may be given as a supplement)

Precautions Antigenic response may not be as great as expected in patients receiving immunosuppressive drug; hypersensitivity reactions may occur; because of potential for febrile reactions, risks and benefits must carefully be considered in patients with history of febrile convulsions; influenza vaccines from previous seasons must not be used; patients with sulfite sensitivity may be affected by this product; concurrent administration of other vaccines (pneumococcal) is acceptable as long as other vaccines are given at a different site; seroconversion does not develop in all persons receiving vaccine; Guillain-Barré syndrome (1978-81 years had the highest incidence of GBS); temporary neurologic disorders

Adverse Reactions
Central nervous system: Malaise, fever

Dermatologic: Hives, angioedema

Local: Local soreness

Neuromuscular & skeletal: Myalgia rarely, Guillain-Barré syndrome

Respiratory: Asthma

Miscellaneous: Rarely anaphylactoid reactions, allergic reactions

Side effects are minor and uneventful in those few who develop them; most reactions occur within 6-12 hours and may last 1-2 days

Drug Interactions Immunosuppressive agents, theophylline, anticoagulants, phenytoin; do not administer within seven days after administration of diphtheria and tetanus toxoids and pertussis vaccine adsorbed (DTP)

Stability Refrigerate at 2°C to 8°C (36°F to 46°F); do not freeze

Usual Dosage Geriatrics and Adults: I.M.: 0.5 mL each year of appropriate vaccine for the year, one dose is all that is necessary; administer in late fall to allow maximum titers to develop by peak epidemic periods usually occurring in early December

Reference Range Less than a fourfold increase in titer; >1:10 IgG and IgM

Patient Information Be aware of possible adverse effects

Nursing Implications Inspect for particulate matter and discoloration prior to administration; for I.M. administration only

(Continued)

Influenza Virus Vaccine *(Continued)*

Additional Information Pharmacy will stock the formulations(s) standardized according to the USPHS requirements for the season. Influenza vaccines from previous seasons must not be used.

Special Geriatric Considerations Limited data on elderly exists due to ethical considerations precluding use of placebo and differences in studies and vaccines; 80% develop a 1:40 HA titer, 70% are completely protected, 90% protected from death; amantadine may be used to prophylax against influenza type A in the following situations:

    High-risk institutionalized patients, both vaccinated and unvaccinated

    Epidemic environment

    Supplement vaccine in those who may have inadequate response (immunosuppressed)

    Those who refuse vaccine

    Those hypersensitive to vaccine or its components

Amantadine dose must be adjusted for renal failure, see Amantadine; administer for 2 weeks in vaccinated patients and 6-12 weeks in unvaccinated patients

Dosage Forms Injection:
Split-virus (Fluogen®; Fluzone®): 0.5 mL, 5 mL
Whole-virus (Fluzone®): 5 mL

References
Bentley DW, "Vaccinations," *Clin Geriatr Med*, 1992, 8(4):745-60.
Gardner P and Schaffner W, "Immunization of Adults," *N Engl J Med*, 1993, 328(17):1252-8.

INH *see* Isoniazid *on page 379*

Inocor® *see* Amrinone Lactate *on page 54*

Insulatard® NPH *see* Insulin Preparations *on this page*

Insulatard® NPH Human *see* Insulin Preparations *on this page*

Insulin Preparations *(in' su lin)*

Brand Names Beef Regular Iletin® II; Humulin® L; Humulin® N; Humulin® R; Humulin® U; Insulatard® NPH; Insulatard® NPH Human; Lente® Iletin®I; Lente® Iletin® II (Beef); Lente® Iletin® II (Pork); Lente® Insulin (Beef); Lente® Purified Pork; Lente® Purified Pork Insulin; Mixtard® 70/30 (Purified Pork); Novolin® 70/30; Novolin® L; Novolin® N; Novolin® R; Novolin® R Penfill; NPH Iletin®I; NPH Insulin (Beef); NPH Purified Pork; Pork NPH Iletin® II; Pork Regular Iletin® II; Regular Iletin® I; Regular Insulin (Pork); Regular Purified Pork; Semilente® Iletin®I; Semilente® Insulin (Beef); Semilente® Purified Pork Human; Ultralente® Iletin®I; Ultralente® Insulin (Beef); Ultralente® Purified Beef

Synonyms Lente; NPH; Semilente; Ultralente

Therapeutic Class Antidiabetic Agent

Use Treatment of insulin-dependent diabetes mellitus, also noninsulin-dependent diabetes mellitus unresponsive to treatment with diet and/or oral hypoglycemics; acute management of hyperkalemia; to assure proper utilization of glucose and reduce glucosuria in nondiabetic patients receiving parenteral nutrition whose glucosuria cannot be adequately controlled with infusion rate adjustments or those who require assistance in achieving optimal caloric intakes

Warnings Any change of insulin should be made cautiously; changing manufacturers, type and/or method of manufacture, may result in the need for a change of dosage; human insulin differs from animal-source insulin

Precautions Any change of insulin should be made cautiously; changing manufacturers, type and/or method of manufacture, may result in the need for a change of dosage; human insulin differs from animal-source insulin

Adverse Reactions
Cardiovascular: Palpitations, tachycardia
Central nervous system: Fatigue, tingling of fingers, mental confusion, loss of consciousness, headache
Dermatologic: Urticaria
Endocrine & metabolic: Hypoglycemia, hypothermia
Gastrointestinal: Hunger, nausea, numbness of mouth
Local: Itching, redness, swelling, stinging, or warmth at injection site, atrophy or hypertrophy of S.C. fat tissue
Neuromuscular & skeletal: Muscle weakness, tremors
Ocular: Transient presbyopia or blurred vision
Miscellaneous: Sweating, anaphylaxis, pallor

Overdosage Symptoms of overdose include tachycardia, anxiety, hunger, tremors, pallor, headache, motor dysfunction, speech disturbances, sweating, palpitations

Drug Interactions See table.

Stability Bottle in use is stable at room temperature up to 1 month; cold (freezing) causes more damage to insulin than room temperatures up to 100°F; avoid direct sunlight; cold injections should be avoided

Mechanism of Action Replacement therapy for persons unable to produce the hormone naturally or in insufficient amounts to maintain glycemic control

Drug Interactions With Insulin Injection

Decrease Hypoglycemic Effect of Insulin	Increase Hypoglycemic Effect of Insulin
Contraceptives, oral	Alcohol
Corticosteroids	Alpha blockers
Dextrothyroxine	Anabolic steroids
Diltiazem	Beta–blockers*
Dobutamine	Clofibrate
Epinephrine	Fenfluramine
Smoking	Guanethidine
Thiazide diuretics	MAO inhibitors
Thyroid hormone	Pentamidine
Niacin	Phenylbutazone
	Salicylates
	Sulfinpyrazone
	Tetracyclines

*Nonselective beta–blockers may delay recovery from hypoglycemic episodes and mask signs/symptoms of hypoglycemia. Cardioselective agents may be alternatives.

Pharmacodynamics Onset and duration of hypoglycemic effects depend upon preparation administered; see table.

Preparation	Onset of Action	Peak	Duration
Regular	30 min	2.5–5 h	5–8 h
Semilente®	1–2 h	3–10 h	10–16 h
Lente®	2.5 h	7–15 h	18–23 h
NPH	90 min	10–20 h	24 h
Ultralente®	4–8 h	10–30 h	>36 h
70/30	30 min		24 h
Isophane/Regular	6	4–8 h	

Usual Dosage Geriatrics and Adults: Dose requires continuous medical supervision; only regular insulin may be given I.V. The daily dose should be divided up depending upon the product used and the patient's response (eg, regular insulin every 4-6 hours); see table; NPH insulin every 12-24 hours.

Adults: S.C.: 0.5-1 unit/kg/day

Dosing adjustment in renal impairment (regular):
Cl_{cr} 10-50 mL/minute: Administer at 75% of normal dose
Cl_{cr} <10 mL/minute: Administer at 25% to 50% of normal dose; monitor blood glucose closely

Monitoring Parameters Plasma or finger stick blood glucose concentrations; hemoglobin A, C (glycosylated Hgb) fructosamine

Reference Range Therapeutic, serum (fasting): 5-20 μU/mL (SI: 35-145 pmol/L)

Test Interactions Increased catecholamines (U); decreased potassium (S)

Patient Information Do not change insulins without physician's approval; know signs and symptoms of hyperglycemia and hypoglycemia and how to respond to them; reinforce proper use and storage; assess patient's ability to drawing and self inject dose, and to accurately perform home blood glucose (finger stick) monitoring

Nursing Implications Patients using human insulin may be less likely to recognize hypoglycemia than if they use uses pork insulin, patients on pork insulin that have low blood sugar exhibit hunger and sweating

Special Geriatric Considerations How "tightly" a geriatric patient's blood glucose should be controlled is controversial; however, a fasting blood sugar of <150 mg/dL is now an acceptable end point. Such a decision should be based on the patient's functional and cognitive status, how well they recognize hypoglycemic or hyperglycemic symptoms and how to respond to them and their other disease states; patients who are unable to accurately draw up their dose will need assistance such as prefilled syringes. Initial doses may require considerations for renal function in elderly with dosing adjusted subsequently based on blood glucose monitoring.

Dosage Forms
Rapid acting:
Regular human (semisynthetic) insulin injection (Novolin® R): 100 units/mL
Regular Pork (purified) insulin injection: 100 units/mL
Regular pork (standard) insulin injection: 100 units/mL
Semilente® beef (standard) insulin injection: 100 units/mL

(Continued)

Insulin Preparations *(Continued)*

Intermediate acting:
NPH human (semisynthetic) insulin injection (Novolin® N): 100 units/mL
NPH pork (purified) insulin injection: 100 units/mL
NPH beef (standard) insulin injection: 100 units/mL
Lente® human (semisynthetic) insulin injection (Novolin® L): 100 units/mL
Lente® pork (purified) insulin injection: 100 units/mL
Lente® beef (standard) insulin injection: 100 units/mL

Long acting:
Ultralente® human (rDNA) insulin injection (Humulin® U): 100 units/mL
Ultralente® beef (standard) insulin injection: 100 units/mL

Combinations:
70% NPH/30% regular human (semisynthetic) insulin injection (Novolin® 70/30): 100 units/mL
70% NPH/30% regular pork (purified) insulin injection (Mixtard® 70/30): 100 units/mL

Note: U-10 (10 units/mL) and U-1 (1 unit/mL) dilutions can be **extemporaneously compounded by pharmacy**

References
Nathan DM, "Insulin Treatment in the Elderly Diabetic Patient," *Clin Geriatr Med*, 1990, 6(4):923-31.
Morley JE and Perry HM 3d, "The Management of Diabetes Mellitus in Older Individuals," *Drugs*, 1991, 41(4):548-65.

Intal® *see* Cromolyn Sodium *on page 190*

Interferon Beta-1b
Brand Names Betaseron®
Synonyms rIFN-b
Therapeutic Class Interferon
Use Reduces the frequency of clinical exacerbations in ambulatory patients with relapsing-remitting multiple sclerosis (MS)

Unlabeled use: Treatment in AIDS, AIDS-related Kaposi's sarcoma, acute non-A/non-B hepatitis; renal cell carcinoma (metastatic), malignant melanoma; cutaneous T-cell lymphoma

Contraindications Hypersensitivity to *E. coli*-derived products, recombinant interferon beta, or albumin
Warnings Depression and suicidal tendency, anxiety, myelosuppression, confusion, depersonalization, emotional lability
Precautions Patients must be instructed on safe use; baseline laboratory tests are recommended periodically throughout treatment (ie, every 3 months); recommended laboratory tests include CBC with differential, platelets, liver function tests
Adverse Reactions Due to the pivotal position of interferon in the immune system, toxicities can affect nearly every organ system; injection site reactions, injection site necrosis, flu-like symptoms, menstrual disorders, depression (with suicidal ideations), somnolence, palpitations, peripheral vascular disorders, hypertension, blood dyscrasias, dyspnea, laryngitis, cystitis, gastrointestinal complaints, photosensitization
Stability Use within 3 hours of reconstitution; store at 2°C to 8°C (36°F to 46°F); discard any unused portions
Mechanism of Action Interferon beta-1b differs from naturally occurring human protein by a single amino acid substitution and the lack of carbohydrate side chains; alters the expression and response to surface antigens and can enhance immune cell activities. Properties of interferon beta-1b that modify biologic responses are mediated by cell surface receptor interactions; mechanism in the treatment of MS is unknown.
Pharmacokinetics Limited data due to small doses used
Time to peak serum concentration: 1-8 hours
Bioavailability: 50%
Half-life: 8 minutes to 4.3 hours
Usual Dosage Geriatrics and Adults: S.C.: 0.25 mg (8 million units) every other day
Administration Inject 1 mL S.C. with a 27-gauge needle; may be injected into arms, thighs, hips, and abdomen
Monitoring Parameters Hemoglobin, liver function, and blood chemistries; stop therapy if absolute neutrophil count (ANC) drops below 750/mm³; may restart therapy at half-dose when ANC returns to above 750/mm³; if LFTs increase to 10 times upper limit of normal or bilirubin increased above 5 times upper limit of normal, therapy should be stopped; restart half-dose when return to normal
Patient Information Patients must be instructed in aseptic technique when injecting themselves, proper disposal of needles and syringes; injection site may develop a reaction, but this does not dictate the stopping of therapy; flu-like symptoms may occur but the use of aspirin or acetaminophen will relieve the symptoms; warn about depression, feelings of suicide, and photosensitivity; report changes in mental state to physician; use sunblock to prevent photosensitivity reactions

Nursing Implications Patient should be informed of possible side effects, especially depression and suicidal ideations; flu-like symptoms such as chills, fever, malaise, sweating, and myalgia are common; see Monitoring Parameters

Additional Information May be available only in small supplies; for information on availability and distribution, call the patient information line at 800-580-3837

Special Geriatric Considerations No specific recommendations necessary for use in the elderly; monitor for CNS adverse effects which may be significant in elderly; see Warnings

Dosage Forms Powder for injection, lyophilized: 0.3 mg [9.6 million IU units]

Intropin® *see Dopamine Hydrochloride on page 239*

Iodoquinol (eye oh doe kwin' ole)
Brand Names Sebaquin® [OTC]; Yodoxin®
Synonyms Diiodohydroxyquin
Therapeutic Class Amebicide
Use Treatment of acute and chronic intestinal amebiasis; asymptomatic cyst passers; *Blastocystis hominis* infections
Contraindications Known hypersensitivity to iodine or iodoquinol; hepatic or renal damage; pre-existing optic neuropathy
Warnings Optic neuritis, optic atrophy, and peripheral neuropathy have occurred following prolonged use; avoid long-term therapy
Precautions Use with caution in patients with thyroid disease or neurological disorders
Adverse Reactions
Central nervous system: Agitation, retrograde amnesia, fever, headache
Dermatologic: Anal pruritus, rash, acne
Endocrine & metabolic: Enlargement of the thyroid
Gastrointestinal: Nausea, vomiting, diarrhea, gastritis
Neuromuscular & skeletal: Peripheral neuropathy, weakness
Ocular: Optic neuritis, optic atrophy, visual impairment
Overdosage Symptoms of overdose include vomiting, diarrhea, abdominal pain, metallic taste, delirium, stupor, collapse, coma
Mechanism of Action Contact amebicide that works in the lumen of the intestine by an unknown mechanism
Pharmacokinetics
Absorption: Oral: Poor and irregular
Metabolism: In the liver
Elimination: High percentage of dose excreted in feces
Usual Dosage Geriatrics and Adults: Oral: 650 mg 3 times/day after meals for 20 days; not to exceed 2 g/day
Administration Tablets may be crushed and mixed with applesauce or chocolate syrup
Test Interactions May increase protein-bound serum iodine concentrations reflecting a decrease in iodine 131 uptake; false-positive ferric chloride test for phenylketonuria
Patient Information Complete full course of therapy; may cause nausea, vomiting, or diarrhea
Nursing Implications See Administration
Special Geriatric Considerations No special considerations for the elderly, however, this agent is no longer a drug of choice; use only if other therapy is contraindicated or has failed. Due to optic nerve damage, use cautiously in the elderly.
Dosage Forms
Shampoo: 3% (120 mL)
Tablet: 210 mg, 650 mg

Iopidine® *see Apraclonidine Hydrochloride on page 56*

Ipecac Syrup (ip' e kak)
Generic Available Yes
Therapeutic Class Antidote, Emetic
Use Treatment of acute oral drug overdosage and in certain poisonings
Contraindications Do not use in unconscious patients, patients with absent gag reflex; ingestion of strong bases or acids, volatile oils; seizures
Warnings Do not confuse ipecac syrup with ipecac fluid extract, which is 14 times more potent; use with caution in patients with cardiovascular disease and bulimics
Precautions May be ineffective in overdoses of antiemetics; may be cardiotoxic if not vomited and allowed to be absorbed
Adverse Reactions
Cardiovascular: Cardiotoxicity
Central nervous system: Lethargy
Gastrointestinal: Protracted vomiting, diarrhea
Neuromuscular & skeletal: Myopathy
Overdosage Symptoms of overdose include diarrhea, persistent vomiting, hypotension, atrial fibrillation

(Continued)

Ipecac Syrup *(Continued)*

Toxicology Activated charcoal to absorb ipecac or perform gastric lavage; support cardiovascular system by symptomatic care

Drug Interactions
Decreased effect with activated charcoal, milk, carbonated beverages
Increased toxicity of phenothiazines (chlorpromazine has been associated with serious dystonic reactions)

Mechanism of Action Irritates the gastric mucosa and stimulates the medullary chemoreceptor trigger zone to induce vomiting

Pharmacodynamics
Onset of emesis: Within 15-30 minutes
Duration: 20-25 minutes; can last longer, 60 minutes in some cases

Usual Dosage Geriatrics and Adults: Oral: 15-30 mL followed by 200-300 mL of water; repeat dose one time if vomiting does not occur within 20 minutes; if vomiting does not occur after second dose, perform gastric lavage

Patient Information Call Poison Center before administering. Patients should be kept active and moving following administration of ipecac; follow dose with 8 oz of water following initial episode; if vomiting, no food or liquids should be ingested for 1 hour

Nursing Implications Do **not** administer to unconscious patients; patients should be kept active and moving following administration of ipecac; if vomiting does not occur after second dose, gastric lavage may be considered to remove ingested substance

Additional Information Patients should be kept active and moving following administration of ipecac; if vomiting does not occur after second dose, gastric lavage may be considered to remove ingested substance

Special Geriatric Considerations See Precautions and Adverse Reactions

Dosage Forms
Syrup:
OTC: 70 mg/mL, 1.5% alcohol (15 mL, 30 mL)
Prescription: 70 mg/mL, 2% alcohol (30 mL, pints, gallons; UD 15 mL & 30 mL)

I-Phrine® Ophthalmic Solution *see* Phenylephrine Hydrochloride *on page 557*

I-Pilocarpine® *see* Pilocarpine *on page 563*

IPOL® *see* Poliovirus Vaccine, Inactivated *on page 574*

Ipran® *see* Propranolol Hydrochloride *on page 605*

Ipratropium Bromide *(i pra troe' pee um)*

Brand Names Atrovent®
Generic Available No
Therapeutic Class Anticholinergic Agent; Bronchodilator
Use Anticholinergic bronchodilator used for the prevention of bronchospasm associated with COPD, bronchitis, and emphysema
Contraindications Hypersensitivity to atropine or its derivatives
Warnings Not indicated for the initial treatment of acute episodes of bronchospasm
Precautions Use with caution in patients with narrow-angle glaucoma, prostatic hypertrophy or bladder neck obstruction
Adverse Reactions Note: Ipratropium is poorly absorbed from the lung, so systemic effects are rare
Cardiovascular: Palpitations
Central nervous system: Nervousness, dizziness, fatigue, headache
Dermatologic: Rash
Gastrointestinal: Nausea, dry mouth
Ocular: Blurred vision
Respiratory: Cough

Overdosage Symptoms of overdose include dry mouth, drying of respiratory secretions, cough, nausea, GI distress, blurred vision or impaired visual accommodation, headache, nervousness

Toxicology Acute overdosage with ipratropium by inhalation is unlikely since it is so poorly absorbed. However, if poisoning occurs it can be treated like any other anticholinergic toxicity. An anticholinergic overdose with severe life-threatening symptoms, may be treated with physostigmine 1-2 mg S.C. or I.V., slowly.

Mechanism of Action Blocks the action of acetylcholine at parasympathetic sites in bronchial smooth muscle causing bronchodilation

Pharmacodynamics
Onset of action: Bronchodilation begins 1-3 minutes after administration with a maximal effect occurring within 1.5-2 hours
Duration: 4-6 hours

Pharmacokinetics
Absorption: Inhalation: Not readily absorbed into the systemic circulation from the surface of the lung or from GI tract
Distribution: 15% of dose reaches the lower airways

Usual Dosage Geriatrics and Adults:

Inhalation: 2 inhalations 4 times/day up to 12 inhalations/24 hours

Nebulization: 500 mcg 3-4 times/day

Monitoring Parameters Pulmonary function tests

Patient Information Temporary blurred vision may occur if sprayed into eyes. Follow instructions for use accompanying the product. Close eyes when administering ipratropium; wait at least one full minute between inhalations

Nursing Implications Teach patients how to use the inhaler; shake inhaler before administering

Additional Information Some patients may require higher doses (4-8 inhalations/dose)

Special Geriatric Considerations Older patients may find it difficult to use the metered dose inhaler. A spacer device may be useful. Ipratropium has not been specifically studied in the elderly, but it is poorly absorbed from the airways and appears to be safe in this population.

Dosage Forms Solution:

Inhalation: 18 mcg/actuation (14 g)

Nebulizing: 0.2% (2.5 mL)

References

Hughes DT, "The Use of Anticholinergic Drugs in Nocturnal Asthma," *Postgrad Med J*, 1987, 63(Suppl 1):47-51.

I-Pred® see Prednisolone on page 584

Iproveratril Hydrochloride see Verapamil Hydrochloride on page 735

IPV see Poliovirus Vaccine, Inactivated on page 574

Irodex® see Iron Dextran Complex on this page

Iron Dextran Complex

Related Information

Antacid Drug Interactions on page 764

Brand Names Feronim®; Hydextran®; Imferon®; Irodex®; K-Feron®; Nor-Feran®; Proferdex®

Generic Available Yes

Therapeutic Class Iron Salt

Use Treatment of microcytic hypochromic anemia resulting from iron deficiency in whom oral administration is infeasible or ineffective

Contraindications Hypersensitivity to iron dextran; all anemias that are not involved with iron deficiency; hemochromatosis, hemolytic anemia

Warnings Deaths associated with parenteral administration following anaphylactic-type reactions have been reported; use only in patients where the iron deficient state is not amenable to oral iron therapy; I.M. injections have been reported to be carcinogenic in rats and mice

Precautions Use with caution in patients with history of asthma, hepatic impairment rheumatoid arthritis; epinephrine should be immediately available to treat hypersensitivity reactions

Adverse Reactions

Cardiovascular: Cardiovascular collapse, hypotension

Central nervous system: Dizziness, fever, headache, chills

Dermatologic: Urticaria

Gastrointestinal: Nausea, metallic taste

Hematologic: Leukocytosis

Local: Pain, staining of skin at the site of I.M. injection, phlebitis, flushing

Neuromuscular & skeletal: Arthralgia

Respiratory: Respiratory difficulty

Miscellaneous: Lymphadenopathy, sweating

Overdosage Symptoms of overdose include lethargy, tarry stools, hypotension, acidosis, pulmonary edema, hyperthermia, convulsions, tachycardia, enlargement of lymph nodes

Toxicology Although rare, if a severe iron overdose (when the serum iron concentration exceeds the total iron-binding capacity) occurs, it may be treated with deferoxamine. Deferoxamine may be administered I.V. (80 mg/kg over 24 hours) or I.M. (40-90 mg/kg every 8 hours). Hypersensitivity reactions should be treated with 0.5 mL of a 1:1000 solution of epinephrine given I.M. or S.C.

Drug Interactions Decreased effect with chloramphenicol

Stability Commercial injection should be stored at room temperature

Stability of parenteral admixture at room temperature (25°C): 3 months

Mechanism of Action The released iron, from the plasma, eventually replenishes the depleted iron stores in the bone marrow where it is incorporated into hemoglobin

Pharmacokinetics

Absorption: I.M.: Prompt, 50% to 90% absorbed, balance slowly absorbed over months

Elimination: By reticuloendothelial system and excreted in urine and feces (via bile)

Usual Dosage Geriatrics and Adults: A 0.5 mL test dose should be given prior to starting iron dextran therapy

(Continued)

ALPHABETICAL LISTING OF DRUGS

Iron Dextran Complex *(Continued)*

Total replacement dosage of iron dextran (mg) = (0.3) (weight in lbs) (100 - 100 x Hgb divided by 14.8)

> I.V.: This dose can be given in its entirety after a minimum 1-hour waiting period has elapsed after the test dose. Individual daily doses of ≤2 mL can be given I.V. or I.M. until the cumulative total dose necessary for replacement has been reached.

Administration Use Z-track technique for I.M. administration (deep into the upper outer quadrant of buttock); may be administered I.V. bolus at rate ≤50 mg/minute or diluted in 250-1000 mL NS and infused over 1-6 hours

Monitoring Parameters Hemoglobin, hematocrit, ferritin, reticulocyte count

Reference Range Therapeutic: Male: 75-175 μg/dL (SI: 13.4-31.3 μmol/L); Female: 65-165 μg/dL (SI: 11.6-29.5 μmol/L); ranges may vary by laboratory

Test Interactions Increased serum iron concentration for 3 weeks

Patient Information Report any unusual systemic or local reactions to your physician; pain on administration

Nursing Implications See Administration

Additional Information Avoid iron injection if oral intake is feasible; a test dose of 0.5 mL I.V. or I.M. should be given to observe for adverse reactions

Special Geriatric Considerations Anemia in the elderly is most often caused by "anemia of chronic disease" or associated with inflammation rather than blood loss. Iron stores are usually normal or increased, with a serum ferritin >50 ng/mL and a decreased total iron binding capacity. Hence, the anemia is not secondary to iron deficiency but the inability of the reticuloendothelial system to use available iron stores. I.V. administration of iron dextran is often preferred over I.M. in the elderly secondary to a decreased muscle mass and the need for daily injections.

Dosage Forms Injection: 50 mg/mL (2 mL, 5 mL, 10 mL)

References

Lipschitz DA, "The Anemia of Chronic Disease," *J Am Geriatr Soc*, 1990, 38(11):1258-64.

ISD *see* Isosorbide Dinitrate *on page 382*

ISDN *see* Isosorbide Dinitrate *on page 382*

ISG *see* Immune Globulin *on page 366*

Ismelin® *see* Guanethidine Sulfate *on page 335*

Ismotic® *see* Isosorbide *on page 382*

Isobamate *see* Carisoprodol *on page 121*

Iso-Bid® *see* Isosorbide Dinitrate *on page 382*

Isoetharine *(eye soe eth' a reen)*

Brand Names Arm-a-Med® Isoetharine; Beta-2®; Bronkometer®; Bronkosol®; Dey-Lute® Isoetharine

Synonyms Isoetharine Hydrochloride; Isoetharine Mesylate

Generic Available Yes

Therapeutic Class Adrenergic Agonist Agent; Bronchodilator

Use Bronchodilator in bronchial asthma and for reversible bronchospasm occurring with bronchitis and emphysema

Contraindications Known hypersensitivity to isoetharine

Warnings Isoetharine hydrochloride solution contains sulfites which may cause allergic reactions in some patients. Use caution in patients with unstable vasomotor symptoms, diabetes, hyperthyroidism, prostatic hypertrophy, or a history of seizures. Also use caution in the elderly and those patients with cardiovascular disorders such as coronary artery disease, arrhythmias, and hypertension.

Precautions Excessive or prolonged use may result in decreased effectiveness

Adverse Reactions

Cardiovascular: Tachycardia, hypertension

Central nervous system: Anxiety, dizziness, restlessness, excitement, headache

Gastrointestinal: Nausea, vomiting

Neuromuscular & skeletal: Tremors (may be more common in the elderly), weakness

Overdosage Symptoms of overdose include nausea, vomiting, hypertension, tremors

Toxicology In cases of overdose, supportive therapy should be instituted, and prudent use of a cardioselective beta-adrenergic blocker (eg, atenolol or metoprolol) should be considered, keeping in mind the potential for induction of bronchoconstriction in an asthmatic individual. Dialysis has not been shown to be of value in the treatment of an overdose with this agent.

Drug Interactions

Decreased effect with beta-blockers

Increased toxicity with other sympathomimetics (eg, epinephrine)

Stability Do not use if solution is discolored or a precipitation is present; compatible with sterile water, 0:45% NaCl, and 0.9% NaCl

Mechanism of Action Relaxes bronchial smooth muscle by action on beta₂-receptors with little effect on heart rate

Pharmacodynamics
Peak effect: Inhalation: Within 5-15 minutes
Duration: 1-4 hours
Pharmacokinetics
Metabolism: In many tissues including the liver and lungs
Elimination: Primarily (90%) as metabolites
Usual Dosage Treatments are usually not repeated more often than every 4 hours, except in severe cases

Geriatrics and Adults:
Aerosol nebulizer: 1-2 inhalations every 4 hours as needed
Hand nebulizer: 3-7 inhalations undiluted every 4 hours as needed
Monitoring Parameters Pulmonary function, blood pressure, pulse
Patient Information Follow instructions for use of nebulizer
Nursing Implications Monitor lung sounds, blood pressure, pulse; instruct patient on use of nebulizer
Additional Information
Isoetharine hydrochloride: Arm-a-Med® isoetharine, Beta-2®, Bronkosol®, Dey-Lute® isoetharine
Isoetharine mesylate: Bronkometer®
Isoetharine has a shorter duration of action than other beta₂ selective agonists; therefore, it is usually not considered a first-line drug of choice
Special Geriatric Considerations See Additional Information. The elderly may find it useful to utilize a spacer device when using a metered dose inhaler. Oral use should be avoided due to the increased incidence of adverse effects.
Dosage Forms
Aerosol, as mesylate: 0.61% (10 mL, 15 mL)
Solution, inhalation, as hydrochloride: 0.062% (4 mL); 0.08% (3.5 mL); 0.190 (2.5 mL, 5 mL); 0.125% (4 mL); 0.14% (3.5 mL); 0.167% (3 mL); 0.17% (3 mL); 0.2% (2.5 mL); 0.25% (2 mL, 3.5 mL); 0.5% (0.5 mL); 1% (0.5 mL, 0.25 mL, 10 mL, 14 mL, 30 mL)

Isoetharine Hydrochloride *see* Isoetharine *on previous page*

Isoetharine Mesylate *see* Isoetharine *on previous page*

Isonate® *see* Isosorbide Dinitrate *on page 382*

Isoniazid (eye soe nye' a zid)
Related Information
Antacid Drug Interactions *on page 764*
Brand Names Laniazid®; Nydrazid®
Synonyms INH; Isonicotinic Acid Hydrazide
Generic Available Yes
Therapeutic Class Antitubercular Agent
Use Treatment of susceptible tuberculosis infections and prophylactically to those individuals exposed to tuberculosis
Contraindications Acute liver disease; hypersensitivity to isoniazid or any component; previous history of hepatic damage during isoniazid therapy
Warnings Severe and sometimes fatal hepatitis may occur or develop even after many months of treatment; patients must report any prodromal symptoms of hepatitis, such as fatigue, weakness, malaise, anorexia, nausea, or vomiting
Precautions Use with caution in patients with renal impairment and chronic liver disease
Adverse Reactions
Central nervous system: Peripheral neuritis, seizure, stupor, dizziness, psychosis, fever, ataxia, depression
Dermatologic: Skin eruptions
Endocrine & metabolic: Hyperglycemia
Gastrointestinal: Nausea, vomiting, epigastric distress
Hematologic: Blood dyscrasias
Hepatic: Hepatitis, elevated liver transaminase levels
Neuromuscular & skeletal: Hyperreflexia
Ocular: Optic neuritis
Otic: Tinnitus
Overdosage Symptoms of overdose include nausea, vomiting, slurred speech, dizziness, blurred vision, hallucinations, stupor, coma, intractable seizures
Toxicology Because of the severe morbidity and high mortality rates with isoniazid overdose, patients who are asymptomatic after an overdose, should be monitored for 4-6 hours. Pyridoxine has been shown to be effective in the treatment of intoxication, especially when seizures occur. Pyridoxine I.V. is administered on a milligram to milligram dose. If the amount of isoniazid ingested is unknown, 5 g of pyridoxine should be given over 3-5 minutes and may be followed by an additional 5 g in 30 minutes.
Drug Interactions
Inhibits the metabolism and increased toxicity of phenytoin, carbamazepine, primidone, warfarin, diazepam (and other hepatically metabolized benzodiazepines), prednisone, disulfiram
(Continued)

Isoniazid (Continued)

Decreased effect/levels of isoniazid with aluminum salts

Stability Protect oral dosage forms from light

Mechanism of Action Unknown, but may include the inhibition of myocolic acid synthesis resulting in disruption of the bacterial cell wall

Pharmacokinetics

Absorption: Oral, I.M.: Rapid and complete

Distribution: Into all body tissues and fluids including the CSF

Protein binding: 10% to 15%

Metabolism: By the liver with decay rate determined genetically by acetylation phenotype

Half-life:

Fast acetylators: 30-100 minutes

Slow acetylators: 2-5 hours; half-life may be prolonged in patients with impaired hepatic function or severe renal impairment

Time to peak: Oral: Peak serum levels occur within 1-2 hours; rate of absorption can be slowed when administered with food

Elimination: In urine (75% to 95%), feces, and saliva

Usual Dosage Oral, I.M.:

Geriatrics and Adults: 5 mg/kg/day given daily (usual dose: 300 mg)

Disseminated disease: 10 mg/kg/day in 1-2 divided doses

Prophylaxis: 300 mg/day given daily

American Thoracic Society and CDC currently recommend twice weekly therapy as part of a short-course regimen (6-9 months) which follows 1-2 months of daily treatment for uncomplicated pulmonary tuberculosis in compliant patients

Geriatrics and Adults: 15 mg/kg/dose (up to 900 mg) twice weekly

Dialyzable (50% to 100%)

Monitoring Parameters Monitor transaminase levels at baseline 1, 3, 6, and 9 months

Reference Range Therapeutic: 1-7 µg/mL (SI: 7-51 µmol/L); Toxic: 20-710 µg/mL (SI: 146-5176 µmol/L)

Test Interactions False-positive urinary glucose with Clinitest®

Patient Information Report any prodromal symptoms of hepatitis (fatigue, weakness, nausea, vomiting, dark urine, or yellowing of eyes) or any burning, tingling, or numbness in the extremities

Nursing Implications Monitor monthly for signs or symptoms of active disease, hepatitis, or other adverse effects

Additional Information Pyridoxine should be given concomitantly in persons with conditions in which neuropathy is common (eg, diabetes, alcoholism, malnutrition)

Special Geriatric Considerations Age has not been shown to affect the pharmacokinetics of INH since acetylation phenotype determines clearance and half-life, acetylation rate does not change significantly with age; most strains of M. tuberculosis found the elderly should be susceptible to INH since most acquired their initial infection prior to INH's introduction

Dosage Forms

Injection: 100 mg/mL (10 mL)

Syrup: 50 mg/5 mL (473 mL)

Tablet: 50 mg, 100 mg, 300 mg

References

Bass JB Jr, Farer LS, Hopewell PC, et al, "Treatment of Tuberculosis and Tuberculosis Infection in Adults and Children," *Am J Respir Crit Care Med*, 1994, 149(5):1359-74.

Kergueris MF, Bourin M, and Larousse C, "Pharmacokinetics of Isoniazid: Influence of Age," *Eur J Clin Pharmacol*, 1986, 30(3):335-40.

Van Scoy RE and Wilkowske CJ, "Antituberculous Agents: Isoniazid, Rifampin, Streptomycin, Ethambutol, and Pyrazinamide," *Mayo Clin Proc*, 1983, 58(4):233-40.

Yoshikawa TT, "Tuberculosis in Aging Adults," *J Am Geriatr Soc*, 1992, 40(2):178-87.

Isonicotinic Acid Hydrazide see Isoniazid on previous page

Isonipecaine Hydrochloride see Meperidine Hydrochloride on page 441

Isoprenaline Hydrochloride see Isoproterenol on this page

Isopro® see Isoproterenol on this page

Isoproterenol (eye soe proe ter' e nole)

Brand Names Arm-a-Med® Isoproterenol; Dey-Dose® Isoproterenol; Dispos-a-Med® Isoproterenol; Isopro®; Isuprel®; Medihaler-Iso®; Norisodrine®; Vapo-Iso®

Synonyms Isoprenaline Hydrochloride; Isoproterenol Hydrochloride; Isoproterenol Sulfate

Generic Available Yes

Therapeutic Class Adrenergic Agonist Agent; Bronchodilator

Use Asthma or COPD (reversible airway obstruction); A-V nodal block; hemodynamically compromised bradyarrhythmias or atropine-resistant bradyarrhythmias, temporary use in third degree A-V block until pacemaker insertion; low cardiac output; vasoconstrictive shock states

Contraindications Angina, pre-existing cardiac arrhythmias (ventricular); tachycardia or A-V block caused by cardiac glycoside intoxication; allergy to sulfites or isoproterenol or other sympathomimetic amines

Warnings Use with caution in congestive heart failure, ischemia, or aortic stenosis

Precautions Geriatric patients, diabetics, renal or cardiovascular disease, hyperthyroidism

Adverse Reactions
Cardiovascular: Hypertension, tachycardia, palpitations, arrhythmias
Central nervous system: Nervousness, restlessness, anxiety, dizziness, headache
Gastrointestinal: Nausea, vomiting
Neuromuscular & skeletal: Tremors

Overdosage Symptoms of overdose include nausea, vomiting, hypertension, tremors

Toxicology In cases of overdose, supportive therapy should be instituted, and prudent use of a cardioselective beta-adrenergic blocker (eg, atenolol or metoprolol) should be considered, keeping in mind the potential for induction of bronchoconstriction in an asthmatic individual. Dialysis has not been shown to be of value in the treatment of an overdose with this agent.

Drug Interactions Increased toxicity: Sympathomimetic agents, general anesthetics

Stability Do not use discolored solutions; limit exposure to heat, light, or air; incompatible with alkaline solutions
Stability of parenteral admixture at room temperature (25°C): 24 hours
Stability of parenteral admixture at refrigeration temperature (4°C): 24 hours

Mechanism of Action Relaxes bronchial smooth muscle by action on $beta_2$-receptors; causes increased heart rate and contractility by action on $beta_1$-receptors

Pharmacokinetics
Metabolism: By conjugation in many tissues including the liver and lungs
Half-life: 2.5-5 minutes
Time to peak serum concentration: Oral: Within 1-2 hours
Elimination: In urine principally as sulfate conjugates

Usual Dosage Geriatrics and Adults:
Bronchodilation, metered dose inhaler: 1-2 inhalations 4-6 times/day
Hand bulb nebulizer: 5-15 inhalations of a 1:200 solution up to 5 times/day
Glossets: S.L.: 10-20 mg every 3-4 hours as needed up to 60 mg/day
A-V nodal block: I.V. infusion: 2-20 mcg/minute

Monitoring Parameters Pulmonary function, blood pressure, pulse

Patient Information Follow instructions accompanying inhaler; do not exceed recommended doses

Nursing Implications Instruct patient on how to use inhaler or nebulizer

Additional Information Isoproterenol is not a drug of first choice in the chronic treatment of asthma because of its $beta_1$ effects.
Isoproterenol hydrochloride: Aerolone®, Dey-Dose® isoproterenol, Dispos-a-Med® isoproterenol, Isopro®, Isuprel®, Norisodrine®, Vapo-Iso®
Isoproterenol sulfate: Medihaler-Iso®

Special Geriatric Considerations See Additional Information; the elderly may find it useful to utilize a spacer device when using a metered dose inhaler

Dosage Forms
Inhalation: 0.5% (1 mL, 10 mL); 1% (1 mL, 10 mL)
Inhalation, aerosol: 0.25% (15 mL, 22.5 mL)
Injection: 0.2 mg/mL (1 mL, 5 mL, 10 mL)
Tablet (Glosset), sublingual: 10 mg, 15 mg

Isosorbide (eye soe sor' bide)

Brand Names Ismotic®

Generic Available No

Therapeutic Class Diuretic, Osmotic; Ophthalmic Agent, Osmotic

Use Short-term emergency treatment of acute angle-closure glaucoma and short-term reduction of intraocular pressure prior to and following intraocular surgery; may be used to interrupt an acute glaucoma attack; preferred agent when need to avoid nausea and vomiting

Contraindications Severe renal disease, anuria, severe dehydration, acute pulmonary edema, severe cardiac decompensation, known hypersensitivity to isosorbide

Warnings Maintain fluid/electrolyte balance with multiple doses; monitor urinary output; if urinary output declines, need to review clinical status

Precautions Use with caution in patients with impending pulmonary edema, and in the elderly; hypernatremia and dehydration may begin to occur after 72 hours of continuous administration; use is not recommended in patients with anuria, severe dehydration

Adverse Reactions

Cardiovascular: Syncope

Central nervous system: Headache, confusion, disorientation, lethargy, vertigo, dizziness, lightheadedness, irritability

Dermatologic: Rash

Endocrine & metabolic: Hypernatremia, hyperosmolarity

Gastrointestinal: Nausea, vomiting, abdominal/gastric discomfort (infrequently)

Miscellaneous: Hiccups

Overdosage Symptoms of overdose include dehydration, hypotension, hypernatremia

Toxicology General supportive care; fluid administration, electrolyte balance, discontinue agent

Mechanism of Action Elevate osmolarity of glomerular filtrate to hinder the tubular resorption of water and increase excretion of sodium and chloride to result in diuresis; creates an osmotic gradient between plasma and ocular fluids

Pharmacodynamics

Onset of action: Within 10-30 minutes

Peak action: 1-1.5 hours

Duration: 5-6 hours

Pharmacokinetics

Distribution: In total body water

Metabolism: Not metabolized

Half-life: 5-9.5 hours

Elimination: By glomerular filtration; see Mechanism of Action

Usual Dosage Geriatrics and Adults: Oral: Initial: 1.5 g/kg with a usual range of 1-3 g/kg 2-4 times/day

Monitoring Parameters Monitor for signs of dehydration, blood pressure, renal output, intraocular pressure reduction

Nursing Implications Palatability may be improved if poured over ice and sipped

Additional Information Each 220 mL contains isosorbide 100 g, sodium 4.6 mEq and potassium 0.9 mEq; hypernatremia and dehydration may begin to occur after 72 hours of continuous administration; palatability may be improved by sipping over cracked ice

Special Geriatric Considerations Use cautiously due to the elderly's predisposition to dehydration and the fact that they frequently have concomitant diseases which may be aggravated by the use of isosorbide; see Contraindications and Precautions

Dosage Forms Solution: 45% (220 mL)

Isosorbide Dinitrate (eye soe sor' bide)

Brand Names Dilitrate®-SR; Iso-Bid®; Isonate®; Isordil®; Isordil® Titradose®; Isotrate®; Sorbitrate®

Synonyms ISD; ISDN

Generic Available Yes

Therapeutic Class Antianginal Agent; Nitrate; Vasodilator, Coronary

Use Prevention and treatment of angina pectoris; for congestive heart failure; to relieve pain, dysphagia, and spasm in esophageal spasm with GE reflux

Contraindications Severe anemia, closed-angle glaucoma, postural hypotension, cerebral hemorrhage, head trauma, hypersensitivity to isosorbide dinitrate or any component

Warnings Do not crush or chew sublingual dosage form; do not crush chewable tablets before administration; use with caution in patients with hypovolemia, glaucoma, increased intracranial pressure, hypotension

Precautions Increased intracranial pressure; do not use sustained-release products in patients with GI hypermotility or malabsorption syndrome; do not stop use abruptly to avoid withdrawal reactions (angina); must gradually reduce daily doses to withdraw; tolerance to vascular effects of nitrates has been demonstrated; see Dosage for recommendation to minimize development of tolerance

Adverse Reactions
>   Cardiovascular: Postural hypotension, cutaneous flushing of head, neck, and clavicular area, tachycardia
>   Central nervous system: Dizziness, vertigo, headache
>   Dermatologic: Rash
>   Gastrointestinal: Nausea, GI upset

Overdosage Symptoms of overdose include hypotension, throbbing headache, palpitations, visual disturbances, flushing, perspiring skin, vertigo, diaphoresis, dizziness, syncope, nausea, vomiting, anorexia, dyspnea, heart block, confusion, fever, paralysis

Toxicology Formation of methemoglobinemia is dose-related and unusual in normal doses; high levels can cause signs and symptoms of hypoxemia; treatment consists of placing patient in recumbent position and administer fluids; alpha-adrenergic vasopressors may be required; treat methemoglobinemia with oxygen and methylene blue at a dose of 1-2 mg/kg I.V. slowly

Drug Interactions May antagonize the anticoagulant effect of heparin; alcohol increases hypotension; aspirin increases serum nitrate concentration; calcium channel blockers increase hypotension

Mechanism of Action Stimulation of intracellular cyclic-GMP results in vascular smooth muscle relaxation of both arterial and venous vasculature. Increased venous pooling decreases left ventricular pressure (preload) and arterial dilatation decreases arterial resistance (afterload). Therefore, this reduces cardiac oxygen demand by decreasing left ventricular pressure and systemic vascular resistance by dilating arteries. Additionally, coronary artery dilation improves collateral flow to ischemic regions; esophageal smooth muscle is relaxed via the same mechanism.

Pharmacodynamics See table.

Dosage Form	Onset of Action	Duration
Sublingual tablet	2–10 min	1–2 h
Chewable tablet	3 min	0.5–2 h
Oral tablet	45–60 min	4–6 h
Sustained release tablet	30 min	6–12 h

Pharmacokinetics
>   Metabolism: Extensive in the liver to conjugated metabolites, including isosorbide 5-mononitrate (active) and 2-mononitrate (active)
>   Half-life:
>>   Parent: 1-4 hours
>>   5-mononitrate: 4 hours
>   Elimination: In urine and feces

Usual Dosage Geriatrics (give lowest recommended daily dose initially and titrate upward) and Adults:
>   Oral: 5-30 mg 3-4 times/day or 40 mg every 6-12 hours in sustained-released dosage form
>   Chewable: 5-10 mg every 2-3 hours
>   Sublingual: 2.5-10 mg every 4-6 hours

>   Tolerance to nitrate effects develops with chronic exposure. Dose escalation does not overcome this effect. Tolerance can only be overcome by short periods of nitrate absence from the body. Short periods (10-12 hours) or nitrate withdrawal help minimize tolerance. General recommendations are to take the last dose of short-acting agents no later than 7 PM; administer 2-3 times/day rather than 4 times/day. Sustained release preparations could be administered at times to allow a 15- to 17-hour interval between first and last daily dose. Example: Give sustained release at 8 AM and 2 PM for a twice daily regimen.

Monitoring Parameters Monitor anginal episodes, orthostatic blood pressures; a decrease of 15 mm Hg pressure systolic and/or 10 mm Hg diastolic or an increase in heart rate of 10 beats/minute from baseline (no drug) indicates approximate maximal cardiodynamic effects to nitrates and end point for dosing

Test Interactions Decreased cholesterol (S)

Patient Information Dispense drug in easy-to-open container; do not chew or crush sublingual or sustained-release dosage form; do not change brands without consulting your pharmacist or physician; patient should be instructed to take sublingual and chewable tablets while sitting down; any angina that persists for more than 20 minutes should be evaluated by a physician immediately

Nursing Implications Do not crush sustained release or sublingual drug product; monitor blood pressure reduction for maximal effect and orthostatic hypotension

(Continued)

ALPHABETICAL LISTING OF DRUGS
Isosorbide Dinitrate *(Continued)*

Special Geriatric Considerations The first dose of nitrates should be taken in a physician's office to observe for maximal cardiovascular dynamic effects (see Monitoring Parameters) and adverse effects (orthostatic blood pressure drop, headache). The use of nitrates for angina may occasionally promote reflux esophagitis. This may require dose adjustments or changing therapeutic agents to correct this adverse effect.

Dosage Forms
Capsule, sustained release: 40 mg
Tablet:
  Chewable: 5 mg, 10 mg
  Oral: 5 mg, 10 mg, 20 mg, 30 mg, 40 mg
  Sublingual: 2.5 mg, 5 mg, 10 mg
  Sustained release: 40 mg

Isotrate® *see* Isosorbide Dinitrate *on page 382*

Isoxazolyl Penicillin *see* Oxacillin Sodium *on page 521*

Isoxsuprine Hydrochloride *(eye sox' syoo preen)*
Brand Names Vasodilan®; Voxsuprine®
Generic Available Yes
Therapeutic Class Vasodilator
Use Considered "possibly effective" for treatment of peripheral vascular diseases, such as arteriosclerosis obliterans and Raynaud's disease
Contraindications Presence of arterial bleeding
Warnings May cause hypotension in elderly
Precautions See Warnings
Adverse Reactions
Cardiovascular: Hypotension, tachycardia, chest pain
Central nervous system: Dizziness
Dermatologic: Rash
Gastrointestinal: Nausea, vomiting, diarrhea, abdominal distress
Neuromuscular & skeletal: Weakness
Overdosage Symptoms of overdose include hypotension, flushing
Toxicology Vasodilation mediated second to alpha-adrenergic stimulation or direct smooth muscle effects; treat with I.V. fluids, alpha-adrenergic pressors may be required
Drug Interactions May enhance effects of other vasodilators/hypotensive agents; use with caution in elderly
Mechanism of Action In studies on normal human subjects, isoxsuprine increases muscle blood flow but skin blood flow is usually unaffected. Isoxsuprine was originally thought to increase muscle blood flow by beta-receptor stimulations. Since beta-receptor blocking drugs do not antagonize its vascular effects, isoxsuprine probably has a direct action on vascular smooth muscle. Isoxsuprine was shown to inhibit prostaglandin synthetase at high serum concentrations; with low concentrations there was an increase in the P-G synthesis. At high doses blood viscosity is lowered and platelet aggregation is inhibited.
Pharmacokinetics
Absorption: Nearly completely
Metabolism: Partially conjugated in the liver
Serum half-life: 1.25 hours mean
Time to peak serum concentration: Oral, I.M.: Within 1 hour
Elimination: Primarily in urine
Usual Dosage Geriatrics and Adults: 10-20 mg 3-4 times/day; start with lower dose in elderly due to potential hypotension
Monitoring Parameters Monitor orthostatic blood pressure
Patient Information May cause skin rash; discontinue use if rash occurs; arise slowly from prolonged sitting or lying
Nursing Implications See Monitoring Parameters and Patient Information
Special Geriatric Considerations Vasodilators have been used to treat dementia upon the premise that dementia is secondary to a cerebral blood flow insufficiency. The hypothesis is that if blood flow could be increased, cognitive function would be increased. This hypothesis is no longer valid. The use of vasodilators for cognitive dysfunction is not recommended or proven by appropriate scientific study.
Dosage Forms
Injection: 10 mg/2 mL (2 mL)
Tablet: 10 mg, 20 mg

References
Erwin WG, "Senile Dementia of the Alzheimer Type," *Clin Pharm*, 1984, 3:497-504.
Higbee MD, "Noncholinergic Approaches to Treating Senile Dementia of the Alzheimer's Type," *Consult Pharm*, 1992, 7(6):635-41.
Waters C, "Cognitive Enhancing Agents: Current Status in the Treatment of Alzheimer's Disease," *Can J Neurol Sci*, 1988, 15:249-56.

Yesavage JA, Tinklenberg JR, Hollister LE, et al, "Vasodilators in Senile Dementias: A Review of the Literature," *Arch Gen Psychiatry*, 1979, 36:220-3.

Ispid® *see* Sodium Sulfacetamide *on page 651*

Isradipine (is ra' di peen)
Related Information
  Calcium Channel Blocking Agents Comparison *on page 806-807*
Brand Names DynaCirc®
Generic Available No
Therapeutic Class Calcium Channel Blocker
Use Management of hypertension, alone or concurrently with thiazide-type diuretics
Contraindications Sinus bradycardia; advanced heart block; ventricular tachycardia; cardiogenic shock, hypotension, congestive heart failure; hypersensitivity to isradipine or any component, hypersensitivity to calcium channel blockers and adenosine; atrial fibrillation or flutter associated with accessory conduction pathways; not to be given within a few hours of I.V. beta-blocking agents
Warnings Hypotension, congestive heart failure, cardiac conduction defects, PVCs, idiopathic hypertrophic subaortic stenosis; may cause platelet inhibition; do not abruptly withdraw (chest pain); hepatic dysfunction, increased angina; increased intracranial pressure with cranial tumors; elderly may have greater hypotensive effect
Precautions Sick sinus syndrome, severe left ventricular dysfunction, congestive heart failure, hepatic impairment, hypertrophic cardiomyopathy (especially obstructive), concomitant therapy with beta-blockers or digoxin, edema
Adverse Reactions
  Cardiovascular: Atrial and ventricular fibrillation, TIAs, stroke, flushing, hypotension, palpitations, A-V block, congestive heart failure, myocardial infarction, tachycardia, abnormal EKG
  Central nervous system: Fatigue, lethargy, dizziness, lightheadedness, drowsiness, disturbed sleep, psychotic symptoms, equilibrium dysfunction, headache, paresthesia, insomnia
  Dermatologic: Rash, pruritus
  Gastrointestinal: Nausea, vomiting, diarrhea, constipation, abdominal pain, dry mouth
  Hematologic: Leukopenia
  Neuromuscular & skeletal: Numbness, leg and feet cramps, weakness
  Ocular: Blurred vision
  Renal: Polyuria, nocturia
  Respiratory: Throat discomfort, shortness of breath, cough
  Miscellaneous: Sweating, peripheral edema
Overdosage Symptoms of overdose include heartblock, hypotension, asystole, nausea, weakness, dizziness, drowsiness, confusion and slurred speech; profound bradycardia and occasionally hyperglycemia
Toxicology Ipecac-induced emesis can hypothetically worsen calcium antagonist toxicity since it can produce vagal stimulation. The potential for seizures precipitously following acute ingestion of large doses of a calcium antagonist may also contraindicate the use of ipecac. Supportive and symptomatic treatment, including I.V. fluids and Trendelenburg positioning, should be initiated as intoxication may cause hypotension. Although calcium (calcium chloride I.V. 1-2 g over 5-10 minutes with repeats as needed) has been used as an "antidote" for acute intoxications, there is limited experience to support its routine use and should be reserved for those cases where definite signs of myocardial depression are evident. Heart block may respond to isoproterenol, glucagon, atropine and/or calcium, although a temporary pacemaker may be required.
Drug Interactions
  Beta-blockers increased cardiac and A-V conduction depression; fentanyl increased volume requirements and hypotension; although the drug is new, other drug interactions not reported to the same degree as older agents; however, should be suspect of any drug interaction reported with other calcium channel blockers
Mechanism of Action Inhibits calcium ion from entering the "slow channels" or select voltage sensitive areas of vascular smooth muscle and myocardium during depolarization; produces a relaxation of coronary vascular smooth muscle and coronary vasodilation; increases myocardial oxygen delivery in patients with vasospastic angina
Pharmacodynamics
  Onset of action: 2 hours
  Peak effect: 2-4 weeks
Pharmacokinetics
  Absorption: Oral: 90% to 95%
  Protein binding: 95%
  Metabolism: In the liver
  Bioavailability: Absolute due to first-pass elimination 15% to 24%
  Half-life: 8 hours
  Time to peak: Serum concentration: 1-1.5 hours
  Elimination: Renal excretion by metabolites (cyclic lactone and monoacids)
(Continued)

Isradipine *(Continued)*

Usual Dosage Geriatrics and Adults: 2.5 mg twice daily; antihypertensive response seen in 2-3 hours; maximal response in 2-4 weeks; increase dose at 2- to 4-week intervals at 2.5-5 mg increments; usual dose range: 5-20 mg/day. **Note**: Most patients show no improvement with doses >10 mg/day except adverse reaction rate increases; therefore, maximal dose in elderly should be 10 mg/day

Monitoring Parameters Heart rate, blood pressure, signs and symptoms of congestive heart failure

Patient Information Notify physician if you experience irregular heartbeat, shortness of breath, swelling, constipation, nausea, hypotension or dizziness; do not stop or interrupt therapy without physician advice

Nursing Implications Do not crush sustained release capsules; see Warnings, Precautions, Monitoring Parameters, and Special Geriatric Considerations

Additional Information Only approved indication is hypertension, but may be used for congestive heart failure; similar to nifedipine in actions, except for fewer side effects

Special Geriatric Considerations Elderly may experience a greater hypotensive response; constipation may be more of a problem in elderly; calcium channel blockers are no more effective in elderly than other therapies; however, they do not cause significant CNS effects which is an advantage over some antihypertensive agents; see Note in Usual Dosage

Dosage Forms Capsule: 2.5 mg, 5 mg

I-Sulfacet® *see* Sodium Sulfacetamide *on page 651*

Isuprel® *see* Isoproterenol *on page 380*

Itraconazole *(i tra koe' na zole)*

Brand Names Sporanox® Oral

Generic Available No

Therapeutic Class Antifungal Agent, Systemic

Use Treatment of susceptible fungal infections in immunocompromised and nonimmunocompromised patients including blastomycosis and histoplasmosis

Contraindications Known hypersensitivity to itraconazole or other azoles; terfenadine

Warnings Coadministration with terfenadine is contraindicated; rare cases of serious cardiovascular adverse event, including death, ventricular tachycardia and torsade de pointes have been observed due to increased terfenadine concentrations induced by itraconazole; patients who develop abnormal liver function tests during itraconazole therapy should be monitored closely for the development of more severe hepatic injury; if clinical signs and symptoms consistent with liver disease develop that may be attributable to itraconazole, itraconazole should be discontinued

Adverse Reactions
Cardiovascular: Hypertension
Central nervous system: Headache, dizziness, insomnia
Dermatologic: Skin rash, exfoliative skin disorders
Endocrine & metabolic: Hypokalemia, adrenal insufficiency, gynecomastia, breast pain (male)
Gastrointestinal: Nausea, vomiting, diarrhea, abdominal pain, anorexia, flatulence
Genitourinary: Impotence
Hepatic: Elevated AST, ALT, or alkaline phosphatase

Toxicology Overdoses are well tolerated; supportive measures and gastric decontamination with ipecac or sodium bicarbonate lavage should be employed; not removed by dialysis

Drug Interactions
Decreased effect: Rifampin, isoniazid, phenytoin, H_2 antagonists, and omeprazole, antacids
Increased effect: May increase cyclosporine levels when high doses used, phenytoin levels, effect of warfarin and sulfonylureas, digoxin levels
Increased toxicity of astemizole, terfenadine (cardiotoxicity)

Pharmacokinetics
Absorption: Rapid and complete
Protein binding: >99%
Metabolism: Hepatic, >97%
Elimination: 85% renally excreted, 40% as inactive metabolites

Usual Dosage Geriatrics and Adults: Oral: 200 mg once daily, if no obvious improvement or there is evidence of progressive fungal disease, increase the dose in 100 mg increments to a maximum of 400 mg/day
Life-threatening: Loading dose: 200 mg 3 times/day (600 mg/day) should be given for the first 3 days

Administration Doses >200 mg/day are given in 2 divided doses; do not administer with antacids

Monitoring Parameters Signs and symptoms of infection, baseline LFTs, recheck LFTs if therapy is to go beyond 2 weeks; see Drug Interactions

Patient Information Take with food; do not take with antacids

Nursing Implications See Administration

Special Geriatric Considerations No specific data for elderly; use does not require alteration in dose or dose intervals; assess patient's ability to self administer, may be difficult in patients with arthritis or limited range of motion

Dosage Forms Capsule: 100 mg

I-Tropine® see Atropine Sulfate on page 65

IUDR see Idoxuridine on page 362

Iveegam® see Immune Globulin on page 366

I-White® Ophthalmic Solution see Phenylephrine Hydrochloride on page 557

Janimine® see Imipramine on page 365

Jenamicin® see Gentamicin Sulfate on page 320

Kabikinase® see Streptokinase on page 656

Kalcinate® see Calcium Gluconate (Parenteral) on page 108

Kanamycin Sulfate (kan a mye' sin)

Related Information

Aminoglycoside Dosing Guidelines on page 753

Brand Names Kantrex®

Therapeutic Class Antibiotic, Aminoglycoside

Use Treatment of susceptible bacterial infection including gram-negative aerobes, gram-positive *Bacillus* as well as some mycobacteria

Oral: Preoperative bowel preparation in the prophylaxis of infections and adjunctive treatment of hepatic coma (oral kanamycin is not indicated in the treatment of systemic infections)

Parenteral: Rarely used in antibiotic irrigations during surgery

Contraindications Hypersensitivity to kanamycin or any component

Warnings Aminoglycosides are associated with significant nephrotoxicity or ototoxicity; the ototoxicity is directly proportional to the amount of drug given and the duration of treatment. Tinnitus or vertigo are indications of vestibular injury and impending bilateral irreversible damage; renal damage is usually reversible. Elderly patients with pre-existing tinnitus or vertigo or known subclinical deafness, those receiving other ototoxic drugs, or those receiving >15 g kanamycin sulfate should be observed very carefully for eighth nerve damage.

Adverse Reactions

Central nervous system: Neuromuscular blockade

Dermatologic: Rash, photosensitivity

Hematologic: Granulocytopenia, agranulocytosis, thrombocytopenia

Otic: Ototoxicity (auditory and vestibular)

Renal: Nephrotoxicity

Overdosage Symptoms of overdose include ototoxicity, nephrotoxicity, and neuromuscular toxicity

Toxicology The treatment of choice following a single acute overdose appears to be the maintenance of good urine output of at least 3 mL/kg/hour. Dialysis is of questionable value in the enhancement of aminoglycoside elimination. If required, hemodialysis is preferred over peritoneal dialysis in patients with normal renal function. Careful hydration may be all that is required to promote diuresis and therefore the enhancement of the drug's elimination.

Drug Interactions

Increased/prolonged effect of depolarizing and nondepolarizing neuromuscular blocking agents

Increased toxicity: Concurrent use of amphotericin may increase nephrotoxicity

Stability Darkening of vials does not indicate loss of potency

Mechanism of Action Interferes with protein synthesis in bacterial cell by binding to ribosomal subunit

Pharmacokinetics

Distribution: V_d: 0.19 L/kg

Half-life: 2-4 hours, increases in anuria to 80 hours; in older adults the mean half-life has been reported to be longer, 2.5 hours in 50-70 years of age and 4.7 hours in 70-90 years of age; the plasma half-life and V_d have also been reported to be increased in elderly bedridden patients

Time to peak: I.M.: Peak serum levels occur within 1-2 hours

Elimination: Entirely in the kidney, principally by glomerular filtration

Usual Dosage

Geriatrics: I.M., I.V.: Initial dose should be 5-7.5 mg/kg based on ideal body weight (except in obese patients); maintenance dose and interval should be adjusted for estimated renal function; dosing interval in most older patients is every 12-24 hours

(Continued)

Kanamycin Sulfate *(Continued)*

Adults:
Infections: 15 mg/kg/day in divided doses every 8-12 hours
Preoperative intestinal antisepsis: Oral: 1 g every 4-6 hours for 36-72 hours

Dialyzable (50% to 100%)

Administration Dilute to 100-200 mL and infuse over 30 minutes; I.M. doses should be given in a large muscle mass (ie, gluteus maximus)

Monitoring Parameters Serum creatinine and BUN every 2-3 days; peak and trough concentrations; hearing

Reference Range

Therapeutic:
Peak: 25-35 μg/mL (SI: 52-72 μmol/L)
Trough: 4-8 μg/mL (SI: 8-16 μmol/L)

Toxic:
Peak: >35 μg/mL (SI: >72 μmol/L)
Trough: >10 μg/mL (SI: >21 μmol/L)

Test Interactions Increased ammonia (B), protein; decreased magnesium

Nursing Implications Aminoglycoside levels in blood taken from Silastic® central catheters can sometime give falsely high readings. Give around-the-clock rather than 4 times/day, 3 times/day, etc (ie, 12-6-12-6, not 9-1-5-9) to promote less variation in peak and trough serum levels; modify dosage in patients with renal impairment; see Administration

Special Geriatric Considerations See Warnings, Pharmacokinetics, and Usual Dosage; kanamycin is not a drug of choice in the elderly since the elderly may have increased adverse effects (renal)

Dosage Forms
Capsule: 500 mg
Injection: 1 g/3 mL

References

Kristensen M, Molholm HJ, Kampmann J, et al, "Letter: Drug Elimination and Renal Function," *J Clin Pharmacol*, 1974, 14(5-6):307-8.

Yasuhara H, Kobayashi S, Sakamoto K, et al, "Pharmacokinetics of Amikacin and Cephalothin in Bedridden Elderly Patients," *J Clin Pharmacol*, 1982, 22:403-9.

Kantrex® *see* Kanamycin Sulfate *on previous page*

Kaochlor® S-F *see* Potassium Chloride *on page 576*

Kaolin and Pectin (kay' oh lin)

Brand Names Kao-Spen® [OTC]; Kapectolin® [OTC]

Synonyms Pectin and Kaolin

Therapeutic Class Antidiarrheal

Use Treatment of uncomplicated diarrhea

Restrictions See Warnings and Precautions

Contraindications Hypersensitivity to kaolin or pectin; fecal impaction, ileus

Warnings Do not use with diarrhea associated with toxigenic bacteria or pseudomembranous colitis

Precautions Use with caution in patients >60 years of age; presence of high fever; do not use in patients predisposed to fecal impaction

Adverse Reactions Gastrointestinal: Constipation, fecal impaction

Overdosage May cause bowel impaction and obstruction

Drug Interactions Oral lincomycin and oral digoxin

Mechanism of Action Controls diarrhea because of its adsorbent action

Usual Dosage Geriatrics and Adults: Oral: 60-120 mL after each loose stool

Monitoring Parameters Monitor for reduction of stools per day and increased consistency; monitor for signs of fluid and electrolyte loss

Patient Information If diarrhea is not controlled in 48 hours, contact a physician

Nursing Implications Shake well before giving

Special Geriatric Considerations Elderly often present bowel impaction with diarrhea. The use of adsorbents in the face of fecal impaction could aggravate this serious condition. Also, diarrhea causes fluid/electrolyte loss which elderly do not tolerate well. Use of adsorbents can cause further loss of fluid/electrolytes.

Dosage Forms Suspension: Kaolin 975 mg and pectin 22 mg per 5 mL

Kaolin and Pectin With Opium (kay' oh lin & pek' tin with oh' pee um)

Brand Names Parepectolin®

Therapeutic Class Antidiarrheal

Use Symptomatic relief of diarrhea

Restrictions C-V

Contraindications Should not be used to treat diarrhea (opium) caused by poisons, toxins, or infectious agents until GI tract has been cleared of causative agent; do not use in patients with hypersensitivity to opium or morphine derivatives

Warnings Do not use with diarrhea associated with toxigenic bacteria or pseudomembranous colitis

Precautions Use with caution in geriatric patients predisposed to fecal impaction/intestinal obstruction; use with caution in patients >60 years of age, presence of high fever

Adverse Reactions Gastrointestinal: Constipation, fecal impaction

Overdosage Symptoms of overdose include constipation, bowel obstruction, fecal impaction; opium absorption may cause signs of narcotic drug use (confusion, lethargy, hypotension, drowsiness, sedation)

Drug Interactions Chloroquine, digoxin, lincomycin, CNS depressants, anticholinergic drugs, disulfiram, MAO inhibitors, metronidazole, procarbazine

Mechanism of Action Opium reduces intestinal motility, relieves tenesmus, cramps, and colic pain secondary to diarrhea. Kaolin and pectin act by adsorbent action.

Pharmacokinetics Absorption: Opium is absorbed from GI tract; kaolin and pectin are not absorbed

Usual Dosage Geriatrics and Adults: Oral: 15-30 mL with each loose bowel movement, not to exceed 120 mL in 12 hours

Patient Information If diarrhea is not controlled in 48 hours, contact a physician

Nursing Implications Monitor for signs of opium (narcotic) action, see Overdosage; shake well before giving

Special Geriatric Considerations Elderly often present bowel impaction with diarrhea. The use of adsorbents in the face of fecal impaction could aggravate this serious condition. Also, diarrhea causes fluid/electrolyte loss which elderly do not tolerate well. Use of adsorbents can cause further loss of fluid/electrolytes. The use of this product in elderly is discouraged due to side effect potential and lack of clinical efficacy for disease process.

Dosage Forms Suspension: Kaolin 5.5 g, pectin 162 mg and opium 15 mg per 30 mL = 3.7 mL paregoric (240 mL)

Kaon® see Potassium Gluconate on page 578

Kaon-CL® see Potassium Chloride on page 576

Kaopectate® Advanced Formula® [OTC] see Attapulgite on page 66

Kao-Spen® [OTC] see Kaolin and Pectin on previous page

Kapectolin® PG see Hyoscyamine, Atropine, Scopolamine, Kaolin, Pectin and Opium on page 358

Kapectolin® [OTC] see Kaolin and Pectin on previous page

Karidium® see Fluoride on page 299

Karigel® see Fluoride on page 299

Kato® see Potassium Chloride on page 576

Kayexalate® see Sodium Polystyrene Sulfonate on page 650

Kaylixir® see Potassium Gluconate on page 578

KCl see Potassium Chloride on page 576

K-Dur® 20 see Potassium Chloride on page 576

Keflet® see Cephalexin Monohydrate on page 142

Keflex® see Cephalexin Monohydrate on page 142

Keflin® see Cephalothin Sodium on page 143

Keftab® see Cephalexin Monohydrate on page 142

Kefurox® see Cefuroxime on page 141

Kefzol® see Cefazolin Sodium on page 127

Kemadrin® see Procyclidine Hydrochloride on page 595

Kenacort® Syrup see Triamcinolone on page 710

Kenacort® Tablet see Triamcinolone on page 710

Kenalog® Injection see Triamcinolone on page 710

Kerlone® see Betaxolol Hydrochloride on page 84

Ketoconazole (kee toe koe' na zole)
Related Information
Antacid Drug Interactions on page 764
Brand Names Nizoral®
Therapeutic Class Antifungal Agent, Systemic; Antifungal Agent, Topical
Use Treatment of susceptible fungal infections, including candidiasis, oral thrush, blastomycosis, histoplasmosis, paracoccidioidomycosis, chronic mucocutaneous candidiasis, as well as certain recalcitrant cutaneous dermatophytoses; used topically for treatment of tinea corporis, tinea cruris, tinea versicolor and cutaneous candidiasis

(Continued)

Ketoconazole *(Continued)*

Investigational use: Advanced prostate cancer

Contraindications Hypersensitivity to ketoconazole or any component; CNS fungal infections (due to poor CNS penetration)

Warnings Has been associated with hepatotoxicity, including some fatalities; perform periodic liver function tests; high doses of ketoconazole may depress adrenocortical function

Precautions Gastric acidity is necessary for the dissolution and absorption of ketoconazole; use with caution in patients with impaired hepatic function; lowers serum testosterone at dose of 800 mg/day and abolishes them at doses of 1600 mg/day; see Drug Interactions

Adverse Reactions

Central nervous system: Severe depression, suicidal tendencies (rare), dizziness, somnolence, fever

Dermatologic: Pruritus, rash

Endocrine & metabolic: Adrenal cortical insufficiency, gynecomastia

Gastrointestinal: Nausea, vomiting, abdominal discomfort, GI bleeding, diarrhea

Genitourinary: Impotence

Hematologic: Thrombocytopenia, leukopenia, hemolytic anemia

Hepatic: Hepatotoxicity

Local: Irritation, stinging

Ocular: Photophobia

Overdosage Symptoms of overdose include dizziness, headache, nausea, vomiting, diarrhea; institute supportive measures (ie, gastric lavage with sodium bicarbonate)

Drug Interactions

Drugs that decrease absorption (raise gastric pH) such as antacids, H_2-receptor blockers

Drugs that decreased serum concentrations of ketoconazole (rifampin, isoniazid)

Drug concentrations that are increased by ketoconazole (phenytoin, cyclosporine, theophylline, terfenadine, warfarin)

Mechanism of Action Alters the permeability of the cell wall; inhibits biosynthesis of triglycerides and phospholipids by fungi; inhibits several fungal enzymes that results in a build-up of toxic concentrations of hydrogen peroxide

Pharmacokinetics

Absorption: Oral: Rapid (~75%)

Distribution: Minimal into the CNS

Protein binding: 93% to 96%

Metabolism: Partially in the liver by enzymes to inactive compounds

Bioavailability: Decreases as pH of the gastric contents increase

Half-life, biphasic:

Initial: 2 hours

Terminal: 8 hours

Time to peak: Peak serum levels occur within 1-2 hours

Elimination: Primarily in feces (57%) with smaller amounts excreted in urine (13%)

Usual Dosage Geriatrics and Adults:

Oral: 200-400 mg/day as a single daily dose for 1-2 weeks for candidiasis and 6 weeks for other mycoses

Shampoo: Apply twice weekly for 4 weeks with at least 3 days between each shampoo

Topical: Rub gently into the affected area 1-2 times/day

Not dialyzable (0% to 5%)

Administration Administer 2 hours prior to antacids or H_2-receptor antagonists to prevent decreased absorption due to the high pH of gastric contents

Monitoring Parameters Signs and symptoms of infection, baseline LFTs; recheck if therapy is to go beyond 2 weeks; serum concentration and subjective response; see Drug Interactions

Reference Range Therapeutic: Peak: 1-4 mg/L; Trough: ≤ 1 mg/L

Patient Information Cream is for topical application to the skin only; avoid contact with the eye; avoid taking antacids or H_2 antagonists at the same time as ketoconazole; may cause headache, dizziness or drowsiness, observe caution when driving or operating machinery; notify physician of GI side effects; dark urine or pale stools occur

Nursing Implications See Administration and Monitoring Parameters

Special Geriatric Considerations See Usual Dosage and Monitoring Parameters

Dosage Forms

Cream: 2% (15 g, 30 g, 60 g)

Shampoo: 2% (120 mL)

Tablet: 200 mg

Ketoprofen *(kee toe proe' fen)*

Brand Names Orudis®

Generic Available No

Therapeutic Class Analgesic, Non-narcotic; Anti-inflammatory Agent; Nonsteroidal Anti-inflammatory Agent (NSAID), Oral

Use Acute or long-term treatment of rheumatoid arthritis and osteoarthritis; mild to moderate pain, sunburn, migraine headache prophylaxis

Contraindications Known hypersensitivity to ketoprofen or other NSAIDs/aspirin

Warnings GI toxicity (bleeding, ulceration, perforation); CNS effects may occur (headaches, confusion, depression); hypersensitivity, anaphylactoid reactions (intermittent tolmetin use more often); renal function decline, acute renal insufficiency, interstitial nephritis, dysuria, cystitis, hematuria, nephrotic syndrome, hyperkalemia in acute renal insufficiency, hyponatremia, papillary necrosis, hepatic function impairment; elderly have increased risk for adverse reactions to NSAIDs; see Special Geriatric Considerations

Precautions Use with caution in patients with congestive heart failure, hypertension, decreased renal or hepatic function, history of GI disease (bleeding or ulcers), or those receiving anticoagulants; perform ophthalmologic evaluation for those who develop eye complaints during therapy (blurred vision, diminished vision, changes in color vision, retinal changes); NSAIDs may mask signs/symptoms of infections; photosensitivity reported

Adverse Reactions

Cardiovascular: Congestive heart failure, angina, hypertension, hypotension, fluid retention, arrhythmias, edema

Central nervous system: Headache, drowsiness, vertigo, dizziness, fatigue, hallucinations, confusion, depression, emotional lability, psychotic behavior, asthenia

Dermatologic: Rash, urticaria, angioedema, Stevens-Johnson syndrome, exfoliative dermatitis, ecchymosis, petechiae, purpura, bruising

Endocrine & metabolic: Hyperglycemia, hypoglycemia, hyperkalemia, gynecomastia, hyponatremia

Gastrointestinal: Dyspepsia, heartburn, nausea, diarrhea, constipation, flatulence, stomatitis, vomiting, abdominal pain, peptic ulcer, GI bleeding, GI perforation, gingival ulcers, pancreatitis, proctitis, paralytic ulcers, colitis, anorexia, weight loss

Genitourinary: Impotence, azotemia

Hematologic: Neutropenia, anemia, agranulocytosis, bone marrow suppression, hemolytic anemia, hemorrhage, inhibition of platelet aggregation

Hepatic: Hepatitis, elevated LFTs, cholestatic jaundice

Neuromuscular & skeletal: Involuntary muscle movements, muscle weakness, tremors

Ocular: Vision changes

Otic: Tinnitus

Renal: Dysuria, polyuria, pyuria, oliguria, anuria, acute renal failure

Respiratory: Exacerbation of asthma, dyspnea

Miscellaneous: Dry mucous membranes, thirst, pyrexia, sweating

Overdosage Symptoms include drowsiness, lethargy, disorientation, confusion, dizziness, numbness, paresthesia, nausea, vomiting, gastric irritation, abdominal pain, headache, tinnitus, sweating, blurred vision, muscle twitching, seizures, coma, acute renal failure, increased BUN and serum creatinine, hypotension, tachycardia, and metabolic acidosis

Toxicology Management of a nonsteroidal anti-inflammatory agent (NSAID) intoxication is primarily supportive and symptomatic. Fluid therapy is commonly effective in managing the hypotension that may occur following an acute NSAID overdose, except when this is due to an acute blood loss. Seizures tend to be very short-lived and often do not require drug treatment although recurrent seizures should be treated with I.V. diazepam. Since many of the NSAIDs undergo enterohepatic cycling, multiple doses of charcoal may be needed to reduce the potential for delayed toxicities.

Drug Interactions

May increase digoxin, methotrexate, and lithium serum concentrations

Aspirin or other salicylates may decrease NSAID serum concentrations

Other NSAIDs may increase adverse GI effects

Increased prothrombin time with anticoagulants

Decreased antihypertensive effects of ACE inhibitors, beta-blockers, and thiazide diuretics

Effects of loop diuretics may decrease

Increased response to sympathomimetics

Probenecid may increase toxicity of NSAIDs by increase in serum concentrations

Diuretics increase risk of acute renal insufficiency

Azotemia may be enhanced in elderly receiving loop diuretics

Mechanism of Action Inhibits prostaglandin synthesis, acts on the hypothalamus heat-regulating center to reduce fever, blocks prostaglandin synthetase action which prevents formation of the platelet-aggregating substance thromboxane A_2; decreases pain receptor sensitivity. Other proposed mechanisms of action are lysosomal stabilization, kinin and leukotriene production, alteration of chemotactic factors, and inhibition of neutrophil activation. This latter mechanism may be the most significant pharmacologic action to reduce inflammation.

Pharmacokinetics

Absorption: Almost completely

Protein binding: >90%

Metabolism: In the liver

Half-life: 1-4 hours

(Continued)

Ketoprofen *(Continued)*

Time to peak serum concentration: Oral: Within 0.5-2 hours

Elimination: Renal excretion (60% to 75% of a dose), primarily as glucuronide conjugates

Usual Dosage Oral:

Geriatrics: Initial: 25-50 mg 3-4 times/day; increase up to 150-300 mg/day (maximum daily dose: 300 mg)

Adults: 50-75 mg 3-4 times/day up to 300 mg/day (maximum)

Monitoring Parameters Monitor response (pain, range of motion, grip strength, mobility, ADL function), inflammation; observe for weight gain, edema; monitor renal function; observe for bleeding, bruising; evaluate gastrointestinal effects (abdominal pain, bleeding, dyspepsia); mental confusion, disorientation, CBC, serum, creatinine, BUN, liver function tests

Test Interactions Increased chloride (S), increased sodium (S)

Patient Information Serious gastrointestinal bleeding can occur as well as ulceration and perforation. Pain may or may not be present. Avoid aspirin and aspirin-containing products while taking this medication. If gastric upset occurs, take with food, milk, or antacid. If gastric adverse effects persist, contact physician. May cause drowsiness, dizziness, blurred vision, and confusion. Use caution when performing tasks which require alertness (eg, driving). Do not take for more than 3 days for fever or 10 days for pain without physician advice.

Nursing Implications See Overdosage, Monitoring Parameters, Patient Information, and Special Geriatric Considerations

Additional Information Dose must be lowest recommended in renal insufficiency. There are no clinical guidelines to predict which NSAID will give response in a particular patient. Trials with each must be initiated until response determined. Consider dose, patient convenience, and cost.

Special Geriatric Considerations Elderly are a high-risk population for adverse effects from nonsteroidal anti-inflammatory agents. As much as 60% of elderly can develop peptic ulceration and/or hemorrhage asymptomatically. The concomitant use of H_2 blockers, omeprazole, and sucralfate is not effective as prophylaxis. Misoprostol is the only prophylactic agent proven effective. Also, concomitant disease and drug use contribute to the risk for GI adverse effects. Use lowest effective dose for shortest period possible. Consider renal function decline with age. Use of NSAIDs can compromise existing renal function especially when Cl_{cr} is $\leq$30 mL/minute. Tinnitus may be a difficult and unreliable indication of toxicity due to age-related hearing loss or eighth cranial nerve damage. CNS adverse effects such as confusion, agitation, and hallucination are generally seen in overdose or high dose situations, but elderly may demonstrate these adverse effects at lower doses than younger adults.

Dosage Forms Capsule: 25 mg, 50 mg, 75 mg

References

Brooks PM, Day RO, "Nonsteroidal Anti-inflammatory Drugs – Differences and Similarities," *N Engl J Med*, 1991, 324(24):1716-25.

Clinch D, Banerjee AK, Ostick G, "Absence of Abdominal Pain in Elderly Patients With Peptic Ulcer," *Age Ageing*, 1984, 13:120-3.

Clive DM, Stoff JS, "Renal Syndromes Associated With Nonsteroidal Anti-inflammatory Drugs," *N Engl J Med*, 1984, 310(9):563-72.

Graham DY, "Prevention of Gastroduodenal Injury Induced by Chronic Nonsteroidal Anti-inflammatory Drug Therapy," *Gastroenterology*, 1989, 96(2 Pt 2 Suppl):675-81.

Gurwitz JH, Avarn J, Ross-Degan D, et al, "Nonsteroidal Anti-Inflammatory Drug-Associated Azotemia in the Very Old," *JAMA*, 1990, 264(4):471-5.

Knodel LC, "Preventing NSAID-Induced Ulcers: The Role of Misoprostol," *Consult Pharm*, 1989, 4:37-41.

Pounder R, "Silent Peptic Ulceration: Deadly Silence or Golden Silence?" *Gastroenterology*, 1989, 96(2 Pt 2 Suppl):626-31.

Ketorolac Tromethamine *(kee' toe role ak)*

Brand Names Acular® Ophthalmic; Toradol®

Generic Available No

Therapeutic Class Analgesic, Non-narcotic; Anti-inflammatory Agent; Nonsteroidal Anti-inflammatory Agent (NSAID), Oral; Nonsteroidal Anti-Inflammatory Agent (NSAID), Parenteral

Use

Oral: Limited duration, as needed, for management of pain

I.M.: Short-term management of pain, up to 5 days

Ophthalmic: Relief of ocular itching secondary to seasonal allergic conjunctivitis

Contraindications In patients who have developed nasal polyps, angioedema, or bronchospastic reactions to other NSAIDs; hypersensitivity to ketorolac or any component of the products used

Warnings The use of ketorolac at recommended doses for more than 5 days is associated with an increased frequency and severity of adverse events; cross-sensitivity to aspirin and other NSAIDs exists; GI toxicity (bleeding, ulceration, perforation); CNS effects may occur (headaches, confusion, depression); hypersensitivity, anaphylactoid reactions (intermittent tolmetin use more often); renal function decline, acute renal insufficiency, interstitial nephritis, dysuria, cystitis, hematuria, nephrotic syndrome, hyperkalemia in acute renal insufficiency, hyponatremia, papillary necrosis, hepatic function impairment; elderly have increased risk for adverse reactions to NSAIDs; see Special Geriatric Considerations

Note: Ophthalmic solution: Use caution if patients wears soft contact lenses; eye irritation, redness, and burning reported; also systemic absorption may lead to adverse effects (ie, bleeding)

Precautions Use extra caution and reduce dosages in the elderly because it is cleared renally somewhat slower and the elderly are also more sensitive to the renal effects of NSAIDs; use with caution in patients with congestive heart failure, hypertension, decreased renal or hepatic function, history of GI disease (bleeding or ulcers), or those receiving anticoagulants; perform ophthalmologic evaluation for those who develop eye complaints during therapy (blurred vision, diminished vision, changes in color vision, retinal changes); NSAIDs may mask signs/symptoms of infections; photosensitivity reported

Adverse Reactions

Cardiovascular: Congestive heart failure, angina, hypertension, hypotension, fluid retention, arrhythmias, edema

Central nervous system: Headache, drowsiness, vertigo, dizziness, fatigue, hallucinations, confusion, depression, emotional lability, psychotic behavior, asthenia

Dermatologic: Rash, urticaria, angioedema, Stevens-Johnson syndrome, exfoliative dermatitis, ecchymosis, petechiae, purpura, bruising

Endocrine & metabolic: Hyperglycemia, hypoglycemia, hyperkalemia, gynecomastia, hyponatremia

Gastrointestinal: Dyspepsia, heartburn, nausea, diarrhea, constipation, pain, flatulence, anorexia, stomatitis, vomiting, abdominal pain, peptic ulcer, GI bleeding, GI perforation, gingival ulcers, pancreatitis, proctitis, paralytic ulcers, colitis, weight loss

Genitourinary: Impotence, azotemia

Hematologic: Postoperative hematomas, wound bleeding (with I.M.), neutropenia, anemia, agranulocytosis, bone marrow suppression, hemolytic anemia, hemorrhage, inhibition of platelet aggregation

Hepatic: Hepatitis, elevated LFTs, cholestatic jaundice

Local: Pain at injection site

Neuromuscular & skeletal: Involuntary muscle movements, muscle weakness, tremors

Ocular: Vision changes, burning, redness, irritation, stinging and burning is transient (40%); allergic reactions (3%), superficial keratitis, ocular infections

Otic: Tinnitus

Renal: Dysuria, polyuria, pyuria, oliguria, anuria, renal impairment, acute renal failure

Respiratory: Exacerbation of asthma, dyspnea

Miscellaneous: Dry mucous membranes, thirst, pyrexia, sweating

Overdosage Symptoms include drowsiness, lethargy, disorientation, confusion, dizziness, numbness, paresthesia, nausea, vomiting, gastric irritation, abdominal pain, headache, tinnitus, sweating, blurred vision, muscle twitching, seizures, coma, acute renal failure, increased BUN and serum creatinine, hypotension, tachycardia, and metabolic acidosis

Toxicology Management of a nonsteroidal anti-inflammatory drug (NSAID) intoxication is primarily supportive and symptomatic. Fluid therapy is commonly effective in managing the hypotension that may occur following an acute NSAID overdose, except when this is due to an acute blood loss. Seizures tend to be very short-lived and often do not require drug treatment although recurrent seizures should be treated with I.V. diazepam. Since many of the NSAIDs undergo enterohepatic cycling, multiple doses of charcoal may be needed to reduce the potential for delayed toxicities; NSAIDs are highly bound to plasma proteins; therefore, hemodialysis and peritoneal dialysis are not useful; if ocular solution is ingested, dilute with oral fluids

Drug Interactions

Cyclosporine; may increase digoxin, methotrexate, and lithium serum concentrations

Aspirin or other salicylates may decrease NSAID serum concentrations

Other nonsteroidal anti-inflammatories may increase adverse GI effects

Increased prothrombin time with anticoagulants

Decreased antihypertensive effects of ACE inhibitors, beta-blockers, and thiazide diuretics

Effects of loop diuretics may be decreased

Increased response to sympathomimetics

Probenecid may increase toxicity of NSAIDs by increase in serum concentrations

Diuretics increase risk of acute renal insufficiency

Azotemia may be increased in elderly receiving loop diuretics

Stability Protect from light

Mechanism of Action Inhibits prostaglandin synthesis by decreasing the activity of the enzyme, cyclo-oxygenase, which results in decreased formation of prostaglandin precursors; acts on the hypothalamus heat-regulating center to reduce fever, blocks prostaglandin synthetase action which prevents formation of the platelet-aggregating

(Continued)

Ketorolac Tromethamine *(Continued)*

substance thromboxane A_2; decreases pain receptor sensitivity. Other proposed mechanisms of action are lysosomal stabilization, kinin and leukotrienes production, alteration of chemotactic factors, and inhibition of neutrophil activation. This latter mechanism may be the most significant pharmacologic action to reduce inflammation. Prostaglandins appear to have a role in the miotic response produced during ocular surgery by constricting the iris sphincter independently of cholinergic response. Ketorolac inhibits the miosis induced during the course of surgery.

Pharmacodynamics

Onset of action: I.M.: Within 10 minutes

Peak effect: Within 75-150 minutes

Duration of action: 6-8 hours

Pharmacokinetics

Absorption: Oral: Well absorbed

Protein binding: 99%

Metabolism: In the liver

Half-life: 2-8 hours, half-life is increased 30% to 50% in elderly

Time to peak serum concentration: Within 30-60 minutes

Elimination: Renal excretion, 61% appearing in urine as unchanged drug

Usual Dosage

Geriatrics and Adults:

Oral: 10 mg every 4-6 hours as needed for limited-duration treatment of pain; do not use chronic doses of 10 mg 4 times/day; maximum daily dose: 40 mg

I.M.: <50 kg: 30 mg loading dose then 15 mg every 6 hours; maximum dose in the first 24 hours: 150 mg with 120 mg/24 hours thereafter; elderly ($\geq$65 years of age) should be dosed upon the limits for those <50 kg; limit duration of use to 5 days

Ophthalmic: Instill 1 drop (0.25 mg) 4 times/day; efficacy has not been proved beyond 1 week of therapy

Adults >50 kg: I.M.: 30-60 mg loading dose then 15-30 mg every 6 hours

Transition from parenteral to oral dosing: Limit maximum dose on day of transition to 120 mg including oral dose; subsequent oral dose should not exceed 40 mg/day

Monitoring Parameters Monitor response (pain, range of motion, grip strength, mobility, ADL function), inflammation; observe for weight gain, edema; monitor renal function (creatinine, BUN); observe for bleeding, bruising; evaluate gastrointestinal effects (abdominal pain, bleeding, dyspepsia); mental confusion, disorientation, CBC, serum, liver function tests

Reference Range Serum concentration: Therapeutic: 0.3-5 μg/mL; Toxic: >5 μg/mL

Test Interactions Increases chloride (S), sodium (S), bleeding time

Patient Information Serious gastrointestinal bleeding can occur as well as ulceration and perforation. Pain may or may not be present. Avoid aspirin and aspirin-containing products while taking this medication. If gastric upset occurs, take with food, milk, or antacid. If gastric adverse effects persist, contact physician. May cause drowsiness, dizziness, blurred vision, and confusion. Use caution when performing tasks which require alertness (eg, driving). Do not take for more than 3 days for fever or 10 days for pain without physician's advice.

Nursing Implications See Overdosage, Monitoring Parameters, Patient Information, and Special Geriatric Considerations

Additional Information First parenteral NSAID for analgesia; 30 mg provides the analgesia comparable to 12 mg of morphine or 100 mg of meperidine; pain relief usually begins within 10 minutes; there are no clinical guidelines to predict which NSAID will give response in a particular patient. Trials with each must be initiated until response determined. Consider dose, patient convenience, and cost.

Special Geriatric Considerations Elderly are a high-risk population for adverse effects from nonsteroidal anti-inflammatory agents. As much as 60% of elderly can develop peptic ulceration and/or hemorrhage asymptomatically. The concomitant use of H_2 blockers, omeprazole, and sucralfate is not effective as prophylaxis. Misoprostol is the only prophylactic agent proven effective. Also, concomitant disease and drug use contribute to the risk for GI adverse effects. Use lowest effective dose for shortest period possible. Consider renal function decline with age. Use of NSAIDs can compromise existing renal function especially when Cl_{cr} is $\leq$30 mL/minute. Tinnitus may be a difficult and unreliable indication of toxicity due to age-related hearing loss or eighth cranial nerve damage. CNS adverse effects such as confusion, agitation, and hallucination are generally seen in overdose or high dose situations, but elderly may demonstrate these adverse effects at lower doses than younger adults; see Pharmacokinetics.

Dosage Forms

Injection, single dose syringes: 15 mg, 30 mg, 60 mg

Solution, ophthalmic: 0.5% (5 mL)

Tablet: 10 mg

References

Brooks PM, Day RO, "Nonsteroidal Anti-inflammatory Drugs – Differences and Similarities," *N Engl J Med*, 1991, 324(24):1716-25.

Clinch D, Banerjee AK, Ostick G, "Absence of Abdominal Pain in Elderly Patients With Peptic Ulcer," *Age Ageing*, 1984, 13:120-3.

Clive DM, Stoff JS, "Renal Syndromes Associated With Nonsteroidal Anti-inflammatory Drugs," *N Engl J Med*, 1984, 310(9):563-72.

Graham DY, "Prevention of Gastroduodenal Injury Induced by Chronic Nonsteroidal Anti-inflammatory Drug Therapy," *Gastroenterology*, 1989, 96(2 Pt 2 Suppl):675-81.

Jallad NS, Garg DC, Martinez JJ, et al, "Pharmacokinetics of Single-Dose Oral and Intramuscular Ketorolac Tromethamine in the Young and Elderly," *J Clin Pharmacol*, 1990, 30(1):76-81.

Knodel LC, "Preventing NSAID-Induced Ulcers: The Role of Misoprostol," *Consult Pharm*, 1989, 4:37-41.

Pounder R, "Silent Peptic Ulceration: Deadly Silence or Golden Silence?" *Gastroenterology*, 1989, 96(2 Pt 2 Suppl):626-31.

Key-Pred® *see* Prednisolone *on page 584*

Key-Pred-SP® *see* Prednisolone *on page 584*

K-Feron® *see* Iron Dextran Complex *on page 377*

Kinesed® *see* Hyoscyamine, Atropine, Scopolamine and Phenobarbital *on page 357*

Klonopin™ *see* Clonazepam *on page 176*

K-Lor™ *see* Potassium Chloride *on page 576*

Klor-con® *see* Potassium Chloride *on page 576*

Kloromin® [OTC] *see* Chlorpheniramine Maleate *on page 152*

Klorvess® *see* Potassium Chloride *on page 576*

Klotrix® *see* Potassium Chloride *on page 576*

K-Lyte/CL® *see* Potassium Chloride *on page 576*

Konakion® *see* Vitamin K and Menadiol *on page 738*

Kondremul® [OTC] *see* Mineral Oil *on page 473*

Konsyl-D® [OTC] *see* Psyllium *on page 610*

Konsyl® [OTC] *see* Psyllium *on page 610*

K-Phos® MF *see* Potassium Phosphate and Sodium Phosphate *on page 580*

K-Phos® Neutral *see* Potassium Phosphate and Sodium Phosphate *on page 580*

K-Phos® No. 2 *see* Potassium Phosphate and Sodium Phosphate *on page 580*

K-Phos® Original *see* Potassium Acid Phosphate *on page 575*

K-Tab® *see* Potassium Chloride *on page 576*

Kwell® *see* Lindane *on page 407*

Kytril® *see* Granisetron *on page 328*

***L*-3-Hydroxytyrosine** *see* Levodopa *on page 402*

Labetalol and Hydrochlorothiazide
(labet' a lole & hye droe klor oh thye' a zide)
Related Information
Hydrochlorothiazide *on page 347*
Labetalol Hydrochloride *on this page*
Brand Names Normozide®; Trandate® HCT
Generic Available No
Therapeutic Class Antihypertensive, Combination
Special Geriatric Considerations Combination products are not recommended for first-line treatment and divided doses of diuretics may increase the incidence of nocturia in the elderly
Dosage Forms Tablet: 25 mg hydrochlorothiazide and 100 mg labetalol; 25 mg hydrochlorothiazide and 200 mg labetalol; 25 mg hydrochlorothiazide and 300 mg labetalol

Labetalol Hydrochloride (la bet' a lole)
Related Information
Beta-Blockers Comparison *on page 804-805*
Brand Names Normodyne®; Trandate®
Synonyms Ibidomide Hydrochloride
Generic Available No
Therapeutic Class Alpha-/Beta- Adrenergic Blocker
Use Treatment of mild to severe hypertension; I.V. for hypertensive emergencies
Contraindications Asthma, cardiogenic shock, uncompensated congestive heart failure, bradycardia, pulmonary edema, or heart block
(Continued)

Labetalol Hydrochloride *(Continued)*

Warnings Orthostatic hypotension may occur with I.V. administration; patient should remain supine during and for up to 3 hours after I.V. administration

Precautions Paradoxical increase in blood pressure has been reported with treatment of pheochromocytoma or clonidine withdrawal syndrome; use with extreme caution in patients with hyper-reactive airway disease, congestive heart failure, diabetes mellitus, hepatic dysfunction

Adverse Reactions

Cardiovascular: Orthostatic hypotension especially with I.V. administration, edema, congestive heart failure, A-V conduction disturbances, bradycardia

Central nervous system: Drowsiness, fatigue, paresthesia, dizziness, behavior disorders, headache

Dermatologic: Tingling in scalp or skin (transient with initiation of therapy), rash

Gastrointestinal: Nausea, dry mouth

Genitourinary: Sexual dysfunction, urinary problems

Neuromuscular & skeletal: Reversible myopathy

Respiratory: Bronchospasm, nasal congestion

Overdosage Symptoms of overdose include hypotension, bradycardia, bronchospasm

Toxicology Sympathomimetics (eg, epinephrine or dopamine), glucagon or a pacemaker can be used to treat the toxic bradycardia, asystole, and/or hypotension. Initially, fluids may be the best treatment for toxic hypotension. Patients should remain supine; serum glucose and potassium should be measured. Use supportive measures: lavage, syrup of ipecac; atenolol may be removed by hemodialysis. I.V. glucose should be administered for hypoglycemia; seizures may be treated with phenytoin or diazepam intravenously; continuous monitoring of blood pressure and EKG is necessary. If PVCs occur, treat with lidocaine or phenytoin; avoid quinidine, procainamide, and disopyramide since these agents further depress myocardial function. Bronchospasm can be treated with theophylline on beta$_2$ agonists (epinephrine).

Drug Interactions

Decreased effect of beta-adrenergic agonists

Increased effect: Cimetidine, other hypotensives

Increased toxicity: Halothane (with I.V. labetalol)

Stability Stable in D$_5$W, saline for 24 hours; incompatible with alkaline solutions; use only solutions that are clear or slightly yellow; may cause a precipitate if exposed to alkaline admixture

Stability of parenteral admixture at room temperature (25°C) and refrigeration temperature (4°C): 24 hours

Mechanism of Action Blocks alpha-, beta$_1$- and beta$_2$-adrenergic receptor sites; elevated renins are reduced

Pharmacodynamics

Onset of action:

Oral: 20 minutes to 2 hours; maximum: 1-4 hours

I.V.: 2-5 minutes; maximum: 5-15 minutes

Duration:

Oral: 8-24 hours (dose-dependent)

I.V.: 2-4 hours

Pharmacokinetics

Distribution: V$_d$: Adults: 3-16 L/kg, mean: 9.4 L/kg; moderately lipid soluble, therefore, it can enter the CNS

Protein binding: 50%

Metabolism: Extensive first-pass effect; metabolized in liver primarily via glucuronide conjugation

Bioavailability: Oral: 25%; increased bioavailability with liver disease, in elderly, and with concurrent cimetidine

Half-life: 6-8 hours

Elimination: In elderly, total body clearance of labetalol is decreased; <5% excreted in urine unchanged

Usual Dosage

Geriatrics: Oral: Initial: 100 mg 1-2 times/day increasing as needed

Adults:

Oral: Initial: 100 mg twice daily, may increase as needed every 2-3 days by 100 mg until desired response is obtained; usual dose: 200-400 mg twice daily; not to exceed 2.4 g/day

I.V.: 20 mg or 1-2 mg/kg whichever is lower, IVP over 2 minutes, may give 40-80 mg at 10-minute intervals, up to 300 mg total dose

I.V. infusion: Initial: 2 mg/minute; titrate to response

Monitoring Parameters Blood pressure, standing and sitting/supine, pulse, mental status; if used in a diabetic patient, monitor glucose carefully; if used in patients with COPD, monitor pulmonary function

Test Interactions False-positive urine catecholamines, VMA if measured by fluorometric or photometric methods; use HPLC or specific catecholamine radioenzymatic technique

Patient Information Do not stop medication without consulting physician; may mask signs and symptoms of hypoglycemia in diabetic patients; sweating will still be present

Special Geriatric Considerations Due to alterations in the beta-adrenergic autonomic nervous system, beta-adrenergic blockade may result in less hemodynamic response than seen in younger adults. Studies indicate that despite decreased sensitivity to the chronotropic effects of beta blockade with age, there appears to be an increased myocardial sensitivity to the negative inotropic effect during stress (ie, exercise). Controlled trials have shown the overall response rate for propranolol to be only 20% to 50% in elderly populations. Therefore, all beta-adrenergic blocking drugs may result in a decreased response as compared to younger adults.

Dosage Forms
Injection: 5 mg/mL (20 mL, 40 mL, 60 mL)
Tablet: 100 mg, 200 mg, 300 mg

LaBID® see Theophylline on page 681

Lacri-Lube® [OTC] see Ocular Lubricant on page 515

Lactinex® [OTC] see Lactobacillus acidophilus and Lactobacillus bulgaricus on this page

Lactobacillus acidophilus and Lactobacillus bulgaricus
(lak toe ba sil' us)
Brand Names Bacid® [OTC]; Lactinex® [OTC]; More-Dophilus® [OTC]; Pro-Bionate® [OTC]; Superdophilus® [OTC]
Generic Available No
Therapeutic Class Antidiarrheal
Use Dietary supplement

Unlabeled uses: Treatment of uncomplicated diarrhea particularly that is caused by antibiotic therapy; re-establishes normal physiologic and bacterial flora of the intestinal tract; see Warnings

Contraindications Allergy to milk or lactose

Warnings Discontinue if high fever present; the FDA has determined that these agents are not generally recognized as safe and effective as antidiarrheal agents

Adverse Reactions Gastrointestinal: Intestinal flatus

Stability Store in the refrigerator (capsules and granules)

Mechanism of Action Creates an environment unfavorable to potentially pathogenic fungi or bacteria through the production of lactic acid, and favors establishment of an aciduric flora, thereby suppressing the growth of pathogenic microorganisms; helps re-establish normal intestinal flora

Pharmacokinetics
Absorption: Oral: Not absorbed
Distribution: Locally, primarily in the colon
Elimination: In feces

Usual Dosage Geriatrics and Adults: Oral:
Capsules: 2 capsules 2-4 times/day
Granules: 1 packet added to or taken with cereal, food, milk, fruit juice, or water, 3-4 times/day
Powder: $1/4$ to 1 teaspoonful 1-3 times/day with liquid
Tablet, chewable: 4 tablets 3-4 times/day; may follow each dose with a small amount of milk, fruit juice, or water
See Additional Information

Administration See Usual Dosage

Monitoring Parameters Monitor for decrease in frequency of stool and increased mass of stool

Patient Information Refrigerate; granules may be added to or taken with cereal, food, milk, fruit juice, or water

Nursing Implications Granules may be added to or given with cereal, food, milk, fruit juice, or water

Additional Information Probionate®, Superdophilus® and Lactinex®, mixed L. acidophilus and L. bulgaricus, More-Dophilus® can be stored at room temperature

Special Geriatric Considerations No specific recommendations due to age; keep in mind that elderly suffer significantly with fluid and electrolyte loss (lethargy, confusion, etc) and diarrhea should be aggressively treated

Dosage Forms
Capsule: 50s, 100s
Granules: 1 g/packet (12 packets/box)
Powder: 12 oz
Tablet, chewable: 50s

Lactulose (lak' tyoo lose)
Brand Names Cephulac®; Cholac®; Chronulac®; Constilac®; Constulose®; Duphalac®; Enulose®; Generlac®; Lactulose PSE®
Therapeutic Class Ammonium Detoxicant; Laxative, Miscellaneous

(Continued)

Lactulose *(Continued)*

Use Adjunct in the prevention and treatment of portal-systemic encephalopathy; treatment of chronic constipation

Contraindications Patients with galactosemia

Warnings Use cautiously in patients undergoing electrocautery procedures due to the accumulation of H_2 gas which may explode when ignited by electrical spark. This complication has not been reported with lactulose; patients should have bowel cleansing done with a nonfermentable agent.

Precautions Use with caution in patients with diabetes mellitus since lactulose contains small amounts of galactose and lactose; monitor periodically for electrolyte imbalance when lactulose is used >6 months or in patients predisposed to electrolyte abnormalities; patients receiving lactulose and an oral anti-infective agent should be monitored for possible inadequate response to lactulose; use with concomitant laxative in initial treatment of portal-systemic encephalopathy may result in early loose stools, incorrectly indicating adequate dose of lactulose

Adverse Reactions
Cardiovascular: Hypotension
Gastrointestinal: Cramping (20%), flatulence, abdominal discomfort, diarrhea, nausea, vomiting
Endocrine & metabolic: Dehydration, electrolyte loss

Overdosage Symptoms of overdose include potassium depletion; manifests by abdominal pain and diarrhea

Drug Interactions Oral neomycin, other antibiotics, laxatives, antacids

Stability Keep solution at room temperature to reduce viscosity; discard solution if cloudy or very dark

Mechanism of Action Prevents absorption of ammonia in colon as a result of bacterial degradation into low molecular weight organic acids which decrease the pH; produces an osmotic effect in the colon with resultant distention promoting peristalsis

Pharmacokinetics
Absorption: Oral: Not absorbed appreciably, this is desirable since the intended site of action is within the colon; requires colonic flora for primary drug activation
Metabolism: By colonic flora to lactic acid and acetic acid
Elimination: Primarily in feces and urine ($\sim$3%)

Usual Dosage Geriatrics and Adults:
Oral:
Acute episodes of portal systemic encephalopathy: 30-45 mL at 1- to 2-hour intervals until laxative effect observed
Laxative: 15-30 mL 1-2 times/day
Chronic therapy: 30-45 mL/dose 3-4 times/day; titrate dose to produce 2-3 soft stools daily

Rectal: 300 mL diluted with 700 mL of water or normal saline, and given via a rectal balloon catheter and retained for 30-60 minutes; may give every 4-6 hours

Monitoring Parameters Monitor for number of stools per day, dehydration, hypotension; measure serum electrolytes with long-term use; monitor serum ammonia concentrations when treating hepatic encephalopathy

Test Interactions Decreased ammonia (B)

Patient Information Lactulose can be taken "as is" or diluted with water, fruit juice or milk, or taken in a food; laxative results may not occur for 24-48 hours; take with a full glass of water

Nursing Implications Dilute lactulose in water, usually 60-120 mL, prior to administering through a gastric or feeding tube; monitor serum ammonia in hepatic disease; see Monitoring Parameters

Additional Information Diarrhea indicates overdosage and responds to dose reduction

Special Geriatric Considerations Elderly are more likely to show CNS signs of dehydration and electrolyte loss than younger adults. Therefore, monitor closely for fluid and electrolyte loss with chronic use. Sorbitol is equally effective as a laxative and less expensive. However, sorbitol **cannot be substituted** in the treatment of hepatic encephalopathy.

Dosage Forms Syrup: 10 g/15 mL (15 mL, 30 mL, 237 mL, 473 mL, 946 mL, 1890 mL)

References
Lederle FA, Busch DL, Mattox KM, et al, "Cost-Effective Treatment of Constipation in the Elderly: A Randomized Double-Blind Comparison of Sorbitol and Lactulose," *Am J Med*, 1990, 89(5):597-601.

Lactulose PSE® *see Lactulose on previous page*

Lamictal® *see Lamotrigine on this page*

Lamisil® *see Terbinafine on page 672*

Lamotrigine (la moe' tri jeen)

Brand Names Lamictal®
Synonyms BW-430C; LTG
Generic Available No

Therapeutic Class Anticonvulsant, Miscellaneous

Use Adjunctive treatment of partial seizures

Unlabeled use: Generalized tonic-clonic seizures in adults, absence, atypical absence, and myoclonic seizures

Contraindications Hypersensitivity to lamotrigine or any of its components

Warnings Dermatologic: Rash develops in ~10% of patients; rash usually occurs in first 4-6 weeks of therapy; occurs more often in patients receiving valproic acid; Stevens-Johnson syndrome, toxic epidermal necrolysis, and angioedema have been reported (0.3% of rashes)

Sudden death is rare (0.0035 deaths/patient year); withdrawal seizures occur when AED is abruptly discontinued. Status epilepticus reported with the use of lamotrigine (7/2343). Multiorgan failure and hepatic failure have been reported. Renal/hepatic dysfunction requires dose reductions and close monitoring.

Elderly: In a single dose study the pharmacokinetics of lamotrigine were similar to those of young adults

Precautions No accepted plasma concentration values have been established for therapeutic effect or toxicity. Use with caution in patients with hepatic failure, renal dysfunction, or drugs (AEDs) affecting lamotrigine clearance. Photosensitivity may occur; patients should take precaution. Since lamotrigine binds to melanin, periodic eye examinations are advised with long-term use. The efficacy of using lamotrigine with valproic acid as a two-drug regimen is not recommended due to a lack of data.

Adverse Reactions

Cardiovascular: Atrial fibrillation, hypertension, myocardial infarction, hypotension (<0.1%)

Central nervous system: Dizziness, sedation, ataxia, insomnia, depression, anxiety, irritability, speech disorder, memory decrease, headache, migraine

Dermatologic: Hypersensitivity rash, angioedema, Stevens-Johnson syndrome

Gastrointestinal: Nausea, vomiting, dyspepsia, gingival hyperplasia, stomatitis, gastritis

Neuromuscular & skeletal: Tremors, arthralgia, back pain, chest pain, myalgia

Ocular: Nystagmus, diplopia, blurred vision

Renal: Hematuria

Respiratory: Rhinitis

Overdosage Signs and symptoms of overdose include coma, dizziness, headache, and somnolence

Toxicology Treatment of overdosage is general supportive care; monitor vital signs, induce emesis if indicated, however, the drug is rapidly absorbed; uncertain if hemodialysis is effective

Drug Interactions

Lamotrigine serum concentrations are decreased by carbamazepine, phenobarbital, primidone, and phenytoin

Increased serum concentrations of carbamazepine epoxide

Lamotrigine serum levels increased by valproic acid (twofold)

Lamotrigine decreases valproic acid serum concentrations

Mechanism of Action Exact mechanism of action is unknown; may stabilize neuronal membranes by inhibiting sodium channels and, thereby, inhibits release of glutamine, an excitatory amino acid; has a weak inhibitory effect on serotonin 5-HT$_3$ receptors

Pharmacokinetics

Distribution: V_d: 1.1 L/kg

Protein binding: 55%

Metabolism: Hepatic and renal

Half-life: 24 hours; increases to 59 hours with concomitant valproic acid therapy; decreases with concomitant phenytoin or carbamazepine therapy to 15 hours

Elimination: Hepatic and renal

Usual Dosage

Initial dose: 50-100 mg/day then titrate to daily maintenance dose of 100-400 mg/day in 1-2 divided daily doses

With concomitant valproic acid therapy: Start initial dose at 25 mg/day then titrate to maintenance dose of 50-200 mg/day in 1-2 divided daily doses

Monitoring Parameters Monitor for therapeutic response and for adverse reactions; no established therapeutic serum concentrations

Reference Range Therapeutic: 2-4 mcg/mL

Patient Information Rash should be reported immediately to physician; patients should be warned of photosensitivity and take precautions (ie, sunscreen use, sunglasses, protective clothing, avoiding sunlight)

Nursing Implications See Precautions and Patient Information

Additional Information Low water solubility

Special Geriatric Considerations No pharmacokinetic differences noted between young adults and elderly; use with caution in elderly with significant renal decline

Dosage Forms Tablet: 25 mg, 100 mg, 150 mg, 200 mg

Lamprene® see Clofazimine Palmitate on page 173

Lanatrate® *see* Ergotamine *on page 261*

Laniazid® *see* Isoniazid *on page 379*

Lanoxicaps® *see* Digoxin *on page 222*

Lanoxin® *see* Digoxin *on page 222*

Larodopa® *see* Levodopa *on page 402*

Larotid® *see* Amoxicillin Trihydrate *on page 49*

Lasix® *see* Furosemide *on page 315*

Lax-Pills® [OTC] *see* Phenolphthalein *on page 556*

/-Bunolol Hydrochloride *see* Levobunolol Hydrochloride *on next page*

L-Deprenyl *see* Selegiline Hydrochloride *on page 640*

L-Dopa *see* Levodopa *on page 402*

Ledercillin® VK *see* Penicillin V Potassium *on page 543*

Legatrin® [OTC] *see* Quinine Sulfate *on page 620*

Lente *see* Insulin Preparations *on page 372*

Lente® Iletin®I *see* Insulin Preparations *on page 372*

Lente® Iletin® II (Beef) *see* Insulin Preparations *on page 372*

Lente® Iletin® II (Pork) *see* Insulin Preparations *on page 372*

Lente® Insulin (Beef) *see* Insulin Preparations *on page 372*

Lente® Purified Pork *see* Insulin Preparations *on page 372*

Lente® Purified Pork Insulin *see* Insulin Preparations *on page 372*

Lescol® *see* Fluvastatin *on page 309*

Leukeran® *see* Chlorambucil *on page 147*

Leuprolide Acetate (loo proe' lide)

Brand Names Lupron®
Synonyms Leuprorelin Acetate
Generic Available No
Therapeutic Class Antineoplastic Agent, Hormone (Gonadotropin Hormone-Releasing Antigen); Gonadotropin Releasing Hormone Analog
Use Palliative treatment of advanced prostate carcinoma, endometriosis

Unlabeled use: Treatment of breast, ovarian, and endometrial cancer; prostatic hypertrophy; leiomyoma uteri

Contraindications Hypersensitivity to leuprolide; gonadotropin-releasing hormone (GnRH); GnRH agonists analogs; undiagnosed abnormal vaginal bleeding
Warnings Tumor flare and bone pain may occur at initiation of therapy; transient weakness and paresthesia of lower limbs, hematuria, and urinary tract obstruction in first week of therapy; animal studies have shown dose-related benign pituitary hyperplasia and benign pituitary adenomas after 2 years of use
Precautions Use with caution in patients hypersensitive to benzyl alcohol; after 6 months use of Depot® leuprolide, vertebral bone density decreased (average 13.5%)
Adverse Reactions

Cardiovascular: Edema, cardiac arrhythmias, EKG changes, elevated blood pressure, hypotension, angina

Central nervous system: Dizziness, paresthesia, lethargy, insomnia, headache, nervousness

Dermatologic: Rash, hair growth

Endocrine & metabolic: Estrogenic effects (gynecomastia, breast tenderness), decreased testicular size, hot flashes

Gastrointestinal: Nausea, vomiting, diarrhea, GI bleed, anorexia, peptic ulcer

Genitourinary: Urinary urgency/frequency, bladder spasm, impotence, decreased libido

Hematologic: Decreased hemoglobin and hematocrit

Neuromuscular & skeletal: Myalgia, pain, bone loss, pelvic fibrosis

Ocular: Blurred vision

Respiratory: Dyspnea, cough, pneumonia, hemoptysis

Miscellaneous: Sweating

Overdosage Animal (rats) data: Dyspnea, decreased activity, injection site irritation
Toxicology General supportive care; decrease dose
Stability Store unopened vials in refrigerator, vial in use can be kept at room temperature for several months with minimal loss of potency; upon reconstitution, the suspension is stable for 24 hours, however the product does not contain a preservative
Mechanism of Action Continuous daily administration results in suppression of ovarian and testicular steroidogenesis due to decreased levels of LH and FSH with subsequent decrease in testosterone (males) and estrogen (females) levels

Pharmacokinetics Serum testosterone levels first increase within 3 days of therapy, then decrease after 2-4 weeks with continued therapy; requires parenteral administration since it is rapidly destroyed within the GI tract

Bioavailability: Not bioavailable if given orally; bioavailability of S.C. and I.V. doses is comparable

Half-life: 3-4.25 hours

Elimination: Not well defined

Usual Dosage Geriatrics and Adults:

Advanced prostatic carcinoma:

I.M. (suspension): 7.5 mg/dose given monthly (28-33)

S.C.: 1 mg/day

Endometriosis: I.M. (Depot®): 3.75 mg/month

Monitoring Parameters Serum levels of testosterone, acid phosphatase; bone density in high-risk patients (osteoporosis, use of Depot® leuprolide)

Patient Information Patient must be taught aseptic technique and S.C. injection technique. Rotate S.C. injection sites frequently. Disease flare (increased bone paint, urinary retention) can briefly occur with initiation of therapy. Store vials under refrigeration but do not freeze. Do not discontinue medication without physician's advice.

Nursing Implications When administering the Depot® form, do not use needles smaller than 22-gauge; reconstitute only with diluent provided; must teach patient injection technique; rotate S.C. injection site frequently; see Monitoring Parameters

Special Geriatric Considerations Leuprolide has the advantage of not increasing risk of atherosclerotic vascular disease, causing swelling of breasts, fluid retention, and thromboembolism as compared to estrogen therapy

Dosage Forms

Injection: 5 mg/mL (2.8 mL)

Powder for injection (Depot-Ped™): 7.5 mg, 11.25 mg, 15 mg

Suspension, Depot®: 3.75 mg/mL; 7.5 mg/mL

Leuprorelin Acetate see Leuprolide Acetate on previous page

Levatol® see Penbutolol Sulfate on page 536

Levobunolol Hydrochloride (lee voe byoo' noe lole)

Related Information

Glaucoma Drug Therapy Comparison on page 810

Brand Names Betagan®

Synonyms l-Bunolol Hydrochloride

Generic Available No

Therapeutic Class Beta-Adrenergic Blocker, Ophthalmic

Use Lower intraocular pressure in chronic open-angle glaucoma or ocular hypertension

Contraindications Known hypersensitivity to levobunolol; bronchial asthma, severe COPD, sinus bradycardia, second or third degree A-V block; cardiac failure, cardiogenic shock

Precautions Use with caution in patients with congestive heart failure, diabetes mellitus, hyperthyroidism, cerebral insufficiency due to systemic absorption

Adverse Reactions

Cardiovascular: Bradycardia, arrhythmia, hypotension

Central nervous system: Dizziness, headache

Dermatologic: Skin rash

Local: Stinging, burning, erythema, itching, alopecia

Ocular: Blepharoconjunctivitis, decreased visual acuity, conjunctivitis, keratitis

Respiratory: Bronchospasm

Overdosage Symptoms of overdose include bradycardia, hypotension, bronchospasm

Toxicology Flush eye(s) with water or normal saline

Drug Interactions Systemic beta-adrenergic blocking agents; ophthalmic epinephrine (increased blood pressure/loss of IOP effect), quinidine (sinus bradycardia), verapamil (bradycardia and asystole have been reported)

Mechanism of Action A nonselective beta-adrenergic blocking agent that most likely lowers intraocular pressure by reducing aqueous humor production and possibly increasing the outflow of aqueous humor

Pharmacodynamics

Onset of action: Following ophthalmic instillation decreases in intraocular pressure (IOP) can be noted within 1 hour

Peak effects: Within 2-6 hours; reductions in IOP can last from 1-7 days

Pharmacokinetics Elimination not well defined

Usual Dosage Geriatrics and Adults: Instill 1 drop in eye(s) 1-2 times/day

Administration Apply finger pressure over nasolacrimal duct to decrease systemic absorption

Monitoring Parameters Intraocular pressure, heart rate, funduscopic exam, visual field testing

Patient Information May sting on instillation, do not touch dropper to eye; visual acuity may be decreased after administration; night vision may be decreased; distance

(Continued)

401

Levobunolol Hydrochloride *(Continued)*

vision may be altered; apply finger pressure between the bridge of the nose and corner of the eye to decrease systemic absorption; assess patient's or caregiver's ability to administer

Nursing Implications See Administration

Additional Information Contains metabisulfite

Special Geriatric Considerations Because systemic absorption does occur with ophthalmic administration, the elderly with other disease states or syndromes that may be affected by a beta-blocker (CHF, COPD, etc) should be monitored closely

Dosage Forms Solution: 0.25%, 0.5% (2 mL, 5 mL, 10 mL, 15 mL)

Levodopa (lee voe doe' pa)

Related Information

Antacid Drug Interactions *on page 764*

Brand Names Dopar®; Larodopa®

Synonyms *L*-3-Hydroxytyrosine; *L*-Dopa

Generic Available No

Therapeutic Class Anti-Parkinson's Agent

Dosage Forms

Capsule: 100 mg, 250 mg, 500 mg

Tablet: 100 mg, 250 mg, 500 mg

Levodopa and Carbidopa (lee voe doe' pa & kar bi doe' pa)

Brand Names Sinemet®

Synonyms Carbidopa and Levodopa

Generic Available No

Therapeutic Class Anti-Parkinson's Agent

Use Treatment of parkinsonian syndrome

Contraindications Narrow-angle glaucoma, MAO inhibitors, hypersensitivity to levodopa, carbidopa, or any component; do not use in patients with malignant melanoma or undiagnosed skin lesions

Precautions Use with caution in patients with history of myocardial infarction, arrhythmias, asthma, wide-angle glaucoma, peptic ulcer disease; sudden discontinuation of levodopa may cause a worsening of Parkinson's disease

Adverse Reactions

Cardiovascular: Orthostatic hypotension, palpitations, cardiac arrhythmias

Central nervous system: Memory loss, nervousness, anxiety, insomnia, fatigue, hallucinations, ataxia, confusion

Gastrointestinal: Nausea, vomiting, GI bleeding, dry mouth

Neuromuscular & skeletal: Dystonic movements, "on-off"

Ocular: Blurred vision

Overdosage Symptoms of overdose include palpitations, arrhythmias, hypotension

Toxicology Treatment is supportive; initiate gastric lavage, administer I.V. fluids judiciously and monitor EKG

Drug Interactions

Decreased effect: Phenytoin, benzodiazepines, tricyclic antidepressants, phenothiazines, haloperidol, reserpine, methyldopa

Increased effect: Antacids

Increased toxicity: Nonselective MAO inhibitors

Mechanism of Action Parkinson's symptoms are due to a lack of striatal dopamine; levodopa circulates in the plasma to the blood-brain-barrier (BBB), where it crosses, to be converted by striatal enzymes to dopamine; carbidopa inhibits the peripheral plasma breakdown of levodopa by inhibiting its decarboxylation, and thereby increases available levodopa at the BBB

Pharmacodynamics Peak effect: Oral: Within 1-2 hours after administration; may take 2-3 weeks to see the full therapeutic effect

Pharmacokinetics

Carbidopa:

Absorption: Oral: 40% to 70%

Protein binding: 36%

Half-life: 1-2 hours

Elimination: Excreted unchanged

Levodopa:

Absorption: May be decreased if given with a high protein meal

Half-life: 1.2-2.3 hours

Elimination: Primarily in urine (80%) as dopamine, norepinephrine, and homovanillic acid

Usual Dosage Oral:

Geriatrics: Initial: 25/100 twice daily, increase as necessary; Sinemet® may be used as initial therapy

Adults: Initial: 25/100 2-4 times/day, increase as necessary to a maximum of 200/2000 mg/day

Conversion from Sinemet® to Sinemet® CR (50/200): (Sinemet® [total daily dose of levodopa] / Sinemet® CR)

300-400 mg / 1 tablet twice daily
500-600 mg / 1½ tablets twice daily or one 3 times/day
700-800 mg / 4 tablets in 3 or more divided doses
900-1000 mg / 5 tablets in 3 or more divided doses

Intervals between doses of Sinemet® CR should be 4-8 hours while awake

Monitoring Parameters Blood pressure, standing and sitting/supine; symptoms of parkinsonism, dyskinesias, mental status

Test Interactions False-positive reaction for urinary glucose with Clinitest®; false-negative reaction using Clinistix®; false-positive urine ketones with Acetest®, Ketostix®, Labstix®

Patient Information Take on an empty stomach if possible; if GI distress occurs, take with meals; rise carefully from lying or sitting position; do not crush or chew sustained release product

Nursing Implications Space doses evenly over the waking hours; do not crush sustained release product

Additional Information 50-100 mg/day of carbidopa is needed to block the peripheral conversion of levodopa to dopamine. "On-off" can be managed by giving smaller, more frequent doses of Sinemet® or adding a dopamine agonist or selegiline; when adding a new agent, doses of Sinemet® should usually be decreased. Protein in the diet should be distributed throughout the day to avoid fluctuations in levodopa absorption. A new algorithm for the treatment of Parkinson's disease recommends initiating levodopa therapy with the sustained-release form.

Special Geriatric Considerations The elderly may be more sensitive to the CNS effects of levodopa

Dosage Forms Tablet:
Sinemet®-10/100: Carbidopa 10 mg and levodopa 100 mg
Sinemet®-25/100: Carbidopa 25 mg and levodopa 100 mg
Sinemet®-25/250: Carbidopa 25 mg and levodopa 250 mg
Sinemet® CR: Carbidopa 25 mg and levodopa 100 mg
Sinemet® CR: Carbidopa 50 mg and levodopa 200 mg

References
Koller WC, Silver DE, and Lieberman A, "An Algorithm for the Management of Parkinson's Disease," *Neurology*, 1994, 44(12):S1-52.

Levo-Dromoran® *see* Levorphanol Tartrate *on this page*

Levorphanol Tartrate (lee vor' fa nole)

Related Information
Narcotic Agonist Comparative Pharmacology *on page 811*
Pharmacokinetics of Narcotic Agonist Analgesics *on page 812*

Brand Names Levo-Dromoran®

Synonyms Levorphan Tartrate

Generic Available Yes: Tablet

Therapeutic Class Analgesic, Narcotic

Use Relief of moderate to severe pain; also used parenterally for preoperative sedation and an adjunct to nitrous oxide/oxygen anesthesia

Restrictions C-II

Contraindications Hypersensitivity to levorphanol or any component

Warnings Levorphanol is not usually recommended for use in the elderly because of its long half-life and, therefore, its tendency to accumulate

Precautions Levorphanol tartrate shares the toxic potentials of opiate agonists, and usual precautions of opiate agonist therapy should be observed

Adverse Reactions
Cardiovascular: Palpitations, hypotension, bradycardia, peripheral vasodilation
Central nervous system: CNS depression, drowsiness, sedation, increased intracranial pressure
Dermatologic: Pruritus
Endocrine & metabolic: Antidiuretic hormone release
Gastrointestinal: Nausea, vomiting, constipation
Genitourinary: Urinary retention
Ocular: Miosis
Respiratory: Respiratory depression
Miscellaneous: Physical and psychological dependence, biliary or urinary tract spasm, histamine release

Overdosage Symptoms of overdose include CNS depression, respiratory depression, miosis, apnea, pulmonary edema, convulsions

Toxicology Naloxone 2 mg I.V. with repeat administration as necessary up to a total of 10 mg

Drug Interactions Increased toxicity: CNS depressants

Stability Store at room temperature, protect from freezing

(Continued)

Levorphanol Tartrate (Continued)

Mechanism of Action Binds to opiate receptors in the CNS, causing inhibition of ascending pain pathways, altering the perception of and response to pain; produces generalized CNS depression

Pharmacodynamics
Onset of action: Oral: 10-60 minutes
Duration: 6-8 hours; enhanced analgesia has been seen in elderly patients on therapeutic dose of narcotics; duration of action may be increased in the elderly

Pharmacokinetics
Metabolism: In the liver
Half-life: 11 hours
Elimination: In urine as glucuronide

Usual Dosage Geriatrics and Adults: Oral, S.C.: 2 mg, up to 3 mg if necessary every 12 hours

Monitoring Parameters Pain relief, respiratory and mental status, blood pressure

Patient Information May cause drowsiness; avoid alcoholic beverages

Nursing Implications Observe patient for oversedation, respiratory depression

Additional Information 2 mg levorphanol I.M. produces analgesia comparable to that produced by 10 mg of morphine I.M.

Special Geriatric Considerations See Warnings; the elderly may be particularly susceptible to the CNS depressant and constipating effects of narcotics; see Pharmacodynamics

Dosage Forms
Injection: 2 mg/mL (1 mL, 10 mL)
Injection (PCA syringe): 0.1 mg/mL (30 mL, 60 mL)
Tablet: 2 mg

Levorphan Tartrate see Levorphanol Tartrate on previous page

Levothroid® see Levothyroxine Sodium on this page

Levothyroxine Sodium (lee voe thye rox' een)

Brand Names Levothroid®; Levoxine®; Synthroid®; Synthrox®; Syroxine®

Synonyms L-Thyroxine Sodium; T₄ Thyroxine Sodium

Generic Available Yes

Therapeutic Class Thyroid Product

Use Replacement or supplemental therapy in hypothyroidism; pituitary TSH suppressants (thyroid nodules, thyroiditis, multinodular goiter, thyroid cancer), thyrotoxicosis, diagnostic suppression tests

Contraindications Recent myocardial infarction or thyrotoxicosis, uncomplicated by hypothyroidism; uncorrected adrenal insufficiency, hypersensitivity to active or extraneous constituents

Warnings Ineffective for weight reduction; high doses may produce serious or even life-threatening toxic effects particularly when used with some anorectic drugs; use cautiously in patients with pre-existing cardiovascular disease (angina, CHD), elderly since they may be more likely to have compromised cardiovascular functions

Precautions Patients with angina pectoris or other cardiovascular disease; adrenal insufficiency, myxedema, diabetes mellitus and insipidus may have symptoms exaggerated or aggravated; thyroid replacement requires periodic assessment of thyroid status. Chronic hypothyroidism predisposes patients to coronary artery disease.

Adverse Reactions
Cardiovascular: Palpitations, tachycardia, cardiac arrhythmias
Central nervous system: Nervousness, tachycardia, cardiac, headache arrhythmias, insomnia, fever
Dermatologic: Hair loss
Endocrine & metabolic: Excessive bone loss with overtreatment (excess thyroid replacement)
Gastrointestinal: Weight loss, increased appetite, diarrhea, abdominal cramps, vomiting
Neuromuscular & skeletal: Tremors
Miscellaneous: Sweating, heat intolerance

Overdosage Chronic excessive use results in signs and symptoms of hyperthyroidism, weight loss, nervousness, sweating, tachycardia, insomnia, heat intolerance, palpitations, vomiting, psychosis, fever, seizures, angina, arrhythmias, and congestive heart failure in those predisposed

Toxicology Reduce dose or temporarily discontinue therapy; normal hypothalamic-pituitary-thyroid axis will return to normal in 6-8 weeks; serum T₄ levels do not correlate well with toxicity; in massive acute ingestion, reduce GI absorption, give general supportive care; treat congestive heart failure with digitalis glycosides; excessive adrenergic activity (tachycardia) require propranolol 1-3 mg I.V. over 10 minutes or 80-160 mg orally/day; fever may be treated with acetaminophen

Drug Interactions
Cholestyramine and colestipol decrease the effect of orally administered thyroid replacement

Estrogens increase TBG, thereby decreasing effect of thyroid replacement

Anticoagulants may increase action

Beta-blocker effect is decreased when patients become euthyroid

Serum digitalis concentrations are reduced in hyperthyroidism or when hypothyroid patients are converted to a euthyroid state

Theophylline levels decrease when hypothyroid patients converted to a euthyroid state

Stability Protect tablets from light; do not mix I.V. solution with other I.V. infusion solutions; reconstituted solutions should be used immediately and any unused portions discarded

Mechanism of Action Exact mechanism of action is unknown; however, it is believed the thyroid hormone exerts its many metabolic effects through control of DNA transcription and protein synthesis; involved in normal metabolism, growth, and development; promotes gluconeogenesis, increases utilization and mobilization of glycogen stores and stimulates protein synthesis, increases basal metabolic rate

Pharmacodynamics

Onset of action:

Oral: Therapeutic effects require 3-5 days

I.V.: Within 6-8 hours, with maximum effect within 24 hours; 4-6 weeks may be required to see maximal effect for each dose

Pharmacokinetics

Absorption: Oral: Erratic, 48% to 79%; T_3 is 95% absorbed

Distribution: 80% of T_3 is derived from monodeiodination of T_4 in the periphery (liver, kidneys, other tissues)

Half-life: 6-7 days for T_4 and 1-2 days for T_3

Time to peak: Peak serum levels occur within 2-4 hours

Elimination: As conjugated forms in feces, bile

Usual Dosage Geriatrics and Adults: Dosage should be individualized and response monitored both clinically and with appropriate laboratory (TSH, T_4); see Additional Information

Oral: 12.5-25 mcg/day to start, then increase by 25-50 mcg/day at intervals of 2-4 weeks; average adult dose: 100-200 mcg/day; many elderly can be safely initiated on 25 mcg/day

I.M., I.V.: 50% of oral dose

Myxedema coma or stupor: I.V.: 200-500 mcg one time, then 100-300 mcg the next day if necessary; normal T_4 levels achieved in 24 hours; T_3 normalizes in 3 days; maintenance: 0.05-1 mg/day; begin oral therapy as soon as patient is stabilized

Thyroid suppression therapy: 2.6 mcg/kg/day for 7-10 days

Monitoring Parameters T_4, TSH, heart rate, blood pressure, clinical signs of hypo- and hyperthyroidism; TSH is the most reliable guide for evaluating adequacy of thyroid replacement dosage. TSH may be elevated during the first few months of thyroid replacement despite patients being clinically euthyroid. In cases where T_4 remains low and TSH is within normal limits, an evaluation of "free" (unbound) T_4 is needed to evaluate further increase in dosage

Reference Range

TSH: 0.4-10 (for those $\geq$80 years) mIU/L

T_4: 4-12 μg/dL (SI: 51-154 nmol/L)

T_3 (RIA) (total T_3): 80-230 ng/dL (SI: 1.2-3.5 nmol/L)

T_4 free (Free T_4): 0.7-1.8 ng/dL (SI: 9-23 pmol/L)

Test Interactions Increased calcium (S); many drugs may have effects on thyroid function tests; para-aminosalicylic acid, aminoglutethimide, amiodarone, barbiturates, carbamazepine, chloral hydrate, clofibrate, colestipol, corticosteroids, danazol, diazepam, estrogens, ethionamide, fluorouracil, I.V. heparin, insulin, lithium, methadone, methimazole, mitotane, nitroprusside, oxyphenbutazone, phenylbutazone, PTU, perphenazine, phenytoin, propranolol, salicylates, sulfonylureas, and thiazides

Patient Information Do not change brands without physician's knowledge; report immediately to physician any chest pain, increased pulse, palpitations, heat intolerance, excessive sweating; do not stop use without physician's advice; replacement therapy will be for life; take as a single dose before breakfast

Nursing Implications I.V. form must be prepared immediately prior to administration; dilute 200 mcg/mL vial with 2 mL of 0.9% sodium chloride injection and shake well until a clear solution is obtained; should not be admixed with other solutions; see Monitoring Parameters, Reference Range, Warnings, and Special Geriatric Considerations

Additional Information Levothroid® tablets contain lactose. To convert doses: Levothyroxine 0.05-0.06 mg is equivalent to 60 mg thyroid USP; 60 mg thyroglobulin; 4.5 mg thyroid strong; 1 grain (60 mg) liotrix

Special Geriatric Considerations Elderly do not have a change in serum thyroxine associated with aging; however, plasma T_3 concentrations are decreased 25% to 40% in elderly. There is not a compensatory rise in thyrotropin suggesting that lower T_3 is not reacted upon as a deficiency by the pituitary. This indicates a slightly lower than normal dosage of thyroid hormone replacement is usually sufficient in older patients

(Continued)

Levothyroxine Sodium *(Continued)*

than in younger adult patients. TSH must be monitored since insufficient thyroid replacement (elevated TSH) is a risk for coronary artery disease and excessive replacement (low TSH) may cause signs of hyperthyroidism and excessive bone loss. Some clinicians suggest levothyroxine is the drug of choice for replacement therapy; see Usual Dosage and Overdosage.

Dosage Forms
Injection: 0.2 mg/vial (6 mL, 10 mL); 0.5 mg (6 mL, 10 mL)
Tablet: 0.025 mg, 0.05 mg, 0.075 mg, 0.088 mg, 0.1 mg, 0.112 mg, 0.125 mg, 0.15 mg, 0.175 mg, 0.2 mg, 0.3 mg

References
Helfand M and Crapo LM, "Monitoring Therapy in Patients Taking Levothyroxine," *Ann Intern Med*, 1990, 113(6):450-4.
Johnson DG and Campbell S, "Hormonal and Metabolic Agents," *Geriatric Pharmacology*, Bressler R and Katz MD, eds, New York, NY: McGraw-Hill, 1993, 427-50.
Sanders LR, "Pituitary, Thyroid, Adrenal and Parathyroid Diseases in the Elderly," *Geriatric Medicine*, 1990, 475-87.
Sawin CT, Geller A, Hershman JM, et al, "The Aging Thyroid. The Use of Thyroid Hormone in Older Persons," *JAMA*, 1989, 261(18):2653-5.
Watts NB, "Use of a Sensitive Thyrotropin Assay for Monitoring Treatment With Levothyroxine," *Arch Intern Med*, 1989, 149(2):309-12.

Levoxine® *see* Levothyroxine Sodium *on page 404*

Levsin® *see* Hyoscyamine Sulfate *on page 359*

Levsinex® *see* Hyoscyamine Sulfate *on page 359*

Lexocort® *see* Hydrocortisone *on page 351*

l-**Hyoscyamine Sulfate** *see* Hyoscyamine Sulfate *on page 359*

Libritabs® *see* Chlordiazepoxide *on page 149*

Librium® *see* Chlordiazepoxide *on page 149*

Lidex® *see* Fluocinonide *on page 299*

Lidex® E *see* Fluocinonide *on page 299*

Lidocaine Hydrochloride *(lye' doe kane)*

Related Information
Drug Levels Commonly Monitored Guidelines *on page 771-772*

Brand Names Anestacon®; Baylocaine®; Dalcaine®; Dilocaine®; Duo-Trach®; LidoPen®; Nervocaine®; Octocaine®; Xylocaine®

Synonyms Lignocaine Hydrochloride

Generic Available Yes

Therapeutic Class Antiarrhythmic Agent, Class IB; Local Anesthetic, Injectable; Local Anesthetic, Topical

Use Local anesthetic and acute treatment of ventricular arrhythmias from myocardial infarction, cardiac manipulation, digitalis intoxication

Contraindications Known hypersensitivity to amide-type local anesthetics; patients with Adams-Stokes syndrome or with severe degree of S-A, A-V, or intraventricular heart block (without a pacemaker); Wolff-Parkinson-White syndrome

Warnings Do not use preparations containing preservatives for spinal or epidural (including caudal) anesthesia

Precautions Hepatic disease, heart failure, marked hypoxia, severe respiratory depression, hypovolemia or shock; incomplete heart block or bradycardia, atrial fibrillation

Adverse Reactions
Cardiovascular: Bradycardia, hypotension, heart block, arrhythmias, cardiovascular collapse
Central nervous system: Lethargy, coma, paresthesias, agitation, slurred speech, seizures, anxiety, euphoria, hallucinations, lightheadedness, nervousness, drowsiness, confusion
Gastrointestinal: Nausea, vomiting
Neuromuscular & skeletal: Twitching, tremors
Ocular: Blurred or double vision
Otic: Tinnitus
Respiratory: Depression or arrest

Overdosage Symptoms of overdose include convulsions, respiratory failure, bradycardia, hypotension, cardiovascular collapse, euphoria, tinnitus

Toxicology Treatment is primarily symptomatic and supportive. Termination of anesthesia by pneumatic tourniquet inflation should be attempted when the agent is administered by infiltration or regional injection. Seizures commonly respond to diazepam, while hypotension responds to I.V. fluids and Trendelenburg positioning. Bradyarrhythmias (when the heart rate is <60) can be treated with I.V., I.M., or S.C. atropine 15 mcg/kg. With the development of metabolic acidosis, I.V. sodium bicarbonate 0.5-2 mEq/kg and ventilatory assistance should be instituted. Methemoglobinemia should be treated with methylene blue 1-2 mg/kg in a 1% sterile aqueous solution I.V. push over 4-6 minutes repeated up to a total dose of 7 mg/kg.

Drug Interactions
Concomitant cimetidine or propranolol may result in increased serum concentrations of lidocaine with resultant toxicity
Procainamide may have enhanced pharmacologic action on myocardium
Succinylcholine may have prolonged neuromuscular blockade
Stability I.V. infusion solutions admixed in D$_5$W are stable for a minimum of 24 hours
Mechanism of Action Class IB antiarrhythmic; suppresses automaticity of conduction tissue, by increasing electrical stimulation threshold of ventricle, HIS-Purkinje system, and spontaneous depolarization of the ventricles during diastole by a direct action on the tissues; blocks both the initiation and conduction of nerve impulses by decreasing the neuronal membrane's permeability to sodium ions which results in inhibition of depolarization with resultant blockade of conduction
Pharmacodynamics
Onset of action (single bolus dose): 45-90 seconds
Duration: 10-20 minutes
Pharmacokinetics
Distribution: V$_d$ alterable by many patient factors, decreased in congestive heart failure and liver disease
Protein binding: 60% to 80%; binds to alpha$_1$-acid glycoprotein
Half-life: Biphasic:
Alpha: 7-30 minutes
Beta: Terminal: Adults: 1.5-2 hours
Metabolism: 90% metabolized in liver; active metabolites monoethylglycinexylidide (MEGX) and glycinexylidide (GX) can accumulate and may cause CNS toxicity
Usual Dosage Geriatrics and Adults:
Topical: Apply to affected area as needed; maximum: 3 mg/kg/dose; do not repeat within 2 hours

Injectable local anesthetic: Varies with procedure, degree of anesthesia needed, vascularity of tissue, duration of anesthesia required, and physical condition of patient; maximum: 4.5 mg/kg/dose; do not repeat within 2 hours
Antiarrhythmic:
I.M.: 300 mg may be repeated in 1-1.5 hours
I.V.: 50-100 mg bolus over 2-3 minutes; may repeat in 5-10 minutes up to 200-300 mg in a 1-hour period; continuous infusion of 20-50 mcg/kg/minute or 1-4 mg/minute; decrease the dose in patients with congestive heart failure, shock, or hepatic disease

Not dialyzable (0% to 5%)
Monitoring Parameters EKG, blood pressure, pulse, paresthesias
Reference Range Therapeutic: 1.5-4.0 µg/mL (SI: 6.4-17.1 µmol/L), up to 6.0 µg/mL (SI: 25.6 µmol/L) if necessary; Toxic: >8 µg/mL (SI: >34.2 µmol/L)
Nursing Implications Local thrombophlebitis may occur in patients receiving prolonged I.V. infusions; pain with I.M. injection
Special Geriatric Considerations Due to decreases in phase I metabolism and possibly decrease in splanchnic perfusion with age, there may be a decreased clearance or increased half-life in elderly and increased risk for CNS side effects and cardiac effects
Dosage Forms
Injection: 0.5% (50 mL); 1% (2 mL, 5 mL, 10 mL, 20 mL, 30 mL, 50 mL); 1.5% (20 mL); 2% (2 mL, 5 mL, 10 mL, 20 mL, 30 mL, 50 mL); 4% (5 mL); 10% (10 mL); 20% (10 mL, 20 mL)
Injection:
I.M. use: 100 mg/mL (3 mL, 5 mL)
Direct I.V.: 10 mg/mL (5 mL, 10 mL); 20 mg/mL (5 mL)
I.V. admixture: 40 mg/mL (25 mL, 30 mL); 100 mg/mL (10 mL); 200 mg/mL (5 mL, 10 mL)
I.V. infusion, D$_5$W: 2 mg/mL (500 mL); 4 mg/mL (250 mL, 500 mL, 1000 mL); 8 mg/mL (250 mL, 500 mL)
Jelly: 2% (30 mL)
Liquid, viscous: 2% (20 mL, 100 mL)
Ointment: 2.5% [OTC]; 5% (35 g)
Solution, topical: 4%

LidoPen® see Lidocaine Hydrochloride on previous page

Lignocaine Hydrochloride see Lidocaine Hydrochloride on previous page

Lindane (lin' dane)
Brand Names Kwell®; Scabene®
Synonyms Benzene Hexachloride; Gamma Benzene Hexachloride; Hexachlorocyclohexane
Generic Available Yes
Therapeutic Class Antiparasitic Agent, Topical; Pediculocide; Scabicidal Agent; Shampoos
(Continued)

Lindane *(Continued)*

Use Treatment of scabies and pediculosis

Contraindications Hypersensitivity to lindane or any component; acutely inflamed skin or raw, weeping surfaces

Warnings Avoid contact with the face, eyes, mucous membranes, and urethral meatus

Precautions Use with caution in patients with existing seizure disorder; avoid contact with the face, eyes, mucous membranes, and urethral meatus

Adverse Reactions Seizures have been reported in geriatric patients 4-5 days after application; serum concentration 1 week after application higher than expected; skin and adipose tissue may act as repositories

Central nervous system: Dizziness, restlessness, ataxia, seizures, headache
Dermatologic: Eczematous eruptions, contact dermatitis
Gastrointestinal: Nausea, vomiting
Hematologic: Aplastic anemia
Hepatic: Hepatitis
Renal: Hematuria
Respiratory: Pulmonary edema

Overdosage Symptoms of overdose include vomiting, restlessness, ataxia, seizures, arrhythmia, pulmonary edema, hematuria, hepatitis

Toxicology Absorbed through skin and mucous membranes and GI tract, has occasionally caused serious CNS, hepatic and renal toxicity when used excessively for prolonged periods, or when accidental ingestion has occurred; diazepam 0.01 mg/kg can be used to control seizures

Drug Interactions Oil based hair dressing may increase toxic potential

Mechanism of Action Directly absorbed by parasites and ova through the exoskeleton; stimulates the nervous system resulting in seizures and death of parasitic arthropods

Pharmacokinetics
Absorption: Up to 13% systemically; stored in body fat
Metabolism: By the liver
Elimination: In urine and feces

Usual Dosage Adults: Topical:
Scabies: Apply a thin layer of lotion and massage it on skin from the neck to the toes. For adults, bathe and remove the drug after 8-12 hours

Pediculosis: 15-30 mL of shampoo is applied and lathered for 4-5 minutes; rinse hair thoroughly and comb with a fine tooth comb to remove nits; repeat treatment in 7 days if lice or nits are still present

Patient Information For topical use only; do not apply to face; avoid getting in eyes, do not bathe prior to application

Nursing Implications Drug should not be administered orally; do not bathe prior to application; apply with rubber gloves

Special Geriatric Considerations Because of the potential for systemic absorption and CNS side effects, lindane should be used with caution; not considered a drug of first choice; consider permethrin or crotamiton agent first

Dosage Forms
Cream: 1% (60 g, 454 g)
Lotion: 1% (60 mL, 473 mL, 4000 mL)
Shampoo: 1% (60 mL, 473 mL, 4000 mL)

Lioresal® *see* Baclofen *on page 74*

Liothyronine Sodium *(lye oh thye' roe neen)*

Brand Names Cytomel®; Triostat™

Synonyms Sodium *L*-Tri-iodothyronine; T_3 Thyronine Sodium

Generic Available Yes

Therapeutic Class Thyroid Product

Use Replacement or supplemental therapy in hypothyroidism, management of nontoxic goiter, chronic lymphocytic thyroiditis, as an adjunct in thyrotoxicosis and as a diagnostic aid

Contraindications Recent myocardial infarction or thyrotoxicosis, uncomplicated by hypothyroidism; uncorrected adrenal insufficiency, hypersensitivity to active or extraneous constituents

Warnings Ineffective for weight reduction; high doses may produce serious or even life-threatening toxic effects particularly when used with some anorectic drugs; use cautiously in patients with pre-existing cardiovascular disease (angina, CHD), elderly since they may be more likely to have compromised cardiovascular function

Precautions Patients with angina pectoris or other cardiovascular disease; adrenal insufficiency, myxedema, diabetes mellitus and insipidus may have symptoms exaggerated or aggravated; thyroid replacement requires periodic assessment of thyroid status. Chronic hypothyroidism predisposes patients to coronary artery disease.

Adverse Reactions
Cardiovascular: Palpitations, tachycardia, cardiac arrhythmias
Central nervous system: Nervousness, headache, insomnia, fever

Dermatologic: Hair loss

Endocrine & metabolic: Excessive bone loss with overtreatment (excess thyroid replacement)

Gastrointestinal: Weight loss, increased appetite, diarrhea, abdominal cramps, vomiting

Neuromuscular & skeletal: Tremors

Miscellaneous: Sweating, heat intolerance

Overdosage Chronic excessive use results in signs and symptoms of hyperthyroidism, weight loss, nervousness, sweating, tachycardia, insomnia, heat intolerance, palpitations, vomiting, psychosis, fever, seizures, angina, arrhythmias, and congestive heart failure in those predisposed

Toxicology Reduce dose or temporarily discontinue therapy; normal hypothalamic-pituitary-thyroid axis will return to normal in 6-8 weeks; serum T_4 levels do not correlate well with toxicity; in massive acute ingestion, reduce GI absorption, give general supportive care; treat congestive heart failure with digitalis glycosides; excessive adrenergic activity (tachycardia) require propranolol 1-3 mg I.V. over 10 minutes or 80-160 mg orally/day; fever may be treated with acetaminophen

Drug Interactions

Cholestyramine and colestipol decrease the effect of orally administered thyroid replacement

Estrogens increase TBG, thereby decreasing effect of thyroid replacement

Anticoagulants may increase action

Beta-blocker effect is decreased when patients become euthyroid

Serum digitalis concentrations are reduced in hyperthyroidism or when hypothyroid patients are converted to a euthyroid state

Theophylline levels decrease when hypothyroid patients converted to a euthyroid state

Stability Store between 2°C to 8°C (36°F to 46°F)

Mechanism of Action The primary active compound is T_3 (tri-iodothyronine), which may be converted from T_4 (thyroxine) and then circulates throughout the body to influence growth and maturation of various tissues; exact mechanism of action is unknown; however, it is believed the thyroid hormone exerts its many metabolic effects through control of DNA transcription and protein synthesis; involved in normal metabolism, growth, and development; promotes gluconeogenesis, increases utilization and mobilization of glycogen stores, and stimulates protein synthesis, increases basal metabolic rate

Pharmacodynamics

Onset of effects: Within 24-72 hours

Duration: 72 hours

Pharmacokinetics

Absorption: Oral: Well absorbed, ~85% to 90%

Metabolism: Liver metabolism to inactive conjugated compounds

Half-life: 1-2 days

Elimination: In urine

Usual Dosage See Additional Information

Hypothyroidism:

Geriatrics: Initial: 5 mcg/day, increase dose 5 mcg/day every 1-2 weeks; usual maintenance dose: 25-75 mcg/day

Adults: Initial: 25 mcg/day; increase by 12.5-25 mcg/day at 1- to 2- week intervals

Nontoxic goiter: 5 mcg/day, increase by 5-10 mcg/day at 1- to 2-week intervals; use 5 mcg increments in elderly

T_3 suppression test: 75-100 mcg/day for 7 days; use lowest dose for elderly

Myxedema: 5 mcg/day; increase 5-10 mcg/day at 1- to 2-week intervals; usual maintenance dose: 50-100 mcg/day; use 5 mcg increments in elderly

Monitoring Parameters T_4, TSH, heart rate, blood pressure, clinical signs of hypo- and hyperthyroidism; TSH is the most reliable guide for evaluating adequacy of thyroid replacement dosage. TSH may be elevated during the first few months of thyroid replacement despite patients being clinically euthyroid. In cases where T_4 remains low and TSH is within normal limits, an evaluation of "free" (unbound) T_4 is needed to evaluate further increase in dosage

Reference Range Free T_3, Serum: 250-390 pg/dL; TSH: 0.4-10 (for those ≥ 80 years of age) mIU/L

Test Interactions Increased calcium (S); many drugs may have effects on thyroid function tests; para-aminosalicylic acid, aminoglutethimide, amiodarone, barbiturates, carbamazepine, chloral hydrate, clofibrate, colestipol, corticosteroids, danazol, diazepam, estrogens, ethionamide, fluorouracil, I.V. heparin, insulin, lithium, methadone, methimazole, mitotane, nitroprusside, oxyphenbutazone, phenylbutazone, PTU, perphenazine, phenytoin, propranolol, salicylates, sulfonylureas, and thiazides

Patient Information Do not change brands without physician's knowledge; report immediately to physician any chest pain, increased pulse, palpitations, heat intolerances, excessive sweating; do not stop use without physician's advice; replacement therapy will be for life; take as a single dose before breakfast

(Continued)

Liothyronine Sodium *(Continued)*

Nursing Implications See Monitoring Parameters, Reference Range, Warnings, and Special Geriatric Considerations

Additional Information Short duration action permits fast dosage changes or diminishes toxicity rapidly; the rapid onset and dissipation of action make this a difficult agent to use in those likely to have adverse effects to thyroid such as elderly; if rapid correction of thyroid is needed, T_3 is preferred but use cautiously and with lower recommended doses. 15-37.5 mcg is equivalent to 0.05-0.06 mg levothyroxine; 60 mg thyroid USP; 45 mg Thyroid Strong®, and 60 mg thyroglobulin

Special Geriatric Considerations Elderly do not have a change in serum thyroxine associated with aging; however, plasma T_3 concentrations are decreased 25% to 40% in elderly. There is not a compensatory rise in thyrotropin suggesting that lower T_3 is not reacted upon as a deficiency by the pituitary. This indicates a slightly lower than normal dosage of thyroid hormone replacement is usually sufficient in older patients than in younger adult patients. TSH must be monitored since insufficient thyroid replacement (elevated TSH) is a risk for coronary artery disease and excessive replacement (low TSH) may cause signs of hyperthyroidism and excessive bone loss; see Usual Dosage and Overdosage.

Dosage Forms Tablet: 5 mcg, 25 mcg

References

Helfand M and Crapo LM, "Monitoring Therapy in Patients Taking Levothyroxine," *Ann Intern Med*, 1990, 113(6):450-4.

Johnson DG and Campbell S, "Hormonal and Metabolic Agents," *Geriatric Pharmacology*, Bressler R and Katz MD, eds, New York, NY: McGraw-Hill, 1993, 427-50.

Sanders LR, "Pituitary, Thyroid, Adrenal and Parathyroid Diseases in the Elderly," *Geriatric Medicine*, 1990, 475-87.

Sawin CT, Geller A, Hershman JM, et al, "The Aging Thyroid. The Use of Thyroid Hormone in Older Persons," *JAMA*, 1989, 261(18):2653-5.

Watts NB, "Use of a Sensitive Thyrotropin Assay for Monitoring Treatment With Levothyroxine," *Arch Intern Med*, 1989, 149(2):309-12.

Liotrix *(lye' oh trix)*

Brand Names Euthroid®; Thyrolar®

Synonyms T_3/T_4 Liotrix

Therapeutic Class Thyroid Hormone

Use Replacement or supplemental therapy in hypothyroidism and thyroid cancer

Contraindications Hypersensitivity to liotrix or any component; recent myocardial infarction or thyrotoxicosis, uncomplicated by hypothyroidism; uncorrected adrenal insufficiency, hypersensitivity to active or extraneous constituents

Warnings Ineffective for weight reduction; high doses may produce serious or even life-threatening toxic effects particularly when used with some anorectic drugs; use cautiously in patients with pre-existing cardiovascular disease (angina, CHD), elderly since they may be more likely to have compromised cardiovascular function

Precautions Patients with angina pectoris or other cardiovascular disease; adrenal insufficiency, myxedema, diabetes mellitus and insipidus may have symptoms exaggerated or aggravated; thyroid replacement requires periodic assessment of thyroid status; TSH is the most reliable guide for evaluating adequacy of thyroid replacement dosage. Chronic hypothyroidism predisposes patients to coronary artery disease.

Adverse Reactions

Cardiovascular: Palpitations, tachycardia, cardiac arrhythmias

Central nervous system: Nervousness, headache, insomnia, fever

Dermatologic: Hair loss

Endocrine & metabolic: Excessive bone loss with overtreatment (excess thyroid replacement)

Gastrointestinal: Weight loss, increased appetite, diarrhea, abdominal cramps, vomiting

Neuromuscular & skeletal: Tremors

Miscellaneous: Sweating, heat intolerance

Overdosage Chronic excessive use results in signs and symptoms of hyperthyroidism, weight loss, nervousness, sweating, tachycardia, insomnia, heat intolerance, palpitations, vomiting, psychosis, fever, seizures, angina, arrhythmias, and congestive heart failure in those predisposed

Toxicology Reduce dose or temporarily discontinue therapy; normal hypothalamic-pituitary-thyroid axis will return to normal in 6-8 weeks; serum T_4 levels do not correlate well with toxicity; in massive acute ingestion, reduce GI absorption, give general supportive care; treat congestive heart failure with digitalis glycosides; excessive adrenergic activity (tachycardia) require propranolol 1-3 mg I.V. over 10 minutes or 80-160 mg orally/day; fever may be treated with acetaminophen

Drug Interactions

Cholestyramine and colestipol decrease the effect of orally administered thyroid replacement

Estrogens increase TBG, thereby decreasing effect of thyroid replacement

Anticoagulants may increase action

Beta-blocker effect is decreased when patients become euthyroid

Serum digitalis concentrations are reduced in hyperthyroidism or when hypothyroid patients are converted to a euthyroid state

Theophylline levels decrease when hypothyroid patients converted to a euthyroid state

Mechanism of Action Liotrix is uniform mixture of synthetic T_4 and T_3 in 4:1 ratio; exact mechanism of action is unknown; however, it is believed the thyroid hormone exerts its many metabolic effects through control of DNA transcription and protein synthesis; involved in normal metabolism, growth, and development; promotes gluconeogenesis, increases utilization and mobilization of glycogen stores and stimulates protein synthesis, increases basal metabolic rate

Pharmacokinetics

Absorption: 50% to 95% from GI tract

Metabolism: Partially in liver, kidneys, and intestines

Half-life: 6-7 days

Time to peak: 12-48 hours

Elimination: In feces and bile as conjugated metabolites

Usual Dosage See Additional Information

Geriatrics: Initial: 15 mg, adjust dose at 2- to 4-week intervals in increments of 15 mg

Adults: Initial: 15-30 mg, adjust dose at 2- to 4-week intervals in increments of 15 mg

Usual maintenance dose: 60-120 mg/day

Thyroid cancer: Doses will be larger than usual maintenance dose

Monitoring Parameters T_4, TSH, heart rate, blood pressure, clinical signs of hypo- and hyperthyroidism; TSH is the most reliable guide for evaluating adequacy of thyroid replacement dosage. TSH may be elevated during the first few months of thyroid replacement despite patients being clinically euthyroid. In cases where T_4 remains low and TSH is within normal limits, an evaluation of "free" (unbound) T_4 is needed to evaluate further increase in dosage

Reference Range

TSH: 0.4-10 (for those $\geq$80 years) mIU/L

T_4: 4-12 μg/dL (SI: 51-154 nmol/L)

T_3 (RIA) (total T_3): 80-230 ng/dL (SI: 1.2-3.5 nmol/L)

T_4 free (Free T_4): 0.7-1.8 ng/dL (SI: 9-23 pmol/L)

Test Interactions Increased calcium (S); many drugs may have effects on thyroid function tests; para-aminosalicylic acid, aminoglutethimide, amiodarone, barbiturates, carbamazepine, chloral hydrate, clofibrate, colestipol, corticosteroids, danazol, diazepam, estrogens, ethionamide, fluorouracil, I.V. heparin, insulin, lithium, methadone, methimazole, mitotane, nitroprusside, oxyphenbutazone, phenylbutazone, PTU, perphenazine, phenytoin, propranolol, salicylates, sulfonylureas, and thiazides

Patient Information Do not change brands without physician's knowledge; report immediately to physician any chest pain, increased pulse, palpitations, heat intolerances, excessive sweating; do not stop use without physician's advice; replacement therapy will be for life; take as a single dose before breakfast

Nursing Implications See Warnings, Monitoring Parameters, Reference Range, and Special Geriatric Considerations

Additional Information Since T_3 is produced by monodeiodination of T_4 in peripheral tissues (80%) and since elderly have decreased T_3 (25% to 40%), little advantage to this product exists and cost is not justified; no advantage over synthetic levothyroxine sodium; 1 grain (60 mg) liotrix is equivalent to 0.05-0.06 mg levothyroxine; 60 mg thyroid USP and thyroglobulin; and 45 mg of Thyroid Strong®

Special Geriatric Considerations Elderly do not have a change in serum thyroxine associated with aging; however, plasma T_3 concentrations are decreased 25% to 40% in elderly. There is not a compensatory rise in thyrotropin suggesting that lower T_3 is not reacted upon as a deficiency by the pituitary. This indicates a slightly lower than normal dosage of thyroid hormone replacement is usually sufficient in older patients than in younger adult patients. TSH must be monitored since insufficient thyroid replacement (elevated TSH) is a risk for coronary artery disease and excessive replacement (low TSH) may cause signs of hyperthyroidism and excessive bone loss; see Usual Dosage and Overdosage.

Dosage Forms Tablet: 30 mg, 60 mg, 120 mg, 180 mg (thyroid equivalent)

References

Helfand M and Crapo LM, "Monitoring Therapy in Patients Taking Levothyroxine," *Ann Intern Med*, 1990, 113(6):450-4.

Johnson DG and Campbell S, "Hormonal and Metabolic Agents," *Geriatric Pharmacology*, Bressler R and Katz MD, eds, New York, NY: McGraw-Hill, 1993, 427-50.

Sanders LR, "Pituitary, Thyroid, Adrenal and Parathyroid Diseases in the Elderly," *Geriatric Medicine*, 1990, 475-87.

Sawin CT, Geller A, Hershman JM, et al, "The Aging Thyroid. The Use of Thyroid Hormone in Older Persons," *JAMA*, 1989, 261(18):2653-5.

Watts NB, "Use of a Sensitive Thyrotropin Assay for Monitoring Treatment With Levothyroxine," *Arch Intern Med*, 1989, 149(2):309-12.

Liquaemin® *see* Heparin *on page 340*

ALPHABETICAL LISTING OF DRUGS

Liquid Paraffin *see* Mineral Oil *on page 473*
Liquid Pred® *see* Prednisone *on page 586*

Lisinopril (lyse in' oh pril)
Brand Names Prinivil®; Zestril®
Generic Available No
Therapeutic Class Angiotensin-Converting Enzyme (ACE) Inhibitors
Use Treatment of hypertension, either alone or in combination with other antihypertensive agents; adjunctive therapy in treatment of CHF (afterload reduction)
Contraindications Hypersensitivity to lisinopril or any component or any ACE inhibitor
Warnings Neutropenia, agranulocytosis, angioedema, decreased renal function (hypertension, renal artery stenosis, congestive heart failure), hepatic dysfunction (elimination, activation), proteinuria, first-dose hypotension (hypovolemia, CHF, dehydrated patients at risk, eg, diuretic use, elderly), elderly (due to renal function changes)
Precautions Use with caution and modify dosage in patients with renal impairment; use with caution in patients with collagen vascular disease, congestive heart failure, hypovolemia, valvular stenosis, hyperkalemia (>5.7 mEq/L), anesthesia
Adverse Reactions
Cardiovascular: Hypotension, tachycardia, arrhythmias, orthostatic blood pressure changes, angina, palpitations, chest pain, syncope, myocardial infarction, CVA, flushing
Central nervous system: Nervousness, depression, confusion, somnolence, fatigue, dizziness, headache, paresthesias, asthenia, insomnia, malaise, vertigo, fever
Dermatologic: Rash, pruritus, urticaria, angioedema
Endocrine & metabolic: Hyperkalemia
Gastrointestinal: Pancreatitis, constipation, anorexia, nausea, vomiting, diarrhea, abdominal pain, dry mouth, dysgeusia, dyspepsia, flatulence, pancreatitis
Genitourinary: Impotence, decreased libido, azotemia (progressive)
Hematologic: Anemia, neutropenia, agranulocytosis
Hepatic: Hepatitis, hepatocellular/cholestatic jaundice
Neuromuscular & skeletal: Myalgia, arthralgia, muscle cramps, arthritis
Ocular: Blurred vision
Renal: Oliguria, proteinuria, increased BUN, serum creatinine
Respiratory: Chronic cough (nonproductive, persistent; more often in women and seen in 15% to 30% of patients), asthma, bronchitis, bronchospasm, dyspnea, sinusitis
Miscellaneous: Loss of taste perception, sweating, peripheral edema
Overdosage Symptoms of overdose include hypotension
Toxicology Following initiation of essential overdose management, toxic symptom treatment and supportive treatment should be initiated. Hypotension usually responds to I.V. fluids or Trendelenburg positioning. If unresponsive to these measures, the use of a parenteral inotrope may be required (eg, norepinephrine 0.1-0.2 mcg/kg/minute titrated to response). Seizures commonly respond to diazepam (I.V. 5-10 mg bolus in adults every 15 minutes if needed up to a total of 30 mg) or to phenytoin or phenobarbital.
Drug Interactions
ACE inhibitors (captopril) and potassium-sparing diuretics → additive hyperkalemic effect
ACE inhibitors (captopril) and indomethacin or nonsteroidal anti-inflammatory agents → reduced antihypertensive response to ACE inhibitors
Allopurinol and ACE inhibitors (captopril) → neutropenia
Antacids and ACE inhibitors → ↓ absorption of ACE inhibitors
Phenothiazines and ACE inhibitors → ↑ ACE inhibitor effect
Probenecid and ACE inhibitors (captopril) → ↑ ACE inhibitors (captopril) levels
Rifampin and ACE inhibitors (enalapril) → ↓ ACE inhibitor effect
Digoxin and ACE inhibitors → ↑ serum digoxin levels
Lithium and ACE inhibitors → ↑ lithium serum levels
Tetracycline and ACE inhibitors (quinapril) → ↓ tetracycline absorption (up to 37%)
Capsaicin may enhance or cause cough associated with ACE inhibitors
Food decreases captopril absorption; rate, but not extent, of ramipril and fosinopril is reduced by concomitant administration with food; food does not reduce absorption of enalapril, lisinopril or benazepril
Mechanism of Action Competitive inhibitor of angiotensin-converting enzyme (ACE); prevents conversion of angiotensin I to angiotensin II, a potent vasoconstrictor; results in lower levels of angiotensin II which causes an increase in plasma renin activity and a reduction in aldosterone secretion; a CNS mechanism may also be involved in hypotensive effect as angiotensin II increases adrenergic outflow from CNS; vasoactive kallikreins may be decreased in conversion to active hormones by ACE inhibitors, thus reducing blood pressure
Pharmacodynamics Oral:
Onset of action: Within 1 hour

Peak effects: Within 6 hours
Duration: 24 hours
Pharmacokinetics
Absorption: Oral: Well absorbed
Protein binding: 25%
Half-life: 11-12 hours
Time to peak: Peak level achieved in 6-7 hours and unaffected by food
Elimination: Almost entirely in urine as unchanged drug (100%)
Usual Dosage
Geriatrics: Initial: 2.5-5 mg/day; increase doses 2.5-5 mg/day at 1- to 2-week intervals; maximum daily dose: 40 mg

Adults: Initial: 10 mg/day; increase doses 5-10 mg/day at 1- to 2-week intervals; maximum daily dose: 40 mg

Patients taking diuretics should have them discontinued 2-3 days prior to initiating lisinopril if possible; restart diuretic after blood pressure is stable if needed; in patients with hyponatremia (<130 mEq/L), start dose at 2.5 mg/day

Dosing adjustment in renal impairment: Cl_{cr} <30 mL/minute: Drug is eliminated (100%) renally; start doses at lowest recommended dose (2.5 mg) and adjust dose at 1- to 2-week intervals based upon blood pressure response
Monitoring Parameters Serum potassium levels, BUN, serum creatinine, WBC
Test Interactions Increased potassium (S); increased serum creatinine/BUN
Patient Information Do not stop therapy except under prescriber advice; notify physician if you develop sore throat, fever, swelling of hands, feet, face, eyes, lips, and tongue; difficult breathing, irregular heartbeats, chest pains, or cough. May cause dizziness, fainting, and lightheadedness, especially in first week of therapy, sit and stand up slowly; may cause changes in taste or rash; do not add a salt substitute (potassium) without advice of physician
Nursing Implications Watch for hypotensive effect within 1-3 hours of first dose or new higher dose; see Precautions, Warnings, Monitoring Parameters, and Special Geriatric Considerations
Special Geriatric Considerations Due to frequent decreases in glomerular filtration (also creatinine clearance) with aging, elderly patients may have exaggerated responses to ACE inhibitors; differences in clinical response due to hepatic changes are not observed. ACE inhibitors may be preferred agents in elderly patients with congestive heart failure and diabetes mellitus. Diabetic proteinuria is reduced and insulin sensitivity is enhanced. In general, the side effect profile is favorable in elderly and causes little or no CNS confusion; use lowest dose recommendations initially.
Dosage Forms Tablet: 2.5 mg, 5 mg, 10 mg, 20 mg, 40 mg
References
McAreavey D and Robertson JIS, "Angiotensin Converting Enzyme Inhibitors and Moderate Hypertension," *Drugs*, 1990, 40(3):326-45.

Lithane® see Lithium on this page

Lithium (lith' ee um)
Related Information
Drug Levels Commonly Monitored Guidelines on page 771-772
Brand Names Cibalith-S®; Eskalith®; Lithane®; Lithobid®; Lithonate®; Lithotabs®
Synonyms Lithium Carbonate; Lithium Citrate
Generic Available Yes
Therapeutic Class Antimanic Agent
Use Treatment of manic episodes in bipolar disorders; prevention of subsequent manic episodes
Contraindications Hypersensitivity to lithium or any component; severe cardiovascular or renal disease
Warnings Lithium toxicity is closely related to serum levels and can occur at therapeutic doses; serum lithium determinations are required to monitor therapy; concomitant use of lithium with thiazide diuretics may decrease renal excretion and enhance lithium toxicity; lithium dosage may need to be reduced by 30%
Precautions Use with caution in patients with cardiovascular or thyroid disease
Adverse Reactions
Cardiovascular: Arrhythmias, sinus node dysfunction
Central nervous system: Sedation, confusion, somnolence, seizures, fatigue, headache, vertigo
Dermatologic: Rash
Endocrine & metabolic: Nephrogenic diabetes insipidus (thirst, polyuria, polydipsia), goiter, hypothyroidism
Gastrointestinal: Nausea, diarrhea, vomiting, dry mouth
Hematologic: Leukocytosis
Neuromuscular & skeletal: Muscle hyperirritability (twitching, fasciculations), tremors, muscle weakness
(Continued)
413

Lithium *(Continued)*

Overdosage Symptoms of overdose include sedation, confusion, tremors, joint pain, visual changes, seizures, coma

Toxicology There is no specific antidote for lithium poisoning. In the acute ingestion, following initiation of essential overdose management, correction of fluid and electrolyte imbalances should be commenced. Activated charcoal may not be effective in adsorbing lithium but is not harmful if used. Theophylline, mannitol and urea have all been shown to decrease serum lithium levels by enhancing its elimination, but hemodialysis is the treatment of choice for severe intoxications.

Drug Interactions
Decreased effect with xanthines (eg, theophylline, caffeine)
Increased effect/toxicity of CNS depressants, iodide salts (increased hypothyroid effect), neuromuscular blockers
Increased toxicity with thiazide diuretics, NSAIDs, haloperidol, phenothiazines (neurotoxicity), carbamazepine, fluoxetine, ACE inhibitors

Mechanism of Action Alters cation transport across cell membrane in nerve and muscle cells and influences reuptake of serotonin and/or norepinephrine

Pharmacokinetics
Distribution: Adults:
V_d: Initial: 0.3-0.4 L/kg
V_{dss}: 0.7-1 L/kg
Half-life: Terminal: 18-24 hours, can increase to more than 36 hours in elderly or patients with renal impairment
Time to peak serum concentration: Oral: Within 0.5-2 hours following absorption (nonsustained release product)
Elimination: 90% to 98% of dose excreted in urine as unchanged drug; other excretory routes include feces (1%) and sweat (4% to 5%)

Usual Dosage Monitor serum concentrations and clinical response (efficacy and toxicity) to determine proper dose. Total daily dose will be decreased in patients with renal impairment. Oral:
Geriatrics: Initial dose: 300 mg twice daily, increase weekly in increments of 300 mg/day, monitoring levels; rarely need to go above 900-1200 mg/day

Adults: 300 mg 3-4 times/day; usual maximum maintenance dose: 2.4 g/day

Dosing adjustment in renal impairment:
Cl_{cr} 10-50 mL/minute: Administer 50% to 75% of normal dose
Cl_{cr} <10 mL/minute: Administer 25% to 50% of normal dose
Dialyzable (50% to 100%)

Monitoring Parameters Lithium levels, fluid status, serum electrolytes, renal function

Reference Range Therapeutic: 0.6-1.2 mEq/L (SI: 0.6-1.2 mmol/L), for acute mania; 0.8-1 mEq/L (SI: 0.8-1 mmol/L) for protection against future episodes in most patients with bipolar disorder. A higher rate of relapse is described in subjects who are maintained below 0.4 mEq/L (SI: 0.4 mmol/L), geriatric patients can usually be maintained at the lower end of the therapeutic range (0.6-0.8 mEq/L); Toxic: >2 mEq/L (SI: >2 mmol/L).

Test Interactions Increased calcium (S), glucose, magnesium, potassium (S); decreased thyroxine (S)

Patient Information Avoid tasks requiring psychomotor coordination until the CNS effects are known, blood level monitoring is required to determine the proper dose; maintain a steady salt and fluid intake especially during the summer months; do not crush or chew slow or controlled release tablets, swallow whole; take with meals

Nursing Implications Give with meals to decrease GI upset, encourage adequate fluid intake, monitor for signs of toxicity; do not crush slow or controlled release tablets

Additional Information 5 mL of lithium citrate syrup contains 8 mEq of lithium and is approximately equivalent to 300 mg of lithium carbonate
Lithium citrate: Cibalith-S®
Lithium carbonate: Eskalith®, Lithane®, Lithobid®, Lithonate®, Lithotabs®

Special Geriatric Considerations Some elderly patients may be extremely sensitive to the effects of lithium; initial doses need to be adjusted for renal function in elderly; thereafter, adjust doses based upon serum concentrations and response; see Usual Dosage and Reference Range

Dosage Forms
Capsule, as carbonate: 150 mg, 300 mg, 600 mg
Syrup, as citrate: 300 mg/5 mL (5 mL, 10 mL, 480 mL)
Tablet, as carbonate: 300 mg
Tablet:
Controlled release, as carbonate: 450 mg
Slow release, as carbonate: 300 mg

References

Foster JF, Gershell WJ, and Goldfarb AI, "Lithium Treatment in the Elderly. I. Clinical Usage," *J Gerontol*, 1977, 32(3):299-302.
Hicks R, Dysken MW, Davis JM, et al, "The Pharmacokinetics of Psychotropic Medication in the Elderly: A Review," *J Clin Psychiatry*, 1981, 42(10):374-85.

Lithium Carbonate *see* Lithium *on page 413*

Lithium Citrate *see* Lithium *on page 413*

Lithobid® *see* Lithium *on page 413*

Lithonate® *see* Lithium *on page 413*

Lithotabs® *see* Lithium *on page 413*

Lixolin® *see* Theophylline *on page 681*

Lo-Aqua® *see* Furosemide *on page 315*

Locoid® *see* Hydrocortisone *on page 351*

Lodine® *see* Etodolac *on page 277*

Lodosyn® *see* Carbidopa *on page 120*

Lodoxamide Tromethamine
Brand Names Alomide®
Therapeutic Class Ophthalmic Agent, Miscellaneous
Use Treatment of vernal keratoconjunctivitis, vernal conjunctivitis, and vernal keratitis
Contraindications Hypersensitivity to any component of product
Warnings Not for injection; not for use in patients wearing soft contact lenses during treatment
Adverse Reactions
    Central nervous system: Headache, dizziness, somnolence
    Dermatologic: Rash
    Gastrointestinal: Nausea, stomach discomfort
    Local: Transient burning, stinging, discomfort
    Ocular: Blurred vision, corneal erosion/ulcer, eye pain, corneal abrasion, blepharitis
    Respiratory: Sneezing, dry nose
Overdosage Symptoms of overdose include feeling of warmth, headache, dizziness, fatigue, sweating, nausea, and loose stools following oral administration
Toxicology Consider emesis in the event of accidental ingestion
Mechanism of Action Mast cell stabilizer that inhibits the *in vivo* type I immediate hypersensitivity reaction to increase cutaneous vascular permeability associated with IgE and antigen-mediated reactions
Pharmacokinetics Absorption: Topical: Very small and undetectable
Usual Dosage Geriatrics and Adults: Instill 1-2 drops in eye(s) 4 times/day for up to 3 months
    Dosage Forms Solution, ophthalmic: 0.1% (10 mL)

Lodrane® *see* Theophylline *on page 681*

Lofene® *see* Diphenoxylate and Atropine *on page 230*

Logen® *see* Diphenoxylate and Atropine *on page 230*

Lomefloxacin Hydrochloride (loe me flox' a sin)
Brand Names Maxaquin®
Therapeutic Class Antibiotic, Quinolone
Use Quinolone antibiotic for skin and skin structure, lower respiratory and urinary tract infections, and sexually transmitted diseases; prophylaxis preoperatively to transurethral procedures
Contraindications Hypersensitivity to lomefloxacin or other members of the quinolone group such as nalidixic acid, oxolinic acid, cinoxacin, norfloxacin, and ciprofloxacin
Warnings Use with caution in patients with epilepsy or other CNS diseases which could predispose them to seizures
Adverse Reactions
    Cardiovascular: Hyper- and hypotension, syncope, bradycardia, tachycardia, arrhythmias, angina, cardiac failure, flushing
    Central nervous system: Fatigue, malaise, seizures, vertigo, paresthesias, headache, dizziness, coma
    Dermatologic: Rash, photosensitivity
    Gastrointestinal: Abdominal pain, nausea, vomiting, flatulence, constipation, tongue discoloration, taste perversion, diarrhea, dry mouth, pseudomembranous colitis
    Hematologic: Thrombocytopenia purpura
    Neuromuscular & skeletal: Tremors, gout, myalgia, leg cramps, hyperkinesia
    Renal: Dysuria, hematuria, micturition disorder, anuria
    Respiratory: Dyspnea
    Miscellaneous: Flu-like symptoms, facial edema, decreased heat tolerance, sweating
Overdosage Symptoms of overdose include acute renal failure, seizures
Toxicology GI decontamination and supportive care; diazepam for seizures; not removed by peritoneal or hemodialysis
Drug Interactions
    Decreased effect: Bismuth subsalicylate, antacids (aluminum, magnesium), iron salts, zinc salts, sucralfate
    (Continued)

Lomefloxacin Hydrochloride *(Continued)*

Increased levels: Probenecid, cimetidine

Increased levels/effect/toxicity: Warfarin, cyclosporine, NSAIDs (increased seizures)

Mechanism of Action Exerts a broad spectrum antimicrobial effect. The primary target of the fluoroquinolones is DNA gyrase (topoisomerase II), an essential bacterial enzyme that maintains the superhelical structure of DNA. DNA gyrase is required for DNA replication and transcription, DNA repair, recombination, and transposition.

Pharmacokinetics

Absorption: Well absorbed

Distribution: V_d: 2.4-3.5 L/kg

Protein binding: 20%

Half-life, elimination: 5-7.5 hours; prolonged to a mean of 12.7 hours in middle age and elderly patients

Elimination: Primarily unchanged in urine

Usual Dosage Geriatrics and Adults: Oral: 400 mg once daily for 10-14 days

Dosing adjustment in renal impairment: $Cl_{cr} > 10$ but <40 mL/minute/1.73 m^2: Give 400 mg first dose, followed by 200 mg/day for a total of 10-14 days

Monitoring Parameters Signs and symptoms of infection, WBC, mental status

Patient Information Take 1 hour before or 2 hours after meals

Special Geriatric Considerations Dosage adjustment not necessary in patients with normal renal function; otherwise follow dosage guidelines in renal impairment; age-associated increase in half-life and decrease in clearance thought to be secondary to age-related changes in renal function; adjust dose for renal function

Dosage Forms Tablet: 400 mg

References

Kovarik JM, Hoepelman AI, Smit JM, et al, "Steady-State Pharmacokinetics and Sputum Penetration of Lomefloxacin in Patients With Chronic Obstructive Pulmonary Disease and Acute Respiratory Tract Infections," *Antimicrob Agents Chemother*, 1992, 36(11):2458-61.

Lomenate® *see* Diphenoxylate and Atropine *on page 230*

Lomodix® *see* Diphenoxylate and Atropine *on page 230*

Lomotil® *see* Diphenoxylate and Atropine *on page 230*

Loniten® *see* Minoxidil *on page 474*

Lonox® *see* Diphenoxylate and Atropine *on page 230*

Loperamide Hydrochloride *(loe per' a mide)*

Brand Names Imodium®; Imodium® A-D Caplets [OTC]; Imodium® A-D Liquid [OTC]

Therapeutic Class Antidiarrheal

Use Treatment of acute diarrhea and chronic diarrhea associated with inflammatory bowel disease; decrease the volume of ileostomy discharge

Unlabeled use: Treatment of traveler's diarrhea in combination with trimethoprim-sulfamethoxazole (3 days of therapy)

Restrictions Imodium® 2 mg capsules are legend

Contraindications Hypersensitivity to loperamide or any component; patients who must avoid constipation; diarrhea resulting from some infections; patients with pseudomembranous colitis; bloody diarrhea

Warnings Should not be used if diarrhea accompanied by high fever, blood in stool, liver disease; may induce toxic megacolon in patients with acute ulcerative colitis; discontinue use in ulcerative colitis if abdominal distention occurs

Precautions Large first-pass metabolism, use with caution in hepatic dysfunction; if clinical improvement is not seen in 48 hours, discontinue use

Adverse Reactions

Central nervous system: Sedation, fatigue, dizziness, drowsiness

Dermatologic: Rash

Gastrointestinal: Nausea, vomiting, constipation, abdominal cramping, dry mouth, abdominal distention

Overdosage Symptoms of overdose include CNS depression, constipation, GI irritation, nausea, vomiting; overdosage is noted when daily doses approximate 60 mg of loperamide

Toxicology Treatment of overdose: Gastric lavage followed by 100 g activated charcoal through a nasogastric tube. Monitor for signs of CNS depression. If they occur, administer naloxone 2 mg I.V.; repeat as necessary. Loperamide has a short duration of action (1-3 hours).

Drug Interactions CNS depressants (antidepressants, antipsychotics, hypnotics, anxiolytics, alcohol) may be enhanced in action

Mechanism of Action Acts directly on intestinal muscles to inhibit peristalsis and prolongs transit time enhancing fluid and electrolyte movement through intestinal mucosa; reduces fecal volume, increases viscosity, and diminishes fluid and electrolyte loss; demonstrates antisecretory activity; exhibits peripheral action

Pharmacodynamics Onset of action: Oral: Occurs within 30-60 minutes

Pharmacokinetics

Absorption: Oral: <40%

Protein binding: 97%

Metabolism: Hepatic metabolism (>50%) to inactive compounds
Half-life: 7-14 hours
Elimination: Fecal and urinary (1%) excretion of metabolites and unchanged drug (30% to 40%)

Usual Dosage Geriatrics and Adults: Oral: Initial: 4 mg (2 capsules), followed by 2 mg after each loose stool, up to 16 mg/day (8 capsules); see Additional Information

Monitoring Parameters Monitor stool frequency and consistency; observe for toxicity with use more than 48 hours

Patient Information Do not take more than 8 capsules/80 mL in 24 hours; may cause drowsiness; use caution when driving; may cause dry mouth; notify physician if diarrhea persists or abdominal distention occurs; if diarrhea does not subside in 2-3 days, consult physician when buying without physician's advice.

Nursing Implications Therapy for chronic diarrhea should not exceed 10 days; if diarrhea persists longer than 48 hours for acute diarrhea, etiology should be examined; monitor stool frequency and consistency

Additional Information If clinical improvement is not achieved after 16 mg/day for 10 days, control is unlikely with further use. Continue use if diet or other treatment does not control.

Special Geriatric Considerations Elderly are particularly sensitive to fluid and electrolyte loss. This generally results in lethargy, weakness, and confusion. Repletion and maintenance of electrolytes and water are essential in the treatment of diarrhea. Drug therapy must be limited in order to avoid toxicity with this agent.

Dosage Forms
Caplet (tablet): 2 mg
Capsule: 2 mg
Liquid: 1 mg/5 mL (60 mL, 90 mL, 120 mL)

Lopid® *see* Gemfibrozil *on page 319*

Lopressor® *see* Metoprolol Tartrate *on page 465*

Lopurin™ *see* Allopurinol *on page 26*

Lorabid™ *see* Loracarbef *on this page*

Loracarbef
Brand Names Lorabid™
Generic Available No
Therapeutic Class Antibiotic, Carbacephem
Use Infections caused by susceptible organisms involving the respiratory tract, acute otitis media, sinusitis, skin and skin structure, bone and joint, and urinary tract and gynecologic

Contraindications Patients with a history of hypersensitivity to loracarbef

Warnings Use with caution in patients with a previous history of hypersensitivity to other cephalosporins; use with caution in patients allergic to other beta-lactams

Adverse Reactions
Cardiovascular: Vasodilation
Central nervous system: Somnolence, nervousness, dizziness, headache
Dermatologic: Skin rashes
Gastrointestinal: Diarrhea, nausea, vomiting, abdominal pain, anorexia, pseudomembranous colitis
Genitourinary: Vaginitis, vaginal moniliasis
Hematologic: Transient thrombocytopenia, leukopenia, eosinophilia
Hepatic: Transient elevations of ALT, AST, and alkaline phosphatase
Renal: Transient elevations of creatinine and BUN

Overdosage Symptoms of overdose include abdominal discomfort, diarrhea

Toxicology Supportive care only

Drug Interactions Increased serum levels with probenecid

Food/Drug Interactions Decreased bioavailability with food

Stability Suspension may be kept at room temperature for 14 days

Mechanism of Action Inhibits bacterial cell wall synthesis by binding to one or more of the penicillin binding proteins (PBPs); inhibits the final transpeptidation step of peptidoglycan synthesis in bacterial cell walls, thus inhibiting cell wall biosynthesis. It is thought that beta-lactam antibiotics inactivate transpeptidase via acylation of the enzyme with cleavage of the CO-N bond of the beta-lactam ring. Upon exposure to beta-lactam antibiotics, bacteria eventually lyse due to ongoing activity of cell wall autolytic enzymes (autolysins and murein hydrolases) while cell wall assembly is arrested.

Pharmacokinetics
Absorption: Oral: Rapid
Half-life, elimination: ~1 hour
Time to peak serum concentration: Oral: Within 1 hour
Elimination: Plasma clearance: ~200-300 mL/minute

(Continued)

Loracarbef *(Continued)*

Usual Dosage Oral:

Geriatrics and Adults:

Uncomplicated urinary tract infections: 200 mg once daily for 7 days

Skin and soft tissue: 200-400 mg every 12-24 hours

Uncomplicated pyelonephritis: 400 mg every 12 hours for 14 days

Dosing comments in renal impairment:

Cl_{cr} ≥50 mL/minute: Give usual dose

Cl_{cr} 10-49 mL/minute: 50% of usual dose at usual interval or usual dose given half as often

Cl_{cr} <10 mL/minute: Give usual dose every 3-5 days

Hemodialysis: Doses should be administered after dialysis sessions

Administration Take on an empty stomach

Monitoring Parameters Signs and symptoms of infection, WBC, mental status

Patient Information Take on an empty stomach at least 1 hour before or 2 hours after meals; complete full course of therapy

Nursing Implications See Administration

Special Geriatric Considerations Half-life slightly prolonged with age, presumably due to the reduced creatinine clearance related to aging; adjust dose for renal function; see Usual Dosage

Dosage Forms

Capsule: 200 mg

Suspension, oral: 100 mg/5 mL; 200 mg/5 mL

References

DeSante KA and Zeckel ML, "Pharmacokinetic Profile of Loracarbef," *Am J Med*, 1992, 92(6A):16S-9S.

Loratadine *(lor at' a deen)*

Brand Names Claritin®

Therapeutic Class Antihistamine

Use Relief of nasal and non-nasal symptoms of seasonal allergic rhinitis

Contraindications Patients hypersensitive to loratadine or any of its components

Warnings Patients with liver impairment should start with a lower dose (10 mg every other day), since their ability to clear the drug will be reduced

Adverse Reactions

Central nervous system: Low incidence of fatigue, dizziness, headache, sedation

No significant anticholinergic effects, though dry mouth has been reported

Overdosage Symptoms of overdose include somnolence, tachycardia, headache

Toxicology No specific antidote is available, treatment is first decontamination, then symptomatic and supportive; loratadine is not eliminated by dialysis

Drug Interactions

Increased toxicity: Procarbazine, other antihistamines, alcohol

Increased plasma concentrations of loratadine and its active metabolite with ketoconazole; erythromycin increases the AUC of loratadine and its active metabolite; no change in $Q-T_c$ interval was seen

Mechanism of Action Long-acting tricyclic antihistamine with selective peripheral histamine H_1-receptor antagonistic properties

Pharmacokinetics

Onset of action: Within 1-3 hours

Peak effect: 8-12 hours

Duration: >24 hours

Absorption: Rapid

Metabolism: Extensive to an active metabolite

Half-life:

Geriatrics: 18.2 hours (6.7-37 hours)

Adults: 12-15 hours

Elimination: In one study, the AUC and peak plasma levels of both loratadine and its active metabolite were approximately 50% higher in elderly patients as compared to younger adults

Usual Dosage Geriatrics and Adults: Oral: 10 mg/day on an empty stomach

Dosing interval in hepatic impairment: 10 mg every other day to start

Monitoring Parameters Relief of symptoms, mental status

Patient Information Drink plenty of water; may cause dry mouth, sedation, drowsiness, and can impair judgment and coordination

Nursing Implications See Monitoring Parameters

Special Geriatric Considerations Loratadine is one of the newer, nonsedating antihistamines; because of its low incidence of side effects, it seems to be a good choice in the elderly. However, there is a wide variation in loratadine half-life reported in the elderly and this should be kept in mind when initiating dosing.

Dosage Forms Tablet: 10 mg

Lorazepam (lor a' ze pam)

Related Information
Antacid Drug Interactions *on page 764*
Anxiolytic/Hypnotic Use in Long-Term Care Facilities *on page 755-756*
Benzodiazepines Comparison *on page 802-803*

Brand Names Ativan®

Generic Available Yes

Therapeutic Class Antianxiety Agent; Benzodiazepine; Hypnotic; Sedative

Use Management of anxiety, status epilepticus, preoperative sedation, and amnesia

Restrictions C-IV

Contraindications Hypersensitivity to lorazepam or any component; there may be a cross-sensitivity with other benzodiazepines; do not use in comatose patients, those with pre-existing CNS depression, narrow-angle glaucoma, severe uncontrolled pain, severe hypotension

Warnings Dilute injection prior to I.V. use with equal volume of compatible diluent (D_5W, 0.9% NaCl, sterile water for injection); do **not** inject intra-arterially, arteriospasm and gangrene may occur; injection contains benzyl alcohol 2%, polyethylene glycol and propylene glycol

Precautions Use caution in patients with renal or hepatic impairment, dementia, myasthenia gravis, Parkinson's disease, or a history of drug dependence

Adverse Reactions
Cardiovascular: Cardiac arrest, hypertension or hypotension, bradycardia, circulatory collapse
Central nervous system: Drowsiness, confusion, dizziness, ataxia, amnesia, slurred speech, paradoxical excitement or rage, transitory hallucinations
Gastrointestinal: Constipation, dry mouth, nausea, vomiting
Genitourinary: Urinary incontinence or retention
Local: Phlebitis, pain with injection
Neuromuscular & skeletal: Impaired coordination
Ocular: Blurred vision, diplopia, nystagmus
Respiratory: Decrease in respiratory rate, apnea, laryngospasm
Miscellaneous: Physical and psychological dependence with prolonged use

Overdosage Symptoms of overdose include somnolence, confusion, coma, and diminished reflexes

Toxicology Treatment for benzodiazepine overdose is supportive; rarely is mechanical ventilation required; flumazenil has been shown to selectively block the binding of benzodiazepines to CNS receptors, resulting in a reversal of benzodiazepine-induced sedation; however, its use may not alter the course of overdose

Drug Interactions Increased toxicity: CNS depressants, alcohol

Stability Intact vials should be refrigerated, protect from light; may be stored at room temperature for up to 2 weeks; do not use discolored or precipitate containing solutions
Stability of parenteral admixture at room temperature (25°C): 4 hours

Mechanism of Action Benzodiazepines appear to potentiate the effects of GABA and other inhibitory neurotransmitters by binding to specific benzodiazepine-receptor sites in various areas of the CNS

Pharmacodynamics
Onset of action: I.M.: Hypnosis occurs in ~20-30 minutes
Duration: 6-8 hours
Studies have shown that the elderly are more sensitive to the effects of benzodiazepines as compared to younger adults

Pharmacokinetics
Absorption: Oral, I.M.: Promptly absorbed
Protein binding: 85%; free fraction may be significantly higher in the elderly
Metabolism: In the liver to inactive compounds with urinary excretion and minimal fecal clearance; metabolism is not significantly affected in the elderly
Half-life: 10-16 hours; one study found the half-life in elderly to be 15.9 hours as compared to 14.1 hours in younger adults

Usual Dosage
Anxiety and sedation: Oral:
Geriatrics: Initial: 0.5-1 mg/day in divided doses; initial dose should not exceed 2 mg/day
Adults: 1-10 mg/day in 2-3 divided doses; usual dose: 2-6 mg/day in divided doses

Insomnia: Oral:
Geriatrics: 0.5-1 mg at bedtime
Adults: 2-4 mg at bedtime

Preoperative: Geriatrics and Adults:
I.M.: 0.05 mg/kg administered 2 hours before surgery; maximum: 4 mg/dose
I.V.: 0.044 mg/kg 15-20 minutes before surgery; usual maximum: 2 mg/dose

Operative amnesia: Geriatrics and Adults: I.V.: up to 0.05 mg/kg; maximum: 4 mg/dose

(Continued)

Lorazepam (Continued)

Status epilepticus: Geriatrics and Adults: I.V.: 4 mg/dose given slowly over 2-5 minutes; may repeat in 10-15 minutes; usual maximum dose: 8 mg

Administration See Warnings

Monitoring Parameters Respiratory, cardiovascular and mental status, symptoms of anxiety

Reference Range Therapeutic: 50-240 ng/mL (SI: 156-746 nmol/L)

Test Interactions May increase the results of liver function tests

Patient Information Avoid alcohol and other CNS depressants; may cause drowsiness; avoid activities needing good psychomotor coordination until CNS effects are known; may cause physical or psychological dependence; avoid abrupt discontinuation after prolonged use

Nursing Implications Keep injectable form in the refrigerator; inadvertent intra-arterial injection may produce arteriospasm resulting in gangrene which may require amputation; emergency resuscitative equipment should be available when administering by I.V.; prior to I.V. use, Ativan® injection must be diluted with an equal amount of compatible diluent; injection must be made slowly with repeated aspiration to make sure the injection is not intra-arterial and that perivascular extravasation has not occurred; do not exceed 2 mg/minute, if given faster, lorazepam may cause respiratory depression; provide safety measures (ie, side rails, night light, and call button); remove smoking materials from area; supervise ambulation

Additional Information I.M. lorazepam is rapidly and completely absorbed and, therefore, may be more predictable as compared to I.M. chlordiazepoxide or diazepam

Special Geriatric Considerations Because lorazepam is relatively short acting with an inactive metabolite, it is a preferred agent to use in elderly patients when a benzodiazepine is indicated; see Pharmacokinetics, Pharmacodynamics, and Usual Dosage

Dosage Forms

Injection: 2 mg/mL (1 mL, 10 mL); 4 mg/mL (1 mL, 10 mL)
Tablet: 0.5 mg, 1 mg, 2 mg

References

Divoll M and Greenblatt DJ, "Effect of Age and Sex on Lorazepam Protein Binding," *J Pharm Pharmacol*, 1982, 34(2):122-3.

Greenblatt DJ, Allen MD, Locniskar A, et al, "Lorazepam Kinetics in the Elderly," *Clin Pharmacol Ther*, 1979, 26(1):103-13.

Lorelco® see Probucol on page 589

Lortab® see Hydrocodone and Acetaminophen on page 350

Losec® see Omeprazole on page 517

Lotensin® see Benazepril Hydrochloride on page 76

Lotrimin® see Clotrimazole on page 180

Lo-Trol® see Diphenoxylate and Atropine on page 230

Lovastatin (loe' va sta tin)

Brand Names Mevacor®

Synonyms Mevinolin; Monacolin K

Generic Available No

Therapeutic Class Antilipemic Agent; HMG-CoA Reductase Inhibitor

Use Adjunct to dietary therapy to decrease elevated serum total and LDL cholesterol concentrations in primary hypercholesterolemia

Contraindications Active liver disease or unexplained persistent elevations of LFTs, hypersensitivity to lovastatin or any component

Warnings Musculoskeletal effects include myopathy (myalgia and/or muscle weakness accompanied by markedly elevated CK concentrations), rash and/or pruritus; hepatocellular carcinomas have been found in mice taking in excess of 300 times the recommended dose based on body weight

Precautions May elevate aminotransferases; LFTs should be performed before and every 4- 6 weeks during the first 12-15 months of therapy and periodically thereafter; serum cholesterol and triglyceride concentrations should be determined prior to and regularly during therapy; use with caution in patients who consume large quantities of alcohol

Adverse Reactions

Central nervous system: Headache, dizziness
Dermatologic: Rash, pruritus
Endocrine & metabolic: Gynecomastia
Gastrointestinal: Flatulence, abdominal pain, cramps, diarrhea pancreatitis, constipation, nausea
Hepatic: Increased LFTs
Neuromuscular & skeletal: Myalgia, muscle cramps, myopathy

Ocular: Blurred vision, myositis

Overdosage Few cases have been reported; no patients were symptomatic and all recovered without adverse effects

Drug Interactions Increased anticoagulant effect of warfarin; concurrent use of niacin, gemfibrozil, erythromycin, and cyclosporine increases the risk of rhabdomyolysis or myopathy

Mechanism of Action Lovastatin acts by competitively inhibiting 3-hydroxy-3-methylglutaryl-coenzyme A reductase (HMG-Co-A reductase), the enzyme that catalyzes the rate-limiting step in cholesterol biosynthesis

Pharmacokinetics

Absorption: Oral, 30%

Protein binding: 95%

Half-life: 1.1-1.7 hours

Time to peak: Peak serum levels occur within 2-4 hours while LDL cholesterol concentration reductions require 3 days of therapy

Elimination: ~80% to 85% of dose excreted in feces and 10% in urine following liver hydrolysis

Usual Dosage Oral:

Geriatrics and Adults: Initial: 20 mg with evening meal (for patients with serum cholesterol >300 mg/dL: 40 mg/day initially), then adjust at 4-week intervals to between 20-80 mg/day; maximum dose: 80 mg/day

Patients taking immunosuppressive drugs: Maximum dose: 20 mg/day

Monitoring Parameters Serum cholesterol (total and fractionated); reduce dose if indicated

Test Interactions Increased ALT, AST, CPK, alkaline phosphatase, bilirubin; altered thyroid function tests

Patient Information Promptly report any unexplained muscle pain, tenderness or weakness, especially if accompanied by malaise or fever; follow prescribed diet; take with meals

Additional Information For explicit guidelines on the risk factors for CHD and when to treat high blood cholesterol, see References.

Special Geriatric Considerations The definition of and, therefore, when to treat hyperlipidemia in the elderly is a controversial issue. The National Cholesterol Education Program recommends that all adults 20 years of age and older maintain a plasma cholesterol of <200 mg/dL. By this definition, 60% of all elderly would be considered to have a borderline high (200-239 mg/dL) or high blood (≥240 mg/dL) elevated cholesterol. However, plasma cholesterol has been shown to be a less reliable predictor of coronary heart disease in the elderly. Therefore, it is the authors' belief that pharmacologic treatment be reserved for those who are unable to obtain a desirable plasma cholesterol level by diet alone and for whom the benefits of treatment are believed to outweigh the potential adverse effects, drug interactions, and cost of treatment.

Dosage Forms Tablet: 10 mg, 20 mg, 40 mg

References

"Summary of the Second Report of the National Cholesterol Education Program (NCEP) Expert Panel on Detection, Evaluation, and Treatment of High Blood Cholesterol in Adults (Adult Treatment Panel II)," *JAMA*, 1993, 269(23):3015-23.

Lovenox® *see* Enoxaparin Sodium *on page 254*

Low-Quel® *see* Diphenoxylate and Atropine *on page 230*

Loxapine (lox' a peen)

Related Information

Antipsychotic Agents Comparison *on page 801*

Antipsychotic Medication Guidelines *on page 754*

Brand Names Loxitane®

Synonyms Loxapine Hydrochloride; Loxapine Succinate; Oxilapine Succinate

Generic Available No

Therapeutic Class Antipsychotic Agent

Use Management of psychotic disorders; nonpsychotic symptoms associated with dementia in elderly, Tourette's syndrome, Huntington's chorea

Contraindications Hypersensitivity to loxapine or any component, avoid use in patients with narrow-angle glaucoma, bone marrow depression, severe liver or cardiac disease; severe CNS depression, coma; subcortical brain damage; circulatory collapse, severe hypotension or hypertension

Warnings

Tardive dyskinesia: Prevalence rate may be 40% in elderly; elderly women especially at risk; embarrassment from dyskinesias may lead to greater social isolation; development of the syndrome and the irreversible nature are proportional to duration and total cumulative dose over time. May be reversible if diagnosed early in therapy; intermittent use of antipsychotics (not proven use) helps decrease total cumulative dose.

EPS: Extrapyramidal reactions are more common in elderly with up to 50% developing these reactions after age 60. These reactions may be more common in dementia

(Continued)

Loxapine *(Continued)*

patients. Drug-induced **Parkinson's syndrome** occurs often. Discontinuation usually resolves symptoms but may take weeks to months (12+) to clear. **Akathisia** is the most common EPS reaction in elderly. The symptoms of motor restlessness are difficult to diagnose in demented elderly; increased nervousness, assertiveness, restlessness with constant movement may indicate this adverse event. Consider decreasing dose if antipsychotic to treat as well as diagnose problem; usually see this reaction within 2-3 months of initiating antipsychotic drug.

Anticholinergic effects: These side effects most common with low potency antipsychotics (eg, thioridazine, chlorpromazine). CNS toxicity occurs more frequently and severely in elderly; increased confusion, memory loss, psychotic behavior, and agitation frequently occur as a consequence of anticholinergic effects to antipsychotic agents. Peripheral anticholinergic action troublesome to elderly; most peripheral anticholinergic effects last only 2-3 weeks; see Adverse Reactions.

Orthostatic hypotension: More common with low potency agents (eg, thioridazine, chlorpromazine, and clozapine) but of concern with all antipsychotic agents; orthostasis due to alpha-receptor blockade by antipsychotic agents. Elderly present many risk factors for orthostatic hypotension: blunted baroreceptor reflexes, decreased vascular tone, decreased vascular volume, and possible presence of cardiac diseases which result in decreased cardiac output.

Sedation: Common side effect with antipsychotic therapy; should not be used as a hypnotic unless insomnia is associated with target behavior symptoms treated with antipsychotic medications; see Special Geriatric Considerations. Anecdotal reports suggesting antipsychotic sedation in nonpsychotic patients is extremely unpleasant due to feelings of depersonalization, derealization, and dysphoria. Due to the long duration of action with antipsychotic drugs, these reactions may last up to 24 hours and result in decreased daytime function.

Cardiac toxicity: Life-threatening arrhythmias have occurred at therapeutic doses of antipsychotics. Thioridazine more commonly demonstrates EKG changes than other antipsychotics; suggested to use high potency antipsychotic agents (ie, haloperidol) in patients with cardiac conduction defects.

Precautions Watch for hypotension when administering I.M. or I.V.; use with caution in patients with cardiovascular disease, seizures, and Parkinson's disease; benefits of therapy must be weighed against risks of therapy

Adverse Reactions

Anticholinergic: Dry mouth (problem for denture user), urinary retention, constipation, adynamic ileus, overflow incontinence, blurred vision

Cardiovascular: Hypotension (especially orthostatic), tachycardia, arrhythmias, abnormal T waves with prolonged ventricular repolarization, EKG changes

Central nervous system: Sedation, drowsiness, restlessness, anxiety, extrapyramidal reactions, dystonic reactions, pseudoparkinsonian signs and symptoms, tardive dyskinesia, neuroleptic malignant syndrome, seizures, altered central temperature regulation

Endocrine & metabolic: Amenorrhea, galactorrhea, gynecomastia

Gastrointestinal: Constipation, adynamic ileus, GI upset, weight gain, dry mouth (problem for denture user), weight gain

Genitourinary: Urinary retention, overflow incontinence, priapism, sexual dysfunction (up to 60%)

Hematologic: Agranulocytosis, leukopenia (usually in patients with large doses for prolonged periods)

Hepatic: Cholestatic jaundice

Ocular: Blurred vision, retinal pigmentation, decreased visual acuity (may be irreversible)

Overdosage Symptoms of overdose include deep sleep, coma, extrapyramidal symptoms, abnormal involuntary muscle movements, hypotension or hypertension; agitation, restlessness, fever, hypothermia or hyperthermia, seizures, cardiac arrhythmias, EKG changes

Toxicology Following initiation of essential overdose management, toxic symptom treatment and supportive treatment should be initiated. Hypotension usually responds to I.V. fluids or Trendelenburg positioning. If unresponsive to these measures the use of a parenteral inotrope may be required (eg, norepinephrine 0.1-0.2 mcg/kg/minute titrated to response). Do not use epinephrine. Seizures commonly respond to diazepam (I.V. 5-10 mg bolus in adults every 15 minutes if needed up to a total of 30 mg) or to phenytoin or phenobarbital. Also critical cardiac arrhythmias often respond to I.V. phenytoin (15 mg/kg up to 1 g), while other antiarrhythmics can be used. Neuroleptics often cause extrapyramidal symptoms (eg, dystonic reactions) requiring management with diphenhydramine 1-2 mg/kg up to a maximum of 50 mg I.M. or I.V. slow push followed by a maintenance dose for 48-72 hours. When these reactions are unresponsive to diphenhydramine, benztropine mesylate I.V. 1-2 mg may be effective. These agents are generally effective within 2-5 minutes.

Drug Interactions

May increase CNS depression with other CNS depressants

Anticonvulsants (phenytoin, carbamazepine, phenobarbital) may decrease serum concentrations of loxapine

May increase CNS disorientation with lithium

Stability Protect from light; dispense in amber or opaque vials

Mechanism of Action Unclear mechanism of action, thought to be similar to chlorpromazine; blocks postsynaptic mesolimbic dopaminergic D_1 and D_2 receptors in the brain; exhibits a strong alpha-adrenergic blocking and anticholinergic effect, depresses the release of hypothalamic and hypophyseal hormones; believed to depress the reticular activating system thus affecting basal metabolism, body temperature, wakefulness, vasomotor tone, and emesis

Pharmacodynamics
Onset of action: Oral: Within 20-30 minutes
Peak effects: 90-180 minutes
Duration: ~12 hours

Pharmacokinetics
Metabolism: Liver metabolism to glucuronide conjugates
Half-life: Biphasic:
Initial: 5 hours
Terminal: 12-19 hours
Elimination: In urine, and to a smaller degree, the feces within 24 hours

Usual Dosage
Geriatrics (nonpsychotic patients, dementia behavior): Initial: 5-10 mg 1-2 times/day; increase dose at 4- to 7-day intervals by 5-10 mg/day; increase dosing intervals (twice daily, 3 times/day, etc) as necessary to control response or side effects; maximum daily dose: 125 mg; gradual increases (titration) may prevent some side effects or their severity.
I.M.: 12.5-25 mg every 4-8 hours; increase dose by 12.5 mg increments if necessary to 50 mg

Adults:
Oral: 10 mg twice daily, increase dose until psychotic symptoms are controlled; usual dose range: 60-100 mg/day in divided doses 2-4 times/day
I.M.: 12.5-50 mg every 4-8 hours

Not dialyzable (0% to 5%)

Monitoring Parameters Orthostatic blood pressures; tremors, gait changes, abnormal movement in trunk, neck, buccal area or extremities; monitor target behaviors for which the agent is given

Patient Information Oral concentrate must be diluted in 2-4 oz of liquid (water, fruit juice, carbonated drinks, milk, or pudding); do not take antacid within 1 hour of taking drug; avoid alcohol; avoid excess sun exposure (use sun block); may cause drowsiness, rise slowly from recumbent position; use of supportive stockings may help prevent orthostatic hypotension

Nursing Implications Injectable is for I.M. use only; dilute the oral concentrate with water or juice before administration; avoid skin contact with oral suspension or solution; may cause contact dermatitis; monitor orthostatic blood pressures 3-5 days after initiation of therapy or a dose increase; observe for tremor and abnormal movement or posturing (extrapyramidal symptoms)

Additional Information
Loxapine hydrochloride: Loxitane® C oral concentrate, Loxitane® IM
Loxapine succinate: Loxitane® capsule

Special Geriatric Considerations See Warnings
Many elderly patients receive antipsychotic medications for inappropriate nonpsychotic behavior. Before initiating antipsychotic medication, the clinician should investigate any possible reversible cause; any stress or stress from any disease can cause acute "confusion" or worsening of baseline nonpsychotic behavior. Most commonly acute changes in behavior are due to increases in drug dose or addition of new drug to regimen; fluid electrolyte loss; infections; and changes in environment.
Any changes in disease status in any organ system can result in behavior changes.

Dosage Forms
Capsule: 5 mg, 10 mg, 25 mg, 50 mg
Concentrate: 25 mg/mL (120 mL dropper bottle)
Injection: 50 mg/mL (1 mL)

Loxapine Hydrochloride see Loxapine on page 421

Loxapine Succinate see Loxapine on page 421

Loxitane® see Loxapine on page 421

Lozol® see Indapamide on page 368

L-PAM see Melphalan on page 440

L-Phenylalanine Mustard see Melphalan on page 440

L-Sarcolysin see Melphalan on page 440

LTG see Lamotrigine on page 398

ALPHABETICAL LISTING OF DRUGS

L-Thyroxine Sodium *see* Levothyroxine Sodium *on page 404*

Ludiomil® *see* Maprotiline Hydrochloride *on page 432*

Lufyllin® *see* Dyphylline *on page 247*

Luminal® *see* Phenobarbital *on page 554*

Lupron® *see* Leuprolide Acetate *on page 400*

Luride® *see* Fluoride *on page 299*

Luride®-SF F Lozi-Tabs® *see* Fluoride *on page 299*

Lyphocin® *see* Vancomycin Hydrochloride *on page 730*

Maalox® [OTC] *see* Aluminum Hydroxide and Magnesium Hydroxide *on page 29*

Maalox® Therapeutic Concentrate [OTC] *see* Aluminum Hydroxide and Magnesium Hydroxide *on page 29*

Maalox® Plus [OTC] *see* Aluminum Hydroxide, Magnesium Hydroxide and Simethicone *on page 31*

Macrodantin® *see* Nitrofurantoin *on page 504*

Magaldrate (mag' al drate)

Brand Names Riopan® [OTC]; Riopan Extra Strength® [OTC]

Synonyms Hydromagnesium aluminate

Generic Available Yes

Therapeutic Class Antacid

Use Symptomatic relief of hyperacidity associated with peptic ulcer, gastritis, peptic esophagitis and hiatal hernia

Restrictions See Precautions and Contraindications

Contraindications Patients with colostomy or an ileostomy, appendicitis, ulcerative colitis, diverticulitis

Warnings Sodium content may be significant for patients with hypertension, renal failure, congestive heart failure; hypermagnesemia may result with renal insufficiency when >50 mEq of magnesium is administered daily; patients with Cl_{cr} <30 mL/minute are at risk for hypermagnesemia

Precautions Aluminum intoxication, osteomalacia, patients with GI hemorrhage; use with caution in patients on low sodium diets (patients with congestive heart failure, edema, hypertension), cirrhosis, and renal failure; magnesium intoxication may occur with renal insufficiency

Adverse Reactions
Endocrine & metabolic: Dehydration or fluid restriction
Gastrointestinal: Constipation, decreased bowel motility, fecal impaction
Miscellaneous: Hemorrhoids

Overdosage
Aluminum: Osteomalacia (bone pain), malaise, weakness, and aluminum intoxication (encephalopathy) may occur in patients with renal insufficiency
Magnesium: CNS depression, confusion, hypotension, muscle weakness, blockage of peripheral neuromuscular transmission; serum >4 mEq/L (4.8 mg/dL): deep tendon reflexes may be depressed; serum ≥10 mEq/L (12 mg/dL): deep tendon reflexes may disappear, respiratory paralysis may occur, heart block may occur

Toxicology Deferoxamine, traditionally used as an iron chelator, has been shown to increase urinary aluminum output. Deferoxamine chelation of aluminum has resulted in improvements of clinical symptoms and bone histology. Deferoxamine, however, remains an experimental treatment for aluminum poisoning and has a significant potential for adverse effects. Hypermagnesemia, toxic symptoms usually present with serum level >4 mEq/L; concurrent hypocalcemia, impaired clotting, somnolence, and disappearance of deep tendon reflexes. Serum level >12 mEq/L may be fatal, serum level ~10 mEq/L may cause complete heart block; I.V. calcium (5-10 mEq) will reverse respiratory depression or heart block; peritoneal dialysis or hemodialysis may be needed

Drug Interactions
Magnesium and aluminum combination compounds decrease the pharmacologic effect of benzodiazepines, captopril, glucocorticosteroids, fluoroquinolones, H_2 antagonists, hydantoins, iron compounds, ketoconazole, penicillamine, phenothiazines, salicylates, tetracyclines, ticlopidine; concomitant use with sodium polystyrene sulfonate may cause metabolic alkalosis in patients with renal insufficiency
Magnesium and aluminum combination compounds increase the pharmacologic effect of levodopa, quinidine, sulfonylureas, valproic acid

Mechanism of Action Neutralize gastric acid and, therefore, increase pH of the stomach and duodenal bulb; with increased pH above 4, the proteolytic activity of pepsin is diminished. Antacids also increase lower esophageal sphincter tone; aluminum ions inhibit gastric emptying by decreasing smooth muscle contraction

Pharmacodynamics Acid-neutralizing capacity varies from product to product; antacids ingested in a fasting state give reduced acidity for 30 minutes; if ingested 1 hour after meals, reduced acidity may be extended for 3 hours

Usual Dosage Geriatrics and Adults: Oral: 480-1080 mg between meals (1-2 hours after meals) and at bedtime

Monitoring Parameters

Aluminum: Monitor phosphorous levels periodically when patient is on chronic therapy; when used as a phosphate binder, dose to achieve a serum phosphate concentration ≤4 mg/100 mL; observe for complaints or bone pain, malaise, and muscular weakness

Magnesium: See Overdosage; observe for signs of mental confusion and increased somnolence

Reference Range

Aluminum: Normal range (serum): 0-6 ng/mL; dialysis patients may attain up to 40 ng/mL without symptoms of toxicity; >100 ng/mL possible CNS toxicity

Magnesium: Normal range (serum): 1.5-2.3 mg/dL (1.25-1.9 mEq/L); toxicity occurs with serum levels >4 mEq/L (4.8 mg/dL)

Test Interactions Decreased inorganic phosphorus

Patient Information Chew tablets thoroughly before swallowing with water; notify physician if relief is not obtained or if signs of bleeding from GI tract occur

Nursing Implications Administer 1-2 hours apart from oral drugs; shake suspensions well; observe for constipation, fecal impaction, diarrhea, and hypophosphatemia; see Monitoring Parameters and Reference Range

Additional Information A chemical entity known as hydroxy magnesium aluminate equivalent to magnesium oxide and aluminum oxide; unlike other magnesium containing antacids, Riopan® is safe to use in renal patients if used cautiously

Special Geriatric Considerations Elderly, due to disease or drug therapy, may be predisposed to diarrhea or constipation. Diarrhea may result in electrolyte imbalance. Decreased renal function (Cl_{cr} <30 mL/minute) may result in toxicity of aluminum or magnesium. Drug interactions must be considered. If possible, give antacid 1-2 hours apart from other drugs. When treating ulcers, consider buffer capacity (mEq/mL) antacid.

Dosage Forms

Suspension: 540 mg/5 mL (360 mL); 1080 mg/5 mL

Tablet: 480 mg

References
Gams JG, "Clinical Significance of Magnesium: A Review," *Drug Intell Clin Pharm*, 1987, 21(3):240-6.

Peterson WL, Sturdevant RAL, Franki HD, et al, "Healing of Duodenal Ulcer With an Antacid Regimen," *N Engl J Med*, 1977, 297(7):341-5.

Magaldrate and Simethicone (mag' al drate)

Related Information

Magaldrate *on previous page*

Simethicone *on page 645*

Brand Names Riopan Plus® [OTC]

Synonyms Simethicone and Magaldrate

Therapeutic Class Antacid; Antiflatulent

Use Relief of hyperacidity associated with peptic ulcer, gastritis, peptic esophagitis and hiatal hernia which are accompanied by symptoms of gas

Restrictions See Precautions and Contraindications

Contraindications Patients with colostomy or an ileostomy, appendicitis, ulcerative colitis, diverticulitis

Warnings Sodium content may be significant for patients with hypertension, renal failure, congestive heart failure; hypermagnesemia may result with renal insufficiency when >50 mEq of magnesium is administered daily; patients with Cl_{cr} <30 mL/minute are at risk for hypermagnesemia

Precautions Aluminum intoxication, osteomalacia, patients with GI hemorrhage; use with caution in patients on low sodium diets (patients with congestive heart failure, edema, hypertension), cirrhosis, and renal failure; magnesium intoxication may occur with renal insufficiency

Adverse Reactions

Endocrine & metabolic: Dehydration or fluid restriction

Gastrointestinal: Constipation, decreased bowel motility, fecal impaction

Miscellaneous: Hemorrhoids

Overdosage

Aluminum: Osteomalacia (bone pain), malaise, weakness, and aluminum intoxication (encephalopathy) may occur in patients with renal insufficiency

Magnesium: CNS depression, confusion, hypotension, muscle weakness, blockage of peripheral neuromuscular transmission serum >4 mEq/L (4.8 mg/dL): deep tendon reflexes may be depressed; serum ≥10 mEq/L (12 mg/dL): deep tendon reflexes may disappear, respiratory paralysis may occur, heart block may occur

Toxicology Deferoxamine, traditionally used as an iron chelator, has been shown to increase urinary aluminum output. Deferoxamine chelation of aluminum has resulted in improvements of clinical symptoms and bone histology. Deferoxamine, however, remains an experimental treatment for aluminum poisoning and has a significant poten-

(Continued)

ALPHABETICAL LISTING OF DRUGS

Magaldrate and Simethicone *(Continued)*

tial for adverse effects. Hypermagnesemia, toxic symptoms usually present with serum level >4 mEq/L; concurrent hypocalcemia, impaired clotting, somnolence, and disappearance of deep tendon reflexes. Serum level >12 mEq/L may be fatal, serum level ~10 mEq/L may cause complete heart block; I.V. calcium (5-10 mEq) will reverse respiratory depression or heart block; peritoneal dialysis or hemodialysis may be needed

Drug Interactions

Magnesium and aluminum combination compounds decrease the pharmacologic effect of benzodiazepines, captopril, glucocorticosteroids, fluoroquinolones, H_2 antagonists, hydantoins, iron compounds, ketoconazole, penicillamine, phenothiazines, salicylates, tetracyclines, ticlopidine; concomitant use with sodium polystyrene sulfonate may cause metabolic alkalosis in patients with renal insufficiency

Magnesium and aluminum combination compounds increase the pharmacologic effect of levodopa, quinidine, sulfonylureas, valproic acid

Mechanism of Action Neutralize gastric acid and, therefore, increase pH of the stomach and duodenal bulb; with increased pH above 4, the proteolytic activity of pepsin is diminished. Antacids also increase lower esophageal sphincter tone; aluminum ions inhibit gastric emptying by decreasing smooth muscle contraction

Pharmacodynamics Acid-neutralizing capacity varies from product to product; antacids ingested in a fasting state give reduced acidity for 30 minutes; if ingested 1 hour after meals, reduced acidity may be extended for 3 hours

Usual Dosage Geriatrics and Adults: Oral: 480-1080 mg between meals (1-2 hours after meals) and at bedtime

Monitoring Parameters

Aluminum: Monitor phosphorous levels periodically when patient is on chronic therapy; when used as a phosphate binder, dose to achieve a serum phosphate concentration ≤4 mg/100 mL; observe for complaints or bone pain, malaise, and muscular weakness

Magnesium: See Overdosage; observe for signs of mental confusion and increased somnolence

Reference Range

Aluminum: Normal range (serum): 0-6 ng/mL; dialysis patients may attain up to 40 ng/mL without symptoms of toxicity; >100 ng/mL possible CNS toxicity

Magnesium: Normal range (serum): 1.5-2.3 mg/dL (1.25-1.9 mEq/L); toxicity occurs with serum levels >4 mEq/L (4.8 mg/dL)

Test Interactions Decreased inorganic phosphorus

Patient Information Notify physician if relief is not obtained or if signs of bleeding from GI tract occur

Nursing Implications Administer 1-2 hours apart from oral drugs; shake suspensions well; observe for constipation, fecal impaction, diarrhea, and hypophosphatemia; see Monitoring Parameters and Reference Range

Additional Information A chemical entity known as hydroxy magnesium aluminate equivalent to magnesium oxide and aluminum oxide; unlike other magnesium containing antacids, Riopan® is safe to use in renal patients if used cautiously

Special Geriatric Considerations Elderly, due to disease or drug therapy, may be predisposed to diarrhea or constipation. Diarrhea may result in electrolyte imbalance. Decreased renal function (Cl_{cr} <30 mL/minute) may result in toxicity of aluminum or magnesium. Drug interactions must be considered. If possible, give antacid 1-2 hours apart from other drugs. When treating ulcers, consider buffer capacity (mEq/mL) antacid.

Dosage Forms Suspension: Magaldrate 480 mg and simethicone 20 mg/5 mL (360 mL)

References

Gams JG, "Clinical Significance of Magnesium: A Review," *Drug Intell Clin Pharm*, 1987, 21(3):240-6.
Peterson WL, Sturdevant RAL, Franki HD, et al, "Healing of Duodenal Ulcer With an Antacid Regimen," *N Engl J Med*, 1977, 297(7):341-5.

Magan® *see* Salicylates (Various Salts) *on page 633*

Magnesia Magma *see* Magnesium Hydroxide *on next page*

Magnesium Citrate *(mag nee' zhum)*

Brand Names Citroma® [OTC]; Citro-Nesia™ [OTC]

Synonyms Citrate of Magnesia

Generic Available Yes

Therapeutic Class Laxative, Saline

Use Evacuate bowel prior to certain surgical and diagnostic procedures or overdose situations

Restrictions See Precautions and Contraindications

Contraindications Renal failure, appendicitis, abdominal pain, intestinal impaction, obstruction or perforation, diabetes mellitus, complications in gastrointestinal tract, patients with colostomy, ileostomy, ulcerative colitis or diverticulitis

Warnings Monitor serum magnesium level, respiratory rate, deep tendon reflex

Precautions Use with caution in patients with impaired renal function, especially if Cl_{cr}

<30 mL/minute (accumulation of magnesium which may lead to magnesium intoxication); use with caution in digitalized patients (may alter cardiac conduction leading to heart block); use with caution in patients with lithium administration; use with caution with neuromuscular blocking agents, CNS depressants

Adverse Reactions
Cardiovascular: Hypotension, heart block
Endocrine & metabolic: Hypermagnesemia
Gastrointestinal: Abdominal cramps, diarrhea, gas formation
Respiratory: Respiratory depression

Overdosage Serious, potentially life-threatening electrolyte disturbances may occur with long-term use or overdosage due to diarrhea; hypermagnesemia may occur; CNS depression, confusion, hypotension, muscle weakness, blockage of peripheral neuromuscular transmission; serum >4 mEq/L (4.8 mg/dL): deep tendon reflexes may be depressed; serum ≥10 mEq/L (12 mg/dL): deep tendon reflexes may disappear, respiratory paralysis may occur, heart block may occur; I.V. calcium (5-10 mEq) will reverse respiratory depression or heart block; in extreme cases, peritoneal dialysis or hemodialysis may be required

Toxicology Toxic symptoms usually present with serum level >4 mEq/L; concurrent hypocalcemia, impaired clotting, somnolence, and disappearance of deep tendon reflexes; serum level >12 mEq/L may be fatal, serum level ~10 mEq/L may cause complete heart block

Drug Interactions
Magnesium compounds decrease the pharmacologic effect of benzodiazepines, chloroquine, glucocorticosteroids, digoxin, H_2 antagonists, hydantoins, iron compounds, nitrofurantoin, penicillamine, phenothiazines, tetracyclines, ticlopidine
Magnesium compounds increase the pharmacologic effect of dicumarol, quinidine, sulfonylureas

Mechanism of Action Promotes bowel evacuation by causing osmotic retention of fluid which distends the colon with increased peristaltic activity

Pharmacodynamics Onset of cathartic action: Oral: Within 1-2 hours

Pharmacokinetics
Absorption: Oral: 15% to 30%
Elimination: Renal

Usual Dosage Geriatrics and Adults: Cathartic: Oral: $^1/_2$ to 1 full bottle (120-240 mL)

Monitoring Parameters See Overdosage

Reference Range Adults: 2.2-2.8 mg/dL ~1.8-2.3 mEq/L

Test Interactions Increased magnesium; decreased protein, calcium (S), decreased potassium (S)

Patient Information Take with a glass of water, fruit juice, or citrus flavored carbonated beverage; report severe abdominal pain to physician

Nursing Implications To increase palatability, manufacturer suggests chilling the solution prior to administration; see Overdosage

Additional Information 3.85-4.71 mEq of magnesium/5 mL

Special Geriatric Considerations Elderly, due to disease or drug therapy, may be predisposed to diarrhea. Diarrhea may result in electrolyte imbalance. Decreased renal function (Cl_{cr} <30 mL/minute) may result in toxicity; monitor for toxicity and Cl_{cr} <30 mL/minute

Dosage Forms Solution: 300 mL

References
Chernow B, Smith J, Rainey TG, et al, "Hypomagnesemia: Implications for the Critical Care Specialist," *Crit Care Med*, 1982, 10(3):193-6.
Gams JG, "Clinical Significance of Magnesium: A Review," *Drug Intell Clin Pharm*, 1987, 21(3):240-6.

Magnesium Hydroxide

Brand Names Phillips'® Milk of Magnesia [OTC]
Synonyms Magnesia Magma; Milk of Magnesia; MOM
Generic Available Yes
Therapeutic Class Antacid; Laxative, Saline; Magnesium Salt
Use Short-term treatment of occasional constipation and symptoms of hyperacidity
Restrictions See Precautions and Contraindications
Contraindications Patients with colostomy or an ileostomy, intestinal obstruction, fecal impaction, renal failure, appendicitis; heart block, myocardial damage, serious renal impairment, hepatitis and Addison's disease
Warnings Hypermagnesemia and toxicity may occur due to decreased renal clearance (Cl_{cr} <30 mL/minute) of absorbed magnesium; monitor serum magnesium level, respiratory rate, deep tendon reflex, renal function when $MgSO_4$ is administered parenterally
Precautions Use with caution in patients with impaired renal function (accumulation of magnesium which may lead to magnesium intoxication); use with caution in digitalized patients (may alter cardiac conduction leading to heart block); use with caution with neuromuscular blocking agents, lithium administration

Adverse Reactions
Cardiovascular: Hypotension
Endocrine & metabolic: Hypermagnesemia

(Continued)

Magnesium Hydroxide *(Continued)*

Gastrointestinal: Diarrhea, abdominal cramps
Neuromuscular & skeletal: Muscle weakness
Respiratory: Respiratory depression

Overdosage May cause severe diarrhea, CNS depression, confusion, hypotension, muscle weakness, blockage of peripheral neuromuscular transmission; serum >4 mEq/L (4.8 mg/dL): deep tendon reflexes may be depressed; serum ≥10 mEq/L (12 mg/dL): deep tendon reflexes may disappear, respiratory paralysis may occur, heart block may occur; I.V. calcium (5-10 mEq) will reverse respiratory depression or heart block; in extreme cases, peritoneal dialysis or hemodialysis may be required

Toxicology Toxic symptoms usually present with serum level >4 mEq/L; concurrent hypocalcemia, impaired clotting, somnolence, and disappearance of deep tendon reflexes; serum level >12 mEq/L may be fatal, serum level ~10 mEq/L may cause complete heart block

Drug Interactions

Magnesium compounds decrease the pharmacologic effect of benzodiazepines, chloroquine, glucocorticosteroids, digoxin, H_2 antagonists, hydantoins, iron compounds, nitrofurantoin, penicillamine, phenothiazines, tetracyclines, ticlopidine

Magnesium compounds increase the pharmacologic effect of dicumarol, quinidine, sulfonylureas

Mechanism of Action Promotes bowel evacuation by causing osmotic retention of fluid which distends the colon with increased peristaltic activity; reacts with hydrochloric acid in stomach to form magnesium chloride

Pharmacodynamics Onset of laxative action: Within 4-8 hours

Pharmacokinetics

Absorption: Absorbed magnesium ions (up to 30%)
Elimination: Usually by kidneys, unabsorbed drug is excreted in feces

Usual Dosage Oral:

Geriatrics: Laxative: 30 mL/day
Adults:
Laxative: 30-60 mL/day or in divided doses
Antacid: 5-15 mL as needed

Monitoring Parameters See Overdosage

Reference Range Adults: 2.2-2.8 mg/dL ~1.8-2.3 mEq/L

Test Interactions Increased magnesium; decreased protein, calcium (S), decreased potassium (S)

Patient Information Dilute dose in water or juice, shake well; chew tablets well

Nursing Implications MOM concentrate is 3 times as potent as regular strength product; monitor for toxicity in patients with decreased renal function; see Special Geriatric Considerations

Additional Information 1.05 g magnesium = ~87 mEq magnesium/30 mL

Special Geriatric Considerations Elderly, due to disease or drug therapy, may be predisposed to diarrhea. Diarrhea may result in electrolyte imbalance. Decreased renal function (Cl_{cr} <30 mL/minute) may result in toxicity; monitor for toxicity.

Dosage Forms

Liquid: 390 mg/5 mL (10 mL, 15 mL, 20 mL, 30 mL, 100 mL, 120 mL, 180 mL, 360 mL, 720 mL)
Suspension, oral: 2.5 g/30 mL (10 mL, 15 mL, 30 mL)
Tablet: 300 mg, 600 mg

References

Chernow B, Smith J, Rainey TG, et al, "Hypomagnesemia: Implications for the Critical Care Specialist," *Crit Care Med*, 1982, 10(3):193-6.

Gams JG, "Clinical Significance of Magnesium: A Review," *Drug Intell Clin Pharm*, 1987, 21(3):240-6.

Magnesium Hydroxide and Aluminum Hydroxide *see* Aluminum Hydroxide and Magnesium Hydroxide *on page 29*

Magnesium Hydroxide and Mineral Oil Emulsion

Related Information

Magnesium Hydroxide *on previous page*
Mineral Oil *on page 473*

Brand Names Haley's M-O® [OTC]

Synonyms MOM/Mineral Oil Emulsion

Generic Available No

Therapeutic Class Laxative, Lubricant; Laxative, Saline

Use Short-term treatment of occasional constipation

Restrictions See Precautions and Contraindications

Contraindications Patients with colostomy or an ileostomy, intestinal obstruction, fecal impaction, renal failure, appendicitis; heart block, myocardial damage, serious renal impairment, hepatitis and Addison's disease

Warnings Hypermagnesemia and toxicity may occur due to decreased renal clearance (Cl_{cr} <30 mL/minute) of absorbed magnesium; monitor serum magnesium level, respiratory rate, deep tendon reflex

Precautions Use with caution in patients with impaired renal function (accumulation of magnesium which may lead to magnesium intoxication); use with caution in digitalized patients (may alter cardiac conduction leading to heart block); use with caution with neuromuscular blocking agents, lithium administration; see Special Geriatric Considerations

Adverse Reactions
Cardiovascular: Hypotension
Endocrine & metabolic: Hypermagnesemia
Gastrointestinal: Diarrhea, abdominal cramps
Neuromuscular & skeletal: Muscle weakness
Respiratory: Respiratory depression

Overdosage May cause severe diarrhea and fluid and electrolyte imbalance, hypermagnesemia

Toxicology Toxic symptoms usually present with serum level >4 mEq/L; concurrent hypocalcemia, impaired clotting, somnolence, and disappearance of deep tendon reflexes; serum level >12 mEq/L may be fatal, serum level ~10 mEq/L may cause complete heart block

Drug Interactions
Magnesium compounds decrease the pharmacologic effect of benzodiazepines, chloroquine, glucocorticosteroids, digoxin, H_2 antagonists, hydantoins, iron compounds, nitrofurantoin, penicillamine, phenothiazines, tetracyclines, ticlopidine
Magnesium compounds increase the pharmacologic effect of dicumarol, quinidine, sulfonylureas

Mechanism of Action Promotes bowel evacuation by causing osmotic retention of fluid which distends colon and therefore increases peristaltic action. Mineral oil retards colonic absorption of fecal water and softens stool

Pharmacodynamics Onset of action: 4-8 hours

Pharmacokinetics
Absorption: Absorbed magnesium ions (up to 30%)
Elimination: Usually by kidneys, unabsorbed drug is excreted in feces

Usual Dosage Geriatrics and Adults: Oral: 5-45 mL at bedtime

Monitoring Parameters See Overdosage

Reference Range Adults: 2.2-2.8 mg/dL ~1.8-2.3 mEq/L

Test Interactions Increased magnesium; decreased protein

Patient Information Shake well; take with full glass of water; report persistent diarrhea or abdominal pains with incidence of blood in stool or vomit

Nursing Implications See Overdosage

Special Geriatric Considerations The use of mineral oil products may be hazardous in elderly with conditions predisposing them to aspiration. Elderly, due to disease or drug therapy, may be predisposed to diarrhea. Diarrhea may result in electrolyte imbalance. Decreased renal function (Cl_{cr} <30 mL/minute) may result in toxicity; monitor for toxicity.

Dosage Forms Suspension: Equivalent to magnesium hydroxide 24 mL/mineral oil emulsion (30 mL unit dose)

References
Chernow B, Smith J, Rainey TG, et al, "Hypomagnesemia: Implications for the Critical Care Specialist," *Crit Care Med*, 1982, 10(3):193-6.
Gams JG, "Clinical Significance of Magnesium: A Review," *Drug Intell Clin Pharm*, 1987, 21(3):240-6.

Magnesium Oxide

Brand Names Mag-Ox 400®; Maox®; Uro-Mag®

Therapeutic Class Antacid

Use Short-term treatment of occasional constipation and symptoms of hyperacidity; treat or prevent hypomagnesemia

Restrictions See Precautions and Contraindications

Contraindications Patients with colostomy or an ileostomy, appendicitis, ulcerative colitis, diverticulitis; heart block, myocardial damage, serious renal impairment, hepatitis and Addison's disease

Warnings Hypermagnesemia and toxicity may occur due to decreased renal clearance (Cl_{cr} <30 mL/minute) of absorbed magnesium; monitor serum magnesium level, respiratory rate, deep tendon reflex

Precautions Use with caution in patients with impaired renal function (accumulation of magnesium which may lead to magnesium intoxication); use with caution in digitalized patients (may alter cardiac conduction leading to heart block); use with caution in patients with lithium administration

Adverse Reactions
Cardiovascular: Hypotension, EKG changes
Central nervous system: Mental depression, coma
Gastrointestinal: Nausea, vomiting
Respiratory: Respiratory depression

Overdosage May cause diarrhea, severe electrolyte imbalance, and hypermagnesemia, CNS depression, confusion, hypotension, muscle weakness, blockage

(Continued)

429

Magnesium Oxide *(Continued)*

of peripheral neuromuscular transmission serum >4 mEq/L (4.8 mg/dL): deep tendon reflexes may be depressed; serum ≥10 mEq/L (12 mg/dL): deep tendon reflexes may disappear, respiratory paralysis may occur, heart block may occur; intravenous calcium (5-10 mEq) will reverse respiratory depression or heart block; in extreme cases, peritoneal dialysis or hemodialysis may be required

Toxicology Toxic symptoms usually present with serum level >4 mEq/L; concurrent hypocalcemia, impaired clotting, somnolence, and disappearance of deep tendon reflexes; serum level >12 mEq/L may be fatal, serum level ~10 mEq/L may cause complete heart block

Drug Interactions

Magnesium compounds decrease the pharmacologic effect of benzodiazepines, chloroquine, glucocorticosteroids, digoxin, H_2 antagonists, hydantoins, iron compounds, nitrofurantoin, penicillamine, phenothiazines, tetracyclines, ticlopidine

Magnesium compounds increase the pharmacologic effect of dicumarol, quinidine, sulfonylureas

Mechanism of Action Promotes bowel evacuation by causing osmotic retention of fluid which distends the colon with increased peristaltic activity when taken orally

Pharmacokinetics

Absorption: Absorbed magnesium is rapidly eliminated by the kidneys; see Special Geriatric Considerations

Elimination: Primarily excreted in feces

Usual Dosage Geriatrics and Adults: Oral:

Antacid: 140 mg to 1.5 g with water or milk 3-4 times/day after meals and at bedtime

Laxative: 2-4 g with full glass of water; cathartic action occurs within 1-2 hours

Monitoring Parameters See Overdosage

Reference Range Adults: 2.2-2.8 mg/dL ~1.8-2.3 mEq/L

Test Interactions Increased magnesium; decreased protein, calcium (S), decreased potassium (S)

Patient Information Chew tablets before swallowing; take with full glass of water; notify physician if relief not obtained or if any signs of bleeding occur (black tarry stools, "coffee ground" vomit)

Nursing Implications Monitor for diarrhea and signs of hypermagnesemia; see Overdosage

Special Geriatric Considerations Elderly, due to disease or drug therapy, may be predisposed to diarrhea. Diarrhea may result in electrolyte imbalance. Decreased renal function (Cl_{cr} <30 mL/minute) may result in toxicity; monitor for toxicity.

Dosage Forms

Capsule: 140 mg

Tablet: 400 mg, 420 mg

References

Chernow B, Smith J, Rainey TG, et al, "Hypomagnesemia: Implications for the Critical Care Specialist," *Crit Care Med*, 1982, 10(3):193-6.

Gams JG, "Clinical Significance of Magnesium: A Review," *Drug Intell Clin Pharm*, 1987, 21(3):240-6.

Magnesium Salicylate *see* Salicylates (Various Salts) *on page 633*

Magnesium Salts (Various Salts)

Brand Names Epsom Salt [OTC]; Magonate® [OTC]; Mg-plus® [OTC]; Slow-Mag® [OTC]

Synonyms Epsom Salts

Generic Available Yes

Therapeutic Class Anticonvulsant, Miscellaneous; Electrolyte Supplement, Parenteral; Laxative, Saline; Magnesium Salt

Use Treatment and prevention of hypomagnesemia; short-term treatment of constipation

Restrictions See Precautions and Contraindications

Contraindications Heart block, myocardial damage, serious renal impairment, hepatitis and Addison's disease

Warnings Monitor serum magnesium level, respiratory rate, deep tendon reflex, renal function when $MgSO_4$ is administered parenterally

Precautions Use with caution in patients with impaired renal function, especially when Cl_{cr} <30 mL/minute (accumulation of magnesium which may lead to magnesium intoxication); use with caution in digitalized patients (may alter cardiac conduction leading to heart block); use with caution with neuromuscular blocking agents, lithium administration

Adverse Reactions

Serum magnesium levels >3 mg/dL:

Central nervous system: Depressed CNS, blocked peripheral neuromuscular transmission leading to anticonvulsant effects

Gastrointestinal: Diarrhea

Serum magnesium levels >5 mg/dL:
  Cardiovascular: Flushing
  Central nervous system: Somnolence
Serum magnesium levels >12.5 mg/dL:
  Cardiovascular: Complete heart block
  Respiratory: Respiratory paralysis

Overdosage Symptoms of overdose include CNS depression, confusion, hypotension, muscle weakness, blockage of peripheral neuromuscular transmission serum >4 mEq/L (4.8 mg/dL): deep tendon reflexes may be depressed; serum ≥10 mEq/L (12 mg/dL): deep tendon reflexes may disappear, respiratory paralysis may occur, heart block may occur; I.V. calcium (5-10 mEq) will reverse respiratory depression or heart block; in extreme cases, peritoneal dialysis or hemodialysis may be required

Toxicology Toxic symptoms usually present with serum level >4 mEq/L; concurrent hypocalcemia, impaired clotting, somnolence, and disappearance of deep tendon reflexes; serum level >12 mEq/L may be fatal, serum level ~10 mEq/L may cause complete heart block

Drug Interactions
  Magnesium compounds decrease the pharmacologic effect of benzodiazepines, chloroquine, glucocorticosteroids, digoxin, H_2 antagonists, hydantoins, iron compounds, nitrofurantoin, penicillamine, phenothiazines, tetracyclines, ticlopidine
  Magnesium compounds increase the pharmacologic effect of dicumarol, quinidine, sulfonylureas

Stability Refrigeration of intact ampuls may result in precipitation or crystallization
  Stability of parenteral admixture at room temperature (25°C): 60 days

Mechanism of Action Promotes bowel evacuation by causing osmotic retention of fluid which distends the colon with increased peristaltic activity when taken orally; parenterally, decreases acetylcholine in motor nerve terminals and acts on myocardium by slowing rate of S-A node impulse formation and prolonging conduction time

Pharmacodynamics
  Onset of action:
    Oral: Within 1-2 hours
    I.M.: Within 60 minutes
    I.V.: Immediately
  Duration:
    I.M.: 3-4 hours
    I.V.: 30 minutes

Pharmacokinetics
  Absorption: Absorbed magnesium is rapidly eliminated by the kidneys; see Special Geriatric Considerations
  Elimination: Primarily excreted in feces

Usual Dosage Dose represented as $MgSO_4$ unless stated otherwise
  Hypomagnesemia: Geriatrics and Adults:
    I.M., I.V.: 1 g every 6 hours for 4 doses or 250 mg/kg over a 4-hour period; for severe hypomagnesemia: 8-12 g $MgSO_4$/day in divided doses has been used
    Oral: 3 g every 6 hours for 4 doses as needed
  Cathartic: Geriatrics and Adults: Oral: 10-30 g
  Dietary supplement: 50-500 mg/day in divided doses
  Hyperalimentation: 8-24 mEq/day
  Hypomagnesemia with hypovolemia: Oral: 200-400 mg/day in divided doses
  Recommended daily allowance: Adults:
    Male: 350-400 mg/day
    Female: 280-300 mg/day

Monitoring Parameters See Overdosage

Reference Range Adults: 2.2-2.8 mg/dL ~1.8-2.3 mEq/L

Test Interactions Increased magnesium; decreased protein, calcium (S), decreased potassium (S)

Patient Information Take in divided doses; report diarrhea (>5 stools/day) or changes in mental function to physician, nurse, or pharmacist

Nursing Implications Monitor blood pressure when administering $MgSO_4$ I.V.; serum magnesium levels should be monitored to avoid overdose; monitor for diarrhea, hypotension, CNS confusion

Additional Information 1 g magnesium = 8.3 mEq (41.1 mmol); see individual agents for magnesium content per dose

Special Geriatric Considerations Elderly, due to disease or drug therapy, may be predisposed to diarrhea. Diarrhea may result in electrolyte imbalance. Decreased renal function (Cl_{cr} <30 mL/minute) may result in toxicity; monitor for toxicity.

Dosage Forms
  Granules, as sulfate: ~40 mEq magnesium/5 g (240 g)
  Injection, as sulfate: 10% = 0.8 mEq/mL (2 mL, 10 mL, 20 mL, 30 mL, 50 mL); 20% = 1.97 mEq/mL (2 mL, 10 mL, 20 mL, 30 mL, 50 mL); 50% = 4 mEq/mL (2 mL, 10 mL, 20 mL, 30 mL, 50 mL)

(Continued)

Magnesium Salts (Various Salts) *(Continued)*

Liquid, as sulfate: 54 mg/5 mL
Tablet, as various salts: 140 mg, 400 mg, 500 mg

References

Chernow B, Smith J, Rainey TG, et al, "Hypomagnesemia: Implications for the Critical Care Specialist," *Crit Care Med*, 1982, 10(3):193-6.
Gams JG, "Clinical Significance of Magnesium: A Review," *Drug Intell Clin Pharm*, 1987, 21(3):240-6.

Magonate® [OTC] *see* Magnesium Salts (Various Salts) *on page 430*

Mag-Ox 400® *see* Magnesium Oxide *on page 429*

Maigret-50® *see* Phenylpropanolamine Hydrochloride *on page 559*

Mallamint® [OTC] *see* Calcium Salts (Oral) *on page 111*

Malotuss [OTC] *see* Guaifenesin *on page 331*

Mandelamine® *see* Methenamine *on page 452*

Mandol® *see* Cefamandole Nafate *on page 126*

Mantoux *see* Tuberculin Purified Protein Derivative *on page 725*

Maox® *see* Magnesium Oxide *on page 429*

Maprotiline Hydrochloride *(ma proe' ti leen)*

Related Information

Antidepressant Agents Comparison *on page 800*

Brand Names Ludiomil®

Generic Available No

Therapeutic Class Antidepressant, Tetracyclic

Use Treatment of depression and anxiety associated with depression

Contraindications Narrow-angle glaucoma, hypersensitivity to maprotiline or any component

Warnings To avoid cholinergic crisis do not discontinue abruptly in patients receiving high doses chronically

Precautions Use with caution in patients with cardiac conduction disturbances, history of hyperthyroidism; an EKG prior to starting therapy is advised

Adverse Reactions

Cardiovascular: Stroke, heart block, tachycardia, orthostatic hypotension
Central nervous system: Seizures, sedation, confusion
Dermatologic: Rash
Gastrointestinal: Constipation, increased appetite and weight gain, extreme dry mouth, weight loss, nausea, vomiting
Genitourinary: Urinary retention, swollen testicles
Neuromuscular & skeletal: Tremors
Ocular: Blurred vision, increased intraocular pressure
Otic: Tinnitus

Overdosage Symptoms of overdose include agitation, confusion, hallucinations, urinary retention, hypothermia, hypotension, tachycardia

Toxicology Following initiation of essential overdose management, toxic symptoms should be treated. Ventricular arrhythmias often respond to phenytoin 15-20 mg/kg with concurrent systemic alkalinization (sodium bicarbonate 0.5-2 mEq/kg I.V.). Arrhythmias unresponsive to this therapy may respond to lidocaine 1 mg/kg I.V. followed by a titrated infusion. Physostigmine (1-2 mg I.V. slowly) may be indicated in reversing cardiac arrhythmias that are due to vagal blockade or for anticholinergic effects. Seizures usually respond to diazepam I.V. boluses (5-10 mg, up to 30 mg). If seizures are unresponsive or recur, phenytoin or phenobarbital may be required.

Drug Interactions

Decreased effect of clonidine and guanethidine; decreased effect with barbiturates, phenytoin, carbamazepines
Increased effect/toxicity of CNS depressants, MAO inhibitors (hyperpyretic crisis), anticholinergics, sympathomimetics, thyroid (increased cardiotoxicity), phenothiazines (seizures), benzodiazepines

Mechanism of Action Traditionally believed to increase the synaptic concentration of norepinephrine in the central nervous system by inhibition of their reuptake by the presynaptic neuronal membrane. However, additional receptor effects have been found including desensitization of adenyl cyclase, down regulation of beta-adrenergic receptors, and down regulation of serotonin receptors.

Pharmacodynamics Onset of therapeutic effects: May take 1-3 weeks before effects are seen; norepinephrine only

Pharmacokinetics

Absorption: Oral: Slow
Protein binding: 88%
Metabolism: Metabolized in the liver to active and inactive compounds
Half-life: 21-25 hours
Time to peak: Peak serum levels occur within 12 hours

Elimination: In urine (70%) and feces (30%)
Geriatrics: After a single 125 mg oral dose in 5 subjects between 75-83 years of age 50% of the dose was absorbed, the average time to peak was 7 hours, and the average elimination half-life was 31.5 hours

Usual Dosage Oral:
Geriatrics: Initial: 25 mg at bedtime, increase by 25 mg every 3 days for inpatients and weekly for outpatients if tolerated; usual maintenance dose: 50-75 mg/day, higher doses may be necessary in nonresponders

Adults: 75 mg/day to start, increase by 25 mg every 2 weeks up to 150-225 mg/day; given in 3 divided doses or in a single daily dose

Monitoring Parameters Sleep, appetite, mood, somatic complaints, mental status, weight, blood pressure and heart rate, urine flow/output

Reference Range Therapeutic: 200-600 ng/mL (SI: 721-2163 nmol/L); not well established

Patient Information Do not drink alcoholic beverages, may cause drowsiness, dry mouth, constipation, blurred vision; rise slowly to avoid dizziness

Nursing Implications Offer patient sugarless hard candy for dry mouth; see Monitoring Parameters

Special Geriatric Considerations See Pharmacokinetics and Usual Dosage; use with caution due to sedation and anticholinergic effects

Dosage Forms Tablet: 25 mg, 50 mg, 75 mg

References
Hrdina PD, Rovei V, Henry JF, et al, "Comparison of Single-Dose Pharmacokinetics of Imipramine and Maprotiline in the Elderly," *Psychopharmacology*, 1980, 70(1):29-34.

Marbaxin® *see* Methocarbamol *on page 454*

Marezine® [OTC] *see* Cyclizine *on page 194*

Marmine® [OTC] *see* Dimenhydrinate *on page 227*

Mar-Pred® *see* Methylprednisolone *on page 461*

Maxair™ *see* Pirbuterol Acetate *on page 570*

Maxaquin® *see* Lomefloxacin Hydrochloride *on page 415*

Maxidex® *see* Dexamethasone *on page 207*

Maxitrol® Ophthalmic *see* Neomycin, Polymyxin B, and Dexamethasone *on page 495*

Maxivate® *see* Betamethasone *on page 82*

Maxolon® *see* Metoclopramide *on page 462*

Maxzide® *see* Hydrochlorothiazide and Triamterene *on page 349*

Maxzide®-25 *see* Hydrochlorothiazide and Triamterene *on page 349*

Measles Virus Vaccine, Live, Attenuated
Related Information
Immunization Guidelines *on page 759-762*

Brand Names Attenuvax®

Synonyms More Attenuated Enders Strain; Rubeola vaccine

Therapeutic Class Vaccine, Live Virus

Use Immunization against measles (rubeola) in persons ≥15 months of age and adults in isolated communities where measles is not endemic

Contraindications Known hypersensitivity to eggs, known hypersensitivity to neomycin, acute respiratory infections, activated tuberculosis, immunosuppressed patients (drug induced or disease)

Warnings Do not give with ISG concurrently

Precautions History of febrile seizures, hypersensitivity reactions may occur if sensitive to eggs, chickens, chicken feathers; do not give with other live vaccines; may depress tuberculin skin testing temporarily

Adverse Reactions
Cardiovascular: Headache
Central nervous system: Fever, rarely encephalitis
Dermatologic: Rarely urticaria
Hematologic: Thrombocytopenia
Local: Burning or stinging, swelling, induration, erythema
Respiratory: Sore throat, coryza
Miscellaneous: Lymphadenopathy

Drug Interactions Whole blood, immune globulin, immunosuppressive drugs, should not be given within 1 month of other live virus vaccines except monovalent or trivalent polio vaccine; may temporarily depress tuberculin skin test sensitivity

Stability Refrigerate at 2°C to 8°C (36°F to 46°F); discard if left at room temperature for over 8 hours

Mechanism of Action 97% respond; antibody levels last 8 years

Usual Dosage Geriatrics and Adults: S.C.: Administer entire volume of reconstituted vaccine in outer aspect of the upper arm

(Continued)

Measles Virus Vaccine, Live, Attenuated *(Continued)*
Monitoring Parameters Monitor for side effects

Nursing Implications Vaccine should not be given I.V.; S.C. injection preferred with a 25-gauge ⅝" needle; federal law requires that the date of administration, the vaccine manufacturer, lot number of vaccine, and the administering person's name, title and address be entered into the patient's permanent medical record

Special Geriatric Considerations Generally not recommended for adults since most have become immune; if from an isolated community where measles is not endemic, may require vaccination, no dose reduction is necessary

Dosage Forms Injection: 1000 TCID$_{50}$ per dose

References
Gardner P and Schaffner W, "Immunization of Adults," *N Engl J Med*, 1993, 328(17):1252-8.

Measurin® [OTC] *see* Aspirin *on page 58*

Meclizine Hydrochloride (mek' li zeen)
Brand Names Antivert®; Antrizine®; Bonine® [OTC]; Dizmiss® [OTC]; Meni-D®; Ru-Vert-M®

Synonyms Meclizine Hydrochloride

Generic Available Yes

Therapeutic Class Antiemetic; Antihistamine

Use Prevention and treatment of nausea, vomiting, and dizziness of motion sickness; management of vertigo with diseases affecting the vestibular system (only "possibly" effective)

Contraindications Hypersensitivity to meclizine, cyclizine, or any component

Precautions Use with caution in patients with angle-closure glaucoma, prostatic hypertrophy, or GI obstruction; elderly may be at risk for anticholinergic side effects such as glaucoma, constipation, urinary retention, confusion

Adverse Reactions
Cardiovascular: Palpitations, tachycardia, hypotension
Central nervous system: Drowsiness, fatigue, restlessness, excitation, insomnia, confusion, euphoria, vertigo, visual hallucinations, auditory hallucinations
Dermatologic: Rash, urticaria
Gastrointestinal: Dry mouth, anorexia, nausea, vomiting, diarrhea, constipation
Genitourinary: Urinary frequency, urinary retention, difficult urination
Ocular: Blurred vision, diplopia
Otic: Tinnitus
Miscellaneous: Dry nose

Overdosage Symptoms of overdose include excitation alternating with drowsiness, respiratory depression, hallucinations

Toxicology There is no specific treatment for an antihistamine overdose, however, most of its clinical toxicity is due to anticholinergic effects. Anticholinesterase inhibitors may be useful by reducing acetylcholinesterase. Anticholinesterase inhibitors include physostigmine, neostigmine, pyridostigmine, and edrophonium. For anticholinergic overdose with severe life-threatening symptoms, physostigmine 1-2 mg I.V., slowly may be given to reverse these effects.

Drug Interactions See Adverse Reactions; may enhance anticholinergic action of drugs with anticholinergic pharmacologic action

Mechanism of Action Has antiemetic, anticholinergic, and antihistaminic activity; has central anticholinergic action by blocking chemoreceptor trigger zone; decreases excitability of the middle ear labyrinth and blocks conduction in the middle ear vestibular-cerebellar pathways

Pharmacodynamics
Onset of action: Oral: Within 30-60 minutes
Duration: 8-24 hours

Pharmacokinetics
Metabolism: Reportedly in the liver
Half-life: 6 hours
Elimination: As metabolites in urine and as unchanged drug in feces

Usual Dosage Geriatrics and Adults: Oral:
Motion sickness: 12.5-25 mg initially 1 hour before travel, repeat dose every 12-24 hours if needed; doses up to 50 mg may be needed

Vertigo: 25-100 mg/day in divided doses

Monitoring Parameters Monitor for CNS anticholinergic side effects in elderly, relief of symptoms

Patient Information May impair ability to perform hazardous tasks; may cause drowsiness; may cause dry mouth, constipation, difficulty urinating, dry eyes

Nursing Implications See Precautions and Special Geriatric Considerations

Special Geriatric Considerations Due to anticholinergic action, use lowest dose in divided doses to avoid side effects and their inconvenience; limit use if possible; may cause confusion or aggravate symptoms of confusion in those with dementia; if vertigo does not respond in 1-2 weeks, it is advised to discontinue use

Dosage Forms
Capsule: 25 mg
Tablet: 12.5 mg, 25 mg, 50 mg

Tablet, chewable: 25 mg

Meclofenamate Sodium (me kloe fen am' ate)

Brand Names Meclomen®

Synonyms Fenamates

Generic Available Yes

Therapeutic Class Analgesic, Non-narcotic; Anti-inflammatory Agent; Nonsteroidal Anti-inflammatory Agent (NSAID), Oral

Use Treatment of inflammatory disorders such as rheumatoid arthritis, mild to moderate pain, osteoarthritis, pain of sunburn, migraine headaches (acute)

Contraindications Active GI bleeding, ulcer disease, hypersensitivity to meclofenamate or other NSAIDs

Warnings GI toxicity (bleeding, ulceration, perforation); CNS effects may occur (headaches, confusion, depression); hypersensitivity, anaphylactoid reactions (intermittent tolmetin use more often); renal function decline, acute renal insufficiency, interstitial nephritis, dysuria, cystitis, hematuria, nephrotic syndrome, hyperkalemia in acute renal insufficiency, hyponatremia, papillary necrosis, hepatic function impairment; elderly have increased risk for adverse reactions to NSAIDs; see Special Geriatric Considerations

Precautions Use with caution in patients with congestive heart failure, hypertension, decreased renal or hepatic function, history of GI disease (bleeding or ulcers), or those receiving anticoagulants; perform ophthalmologic evaluation for those who develop eye complaints during therapy (blurred vision, diminished vision, changes in color vision, retinal changes); NSAIDs may mask signs/symptoms of infections; photosensitivity reported

Adverse Reactions

Cardiovascular: Congestive heart failure, angina, hypertension, hypotension, fluid retention, arrhythmias, edema

Central nervous system: Headache, drowsiness, vertigo, dizziness, fatigue, hallucinations, confusion, depression, emotional lability, psychotic behavior, asthenia

Dermatologic: Rash, urticaria, angioedema, Stevens-Johnson syndrome, exfoliative dermatitis, ecchymosis, petechiae, purpura, bruising

Endocrine & metabolic: Hyperglycemia, hypoglycemia, hyperkalemia, gynecomastia, hyponatremia

Gastrointestinal: Dyspepsia, heartburn, nausea, diarrhea, constipation, flatulence, stomatitis, vomiting, abdominal pain, peptic ulcer, GI bleeding, GI perforation, gingival ulcers, pancreatitis, proctitis, paralytic ulcers, colitis, anorexia, weight loss

Genitourinary: Impotence, azotemia

Hematologic: Neutropenia, anemia, agranulocytosis, bone marrow suppression, hemolytic anemia, hemorrhage, inhibition of platelet aggregation

Hepatic: Hepatitis, elevated LFTs, cholestatic jaundice

Neuromuscular & skeletal: Involuntary muscle movements, muscle weakness, tremors

Ocular: Vision changes

Otic: Tinnitus

Renal: Dysuria, polyuria, pyuria, oliguria, anuria, acute renal failure

Respiratory: Exacerbation of asthma, dyspnea

Miscellaneous: Dry mucous membranes, thirst, pyrexia, sweating

Overdosage Symptoms of overdose include drowsiness, lethargy, disorientation, confusion, dizziness, numbness, paresthesia, nausea, vomiting, gastric irritation, abdominal pain, headache, tinnitus, sweating, blurred vision, muscle twitching, seizures, coma, acute renal failure, increased BUN and serum creatinine, hypotension, tachycardia, and metabolic acidosis

Toxicology Management of a nonsteroidal anti-inflammatory agent (NSAID) intoxication is primarily supportive and symptomatic. Fluid therapy is commonly effective in managing the hypotension that may occur following an acute NSAID overdose, except when this is due to an acute blood loss. Seizures tend to be very short-lived and often do not require drug treatment although recurrent seizures should be treated with I.V. diazepam. Since many of the NSAIDs undergo enterohepatic cycling, multiple doses of charcoal may be needed to reduce the potential for delayed toxicities. Dialysis may be required to correct serious azotemia/electrolyte shift.

Drug Interactions

May increase digoxin, methotrexate, and lithium serum concentrations

Aspirin or other salicylates may decrease NSAID serum concentrations

Other NSAIDs may increase adverse GI effects

Increased prothrombin time with anticoagulants

Decreased antihypertensive effects of ACE inhibitors, beta-blockers, and thiazide diuretics

Increased response to sympathomimetics

Probenecid may increase toxicity of NSAIDs by increase in serum concentrations

Effects of loop diuretics may decrease

Diuretics may increase the risk of acute renal insufficiency

Azotemia may be increased in elderly receiving loop diuretics

Mechanism of Action Inhibits prostaglandin synthesis, acts on the hypothalamus

(Continued)

435

Meclofenamate Sodium *(Continued)*

heat-regulating center to reduce fever, blocks prostaglandin synthetase action which prevents formation of the platelet-aggregating substance thromboxane A_2; decreases pain receptor sensitivity. Other proposed mechanisms of action are lysosomal stabilization, kinin and leukotriene production, alteration of chemotactic factors, and inhibition of neutrophil activation. This latter mechanism may be the most significant pharmacologic action to reduce inflammation.

Pharmacodynamics
Onset of analgesia: 30 minutes to 1 hour
Duration of action: 2-4 hours
Onset of anti-inflammatory action: 3-4 days
Peak effect: 2-3 weeks

Pharmacokinetics
Protein binding: 99%
Half-life: 2-3.3 hours
Time to peak: Oral: Peak serum levels occur within 30-90 minutes
Elimination: Principally in urine and in feces as glucuronide conjugates

Usual Dosage Geriatrics and Adults: Oral: Initial:
Mild to moderate pain: 50 mg every 4-6 hours; increases to 100 mg may be required; maximum dose: 400 mg

Rheumatoid arthritis and osteoarthritis: 50 mg every 4-6 hours; increase, over weeks, to 200-400 mg/day in 3-4 divided doses; do not exceed 400 mg/day; maximal benefit for any dose may not be seen for 2-3 weeks

Monitoring Parameters Monitor response (pain, range of motion, grip strength, mobility, ADL function), inflammation; observe for weight gain, edema; monitor renal function; observe for bleeding, bruising; evaluate gastrointestinal effects (abdominal pain, bleeding, dyspepsia); mental confusion, disorientation, CBC, serum, creatinine, BUN, liver function tests

Test Interactions Increased chloride (S), increased sodium (S)

Patient Information Serious gastrointestinal bleeding can occur as well as ulceration and perforation. Pain may or may not be present. Avoid aspirin and aspirin-containing products while taking this medication. If gastric upset occurs, take with food, milk, or antacid. If gastric adverse effects persist, contact physician. May cause drowsiness, dizziness, blurred vision, and confusion. Use caution when performing tasks which require alertness (eg, driving). Do not take for more than 3 days for fever or 10 days for pain without physician advice.

Nursing Implications See Overdosage, Monitoring Parameters, Patient Information, and Special Geriatric Considerations

Additional Information There are no clinical guidelines to predict which NSAID will give response in a particular patient. Trials with each must be initiated until response determined. Consider dose, patient convenience, and cost.

Special Geriatric Considerations Elderly are a high-risk population for adverse effects from nonsteroidal anti-inflammatory agents. As much as 60% of elderly can develop peptic ulceration and/or hemorrhage asymptomatically. The concomitant use of H_2 blockers, omeprazole, and sucralfate is not effective as prophylaxis. Misoprostol is the only prophylactic agent proven effective. Also, concomitant disease and drug use contribute to the risk for GI adverse effects. Use lowest effective dose for shortest period possible. Consider renal function decline with age. Use of NSAIDs can compromise existing renal function especially when Cl_{cr} is $\leq$30 mL/minute. Tinnitus may be a difficult and unreliable indication of toxicity due to age-related hearing loss or eighth cranial nerve damage. CNS adverse effects such as confusion, agitation, and hallucination are generally seen in overdose or high dose situations, but elderly may demonstrate these adverse effects at lower doses than younger adults.

Dosage Forms Capsule: 50 mg, 100 mg

References
Brooks PM, Day RO, "Nonsteroidal Anti-inflammatory Drugs – Differences and Similarities," *N Engl J Med*, 1991, 324(24):1716-25.
Clinch D, Banerjee AK, Ostick G, "Absence of Abdominal Pain in Elderly Patients With Peptic Ulcer," *Age Ageing*, 1984, 13:120-3.
Clive DM, Stoff JS, "Renal Syndromes Associated With Nonsteroidal Anti-inflammatory Drugs," *N Engl J Med*, 1984, 310(9):563-72.
Graham DY, "Prevention of Gastroduodenal Injury Induced by Chronic Nonsteroidal Anti-inflammatory Drug Therapy," *Gastroenterology*, 1989, 96(2 Pt 2 Suppl):675-81.
Gurwitz JH, Avarn J, Ross-Degan D, et al, "Nonsteroidal Anti-Inflammatory Drug-Associated Azotemia in the Very Old," *JAMA*, 1990, 264(4):471-5.
Knodel LC, "Preventing NSAID-Induced Ulcers: The Role of Misoprostol," *Consult Pharm*, 1989, 4:37-41.
Pounder R, "Silent Peptic Ulceration: Deadly Silence or Golden Silence?" *Gastroenterology*, 1989, 96(2 Pt 2 Suppl):626-31.

Meclomen® *see* Meclofenamate Sodium *on previous page*

Meclozine Hydrochloride *see* Meclizine Hydrochloride *on page 434*

Medihaler-Epi® *see* Epinephrine *on page 256*

Medihaler Ergotamine® *see* Ergotamine *on page 261*

Medihaler-Iso® *see* Isoproterenol *on page 380*

Medilax® [OTC] *see* Phenolphthalein *on page 556*

Medipren® [OTC] *see* Ibuprofen *on page 360*

Medi-Tuss® AC *see* Guaifenesin and Codeine *on page 332*

Medi-Tuss® [OTC] *see* Guaifenesin *on page 331*

Medralone® *see* Methylprednisolone *on page 461*

Medrol® *see* Methylprednisolone *on page 461*

Medroxyprogesterone Acetate (me drox' ee proe jess' te rone)

Brand Names Amen®; Curretab®; Cycrin®; Depo-Provera®; Provera®

Synonyms Acetoxymethylprogesterone; Methylacetoxyprogesterone

Therapeutic Class Contraceptive, Progestin Only; Progestin

Use Endometrial carcinoma or renal carcinoma as well as secondary amenorrhea or abnormal uterine bleeding due to hormonal imbalance

Unlabeled use: Treatment of menopausal symptoms, to stimulate respiration in obstructive sleep apnea, and to induce endometrial shedding in postmenopausal women taking estrogens.

Contraindications Thrombophlebitis; hypersensitivity to medroxyprogesterone or any component; cerebral apoplexy, undiagnosed vaginal bleeding, liver dysfunction

Precautions Use with caution in patients with depression, diabetes, epilepsy, asthma, migraines, renal or cardiac dysfunction; pretreatment exams should include PAP smear, physical exam of breasts and pelvic areas. May increase serum cholesterol, LDL, decrease HDL and triglycerides

Adverse Reactions

Cardiovascular: Edema, thromboembolic disorders

Central nervous system: Depression, dizziness, nervousness

Dermatologic: Melasma, chloasma, urticaria, acne

Endocrine & metabolic: Breakthrough bleeding, breast tenderness

Gastrointestinal: Weight gain

Hepatic: Cholestatic jaundice

Toxicology Toxicity is unlikely following single exposures of excessive doses, and supportive treatment is adequate in most cases

Drug Interactions Aminoglutethimide may decrease the effects by increasing hepatic metabolism

Mechanism of Action Inhibits secretion of pituitary gonadotropins, which prevents follicular maturation and ovulation, stimulates growth of mammary tissue, and transform proliferative endometrium into secretory endometrium

Pharmacokinetics

Absorption: I.M.: Slow

Metabolism: Oral: In the liver

Elimination: In urine and feces

Usual Dosage Geriatrics and Adults: Oral:

Accompanying postmenopausal estrogen therapy, postmenopausal: 2.5-10 mg the last 10-13 days of estrogen dosing each month or daily

Abnormal uterine bleeding: 5-10 mg for 5-10 days starting on day 16 or 21 of cycle

Endometrial or renal carcinoma: I.M.: 400-1000 mg/week

Monitoring Parameters In diabetics, glucose tolerance may be decreased

Test Interactions Altered thyroid and liver function tests

Patient Information Take this medicine only as directed; do not take more of it and do not take it for a longer period of time; drug will induce menstrual bleeding in women with an intact uterus; take with food if GI upset occurs

Nursing Implications Patients should receive a copy of the patient labeling for the drug

Special Geriatric Considerations See Usual Dosage and Patient Information

Dosage Forms

Injection, suspension: 100 mg/mL (5 mL); 400 mg/mL (1 mL, 2.5 mL, 10 mL)

Tablet: 2.5 mg, 5 mg, 10 mg

Mefenamic Acid (me fe nam' ik)

Brand Names Ponstel®

Generic Available No

Therapeutic Class Analgesic, Non-narcotic; Nonsteroidal Anti-inflammatory Agent (NSAID), Oral

Use Short-term relief of mild to moderate pain, sunburn, migraine headache (acute)

Contraindications Known hypersensitivity to mefenamic acid or other NSAIDs

Warnings GI toxicity (bleeding, ulceration, perforation); CNS effects may occur (headaches, confusion, depression); hypersensitivity, anaphylactoid reactions (intermittent

(Continued)

Mefenamic Acid *(Continued)*

tolmetin use more often); renal function decline, acute renal insufficiency, interstitial nephritis, dysuria, cystitis, hematuria, nephrotic syndrome, hyperkalemia in acute renal insufficiency, hyponatremia, papillary necrosis, hepatic function impairment; elderly have increased risk for adverse reactions to NSAIDs; see Special Geriatric Considerations

Precautions Use with caution in patients with congestive heart failure, hypertension, decreased renal or hepatic function, history of GI disease (bleeding or ulcers), or those receiving anticoagulants; perform ophthalmologic evaluation for those who develop eye complaints during therapy (blurred vision, diminished vision, changes in color vision, retinal changes); NSAIDs may mask signs/symptoms of infections; photosensitivity reported

Adverse Reactions

Cardiovascular: Congestive heart failure, angina, hypertension, hypotension, fluid retention, arrhythmias, edema

Central nervous system: Headache, drowsiness, vertigo, dizziness, fatigue, hallucinations, confusion, depression, emotional lability, psychotic behavior, asthenia

Dermatologic: Rash, urticaria, angioedema, Stevens-Johnson syndrome, exfoliative dermatitis, ecchymosis, petechiae, purpura, bruising

Endocrine & metabolic: Hyperglycemia, hypoglycemia, hyperkalemia, gynecomastia, hyponatremia

Gastrointestinal: Dyspepsia, heartburn, nausea, diarrhea, constipation, flatulence, stomatitis, vomiting, abdominal pain, peptic ulcer, GI bleeding, GI perforation, gingival ulcers, pancreatitis, proctitis, paralytic ulcers, colitis, anorexia, weight loss

Genitourinary: Impotence, azotemia

Hematologic: Neutropenia, anemia, agranulocytosis, bone marrow suppression, hemolytic anemia, hemorrhage, inhibition of platelet aggregation

Hepatic: Hepatitis, elevated LFTs, cholestatic jaundice

Neuromuscular & skeletal: Involuntary muscle movements, muscle weakness, tremors

Ocular: Vision changes

Otic: Tinnitus

Renal: Dysuria, polyuria, pyuria, oliguria, anuria, acute renal failure

Respiratory: Exacerbation of asthma, dyspnea

Miscellaneous: Dry mucous membranes, thirst, pyrexia, sweating

Overdosage Symptoms include drowsiness, lethargy, disorientation, confusion, dizziness, numbness, paresthesia, nausea, vomiting, gastric irritation, abdominal pain, headache, tinnitus, sweating, blurred vision, muscle twitching, seizures, coma, acute renal failure, increased BUN and serum creatinine, hypotension, tachycardia, and metabolic acidosis

Toxicology Management of a nonsteroidal anti-inflammatory agent (NSAID) intoxication is primarily supportive and symptomatic. Fluid therapy is commonly effective in managing the hypotension that may occur following an acute NSAID overdose, except when this is due to an acute blood loss. Seizures tend to be very short-lived and often do not require drug treatment although recurrent seizures should be treated with I.V. diazepam. Since many of the NSAIDs undergo enterohepatic cycling, multiple doses of charcoal may be needed to reduce the potential for delayed toxicities.

Drug Interactions

May increase digoxin, methotrexate, and lithium serum concentrations

Aspirin or other salicylates may decrease NSAID serum concentrations

Other NSAIDs may increase adverse GI effects

Increased prothrombin time with anticoagulants

Decreased antihypertensive effects of ACE inhibitors, beta-blockers, and thiazide diuretics

Increased response to sympathomimetics

Probenecid may increase toxicity of NSAIDs by increase in serum concentrations

Effects of loop diuretics may decrease

Diuretics may increase the risk of acute renal insufficiency

Azotemia may be increased in elderly receiving loop diuretics

Mechanism of Action Inhibits prostaglandin synthesis, acts on the hypothalamus heat-regulating center to reduce fever, blocks prostaglandin synthetase action which prevents formation of the platelet-aggregating substance thromboxane A_2; decreases pain receptor sensitivity. Other proposed mechanisms of action are lysosomal stabilization, kinin and leukotriene production, alteration of chemotactic factors, and inhibition of neutrophil activation. This latter mechanism may be the most significant pharmacologic action to reduce inflammation.

Pharmacodynamics

Peak effect: Oral: Within 2-4 hours

Duration: Up to 6 hours

Pharmacokinetics

Protein binding: High (>90%)

Metabolism: Conjugated in the liver

Half-life: 3.5 hours

Elimination: In urine (50%) and feces as unchanged drug and metabolites

Usual Dosage Geriatrics and Adults: Oral: 500 mg to start then 250 mg every 6 hours as needed; maximum therapy: 1 week; maximum dose: 1000 mg/day

Monitoring Parameters Monitor for pain relief, gastric adverse effects, bleeding, confusion; renal function

Test Interactions Increased chloride (S), increased sodium (S), positive Coombs' [direct]

Patient Information Serious gastrointestinal bleeding can occur as well as ulceration and perforation. Pain may or may not be present. Avoid aspirin and aspirin-containing products while taking this medication. If gastric upset occurs, take with food, milk, or antacid. If gastric adverse effects persist, contact physician. May cause drowsiness, dizziness, blurred vision, and confusion. Use caution when performing tasks which require alertness (eg, driving). Do not take for more than 3 days for fever or 10 days for pain without physician advice.

Nursing Implications See Overdosage, Monitoring Parameters, Patient Information, and Special Geriatric Considerations

Additional Information There are no clinical guidelines to predict which NSAID will give response in a particular patient. Trials with each must be initiated until response determined. Consider dose, patient convenience, and cost.

Special Geriatric Considerations Elderly are a high-risk population for adverse effects from nonsteroidal anti-inflammatory agents. As much as 60% of elderly can develop peptic ulceration and/or hemorrhage asymptomatically. The concomitant use of H_2 blockers, omeprazole, and sucralfate is not effective as prophylaxis. Misoprostol is the only prophylactic agent proven effective. Also, concomitant disease and drug use contribute to the risk for GI adverse effects. Use lowest effective dose for shortest period possible. Consider renal function decline with age. Use of NSAIDs can compromise existing renal function especially when Cl_{cr} is ≤ 30 mL/minute. Tinnitus may be a difficult and unreliable indication of toxicity due to age-related hearing loss or eighth cranial nerve damage. CNS adverse effects such as confusion, agitation, and hallucination are generally seen in overdose or high dose situations, but elderly may demonstrate these adverse effects at lower doses than younger adults.

Dosage Forms Capsule: 250 mg

References

Brooks PM, Day RO, "Nonsteroidal Anti-inflammatory Drugs – Differences and Similarities," *N Engl J Med*, 1991, 324(24):1716-25.

Clinch D, Banerjee AK, Ostick G, "Absence of Abdominal Pain in Elderly Patients With Peptic Ulcer," *Age Ageing*, 1984, 13:120-3.

Clive DM, Stoff JS, "Renal Syndromes Associated With Nonsteroidal Anti-inflammatory Drugs," *N Engl J Med*, 1984, 310(9):563-72.

Graham DY, "Prevention of Gastroduodenal Injury Induced by Chronic Nonsteroidal Anti-inflammatory Drug Therapy," *Gastroenterology*, 1989, 96(2 Pt 2 Suppl):675-81.

Gurwitz JH, Avarn J, Ross-Degan D, et al, "Nonsteroidal Anti-Inflammatory Drug-Associated Azotemia in the Very Old," *JAMA*, 1990, 264(4):471-5.

Knodel LC, "Preventing NSAID-Induced Ulcers: The Role of Misoprostol," *Consult Pharm*, 1989, 4:37-41.

Pounder R, "Silent Peptic Ulceration: Deadly Silence or Golden Silence?" *Gastroenterology*, 1989, 96(2 Pt 2 Suppl):626-31.

Mefoxin® see Cefoxitin Sodium on page 134

Megace® see Megestrol Acetate on this page

Megacillin® see Penicillin G Benzathine, Parenteral on page 539

Megestrol Acetate (me jess' trole)

Brand Names Megace®

Generic Available Yes

Therapeutic Class Antineoplastic Agent, Hormone (Gonadotropin Hormone-Releasing Antigen); Progestin

Use Palliative treatment of breast and endometrial carcinomas

Unlabeled use: Appetite stimulation and promotion of weight gain in cachexia

Contraindications Hypersensitivity to megestrol or any component

Warnings The use in other types of neoplastic disease is not recommended.

Precautions Use with caution in patients with a history of thrombophlebitis

Adverse Reactions

Cardiovascular: Deep vein thrombophlebitis, edema

Central nervous system: Carpal tunnel syndrome

Dermatologic: Alopecia, rash

Endocrine & metabolic: Vaginal bleeding and discharge, hyperglycemia

Gastrointestinal: Weight gain, nausea, vomiting

Respiratory: Hyperpnea, dyspnea, pulmonary embolism

Miscellaneous: Tumor flare

Mechanism of Action Megestrol is an antineoplastic progestin thought to act through an antileutenizing effect mediated via the pituitary

Pharmacokinetics

Absorption: Oral: Well absorbed

Metabolism: Completely in the liver to free steroids and glucuronide conjugates

(Continued)

Megestrol Acetate *(Continued)*

Time to peak: Oral: Peak serum levels occur within 1-3 hours

Usual Dosage Geriatrics and Adults: Oral:

Breast carcinoma: 40 mg 4 times/day

Endometrial carcinoma: 40-320 mg/day in divided doses

Use for 2 continuous months to determine efficacy; maximum doses used have been up to 800 mg/day

Monitoring Parameters Monitor for tumor response; observe for signs of thromboembolic phenomena

Patient Information Report any calf pain, difficulty breathing, or vaginal bleeding to physician; may cause abdominal pain, headache, nausea, vomiting, breast tenderness; notify physician if these persist

Nursing Implications Monitor for thromboembolism; see Adverse Reactions

Special Geriatric Considerations Elderly females may have vaginal bleeding or discharge and need to be forewarned of this side effect and inconvenience. No specific changes in dose are required for elderly.

Dosage Forms Tablet: 20 mg, 40 mg

Mellaril® *see* Thioridazine *on page 684*

Mellaril-S® *see* Thioridazine *on page 684*

Melphalan (mel' fa lan)

Brand Names Alkeran®

Synonyms L-PAM; L-Phenylalanine Mustard; L-Sarcolysin

Generic Available No

Therapeutic Class Antineoplastic Agent, Alkylating Agent (Nitrogen Mustard)

Use Palliative treatment of multiple myeloma and nonresectable epithelial ovarian carcinoma; neuroblastoma, rhabdomyosarcoma; breast cancer; limb perfusion in malignant melanoma

Contraindications Hypersensitivity to melphalan or any component; severe bone marrow depression; patients whose disease was resistant to prior therapy

Warnings The U.S. Food and Drug Administration (FDA) currently recommends that procedures for proper handling and disposal for antineoplastic agents be considered. Is potentially mutagenic, carcinogenic, and teratogenic; produces amenorrhea.

Precautions Reduce dosage or discontinue therapy if total leukocyte count <3000/mm³ or platelet count <100,000/mm³; use with caution in patients with bone marrow suppression and impaired renal function

Adverse Reactions

Cardiovascular: Vasculitis

Dermatologic: Alopecia, rash, pruritus, vesiculation of skin

Endocrine & metabolic: Leukopenia, thrombocytopenia, anemia, agranulocytosis, hemolytic anemia

Gastrointestinal: Nausea, vomiting, diarrhea, stomatitis

Genitourinary: Bladder irritation, hemorrhagic cystitis

Local: Burning and discomfort at injection site

Respiratory: Pulmonary fibrosis

Overdosage Symptoms of overdose include hypocalcemia, pulmonary fibrosis

Toxicology General supportive measures; monitor CBC 3-6 weeks; transfusions as needed; no known antidote available

Drug Interactions Cyclosporine

Stability Store at room temperature; protect from light; do not refrigerate; use within 1 hour of reconstitution; dispense in glass

Mechanism of Action Alkylating agent that inhibits DNA and RNA synthesis via formation of carbonium ions; cross-links strands of DNA

Pharmacokinetics

Absorption: Oral: Variable and incomplete

Half-life: Terminal: 90 minutes

Time to peak: Peak serum levels have been reported to occur within 2 hours; food interferes with absorption

Elimination: 10% to 15% of dose excreted unchanged in urine; after oral administration, 20% to 50% is excreted in stool

Usual Dosage Oral (refer to individual protocols):

Geriatrics: See adult dose; no specific recommendations for creatinine clearance changes with age

Adults:

Multiple myeloma: 6 mg/m²/day for 5 days, repeat every 6 weeks, or 0.1 mg/kg/day for 2-3 weeks; maintenance dose: 2-4 mg/day when bone marrow has recovered; see Precautions

Ovarian carcinoma: 0.2 mg/kg/day for 5 days, repeat in 4-5 weeks

Monitoring Parameters See Precautions; observe for signs of infection or bleeding

Test Interactions False-positive Coombs' test [direct]

Patient Information Any signs of infection, easy bruising or bleeding, shortness of breath, or painful or burning urination should be brought to physician's attention. Nausea, vomiting, or hair loss sometimes occur

Nursing Implications Protect tablets from light; monitor WBCs and platelets; observe for infections and bleeding; see Warnings and Additional Information

Additional Information

Myelosuppressive effects:

WBC: Moderate

Platelets: Moderate

Onset (days): 7

Nadir (days): 10-18

Recovery (days): 42-50

Special Geriatric Considerations Toxicity to immunosuppressives is increased in elderly. Start with lowest recommended adult doses. Signs of infection, such as fever and WBC rise, may not occur. Lethargy and confusion may be more prominent signs of infection.

Dosage Forms Tablet: 2 mg

References

Hutchins LF and Lipschitz DA, "Cancer, Clinical Pharmacology, and Aging," *Clin Geriatr Med*, 1987, 3(3):483-503.

Kaplan HG, "Use of Cancer Chemotherapy in the Elderly," *Drug Treatment in the Elderly*, Vestal RE, ed, Boston, MA: ADIS Health Science Press, 1984, 338-49.

Menadiol and Vitamin K *see* Vitamin K and Menadiol *on page 738*

Menadol® [OTC] *see* Ibuprofen *on page 360*

Meni-D® *see* Meclizine Hydrochloride *on page 434*

Mepacrine Hydrochloride *see* Quinacrine Hydrochloride *on page 615*

Meperidine Hydrochloride (me per' i deen)

Related Information

Narcotic Agonist Comparative Pharmacology *on page 811*

Pharmacokinetics of Narcotic Agonist Analgesics *on page 812*

Brand Names Demerol®; Pethadol®

Synonyms Isonipecaine Hydrochloride; Pethidine Hydrochloride

Generic Available Yes

Therapeutic Class Analgesic, Narcotic

Use Management of moderate to severe pain; adjunct to anesthesia and preoperative sedation

Restrictions C-II

Contraindications Hypersensitivity to meperidine or any component; patients receiving MAO inhibitors presently or in the past 14 days

Warnings Some preparations contain sulfites which may cause allergic reaction; use with caution in patients with renal failure or seizure disorders or those receiving high dose meperidine: normeperidine (an active metabolite and CNS stimulant) may accumulate and precipitate twitches, tremors, or seizures

Precautions Use with caution in patients with pulmonary, hepatic, or renal disorders; patients with tachycardias, biliary colic, or increased intracranial pressure

Adverse Reactions

Cardiovascular: Palpitations, hypotension, bradycardia, peripheral vasodilation, tachycardia

Central nervous system: CNS depression, dizziness, drowsiness, sedation, increased intracranial pressure

Dermatologic: Pruritus

Endocrine & metabolic: Antidiuretic hormone release

Gastrointestinal: Nausea, vomiting, constipation

Neuromuscular & skeletal: Metabolite normeperidine may precipitate tremors or seizures

Ocular: Miosis

Respiratory: Respiratory depression

Miscellaneous: Physical and psychological dependence, biliary or urinary tract spasm, histamine release

Overdosage Symptoms of overdose include CNS depression, respiratory depression, mydriasis, bradycardia, pulmonary edema, chronic tremors, CNS excitability, seizures

Toxicology Treatment of an overdose includes support of the patient's airway, establishment of an I.V. line and administration of naloxone 2 mg I.V. with repeat administration as necessary up to a total of 10 mg

Drug Interactions

Decreased effect with phenytoin (increased toxicity of meperidine concurrently)

Increased effect/toxicity of isoniazid; increased effect/toxicity with MAO inhibitors (can be fatal), serotonin reuptake inhibitors (eg, fluoxetine), CNS depressants, TCAs, phenothiazines, barbiturates, amphetamines, cimetidine

Stability Protect oral dosage forms from light

Mechanism of Action Binds to opiate receptors in the CNS, causing inhibition of as-

(Continued)

441

Meperidine Hydrochloride *(Continued)*

cending pain pathways, altering the perception of and response to pain; produces generalized CNS depression

Pharmacodynamics
Onset of action:
Oral, S.C., I.M.: Within 10-15 minutes
I.V.: Effects within 5 minutes
Peak effects: Oral, S.C., I.M.: Within 1 hour
Duration: Oral, S.C., I.M.: 2-4 hours
Enhanced analgesia has been seen in elderly patients on therapeutic doses of narcotics; duration of action may be increased in the elderly

Pharmacokinetics
Distribution: V_d: Increased in elderly
Protein binding: 65% to 75%; decreased in elderly
Metabolism: In liver
Bioavailability: ~50% to 60%, increased bioavailability with liver disease
Half-life:
Adults:
Terminal: 2.5-4 hours
Terminal in liver disease: 7-11 hours
Elderly: 7 hours
Normeperidine (active metabolite): 15-30 hours; normeperidine half-life is dependent on renal function and can accumulate with high doses or in patients with decreased renal function
Time to peak serum concentration: Longer in elderly
Elimination: ~5% meperidine eliminated unchanged in urine

Usual Dosage Doses should be titrated to appropriate analgesic effect; when changing route of administration, note that oral doses are about half as effective as parenteral dose.

Geriatrics:
Oral: 50 mg every 4 hours
I.M.: 25 mg every 4 hours

Adults: Oral, I.M., I.V.: S.C.: 50-150 mg/dose every 3-4 hours as needed

Dosing adjustment in renal impairment:
Cl_{cr} 10-50 mL/minute: Administer at 75% of normal dose
Cl_{cr} <10 mL/minute: Administer at 50% of normal dose

Dosing adjustment/comments in hepatic disease: Increased narcotic effect in cirrhosis; reduction in dose more important for oral than I.V. route

Monitoring Parameters Pain relief, respiratory and mental status, blood pressure

Reference Range Therapeutic: 70-500 ng/mL (SI: 283-2020 nmol/L); Toxic: >1000 ng/mL (SI: >4043 nmol/L)

Patient Information Will cause drowsiness; avoid alcoholic beverages

Nursing Implications Observe patient for excessive sedation, CNS depression, seizures; if I.V. administration is required, inject very slowly using a diluted solution

Special Geriatric Considerations Meperidine is not recommended as a drug of first choice for the treatment of chronic pain in the elderly due to the accumulation of its metabolite, normeperidine; for acute pain, its use should be limited to 1-2 doses; see Warnings, Adverse Reactions, and Pharmacodynamics

Dosage Forms
Injection:
Multiple dose vials: 50 mg/mL (30 mL); 100 mg/mL (20 mL)
Single dose: 10 mg/mL (5 mL, 10 mL, 30 mL); 25 mg/dose (0.5 mL, 1 mL); 50 mg/dose (1 mL); 75 mg/dose (1 mL, 1.5 mL); 100 mg/dose (1 mL)
Syrup: 50 mg/5 mL (500 mL)
Tablet: 50 mg, 100 mg

References
Ferrell BA, "Pain Management in Elderly People," *J Am Geriatr Soc*, 1991, 39(1):64-73.

Mephenytoin *(me fen' i toyn)*

Brand Names Mesantoin®

Synonyms Methoin; Methylphenylethylhydantoin; Phenantoin

Therapeutic Class Anticonvulsant, Hydantoin

Use Treatment of tonic-clonic and partial seizures in patients who are uncontrolled with less toxic anticonvulsants

Contraindications Hypersensitivity to mephenytoin or any component

Warnings Fatal irreversible aplastic anemia has occurred

Precautions Abrupt withdrawal may precipitate seizures

Adverse Reactions
Central nervous system: Sedation, ataxia, nervousness, mental confusion
Dermatologic: Rash, erythema multiforme, alopecia
Endocrine & metabolic: Nausea, vomiting, insomnia

Gastrointestinal: Weight gain

Hematologic: Neutropenia, leukopenia, thrombocytopenia, agranulocytosis, anemia

Hepatic: Hepatitis

Neuromuscular & skeletal: Tremors

Ocular: Diplopia, photophobia

Miscellaneous: Hodgkin's disease-like syndrome, serum sickness

Overdosage Symptoms of overdose include restlessness, dizziness, drowsiness, nausea, vomiting, nystagmus, ataxia, dysarthria, tremor, slurred speech, hypotension, respiratory depression, coma

Drug Interactions

Increased hydantoin effects (inhibited metabolism) seen with allopurinol, amiodarone, benzodiazepines, chloramphenicol, cimetidine, fluconazole, isoniazid, metronidazole, miconazole, omeprazole, phenacemide, phenylbutazone, succinimides, sulfonamides, trimipramine, valproic acid

The following displace hydantoin anticonvulsants and increase effects: Salicylates, tricyclic antidepressants, valproic acid; other agents increasing effects of hydantoins include ibuprofen, chlorpheniramine, phenothiazines

Decreased effects of hydantoin by increased metabolism with barbiturates, carbamazepine, diazoxide, rifampin, theophylline

Decreased absorption with antacids, sucralfate

Decreased hydantoin effect with folic acid, influenza vaccine, loxapine, nitrofurantoin, pyridoxine

Mechanism of Action Stabilizes neuronal membranes and decreases seizure activity by increasing efflux or decreasing influx of sodium ions across cell membranes in the motor cortex during generation of nerve impulses; prolongs effective refractory period and suppresses ventricular pacemaker automaticity, shortens action potential in the heart

Pharmacodynamics

Onset of action: 30 minutes

Duration of action: 24-48 hours

Pharmacokinetics

Absorption: Oral: Rapid

Metabolism: In the liver

Half-life: 144 hours

Elimination: In urine

Usual Dosage Adults: Oral: Initial dose: 50-100 mg/day given daily; increase by 50-100 mg at weekly intervals; usual maintenance dose: 200-600 mg/day in 3 divided doses; maximum: 800 mg/day

Reference Range 10-20 μg/mL; **Note:** Some clinicians now recommend 5-20 μg/mL

Test Interactions Increased alkaline phosphatase (S); decreased calcium (S)

Nursing Implications Monitor CBC and platelets

Additional Information Usually listed in combination with other anticonvulsants

Special Geriatric Considerations Elderly may have reduced hepatic clearance due to age decline in phase I metabolism

Dosage Forms Tablet: 100 mg

Mephyton® see Vitamin K and Menadiol on page 738

Meprobamate (me proe ba' mate)

Related Information

Anxiolytic/Hypnotic Use in Long-Term Care Facilities on page 755-756

Brand Names Equanil®; Meprospan®; Miltown®; Neuramate®

Generic Available Yes

Therapeutic Class Antianxiety Agent

Use Management of anxiety disorders

Restrictions C-IV

Contraindications Acute intermittent porphyria; hypersensitivity to meprobamate or any component; do not use in a comatose patient or in those with pre-existing CNS depression

Warnings Physical and psychological dependence and abuse may occur; use with caution in patients with renal or hepatic impairment, or with a history of seizures

Precautions Allergic reaction may occur in patients with history of dermatological condition (usually by fourth dose)

Adverse Reactions

Cardiovascular: Palpitations, tachycardia, arrhythmias, syncope

Central nervous system: Drowsiness, ataxia, slurred speech, dizziness

Gastrointestinal: Nausea, vomiting, diarrhea

Overdosage Symptoms of overdose include drowsiness, lethargy, ataxia, coma, hypotension, shock, death

Toxicology Treatment is supportive following attempts to enhance drug elimination. Hypotension should be treated with I.V. fluids and/or Trendelenburg positioning. Dialysis and hemoperfusion have not demonstrated significant reductions in blood drug concentrations.

(Continued)

Meprobamate *(Continued)*

Drug Interactions Increased toxicity: CNS depressants, alcohol

Mechanism of Action Precise mechanisms is not yet clear, but many effects have been ascribed to its central depressant actions

Pharmacodynamics Onset of action: Oral: Following administration sedation occurs within 60 minutes

Pharmacokinetics
Metabolism: Promptly in the liver
Half-life: 10 hours
Elimination: In urine (8% to 20% as unchanged drug) and in feces (10% as metabolites)

Usual Dosage Oral:
Geriatrics (use lowest effective dose): Initial: 200 mg 2-3 times/day
Adults: 400 mg 3-4 times/day, up to 2400 mg/day

Moderately dialyzable (20% to 50%)

Monitoring Parameters Mental status

Reference Range Therapeutic: 6-12 µg/mL (SI: 28-55 µmol/L); Toxic: >60 µg/mL (SI: >275 µmol/L)

Patient Information May cause drowsiness; avoid alcoholic beverages

Nursing Implications Monitor mental status; assist with ambulation

Special Geriatric Considerations Meprobamate is not considered a drug of choice in the elderly because of its potential to cause physical and psychological dependence; interpretive guidelines from the Health Care Financing Administration (HCFA) strongly discourage the use of meprobamate in residents of long-term care facilities

Dosage Forms Tablet: 200 mg, 400 mg

Meprolone® *see* Methylprednisolone *on page 461*

Mepron™ *see* Atovaquone *on page 64*

Meprospan® *see* Meprobamate *on previous page*

Mercaptopurine *(mer kap toe pyoor' een)*

Brand Names Purinethol®

Synonyms 6-Mercaptopurine; 6-MP

Generic Available No

Therapeutic Class Antineoplastic Agent, Antimetabolite; Antineoplastic Agent, Purine

Use Treatment of leukemias; Crohn's disease; ulcerative colitis; other collagen vascular diseases

Contraindications Hypersensitivity to mercaptopurine or any component; severe liver disease; severe bone marrow depression; patients whose disease showed prior resistance to mercaptopurine or thioguanine

Warnings The U.S. Food and Drug Administration (FDA) currently recommends that procedures for proper handling and disposal of antineoplastic agents be considered. Mercaptopurine may be potentially carcinogenic

Precautions Adjust dosage in patients with renal impairment or hepatic failure; patients who receive allopurinol concurrently should have the mercaptopurine dose reduced $\frac{1}{3}$ to $\frac{1}{4}$ of the usual dose

Adverse Reactions
Dermatologic: Rash
Endocrine & metabolic: Hyperuricemia
Gastrointestinal: Mild nausea or vomiting, diarrhea, stomatitis
Hematologic: Myelosuppression
Hepatic: Hepatotoxicity (occurs most frequently with doses greater than 2.5 mg/kg/day)
Renal: Renal toxicity (oliguria, hematuria)
Miscellaneous: Drug fever

Overdosage Symptoms of overdose include bone marrow depression, nausea, vomiting, diarrhea, hepatic necrosis, gastroenteritis

Toxicology No known pharmacologic antagonist for mercaptopurine

Drug Interactions Allopurinol may potentiate the effect of bone marrow suppression (inhibits xanthine oxidase); trimethoprim and sulfamethoxazole may enhance bone marrow suppression of mercaptopurine

Mechanism of Action Purine antagonist which inhibits DNA and RNA synthesis through pseudofeedback inhibition of the first step of purine synthesis which disrupts biosynthesis of purine nucleotides

Pharmacokinetics
Absorption: Variable and incomplete (16% to 50%)
Protein binding: 19%
Metabolism: Undergoes first-pass metabolism in the GI mucosa and liver; metabolized in the liver to sulfate conjugates, 6-thiouric acid and other inactive compounds
Half-life (adults): 47 minutes
Time to peak concentrations: Within 2 hours

Elimination: Prompt excretion in urine

Usual Dosage Oral (refer to individual protocols):

Geriatrics: Due to renal decline with age, start with lower recommended doses for adults

Adults:

Induction: 2.5-5 mg/kg/day or 80-100 mg/m^2/day given once daily

Maintenance: 1.5-2.5 mg/kg/day; calculate doses to nearest 25 mg daily dosage

Monitoring Parameters Monitor leukocyte count and platelets

Test Interactions Increased potassium (S)

Patient Information Do not take with meals; nausea and vomiting are rare with usual doses; report to physician if fever, sore throat, bleeding, bruising, shortness of breath, or painful urination occurs; hair loss occurs sometimes

Nursing Implications Adjust dosage in patients with renal insufficiency to lowest recommended dose; monitor dose response with WBC and platelet counts; observe for signs of infection and bleeding or bruising; see Additional Information

Additional Information Myelosuppressive effects:

WBC: Moderate

Platelets: Moderate

Onset (days): 7-10

Nadir (days): 14

Recovery (days): 21

Special Geriatric Considerations Toxicity to immunosuppressives is increased in elderly. Start with lowest recommended adult doses. Signs of infection, such as fever and WBC rise, may not occur. Lethargy and confusion may be more prominent signs of infection.

Dosage Forms Tablet: 50 mg

References

Hutchins LF and Lipschitz DA, "Cancer, Clinical Pharmacology, and Aging," *Clin Geriatr Med*, 1987, 3(3):483-503.

Kaplan HG, "Use of Cancer Chemotherapy in the Elderly," *Drug Treatment in the Elderly*, Vestal RE, ed, Boston, MA: ADIS Health Science Press, 1984, 338-49.

6-Mercaptopurine *see* Mercaptopurine *on previous page*

Meruvax® II *see* Rubella Virus Vaccine, Live *on page 632*

Mesalamine (me sal' a meen)

Brand Names Asacol®; Rowasa®

Synonyms 5-Aminosalicylic Acid; 5-ASA; Fisalamine; Mesalazine

Therapeutic Class 5-Aminosalicylic Acid Derivative; Anti-inflammatory Agent, Rectal

Use Treatment of ulcerative colitis, proctosigmoiditis, and proctitis

Contraindications Known hypersensitivity to mesalamine, sulfites, sulfasalazines, or salicylates

Warnings Reported to produce intolerance or exacerbation of colitis (3%) in some patients; paracolitis reported in some patients when using mesalamine; renal impairment has occurred in some patients

Precautions Pericarditis should be considered in patients with chest pain; pancreatitis should be considered in any patient with new abdominal complaints; sulfite hypersensitivity

Adverse Reactions

Central nervous system: Malaise, dizziness, asthenia, chills, depression, anxiety, fever

Dermatologic: Rash, pruritus

Gastrointestinal: Abdominal pain, cramps, diarrhea, dyspepsia, eructation, nausea, vomiting, discomfort, headache, flatulence, pancreatitis, dry mouth, tenesmus, taste alterations

Genitourinary: Urinary urgency, epididymitis

Hematologic: Agranulocytosis, leukopenia

Neuromuscular & skeletal: Peripheral neuropathy, arthralgia, back pain, hypertonia, pain, tremors

Ocular: Eye pain

Otic: Tinnitus

Renal: Dysuria, hematuria

Respiratory: Pharyngitis, chest pain, asthma exacerbation, rhinitis, sinusitis

Miscellaneous: Lymphadenopathy, flu symptoms

Overdosage Symptoms of overdose include renal function impairment

Toxicology Treat with emesis, gastric lavage, and follow with activated charcoal slurry

Stability Unstable in presence of water or light; once foil has been removed, unopened bottles have an expiration of 1 year following the date of manufacture

Mechanism of Action Mesalamine (5-aminosalicylic acid) is the active component of sulfasalazine; the specific mechanism of action of mesalamine is unknown; however, it is thought that it modulates chemical mediators of the inflammatory response, especially leukotrienes; action appears topical rather than systemic

(Continued)

Mesalamine *(Continued)*

Pharmacokinetics

Absorption: Rectal: ~15%, this is variable and dependent upon retention time, underlying GI disease, and colonic pH

Metabolism: In the liver by acetylation to acetyl-5-aminosalicylic acid (active), and to glucuronide conjugates; intestinal metabolism may also occur

Half-life:

5-ASA: 30-90 minutes

acetyl 5-ASA: 5-10 hours

Time to peak: Peak serum levels occur within 4-7 hours

Elimination: Most metabolites are excreted in urine with <2% appearing in feces

Usual Dosage Geriatrics and Adults:

Oral: 800 mg 3 times/day for 6 weeks

Retention enema: 60 mL (4 g) at bedtime, retained overnight, ~8 hours for 3-6 weeks

Rectal: Insert 1 suppository (500 mg) in rectum twice daily for 3-6 weeks

Monitoring Parameters Renal status (serum creatinine); stool frequency; GI symptoms; sigmoidoscopy

Test Interactions Elevations in AST, ALT, alkaline phosphatase, serum creatine, BUN

Patient Information Retain enemas for 8 hours or as long as practical; shake well before administering; (oral) do not chew or break tablets; (suppositories) remove foil wrapper, avoid excessive handling; shake suspension well

Nursing Implications Provide patient with copy of mesalamine administration instructions; monitor renal status and bowel function/status

Special Geriatric Considerations Elderly may have difficulty administering and retaining rectal suppositories. Given renal function decline with aging, monitor serum creatinine often during therapy.

Dosage Forms

Suppository, rectal: 500 mg

Suspension, rectal: 4 g/60 mL

Tablet, delayed release: 400 mg

Mesalazine *see Mesalamine on previous page*

Mesantoin® *see Mephenytoin on page 442*

Mesoridazine Besylate *(mez oh rid' a zeen)*

Related Information

Antacid Drug Interactions *on page 764*

Antipsychotic Agents Comparison *on page 801*

Antipsychotic Medication Guidelines *on page 754*

Brand Names Serentil®

Generic Available No

Therapeutic Class Antipsychotic Agent; Phenothiazine Derivative

Use Management of manifestations of psychotic disorders; depressive neurosis; alcohol withdrawal; nausea and vomiting; nonpsychotic symptoms associated with dementia in elderly, Tourette's syndrome; Huntington's chorea; spiromatic torticollis and Reye's syndrome; see Special Geriatric Considerations

Contraindications Hypersensitivity to mesoridazine or any component, cross-sensitivity with other phenothiazines may exist; avoid use in patients with narrow-angle glaucoma, bone marrow depression, severe liver or cardiac disease; subcortical brain damage, circulatory collapse, severe hypotension or hypertension

Warnings

Tardive dyskinesia: Prevalence rate may be 40% in elderly; elderly women especially at risk; embarrassment from dyskinesias may lead to greater social isolation; development of the syndrome and the irreversible nature are proportional to duration and total cumulative dose over time. May be reversible if diagnosed early in therapy; intermittent use of antipsychotics (not proven use) helps decrease total cumulative dose.

EPS: Extrapyramidal reactions are more common in elderly with up to 50% developing these reactions after age 60. These reactions may be more common in dementia patients. Drug-induced **Parkinson's syndrome** occurs often. Discontinuation usually resolves symptoms but may take weeks to months (12+) to clear. **Akathisia** is the most common EPS reaction in elderly. The symptoms of motor restlessness are difficult to diagnose in demented elderly; increased nervousness, assertiveness, restlessness with constant movement may indicate this adverse event. Consider decreasing dose if antipsychotic to treat as well as diagnose problem; usually see this reaction within 2-3 months of initiating antipsychotic drug.

Anticholinergic effects: These side effects most common with low potency antipsychotics (eg, thioridazine, chlorpromazine). CNS toxicity occurs more frequently and severely in elderly; increased confusion, memory loss, psychotic behavior, and agitation frequently occur as a consequence of anticholinergic effects to antipsychotic agents. Peripheral anticholinergic action troublesome to elderly; most peripheral anticholinergic effects last only 2-3 weeks; see Adverse Reactions.

Orthostatic hypotension: More common with low potency agents (eg, thioridazine, chlorpromazine, and clozapine) but of concern with all antipsychotic agents; orthostasis due to alpha-receptor blockade by antipsychotic agents. Elderly present many risk factors for orthostatic hypotension: blunted baroreceptor reflexes, decreased vascular tone, decreased vascular volume, and possible presence of cardiac diseases which result in decreased cardiac output.

Sedation: Common side effect with antipsychotic therapy; should not be used as a hypnotic unless insomnia is associated with target behavior symptoms treated with antipsychotic medications; see Special Geriatric Considerations. Anecdotal reports suggesting antipsychotic sedation in nonpsychotic patients is extremely unpleasant due to feelings of depersonalization, derealization, and dysphoria. Due to the long duration of action with antipsychotic drugs, these reactions may last up to 24 hours and result in decreased daytime function.

Cardiac toxicity: Life-threatening arrhythmias have occurred at therapeutic doses of antipsychotics. Thioridazine more commonly demonstrates EKG changes than other antipsychotics; suggested to use high potency antipsychotic agents (ie, haloperidol) in patients with cardiac conduction defects.

Precautions Use with caution in patients with cardiovascular disease, seizures, and Parkinson's disease; benefits of therapy must be weighed against risks of therapy

Adverse Reactions

Cardiovascular: Orthostatic hypotension, tachycardia, arrhythmias, abnormal T waves with prolonged ventricular repolarization, EKG changes

Central nervous system: Sedation, drowsiness, restlessness, anxiety, extrapyramidal reactions, pseudoparkinsonian signs and symptoms, tardive dyskinesia, neuroleptic malignant syndrome, seizures, altered central temperature regulation

Dermatologic: Hyperpigmentation, pruritus, rash, photosensitivity

Endocrine & metabolic: Amenorrhea, galactorrhea, gynecomastia

Gastrointestinal: GI upset, dry mouth (problem for denture users), constipation, adynamic ileus, weight gain

Genitourinary: Urinary retention, overflow incontinence, priapism, sexual dysfunction (up to 60%), impotence

Hematologic: Agranulocytosis, leukopenia (usually in patients with large doses for prolonged periods), thrombocytopenia, hemolytic anemia, eosinophilia

Hepatic: Cholestatic jaundice (rare)

Ocular: Retinal pigmentation, blurred vision

Miscellaneous: Anaphylactoid reactions

Sedation and anticholinergic effects are more pronounced than extrapyramidal effects

Overdosage Symptoms of overdose include deep sleep, coma, extrapyramidal symptoms, abnormal involuntary muscle movements, hypotension or hypertension; agitation, restlessness, fever, hypothermia or hyperthermia, seizures, cardiac arrhythmias, EKG changes

Toxicology Following initiation of essential overdose management, toxic symptom treatment and supportive treatment should be initiated. Hypotension usually responds to I.V. fluids or Trendelenburg positioning. If unresponsive to these measures the use of a parenteral inotrope may be required (eg, norepinephrine 0.1-0.2 mcg/minute titrated to response). Do not use epinephrine. Seizures commonly respond to diazepam (I.V. 5-10 mg bolus every 15 minutes if needed up to a total of 30 mg) or to phenytoin or phenobarbital. Also critical cardiac arrhythmias often respond to I.V. phenytoin (15 mg/kg up to 1 g), while other antiarrhythmics can be used. Neuroleptics often cause extrapyramidal symptoms (eg, dystonic reactions) requiring management with diphenhydramine 1-2 mg/kg up to a maximum of 50 mg I.M. or I.V. slow push followed by a maintenance dose for 48-72 hours. When these reactions are unresponsive to diphenhydramine, benztropine mesylate I.V. 1-2 mg may be effective. These agents are generally effective within 2-5 minutes.

Drug Interactions

Alcohol may increase CNS sedation

Anticholinergic agents may decrease pharmacologic effects; increase anticholinergic side effects; may enhance tardive dyskinesia

Aluminum salts may decrease absorption of phenothiazines

Barbiturates may decrease phenothiazine serum concentrations

Bromocriptine may have decreased efficacy when administered with phenothiazines

Guanethidine's hypotensive effect is decreased by phenothiazines

Lithium administration with phenothiazines may increase disorientation

Meperidine and phenothiazine coadministration increases sedation and hypotension

Methyldopa administration with phenothiazine (trifluoperazine) may significantly increase blood pressure

Norepinephrine, epinephrine have decreased pressor effect when administered with chlorpromazine; therefore, be aware of possible decreased effectiveness or when any phenothiazine is used

Phenytoin serum concentrations may increase or decrease with phenothiazines; tricyclic antidepressants may have increased serum concentrations with concomitant administration with phenothiazines

(Continued)

Mesoridazine Besylate *(Continued)*

Propranolol administered with phenothiazines may increase serum concentrations of both drugs

Valproic acid may have increased half-life when administered with phenothiazines (chlorpromazine)

Stability Protect all dosage forms from light, clear or slightly yellow solutions may be used; should be dispensed in amber or opaque vials/bottles. Solutions may be diluted or mixed with fruit juices or other liquids but must be administered immediately after mixing; do not prepare bulk dilutions or store bulk dilutions.

Mechanism of Action Blocks postsynaptic mesolimbic dopaminergic D_1 and D_2 receptors in the brain; exhibits a strong alpha-adrenergic blocking and anticholinergic effect, depresses the release of hypothalamic and hypophyseal hormones; believed to depress the reticular activating system thus affecting basal metabolism, body temperature, wakefulness, vasomotor tone, and emesis

Pharmacokinetics

Absorption: Oral: May be affected by the inherent anticholinergic action on the gastrointestinal tissue causing variable absorption. Absorption from tablets is erratic with less variation seen with solutions. These agents are widely distributed in tissues with CNS concentrations exceeding that of plasma due to their lipophilic characteristics.

Protein binding: Antipsychotic agents are bound 90% to 99% to plasma proteins; highly bound to brain and lung tissue and other tissues with a high blood perfusion

Half-life: Elimination half-lives of antipsychotics range from 20-40 hours which may be extended in elderly due to decline in oxidative hepatic reactions (phase I) with age

Time to peak: Peak concentrations between 2-4 hours

Elimination: Excretion occurs through hepatic metabolism (oxidation) where numerous active metabolites are produced; active metabolites excreted in urine

The biologic effect of a single dose persists for 24 hours. When the patient has accommodated to initial side effects (sedation), once daily dosing is possible due to the long half-life of antipsychotics.

Steady-state plasma levels are achieved in 4-7 days; therefore, if possible, do not make dose adjustments more than once in a 7-day period. Due to the long half-lives of antipsychotics, as needed (PRN) use is ineffective since repeated doses are necessary to achieve therapeutic tissue concentrations in the CNS.

Usual Dosage

Geriatrics (nonpsychotic patients, dementia behavior): Oral: Initial: 10 mg 1-2 times/day; if <10 mg/day desires, consider administering 10 mg every other day (qod); increase dose at 4- to 7-day intervals by 10-25 mg/day; increase dose intervals (bid, tid, etc) as necessary to control response or side effects; maximum daily dose: 250 mg; gradual increases (titration) may prevent some side effects or decrease their severity

Geriatrics and Adults: I.M.: Initial: 25 mg; repeat doses in 30-60 minutes if necessary; dose range: 25-200 mg/day. Elderly usually require less than maximal daily dose.

Adults: Oral: Initial: 25 mg for most patients; may repeat dose in 30-60 minutes, if necessary; usual optimum dosage range: 25-200 mg/day. Concentrate may be diluted just prior to administration with distilled water, acidified tap water, orange or grape juice; do not prepare and store bulk dilutions.

Not dialyzable (0% to 5%)

Monitoring Parameters Orthostatic blood pressures; tremors, gait changes, abnormal movement in trunk, neck, buccal area or extremities; monitor target behaviors for which the agent is given

Test Interactions Increased cholesterol (S), increased glucose; decreased uric acid (S)

Patient Information Oral concentrate must be diluted in 2-4 oz of liquid (water, fruit juice, carbonated drinks, milk, or pudding); do not take antacid within 1 hour of taking drug; avoid alcohol; avoid excess sun exposure (use sun block); may cause drowsiness, rise slowly from recumbent position; use of supportive stockings may help prevent orthostatic hypotension

Nursing Implications Watch for hypotension when administering I.M. or I.V.; dilute the oral concentrate with water or juice before administration; avoid skin contact with oral solution; may cause contact dermatitis; monitor orthostatic blood pressures 3-5 days after initiation of therapy or a dose increase; observe for tremor and abnormal movement or posturing (extrapyramidal symptoms)

Special Geriatric Considerations See Warnings

Many elderly patients receive antipsychotic medications for inappropriate nonpsychotic behavior. Before initiating antipsychotic medication, the clinician should investigate any possible reversible cause; any stress or stress from any disease can cause acute "confusion" or worsening of baseline nonpsychotic behavior. Most commonly acute changes in behavior are due to increases in drug dose or addition of new drug to regimen; fluid electrolyte loss; infections; and changes in environment.

Any changes in disease status in any organ system can result in behavior changes.

Dosage Forms

Injection: 25 mg/mL (1 mL)

Liquid: 25 mg/mL

Tablet: 10 mg, 25 mg, 50 mg

Mestinon® *see* Pyridostigmine Bromide *on page 612*

Metacortandralone *see* Prednisolone *on page 584*

Metamucil® [OTC] *see* Psyllium *on page 610*

Metamucil® Instant Mix [OTC] *see* Psyllium *on page 610*

Metaprel® *see* Metaproterenol Sulfate *on this page*

Metaproterenol Sulfate (met a proe ter' e nol)

Brand Names Alupent®; Arm-a-Med® Metaproterenol; Dey-Dose® Metaproterenol; Metaprel®; Prometa®

Synonyms Orciprenaline Sulfate

Generic Available Yes (except inhaler)

Therapeutic Class Adrenergic Agonist Agent; Beta-2-Adrenergic Agonist Agent; Bronchodilator

Use Bronchodilator in reversible airway obstruction due to asthma or COPD

Contraindications Hypersensitivity to metaproterenol or any component; pre-existing cardiac arrhythmias associated with tachycardia

Warnings Use caution in patients with unstable vasomotor symptoms, diabetes, hyperthyroidism, prostatic hypertrophy, or a history of seizures; also use caution in the elderly and those patients with cardiovascular disorders such as coronary artery disease, arrhythmias, and hypertension

Precautions Excessive use may result in tolerance; deaths have been reported after excessive use; though the exact cause is unknown, cardiac arrest after a severe asthmatic crisis is suspected

Adverse Reactions
Cardiovascular: Tachycardia, palpitations, elevation or depression of blood pressure
Central nervous system: Nervousness, CNS stimulation, hyperactivity, insomnia
Gastrointestinal: GI upset
Neuromuscular & skeletal: Tremors (may be more common in the elderly)

Overdosage Symptoms of overdose include tremor, dizziness, nervousness, headache, nausea, coughing, seizures, angina, hypertension

Toxicology In cases of overdose, supportive therapy should be instituted, and prudent use of a cardioselective beta-adrenergic blocker (eg, atenolol or metoprolol) should be considered, keeping in mind the potential for induction of bronchoconstriction in an asthmatic individual. Dialysis has not been shown to be of value in the treatment of an overdose with this agent.

Drug Interactions
Decreased therapeutic effect: Beta-adrenergic blockers (eg, propranolol)
Increased therapeutic effect: Inhaled ipratropium → ↑ duration of bronchodilation, nifedipine → ↑ FEV-1
Increased toxicity (cardiovascular): MAO inhibitors, tricyclic antidepressants, sympathomimetic agents (eg, amphetamine, dopamine, dobutamine), inhaled anesthetics (eg, enflurane)

Stability Store in tight, light-resistant container

Mechanism of Action Relaxes bronchial smooth muscle by action on beta$_2$-receptors with little effect on heart rate

Pharmacodynamics
Onset of action: Oral: Bronchodilation occurs within 15 minutes; following inhalation these effects occur within 5 minutes
Peak effect: Within 1 hour
Duration of action: Similar (~3-4 hours) regardless of route administered

Pharmacokinetics
Absorption: Oral: 40% from GI tract
Metabolism: In the liver
Elimination: Via kidneys as metabolites

Usual Dosage
Oral:
Geriatrics: Initial: 10 mg 3-4 times/day increasing as necessary up to 20 mg 3-4 times/day
Adults: 20 mg 3-4 times/day

Nebulizer: Geriatrics and Adults: 5-20 breaths of full strength 5% metaproterenol **or** 0.2-0.3 mL of 5% metaproterenol in 2.5-3 mL normal saline nebulized every 4-6 hours (can be given more frequently according to need)

Inhalation, metered dose: Geriatrics and Adults: 2-3 inhalations every 3-4 hours to a maximum of 12 inhalations/day

Monitoring Parameters Pulmonary function, blood pressure, pulse

Patient Information Do not exceed recommended dosage – excessive use may lead to adverse effects or loss of effectiveness. Follow instructions accompanying inhaler. If more than one inhalation per dose is necessary, wait at least 1 full minute between

(Continued)

Metaproterenol Sulfate *(Continued)*

inhalations – second inhalation is best delivered after 10 minutes for Alupent®. May cause nervousness, restlessness, insomnia – if these effects continue after dosage reduction, notify physician. Also notify physician if palpitations, tachycardia, chest pain, muscle tremors, dizziness, headache, flushing or if breathing difficulty persists.

Nursing Implications Before using, the inhaler must be shaken well; assess lung sounds, pulse, and blood pressure before administration and during peak of medication; observe patient for wheezing after administration, if this occurs, call physician

Additional Information Metaproterenol has more beta₁ activity than other sympathomimetics such as albuterol and, therefore, may no longer be the beta agonist of first choice

Special Geriatric Considerations See Additional Information. The elderly may find it useful to utilize a spacer device when using a metered dose inhaler. Oral use should be avoided due to the increased incidence of adverse effects.

Dosage Forms
Aerosol: 0.65 mg/dose (15 mL)
Solution, inhalation: 0.4% (2.5 mL); 0.6% (2.5 mL); 5% (10 mL, 30 mL)
Syrup: 10 mg/5 mL (480 mL)
Tablet: 10 mg, 20 mg

Methadone Hydrochloride (meth' a done)

Related Information
Narcotic Agonist Comparative Pharmacology *on page 811*
Pharmacokinetics of Narcotic Agonist Analgesics *on page 812*
Brand Names Dolophine®; Methadose®
Generic Available Yes
Therapeutic Class Analgesic, Narcotic
Use Management of severe pain, used in narcotic detoxification maintenance programs
Restrictions C-II
Contraindications Hypersensitivity to methadone or any component
Warnings Tablets are to be used only for oral administration and **must not** be used for injection
Precautions Cumulative effect of methadone, dose and frequency should be titrated for optimal response
Adverse Reactions
Cardiovascular: Palpitations, hypotension, bradycardia, peripheral vasodilation
Central nervous system: CNS depression, increased intracranial pressure
Dermatologic: Pruritus
Endocrine & metabolic: Antidiuretic hormone release
Gastrointestinal: Nausea, vomiting, constipation
Ocular: Miosis
Respiratory: Respiratory depression
Miscellaneous: Physical and psychological dependence, histamine release, biliary or urinary tract spasm
Overdosage Symptoms of overdose include respiratory depression, CNS depression, miosis, hypothermia, circulatory collapse, convulsions
Toxicology Naloxone 2 mg I.V. with repeat administration as necessary up to a total of 10 mg
Drug Interactions
Decreased effect with phenytoin (increased withdrawal), rifampin (→ withdrawal), pentazocine (→ withdrawal)
Increased effect/toxicity with CNS depressants, phenothiazines, TCAs, MAO inhibitors
Mechanism of Action Binds to opiate receptors in the CNS, causing inhibition of ascending pain pathways, altering the perception of and response to pain; produces generalized CNS depression
Pharmacodynamics
Onset of action:
Oral: Within 30-60 minutes
Parenteral: Within 10-20 minutes
Duration: Oral: 6-8 hours; after repeated oral doses, duration of effect increases to 22-48 hours; enhanced analgesia has been seen in elderly patients on therapeutic doses of narcotics; duration of action may be increased in the elderly
Peak effects: Within 1-2 hours
Pharmacokinetics
Protein binding: 80% to 85%
Metabolism: Liver metabolism (N-demethylation)
Half-life:
Elderly: >36 hours
Adults: 15-29 hours, half-life may be prolonged with alkaline pH
Elimination: In urine (<10% as unchanged drug); increased renal excretion with urine pH <6

Usual Dosage Doses should be titrated to appropriate effects:
Geriatrics: Oral, I.M.: 2.5 mg every 8-12 hours

Adults: Analgesia: Oral, I.M., I.V., S.C.: 2.5-10 mg every 3-8 hours as needed, up to 5-20 mg every 6-8 hours

Dosing interval in renal impairment:
Cl_{cr} >50 mL/minute: Administer every 6 hours
Cl_{cr} 10-50 mL/minute: Administer every 8 hours
Cl_{cr} <10 mL/minute: Administer every 8-12 hours

Monitoring Parameters Pain relief, respiratory and mental status, blood pressure

Reference Range Therapeutic: 100-400 ng/mL (SI: 0.32-1.29 μmol/L); Toxic: >2 μg/mL (SI: >6.46 μmol/L)

Test Interactions Increased thyroxine (S), increased aminotransferase [ALT (SGPT)/ AST (SGOT)] (S)

Patient Information May cause drowsiness, avoid alcohol and other CNS depressants

Nursing Implications Observe patient for excessive sedation, respiratory depression, implement safety measures, assist with ambulation

Special Geriatric Considerations Because of its long half-life and risk of accumulation, methadone is not considered a drug of first choice in the elderly; the elderly may be particularly susceptible to the CNS depressant and constipating effects of narcotics; see Usual Dosage; adjust dose for renal function

Dosage Forms
Injection: 10 mg/mL (1 mL, 10 mL, 20 mL)
Solution:
Oral: 5 mg/5 mL (5 mL, 500 mL); 10 mg/5 mL (500 mL)
Oral, concentrate: 10 mg,mL (30 mL)
Tablet: 5 mg, 10 mg

References
Ferrell BA, "Pain Management in Elderly People," *J Am Geriatr Soc*, 1991, 39(1):64-73.

Methadose® *see* Methadone Hydrochloride *on previous page*

Methaminodiazepoxide Hydrochloride *see* Chlordiazepoxide *on page 149*

Methazolamide (meth a zoe' la mide)
Related Information
Glaucoma Drug Therapy Comparison *on page 810*

Brand Names Neptazane®

Generic Available No

Therapeutic Class Carbonic Anhydrase Inhibitor; Diuretic, Carbonic Anhydrase Inhibitor

Use Adjunctive treatment of open-angle or secondary glaucoma; short-term therapy of narrow-angle glaucoma when delay of surgery is desired

Contraindications Marked kidney or liver dysfunction, severe pulmonary obstruction, hypersensitivity to methazolamide or any component

Precautions Sulfonamide-type reactions, melena, anorexia, nausea, vomiting, constipation, hematuria, glycosuria, urinary frequency, renal colic, renal calculi, crystalluria, polyuria, hepatic insufficiency, various CNS effects, transient myopia, bone marrow depression, thrombocytopenia/purpura, hemolytic anemia, leukopenia, pancytopenia, agranulocytosis, urticaria, pruritus, rash, Stevens-Johnson syndrome, weight loss, fever, acidosis

Adverse Reactions
Central nervous system: Paresthesias, fever, depression, drowsiness, dizziness, malaise
Dermatologic: Rash
Endocrine & metabolic: Hyperchloremic metabolic acidosis, hypokalemia
Gastrointestinal: GI irritation, anorexia
Genitourinary: Increased urination
Hematologic: Bone marrow suppression
Renal: Crystalluria, dysuria

Drug Interactions Increased lithium excretion and altered excretion of other drugs by alkalinization of the urine, such as amphetamines, quinidine, procainamide, methenamine, phenobarbital, salicylates; hypokalemia may be compounded with concurrent diuretic use or steroids; primidone absorption may be delayed; digitalis toxicity may occur if hypokalemia is untreated

Mechanism of Action Reversible inhibition of the enzyme carbonic anhydrase resulting in decreased intraocular pressure; noncompetitive inhibition of the enzyme carbonic anhydrase; thought that carbonic anhydrase is located at the luminal border of cells of the proximal tubule. When the enzyme is inhibited, there is an increase in urine volume and a change to an alkaline pH with a subsequent decrease in the excretion of titratable acid and ammonia.

(Continued)

451

Methazolamide *(Continued)*

Pharmacodynamics
Onset of action: 2-4 hours
Peak effect: 6-8 hours
Duration: 10-18 hours

Pharmacokinetics
Absorption: Slow from GI tract
Distribution: Well into tissue
Protein binding: ~55%
Half-life: ~14 hours
Elimination: ~25% excreted unchanged in urine

Usual Dosage Geriatrics and Adults: Oral: 50-100 mg 2-3 times/day

Monitoring Parameters Intraocular pressure, potassium, serum bicarbonate, sodium

Test Interactions Increased chloride (S)

Patient Information Take with food; ability to perform tasks requiring mental alertness and/or physical coordination may be impaired; report numbness or tingling of extremities to physician

Nursing Implications May cause an alteration in taste, especially when drinking carbonated beverages

Special Geriatric Considerations Malaise and complaints of tiredness and myalgia are signs of excessive dosing and acidosis in the elderly

Dosage Forms Tablet: 25 mg, 50 mg

Methenamine *(meth en' a meen)*

Brand Names Hiprex®; Mandelamine®; Urex®; Urised®

Synonyms Hexamethylenetetramine

Generic Available Yes

Therapeutic Class Antibiotic, Miscellaneous

Use Prophylaxis or suppression of recurrent urinary tract infections; urinary tract discomfort secondary to hypermotility

Contraindications Severe dehydration, renal insufficiency, hepatic insufficiency in patients receiving hippurate salt, hypersensitivity to methenamine or any component

Warnings Doses ≥8 g/day for prolonged periods may lead to bladder irritation, dysuria, and frequent micturition; an acidic urine (pH ≤6) must be present or the drug will not be effective; methenamine mandelate suspensions have a vegetable oil base which if aspirated may result in a lipid pneumonitis

Precautions Patients with liver dysfunction should have periodic liver function tests; gout (precipitation of uric acid crystals in the urine)

Adverse Reactions
Central nervous system: Headache
Dermatologic: Rash, pruritus
Gastrointestinal: Nausea, vomiting, diarrhea, abdominal cramping, anorexia
Genitourinary: Hematuria, bladder irritation
Hepatic: Elevation in AST and ALT
Renal: Dysuria, crystalluria

Toxicology Well tolerated GI decontamination and supportive care

Drug Interactions Sulfonamides (may precipitate); sodium bicarbonate and acetazolamide will decrease effect secondary to alkalinization of urine

Stability Protect from excessive heat

Mechanism of Action Methenamine is hydrolyzed to formaldehyde and ammonia in acidic urine; formaldehyde has nonspecific bactericidal action

Pharmacokinetics
Absorption: Readily from GI tract; 10% to 30% of drug will be hydrolyzed by gastric juices unless it is protected by an enteric coating
Metabolism: ~10% to 25% is metabolized in the liver
Half-life: 3-6 hours
Elimination: Occurs via glomerular filtration and tubular secretion with ~70% to 90% of dose excreted unchanged in urine within 24 hours

Usual Dosage Geriatrics and Adults: Oral:
Hippurate: 1 g twice daily
Mandelate: 1 g 4 times/day after meals and at bedtime
Must be accompanied by 1 g of ascorbic acid (vitamin C) 4 times (or more)/day

Monitoring Parameters Urinalysis, periodic liver function tests in patients, temperature

Test Interactions False increase in catecholamines, vanillylmandelic acid, and 17-hydroxycorticosteroids in urine; false decrease in 5-hydroxyindoleacetic acid

Patient Information Take with ascorbic acid to acidify urine and avoid intake of alkalinizing agents (sodium bicarbonate, antacids); take with food to minimize GI upset; drink plenty of fluids to ensure adequate urine flow; complete full course of therapy; notify physician of rash or if side effects persist or are bothersome

Nursing Implications Give around-the-clock to promote less variation in peak and trough serum levels

Additional Information Hippurate salt should not be used to treat infections outside of the lower urinary tract

Special Geriatric Considerations See Warnings; methenamine has little, if any, role in the treatment or prevention of infections in patients with indwelling urinary (Foley®) catheters; furthermore, in noncatheterized patients, more effective antibiotics are available for the prevention or treatment of urinary tract infections; the influence of decreased renal function on the pharmacologic effects of methenamine results are unknown

Dosage Forms

Granules (orange flavor): 1 g (56s)

Suspension, oral, as mandelate (Mandelamine®): 250 mg/5 mL (coconut flavor), 500 mg/5 mL (cherry flavor)

Tablet, as hippurate (Hiprex®, Urex®): 1 g (Hiprex® contains tartrazine dye)

Tablet, as mandelate, enteric coated (Mandelamine®): 250 mg, 500 mg, 1 g

References

Vainrub B and Musher DM, "Lack of Effect of Methenamine in Suppression of, or Prophylaxis Against, Chronic Urinary Tract Infection," *Antimicrob Agents Chemother*, 1977, 12:625-9.

Methicillin Sodium (meth i sill' in)

Brand Names Staphcillin®

Synonyms Dimethoxyphenyl Penicillin Sodium; Sodium Methicillin

Therapeutic Class Antibiotic, Penicillin

Use Treatment of susceptible bacterial infections such as osteomyelitis, septicemia, endocarditis, and CNS infections due to penicillinase-producing strains of *Staphylococcus*

Contraindications Known hypersensitivity to methicillin or any penicillin

Precautions Modify dosage in patients with renal impairment; use with caution in cephalosporin allergic patients

Adverse Reactions

Central nervous system: Fever

Dermatologic: Rash

Hematologic: Eosinophilia, anemia leukopenia, neutropenia, thrombocytopenia

Local: Phlebitis

Renal: Nephrotoxicity (interstitial nephritis), hemorrhagic cystitis

Miscellaneous: Serum sickness like reactions

Overdosage Symptoms of overdose include neuromuscular hypersensitivity, seizure

Toxicology Many beta-lactam-containing antibiotics have the potential to cause neuromuscular hyperirritability or convulsive seizures. Hemodialysis may be helpful to aid in the removal of the drug from the blood, otherwise most treatment is supportive or symptom directed.

Drug Interactions Probenecid may increase levels

Stability Reconstituted solution is stable for 24 hours at room temperature and 4 days when refrigerated; discard solutions if it has a distinctive hydrogen sulfide odor and/or color turns to a deep orange; incompatible with aminoglycosides and tetracyclines

Mechanism of Action Interferes with bacterial cell wall synthesis during active multiplication causing cell death and resultant bactericidal activity against susceptible bacteria

Pharmacokinetics

Protein binding: 40%

Half-life: Adults with normal renal function: 0.4-0.5 hours

Time to peak serum concentration:

I.M.: Within 30-60 minutes

I.V. infusion: Within 5 minutes

Elimination: ~60% to 70% of dose is eliminated unchanged in urine within 4 hours, by tubular secretion and glomerular filtration

Usual Dosage I.M., I.V.: Geriatrics and Adults: 4-12 g/day in divided doses every 4-6 hours

Dosing interval in renal impairment: Cl_{cr} <10 mL/minute: Do not exceed 2 g/12 hours

Not dialyzable (0% to 5%)

Administration Can be administered IVP at a rate not to exceed 200 mg/minute or intermittent infusion over 20-30 minutes; final concentration for administration should not exceed 20 mg/mL

Monitoring Parameters Renal function, signs and symptoms of infection, temperature

Test Interactions Positive Coombs' test [direct]

Nursing Implications See Administration

Special Geriatric Considerations Because of its greater potential for interstitial nephritis, methicillin is not the parenteral antistaphylococcal agent of choice; either nafcillin or oxacillin are preferred alternatives; adjust dose for renal function

Dosage Forms Injection: 1 g, 4 g, 6 g, 10 g

Methimazole (meth im' a zole)

Brand Names Tapazole®

Synonyms Thiamazole

Generic Available No

Therapeutic Class Antithyroid Agent

Use Palliative treatment of hyperthyroidism, to return the hyperthyroid patient to a normal metabolic state prior to thyroidectomy, and to control thyrotoxic crisis that may accompany thyroidectomy

Contraindications Hypersensitivity to methimazole or any component

Warnings Use of antithyroid drugs may cause agranulocytosis, thyroid, hyperplasia, thyroid carcinoma

Precautions Use with extreme caution in patients receiving other drugs known to cause agranulocytosis, patients >40 years of age; avoid doses >40 mg/day

Adverse Reactions

Cardiovascular: Edema, cutaneous vasculitis, periarteritis

Central nervous system: Headache, drowsiness, paresthesia, CNS stimulation, depression, neuritis, vertigo

Dermatologic: Rash, urticaria, pruritus, exfoliative dermatitis

Gastrointestinal: Nausea, vomiting, loss of taste

Hematologic: Aplastic anemia, agranulocytosis, thrombocytopenia, bleeding

Hepatic: Jaundice, hepatitis

Neuromuscular & skeletal: Arthralgia

Renal: Nephritis

Miscellaneous: Drug fever, lupus-like syndrome

Overdosage Symptoms of overdose include nausea, vomiting, arthralgia, pancytopenia, and signs of hypothyroidism

Toxicology General supportive care; monitor bone marrow response

Stability Protect from light

Mechanism of Action Inhibits the synthesis of thyroid hormones by blocking the oxidation of iodine in the thyroid gland, blocking iodine's ability to combine with tyrosine to form thyroxine and tri-iodothyronine (T_3); does not inactivate circulating T_4 and T_3

Pharmacodynamics

Onset of action: Oral: Within 30-40 minutes

Duration: 2-4 hours

Pharmacokinetics

Half-life: 4-13 hours

Elimination: Renally with ~12% excreted in urine within 24 hours and remainder hepatically metabolized

Usual Dosage Geriatrics and Adults: Oral: Initial: 15 mg/day (doses best given in divided doses at 8-hour intervals); more severe disease may require doses from 30-60 mg/day; maintenance: 5-15 mg/day

Monitoring Parameters Monitor signs of hypo- and hyperthyroidism, T_4, T_3, TSH, CBC

Test Interactions Increased prothrombin (S)

Patient Information Take with meals; do not exceed prescribed dosage; take at regular intervals around-the-clock; notify physician or pharmacist if fever, sore throat, unusual bleeding or bruising, headache, or general malaise occurs

Nursing Implications See Warnings, Precautions, Monitoring Parameters, and Special Geriatric Considerations

Additional Information Periodic blood counts are recommended with chronic therapy; see Warnings

Special Geriatric Considerations The use of antithyroid thioamides is as effective in elderly as they are in younger adults; however, the expense, potential adverse effects, and inconvenience (compliance, monitoring) make them undesirable. The use of radioiodine due to ease of administration and less concern for long-term side effects and reproduction problems (some older males) makes it a more appropriate therapy.

Dosage Forms Tablet: 5 mg, 10 mg

References

Johnson DG and Campbell S, "Hormonal and Metabolic Agents," *Geriatric Pharmacology*, Bressler R and Katz MD, eds, New York, NY: McGraw-Hill, 1993, 427-50.

Raby C, Lagorce JF, Jambut-Absil AC, et al, "The Mechanism of Action of Synthetic Antithyroid Drugs: Iodine Complexation During Oxidation of Iodide," *Endocrinology*, 1990, 126(3):1683-91.

Methocarbamol (meth oh kar' ba mole)

Brand Names Delaxin®; Marbaxin®; Robaxin®; Robomol®

Generic Available Yes

Therapeutic Class Skeletal Muscle Relaxant

Use Treatment of muscle spasm associated with acute painful musculoskeletal conditions; supportive therapy in tetanus

Contraindications Renal impairment (I.V. only), hypersensitivity to methocarbamol or any component

Precautions Do not exceed 3 g/day I.V./I.M. for more than 3 consecutive days except in the treatment of tetanus; use I.V. form cautiously in epileptic patients

Adverse Reactions I.V. only: In excessive doses, renal impairment has occurred due to the polyethylene glycol base

Cardiovascular: Syncope, hypotension, bradycardia
Central nervous system: Lightheadedness, dizziness, drowsiness, seizures (I.V. only)
Gastrointestinal: Nausea
Ocular: Conjunctivitis, blurred vision
Renal: Renal impairment
Respiratory: Nasal congestion (I.V. only)
Miscellaneous: Allergic manifestations

Overdosage Symptoms of overdose include CNS depression, coma

Toxicology Treatment is supportive following attempts to enhance drug elimination. Hypotension should be treated with I.V. fluids and/or Trendelenburg positioning. Dialysis and hemoperfusion and osmotic diuresis have all been useful in reducing serum drug concentrations. The patient should be observed for possible relapses due to incomplete gastric emptying.

Drug Interactions Increased effect/toxicity: Alcohol, CNS depressants

Mechanism of Action Causes skeletal muscle relaxation by reducing the transmission of impulses from the spinal cord to skeletal muscle

Pharmacodynamics Onset of action: Oral: Muscle relaxation reportedly occurs within 30 minutes

Pharmacokinetics
Metabolism: In the liver
Half-life: 1-2 hours
Time to peak serum concentration: ~2 hours
Elimination: Renal

Usual Dosage
Geriatrics: Oral: 500 mg 4 times/day
Adults: Muscle spasm:
Oral: 1.5 g 4 times/day for 2-3 days, then decrease to 4-4.5 g/day in 3-6 divided doses
I.M., I.V.: 1 g every 8 hours if oral not possible for a maximum of 3 days

Administration
I.M. administration: No more than 500 mg (5 mL)/dose should be injected in each gluteal region
I.V. administration: Infuse over 3-4 hours or give IVP no faster than 300 mg/minute

Monitoring Parameters Relief of symptoms, mental status; blood pressure, pulse in I.V. administration

Patient Information May cause drowsiness, impair judgment or coordination; avoid alcohol or other CNS depressants; may turn urine brown, black, or green; notify physician of rash, itching, or nasal congestion

Nursing Implications See Administration; the parenteral form is hypertonic and causes irritation; avoid extravasation. During the infusion, the patient should be recumbent to minimize adverse reactions; patient should remain recumbent for 15 minutes after the end of the infusion.

Special Geriatric Considerations There is no specific information on the use of skeletal muscle relaxants in the elderly. Methocarbamol has a short half-life, so it may be considered one of the safer agents in this class.

Dosage Forms
Injection: 100 mg/mL (10 mL)
Tablet: 500 mg, 750 mg

Methoin see Mephenytoin on page 442

Methotrexate (meth oh trex' ate)
Related Information
Drug Levels Commonly Monitored Guidelines on page 771-772
Brand Names Folex®; Folex® PFS; Mexate®; Rheumatrex®
Synonyms Amethopterin; MTX
Generic Available Yes
Therapeutic Class Antineoplastic Agent, Antimetabolite
Use Treatment of trophoblastic neoplasms, leukemias, psoriasis, rheumatoid arthritis, osteosarcoma, non-Hodgkin's lymphoma, breast cancer, lung cancer
Contraindications Hypersensitivity to methotrexate or any component; severe renal or hepatic impairment; pre-existing profound bone marrow depression in patients with psoriasis or rheumatoid arthritis; alcoholism, alcoholic liver disease; AIDS, pre-existing blood dyscrasia
Warnings The U.S. Food and Drug Administration (FDA) currently recommends that procedures for proper handling and disposal of antineoplastic agents be considered. Because of the possibility of severe toxic reactions, fully inform patient of the risks involved; may cause hepatotoxicity, fibrosis and cirrhosis, along with marked bone marrow depression; death from intestinal perforation may occur

(Continued)
455

Methotrexate *(Continued)*

Precautions May cause photosensitivity type reaction; reduce dosage in patients with renal or hepatic impairment, ascites, and pleural effusion; use with caution in patients with peptic ulcer disease, ulcerative colitis, pre-existing bone marrow suppression and immunodeficiency syndrome

Adverse Reactions
Cardiovascular: Vasculitis
Central nervous system: Malaise, fatigue, fever, chills, dizziness, encephalopathy, headaches, seizures, confusion
Dermatologic: Alopecia, rash, photosensitivity, depigmentation or hyperpigmentation of skin
Endocrine & metabolic: Rarely diabetes
Gastrointestinal: Ulcerative stomatitis, nausea, abdominal distress, vomiting, diarrhea, anorexia, stomatitis, enteritis
Hematologic: Leukopenia, myelosuppression, anemia, hemorrhage
Hepatic: Hepatotoxicity
Neuromuscular & skeletal: Rarely arthralgia
Ocular: Blurred vision
Renal: Renal failure, cystitis
Miscellaneous: Decreased resistance to infection, rarely anaphylaxis

Overdosage Symptoms of overdose include bone marrow depression, nausea, vomiting, alopecia, melena, diarrhea

Toxicology Antidote: Leucovorin. Leucovorin should be administered as soon as toxicity is seen; administer 10 mg/m² orally or parenterally; follow with 10 mg/m² orally every 6 hours for 72 hours. After 24 hours following methotrexate administration, if the serum creatinine is ≥50% premethotrexate serum creatinine, increase leucovorin dose to 100 mg/m² every 3 hours until serum MTX level is <5 x 10⁻⁸M. Hydration and alkalinization may be used to prevent precipitation of MTX or MTX metabolites in the renal tubules. Toxicity in low dose range is negligible, but may present mucositis and mild bone marrow suppression.

Drug Interactions Nonsteroidal anti-inflammatory drugs (NSAIDs) and salicylates (may suppress MTX's clearance), sulfonamides, live virus vaccines, pyrimethamine, phenytoin, 5-FU; probenecid decreased renal elimination of MTX; phenytoin serum concentrations may decrease

Stability Store intact vials at room temperature; intrathecal solutions should be diluted immediately prior to use; reconstituted solutions remain stable for 4 weeks at room temperature and 3 months when refrigerated; protect from light

Mechanism of Action An antimetabolite that inhibits DNA synthesis and cell reproduction in cancerous cells; interferes with the conversion of folic acid to tetrahydrofolic acid by binding to the enzyme dihydrofolate reductase

Pharmacokinetics
Absorption: Oral: Rapid; well absorbed orally at low doses (<30 mg/m²); incomplete absorption after large doses; completely absorbed after I.M. injection
Protein binding: 50%; does not achieve therapeutic concentrations in the CSF; sustained concentrations are retained in the kidney and liver
Half-life: 8-15 hours with high doses (>30 mg/m²) and 3-10 hours with low doses (<30 mg/m²)
Time to peak: Peak serum levels occur within 1-2 hours; peak serum levels occur 30-60 minutes after parenteral injection
Elimination: Small amounts excreted in feces; primarily excreted in urine (90%) via glomerular filtration and active transport

Usual Dosage Refer to individual protocols
Geriatrics:
Rheumatoid arthritis/psoriasis: Initial: 5 mg once weekly; if nausea occurs, split dose to 2.5 mg every 12 hours for the day of administration; dose may be increased to 7.5 mg/week based upon response; not to exceed 20 mg/week
Neoplastic disease: Refer to specific disease protocols

Adults:
Trophoblastic neoplasms: Oral, I.M.: 15-30 mg/day for 5 days, repeat in 7 days for 3-5 courses; creatinine clearance must be >60 mL/minute before starting therapy
Rheumatoid arthritis: Oral: 7.5 mg once weekly or 2.5 mg every 12 hours for 3 doses/week; not to exceed 20 mg/week

Dosing interval in renal impairment:
Cl_cr 10-50 mL/minute: Reduce dose 50%
Cl_cr <10 mL/minute: Avoid use
Not dialyzable (0% to 5%)

Monitoring Parameters For prolonged use (especially rheumatoid arthritis, psoriasis) a baseline liver biopsy, repeated at each 1-1.5 g cumulative dose interval, should be performed. WBC and platelet counts every 4 weeks; CBC and creatinine, LFTs every 3-4 months; chest x-ray

Reference Range Therapeutic range is dependent upon therapeutic approach. "High-dose" regimens produce drug levels between 10⁻⁶M and 10⁻⁷M 24-72 hours after drug infusion. Toxic: low-dose therapy: >9.1 ng/mL (SI: >20 nmol/L); high-dose therapy: >454 ng/mL (SI: >1000 nmol/L).

Test Interactions Increased potassium (S)

Patient Information Any signs of infection (fever, chills, sore throat), easy bruising or bleeding, shortness of breath, black tarry stools, yellow discoloration of skin or eyes, bloody or dark urine, joint pain, swelling, or painful or burning urination should be brought to physician's attention. Nausea, vomiting, or hair loss sometimes occur. Food may delay absorption; take on empty stomach; avoid alcohol, prolonged sun exposure; may cause loss of appetite.

Nursing Implications For intrathecal use, mix methotrexate without preservative with Elliott's B solution to concentration no greater than 2 mg/mL; see Patient Information and Monitoring Parameters

Additional Information
Myelosuppressive effects:
WBC: Mild
Platelets: Moderate
Onset (days): 7
Nadir (days): 10
Recovery (days): 21
Sodium content of 100 mg injection: 20 mg (0.86 mEq)
Sodium content of 100 mg (low sodium) injection: 15 mg (0.65 mEq)

Special Geriatric Considerations Toxicity to methotrexate or any immunosuppressive is increased in elderly. Must monitor carefully. For rheumatoid arthritis and psoriasis, immunosuppressive therapy should only be used when disease is active and less toxic, traditional therapy is ineffective. Recommended doses should be reduced when initiating therapy in elderly due to possible decreased metabolism, reduced renal function, and presence of interacting diseases and drugs.

Dosage Forms
Injection, as sodium: 2.5 mg/mL (2 mL); 25 mg/mL (2 mL, 4 mL, 8 mL)
Injection, as sodium, preservative free: 25 mg (2 mL, 4 mL, 8 mL)
Powder, for injection, as sodium: 20 mg, 25 mg, 50 mg, 100 mg, 250 mg, 1 g
Tablet: 2.5 mg
Tablet, dose pack: 2.5 mg (4 cards with 3 tablets each)

References
Hutchins LF and Lipschitz DA, "Cancer, Clinical Pharmacology, and Aging," *Clin Geriatr Med*, 1987, 3(3):483-503.
Kaplan HG, "Use of Cancer Chemotherapy in the Elderly," *Drug Treatment in the Elderly*, Vestal RE, ed, Boston, MA: ADIS Health Science Press, 1984, 338-49.

Methsuximide (meth sux' i mide)

Brand Names Celontin®

Generic Available No

Therapeutic Class Anticonvulsant, Succinimide

Use Control of absence (petit mal) seizures; useful adjunct in refractory, partial complex (psychomotor) seizures

Contraindications Known hypersensitivity to methsuximide or other succinimides

Warnings Blood dyscrasias have occurred; can cause hepatic and renal dysfunction; may result in drug-induced lupus erythematosus

Precautions Use with caution in patients with hepatic or renal disease; avoid abrupt withdrawal of methsuximide; succinimides may exacerbate grand mal seizures

Adverse Reactions
Central nervous system: Drowsiness, ataxia, dizziness, nervousness, headache, insomnia, lethargy, mental confusion, depression, sleep disturbances, aggressiveness
Dermatologic: Urticaria, pruritic rash, Stevens-Johnson syndrome
Gastrointestinal: Gum hypertrophy, nausea, vomiting, abdominal pain, anorexia, diarrhea, constipation
Genitourinary: Urinary frequency
Hematologic: Eosinophilia, leukopenia, agranulocytosis, granulocytopenia, bone marrow suppression, pancytopenia, monocytosis
Ocular: Periorbital edema
Miscellaneous: Hiccups

Overdosage Symptoms of overdose include dizziness, ataxia, stupor, coma, confusion, sleepiness, flaccid muscles, shallow respirations, hypotension, nausea, vomiting; chronic overdosage includes skin rash, confusion, ataxia, dizziness, drowsiness, depression, irritability, hepatic dysfunction, hematologic changes, nausea, vomiting, muscular weakness

Toxicology General supportive care; charcoal hemoperfusion and dialysis may be helpful

Drug Interactions Succinimides increase hydantoin serum concentrations, decreased primidone levels and either increased or decreased valproic acid levels

Stability Protect from high temperature

Mechanism of Action Increases the seizure threshold and suppresses paroxysmal

(Continued)

Methsuximide *(Continued)*

spike-and-wave pattern in absence seizures; depresses nerve transmission in the motor cortex

Pharmacokinetics
Methsuximide is rapidly demethylated in the liver to N-desmethylmethsuximide (active metabolite)
Half-life: 2-4 hours
Time to peak: Oral: Peak serum levels occur within 1-3 hours
Elimination: <1% excreted in urine as unchanged drug

Usual Dosage Geriatrics and Adults: Oral: 300 mg/day for the first week; may increase by 300 mg/day at weekly intervals up to 1.2 g in 2-4 divided doses/day

Monitoring Parameters Monitor serum levels, CBC, renal function, LFTs

Reference Range Therapeutic: 10-40 μg/mL (SI: 53-212 μmol/L); Toxic: >40 μg/mL (SI: >212 μmol/L)

Test Interactions Increased alkaline phosphatase (S); decreased calcium (S)

Patient Information May cause drowsiness; periodic blood test monitoring required; if stomach upset occurs, take with food; do not stop medication without physician's advice; notify physician if skin rash, joint pain, fever, sore throat, dizziness, or blurred vision occur

Nursing Implications See Monitoring Parameters

Special Geriatric Considerations No specific data for elderly. This drug is rarely used in elderly, however, if it is used for partial complex seizure control, monitor closely; see Monitoring Parameters

Dosage Forms Capsule: 150 mg, 300 mg

Methylacetoxyprogesterone *see* Medroxyprogesterone Acetate
on page 437

Methyldopa (meth ill doe' pa)

Brand Names Aldomet®
Generic Available Yes
Therapeutic Class Alpha-Adrenergic Inhibitors, Central
Use Management of moderate to severe hypertension
Contraindications Hypersensitivity to methyldopa or any component; (oral suspension contains benzoic acid and sodium bisulfite; injection contains sodium bisulfite); liver disease, pheochromocytoma
Warnings May rarely produce hemolytic anemia and liver disorders; positive Coombs' test occurs in 10% to 20% of patients; perform periodic CBCs
Precautions Sedation (usually transient) may occur during initial therapy or whenever the dose is increased. Use with caution in patients with previous liver disease or dysfunction, the active metabolites of methyldopa accumulate in uremia. Patients with impaired renal function may respond to smaller doses. Elderly patients may experience syncope (avoid by giving smaller doses). Tolerance may occur usually between the second and third month of therapy. Adding a diuretic or increasing the dosage of methyldopa frequently restores blood pressure control.

Adverse Reactions
Cardiovascular: Orthostatic hypotension, bradycardia, edema
Central nervous system: Drowsiness, sedation, vertigo, headache, depression, memory lapse, fever
Dermatologic: Rash
Endocrine & metabolic: Sodium retention, gynecomastia
Gastrointestinal: Nausea, vomiting, diarrhea, dry mouth, "black" tongue, weight gain
Genitourinary: Sexual dysfunction
Hematologic: Hemolytic anemia, positive Coombs' test, leukopenia
Hepatic: Hepatitis, increased liver enzymes, jaundice, cirrhosis
Neuromuscular & skeletal: Weakness
Respiratory: Nasal congestion

Overdosage Symptoms of overdose include hypotension, sedation, bradycardia, dizziness, constipation or diarrhea, flatus, nausea, vomiting
Toxicology Hypotension usually responds to I.V. fluids or Trendelenburg positioning. If unresponsive to these measures the use of a parenteral vasoconstrictor may be required (eg, norepinephrine 0.1-0.2 mcg/kg/minute titrated to response). Treatment is primarily supportive and symptomatic.
Drug Interactions
Increased effect of tolbutamide, levodopa (and hypotension)
Increased toxicity of lithium, haloperidol (CNS effect), sympathomimetics (hypertension)
Stability Injectable dosage form is most stable at acid to neutral pH; stability of parenteral admixture at room temperature (25°C): 24 hours
Mechanism of Action Metabolized to alpha-methyl norepinephrine which lowers arterial pressure by the stimulation of central inhibitory alpha-adrenergic receptors, false neurotransmission, or reduction of plasma renin activity

Pharmacodynamics
  Peak hypotensive effect: Oral, parenteral: Within 3-6 hours
  Duration: 12-24 hours
Pharmacokinetics
  Protein binding: <15%
  Metabolism: Intestinally and in the liver with most (85%) metabolites appearing in urine within 24 hours
  Half-life: 75-80 minutes
  Elimination: Most (85%) metabolites appearing in urine within 24 hours
Usual Dosage
  Geriatrics: Oral: Initial: 125 mg 1-2 times/day; increase by 125 mg every 2-3 days as needed

  Adults:
    Oral: Initial: 250 mg 2-3 times/day; increase every 2 days as needed; usual dose 500 mg to 2 g/day in 2-4 divided doses; maximum: 3 g/day
    I.V.: 250-1000 mg every 6-8 hours

  Slightly dialyzable (5% to 20%)
Administration Infuse over 30-60 minutes
Monitoring Parameters Blood pressure (standing and sitting/lying down), weight, symptoms of fluid retention
Reference Range Therapeutic: 1-5 μg/mL (SI: 4.7-23.7 μmol/L); Toxic: >7 μg/mL (SI: >33 μmol/L)
Test Interactions Methyldopa interferes with the following laboratory tests: urinary uric acid, serum creatinine (alkaline picrate method), AST (colorimetric method), and urinary catecholamines (falsely high levels)
Patient Information May cause transient drowsiness; may cause urine discoloration; notify physician of unexplained prolonged general tiredness, fever or jaundice; rise slowly from sitting/lying position
Nursing Implications Transient sedation or depression may be common for first 72 hours of therapy; usually disappears over time
Special Geriatric Considerations Because of its CNS effects, methyldopa is not considered a drug of first choice in the elderly
Dosage Forms
  Injection, as methyldopate hydrochloride: 50 mg/mL (5 mL, 10 mL)
  Suspension, oral: 250 mg/5 mL (5 mL, 473 mL)
  Tablet: 125 mg, 250 mg, 500 mg

Methyldopa and Hydrochlorothiazide (meth ill doe' pa)
Related Information
  Hydrochlorothiazide *on page 347*
  Methyldopa *on previous page*
Brand Names Aldoril®
Synonyms Hydrochlorothiazide and Methyldopa
Generic Available Yes
Therapeutic Class Antihypertensive, Combination
Special Geriatric Considerations Combination products are not recommended for first-line therapy and divided doses of diuretics may increase the incidence of nocturia in the elderly
Dosage Forms Tablet (Aldoril®):
  15: Methyldopa 250 mg and hydrochlorothiazide 15 mg
  25: Methyldopa 250 mg and hydrochlorothiazide 25 mg
  D30: Methyldopa 500 mg and hydrochlorothiazide 30 mg
  D50: Methyldopa 500 mg and hydrochlorothiazide 50 mg

Methylmorphine *see* Codeine *on page 183*

Methylone® *see* Methylprednisolone *on page 461*

Methylphenidate Hydrochloride (meth ill fen' i date)
Brand Names Ritalin®; Ritalin-SR®
Generic Available Yes
Therapeutic Class Central Nervous System Stimulant, Nonamphetamine
Use Treatment of attention deficit disorder and symptomatic management of narcolepsy

  Unlabeled use: Depression in the elderly, poststroke, and cancer patients
Restrictions C-II
Contraindications Hypersensitivity to methylphenidate or any component; glaucoma; motor tics; Tourette's syndrome; patients with marked agitation, tension, and anxiety
Warnings Has high potential for abuse, may lower seizure disorder
Precautions Use with caution in patients with hypertension, seizures
Adverse Reactions
  Cardiovascular: Tachycardia, hypertension, hypotension, palpitation, cardiac arrhythmias
(Continued)

459

Methylphenidate Hydrochloride *(Continued)*

Central nervous system: Nervousness, insomnia, dizziness, drowsiness, movement disorders, precipitation of Tourette's syndrome, and toxic psychosis (rare), fever, headache; may produce sedation paradoxically

Dermatologic: Rash

Gastrointestinal: Anorexia, nausea, abdominal pain, weight loss

Hematologic: Thrombocytopenia

Ocular: Visual disturbances (rare)

Miscellaneous: Hypersensitivity reactions

Overdosage Symptoms of overdose include vomiting, agitation, tremors, hyperpyrexia, muscle twitching, hallucinations, tachycardia, mydriasis, sweating, palpitations

Toxicology There is no specific antidote for methylphenidate intoxication and the bulk of the treatment is supportive. Hyperactivity and agitation usually respond to reduced sensory input, however with extreme agitation haloperidol (2-5 mg I.M. for adults) may be required. Hyperthermia is best treated with external cooling measures, or when severe or unresponsive, muscle paralysis with pancuronium may be needed. Hypertension is usually transient and generally does not require treatment unless severe. For diastolic blood pressures greater than 110mm Hg. a nitroprusside infusion should be initiated. Seizures usually respond to diazepam I.V. and/or phenytoin maintenance regimens.

Drug Interactions May increase serum concentrations of tricyclic antidepressants, warfarin, phenytoin, phenobarbital and primidone; MAO inhibitors may potentiate effects of methylphenidate; effects of guanethidine, bretylium may be antagonized by methylphenidate; selegiline possible added stimulant effects

Mechanism of Action Appears to stimulate the cerebral cortex and subcortical structures similar to amphetamines; exact mechanism is not well defined

Pharmacodynamics

Immediate-release tablet:

Peak cerebral stimulation: Within 2 hours

Duration: 3-6 hours

Sustained-release tablet:

Peak effect: Within 4-7 hours

Duration: 8 hours

Pharmacokinetics

Absorption: Slow and incomplete from GI tract

Metabolism: In the liver via hydroxylation to ritolinic acid

Half-life: 2-4 hours

Elimination: In urine as metabolites and unchanged drug with 45% to 50% excreted in feces via bile

Usual Dosage Geriatrics and Adults:

Narcolepsy: 10 mg 2-3 times/day, up to 60 mg/day

Depression: Initial: 2.5 mg every morning before 9 AM; dosage may be increased by 2.5-5 mg every 2-3 days as tolerated until maximum of 20 mg/day; dosage may be divided (ie, 7 AM and 12 noon), but should not be given after noon. Do not use the sustained release product.

Administration Do not crush or allow patient to chew sustained release dosage form; dosing should be completed by 12 noon

Monitoring Parameters Blood pressure, heart rate, signs and symptoms of depression

Patient Information Last daily dose should be given several hours before retiring; notify physician if headache, palpitations, nervousness, dizziness, or skin rash occurs; do not crush or chew sustained release form

Nursing Implications See Administration

Additional Information Discontinue periodically to re-evaluate or if no improvement occurs within 1 month

Special Geriatric Considerations Methylphenidate is often useful in treating elderly patients who are discouraged, withdrawn, apathetic, or disinterested in their activities. In particular, it is useful in patients who are starting a rehabilitation program but have resigned themselves to fail; these patients may not have a major depressive disorder; will not improve memory or cognitive function; use with caution in patients with dementia who may have increased agitation and confusion. See Usual Dosage and Adverse Reactions.

Dosage Forms

Tablet: 5 mg, 10 mg, 20 mg

Tablet, sustained release: 20 mg

References

Gurian B and Rosowsky E, "Low-Dose Methylphenidate in the Very Old," *J Geriatr Psychiatry Neurol,* 1990, 3(3):152-4.

Katon W and Raskind M, "Treatment of Depression in the Medically Ill Elderly With Methylphenidate," *Am J Psychiatry,* 1980, 137:963-5.

Lazarus LW, Moberg PJ, Langsley PR, et al, "Methylphenidate and Nortriptyline in the Treatment of Poststroke Depression: A Retrospective Comparison," *Arch Phys Med Rehabil,* 1994, 75(4):403-6.

Methylphenyl *see* Oxacillin Sodium *on page 521*

Methylphenylethylhydantoin *see* Mephenytoin *on page 442*

Methylphytyl Napthoquinone *see* Vitamin K and Menadiol *on page 738*

Methylprednisolone (meth ill pred niss' oh lone)

Related Information

Antacid Drug Interactions *on page 764*

Corticosteroids Comparison, Systemic *on page 808*

Brand Names A-methaPred®; depMedalone®; Depoject®; Depo-Medrol®; Depopred®; Duralone®; Mar-Pred®; Medralone®; Medrol®; Meprolone®; Methylone®; Solu-Medrol®

Synonyms 6-α-Methylprednisolone; Methylprednisolone Acetate; Methylprednisolone Sodium Succinate

Generic Available Yes

Therapeutic Class Adrenal Corticosteroid; Anti-inflammatory Agent; Corticosteroid, Systemic; Corticosteroid, Topical (Low Potency)

Use Primarily as an anti-inflammatory or immunosuppressant agent in the treatment of a variety of diseases including those of hematologic, allergic, inflammatory, neoplastic, and autoimmune origin

Contraindications Hypersensitivity to methylprednisolone or any component; administration of live virus vaccines; systemic fungal infections

Precautions Use with caution in patients with hypothyroidism, cirrhosis, hypertension, congestive heart failure, nonspecific ulcerative colitis, thromboembolic disorders; patients at increased risk for peptic ulcer disease; gradually taper dose to withdraw therapy

Adverse Reactions

Cardiovascular: Edema, hypertension, accelerated atherogenesis

Central nervous system: Vertigo, seizures, psychoses, pseudotumor cerebri, headache

Dermatologic: Acne, skin atrophy, impaired wound healing

Endocrine & metabolic: Cushing's syndrome, pituitary-adrenal axis suppression, growth suppression, glucose intolerance, hypokalemia, alkalosis, postmenopausal bleeding, hot flashes

Gastrointestinal: Peptic ulcer, nausea, vomiting

Neuromuscular & skeletal: Muscle weakness, osteoporosis, fractures

Ocular: Cataracts, glaucoma

Toxicology When consumed in excessive quantities for prolonged periods, systemic hypercorticism and adrenal suppression may occur; in those cases, discontinuation and withdrawal of the corticosteroid should be done judiciously

Drug Interactions

Steroids decrease the effect of anticholinesterases, isoniazid, salicylates, insulin, oral hypoglycemics

Decreased effect: Barbiturates, phenytoin, rifampin

Increased effect (hypokalemia) of potassium-depleting diuretics

Increased risk of digoxin toxicity (due to hypokalemia)

Increased effect: Estrogens, ketoconazole

Stability

Stability of parenteral admixture (Solu-Medrol®) at room temperature (25°C): 24 hours

Stability of parenteral admixture (Solu-Medrol®) at refrigeration temperature (4°C): 24 hours

Mechanism of Action Decreases inflammation by suppression of migration of polymorphonuclear leukocytes and reversal of increased capillary permeability

Pharmacodynamics Time to obtain peak effects and the duration of these effects is dependent upon the route of administration; see table.

Route	Peak Effect	Duration
Oral	1–2 h	30–36 h
I.M.	4–8 d	1–4 wk
Intra–articular	1 wk	1–5 wk

Pharmacokinetics A single dose study found a slower methylprednisolone clearance in older volunteers compared to younger ones

Distribution: V_d: 0.7 L/kg

Half-life: 3-3.5 hours

Usual Dosage Only sodium succinate salt may be given I.V.

Geriatrics: Use the lowest effective dose

(Continued)

461

Methylprednisolone *(Continued)*

Adults:

Anti-inflammatory or immunosuppressive: Oral: 2-60 mg/day in 1-4 divided doses to start, followed by gradual reduction in dosage to the lowest possible level consistent with maintaining an adequate clinical response

I.M. (sodium succinate): 10-80 mg/day once daily

I.M. (acetate): 40-120 mg every 1-2 weeks

I.V. (sodium succinate): 10-40 mg over a period of several minutes and repeated I.V. or I.M. at intervals depending on clinical response; when high dosages are needed, give 30 mg/kg over a period of 10-20 minutes and may be repeated every 4-6 hours for 48 hours

Status asthmaticus: I.V. (sodium succinate): Loading dose: 2 mg/kg/dose, then 0.5-1 mg/kg/dose every hours for up to 5 days

Lupus nephritis:

I.V. (sodium succinate): 1 g/day for 3 days

Intra-articular (acetate): 4-80 mg every 1-5 weeks

Intralesional (acetate): 20-60 mg every 1-5 weeks

Topical: Apply sparingly 2-4 times/day

Note: Alternate day dosing may be attempted in some disease states

Slightly dialyzable (5% to 20%)

Administration Succinate: I.V. push over 1-15 minutes; intermittent infusion over 15-60 minutes; maximum concentration: IVP: 125 mg/mL

Monitoring Parameters Blood pressure, blood glucose, electrolytes, symptoms of fluid retention

Test Interactions Increased amylase (S), chloride (S), increased cholesterol (S), increased glucose, increased protein, increased sodium (S); decreased calcium (S), decreased chloride (S), decreased potassium (S), decreased thyroxine (S)

Patient Information Do not discontinue or decrease the drug without contacting your physician; carry an identification card or bracelet advising that you are on steroids; may take with meals to decrease GI upset; apply topical product sparingly

Nursing Implications Give with meals to decrease GI upset; see Administration and Usual Dosage

Additional Information Sodium content of 1 g sodium succinate injection: 2.01 mEq; 53 mg of sodium succinate salt is equivalent to 40 mg of methylprednisolone base

Methylprednisolone acetate: Depo-Medrol®; methylprednisolone sodium succinate: Solu-Medrol®

Special Geriatric Considerations Because of the risk of adverse effects, systemic corticosteroids should be used cautiously in the elderly, in the smallest possible dose, and for the shortest possible time.

Dosage Forms

Injection, as sodium succinate: 40 mg (1 mL, 3 mL); 125 mg (2 mL, 5 mL); 500 mg (1 mL, 4 mL, 8 mL, 20 mL); 1000 mg (1 mL, 8 mL, 16 mL, 50 mL); 2000 mg (30.6 mL)

Injection, as acetate: 20 mg/mL (5 mL, 10 mL); 40 mg,mL (1 mL, 5 mL, 10 mL); 80 mg/mL (1 mL, 5 mL)

Ointment, topical, as acetate: 0.25% (30 g); 1% (30 g)

Tablet: 2 mg, 4 mg, 8 mg, 16 mg, 24 mg, 32 mg

Tablet, dose pack: 4 mg (21's)

References

Tornatore KM, Logue G, Venuto RC, et al, "Pharmacokinetics of Methylprednisolone in Elderly and Young Healthy Males," *J Am Geriatr Soc,* 1994, 42(10):1118-22.

6-α-Methylprednisolone *see* Methylprednisolone *on previous page*

Methylprednisolone Acetate *see* Methylprednisolone *on previous page*

Methylprednisolone Sodium Succinate *see* Methylprednisolone *on previous page*

Meticorten® *see* Prednisone *on page 586*

Metimyd® *see* Sodium Sulfacetamide and Prednisolone Acetate *on page 652*

Metoclopramide *(met oh kloe pra' mide)*

Brand Names Maxolon®; Octamide® PFS; Reglan®

Generic Available Yes

Therapeutic Class Antiemetic

Use Symptomatic treatment of diabetic gastric stasis, hiccups, gastroesophageal reflux; prevention of nausea associated with chemotherapy or postsurgery and facilitates intubation of the small intestine

Contraindications Hypersensitivity to metoclopramide or any component; GI obstruction, perforation or hemorrhage; pheochromocytoma, history of seizure disorder

Warnings Extrapyramidal reactions (0.2% to 1%), depression; may exacerbate seizures in seizure patients

Precautions Use with caution in patients with Parkinson's disease; dosage and/or frequency of administration should be modified in response to degree of renal impairment; hypoglycemia may be precipitated in patients with gastroparesis when insulin is used for glycemic control; may cause drowsiness, therefore use caution performing hazardous tasks (eg, driving)

Adverse Reactions

Cardiovascular: Transient hypertension, hypotension, supraventricular tachycardia, bradycardia

Central nervous system: Drowsiness, fatigue, lassitude, mental depression, suicidal thoughts, restlessness, anxiety, agitation, extrapyramidal reaction, confusion, hallucinations, dizziness, headache, insomnia, Parkinson-like symptoms, tardive dyskinesia, akathisia, seizures, dystonia, neuroleptic malignant syndrome

Dermatologic: Rash, urticaria

Endocrine & metabolic: Nipple tenderness and gynecomastia in males, fluid retention (transient aldosterone increase)

Gastrointestinal: Constipation, diarrhea, nausea, glossal edema

Genitourinary: Impotence, incontinence

Hematologic: Methemoglobinemia, neutropenia, leukopenia, agranulocytosis

Neuromuscular & skeletal: Myoclonus

Ocular: Visual disturbances

Respiratory: Bronchospasm, laryngeal edema

Overdosage Symptoms of overdose include drowsiness, ataxia, extrapyramidal reactions, seizures, disorientation, muscle hypertonia, irritability, and agitation are common

Toxicology Metoclopramide often causes extrapyramidal symptoms (eg, dystonic reactions) requiring management with diphenhydramine 1-2 mg/kg (adults) up to a maximum of 50 mg I.M. or I.V. slow push followed by a maintenance dose for 48-72 hours. When these reactions are unresponsive to diphenhydramine, benztropine mesylate I.V. 1-2 mg (adults) may be effective. These agents are generally effective within 2-5 minutes.

Drug Interactions

Increases rate of absorption of alcohol

May decrease bioavailability of cimetidine (H$_2$ blockers)

May decrease absorption of digoxin due to increased transit time

Levodopa may decrease effects of metoclopramide on gastrointestinal tract

May increase effect of levodopa in Parkinson's disease

Metoclopramide increases effect of MAO inhibitors

Anticholinergic drugs may decrease effects of metoclopramide

Stability Protection of dilutions do not require light protection if used within 24 hours

Stability of parenteral admixture at room temperature (25°C): 2 days

Stability of parenteral admixture at refrigeration temperature (4°C): 2 days

Mechanism of Action Blocks dopamine receptors in chemoreceptor trigger zone of the CNS; enhances the response to acetylcholine of tissue in upper GI tract causing enhanced motility and accelerated gastric emptying without stimulating secretions

Pharmacodynamics

Onset of action:

Oral: Within 30-60 minutes

I.V.: Within 1-3 minutes

Duration: 1-2 hours, regardless of route administered

Pharmacokinetics

Protein binding: 30%

Half-life: 4-7 (half-life and clearance may be dose-dependent)

Elimination: Primarily as unchanged drug in urine and feces

Usual Dosage

Antiemetic (chemotherapy-induced emesis): Geriatrics and Adults:

I.V.: 1-2 mg/kg/dose every 2-4 hours or (postsurgery); direct I.V. administration should be given slowly over 1-2 minutes

I.M.: 10-20 mg (near end of surgery)

Diabetic gastroparesis:

Geriatrics:

Oral: Initial: 5 mg 30 minutes before meals and at bedtime for 2-8 weeks; increase if necessary to 10 mg doses

I.V.: Initiate at 5 mg over 1-2 minutes; increase to 10 mg if necessary

Adults:

Oral: 10 mg 30 minutes before meals and at bedtime for 2-8 weeks

I.V. (for severe symptoms): 10 mg over 1-2 minutes; 10 days of I.V. therapy may be necessary for best response

Gastroesophageal reflux: Oral:

Geriatrics: 5 mg 4 times/day, 30 minutes before meals and at bedtime; increase dose to 10 mg 4 times/day if no response at lower dose

Adults: 10-15 mg 4 times/day, 30 minutes before meals and at bedtime; single doses of 20 mg are occasionally needed for provoking situations

(Continued)

Metoclopramide (Continued)

Postoperative nausea and vomiting: I.M.:
Geriatrics: 5 mg near end of surgery; may repeat dose if necessary
Adults: 10 mg near end of surgery; 20 mg doses can be used

Dosing adjustment in renal impairment: Since elimination is primarily renal, patients with Cl_{cr} <40 mL/minute should have therapy initiated at $1/2$ the recommended **adult** dose; see Additional Information

Not dialyzable (0% to 5%)

Monitoring Parameters Monitor for dystonic reactions; monitor for signs of hypoglycemia in patients using insulin and those being treated for gastroparesis; monitor for agitation and irritable confusion

Test Interactions Increased aminotransferase [ALT (SGPT)/AST (SGOT)] (S), increased amylase (S)

Patient Information May impair mental alertness or physical coordination; produces drowsiness, dizziness; avoid alcohol, barbiturates or other CNS depressants; take medication 30 minutes before meals; notify physician if any abnormal muscle movements occur

Nursing Implications Parenteral doses of up to 10 mg should be given I.V. push over 1-2 minutes; rapid boluses cause transient anxiety and restlessness followed by drowsiness; higher doses to be given IVPB; see Monitoring Parameters and Special Geriatric Considerations

Additional Information Infuse over at least 15 minutes. For patients who may need rectal administration, an extemporaneous suppository may be prepared with 5 pulverized tablets in polyethylene glycol. Administer 1 suppository 30-60 minutes before meals and at bedtime; use $1/2$ for elderly

Special Geriatric Considerations Elderly are more likely to develop dystonic reactions than younger adults; use lowest recommended doses initially; must consider renal function (estimate creatinine clearance); it is recommended to do involuntary movement assessments on elderly using this medication at high dose and in long-term; see Dosage

Dosage Forms
Injection: 5 mg/mL (2 mL, 10 mL, 30 mL, 50 mL, 100 mL)
Syrup, sugar-free: 5 mg/5 mL (10 mL, 480 mL)
Tablet: 5 mg, 10 mg

Metolazone (me tole' a zone)

Brand Names Mykrox®; Zaroxolyn®

Generic Available No

Therapeutic Class Diuretic, Miscellaneous

Use Management of mild to moderate hypertension; treatment of edema in congestive heart failure and nephrotic syndrome; impaired renal function

Contraindications Hypersensitivity to metolazone or any component; cross-sensitivity with other thiazides and sulfonamides may occur; patients with hepatic coma

Warnings Mykrox® is **not** therapeutically equivalent to Zaroxolyn® and they should not be interchanged for one another

Precautions When metolazone is used in combination with other diuretics, there is an increased risk of azotemia and electrolyte depletion, particularly in the elderly; monitor closely

Adverse Reactions
Cardiovascular: Palpitations, chest pain, orthostatic hypotension
Central nervous system: Vertigo, headache, chills
Dermatologic: Rash, photosensitivity
Endocrine & metabolic: Hypokalemia, hyponatremia, hypochloremia, metabolic alkalosis, hyperglycemia, hyperuricemia
Gastrointestinal: Abdominal bloating, GI irritation
Genitourinary: Prerenal azotemia
Hematologic: Aplastic anemia, hemolytic anemia, leukopenia, agranulocytosis, thrombocytopenia (all rare)
Renal: Polyuria

Overdosage Symptoms of overdose include electrolyte depletion, volume depletion, hypotension, dehydration, circulatory collapse

Toxicology Following GI decontamination, treatment is supportive; hypotension responds to fluids and Trendelenburg position

Drug Interactions
Decreased effect of oral hypoglycemics; decreased absorption with cholestyramine and colestipol
Increased effect with loop diuretics and other antihypertensives
Increased toxicity/levels of lithium; when given with digoxin, diuretic-induced hypokalemia increases the risk of digoxin toxicity

Mechanism of Action Inhibits sodium reabsorption in the distal tubules causing increased excretion of sodium and water as well as potassium and hydrogen ions; does not substantially decrease glomerular filtration rate or renal plasma flow

Pharmacodynamics Irrespective of formulation, diuresis occurs within 60 minutes and continues for 12-24 hours

Pharmacokinetics
Absorption: Oral: Incomplete
Protein binding: 95%
Metabolism: Enterohepatic recycled
Bioavailability: Mykrox® reportedly has the highest bioavailability
Half-life: 6-20 hours, renal function dependent
Elimination: 80% to 95% in urine

Usual Dosage Oral:
Zaroxolyn®:
Geriatrics: Initial: 2.5 mg/day or every other day
Adults:
Edema: 5-20 mg/dose every 24 hours
Hypertension: 2.5-5 mg/dose every 24 hours

Mykrox®: Geriatrics and Adults: 0.5 mg once daily; may increase to 1 mg if response is inadequate; do not use more than 1 mg/day

Not dialyzable (0% to 5%)

Monitoring Parameters Blood pressure both standing and sitting/supine, serum electrolytes, renal function, weight, I & O

Test Interactions Increased ammonia (B), increased amylase (S), increased calcium (S), increased chloride (S), increased cholesterol (S), increased glucose, increased uric acid (S); decreased chloride (S), decreased magnesium, decreased potassium (S), decreased sodium (S)

Patient Information Take in the morning, may be taken with food or milk; take the last dose of multiple doses no later than 6 PM unless instructed otherwise; may cause increased sensitivity to sunlight

Nursing Implications See Monitoring Parameters; check patient for orthostasis

Additional Information 5 mg is approximately equivalent to 50 mg of hydrochlorothiazide; may be effective in patients with glomerular filtration rate of <20 mL/minute; metolazone is often used in combination with a loop diuretic in patients who are unresponsive to the loop diuretic alone

Special Geriatric Considerations See Precautions, Usual Dosage, and Additional Information

Dosage Forms Tablet:
Zaroxolyn®: 2.5 mg, 5 mg, 10 mg
Mykrox®: 0.5 mg

Metoprolol Tartrate (me toe' proe lole)
Related Information
Beta-Blockers Comparison *on page 804-805*
Brand Names Lopressor®
Therapeutic Class Beta-Adrenergic Blocker
Use Treatment of hypertension and angina pectoris; prevention of myocardial infarction

Unlabeled use: Treatment of ventricular arrhythmias, atrial ectopy, migraine prophylaxis, essential tremor, aggressive behavior; diastolic congestive heart failure

Contraindications Hypersensitivity to beta-blocking agents, uncompensated congestive heart failure; cardiogenic shock; bradycardia (heart rate <45 bpm) or heart block; sinus node dysfunction; A-V conduction abnormalities, systolic blood pressure <100 mm Hg; although metoprolol primarily blocks beta₁-receptors, high doses can result in beta₂-receptor blockage; therefore, use with caution in elderly with bronchospastic lung disease.

Warnings Abrupt withdrawal of beta-blockers may result in an exaggerated cardiac beta-adrenergic responsiveness. Symptomatology has included reports of tachycardia, hypertension, ischemia, angina, myocardial infarction, and sudden death. It is recommended that patients be tapered gradually off of beta-blockers over a 2-week period rather than via abrupt discontinuation.

Precautions Administer to CHF patients with caution; administer with caution to patients with bronchospastic disease, diabetes mellitus, hyperthyroidism, myasthenia gravis, impaired hepatic and renal function decline, and severe peripheral vascular disease. Abrupt withdrawal of the drug should be avoided, drug should be discontinued over 2 weeks.

Adverse Reactions
Cardiovascular: Persistent bradycardia, hypotension, chest pain, edema, heart failure, Raynaud's phenomena
Central nervous system: Fatigue, dizziness, insomnia, lethargy, nightmares, depression, confusion, headache, cold extremities
Gastrointestinal: Constipation, diarrhea, nausea
Genitourinary: Impotence

Overdosage Symptoms of overdose include bradycardia, hypotension, heart failure, bronchospasm; see Toxicology

(Continued)

465

Metoprolol Tartrate *(Continued)*

Toxicology Sympathomimetics (eg, epinephrine or dopamine), glucagon or a pacemaker can be used to treat the toxic bradycardia, asystole, and/or hypotension. Initially, fluids may be the best treatment for toxic hypotension. Patients should remain supine; serum glucose and potassium should be measured. Use supportive measures: lavage, syrup of ipecac; not significantly removed by dialysis I.V. glucose should be administered for hypoglycemia; seizures may be treated with phenytoin or diazepam intravenously; continuous monitoring of blood pressure and EKG is necessary. If PVCs occur, treat with lidocaine or phenytoin; avoid quinidine, procainamide, and disopyramide since these agents further depress myocardial function. Bronchospasm can be treated with theophylline on beta$_2$ agonists (epinephrine).

Drug Interactions

Pharmacologic action of beta-antagonists may be decreased by aluminum compounds, calcium salts, barbiturates, cholestyramine, colestipol, NSAIDs, penicillins (ampicillin), rifampin, salicylates, sulfinpyrazone, thyroid hormones; hypoglycemic effect of sulfonylureas may be blunted

Pharmacologic effect of beta-antagonists may be enhanced with concomitant use of calcium channel blockers, oral contraceptives, flecainide (bioavailability and effect of flecainide also enhanced), haloperidol (hypotensive effects of both drugs), H$_2$ antagonists (decreased metabolism), hydralazine (both drugs hypotensive effects increased), loop diuretics (increased serum levels of beta-blockers except atenolol), MAO inhibitors, phenothiazines, propafenone, quinidine, quinolones, thioamines; beta-blockers may decrease clearance of acetaminophen; beta-blockers may increase anticoagulant effects of warfarin (propranolol); benzodiazepine effects enhanced by the lipophilic beta-blockers (atenolol does not interact); significant and fatal increases in blood pressure have occurred after decrease in dose or discontinuation of clonidine in patients receiving both clonidine and beta-blockers together (reduce doses of each cautiously with small decreases); peripheral ischemia of ergot alkaloids enhanced by beta-blockers; beta-blockers increase serum concentration of lidocaine; beta-blockers increase hypotensive effect of prazosin

Mechanism of Action Competitively blocks beta$_1$-receptors, with little or no effect on beta$_2$-receptors except in high doses; does not exhibit any membrane stabilizing or intrinsic sympathomimetic activity; has moderate lipid solubility, therefore, will penetrate blood-brain barrier

Pharmacodynamics

Peak effects: Oral: Within 1.5-4 hours

Duration: 10-20 hours

Pharmacokinetics

Absorption: 95%

Protein binding: 8%

Metabolism: Significant first-pass metabolism; extensively metabolized in the liver

Bioavailability: Oral: 40% to 50%

Half-life: 3-4 hours

Elimination: In urine (3% to 10% as unchanged drug)

Usual Dosage

Geriatrics: Initial: 25 mg/day; usual dose range: 25-300 mg/day

Adults:

Oral: 100-450 mg/day in 1-2 divided doses

I.V.: 5 mg every 2 minutes for 3 doses in early treatment of myocardial infarction

Monitoring Parameters Blood pressure, orthostatic hypotension, heart rate, CNS effects

Test Interactions Increased cholesterol (S), increased glucose

Patient Information Do not discontinue medication abruptly, sudden stopping of medication may precipitate or cause angina; consult pharmacist or physician before taking with other adrenergic drugs (eg, cold medications); notify physician if any of the following symptoms occur: difficult breathing, night cough, swelling of extremities, slow pulse, dizziness, lightheadedness, confusion, depression, skin rash, fever, sore throat, unusual bleeding or bruising; may produce drowsiness, dizziness, lightheadedness, blurred vision, confusion; use with caution while driving or performing tasks requiring alertness; may mask signs of hypoglycemia in diabetics; may be taken without regard to meals

Nursing Implications Monitor hemodynamic status carefully after acute MI, monitor orthostatic blood pressures, apical and peripheral pulse and mental status changes (ie, confusion, depression)

Special Geriatric Considerations Due to alterations in the beta-adrenergic autonomic nervous system, beta-adrenergic blockade may result in less hemodynamic response than seen in younger adults. Studies indicate that despite decreased sensitivity to the chronotropic effects of beta blockade with age, there appears to be an increased myocardial sensitivity to the negative inotropic effect during stress (ie, exercise). Controlled trials have shown the overall response rate for propranolol to be only 20% to 50% in elderly populations. Therefore, all beta-adrenergic blocking drugs may result in a decreased response as compared to younger adults.

Dosage Forms
    Injection: 1 mg/mL (5 mL)
    Tablet: 50 mg, 100 mg
References
    Aagaard GN, "Treatment of Hypertension in The Elderly," *Drug Treatment in the Elderly*, Vestal RE, ed, Boston, MA: ADIS Health Science Press, 1984, 77.

Metreton® *see* Prednisolone *on page 584*

Metric® *see* Metronidazole *on this page*

MetroGel® *see* Metronidazole *on this page*

Metro I.V.® *see* Metronidazole *on this page*

Metronidazole (me troe ni' da zole)

Brand Names Flagyl®; Metric®; MetroGel®; Metro I.V.®; Protostat®
Generic Available Yes
Therapeutic Class Amebicide; Antibiotic, Anaerobic; Antibiotic, Topical; Antiprotozoal
Use Treatment of susceptible anaerobic bacterial and protozoal infections in the following conditions: amebiasis, symptomatic and asymptomatic trichomoniasis; skin and skin structure infections; CNS infections; intra-abdominal infections; systemic anaerobic infections; topically for the treatment of acne rosacea pressure sores; treatment of antibiotic-associated pseudomembranous colitis (AAPC)
Contraindications Hypersensitivity to metronidazole or any component
Warnings Has been shown to be carcinogenic in rodents
Precautions Use with caution in patients with liver impairment, blood dyscrasias; reduce dosage in patients with severe liver impairment, CNS disease, and severe renal failure (GFR <10 mL/minute)
Adverse Reactions
    Cardiovascular: Thrombophlebitis
    Central nervous system: Dizziness, confusion, seizures, headache
    Dermatologic: Rash
    Endocrine & metabolic: Disulfiram-type reaction with alcohol
    Gastrointestinal: Metallic taste, nausea, dry mouth, diarrhea, furry tongue
    Hematologic: Leukopenia
    Neuromuscular & skeletal: Peripheral neuropathy
Overdosage Symptoms of overdose include nausea, vomiting, ataxia, seizures, peripheral neuropathy
Drug Interactions
    Alcohol (disulfiram-like GI reaction), disulfiram (psychosis and confusion), warfarin and other coumarin derivatives (increased anticoagulant effect)
    Metronidazole may decrease the clearance of phenytoin and lithium and increase their serum concentrations and half-lives
    Phenobarbital may increase metronidazole's metabolism
    Cimetidine may decrease metronidazole's metabolism
Stability Reconstituted solution is stable for 96 hours when refrigerated; for I.V. infusion in NS or D_5W and neutralized (with sodium bicarbonate), solution is stable for 24 hours at room temperature; do not refrigerate neutralized solution because a precipitate will occur
Mechanism of Action Reduced to a product which interacts with DNA to cause a loss of helical DNA structure and strand breakage resulting in inhibition of protein synthesis and cell death in susceptible organisms
Pharmacokinetics
    Absorption: Oral: Well absorbed
    Protein binding: <20%
    Metabolism: 30% to 60% in the liver
    Half-life, normal: 6-8 hours (half-life increases with hepatic impairment)
    Time to peak: Peak serum levels occur within 1-2 hours
    Elimination: Final excretion via urine (20% as unchanged drug) and feces (6% to 15%).
    Following a single 500 mg oral dose, serum levels and AUCs were increased, total clearance and V_d reduced in subject >70 years compared to younger subjects (20-25 years); the decreased V_d was attributed to a significant decrease in red blood cell binding
    Drug is extensively removed by hemodialysis and peritoneal dialysis; dosage adjustment is not necessary for mild to moderate renal insufficiency
Usual Dosage
    Geriatrics: Use the lower end of the dosing recommendations for adults; do not give as single dose as efficacy has not been established

    Adults:
        Amebiasis: Oral: 500-750 mg every 8 hours
        Other parasitic infections: Oral: 250 mg every 8 hours or 2 g as a single dose
        Anaerobic infections: Oral, I.V.: 30 mg/kg/day in divided doses every 6 hours; not to exceed 4 g/day

(Continued)

Metronidazole *(Continued)*

AAPC: Oral: 250-500 mg 3-4 times/day for 10-14 days
Topical: Apply a thin film twice daily to affected areas
Vaginal: One applicatorful in vagina each morning and evening, as needed

Dosing interval in renal impairment: No change necessary unless Cl_{cr} <10 mL/minute
Dialyzable (50% to 100%)

Monitoring Parameters Signs and symptoms of infection; diarrhea

Test Interactions May cause falsely decreased AST and ALT levels

Patient Information Urine may be discolored to a dark or reddish-brown; do not take alcohol for at least 24 hours after the last dose; avoid beverage alcohol during therapy; may cause metallic taste; may be taken with food to minimize stomach upset

Nursing Implications Even though metronidazole can be detected in the blood after **topical** application, no antabuse-like reactions have been reported; avoid contact between the drug and aluminum in the infusion set

Additional Information Sodium content of 500 mg (I.V.): 322 mg (14 mEq)

Special Geriatric Considerations See Pharmacokinetics and Usual Dosage

Dosage Forms
Gel, topical: 0.75% (30 g)
Injection, ready to use: 5 mg/mL (100 mL)
Powder, for injection: 500 mg
Tablet: 250 mg, 500 mg

References
Ludwig E, Csiba A, Magyar T, et al, "Age-Associated Pharmacokinetic Changes of Metronidazole," *Int J Clin Pharmacol Ther Toxicol*, 1983, 21(2):87-91.
"Treatment of *Clostridium difficile* Diarrhea," *Med Lett Drugs Ther*, 1989, 31(803):94-5.

Mevacor® *see* Lovastatin *on page 420*

Mevinolin *see* Lovastatin *on page 420*

Mexate® *see* Methotrexate *on page 455*

Mexiletine (mex' i le teen)

Brand Names Mexitil®
Generic Available No
Therapeutic Class Antiarrhythmic Agent, Class IB
Use Management of life-threatening ventricular arrhythmias

Unlabeled use: Diabetic neuropathy associated pain and paresthesias

Contraindications Cardiogenic shock, second or third degree heart block, hypersensitivity to mexiletine or any component

Warnings Exercise extreme caution in patients with pre-existing sinus node dysfunction; mexiletine can worsen CHF, bradycardias, and other arrhythmias; mexiletine, like other antiarrhythmic agents, is proarrhythmic; cost studies indicate a trend toward increased mortality with antiarrhythmics in the face of cardiac disease (myocardial infarction); elevation of AST/ALT; hepatic necrosis reported; leukopenia, agranulocytopenia, and thrombocytopenia; seizures; alterations in urinary pH may change urinary excretion; electrolyte disturbances (hypokalemia, hyperkalemia, etc) after drug response

Precautions A-V second or third degree block, sinus node dysfunction, intraventricular conduction abnormalities; follow closely in patients with liver disease, seizure disorder; avoid drugs or diets that greatly alter urinary pH; mexiletine can worsen arrhythmias; hepatic impairment prolongs half-life; elevations of AST; use with caution in patients with severe congestive heart failure, hypotension

Adverse Reactions
Cardiovascular: Edema, palpitations, bradycardia, chest pain, syncope, hypotension, atrial or ventricular arrhythmias
Central nervous system: Dizziness, confusion, paresthesia, lightheadedness, nervousness, fatigue, depression, memory loss, psychosis, seizures, ataxia
Dermatologic: Rash, dry skin
Gastrointestinal: Nausea, vomiting, diarrhea, heartburn, abdominal pain
Genitourinary: Urinary retention
Hematologic: Rarely thrombocytopenia, rarely positive antinuclear antibody
Hepatic: Rarely hepatitis
Neuromuscular & skeletal: Coordination difficulties, arthralgia, tremors, weakness
Ocular: Diplopia, blurred vision
Otic: Tinnitus
Respiratory: Dyspnea
Miscellaneous: Hiccups

Toxicology Utilize general supportive therapy and general poisoning management if necessary; gastric lavage followed by charcoal administration indicated; atropine may be used for mexiletine-induced bradycardia; acidify urine to elimination; hemodialysis does not eliminate

Drug Interactions
Phenobarbital, phenytoin, rifampin, and other hepatic enzyme inducers may lower mexiletine plasma levels

Cimetidine may increase mexiletine levels

Antacids, narcotics, metoclopramide, or anticholinergics may decrease rate of absorption

Metoclopramide may increase rate of absorption; drugs or diets which affect urine pH can increase or decrease excretion of mexiletine

Theophylline levels increased; caffeine clearance decreased

Mechanism of Action Class IB antiarrhythmic, structurally related to lidocaine, which may cause increase in systemic vascular resistance and decrease in cardiac output; no significant negative inotropic effect; inhibits inward sodium current, decreasing phase O, and effective refractory period

Pharmacodynamics Onset of action: Oral: Within 30 minutes to 2 hours

Pharmacokinetics
Absorption: Elderly have a slightly slower rate of absorption but extent of absorption is the same as young adults

Distribution: V_d: 5-7 L/kg

Protein binding: 50% to 70%

Metabolism: Extensive first-pass metabolism; extensively metabolized in liver (some minor active metabolites)

Bioavailability: Oral: 88%

Half-life: Adults: 10-14 hours (average: 14.4 hours elderly, 12 hours in younger adults); increase in half-life with hepatic or heart failure

Time to peak: Peak levels attained in 2-3 hours

Elimination: 10% to 15% excreted unchanged in urine; urinary acidification increases excretion, alkalinization decreases excretion

Usual Dosage Geriatrics and Adults: Oral: Initial: 200 mg every 8 hours (may load with 400 mg if necessary); adjust dose every 2-3 days; usual dose: 200-300 mg every 8 hours; maximum dose: 1.2 g/day (some patients respond to every 12-hour dosing); patients with hepatic impairment or CHF may require dose reduction; when switching from another antiarrhythmic, initiate a 200 mg dose 6-12 hours after stopping former agents, 3-6 hours after stopping procainamide

Monitoring Parameters EKG, blood pressure, pulse, serum concentrations

Reference Range Therapeutic: 0.5-2 μg/mL; Potentially toxic: >2 μg/mL

Test Interactions Abnormal liver function test, positive ANA, thrombocytopenia

Patient Information Take with food; notify physician of side effects such as jaundice, fever, palpitations, dizziness, tremor, heartburn, and sore throat

Nursing Implications Give around-the-clock rather than 4 times/day, 3 times/day, etc (ie, 12-6-12-6, not 9-1-5-9) to promote less variation in peak and trough serum levels

Additional Information I.V. form under investigation

Special Geriatric Considerations No specific changes in dose are necessary; see Pharmacokinetics

Dosage Forms Capsule: 150 mg, 200 mg, 250 mg

References
Fenster PE and Nolan PE, "Antiarrhythmic Drugs," *Geriatric Pharmacology*, Bressler R and Katz MD, eds, New York, NY: McGraw-Hill, 1993, 6:105-49.

Mexitil® *see* Mexiletine *on previous page*

Mezlin® *see* Mezlocillin Sodium *on this page*

Mezlocillin Sodium (mez loe sill' in)
Brand Names Mezlin®
Therapeutic Class Antibiotic, Penicillin
Use Treatment of infections caused by susceptible gram-negative aerobic bacilli (*Klebsiella*, *Proteus*, *Escherichia coli*, *Enterobacter*, *Pseudomonas aeruginosa*, *Serratia*) involving the skin and skin structure, bone and joint, respiratory tract, urinary tract, gastrointestinal tract, as well as septicemia

Contraindications Hypersensitivity to mezlocillin or any component or penicillins
Warnings If bleeding occurs during therapy, mezlocillin should be discontinued
Precautions If bleeding occurs during therapy, mezlocillin should be discontinued; dosage modification required in patients with impaired renal function; use with caution in patients with renal impairment or biliary obstruction; use with caution in patients with cephalosporin allergy
Adverse Reactions
Cardiovascular: Thrombophlebitis
Central nervous system: Seizures, dizziness, fever, headache
Dermatologic: Rash, exfoliative dermatitis
Endocrine & metabolic: Hypokalemia, hypernatremia
Gastrointestinal: Diarrhea
Genitourinary: Elevated serum creatinine and BUN
Hematologic: Eosinophilia, hemolytic anemia, neutropenia, leukopenia, thrombocytopenia, prolonged bleeding time, positive Coombs' direct test
(Continued)

Mezlocillin Sodium *(Continued)*

Hepatic: Elevated liver enzymes
Renal: Interstitial nephritis
Miscellaneous: Serum sickness-like reaction

Overdosage Symptoms of overdose include neuromuscular hypersensitivity, seizure

Toxicology Many beta-lactam-containing antibiotics have the potential to cause neuro-muscular hyperirritability or convulsive seizures. Hemodialysis may be helpful to aid in the removal of the drug from the blood, otherwise most treatment is supportive or symptom directed.

Drug Interactions Aminoglycosides (synergy), probenecid (decreased clearance), vecuronium (prolonged duration of action), heparin (increased risk of bleeding)

Stability Reconstituted solution is stable for 48 hours at room temperature and 7 days when refrigerated; for I.V. infusion in NS or D_5W solution is stable for 48 hours at room temperature, 7 days when refrigerated or 28 days when frozen; after freezing, thawed solution is stable for 48 hours at room temperature or 7 days when refrigerated; if precipitation occurs under refrigeration, warm in water bath (37°C) for 20 minutes and shake well

Mechanism of Action Interferes with bacterial cell wall synthesis during active multiplication causing cell death and resultant bactericidal activity against susceptible bacteria

Pharmacokinetics

Absorption: I.M.: 63%
Distribution: Into bile, heart, peritoneal fluid, sputum, bone; does not cross the blood-brain barrier well unless meninges are inflamed
Protein binding: 30%
Metabolism: Minimal
Half-life: 50-70 minutes (dose dependent), half-life increased in renal impairment
Time to peak serum concentrations:
    I.M.: Within 45-90 minutes
    I.V. infusion: Within 5 minutes
Elimination: Principally as unchanged drug in urine, also excreted via bile
The pharmacokinetics of mezlocillin in the elderly have not been shown to be significantly altered with increased age

Usual Dosage Geriatrics and Adults: I.M., I.V.:
For uncomplicated urinary tract infection: 1.5-2 g every 6 hours; serious infections: 3-4 g every 4-6 hours

Acute, uncomplicated gonococcal urethritis: 1-2 g, plus 1 g probenecid at time of dose or up to 30 minutes before

Dosing interval in renal impairment:
Cl_{cr} 10-30 mL/minute: Administer every 6-8 hours
Cl_{cr} <10 mL/minute: Administer every 8-12 hours
Moderately dialyzable (20% to 50%)

Dosing adjustment in hepatic impairment: Reduce dose by 50%

Monitoring Parameters Signs and symptoms of infection, electrolytes

Test Interactions False-positive direct Coombs'; false-positive urinary protein

Patient Information Notify physician if diarrhea develops within 2 weeks after completion of therapy

Nursing Implications Give around-the-clock rather than 4 times/day, 3 times/day, etc (ie, 12-6-12-6, not 9-1-5-9) to promote less variation in peak and trough serum levels; dosage modification required in patients with impaired renal function; give I.M. injections in large muscle mass, not more than 2 g/injection. I.M. injections given over 12-15 seconds will be less painful.

Additional Information Minimum volume: 50 mL D_5W (concentration should not exceed 1 g/10 mL); sodium content of 1 g: 42.6 mg (1.85 mEq)

Special Geriatric Considerations See Pharmacokinetics; mezlocillin and the other antipseudomonal infections should be used in combination with another antibiotic for the treatment of mixed infections or against gram-negative bacilli such as *P. aeruginosa* (ie, with an aminoglycoside); sodium content is the lowest of the penicillins; adjust dose for renal function

Dosage Forms Injection: 1 g, 2 g, 3 g, 4 g, 20 g

References

Meyers BR, Mendelson MH, Srulevitch-Chin E, et al, "Pharmacokinetic Properties of Mezlocillin in Ambulatory Elderly Subjects," *J Clin Pharmacol*, 1987, 27(9):678-81.
Yoshikawa TT, "Antimicrobial Therapy for the Elderly Patient," *J Am Geriatr Soc*, 1990, 38(12):1353-72.

Mg-plus® [OTC] *see* Magnesium Salts (Various Salts) *on page 430*
Micatin® [OTC] *see* Miconazole *on this page*

Miconazole *(mi kon' a zole)*

Brand Names Micatin® [OTC]; Monistat™; Monistat-Derm™; Monistat iv™
Synonyms Miconazole Nitrate
Generic Available Yes

Therapeutic Class Antifungal Agent, Topical; Antifungal Agent, Vaginal

Use

Topical: Treatment of vulvovaginal candidiasis and a variety of skin and mucous membrane fungal infections

I.V.: Treatment of severe systemic fungal infections and fungal meningitis that are refractory to standard treatment

Contraindications Hypersensitivity to miconazole, fluconazole, ketoconazole, or polyoxyl 35 castor oil or any component

Precautions Administer I.V. with caution to patients with hepatic insufficiency, cardiorespiratory arrest or anaphylaxis, tachycardia, or arrhythmias with too rapid injection

Adverse Reactions

Cardiovascular: Tachycardia (I.V.), arrhythmias (I.V.)

Central nervous system: Arachnoiditis (I.T.), 8th cranial nerve palsy (I.T.), headache

Dermatologic: Maceration, hives, rash, pruritus (I.V.)

Endocrine & metabolic: Hyperlipidemia with rapid infusion (I.V.)

Gastrointestinal: Nausea (I.V.), vomiting (I.V.), diarrhea (I.V.)

Genitourinary: Pelvic cramps

Hematologic: Transient anemia (I.V.), thrombocytopenia

Local: Irritation, burning, itching, phlebitis

Miscellaneous: Anaphylactoid reactions (I.V.)

Overdosage Symptoms of overdose include nausea, vomiting, drowsiness

Drug Interactions Warfarin (increased anticoagulant effect), amphotericin B (decreased antifungal effect of both agents), phenytoin (levels may be increased)

Stability Protect from heat; darkening of solution indicates deterioration

Stability of parenteral admixture at room temperature (25°C): 2 days

Mechanism of Action Inhibits biosynthesis of ergosterol, damaging the fungal cell wall membrane, which increases permeability causing leaking of nutrients

Pharmacokinetics Multiphasic degradation

Protein binding: 91% to 93%

Metabolism: In the liver

Half-life:

Initial: 40 minutes

Secondary: 126 minutes

Terminal: 24 hours

Elimination: ~50% in feces and <1% in urine as unchanged drug

Usual Dosage Geriatrics and Adults:

Topical: Apply twice daily

Vaginal: Insert contents of one applicator of vaginal cream (100 mg) or 100 mg suppository at bedtime for 7 days, or 200 mg suppository at bedtime for 3 days

Bladder candidal infections: 200 mg diluted solution instilled in the bladder

I.V.: Initial: 200 mg, then 1.2-3.6 g/day divided every 8 hours for 1-20 weeks depending upon organism

I.T.: 20 mg every 1-2 days

Not dialyzable (0% to 5%)

Administration Administer I.V. dose over 2 hours; give around-the-clock rather than 4 times/day, 3 times/day, etc (ie, 12-6-12-6, not 9-1-5-9) to promote less variation in peak and trough serum levels

Monitoring Parameters Signs and symptoms of infection

Test Interactions Increased protein

Patient Information Avoid contact with the eyes; if no response after several weeks of therapy, contact physician

Nursing Implications See Administration

Additional Information

Miconazole: Monistat i.v.™

Miconazole nitrate: Micatin®, Monistat™, Monistat-Derm™

Special Geriatric Considerations No specific data for elderly; use does not require alteration in dose or dose intervals; assess patient's ability to self administer, may be difficult in patients with arthritis or limited range of motion

Dosage Forms

Cream:

Topical, as nitrate: 2% (15 g, 30 g, 85 g)

Vaginal, as nitrate: 2% (47 g = 7 doses)

Injection: 10 mg/mL (20 mL)

Lotion, as nitrate: 2% (30 mL, 60 mL)

Powder, topical: 2% (45 g, 90 g)

Spray: 2% (105 mL)

Suppository, vaginal, as nitrate: 100 mg (7's); 200 mg (3's)

Miconazole Nitrate *see* Miconazole *on previous page*

Micrin® *see* Hydrochlorothiazide *on page 347*

Micro-K® *see* Potassium Chloride *on page 576*

Micronase® *see* Glyburide *on page 324*

ALPHABETICAL LISTING OF DRUGS

microNefrin® *see* Epinephrine *on page 256*
Midamor® *see* Amiloride Hydrochloride *on page 38*

Midazolam Hydrochloride (mid' ay zoe lam)
Related Information
  Antacid Drug Interactions *on page 764*
Brand Names Versed®
Generic Available No
Therapeutic Class Benzodiazepine; Hypnotic; Sedative
Use Preoperative sedation and provide conscious sedation prior to diagnostic or radiographic procedures
Restrictions C-IV
Contraindications Hypersensitivity to midazolam or any component, cross-sensitivity with other benzodiazepines may occur; uncontrolled pain; existing CNS depression; shock; narrow-angle glaucoma
Warnings Midazolam may cause respiratory depression/arrest; deaths and hypoxic encephalopathy have resulted when these were not promptly recognized and treated appropriately. The danger of apnea or underventilation is greater in the elderly; the peak effect may take longer; reduce dosage increments and slow the rate of injection.
Precautions Use with caution in patients with congestive heart failure, renal impairment, pulmonary disease, hepatic dysfunction
Adverse Reactions
  Cardiovascular: Cardiac arrest, hypotension, bradycardia
  Central nervous system: Drowsiness, ataxia, amnesia, dizziness, paradoxical excitement, sedation, headache
  Gastrointestinal: Nausea, vomiting
  Local: Pain and local reactions at injection site (severity less than diazepam)
  Ocular: Blurred vision, diplopia
  Respiratory: Respiratory depression, apnea, laryngospasm, bronchospasm
  Miscellaneous: Physical and psychological dependence with prolonged use, hiccups
Overdosage Symptoms of overdose include sedation, confusion, impaired coordination, diminished reflexes, and coma
Toxicology Treatment for benzodiazepine overdose is supportive; rarely is mechanical ventilation required; flumazenil has been shown to selectively block the binding of benzodiazepines to CNS receptors, resulting in a reversal of benzodiazepine-induced sedation; however, its use may not alter the course of overdose
Drug Interactions
  Decreased effect: Theophylline may antagonize the sedative effects of midazolam
  Increased toxicity: CNS depressants, → ↑ sedation and respiratory depression; doses of anesthetic agents should be reduced when used in conjunction with midazolam; cimetidine may increase midazolam serum concentrations
Stability Admixtures do not require protection from light for short-term storage
Mechanism of Action Benzodiazepines appear to potentiate the effects of GABA and other inhibitory neurotransmitters by binding to specific benzodiazepine-receptor sites in various areas of the CNS
Pharmacodynamics
  Sedation onset:
    I.M.: Within 15 minutes
    I.V. within 1-5 minutes
  Peak effects: I.M.: 30-60 minutes
  Duration: I.M.: Mean: 2 hours, up to 6 hours
Pharmacokinetics
  Distribution: V_d: 0.8-2.5 L/kg; increased V_d with congestive heart failure and chronic renal failure; slightly increased V_d in the elderly
  Protein binding: 95%
  Metabolism: Extensive in the liver (microsomally)
  Half-life: Elimination: 1-4 hours; increased half-life with cirrhosis, congestive heart failure, obesity, elderly (5.6 ± 4.8 hours); some elderly males had a marked increase in elimination half-life
  Elimination: Excreted as glucuronide conjugated metabolites in urine, ~2% to 10% is excreted in feces
  Pharmacokinetics in elderly males were less predictable than in elderly females
Usual Dosage
  Geriatrics: Conscious sedation: Initial: 1 mg slow I.V.; give no more than 1.5 mg in a 2-minute period; if additional titration is needed, give no more than 1 mg over 2 minutes, waiting another 2 or more minutes to evaluate sedative effect; total dose >3.5 mg is rarely necessary

  Adults:
    Preoperative sedation: I.M.: 0.07-0.08 mg/kg 30-60 minutes presurgery; usual dose: 5 mg; lower doses may suffice in the elderly
    Conscious sedation: I.V.: Initial: 0.5-2 mg slow I.V. over at least 2 minutes; slowly titrate to effect by repeating doses every 2-3 minutes if needed; usual total dose: 2.5-5 mg

Administration See Usual Dosage

Monitoring Parameters Respiratory, cardiovascular and mental status

Patient Information May cause drowsiness; do not drive or operate hazardous machinery until the effects of the drug are gone or until the day after administration

Additional Information Healthy adults <60 years of age: Some patients respond to doses as low as 1 mg; no more than 2.5 mg should be administered over a period of 2 minutes. Additional doses of midazolam may be administered after a 2-minute waiting period and evaluation of sedation after each dose increment. A total dose of greater than 5 mg is generally not needed. If narcotics or other CNS depressants are administered concomitantly, the midazolam dose should be reduced by 30%.

Special Geriatric Considerations In the elderly if concomitant CNS depressant medications are used, the midazolam dose will be at least 50% less than doses used in healthy, young, unpremedicated patients; see Warnings and Pharmacokinetics

Dosage Forms Injection: 1 mg/mL (2 mL, 5 mL, 10 mL); 5 mg/mL (1 mL, 2 mL, 5 mL, 10 mL)

References

Kanto J, Aaltonen L, Himberg JJ, et al, "Midazolam as an Intravenous Induction Agent in the Elderly: A Clinical and Pharmacokinetic Study," *Anesth Analg*, 1986, 65(1):15-20.

Servin F, Enriquez I, Fournet M, et al, "Pharmacokinetics of Midazolam Used as an Intravenous Induction Agent for Patients Over 80 Years of Age," *Eur J Anaesthesiol*, 1987, 4(1):1-7.

Midol® 200 [OTC] see Ibuprofen *on page 360*

Migergot® see Ergotamine *on page 261*

Milkinol® [OTC] see Mineral Oil *on this page*

Milk of Magnesia see Magnesium Hydroxide *on page 427*

Miltown® see Meprobamate *on page 443*

Mineral Oil

Brand Names Agoral® Plain [OTC]; Fleet® Mineral Oil Enema [OTC]; Kondremul® [OTC]; Milkinol® [OTC]; Neo-Cultol® [OTC]; Zymenol® [OTC]

Synonyms Heavy Mineral Oil; Liquid Paraffin; White Mineral Oil

Generic Available Yes

Therapeutic Class Laxative, Lubricant

Use Temporary relief of constipation, relief of fecal impaction, preparation for bowel studies or surgery

Contraindications Patients with colostomy or an ileostomy, appendicitis, ulcerative colitis, diverticulitis

Warnings Lipid pneumonitis results from aspiration of mineral oil which usually occurs in patients who are in a supine (debilitated) position. Elderly patients are particularly at risk, especially if they have any condition which interferes with swallowing or epiglottal function (eg, strokes, Parkinson's disease, Alzheimer's disease, esophageal dysmotility).

Precautions Lipid pneumonitis

Adverse Reactions

Gastrointestinal: Nausea, vomiting, diarrhea, abdominal cramps

Respiratory: Lipid pneumonitis with aspiration

Miscellaneous: Large doses may cause anal leakage causing anal itching, irritation, hemorrhoids, perianal discomfort, soiling of clothes

Drug Interactions May impair absorption of fat-soluble vitamins (A,D,K,E), oral contraceptives, coumarin, sulfonamides; administration of surfactants (docusate) with mineral oil may increase mineral oil absorption and therefore enhance toxic potential of mineral oil resulting in a foreign body reaction in lymphoid tissue

Mechanism of Action Eases passage of stool by decreasing water absorption and lubricating the intestine; retards colonic absorption of water

Pharmacodynamics Onset of action: ~6-8 hours; effect on bowel function is generally seen after 2-3 days of use

Pharmacokinetics

Distribution: Site of action is the colon

Elimination: In feces

Usual Dosage Geriatrics and Adults:

Oral: 15-45 mL/day once daily or in divided doses

Rectal: Retention enema, contents of one enema (range 60-150 mL)/day as a single dose

Monitoring Parameters Monitor for response: Stool frequency, consistency. Avoid use in patients who may aspirate.

Patient Information Do not take with food or meals; do not use if experiencing abdominal pain, nausea, or vomiting; do not take while reclining in bed, sit up; do **not** give just before bedtime; wear protective undergarments

Nursing Implications Administer on an empty stomach; avoid administration in a reclining position; sit patient up

Additional Information Do not give with food or meals because of the risk of aspiration; prolonged administration of mineral oil may decrease absorption of lipid-soluble vitamins A, D, E, and K. Light sterile mineral oils are not for injection.

(Continued)

Mineral Oil *(Continued)*

Special Geriatric Considerations See Warnings. Other therapies should be attempted before using mineral oil to relieve constipation and to avoid complications; doses, if used, should begin low and may be used as infrequently as possible

Dosage Forms
Emulsion: 1.4 g/5 mL (480 mL); 2.5 mL/5 mL (420 mL); 2.75 mL/5 mL (480 mL); 4.75 mL/5 mL (240 mL)
Jelly: 2.75 mL/5 mL (180 mL)
Liquid: 500 mL, 1000 mL, 4000 mL
Liquid, rectal: 133 mL

Minipress® *see Prazosin Hydrochloride on page 582*

Minitran® *see Nitroglycerin on page 505*

Minocin® *see Minocycline Hydrochloride on this page*

Minocin® IV *see Minocycline Hydrochloride on this page*

Minocycline Hydrochloride *(mi noe sye' kleen)*

Brand Names Minocin®; Minocin® IV
Therapeutic Class Antibiotic, Tetracycline Derivative
Use Treatment of susceptible bacterial infections of both gram-negative and gram-positive organisms; acne
Contraindications Hypersensitivity to minocycline or any component or tetracycline
Precautions Should be avoided in renal insufficiency; photosensitivity reactions can occur with minocycline, superinfection
Adverse Reactions
Central nervous system: Lightheadedness, vertigo, dizziness
Dermatologic: Skin rashes, photosensitivity, pigmentation of nails, exfoliative dermatitis
Endocrine & metabolic: Diabetes insipidus
Gastrointestinal: Nausea, vomiting, esophagitis, anorexia, abdominal cramps, diarrhea
Genitourinary: Azotemia
Renal: Acute renal failure
Overdosage Symptoms of overdose include photosensitivity, diabetes insipidus, nausea, anorexia, diarrhea
Drug Interactions
Decreased effect with antacids (aluminum, calcium, zinc, or magnesium), bismuth salts, sodium bicarbonate, barbiturates, carbamazepine, hydantoins; decreased effect of oral contraceptives
Increased effect of warfarin
Mechanism of Action Inhibits bacterial protein synthesis by binding with the 30S and possibly the 50S ribosomal subunit(s) of susceptible bacteria, cell wall synthesis is not affected
Pharmacokinetics
Absorption: Well absorbed following administration
Protein binding: 70% to 75%
Half-life: 15 hours
Elimination: Majority of dose deposits for extended periods in fat and eventually is cleared renally
Usual Dosage Geriatrics and Adults:
Infection: Oral, I.V.: 200 mg stat, 100 mg every 12 hours
Acne: Oral: 50 mg 1-3 times/day

Not dialyzable (0% to 5%)
Monitoring Parameters Signs and symptoms of infection
Test Interactions Increased catecholamines (U), increased uric acid (S); decreased urea nitrogen (B)
Patient Information Complete full course of therapy; use caution if vertigo, dizziness, and driving or operation of machinery; may be taken with food or milk; avoid prolonged exposure to sunlight or tanning equipment
Special Geriatric Considerations Minocycline has not been studied in the elderly but its CNS effects may limit its use, see Adverse Reactions; dose reduction for renal function not necessary
Dosage Forms
Capsule: 50 mg, 100 mg
Injection: 100 mg
Suspension, oral: 50 mg/5 mL (60 mL)

Minodyl® *see Minoxidil on this page*

Minoxidil *(mi nox' i dill)*

Brand Names Loniten®; Minodyl®; Rogaine®
Generic Available Yes: Tablet
Therapeutic Class Vasodilator

ALPHABETICAL LISTING OF DRUGS

Use Management of severe hypertension; treatment of male pattern baldness (alopecia androgenetica)

Contraindications Pheochromocytoma, hypersensitivity to minoxidil or any component

Precautions Use with caution in patients with coronary artery disease or with recent myocardial infarction, pulmonary hypertension, significant renal dysfunction, congestive heart failure

Adverse Reactions

Cardiovascular: Edema, congestive heart failure, tachycardia, angina, pericardial effusion, tamponade, EKG changes

Central nervous system: Dizziness, fatigue, headache

Dermatologic: Hypertrichosis (commonly occurs within 1-2 months of therapy), coarsening facial features, dermatologic reactions, rash, Stevens-Johnson syndrome, sunburn

Endocrine & metabolic: Sodium and water retention

Gastrointestinal: Weight gain

Local: Topical burning, itching

Respiratory: Pulmonary hypertension/edema

Overdosage Symptoms of overdose include hypotension, tachycardia

Toxicology Hypotension usually responds to I.V. fluids or Trendelenburg positioning. If unresponsive to these measures the use of a parenteral vasoconstrictor may be required (eg, norepinephrine 0.1-0.2 mcg/kg/minute titrated to response). Treatment is primarily supportive and symptomatic.

Drug Interactions Increased effect: Other hypotensive agents, hypotensive diuretics; concurrent administration with guanethidine may cause profound orthostatic hypotensive effects

Mechanism of Action Produces vasodilation by directly relaxing arteriolar smooth muscle, with little effect on veins, effects may be mediated by cyclic AMP; stimulation of hair growth is secondary to vasodilation, increased cutaneous blood flow and stimulation of resting hair follicles

Pharmacodynamics

Onset of action: Oral: Hypotensive effects occur within 30 minutes

Peak effects: Within 2-8 hours

Duration: Up to 2-5 days

Pharmacokinetics

Protein binding: None

Metabolism: 88% primarily via glucuronidation

Bioavailability: Oral: 90%

Half-life: 3.5-4.2 hours

Elimination: 12% unchanged in urine

Usual Dosage

Geriatrics: Oral: Initial: 2.5 mg once daily, increase gradually

Adults:

Hypertension: Oral: Initial: 5 mg once daily, increase gradually every 3 days; usual dose: 10-40 mg/day in 1-2 divided doses; maximum: 100 mg/day

Alopecia: Apply twice daily

Dialyzable (50% to 100%)

Monitoring Parameters Blood pressure, standing and sitting/supine, fluid and electrolyte status, signs and symptoms of congestive heart failure, weight

Patient Information Topical product must be used every day. Minoxidil is usually taken with at least two other antihypertensive medications. Take all medications as prescribed; do not discontinue except on advice of physician. Notify the physician if any of the following occur: heart rate ≥20 beats per minute over normal; rapid weight gain >5 pounds (2 kg); unusual swelling of extremities, face, or abdomen; breathing difficulty, especially when lying down; new or aggravated angina symptoms (chest, arm or shoulder pain); severe indigestion; dizziness, lightheadedness or fainting; nausea or vomiting may occur.

Nursing Implications May cause hirsutism or hypertrichosis; see Monitoring Parameters

Additional Information Usually given in combination with a diuretic and beta-blocker

Special Geriatric Considerations See Precautions and Adverse Reactions

Dosage Forms

Solution, topical: 2% = 20 mg/metered dose (60 mL)

Tablet: 2.5 mg, 10 mg

Miochol® see Acetylcholine Chloride *on page 20*

Miostat® see Carbachol *on page 116*

Misoprostol (mye soe prost' ole)

Brand Names Cytotec®

Generic Available No

Therapeutic Class Prostaglandin

(Continued)

Misoprostol *(Continued)*

Use Prevention of NSAID-induced gastric ulcers

Unlabeled use: Treatment of duodenal and gastric ulcers

Contraindications Hypersensitivity to misoprostol, prostaglandins, or any component

Warnings Renal function impairment may increase half-life; does not prevent NSAID-induced duodenal ulcers; elderly have an increased AUC in studies

Precautions Diarrhea (13% to 40%) is dose related; diarrhea usually occurs in first 2 weeks; diarrhea is usually self-limited but may require dose reduction or discontinuation; see Additional Information

Adverse Reactions

Cardiovascular: Headache

Endocrine & metabolic: Postmenopausal vaginal bleeding

Gastrointestinal: Diarrhea (transient), abdominal pain, nausea, dyspepsia, vomiting, constipation, flatulence

Overdosage Symptoms of overdose include sedation, tremor, convulsions, dyspnea, abdominal pain, diarrhea, hypotension, bradycardia

Toxicology General supportive care; not dialyzable

Drug Interactions Antacids and food diminish absorption; antacids may enhance diarrhea

Mechanism of Action Misoprostol is a synthetic prostaglandin E_1 analog that replaces the protective prostaglandins consumed with prostaglandin-inhibiting therapies (eg, nonsteroidal anti-inflammatory drugs)

Pharmacokinetics

Absorption: Oral: Rapid

Half-life (parent and metabolite combined): 1.5 hours

Time to peak: Peak serum levels (of active metabolite) occur within 15-30 minutes

Rapidly de-esterified to misoprostol acid

Elimination: In urine (64% to 73% in 24 hours) and feces (15% in 24 hours)

Since elderly have decreased clearance (increased AUC), it may be necessary to reduce dose to 100 mcg 4 times/day

Usual Dosage Oral:

Geriatrics: 100-200 mcg 4 times/day with food; if 200 mcg 4 times/day not tolerated, reduce to 100 mcg 4 times/day or 200 mcg twice daily with food. **Note:** To avoid the diarrhea potential, doses can be initiated at 100 mcg/day and increased 100 mcg/day at 3-day intervals until desired dose is achieved; also, recommend administering with food to decrease diarrhea incidence; see Special Geriatric Considerations

Adults: 200 mcg 4 times/day with food or 100 mcg 4 times/day or 200 mcg twice daily with food if not tolerated

Monitoring Parameters Monitor for diarrhea, stool occult blood; gastroscopy may be preferred

Patient Information May cause diarrhea when first being used (within 2 weeks); diarrhea incidence and severity may be decreased by taking with food and at bedtime

Nursing Implications Incidence of diarrhea may be lessened by having patient take dose right after meals and at bedtime; see Monitoring Parameters

Additional Information Although food may decrease absorption, the clinical significance is unknown; administration with food may decrease diarrhea

Special Geriatric Considerations Elderly, due to extensive use of NSAIDs and the high percentage of asymptomatic hemorrhage and perforation from NSAIDs, are at risk for NSAID-induced ulcers and may be candidates for misoprostol use. However, routine use for prophylaxis is not justified. Patients must be selected upon demonstration that they are at risk for NSAID-induced lesions. Misoprostol should not be used as a first-line therapy for gastric or duodenal ulcers.

Dosage Forms Tablet: 100 mcg, 200 mcg

References

Walt RP, "Misoprostol for the Treatment of Peptic Ulcer and Anti-inflammatory Drug-Induced Gastroduodenal Ulceration," *N Engl J Med*, 1992, 327(22):1575-80.

Mitrolan® Chewable Tablet [OTC] *see* Calcium Polycarbophil *on page 110*

Mixtard® 70/30 (Purified Pork) *see* Insulin Preparations *on page 372*

Moban® *see* Molindone Hydrochloride *on next page*

Mobidin® *see* Salicylates (Various Salts) *on page 633*

Modane® Plus [OTC] *see* Docusate and Phenolphthalein *on page 238*

Modane® [OTC] *see* Phenolphthalein *on page 556*

Modane® Mild [OTC] *see* Phenolphthalein *on page 556*

Modane® Bulk [OTC] *see* Psyllium *on page 610*

Modified Shohl's Solution *see* Sodium Citrate and Citric Acid *on page 649*

Moduretic® *see* Amiloride and Hydrochlorothiazide *on page 38*

Moi-Stir® [OTC] *see* Saliva Substitute *on page 636*

Molindone Hydrochloride (moe lin' done)
Related Information
Antipsychotic Agents Comparison *on page 801*
Antipsychotic Medication Guidelines *on page 754*
Brand Names Moban®
Generic Available No
Therapeutic Class Antipsychotic Agent
Use Management of psychotic disorders; nonpsychotic symptoms associated with dementia in elderly, Tourette's syndrome, Huntington's chorea; see Special Geriatric Considerations
Contraindications Narrow-angle glaucoma, bone marrow depression, CNS depression, liver or cardiac disease, subcortical brain damage; circulatory collapse, severe hypotension or hypertension, hypersensitivity to molindone or any component
Warnings
Tardive dyskinesia: Prevalence rate may be 40% in elderly; elderly women especially at risk; embarrassment from dyskinesias may lead to greater social isolation; development of the syndrome and the irreversible nature are proportional to duration and total cumulative dose over time. May be reversible if diagnosed early in therapy; intermittent use of antipsychotics (not proven use) helps decrease total cumulative dose.

EPS: Extrapyramidal reactions are more common in elderly with up to 50% developing these reactions after age 60. These reactions may be more common in dementia patients. Drug-induced **Parkinson's syndrome** occurs often. Discontinuation usually resolves symptoms but may take weeks to months (12+) to clear. **Akathisia** is the most common EPS reaction in elderly. The symptoms of motor restlessness are difficult to diagnose in demented elderly; increased nervousness, assertiveness, restlessness with constant movement may indicate this adverse event. Consider decreasing dose if antipsychotic to treat as well as diagnose problem; usually see this reaction within 2-3 months of initiating antipsychotic drug.

Anticholinergic effects: These side effects most common with low potency antipsychotics (eg, thioridazine, chlorpromazine). CNS toxicity occurs more frequently and severely in elderly; increased confusion, memory loss, psychotic behavior, and agitation frequently occur as a consequence of anticholinergic effects to antipsychotic agents. Peripheral anticholinergic action troublesome to elderly; most peripheral anticholinergic effects last only 2-3 weeks; see Adverse Reactions.

Orthostatic hypotension: More common with low potency agents (eg, thioridazine, chlorpromazine, and clozapine) but of concern with all antipsychotic agents; orthostasis due to alpha-receptor blockade by antipsychotic agents. Elderly present many risk factors for orthostatic hypotension: blunted baroreceptor reflexes, decreased vascular tone, decreased vascular volume, and possible presence of cardiac diseases which result in decreased cardiac output.

Sedation: Common side effect with antipsychotic therapy; should not be used as a hypnotic unless insomnia is associated with target behavior symptoms treated with antipsychotic medications; see Special Geriatric Considerations. Anecdotal reports suggesting antipsychotic sedation in nonpsychotic patients is extremely unpleasant due to feelings of depersonalization, derealization, and dysphoria. Due to the long duration of action with antipsychotic drugs, these reactions may last up to 24 hours and result in decreased daytime function.

Cardiac toxicity: Life-threatening arrhythmias have occurred at therapeutic doses of antipsychotics. Thioridazine more commonly demonstrates EKG changes than other antipsychotics; suggested to use high potency antipsychotic agents (ie, haloperidol) in patients with cardiac conduction defects.
Precautions Use with caution in patients with severe cardiovascular disease, seizures, and Parkinson's disease; benefits of therapy must be weighed against risks
Adverse Reactions
Cardiovascular: Hypotension, tachycardia, arrhythmias
Central nervous system: Sedation, drowsiness, restlessness, anxiety, extrapyramidal reactions, pseudoparkinsonian signs and symptoms, seizures, altered central temperature regulation, neuroleptic malignant syndrome (NMS)
Dermatologic: Hyperpigmentation, pruritus, rash, photosensitivity
Endocrine & metabolic: Amenorrhea, galactorrhea, gynecomastia
Gastrointestinal: Dry mouth, constipation, GI upset, weight gain
Genitourinary: Urinary retention
Hematologic: Agranulocytosis (more often in women between fourth and tenth weeks of therapy), leukopenia (usually in patients with large doses for prolonged periods)
Ocular: Blurred vision, retinal pigmentation
Overdosage Symptoms of overdose include deep sleep, coma, extrapyramidal symptoms, abnormal involuntary muscle movements, hypotension or hypertension; agitation, restlessness, fever, hypothermia or hyperthermia, seizures, cardiac arrhythmias, EKG changes
(Continued)

477

Molindone Hydrochloride *(Continued)*

Toxicology Following initiation of essential overdose management, toxic symptom treatment and supportive treatment should be initiated. Hypotension usually responds to I.V. fluids or Trendelenburg positioning. If unresponsive to these measures the use of a parenteral inotrope may be required (eg, norepinephrine 0.1-0.2 mcg/kg/ minute titrated to response). Do not use epinephrine. Seizures commonly respond to diazepam (I.V. 5-10 mg bolus in adults every 15 minutes if needed up to a total of 30 mg) or to phenytoin or phenobarbital. Also critical cardiac arrhythmias often respond to I.V. phenytoin (15 mg/kg up to 1 g), while other antiarrhythmics can be used. Neuroleptics often cause extrapyramidal symptoms (eg, dystonic reactions) requiring management with diphenhydramine 1-2 mg/kg up to a maximum of 50 mg I.M. or I.V. slow push followed by a maintenance dose for 48-72 hours. When these reactions are unresponsive to diphenhydramine, benztropine mesylate I.V. 1-2 mg may be effective. These agents are generally effective within 2-5 minutes.

Drug Interactions Administration with CNS depressants will increase CNS depression; may block (weak) antihypertensive effects of guanethidine; anticonvulsants (phenytoin, carbamazepine, and phenobarbital) may decrease serum concentrations of molindone

Stability Protect from light; dispense in amber or opaque vials

Mechanism of Action Mechanism of action is similar to that of chlorpromazine; however, it produces more extrapyramidal effects and less sedation than chlorpromazine; blocks postsynaptic mesolimbic dopaminergic D_1 and D_2 receptors in the brain; exhibits a strong alpha-adrenergic blocking and anticholinergic effect, depresses the release of hypothalamic and hypophyseal hormones; believed to depress the reticular activating system thus affecting basal metabolism, body temperature, wakefulness, vasomotor tone, and emesis

Pharmacodynamics Duration of action: 24-36 hours

Pharmacokinetics

Absorption: Oral: May be affected by the inherent anticholinergic action on the gastrointestinal tissue causing variable absorption. Absorption from tablets is erratic with less variation seen with solutions. These agents are widely distributed in tissues with CNS concentrations exceeding that of plasma due to their lipophilic characteristics.

Protein binding: Antipsychotic agents are bound 90% to 99% to plasma proteins; highly bound to brain and lung tissue and other tissues with a high blood perfusion.

Metabolism: Metabolized in the liver

Time to peak: Following oral administration peak serum levels occur within 90 minutes; peak concentrations between 2-4 hours

Elimination: Principally excreted in the urine and feces (90% within 24 hours); <2% to 3% excreted unmetabolized; eliminated through hepatic metabolism (oxidation) where numerous active metabolites are produced; active metabolites excreted in urine; elimination half-lives of antipsychotics ranges from 20-40 hours which may be extended in elderly due to decline in oxidative hepatic reactions (phase I) with age.

The biologic effect of a single dose persists for 24 hours. When the patient has accommodated to initial side effects (sedation), once daily dosing is possible due to the long half-life of antipsychotics.

Steady-state plasma levels are achieved in 4-7 days; therefore, if possible, do not make dose adjustments more than once in a 7-day period. Due to the long half-lives of antipsychotics, as needed (PRN) use is ineffective since repeated doses are necessary to achieve therapeutic tissue concentrations in the CNS.

Usual Dosage Oral:

Geriatrics (nonpsychotic patients, dementia behavior): Initial: 5-10 mg 1-2 times/day; increase at 4- to 7-day intervals by 5-10 mg/day; increase dosing intervals (bid, tid, etc) as necessary to control response or side effects; maximum daily dose: 112 mg; gradual increases (titration) may prevent some side effects or decrease their severity

Adults: 50-75 mg/day; up to 225 mg/day

Monitoring Parameters Orthostatic blood pressures; tremors, gait changes, abnormal movement in trunk, neck, buccal area or extremities; monitor target behaviors for which the agent is given

Patient Information May cause drowsiness; avoid alcoholic beverages; do not take within 1 hour of taking antacids; rise slowly from recumbent position; use of supportive stockings may prevent orthostatic hypotension

Nursing Implications Monitor orthostatic blood pressures 3-5 days after initiation of therapy or after a dose increase; observe for tremor and abnormal movement or posturing (extrapyramidal symptoms)

Special Geriatric Considerations See Warnings

Many elderly patients receive antipsychotic medications for inappropriate nonpsychotic behavior. Before initiating antipsychotic medication, the clinician should investigate any possible reversible cause; any stress or stress from any disease can cause acute "confusion" or worsening of baseline nonpsychotic behavior. Most commonly acute changes in behavior are due to increases in drug dose or addition of new drug to regimen, fluid electrolyte loss, infections, and changes in environment.

Any changes in disease status in any organ system can result in behavior changes.
Dosage Forms Tablet: 5 mg, 10 mg, 25 mg

Mol-Iron® [OTC] *see* Ferrous Sulfate *on page 289*

MOM *see* Magnesium Hydroxide *on page 427*

Mometasone Furoate (moe met' a sone)
Related Information
Corticosteroids Comparison, Topical *on page 809*
Brand Names Elocon® Topical
Generic Available No
Therapeutic Class Corticosteroid, Topical (Medium Potency)
Use Relief of the inflammatory and pruritic manifestations of corticosteroid-responsive dermatoses
Contraindications Hypersensitivity to mometasone or any component; fungal, viral, or tubercular skin lesions; herpes simplex or zoster
Precautions Systemic absorption of topical corticosteroids has produced reversible HPA axis suppression. This is more likely to occur when the preparation is used on large surfaces or denuded areas for prolonged periods of time or with an occlusive dressing.
Adverse Reactions
Dermatologic: Acne, hypopigmentation, allergic dermatitis, maceration of the skin, skin atrophy
Endocrine & metabolic: HPA suppression, Cushing's syndrome, growth retardation
Local: Burning, itching, irritation, dryness, folliculitis, hypertrichosis
Miscellaneous: Secondary infection
Mechanism of Action Topical corticosteroids have anti-inflammatory, antipruritic, vasoconstrictive, and antiproliferative actions
Usual Dosage Geriatrics and Adults: Topical: Apply sparingly to area once daily, do not use occlusive dressings
Monitoring Parameters Relief of symptoms
Patient Information Use only as prescribed and for no longer than the period prescribed; apply sparingly in a thin film and rub in lightly; avoid contact with eyes; notify physician if condition persists or worsens
Nursing Implications Use sparingly
Additional Information Considered a moderate-potency steroid; may be used for a limited time on the face; prolonged use may cause atrophic changes
Special Geriatric Considerations See Precautions; due to age-related changes in skin, limit use of topical glucocorticosteroids
Dosage Forms
Cream: 0.1% (15 g, 45 g)
Lotion: 0.1% (30 mL, 60 mL)
Ointment, topical: 0.1% (15 g, 45 g)

MOM/Mineral Oil Emulsion *see* Magnesium Hydroxide and Mineral Oil Emulsion *on page 428*

Monacolin K *see* Lovastatin *on page 420*

Monistat™ *see* Miconazole *on page 470*

Monistat-Derm™ *see* Miconazole *on page 470*

Monistat iv™ *see* Miconazole *on page 470*

Monocid® *see* Cefonicid Sodium *on page 130*

Mono-Gesic® *see* Salsalate *on page 637*

Monopril® *see* Fosinopril *on page 313*

More Attenuated Enders Strain *see* Measles Virus Vaccine, Live, Attenuated *on page 433*

More-Dophilus® [OTC] *see* Lactobacillus acidophilus and Lactobacillus bulgaricus *on page 397*

Moricizine Hydrochloride (mor i' siz een)
Brand Names Ethmozine®
Generic Available No
Therapeutic Class Antiarrhythmic Agent, Class I
Use Treatment of ventricular tachycardia and life-threatening ventricular arrhythmias

Unlabeled use: Moricizine 600-900 mg/day may be effective in treatment of PVCs, complete and nonsustained ventricular tachycardia
Contraindications Pre-existing second or third degree A-V block and in patients with right bundle-branch block when associated with left hemiblock, unless pacemaker is present; cardiogenic shock; known hypersensitivity to the drug
(Continued)

ALPHABETICAL LISTING OF DRUGS

Moricizine Hydrochloride *(Continued)*

Warnings Considering the known proarrhythmic properties and lack of evidence of improved survival for any antiarrhythmic drug in patients with life-threatening arrhythmias, it is prudent to reserve the use for patients with life-threatening ventricular arrhythmias; CAST II trial demonstrated a trend towards decreased survival for patients treated with moricizine; proarrhythmic effects occur as with other antiarrhythmic agents; hypokalemia, hyperkalemia, hypomagnesemia may effect response to class I agents; use with caution in patients with sick sinus syndrome, hepatic, and renal impairment

Precautions Use with caution in patients with hepatic or renal insufficiency since increases in half-life may occur; EKG changes may occur due to conduction abnormalities from changes in A-V node conduction; congestive heart failure may be aggravated; may alter pacemaker threshold sensitivity; drug fever

Adverse Reactions
  Cardiovascular: Proarrhythmia, syncope, cardiac arrest, myocardial infarction, chest pain, CHF, cardiac death, hypotension, bradycardia, thromboembolism
  Central nervous system: Dizziness, headache, fatigue, paresthesia, anxiety, depression, agitation, seizure, coma, euphoria, dyskinesia, hallucinations, speech difficulties, confusion, loss of memory, vertigo, somnolence, gait disturbances, akathisia, fever
  Dermatologic: Rash, pruritus, dry skin, urticaria
  Gastrointestinal: Anorexia, bitter taste, abdominal pain, ileus, vomiting, diarrhea, flatulence, dry mouth
  Genitourinary: Urinary incontinence, impotence
  Neuromuscular & skeletal: Tremors, muscle skeletal pain
  Ocular: Nystagmus, periorbital edema, blurred vision, eye pain, diplopia
  Otic: Tinnitus
  Respiratory: Dyspnea, hyperventilation, cough, pharyngitis, apnea, pulmonary embolism, asthma
  Miscellaneous: Temperature intolerance, swelling of lips and tongue, sweating, hypothermia

Overdosage Symptoms of overdose include emesis, lethargy, hypotension, conduction disturbances, sinus arrest, arrhythmias

Toxicology General supportive care; gastric lavage may be helpful

Drug Interactions
  Theophylline levels decreased
  Cimetidine increases moricizine levels
  Digoxin and propranolol have increased cardiac effects

Mechanism of Action Reduces the fast inward current carried by sodium ions, shortens Phase I and Phase II repolarization, resulting in decreased action potential duration and effective refractory period

Pharmacokinetics
  Protein binding, plasma: 95%
  Metabolism: Undergoes significant first-pass metabolism (38%)
  Half-life:
    Normal patients: 3-4 hours
    Cardiac disease patients: 6-13 hours
  Elimination: 56% excreted in feces and 39% in urine, some enterohepatic recycling occurs

Usual Dosage Geriatrics and Adults: Hospitalization required to start therapy. Oral: 200-300 mg every 8 hours, adjust dosage at 150 mg/day at 3-day intervals; to switch from another antiarrhythmic agent to moricizine, start moricizine 6-12 hours after last dose of former agent; may need 24-hour postdose with flecainide; see Additional Information

  Dosing adjustment in renal and hepatic impairment: Initial dose: 600 mg or less/day

Monitoring Parameters Holter monitoring may be considered; monitor pulse, EKG, and blood pressure

Patient Information Take as directed; do not change dose except from advice of your physician; report any chest pain and irregular heartbeats

Nursing Implications Giving 30 minutes after a meal delays the rate of absorption, resulting in lower peak plasma concentrations

Additional Information For transferring a patient from another antiarrhythmic agent, discontinue previous antiarrhythmic for 1-2 half-lives before starting moricizine; if this cannot be done, hospitalize patient to make transfer

Special Geriatric Considerations Due to moricizine binding to plasma albumin and alpha-glycoprotein, other highly bound drugs may displace moricizine; since elderly may require multiple drugs, caution with highly bound drugs is necessary; consider changes in renal and hepatic function with age and monitor closely since half-life may be prolonged

Dosage Forms Tablet: 200 mg, 250 mg, 300 mg

References
Fenster PE and Nolan PE, "Antiarrhythmic Drugs," *Geriatric Pharmacology*, Bressler R and Katz MD, eds, New York, NY: McGraw-Hill, 1993, 6:105-49.

Morphine Sulfate (mor' feen)

Related Information

Narcotic Agonist Comparative Pharmacology *on page 811*

Pharmacokinetics of Narcotic Agonist Analgesics *on page 812*

Brand Names Astramorph™ PF; Duramorph®; MS Contin®; MSIR®; OMS®; RMS®; Roxanol™; Roxanol SR™

Synonyms MS

Generic Available Yes

Therapeutic Class Analgesic, Narcotic

Use Relief of moderate to severe acute and chronic pain; pain of myocardial infarction; relieves dyspnea of acute left ventricular failure and pulmonary edema; preanesthetic medication

Restrictions C-II

Contraindications Known hypersensitivity to morphine sulfate; increased intracranial pressure; severe respiratory depression; severe liver or renal insufficiency

Warnings Some preparations contain sulfites which may cause allergic reactions

Precautions Use with caution in patients with hypersensitivity reactions to other phenanthrene derivative opioid agonists (codeine, hydrocodone, hydromorphone, levorphanol, oxycodone, oxymorphone)

Adverse Reactions

Cardiovascular: Palpitations, hypotension, bradycardia, peripheral vasodilation

Central nervous system: CNS depression, increased intracranial pressure

Dermatologic: Pruritus

Endocrine & metabolic: Antidiuretic hormone release

Gastrointestinal: Nausea, vomiting, constipation

Ocular: Miosis

Respiratory: Respiratory depression

Miscellaneous: Physical and psychological dependence, biliary or urinary tract spasm, histamine release

Overdosage Symptoms of overdose include respiratory depression, miosis, hypotension, bradycardia, apnea, pulmonary edema

Toxicology Treatment of an overdose includes support of the patient's airway, establishment of an I.V. line and administration of naloxone 2 mg I.V. with repeat administration as necessary up to a total of 10 mg.

Drug Interactions Increased toxicity: CNS depressants, phenothiazines, tricyclic antidepressants

Stability Refrigerate suppositories; do not freeze; degradation depends on pH and presence of oxygen; relatively stable in pH 4 and below; darkening of solutions indicate degradation; usual concentration for continuous I.V. infusion = 0.1-1 mg/mL in D_5W

Mechanism of Action Binds to opiate receptors in the CNS, causing inhibition of ascending pain pathways, altering the perception of and response to pain; produces generalized CNS depression

Pharmacodynamics Enhanced analgesia has been seen in elderly patients on therapeutic doses of narcotics; duration of action may be prolonged in the elderly; see table.

Dosage	Analgesia	
Form/Route	Peak	Duration
Tablets	1 h	4–5 h
Oral solution	1 h	4–5 h
Extended release tablets	1 h	8–12 h
Suppository	20–60 min	3–7 h
Subcutaneous injection	50–90 min	4–5 h
I.M. injection	30–60 min	4–5 h
I.V. injection	20 min	4–5 h

Pharmacokinetics

Absorption: Oral: Variable

Distribution: V_d: Decreased in elderly

Metabolism: In the liver via glucuronide conjugation

Half-life: 2-4 hours

Elimination: 6% to 10% excreted unchanged in urine; total body clearance decreased in elderly

Usual Dosage Doses should be titrated to appropriate effect; when changing routes of administration in chronically treated patients, note that oral doses are ~$1/3$ to $1/6$ as effective as parenteral dose

(Continued)

481

ALPHABETICAL LISTING OF DRUGS
Morphine Sulfate *(Continued)*

Geriatrics and Adults:

Oral: Prompt release: 10-30 mg every 4 hours as needed; controlled release: 15-30 mg every 8-12 hours

I.M., I.V., S.C.: 2.5-20 mg/dose every 2-6 hours as needed; usual: 10 mg/dose every 4 hours as needed. Initial I.M. dose for geriatric patients: 2.5-5 mg every 4-6 hours

I.V., S.C. continuous infusion: 0.8-10 mg/hour; may increase depending on pain relief/adverse effects; usual range up to 80 mg/hour

Rectal: 10-20 mg every 4 hours

Epidural: Initial: 5 mg in lumbar region; if inadequate pain relief within 1 hour, give 1-2 mg, maximum: 10 mg/24 hours; geriatric patients: <5 mg may provide satisfactory pain relief

Intrathecal ($^1/_{10}$ of epidural dose): 0.2-1 mg/dose; repeat doses **not** recommended; use extreme caution in geriatric patients

Monitoring Parameters Pain relief, respiratory and mental status, blood pressure

Reference Range Therapeutic: Surgical anesthesia: 65-80 ng/mL (SI: 227-280 nmol/L); Toxic: 200-5000 ng/mL (SI: 700-17,500 nmol/L)

Test Interactions Increased aminotransferase [ALT (SGPT)/AST (SGOT)] (S)

Patient Information May cause drowsiness; avoid alcoholic beverages; do not crush controlled release tablet

Nursing Implications Do not crush controlled release tablet; observe patient for excessive sedation, respiratory depression

Additional Information Because of its variety of dosage forms, morphine is particularly useful in the treatment of terminal pain. Serum concentrations >20 ng/dL may cause seizures; when converting from immediate release to controlled release morphine, the conversion is on a mg for mg basis. Immediate release morphine (oral, I.M., or S.C.) may be used for breakthrough pain until the dosage is adjusted.

Special Geriatric Considerations The elderly may be particularly susceptible to the CNS depressant and constipating effects of narcotics; see Pharmacodynamics and Pharmacokinetics

Dosage Forms

Injection: 0.5 mg/mL (10 mL); 1 mg/mL (10 mL, 30 mL, 60 mL); 2 mg/mL (1 mL, 2 mL, 60 mL); 3 mg/mL (50 mL); 4 mg/mL (1 mL, 2 mL); 5 mg/mL (1 mL, 30 mL); 8 mg/mL (1 mL, 2 mL); 10 mg/mL (1 mL, 2 mL, 10 mL); 15 mg/mL (1 mL, 2 mL, 20 mL)

Injection, preservative free: 0.5 mg/mL (2 mL, 10 mL); 1 mg/mL (2 mL, 10 mL)

Injection, I.V. via PCA pump: 1 mg/mL (10 mL, 30 mL, 60 mL); 5 mg/mL (30 mL)

Injection for I.V. infusion preparation: 25 mg/mL (4 mL, 10 mL, 20 mL)

Solution, oral: 10 mg/5 mL (5 mL, 10 mL, 100 mL, 120 mL, 500 mL); 20 mg/5 mL (5 mL, 100 mL, 120 mL, 500 mL)

Suppositories, rectal: 5 mg, 10 mg, 20 mg, 30 mg

Tablet: 15 mg, 30 mg

Tablet:

Controlled release: 15 mg, 30 mg, 60 mg, 100 mg

Soluble: 10 mg, 15 mg, 30 mg

References
Ferrell BA, "Pain Management in Elderly People," *J Am Geriatr Soc*, 1991, 39(1):64-73.
Kaiko RF, "Age and Morphine Analgesia in Cancer Patients With Postoperative Pain," *Clin Pharmacol Ther*, 1980, 28(6):823-6.
Kaiko RF, Wallenstein SL, Rogers AG, et al, "Narcotics in the Elderly," *Med Clin North Am*, 1982, 66(5):1079-89.

Motrin® *see* Ibuprofen *on page 360*

Motrin® IB [OTC] *see* Ibuprofen *on page 360*

6-MP *see* Mercaptopurine *on page 444*

MS *see* Morphine Sulfate *on previous page*

MS Contin® *see* Morphine Sulfate *on previous page*

MSIR® *see* Morphine Sulfate *on previous page*

MTX *see* Methotrexate *on page 455*

Mupirocin *(myoo peer' oh sin)*

Brand Names Bactroban®

Synonyms Pseudomonic Acid A

Therapeutic Class Antibiotic, Topical

Use Topical treatment of impetigo due to *Staphylococcus aureus*, beta-hemolytic *Streptococcus*, and *S. pyogenes*

Contraindications Known hypersensitivity to mupirocin or polyethylene glycol

Warnings Potentially toxic amounts of polyethylene glycol contained in the vehicle may be absorbed percutaneously in patients with extensive burns or open wounds; prolonged use may result in overgrowth of nonsusceptible organisms

Precautions Use with caution in patients with impaired renal function

Adverse Reactions

Cardiovascular: Swelling

Dermatologic: Pruritus, rash, erythema, dry skin

Local: Burning, stinging, pain, tenderness

Stability Do not mix with Aquaphor®, coal tar solution, or salicylic acid

Mechanism of Action Binds to bacterial isoleucyl transfer-RNA synthetase resulting in the inhibition of protein and RNA synthesis

Pharmacokinetics

Absorption: Topical: Penetrates outer layers of skin; systemic absorption is minimal through intact skin

Protein binding: 95%

Metabolism: Extensive, principally in the liver and skin to monic acid

Half-life: 17-36 minutes

Elimination: In urine

Usual Dosage Geriatrics and Adults: Topical: Apply small amount 2-5 times/day for 5-14 days

Patient Information For topical use only; do not apply into the eye

Additional Information Contains polyethylene glycol vehicle

Special Geriatric Considerations Not for treatment of pressure sores; see Warnings

Dosage Forms Ointment: 2% (15 g)

References

Goldfarb J, Crenshaw D, O'Horo J, et al, "Randomized Clinical Trial of Topical Mupirocin Versus Oral Erythromycin for Impetigo," *Antimicrob Agents Chemother*, 1988, 32(12):1780-3.

Murine® Ear Drops [OTC] *see* Carbamide Peroxide *on page 119*

Murine® Plus [OTC] *see* Tetrahydrozoline Hydrochloride *on page 680*

Muro 128® Ophthalmic [OTC] *see* Sodium Chloride *on page 648*

Myambutol® *see* Ethambutol Hydrochloride *on page 273*

Mycelex® *see* Clotrimazole *on page 180*

Mycelex®-G *see* Clotrimazole *on page 180*

Mycobutin® Oral *see* Rifabutin *on page 627*

Mycogen II Topical *see* Nystatin and Triamcinolone *on page 514*

Mycolog®-II Topical *see* Nystatin and Triamcinolone *on page 514*

Myconel® Topical *see* Nystatin and Triamcinolone *on page 514*

Mycostatin® *see* Nystatin *on page 513*

Mydfrin® Ophthalmic Solution *see* Phenylephrine Hydrochloride *on page 557*

Mykinac® *see* Nystatin *on page 513*

Mykrox® *see* Metolazone *on page 464*

Mylanta®-II [OTC] *see* Aluminum Hydroxide, Magnesium Hydroxide and Simethicone *on page 31*

Mylanta® [OTC] *see* Aluminum Hydroxide, Magnesium Hydroxide and Simethicone *on page 31*

Myleran® *see* Busulfan *on page 100*

Mylicon®-80 [OTC] *see* Simethicone *on page 645*

Mylicon® [OTC] *see* Simethicone *on page 645*

Myochrysine® *see* Gold Sodium Thiomalate *on page 327*

Myotonachol™ *see* Bethanechol Chloride *on page 85*

Myphetapp® [OTC] *see* Brompheniramine and Phenylpropanolamine *on page 94*

Mysoline® *see* Primidone *on page 587*

Mytrex® F Topical *see* Nystatin and Triamcinolone *on page 514*

Mytussin® AC *see* Guaifenesin and Codeine *on page 332*

Mytussin® [OTC] *see* Guaifenesin *on page 331*

Mytussin® DM [OTC] *see* Guaifenesin and Dextromethorphan *on page 332*

Nabumetone

Brand Names Relafen®

Generic Available No

Therapeutic Class Nonsteroidal Anti-inflammatory Agent (NSAID), Oral

Use Management of osteoarthritis and rheumatoid arthritis

Unlabeled use: Sunburn, mild to moderate pain

Contraindications Hypersensitivity to nabumetone, any component, aspirin or other nonsteroidal anti-inflammatory drugs (NSAIDs), salicylate allergy

Warnings GI toxicity (bleeding, ulceration, perforation); CNS effects may occur (headaches, confusion, depression); hypersensitivity, anaphylactoid reactions (intermittent

(Continued)

Nabumetone *(Continued)*

tolmetin use more often); renal function decline, acute renal insufficiency, interstitial nephritis, dysuria, cystitis, hematuria, nephrotic syndrome, hyperkalemia in acute renal insufficiency, hyponatremia, papillary necrosis, hepatic function impairment; elderly have increased risk for adverse reactions to NSAIDs; see Special Geriatric Considerations

Precautions Use with caution in patients with congestive heart failure, hypertension, decreased renal or hepatic function, history of GI disease (bleeding or ulcers), or those receiving anticoagulants; perform ophthalmologic evaluation for those who develop eye complaints during therapy (blurred vision, diminished vision, changes in color vision, retinal changes); NSAIDs may mask signs/symptoms of infections; photosensitivity reported

Adverse Reactions

Cardiovascular: Congestive heart failure, angina, hypertension, hypotension, fluid retention, arrhythmias, edema

Central nervous system: Headache, drowsiness, vertigo, dizziness, fatigue, hallucinations, confusion, depression, emotional lability, psychotic behavior, asthenia

Dermatologic: Rash, urticaria, angioedema, Stevens-Johnson syndrome, exfoliative dermatitis, ecchymosis, petechiae, purpura, bruising

Endocrine & metabolic: Hyperglycemia, hypoglycemia, hyperkalemia, gynecomastia, hyponatremia

Gastrointestinal: Dyspepsia, heartburn, nausea, diarrhea, constipation, flatulence, stomatitis, vomiting, abdominal pain, peptic ulcer, GI bleeding, GI perforation, gingival ulcers, pancreatitis, proctitis, paralytic ulcers, colitis, anorexia, weight loss

Genitourinary: Impotence, azotemia

Hematologic: Neutropenia, anemia, agranulocytosis, bone marrow suppression, hemolytic anemia, hemorrhage, inhibition of platelet aggregation

Hepatic: Hepatitis, elevated LFTs, cholestatic jaundice

Neuromuscular & skeletal: Involuntary muscle movements, muscle weakness, tremors

Ocular: Vision changes

Otic: Tinnitus

Renal: Dysuria, polyuria, pyuria, oliguria, anuria, acute renal failure

Respiratory: Exacerbation of asthma, dyspnea

Miscellaneous: Dry mucous membranes, thirst, pyrexia, sweating

Toxicology Management of a nonsteroidal anti-inflammatory agent (NSAID) intoxication is primarily supportive and symptomatic. Fluid therapy is commonly effective in managing the hypotension that may occur following an acute NSAID overdose, except when this is due to an acute blood loss. Seizures tend to be very short-lived and often do not require drug treatment although recurrent seizures should be treated with I.V. diazepam. Since many of the NSAIDs undergo enterohepatic cycling, multiple doses of charcoal may be needed to reduce the potential for delayed toxicities. NSAIDs are highly bound to plasma proteins, therefore hemodialysis and peritoneal dialysis are not useful.

Drug Interactions

May increase digoxin, methotrexate, and lithium serum concentrations

Aspirin or other salicylates may decrease NSAID serum concentrations

Other NSAIDs may increase adverse GI effects

Increased prothrombin time with anticoagulants

Decreased antihypertensive effects of ACE inhibitors, beta-blockers, and thiazide diuretics

Effects of loop diuretics may decrease

Increased response to sympathomimetics

Probenecid may increase toxicity of NSAIDs by increase in serum concentrations

Diuretics may increase risk for acute renal insufficiency

Azotemia may be enhanced in elderly receiving loop diuretics

Mechanism of Action Inhibits prostaglandin synthesis, acts on the hypothalamus heat-regulating center to reduce fever, blocks prostaglandin synthetase action which prevents formation of the platelet-aggregating substance thromboxane A_2; decreases pain receptor sensitivity. Other proposed mechanisms of action are lysosomal stabilization, kinin and leukotriene production, alteration of chemotactic factors, and inhibition of neutrophil activation. This latter mechanism may be the most significant pharmacologic action to reduce inflammation.

Pharmacokinetics

Absorption: From the stomach and small intestine

Distribution: Readily into most body fluids and tissues; aspirin is hydrolyzed to salicylate (active) by esterases in the GI mucosa, red blood cells, synovial fluid and blood

Metabolism: Metabolism of salicylate occurs primarily by hepatic microsomal enzymes

Half-life, aspirin: 15-20 minutes

Metabolic pathways are saturable such that salicylates half-life is dose-dependent ranging from 3 hours at lower doses (300-600 mg), 5-6 hours (after 1 g) and 15-30 hours with higher doses; in therapeutic anti-inflammatory doses, half-lives generally range from 6-12 hours

Time to peak: Peak plasma levels appear in about 1-2 hours

Usual Dosage Geriatrics and Adults: Initial: 1000 mg as a single dose daily; dose can be increased to 1500-2000 mg/day; total dose may be divided into 2 doses daily; do not exceed 2000 mg/day

Monitoring Parameters Monitor response (pain, range of motion, grip strength, mobility, ADL function), inflammation; observe for weight gain, edema; monitor renal function; observe for bleeding, bruising; evaluate gastrointestinal effects (abdominal pain, bleeding, dyspepsia); mental confusion, disorientation, CBC, serum, creatinine, BUN, liver function tests

Patient Information Serious gastrointestinal bleeding can occur as well as ulceration and perforation. Pain may or may not be present. Avoid aspirin and aspirin-containing products while taking this medication. If gastric upset occurs, take with food, milk, or antacid. If gastric adverse effects persist, contact physician. May cause drowsiness, dizziness, blurred vision, and confusion. Use caution when performing tasks which require alertness (eg, driving). Do not take for more than 3 days for fever or 10 days for pain without physician advice.

Nursing Implications See Monitoring Parameters, Overdosage, Patient Information, and Special Geriatric Considerations

Additional Information There are no clinical guidelines to predict which NSAID will give response in a particular patient. Trials with each must be initiated until response determined. Consider dose, patient convenience, and cost.

Special Geriatric Considerations Elderly are a high-risk population for adverse effects from nonsteroidal anti-inflammatory agents. As much as 60% of elderly can develop peptic ulceration and/or hemorrhage asymptomatically. The concomitant use of H_2 blockers, omeprazole, and sucralfate is not effective as prophylaxis. Misoprostol is the only prophylactic agent proven effective. Also, concomitant disease and drug use contribute to the risk for GI adverse effects. Use lowest effective dose for shortest period possible. Consider renal function decline with age. Use of NSAIDs can compromise existing renal function especially when Cl_{cr} is ≤ 30 mL/minute. Tinnitus may be a difficult and unreliable indication of toxicity due to age-related hearing loss or eighth cranial nerve damage. CNS adverse effects such as confusion, agitation, and hallucination are generally seen in overdose or high dose situations, but elderly may demonstrate these adverse effects at lower doses than younger adults.

Dosage Forms Tablet: 500 mg, 750 mg

References
Brooks PM, Day RO, "Nonsteroidal Anti-inflammatory Drugs – Differences and Similarities," *N Engl J Med*, 1991, 324(24):1716-25.

Clinch D, Banerjee AK, Ostick G, "Absence of Abdominal Pain in Elderly Patients With Peptic Ulcer," *Age Ageing*, 1984, 13:120-3.

Clive DM, Stoff JS, "Renal Syndromes Associated With Nonsteroidal Anti-inflammatory Drugs," *N Engl J Med*, 1984, 310(9):563-72.

Graham DY, "Prevention of Gastroduodenal Injury Induced by Chronic Nonsteroidal Anti-inflammatory Drug Therapy," *Gastroenterology*, 1989, 96(2 Pt 2 Suppl):675-81.

Gurwitz JH, Avarn J, Ross-Degan D, et al, "Nonsteroidal Anti-Inflammatory Drug-Associated Azotemia in the Very Old," *JAMA*, 1990, 264(4):471-5.

Knodel LC, "Preventing NSAID-Induced Ulcers: The Role of Misoprostol," *Consult Pharm*, 1989, 4:37-41.

Pounder R, "Silent Peptic Ulceration: Deadly Silence or Golden Silence?" *Gastroenterology*, 1989, 96:(2 Pt 2 Suppl)626-31.

N-Acetyl-P-Aminophenol see Acetaminophen *on page 13*

NaCl see Sodium Chloride *on page 648*

Nadolol (nay doe' lole)
Related Information
Beta-Blockers Comparison *on page 804-805*
Brand Names Corgard®
Therapeutic Class Antianginal Agent; Beta-Adrenergic Blocker
Use Treatment of hypertension and angina pectoris

Unlabeled use: Prevention of myocardial infarction, prophylaxis of migraine headaches, ventricular arrhythmia treatment, essential tremor, lithium-induced tremor, Parkinson's tremor, aggressive behavior, antipsychotic-induced tremor, anxiety, esophageal varices bleeding, and increased intraocular pressure; diastolic congestive heart failure

Contraindications Uncompensated congestive heart failure, cardiogenic shock, bradycardia or heart block, bronchial asthma, bronchospasms, hypersensitivity to beta-blocking agents, diabetes mellitus

Warnings Abrupt withdrawal of beta-blockers may result in an exaggerated cardiac beta-adrenergic responsiveness. Symptomatology has included reports of tachycardia, hypertension, ischemia, angina, myocardial infarction, and sudden death. It is recommended that patients be tapered gradually off of beta-blockers over a 2-week period rather than via abrupt discontinuation.

Precautions Increase dosing interval in patients with renal dysfunction; administer with caution to patients with bronchospastic disease, diabetes mellitus, hyperthyroidism,

(Continued)

Nadolol (Continued)

myasthenia gravis, and renal function decline and severe peripheral vascular disease; abrupt withdrawal of the drug should be avoided, drug should be discontinued over 2 weeks

Adverse Reactions Other adverse effects similar to other beta-blockers

Cardiovascular: Persistent bradycardia, hypotension, chest pain, edema, heart failure, Raynaud's phenomena

Central nervous system: Depression, confusion, dizziness, fatigue, insomnia, lethargy, nightmares, headache

Gastrointestinal: Constipation, diarrhea, nausea

Genitourinary: Impotence

Miscellaneous: Cold extremities

Overdosage Symptoms of overdose include bronchospasm, bradycardia, heart failure, hypotension; see Toxicology

Toxicology Sympathomimetics (eg, epinephrine or dopamine), glucagon, or a pacemaker can be used to treat the toxic bradycardia, asystole, and/or hypotension; initially fluids may be the best treatment for toxic hypotension; patients should remain supine; serum glucose and potassium should be measured; use supportive measures: lavage, syrup of ipecac. Nadolol may be removed by hemodialysis. I.V. glucose should be administered for hypoglycemia; seizures may be treated with phenytoin or diazepam intravenously; continuous monitoring of blood pressure and EKG is necessary. If PVCs occur, treat with lidocaine or phenytoin; avoid quinidine, procainamide, and disopyramide since these agents further depress myocardial function; bronchospasm can be treated with theophylline or beta$_2$ agonists (epinephrine).

Drug Interactions

Pharmacologic action of beta-antagonists may be decreased by aluminum compounds, calcium salts, barbiturates, cholestyramine, colestipol, NSAIDs, penicillins (ampicillin), rifampin, salicylates, sulfinpyrazone, thyroid hormones; hypoglycemic effect of sulfonylureas may be blunted

Pharmacologic effect of beta-antagonists may be enhanced with concomitant use of calcium channel blockers, oral contraceptives, flecainide (bioavailability and effect of flecainide also enhanced), haloperidol (hypotensive effects of both drugs), H$_2$ antagonists (decreased metabolism), hydralazine (both drugs hypotensive effects increased), loop diuretics (increased serum levels of beta-blockers except atenolol), MAO inhibitors, phenothiazines, propafenone, quinidine, quinolones, thioamines; beta-blockers may decrease clearance of acetaminophen; beta-blockers may increase anticoagulant effects of warfarin (propranolol); benzodiazepine effects enhanced by the lipophilic beta-blockers (atenolol does not interact); significant and fatal increases in blood pressure have occurred after decrease in dose or discontinuation of clonidine in patients receiving both clonidine and beta-blockers together (reduce doses of each cautiously with small decreases); peripheral ischemia of ergot alkaloids enhanced by beta-blockers; beta-blockers increase serum concentration of lidocaine; beta-blockers increase hypotensive effect of prazosin

Mechanism of Action Competitively blocks response to beta$_1$- and beta$_2$-adrenergic stimulation; does not exhibit any membrane stabilizing or intrinsic sympathomimetic activity; low lipid solubility, therefore, little penetration through blood-brain barrier

Pharmacodynamics Duration of effect: 24 hours

Pharmacokinetics

Absorption: Oral: 30% to 50%

Protein binding: 28%

Half-life: Adults: 20-24 hours; increased half-life with decreased renal function

Time to peak: Oral: Peak serum levels occur within 2-4 hours and persist for 17-24 hours

Elimination: Renally eliminated unchanged. Since geriatric patients will have reduced renal function, correct for Cl$_{cr}$

Usual Dosage

Geriatrics: Initial: 20 mg/day; increase doses 20 mg/increase; usual dose range: 20-240 mg

Adults: Initial: 40 mg once daily; increase gradually; usual dosage: 40-80 mg/day; may need up to 240-320 mg/day; doses as high as 640 mg/day have been used

Dosing interval in renal impairment:

Cl$_{cr}$ >50 mL/minute: Administer every 24 hours

Cl$_{cr}$ 31-50 mL/minute: Administer every 24-36 hours

Cl$_{cr}$ 10-30 mL/minute: Administer every 24-48 hours

Cl$_{cr}$ <10 mL/minute: Administer every 40-60 hours

Moderately dialyzable (20% to 50%)

Monitoring Parameters Blood pressure, orthostatic hypotension, heart rate, CNS effects

Test Interactions Increased cholesterol (S), glucose, triglycerides, potassium, uric acid; decreased HDL

Patient Information Do not discontinue medication abruptly, sudden stopping of medication may precipitate or cause angina; consult pharmacist or physician before taking with other adrenergic drugs (eg, cold medications); notify physician if any of the following symptoms occur: difficult breathing, night cough, swelling of extremities, slow pulse, dizziness, lightheadedness, confusion, depression, skin rash, fever, sore throat, unusual bleeding or bruising; may produce drowsiness, dizziness, lightheadedness, blurred vision, confusion; use with caution while driving or performing tasks requiring alertness; may mask signs of hypoglycemia in diabetics; may be taken without regard to meals

Nursing Implications Advise against abrupt withdrawal; monitor orthostatic blood pressures, apical and peripheral pulse and mental status changes (ie, confusion, depression)

Special Geriatric Considerations Due to alterations in the beta-adrenergic autonomic nervous system, beta-adrenergic blockade may result in less hemodynamic response than seen in younger adults. Studies indicate that despite decreased sensitivity to the chronotropic effects of beta blockade with age, there appears to be an increased myocardial sensitivity to the negative inotropic effect during stress (ie, exercise). Controlled trials have shown the overall response rate for propranolol to be only 20% to 50% in elderly populations. Therefore, all beta-adrenergic blocking drugs may result in a decreased response as compared to younger adults. Must adjust dose for renal function, see Precautions and Usual Dosage.

Dosage Forms Tablet: 20 mg, 40 mg, 80 mg, 120 mg, 160 mg

References

Aagaard GN, "Treatment of Hypertension in The Elderly," *Drug Treatment in the Elderly*, Vestal RE, ed, Boston, MA: ADIS Health Science Press, 1984, 77.

Nafazair® see Naphazoline Hydrochloride on page 492

Nafcil™ see Nafcillin Sodium on this page

Nafcillin Sodium (naf sill' in)

Brand Names Nafcil™; Nallpen®; Unipen®

Synonyms Ethoxynaphthamido Penicillin Sodium; Sodium Nafcillin

Generic Available Yes

Therapeutic Class Antibiotic, Penicillin

Use Treatment of susceptible bacterial infections such as osteomyelitis, cellulitis, septicemia, endocarditis, and CNS infections due to penicillinase-producing strains of *Staphylococcus*

Contraindications Hypersensitivity to nafcillin or any component or penicillins

Precautions Extravasation of I.V. infusions should be avoided; modification of dosage is necessary in patients with both severe renal and hepatic impairment; patients with a cephalosporin allergy (anaphylaxis)

Adverse Reactions
Cardiovascular: Thrombophlebitis
Central nervous system: Fever
Dermatologic: Skin rash
Gastrointestinal: Nausea, diarrhea
Hematologic: Neutropenia
Local: Pain
Renal: Rare acute interstitial nephritis
Miscellaneous: Hypersensitivity reactions

Overdosage Symptoms of overdose include neuromuscular hypersensitivity, seizure

Toxicology Many beta-lactam-containing antibiotics have the potential to cause neuromuscular hyperirritability or convulsive seizures. Hemodialysis may be helpful to aid in the removal of the drug from the blood, otherwise most treatment is supportive or symptom directed.

Drug Interactions
Decreased effect of warfarin possible
Increased risk of bleeding with heparin, increased effect with probenecid

Stability Refrigerate oral suspension after reconstitution; discard after 7 days; reconstituted parenteral solution is stable for 3 days at room temperature and 7 days when refrigerated or 12 weeks when frozen; for I.V. infusion in NS or D_5W, solution is stable for 24 hours at room temperature and 96 hours when refrigerated

Mechanism of Action Interferes with bacterial cell wall synthesis during active multiplication causing cell death and resultant bactericidal activity against susceptible bacteria

Pharmacokinetics
Absorption: Oral: Poor and erratic
Protein binding: 90%
Half-life: Adults with normal renal and hepatic function: 0.5-1.5 hours
Time to peak: Peak serum levels occur within 2 hours; peak serum levels occur 30-60 minutes after an I.M. dose
Elimination: Primarily in bile, and 10% to 30% in urine as unchanged drug; undergoes enterohepatic recycling

Usual Dosage Geriatrics and Adults:
Oral: 250-500 mg every 4-6 hours, up to 1 g every 4-6 hours for more severe infections
I.M.: 500 mg every 4-6 hours

(Continued)

Nafcillin Sodium *(Continued)*

I.V.: 500 mg to 2 g every 4-6 hours

Dosing interval in renal impairment: No change necessary
Not dialyzable (0% to 5%)

Administration Give around-the-clock rather than 4 times/day, 3 times/day, etc (ie, 12-6-12-6, not 9-1-5-9) to promote less variation in peak and trough serum levels; burning on I.V. administration may be decreased by further diluting the preparation to 250 mL NS or D₅W

Monitoring Parameters Watch for signs or symptoms of fluid overload or retention in patients with congestive heart failure; pain/burning with administration

Test Interactions False-positive urinary and serum proteins

Patient Information Report any diarrhea that develops within 2 weeks of completion of therapy to your physician or pharmacist; complete full course of therapy

Nursing Implications See Administration

Additional Information Due to its poor oral absorption, patients switched from I.V. to oral treatment should be given a more suitable oral alternative such as dicloxacillin or cloxacillin

Sodium content of 1 g: 66.7 mg (2.9 mEq)

Special Geriatric Considerations Nafcillin has not been studied exclusively in the elderly, however, given its route of elimination, dosage adjustments based upon age and renal function is not necessary

Dosage Forms
Capsule: 250 mg
Injection: 500 mg, 1 g, 2 g, 4 g, 10 g
Powder for oral solution: 250 mg/5 mL (100 mL)
Tablet: 500 mg

Naftifine Hydrochloride (naf' ti feen)

Brand Names Naftin® Topical
Generic Available No
Therapeutic Class Antifungal Agent, Topical
Use Topical treatment of tinea cruris (jock itch), tinea corporis (ring worm), and tinea pedis (athlete's foot)
Contraindications Hypersensitivity to any component
Warnings For external use only
Adverse Reactions
Dermatologic: Dryness, erythema, itching
Local: Irritation, burning, stinging
Mechanism of Action Synthetic, broad-spectrum antifungal agent in the allylamine class; topical antifungals totally unrelated to the imidazole compounds. As with all allylamine derivatives, most active when the allylamine double bond has the transorientation; the corresponding cis-isomer is much less active. The drug appears to have both fungistatic and fungicidal activity with no systemic adverse effects. Exhibits antifungal activity by selectively inhibiting the enzyme squalene epoxidase in a dose-dependent manner. As a result of this inhibitor, the primary sterol, ergosterol, within the fungal membrane is not synthesized.
Pharmacokinetics
Absorption: Systemic, 6% for cream, ≤4% for gel
Half-life: 2-3 days
Elimination: Metabolites excreted in urine and feces
Usual Dosage Geriatrics and Adults: Topical: Apply twice daily
Patient Information External use only; avoid eyes, mouth, and other mucous membranes; do not use occlusive dressings unless directed to do so; discontinue if irritation or sensitivity develops; wash hands after application
Nursing Implications See Patient Information
Special Geriatric Considerations No specific recommendations for use in the elderly
Dosage Forms
Cream: 1% (15 g, 30 g, 60 g)
Gel, topical: 1% (20 g, 40 g, 60 g)

Naftin® Topical *see* Naftifine Hydrochloride *on this page*

NaHCO₃ *see* Sodium Bicarbonate *on page 646*

Nalbuphine Hydrochloride (nal' byoo feen)

Related Information
Pharmacokinetics of Narcotic Agonist Analgesics *on page 812*
Brand Names Nubain®
Generic Available Yes
Therapeutic Class Analgesic, Narcotic
Use Relief of moderate to severe pain

Contraindications Hypersensitivity to nalbuphine or any component

Warnings Use with caution in patients with drug dependence (may experience withdrawal symptoms), head trauma or increased intracranial pressure, decreased hepatic or renal function

Precautions Use with caution in patients with recent myocardial infarction, biliary tract surgery, or sulfite sensitivity; may produce respiratory depression

Adverse Reactions
  Cardiovascular: Hypotension, flushing
  Central nervous system: CNS depression, dizziness, hallucinations
  Dermatologic: Urticaria
  Gastrointestinal: Nausea, vomiting, anorexia, dry mouth
  Respiratory: Pulmonary edema, respiratory depression

Overdosage Symptoms of overdose include CNS depression, respiratory depression, miosis, hypotension, bradycardia

Toxicology Treatment of an overdose includes support of the patient's airway, establishment of an I.V. line and administration of naloxone 2 mg I.V. with repeat administration as necessary up to a total of 10 mg

Drug Interactions Increased toxicity: Barbiturates, anesthetics

Mechanism of Action Binds to opiate receptors in the CNS, causing inhibition of ascending pain pathways, altering the perception of and response to pain; produces generalized CNS depression

Pharmacodynamics
  Peak effect and serum levels:
    I.M.: Within 30 minutes
    I.V.: Within 1-3 minutes

Pharmacokinetics
  Metabolism: In the liver
  Half-life: 3.5-5 hours
  Elimination: Metabolites excreted primarily in feces (via bile) and in urine ($\sim$7%)

Usual Dosage Geriatrics and Adults: I.M., I.V., S.C.: 10 mg/70 kg every 3-6 hours

Monitoring Parameters Relief of pain, respiratory and mental status, blood pressure

Patient Information May cause drowsiness; avoid CNS depressants and alcohol

Nursing Implications Observe patient for excessive sedation, respiratory depression, signs of narcotic withdrawal

Special Geriatric Considerations See Precautions; the elderly may be particularly susceptible to CNS effects; monitor closely

Dosage Forms Injection: 10 mg/mL (1 mL, 10 mL); 20 mg/mL (1 mL, 10 mL)

Naldecon® Senior EX [OTC] *see* Guaifenesin *on page 331*

Nalfon® *see* Fenoprofen Calcium *on page 282*

Nalidixic Acid (nal i dix' ik)

Brand Names NegGram®; Wintomylon®

Synonyms Nalidixinic Acid

Generic Available Yes

Therapeutic Class Antibiotic, Quinolone

Use Urinary tract infections

Contraindications History of convulsive disorders, hypersensitivity to nalidixic acid or any component

Warnings Has been shown to cause cartilage degeneration in immature animals

Precautions Usefulness may be limited by the emergence of bacterial resistance; use with caution in patients with impaired hepatic or renal function

Adverse Reactions
  Central nervous system: Malaise, drowsiness, vertigo, confusion, toxic psychosis, convulsions, fever, headache, increased intracranial pressure, dizziness, chills
  Dermatologic: Rash, urticaria, photosensitivity
  Endocrine & metabolic: Metabolic acidosis
  Gastrointestinal: Nausea, vomiting
  Hematologic: Leukopenia, thrombocytopenia
  Hepatic: Hepatotoxicity
  Ocular: Visual disturbances

Overdosage Symptoms of overdose include nausea, vomiting, toxic psychosis, convulsions, increased intracranial pressure, metabolic acidosis

Drug Interactions Warfarin (increased anticoagulant effect due to displacement from albumin binding sites), antacids (decreased nalidixic acid absorption)

Mechanism of Action Inhibits DNA polymerization in late stages of chromosomal replication

Pharmacokinetics Achieves significant antibacterial concentrations only in the urinary tract
  Protein binding: 90%.
  Metabolism: Partially in the liver

(Continued)

Nalidixic Acid *(Continued)*

Half-life: 6-7 hours (increases significantly with renal impairment)

Time to peak: Oral: Peak serum levels occur within 1-2 hours

Elimination: In urine as unchanged drug and 80% as metabolites; small amounts appear in feces

In one study, nalidixic acid's half-life (11.5 hours) and V_d (.55 L/kg) were significantly greater and its total body clearance significantly decreased (2.9 L/hour) in older volunteers compared to younger volunteers, 2.7 hours, 0.47 L/kg, and 8.3 L/hour, respectively

Usual Dosage Geriatrics and Adults: Oral: 1 g 4 times/day for 2 weeks; then suppressive therapy of 500 mg 4 times/day

Dosing comments in renal impairment: Cl_{cr} <50 mL/minute: Avoid use

Administration Give around-the-clock rather than 4 times/day, 3 times/day, etc (ie, 12-6-12-6, not 9-1-5-9) to promote less variation in peak and trough serum levels

Monitoring Parameters Signs and symptoms of infection

Test Interactions False-positive urine glucose with Clinitest®, false increase in urinary VMA

Patient Information Avoid undue exposure to direct sunlight; take 1 hour before meals; complete full course of therapy

Nursing Implications See Administration

Special Geriatric Considerations See Pharmacokinetics, Precautions, and Usual Dosage; calculate an estimated creatinine clearance to determine if use is appropriate

Dosage Forms

Suspension, oral: 250 mg/5 mL (473 mL)

Tablet: 250 mg, 500 mg, 1 g

References

Barbeau G, Belanger PM, "Pharmacokinetics of Nalidixic Acid in Old and Young Volunteers," *J Clin Pharmacol*, 1982, 22(10):490-6.

Nalidixinic Acid *see* Nalidixic Acid *on previous page*

Nallpen® *see* Nafcillin Sodium *on page 487*

***N*-allylnoroxymorphine Hydrochloride** *see* Naloxone Hydrochloride *on this page*

Naloxone Hydrochloride (nal ox' one)

Brand Names Narcan®

Synonyms *N*-allylnoroxymorphine Hydrochloride

Generic Available Yes

Therapeutic Class Antidote, Narcotic Agonist

Use Reverses CNS and respiratory depression in suspected narcotic overdose; coma of unknown etiology; used investigationally for shock, PCP and alcohol ingestion, and Alzheimer's disease

Contraindications Hypersensitivity to naloxone or any component

Warnings May precipitate withdrawal symptoms in patients addicted to opiates, including hypertension, sweating, agitation, irritability

Precautions Use with caution in patients with cardiovascular disease; excessive dosages should be avoided after use of opiates in surgery, because naloxone may cause an increase in blood pressure and reversal of anesthesia

Adverse Reactions

Cardiovascular: Hypertension, hypotension, tachycardia, ventricular arrhythmias, cardiac arrest

Central nervous system: Insomnia, irritability, anxiety

Dermatologic: Rash

Gastrointestinal: Nausea, vomiting

Miscellaneous: Sweating

Overdosage Symptoms of overdose include excitation, hypotension, hypertension, pulmonary edema, arrhythmias

Toxicology Naloxone is the drug of choice for respiratory depression that is known or suspected to be caused by an overdose of an opiate or opioid. **Caution:** Naloxone's effects are due to its action on narcotic reversal, not due to any direct effect upon opiate receptors. Therefore, adverse events occur secondarily to reversal (withdrawal) of narcotic analgesia and sedation, which can cause severe reactions.

Drug Interactions Decreased effect of narcotic analgesics

Stability Protect from light; stable in 0.9% NaCl and D_5W at 4 mcg/mL for 24 hours; do not mix with alkaline solutions

Mechanism of Action Competes and displaces narcotics at narcotic receptor sites

Pharmacodynamics

Onset of action:

I.V.: Within 2 minutes

S.C., I.M., E.T.: Within 2-5 minutes

Duration of effect: 20-60 minutes; shorter than that of most opioids, therefore, repeated doses are usually needed

Pharmacokinetics
Metabolism: Primarily by glucuronidation in the liver
Half-life: 1-1.5 hours
Elimination: In urine as metabolites

Usual Dosage Continuous infusion: I.V.: If continuous infusion is required, calculate dosage/hour based on effective intermittent dose used and duration of adequate response seen, titrate dose

Geriatrics and Adults: Postoperative narcotic depression (partial reversal): I.V.: 0.1-0.2 mg at 2- to 3-minute intervals to desired degree of reversal; may require repeat doses within 1 or 2 hours

Monitoring Parameters Blood pressure, pulse, mental status

Nursing Implications Monitor patients for signs of narcotic reversal; too rapid a reversal of narcotic depression may result in nausea, vomiting, sweating, tachycardia, increased blood pressure, and tremulousness

Additional Information In Talwin® Nx to prevent abuse of tablets via parenteral administration

Special Geriatric Considerations In small trials, naloxone has shown temporary improvement in Alzheimer's disease; however, is not recommended for treatment

Dosage Forms
Injection: 0.4 mg/mL (1 mL, 2 mL, 10 mL); 1 mg/mL (2 mL, 10 mL)
Injection, neonatal: 0.02 mg/mL (2 mL)

References
Waters C, "Cognitive Enhancing Agents: Current Status in the Treatment of Alzheimer's Disease," *Can J Neurol Sci*, 1988, 15(3):249-56.

Naphazoline and Antazoline (naf az' oh leen)
Related Information
Naphazoline Hydrochloride *on next page*
Brand Names Vasocon-A®
Therapeutic Class Ophthalmic Agent, Vasoconstrictor
Use Topical ocular congestion, irritation and itching
Contraindications Narrow-angle glaucoma, known hypersensitivity to naphazoline or antazoline
Precautions Use with caution in patients with hypothyroidism, heart disease, hypertension or diabetes mellitus
Adverse Reactions
Cardiovascular: Systemic cardiovascular stimulation, hypertension
Central nervous system: Nervousness, dizziness, headache
Gastrointestinal: Nausea
Local effects: Transient stinging, nasal mucosa irritation, dryness, sneezing, rebound congestion
Neuromuscular & skeletal: Weakness
Ocular: Pupillary dilation, increase in intraocular pressure, mydriasis, blurring of vision
Miscellaneous: Sweating
Overdosage Symptoms of overdose include drowsiness, decreased body temperature, bradycardia, short-life hypotension, coma
Toxicology Following initiation of essential overdose management, toxic symptoms should be treated. The patient should be kept warm and monitored for alterations in vital functions. Seizures commonly respond to diazepam (5-10 mg I.V. bolus) every 15 minutes if needed up to a total of 30 mg or to phenytoin or phenobarbital.
Drug Interactions MAO inhibitors
Stability Store in tight, light-resistant containers
Usual Dosage Geriatrics and Adults: Instill 1-2 drops every 3-4 hours
Patient Information Discontinue drug and consult physician if ocular pain or visual changes occur, ocular redness or irritation, or condition worsens or persists for more than 72 hours
Nursing Implications Do not use discolored solutions
Special Geriatric Considerations Evaluate patient's ability to self-administer; use with caution in patients with cardiovascular disease
Dosage Forms Solution: Naphazoline hydrochloride 0.05% and antazoline phosphate 0.5% (15 mL)

Naphazoline and Pheniramine
Related Information
Naphazoline Hydrochloride *on next page*
Brand Names Naphcon-A®
Synonyms Pheniramine and Naphazoline
Therapeutic Class Ophthalmic Agent, Vasoconstrictor
Use Topical ocular vasoconstrictor
(Continued)

Naphazoline and Pheniramine *(Continued)*

Contraindications Hypersensitivity to naphazoline, pheniramine or any component

Warnings Topical antihistamines are potential sensitizers and may produce local sensitivity reactions; because they may produce angle closure, use with caution in persons with a narrow angle or history of glaucoma; use with caution in patients with hypothyroidism, heart disease, hypertension or diabetes mellitus; rebound congestion may occur with extended use

Adverse Reactions

Cardiovascular: Systemic cardiovascular stimulation, hypertension

Central nervous system: Nervousness, dizziness, headache

Gastrointestinal: Nausea

Local effects: Transient stinging, nasal mucosa irritation, dryness, sneezing, rebound congestion

Neuromuscular & skeletal: Weakness

Ocular: Pupillary dilation, increase in intraocular pressure, mydriasis, blurring of vision

Miscellaneous: Sweating

Drug Interactions MAO inhibitors

Usual Dosage Geriatrics and Adults: 1-2 drops every 3-4 hours

Patient Information Discontinue drug and consult physician if ocular pain or visual changes occur, ocular redness or irritation, or condition worsens or persists more than 72 hours

Special Geriatric Considerations Evaluate patient's ability to self-administer; use cautiously in patients with cardiovascular disease

Dosage Forms Solution, ophthalmic: Naphazoline hydrochloride 0.025% and pheniramine 0.3% (15 mL)

Naphazoline Hydrochloride *(naf az' oh leen)*

Brand Names AK-Con®; Albalon® Liquifilm®; Allerest® Eye Drops [OTC]; Clear Eyes® [OTC]; Comfort® [OTC]; Degest® 2 [OTC]; Estivin® II [OTC]; I-Naphline®; Nafazair®; Naphcon® [OTC]; Naphcon Forte®; Ocu-Zoline®; Opcon®; Privine® [OTC]; VasoClear® [OTC]; Vasocon Regular®

Generic Available Yes

Therapeutic Class Adrenergic Agonist Agent, Ophthalmic; Decongestant, Nasal; Nasal Agent, Vasoconstrictor; Ophthalmic Agent, Vasoconstrictor

Use Topical ocular vasoconstrictor; will temporarily relieve congestion, itching, and minor irritation, and to control hyperemia in patients with superficial corneal vascularity

Contraindications Hypersensitivity to naphazoline or any component, narrow-angle glaucoma, prior to peripheral iridectomy (in patients susceptible to angle block)

Precautions Rebound congestion may occur with extended use; use with caution in the presence of hypertension, diabetes, hyperthyroidism, heart disease, coronary artery disease, cerebral arteriosclerosis, or long-standing bronchial asthma

Adverse Reactions

Cardiovascular: Systemic cardiovascular stimulation, hypertension

Central nervous system: Nervousness, dizziness, headache

Gastrointestinal: Nausea

Local effects: Transient stinging, nasal mucosa irritation, dryness, sneezing, rebound congestion

Neuromuscular & skeletal: Weakness

Ocular: Pupillary dilation, increase in intraocular pressure, mydriasis, blurring of vision

Miscellaneous: Sweating

Overdosage Symptoms of overdose include CNS depression, hypothermia, bradycardia, cardiovascular collapse, coma

Toxicology Following initiation of essential overdose management, toxic symptoms should be treated. The patient should be kept warm and monitored for alterations in vital functions. Seizures commonly respond to diazepam (5-10 mg I.V. bolus every 15 minutes if needed up to a total of 30 mg) or to phenytoin or phenobarbital.

Drug Interactions Anesthetics (discontinue mydriatic prior to use of anesthetics that sensitize the myocardium to sympathomimetics, ie, cyclopropane, halothane), MAO inhibitors, tricyclic antidepressants → hypertensive reactions

Stability Store in tight, light-resistant containers

Mechanism of Action Stimulates alpha-adrenergic receptors in the arterioles of the conjunctiva and the nasal mucosa to produce vasoconstriction

Pharmacodynamics

Onset of action: Following topical administration, decongestion occurs within 10 minutes

Duration: 2-6 hours

Pharmacokinetics Elimination is not well defined

Usual Dosage Geriatrics and Adults:

Nasal: 2 drops or sprays in each nostril no more than every 3 hours (drops) or 4-6 hours (spray) as needed

Ophthalmic (0.01% to 0.1%): Instill 1-2 drops into conjunctival sac of affected eye(s) every 3-4 hours; therapy generally should not exceed 3-4 days

Monitoring Parameters Blood pressure in hypertensives

Patient Information Do not use discolored solutions; discontinue eye drops if visual changes or ocular pain occur; do not use nasal products for >3 days without physician's consent

Nursing Implications Rebound congestion can result with continued use beyond 3 days

Special Geriatric Considerations Evaluate patient's ability to self-administer; use cautiously in patients with cardiovascular disease

Dosage Forms Solution:
Nasal:
Drops: 0.05% (20 mL)
Spray: 0.05% (15 mL)
Ophthalmic: 0.012% (7.5 mL, 30 mL); 0.02% (15 mL); 0.025% (15 mL); 0.03% (15 mL); 0.1% (15 mL, 480 mL)

Naphcon-A® see Naphazoline and Pheniramine on page 491

Naphcon Forte® see Naphazoline Hydrochloride on previous page

Naphcon® [OTC] see Naphazoline Hydrochloride on previous page

Naprosyn® see Naproxen on this page

Naproxen (na prox' en)

Brand Names Aleve® [OTC]; Anaprox®; Naprosyn®

Synonyms Naproxen Sodium

Generic Available No

Therapeutic Class Analgesic, Non-narcotic; Anti-inflammatory Agent; Nonsteroidal Anti-inflammatory Agent (NSAID), Oral

Use Management of inflammatory disease and rheumatoid disorders, osteoarthritis; ankylosing spondylitis, tendonitis, bursitis, acute gout; mild to moderate pain; dysmenorrhea; fever, sunburn, migraine headache (acute, prophylaxis)

Contraindications Hypersensitivity to naproxen, aspirin, or other nonsteroidal anti-inflammatory drugs (NSAIDs)

Warnings GI toxicity (bleeding, ulceration, perforation); CNS effects may occur (headaches, confusion, depression); hypersensitivity, anaphylactoid reactions (intermittent tolmetin use more often); renal function decline, acute renal insufficiency, interstitial nephritis, dysuria, cystitis, hematuria, nephrotic syndrome, hyperkalemia in acute renal insufficiency, hyponatremia, papillary necrosis, hepatic function impairment; elderly have increased risk for adverse reactions to NSAIDs; see Special Geriatric Considerations

Precautions Use with caution in patients with congestive heart failure, hypertension, decreased renal or hepatic function, history of GI disease (bleeding or ulcers), or those receiving anticoagulants; perform ophthalmologic evaluation for those who develop eye complaints during therapy (blurred vision, diminished vision, changes in color vision, retinal changes); NSAIDs may mask signs/symptoms of infections; photosensitivity reported

Adverse Reactions
Cardiovascular: Congestive heart failure, angina, hypertension, hypotension, fluid retention, arrhythmias, edema
Central nervous system: Headache, drowsiness, vertigo, dizziness, fatigue, hallucinations, confusion, depression, emotional lability, psychotic behavior, asthenia
Dermatologic: Rash, urticaria, angioedema, Stevens-Johnson syndrome, exfoliative dermatitis, ecchymosis, petechiae, purpura, bruising
Endocrine & metabolic: Hyperglycemia, hypoglycemia, hyperkalemia, gynecomastia, hyponatremia
Gastrointestinal: Dyspepsia, heartburn, nausea, diarrhea, constipation, flatulence, stomatitis, vomiting, abdominal pain, peptic ulcer, GI bleeding, GI perforation, gingival ulcers, pancreatitis, proctitis, paralytic ulcers, colitis, anorexia, weight loss
Genitourinary: Impotence, azotemia
Hematologic: Neutropenia, anemia, agranulocytosis, bone marrow suppression, hemolytic anemia, hemorrhage, inhibition of platelet aggregation
Hepatic: Hepatitis, elevated LFTs, cholestatic jaundice
Neuromuscular & skeletal: Involuntary muscle movements, muscle weakness, tremors
Ocular: Vision changes
Otic: Tinnitus
Renal: Dysuria, polyuria, pyuria, oliguria, anuria, acute renal failure
Respiratory: Exacerbation of asthma, dyspnea
Miscellaneous: Dry mucous membranes, thirst, pyrexia, sweating

Overdosage Symptoms include drowsiness, lethargy, disorientation, confusion, dizziness, numbness, paresthesia, nausea, vomiting, gastric irritation, abdominal pain, headache, tinnitus, sweating, blurred vision, muscle twitching, seizures, coma, acute renal failure, increased BUN and serum creatinine, hypotension, tachycardia, and metabolic acidosis

(Continued)

Naproxen *(Continued)*

Toxicology Management of a nonsteroidal anti-inflammatory agent (NSAID) intoxication is primarily supportive and symptomatic. Fluid therapy is commonly effective in managing the hypotension that may occur following an acute NSAID overdose, except when this is due to an acute blood loss. Seizures tend to be very short-lived and often do not require drug treatment although recurrent seizures should be treated with I.V. diazepam. Since many of the NSAIDs undergo enterohepatic cycling, multiple doses of charcoal may be needed to reduce the potential for delayed toxicities.

Drug Interactions
May increase digoxin, methotrexate, and lithium serum concentrations
Aspirin or other salicylates may decrease NSAID serum concentrations
Other NSAIDs may increase adverse GI effects
Increased prothrombin time with anticoagulants
Decreased antihypertensive effects of ACE inhibitors, beta-blockers, and thiazide diuretics
Effects of loop diuretics may decrease
Increased response to sympathomimetics
Probenecid may increase toxicity of NSAIDs by increase in serum concentrations
Diuretics may increase risk of acute renal insufficiency
May enhance azotemia in elderly receiving loop diuretics

Mechanism of Action Inhibits prostaglandin synthesis, acts on the hypothalamus heat-regulating center to reduce fever, blocks prostaglandin synthetase action which prevents formation of the platelet-aggregating substance thromboxane A_2; decreases pain receptor sensitivity. Other proposed mechanisms of action for salicylate anti-inflammatory action are lysosomal stabilization, kinin and leukotriene production, alteration of chemotactic factors, and inhibition of neutrophil activation. This latter mechanism may be the most significant pharmacologic action to reduce inflammation.

Pharmacodynamics
Analgesia:
Onset of action: 1 hour
Duration: Up to 7 hours
Anti-inflammatory:
Onset of action: Within 2 weeks
Peak: 2-4 weeks

Pharmacokinetics
Absorption: Oral: Almost 100%
Protein binding: High (>90%); increased free fraction in the elderly
Half-life: 12-15 hours
Time to peak: Peak serum levels occur within 1-2 hours for sodium salt and 2-4 hours for plain naproxen

Usual Dosage Geriatrics and Adults: Oral (as naproxen):
Rheumatoid arthritis, osteoarthritis, and ankylosing spondylitis: 500-1000 mg/day in 2 divided doses; maximum, plain: 1500 mg; maximum, sodium salt: 1375 mg

Mild to moderate pain: Initial: 500 mg, then 250 mg every 6-8 hours; maximum: 1250 mg/day; Aleve® : 225 mg every 8 hours

Monitoring Parameters Monitor response (pain, range of motion, grip strength, mobility, ADL function), inflammation; observe for weight gain, edema; monitor renal function (serum creatinine, BUN); observe for bleeding, bruising; evaluate gastrointestinal effects (abdominal pain, bleeding, dyspepsia); mental confusion, disorientation, CBC, liver function tests

Test Interactions Increased chloride (S), increased sodium (S)

Patient Information Serious gastrointestinal bleeding can occur as well as ulceration and perforation. Pain may or may not be present. Avoid aspirin and aspirin-containing products while taking this medication. If gastric upset occurs, take with food, milk, or antacid. If gastric adverse effects persist, contact physician. May cause drowsiness, dizziness, blurred vision, and confusion. Use caution when performing tasks which require alertness (eg, driving). Do not take for more than 3 days for fever or 10 days for pain without physician's advice.

Nursing Implications Administer with food, milk, or antacids to decrease GI adverse effects; monitor for occult blood loss, periodic ophthalmologic exams

Additional Information There are no clinical guidelines to predict which NSAID will give response in a particular patient. Trials with each must be initiated until response determined. Consider dose, patient convenience, and cost.

Special Geriatric Considerations Elderly are a high-risk population for adverse effects from nonsteroidal anti-inflammatory agents. As much as 60% of elderly can develop peptic ulceration and/or hemorrhage asymptomatically. The concomitant use of H_2 blockers, omeprazole, and sucralfate is not effective as prophylaxis. Misoprostol is the only prophylactic agent proven effective. Also, concomitant disease and drug use contribute to the risk for GI adverse effects. Use lowest effective dose for shortest period possible. Consider renal function decline with age. Use of NSAIDs can compromise existing renal function especially when Cl_{cr} is ≤30 mL/minute. Tinnitus may be

494

a difficult and unreliable indication of toxicity due to age-related hearing loss or eighth cranial nerve damage. CNS adverse effects such as confusion, agitation, and hallucination are generally seen in overdose or high-dose situations, but elderly may demonstrate these adverse effects at lower doses than younger adults.

Dosage Forms
Suspension, oral: 125 mg/5 mL (480 mL)
Tablet, as sodium: 275 mg, 550 mg
Tablet: 225 mg [OTC], 250 mg, 375 mg, 500 mg

References
Brooks PM, Day RO, "Nonsteroidal Anti-inflammatory Drugs – Differences and Similarities," *N Engl J Med*, 1991, 324(24):1716-25.
Clinch D, Banerjee AK, Ostick G, "Absence of Abdominal Pain in Elderly Patients With Peptic Ulcer," *Age Ageing*, 1984, 13:120-3.
Clive DM, Stoff JS, "Renal Syndromes Associated With Nonsteroidal Anti-inflammatory Drugs," *N Engl J Med*, 1984, 310(9):563-72.
Graham DY, "Prevention of Gastroduodenal Injury Induced by Chronic Nonsteroidal Anti-inflammatory Drug Therapy," *Gastroenterology*, 1989, 96(2 Pt 2 Suppl):675-81.
Gurwitz JH, Avarn J, Ross-Degan D, et al, "Nonsteroidal Anti-Inflammatory Drug-Associated Azotemia in the Very Old," *JAMA*, 1990, 264(4):471-5.
Knodel LC, "Preventing NSAID-Induced Ulcers: The Role of Misoprostol," *Consult Pharm*, 1989, 4:37-41.
Pounder R, "Silent Peptic Ulceration: Deadly Silence or Golden Silence?" *Gastroenterology*, 1989, 96:(2 Pt 2 Suppl)626-31.

Naproxen Sodium *see* Naproxen *on page 493*

Narcan® *see* Naloxone Hydrochloride *on page 490*

Narcotic Agonist Comparative Pharmacology *see page 811*

Nardil® *see* Phenelzine Sulfate *on page 553*

Nasahist B® *see* Brompheniramine Maleate *on page 95*

Nasalcrom® *see* Cromolyn Sodium *on page 190*

Nasalide® *see* Flunisolide *on page 297*

Nasal Relief® [OTC] *see* Oxymetazoline Hydrochloride *on page 530*

Naturacil® [OTC] *see* Psyllium *on page 610*

Navane® *see* Thiothixene *on page 687*

ND-Stat® *see* Brompheniramine Maleate *on page 95*

Nebcin® *see* Tobramycin *on page 699*

NebuPent™ *see* Pentamidine Isethionate *on page 544*

NegGram® *see* Nalidixic Acid *on page 489*

Nembutal® *see* Pentobarbital *on page 547*

Neo-Calglucon® [OTC] *see* Calcium Salts (Oral) *on page 111*

Neo-Cultol® [OTC] *see* Mineral Oil *on page 473*

Neofed® [OTC] *see* Pseudoephedrine *on page 609*

Neoloid® [OTC] *see* Castor Oil *on page 124*

Neomycin, Polymyxin B, and Dexamethasone
(dex a meth' a sone)
Brand Names AK-Trol® Ophthalmic; Dexacidin® Ophthalmic; Dexasporin® Ophthalmic; Infectrol® Ophthalmic; Maxitrol® Ophthalmic; Ocu-Trol® Ophthalmic
Generic Available Yes
Therapeutic Class Antibiotic, Ophthalmic
Use Steroid-responsive inflammatory ocular conditions in which a corticosteroid is indicated and where bacterial infection or a risk of bacterial infection exists
Contraindications Hypersensitivity to dexamethasone, polymyxin B, neomycin or any component; herpes simplex, vaccinia, and varicella
Warnings Prolonged use may result in glaucoma, defects in visual acuity, posterior subcapsular cataract formation, and secondary ocular infections
Adverse Reactions
Dermatologic: Contact dermatitis, cutaneous sensitization (sensitivity to topical neomycin has been reported to occur in 5% to 15% of patients)
Local: Pain, stinging
Ocular: Development of glaucoma, cataract, increased intraocular pressure, optic nerve damage, visual defects, blurred vision
Miscellaneous: Delayed wound healing, increased incidence to secondary infections
Mechanism of Action Interferes with bacterial protein synthesis by binding to 30S ribosomal subunits; binds to phospholipids, alters permeability, and damages the bacterial cytoplasmic membrane permitting leakage of intracellular constituents; decreases inflammation by suppression of migration of polymorphonuclear leukocytes and reversal of increased capillary permeability; suppresses normal immune response
(Continued)

Neomycin, Polymyxin B, and Dexamethasone *(Continued)*

Usual Dosage Geriatrics and Adults: Ophthalmic:

Ointment: Place a small amount (~$\frac{1}{2}$") in the affected eye 3-4 times/day or apply at bedtime as an adjunct with drops

Solution: Instill 1-2 drops into affected eye(s) every 3-4 hours; in severe disease, drops may be used hourly and tapered to discontinuation

Administration Shake well before using; tilt head back, place medication in conjunctival sac, and close eyes; apply finger pressure on lacrimal sac for 1 minute following instillation

Monitoring Parameters Intraocular pressure with use >10 days

Patient Information For the eye; shake well before using; do not touch dropper to eye; notify physician if condition worsens or does not improve in 3-4 days

Nursing Implications See Administration

Special Geriatric Considerations Assess patients ability to self-administer; see Monitoring Parameters

Dosage Forms Ophthalmic:

Ointment: Neomycin sulfate 3.5 mg, polymyxin b sulfate 10,000 units, and dexamethasone 0.1% per g (3.5 g)

Suspension: Neomycin sulfate 3.5 mg, polymyxin b sulfate 10,000 units, and dexamethasone 0.1% per mL (5 mL)

Neopap® [OTC] *see* Acetaminophen *on page 13*

Neoquess® Injection *see* Dicyclomine Hydrochloride *on page 215*

Neoquess® Tablet *see* Hyoscyamine Sulfate *on page 359*

Neosar® *see* Cyclophosphamide *on page 196*

Neo-Synephrine® 12 Hour Nasal Solution [OTC] *see* Oxymetazoline Hydrochloride *on page 530*

Neo-Synephrine® Ophthalmic Solution *see* Phenylephrine Hydrochloride *on page 557*

Neo-Synephrine® Nasal Solution [OTC] *see* Phenylephrine Hydrochloride *on page 557*

Neothylline® *see* Dyphylline *on page 247*

Nephro-Calci® [OTC] *see* Calcium Salts (Oral) *on page 111*

Neptazane® *see* Methazolamide *on page 451*

Nervocaine® *see* Lidocaine Hydrochloride *on page 406*

Nestrex® *see* Pyridoxine Hydrochloride *on page 613*

Netilmicin Sulfate *(ne til mye' sin)*

Brand Names Netromycin®

Synonyms I-N-Ethyl Sisomicin

Therapeutic Class Antibiotic, Aminoglycoside

Use Short-term treatment of serious or life-threatening infections including septicemia, peritonitis, intra-abdominal abscess, lower respiratory tract infections, urinary tract infections, skin, bone and joint infections caused by sensitive *Pseudomonas aeruginosa, Escherichia coli, Proteus, Klebsiella, Serratia, Enterobacter, Citrobacter,* and *Staphylococcus*

Contraindications Known hypersensitivity to netilmicin (aminoglycosides, bisulfites)

Warnings

Use with caution in patients with pre-existing renal insufficiency, vestibular or cochlear impairment, myasthenia gravis, hypocalcemia, conditions which depress neuromuscular transmission

Parenteral aminoglycosides are associated with nephrotoxicity or ototoxicity; the ototoxicity may be proportional to the amount of drug given and the duration of treatment; tinnitus or vertigo are indications of vestibular injury and impending hearing loss; renal damage is usually reversible

Adverse Reactions

Dermatologic: Rash

Gastrointestinal: Pseudomembranous colitis

Neuromuscular & skeletal: Neuromuscular blockade

Otic: Ototoxicity

Renal: Nephrotoxicity

Respiratory: Respiratory depression

Overdosage Symptoms of overdose include ototoxicity, nephrotoxicity, and neuromuscular toxicity

Toxicology Serum level monitoring is recommended. Symptoms of overdose include ototoxicity, nephrotoxicity, and neuromuscular toxicity. Treatment of choice following a single acute overdose appears to be the maintenance of good urine output of at least 3 mL/kg/hour. Dialysis is of questionable value in the enhancement of aminoglycoside elimination. If required, hemodialysis is preferred over peritoneal dialysis in patients with normal renal function. Careful hydration may be all that is required to promote diuresis and, therefore, the enhancement of the drug's elimination. Chelation with penicillins is experimental.

Drug Interactions
Increased/prolonged effect of depolarizing and nondepolarizing neuromuscular blocking agents
Increased toxicity: Concurrent use of amphotericin, vancomycin, ethacrynic acid, or furosemide may increase nephrotoxicity

Mechanism of Action Interferes with protein synthesis in bacterial cell by binding to ribosomal subunit

Pharmacokinetics
Absorption: I.M.: Well absorbed
Distribution: V_d: 0.16-0.34 L/kg
Half-life: 2-3 hours (age and renal function dependent)
Time to peak: Peak serum levels occur within 30-60 minutes
Elimination: By glomerular filtration; since clearance is dependent upon renal function, the clearance has been found to decrease with age and the half-life increase

Usual Dosage
Dosage should be based on an estimate of ideal body weight. All patients receiving I.M. or I.V. dosing should receive 1.5-2 mg/kg based on ideal body weight as a loading dose regardless of renal function, then give 3-5 mg/kg in 3 divided doses or as indicated by adjustment for renal function.
Geriatrics and Adults:
Intrathecal: 4-8 mg/day
I.M., I.V.: 1-5 mg/kg/day in 1-2 divided doses.

Dosing adjustment in renal impairment: 2 mg/kg (2-3 serum level measurements should be obtained after the initial dose to measure the half-life in order to determine the frequency of subsequent doses)
Dialyzable (50% to 100%)
Some patients may require larger or more frequent doses (eg, every 6 hours) if serum levels document the need (ie, cystic fibrosis or febrile granulocytopenic patients)
Topical: Apply 1-4 times/day to affected area
Ophthalmic:
Ointment: Instill $\frac{1}{2}$" (1.25 cm) 2-3 times/day to every 3-4 hours
Solution: Instill 1-2 drops every 2-4 hours

Dosing adjustment/comments in hepatic disease: Monitor plasma concentrations

Monitoring Parameters Urinalysis, urine output, BUN, serum creatinine; hearing should be tested before, during, and after treatment; particularly in those at risk for ototoxicity or who will be receiving prolonged therapy (>2 weeks). Obtain peak levels 30 minutes after the end of a 30-minute infusion trough levels are drawn within 30 minutes before the next dose.

Reference Range
Therapeutic:
Peak: 4-8 µg/mL (SI: 8-17 µmol/L)
Trough: <2 µg/mL (SI: 4 µmol/L) (depends in part on the minimal inhibitory concentration of drug against organism being treated)
Toxic:
Peak: >12 µg/mL (SI: >21 µmol/L)
Trough: >2 µg/mL (SI: >8.4 µmol/L)

Test Interactions Increased protein; decreased magnesium

Nursing Implications Aminoglycoside levels measured in blood taken from Silastic® central catheters can sometimes give falsely high readings

Special Geriatric Considerations The aminoglycosides are important therapeutic interventions for infections due to susceptible organisms and as empiric therapy in seriously ill patients. Their use is not without risk of toxicity; however, these risks can be minimized if initial dosing is adjusted for estimated renal function and appropriate monitoring performed.

Dosage Forms Injection: 100 mg/mL

References
Welling PG, Baumueller A, Lau CC, et al, "Netilmicin Pharmacokinetics After Single Intravenous Doses to Elderly Male Patients," *Antimicrob Agents Chemother*, 1977, 12:328-34.

Netromycin® see Netilmicin Sulfate *on previous page*

Neupogen® Injection see Filgrastim *on page 290*

Neuramate® see Meprobamate *on page 443*

Neurontin® see Gabapentin *on page 317*

Neurosyn® see Primidone *on page 587*

Neut® see Sodium Bicarbonate *on page 646*

Neutra-Phos® *see* Potassium Phosphate and Sodium Phosphate
on page 580

Neutra-Phos®-K *see* Potassium Phosphate *on page 579*

Neutrexin™ *see* Trimetrexate Glucuronate *on page 721*

NGT® Topical *see* Nystatin and Triamcinolone *on page 514*

Niacels™ [OTC] *see* Niacin *on this page*

Niacin (nye′ a sin)

Brand Names Niac® [OTC]; Niacels™ [OTC]; Niaplus™ [OTC]; Nicobid® [OTC]; Nicolar® [OTC]; Nicotinex [OTC]; Slo-Niacin® [OTC]

Synonyms Nicotinic Acid; Vitamin B_3

Generic Available Yes

Therapeutic Class Antilipemic Agent; Vitamin, Water Soluble

Use Adjunctive treatment of hyperlipidemias; peripheral vascular disease and circulatory disorders; treatment of pellagra; dietary supplement

Unlabeled use: Hypercholesterolemia

Contraindications Liver disease, peptic ulcer, severe hypotension, known hypersensitivity to niacin, hemorrhaging

Precautions Monitor liver function tests and blood glucose; may elevate uric acid levels; use with caution in patients predisposed to gout, tartrazine sensitivity

Adverse Reactions

Cardiovascular: Hypotension, tachycardia, syncope, vasovagal attacks, flushing

Central nervous system: Dizziness, headache

Dermatologic: Pruritus, burning, tingling skin, increased sebaceous gland activity; starting low doses and slowly increasing the nicotinic acid dose greatly reduces the potential for severe flushing or itching reactions; the table lists a titration approach that is useful in reducing these reactions

First week	50 mg twice daily
Second week	100 mg twice daily
Third week	200 mg twice daily
Fourth week	250 mg twice daily
Fifth week	500 mg twice daily
Sixth week	1 g twice daily
Seventh week	1.5 g twice daily

Gastrointestinal: GI upset, nausea, vomiting, heartburn, diarrhea

Hepatic: Abnormal liver function tests, jaundice, chronic liver damage

Ocular: Blurred vision

Overdosage Symptoms of overdose include flushing, GI distress, pruritus

Drug Interactions

Adrenergic-blocking agents may have additive vasodilating effect and may produce postural hypotension

Sulfinpyrazone's uricosuric effect may be inhibited

Probenecid's uricosuric effect may be inhibited

Decreased effect of oral hypoglycemics

Decreased toxicity (flush) with aspirin; increased toxicity with lovastatin (myopathy) and possibly with other HMG-CoA reductase inhibitors

Mechanism of Action A component of two coenzymes which is necessary for tissue respiration, lipid metabolism, and glycogenolysis; inhibits the synthesis of very low density lipoproteins

Pharmacodynamics

Onset of action: Vasodilation occurs within 20 minutes

Duration: 20-60 minutes (extended release preparations persist for 8-10 hours)

Pharmacokinetics

Metabolism: Depending upon the dose, niacin converts to niacinamide; following this conversion, niacinamide is metabolized in the liver

Half-life: 45 minutes

Elimination: In urine

Usual Dosage Geriatrics and Adults: Oral:

Hyperlipidemia: 3-6 g/day in 3 divided doses with or after meals

Pellagra: 50 mg 3-10 times/day, maximum: 500 mg/day

Niacin deficiency: 10-20 mg/day, maximum: 100 mg/day

Monitoring Parameters Fractionated cholesterol

Test Interactions False elevations in some fluorometric determinations of urinary catecholamines; false-positive urine glucose (Benedict's reagent)

Patient Information May experience transient cutaneous flushing and sensation of warmth, especially of face and upper body; itching or tingling, and headache may occur; may cause GI upset, take with food; if dizziness occurs, avoid sudden changes in posture

Nursing Implications Can cause muscle damage leading to muscle aches and cramps; monitor blood glucose concentration, liver function tests in patients on large doses and long-term therapy

Additional Information If flushing is bothersome or persistent, 325 mg of aspirin 30 minutes before each dose or increasing the dose slowly with weekly increase may minimize this reaction; for explicit guidelines on the risk factors for CHD and when to treat high blood cholesterol, see References; due to liver function test abnormalities induced by sustained release niacin, these dosage forms are not currently recommended

Special Geriatric Considerations The definition of and, therefore, when to treat hyperlipidemia in the elderly is a controversial issue. The National Cholesterol Education Program recommends that all adults 20 years of age and older maintain a plasma cholesterol of <200 mg/dL. By this definition, 60% of all elderly would be considered to have a borderline high (200-230 mg/dL) or high blood (≥240 mg/dL) elevated plasma cholesterol. However, plasma cholesterol has been shown to be a less reliable predictor of coronary heart disease in the elderly. Therefore, it is the authors' belief that pharmacologic treatment be reserved for those who are unable to obtain a desirable plasma cholesterol level by diet alone and for whom the benefits of treatment are believed to outweigh the potential adverse effects, drug interactions, and cost of treatment; see Additional Information

Dosage Forms
Capsule: 125 mg, 250 mg, 500 mg
Capsule, timed release: 125 mg, 250 mg, 300 mg, 400 mg, 500 mg
Elixir: 50 mg/5 mL (473 mL, 4000 mL)
Injection: 100 mg/mL (30 mL)
Tablet: 25 mg, 50 mg, 100 mg, 250 mg, 500 mg
Tablet, timed release: 250 mg, 500 mg, 750 mg

References
"Summary of the Second Report of the National Cholesterol Education Program (NCEP) Expert Panel on Detection, Evaluation, and Treatment of High Blood Cholesterol in Adults (Adult Treatment Panel II)," *JAMA*, 1993, 269(23):3015-23.

Niacinamide (nye a sin' a mide)

Synonyms Nicotinamide; Vitamin B_3
Generic Available Yes
Therapeutic Class Vitamin, Water Soluble
Use Prophylaxis and treatment of pellagra
Contraindications Liver disease, peptic ulcer, severe hypotension, known hypersensitivity to niacin
Warnings Large doses should be administered with caution to patients with gallbladder disease, jaundice; liver disease, or diabetes; use with caution in patients predisposed to gout; some products may contain tartrazine

Adverse Reactions
Cardiovascular: Flushing, tachycardia
Central nervous system: Headache, paresthesias
Dermatologic: Pruritus, increased sebaceous gland activity, skin rash
Gastrointestinal: Vomiting, flatulence
Ocular: Blurred vision
Respiratory: Wheezing

Overdosage Symptoms of overdose include flushing, GI distress, pruritus
Mechanism of Action A component of two coenzymes which is necessary for tissue respiration, lipid metabolism, and glycogenolysis

Pharmacokinetics
Absorption: Rapid from GI tract
Metabolism: In the liver
Half-life: 45 minutes
Time to peak: Peak serum level 20-70 minutes
Elimination: In urine

Usual Dosage Geriatrics and Adults: Oral: 50 mg 3-10 times/day
Pellagra: 300-500 mg/day

Test Interactions False elevations of urinary catecholamines
Special Geriatric Considerations Should not be confused with niacin; see Usual Dosage

Dosage Forms
Injection: 100 mg/mL (2 mL)
Tablet: 50 mg, 100 mg, 500 mg

Niac® [OTC] *see Niacin on previous page*

Niaplus™ [OTC] *see* Niacin *on page 498*

Nicardipine Hydrochloride (nye kar' de peen)

Related Information
Calcium Channel Blocking Agents Comparison *on page 806-807*

Brand Names Cardene®

Generic Available No

Therapeutic Class Antianginal Agent; Calcium Channel Blocker

Use Chronic stable angina; management of essential hypertension

Unlabeled use: CHF

Contraindications Severe hypotension or second and third degree heart block; sinus bradycardia; advanced heart block; ventricular tachycardia; cardiogenic shock, hypotension, CHF; hypersensitivity to nicardipine or any component, calcium channel blockers, and adenosine; atrial fibrillation or flutter associated with accessory conduction pathways; not to be given within a few hours of I.V. beta-blocking agents

Warnings Hypotension, CHF; cardiac conduction defects, PVCs, idiopathic hypertrophic subaortic stenosis; may cause platelet inhibition; do not abruptly withdraw (chest pain); hepatic dysfunction, increased angina, increased intracranial pressure with cranial tumors; elderly may have greater hypotensive effect

Precautions Sick sinus syndrome, severe left ventricular dysfunction, CHF, hepatic or renal impairment, hypertrophic cardiomyopathy (especially obstructive), concomitant therapy with beta-blockers or digoxin, edema

Adverse Reactions
Cardiovascular: Sustained tachycardia, myocardial infarction, increased angina, palpitations, peripheral vascular disease, atypical chest pain, chest pain, flushing, syncope, bradycardia, ventricular extrasystoles
Central nervous system: Dizziness, lightheadedness, nervousness, psychotic symptoms, malaise, anxiety, equilibrium difficulty, headache, paresthesia, somnolence, insomnia, disturbed dreams, confusion
Dermatologic: Rash
Gastrointestinal: Nausea, constipation, abdominal discomfort and pain, vomiting, dry mouth
Genitourinary: Polyuria, nocturia
Neuromuscular & skeletal: Arthralgia, hyperkinesia, weakness
Ocular: Blurred vision
Otic: Tinnitus
Respiratory: Shortness of breath, sore throat
Miscellaneous: Nasal congestion, infection, allergic reactions, peripheral edema

Overdosage Symptoms of overdose include hypotension, bradycardia, A-V block, hepatic necrosis

Toxicology Ipecac-induced emesis can hypothetically worsen calcium antagonist toxicity, since it can produce vagal stimulation. The potential for seizures precipitously following acute ingestion of large doses of a calcium antagonist may also contraindicate the use of ipecac. Supportive and symptomatic treatment, including I.V. fluids and Trendelenburg positioning, should be initiated as intoxication may cause hypotension. Although calcium (calcium chloride I.V. 1-2 g in adults over 5-10 minutes with repeats as needed) has been used as an "antidote" for acute intoxications, there is limited experience to support its routine use and should be reserved for those cases where definite signs of myocardial depression are evident. Heart block may respond to isoproterenol, glucagon, atropine and/or calcium although a temporary pacemaker may be required.

Drug Interactions
Beta-blockers increased cardiac and A-V conduction depression
Fentanyl increased volume requirements and hypotension; although this drug is new, other drug interactions not reported to the same degree as older agents; however, should be suspect of any drug interaction reported with other calcium channel blockers

Stability I.V. ampuls must be diluted; dilute each ampul in 240 mL to result in 250 mL of 0.1 mg/mL nicardipine; compatible with D_5W, $D_5\frac{1}{2}NS$, D_5NS, and D_5W with 40 mEq potassium chloride; 0.45% and 0.9% NS; **do not** mix with 5% sodium bicarbonate and lactated Ringer's solution; store at room temperature; protect from light; stable for 24 hours at room temperature

Mechanism of Action Inhibits calcium ion from entering the "slow channels" or select voltage-sensitive areas of vascular smooth muscle and myocardium during depolarization, producing a relaxation of coronary vascular smooth muscle and coronary vasodilation; increases myocardial oxygen delivery in patients with vasospastic angina

Pharmacokinetics
Absorption: Oral: Well absorbed, ~100%
Protein binding: 95%
Metabolism: Extensive first-pass metabolism; only metabolized in the liver
Bioavailability: Absolute, 35%
Half-life: 2-4 hours

Time to peak: Peak serum levels occur within 20-120 minutes and an onset of hypotension occurs within 20 minutes

Elimination: As metabolites in urine

Usual Dosage Geriatrics and Adults:

Angina (immediate release): 20 mg 3 times/day; usual range: 60-120 mg/day; increase dose at 3-day intervals

Hypertension: 20 mg 3 times/day; usual range: 60-120 mg/day; maximum blood pressure effect seen in 1-2 hours of administration
Sustained release: 30 mg twice daily
I.V.: Individualize dose
I.V. to oral equivalence:
20 mg every 8 hours orally = 0.5 mg/hour I.V.
30 mg every 8 hours orally = 1.2 mg/hour I.V.
40 mg every 8 hours orally = 2.2 mg/hour I.V.

Monitoring Parameters Heart rate, signs and symptoms of CHF; monitor blood pressure 1, 2, and 8 hours after dosing; measure sustained release blood pressure at 2, 4, and 6 hours after dosing

Reference Range Therapeutic: 28-50 ng/mL

Patient Information Sustained release products should be taken with food and not crushed; limit caffeine intake; avoid alcohol; notify physician if angina pain is not reduced when taking this drug, irregular heartbeat, shortness of breath, swelling, dizziness, constipation, nausea, or hypotension occur; do not stop therapy without advice of physician

Nursing Implications Do not crush sustained release capsules; see Warnings, Precautions, Monitoring Parameters, and Special Geriatric Considerations

Special Geriatric Considerations Elderly may experience a greater hypotensive response; constipation may be more of a problem in elderly; calcium channel blockers are no more effective in elderly than other therapies; however, they do not cause significant CNS effects which is an advantage over some antihypertensive agents.

Dosage Forms
Capsule: 20 mg, 30 mg
Capsule, sustained release: 30 mg, 45 mg, 60 mg
Injection: 2.5 mg/mL (10 mL vial)

Nicobid® [OTC] *see Niacin on page 498*

Nicolar® [OTC] *see Niacin on page 498*

Nicotinamide *see Niacinamide on page 499*

Nicotinex [OTC] *see Niacin on page 498*

Nicotinic Acid *see Niacin on page 498*

Nidryl® [OTC] *see Diphenhydramine Hydrochloride on page 228*

Nifedipine (nye fed' i peen)
Related Information
Calcium Channel Blocking Agents Comparison *on page 806-807*
Brand Names Adalat®; Adalat® CC; Procardia®; Procardia XL®
Generic Available Yes: Capsule
Therapeutic Class Antianginal Agent; Calcium Channel Blocker
Use Angina (vasospastic, chronic stable), hypertrophic cardiomyopathy, hypertension (sustained release only), pulmonary hypertension

Unlabeled use: Migraine headache, Raynaud's syndrome, CHF

Contraindications Known hypersensitivity to nifedipine or any other calcium channel blocker and adenosine; sick sinus syndrome, second or third degree A-V block, hypotension (<90 mm Hg systolic)

Warnings Monitor EKG and blood pressure closely in patients receiving I.V. therapy; hypotension, CHF; cardiac conduction defects, PVCs, idiopathic hypertrophic subaortic stenosis; may cause platelet inhibition; do not abruptly withdraw (chest pain); hepatic dysfunction, renal function impairment, increased angina, increased intracranial pressure with cranial tumors; elderly may have greater hypotensive effect

Precautions May increase frequency, duration, and severity of angina during initiation of therapy; use with caution in patients with congestive heart failure or aortic stenosis (especially with concomitant beta-adrenergic blocker); sick sinus syndrome, severe left ventricular dysfunction, hepatic impairment, hypertrophic cardiomyopathy (especially obstructive), concomitant therapy with beta-blockers or digoxin, edema

Adverse Reactions
Cardiovascular: Flushing, hypotension, tachycardia, palpitations, syncope, headache, facial edema, CHF, increased angina
Central nervous system: Dizziness, fever, giddiness, ataxia, migraine, chills
Dermatologic: Dermatitis, urticaria, petechiae, bruising, Stevens-Johnson syndrome, hair loss, pruritus, rash, urticaria, erythema multiforme, purpura
Endocrine & metabolic: Gynecomastia, hyperglycemia, gout, breast pain, hypokalemia

(Continued)

Nifedipine *(Continued)*

Gastrointestinal: Nausea, diarrhea, constipation (especially elderly), gingival hyperplasia, weight gain, gastroesophageal reflux, melena, eructation

Genitourinary: Polyuria, nocturia, dysuria, hematuria

Hematologic: Thrombocytopenia, leukopenia, anemia, hematomas

Neuromuscular & skeletal: Joint stiffness, arthritis with increased ANA, muscle cramps, joint pain

Ocular: Blurred vision, transient blindness, periorbital edema

Respiratory: Shortness of breath, rhinitis, sinusitis, nasal congestion

Miscellaneous: Sweating, peripheral edema, epistaxis

Overdosage Symptoms of overdose include peripheral vasodilation, heartblock, hypotension, asystole, nausea, weakness, dizziness, drowsiness, confusion and slurred speech; profound bradycardia and occasionally hyperglycemia

Toxicology Ipecac-induced emesis can hypothetically worsen calcium antagonist toxicity, since it can produce vagal stimulation. The potential for seizures precipitously following acute ingestion of large doses of a calcium antagonist may also contraindicate the use of ipecac. Supportive and symptomatic treatment, including I.V. fluids and Trendelenburg positioning, should be initiated as intoxication may cause hypotension. Although calcium (calcium chloride I.V. 1-2 g in adults over 5-10 minutes with repeats as needed) has been used as an "antidote" for acute intoxications, there is limited experience to support its routine use and should be reserved for those cases where definite signs of myocardial depression are evident. Heart block may respond to isoproterenol, glucagon, atropine and/or calcium although a temporary pacemaker may be required.

Drug Interactions

Beta-blockers may increase cardiovascular adverse effects

Anesthetic doses of fentanyl → hypotension

Cimetidine and ranitidine may increase bioavailability

Cimetidine may increase nifedipine serum concentration

Nifedipine may increase phenytoin and possibly digoxin serum concentrations

Nifedipine may increase pharmacologic action of theophylline

Nifedipine may alter response and serum levels of quinidine

Mechanism of Action Inhibits calcium ion from entering the "slow channels" or select voltage-sensitive areas of vascular smooth muscle and myocardium during depolarization, producing a relaxation of coronary vascular smooth muscle and coronary vasodilation; increases myocardial oxygen delivery in patients with vasospastic angina

Pharmacodynamics

Onset of action:

Oral: Within 20 minutes

S.L.: Within 1-5 minutes

Pharmacokinetics

Protein binding: 92% to 98% (concentration-dependent)

Metabolism: In the liver to inactive metabolites

Bioavailability:

Capsules: 45% to 75%

Sustained release: 65% to 86%

Half-life:

Normal adults: 2-5 hours

Cirrhosis: 7 hours

Elimination: In urine

Usual Dosage Geriatrics and Adults: Initial: 10 mg 3 times/day as capsules or 30-60 mg once daily as sustained release tablet; maintenance: 10-30 mg 3-4 times/day (capsules); titrate over a 7- to 14-day period; maximum: 180 mg/24 hours (capsules) or 120 mg/day (sustained release), increase sustained release at 7- to 14-day intervals

Monitoring Parameters Heart rate, blood pressure, signs and symptoms of CHF, peripheral edema

Reference Range Therapeutic: 25-100 ng/mL

Patient Information Sustained release products should be taken with food and not crushed or chewed; limit caffeine intake; avoid alcohol; notify physician if angina pain is not reduced when taking this drug, irregular heartbeat, shortness of breath, swelling, dizziness, constipation, nausea, or hypotension occur; do not stop therapy without advice of physician; the shell of the sustained-release tablet may appear intact in the stool; this is no cause for concern

Nursing Implications May cause some patients to urinate frequently at night; may cause inflamed gums; capsule may be punctured and drug solution administered sublingually or orally to reduce blood pressure in recumbent patient; see Warnings, Precautions, Adverse Reactions, and Special Geriatric Considerations

Additional Information Capsule may be punctured and drug solution administered sublingually to reduce blood pressure

Special Geriatric Considerations Elderly may experience a greater hypotensive response; constipation may be more of a problem in elderly; calcium channel blockers are no more effective in elderly than other therapies; however, they do not cause significant CNS effects which is an advantage over some antihypertensive agents.

Dosage Forms
Capsule, liquid-filled: 10 mg, 20 mg
Tablet, sustained release: 30 mg, 60 mg, 90 mg

References
Rosen WJ and Johnson CE, "Evaluation of Five Procedures for Measuring Nonstandard Doses of Nifedipine Liquid," *Am J Hosp Pharm,* 1989, 46(11):2313-7.

Nilstat® *see* Nystatin *on page 513*

Nimodipine (nye moe' di peen)
Related Information
Calcium Channel Blocking Agents Comparison *on page 806-807*
Brand Names Nimotop®
Therapeutic Class Calcium Channel Blocker
Use Improvement of neurological deficits due to spasm following subarachnoid hemorrhage from ruptured congenital intracranial aneurysms who are in good neurological condition postictus

Unlabeled use: Migraine headache

Contraindications Sinus bradycardia; advanced heart block; ventricular tachycardia; cardiogenic shock, hypotension, CHF; hypersensitivity to nimodipine or any component, calcium channel blockers, and adenosine; atrial fibrillation or flutter associated with accessory conduction pathways; not to be given within a few hours of I.V. beta-blocking agents

Warnings Hypotension, CHF; cardiac conduction defects, PVCs, idiopathic hypertrophic subaortic stenosis; may cause platelet inhibition; do not abruptly withdraw (chest pain); hepatic dysfunction, increased angina, decreased neuromuscular transmission with Duchenne's muscular dystrophy; increased intracranial pressure with cranial tumors; elderly may have greater hypotensive effect

Adverse Reactions
Cardiovascular: Hypotension, bradycardia, first, second, or third degree A-V block, worsening heart failure, palpitations, CHF, myocardial infarction, angina, tachycardia
Central nervous system: Headache, fatigue, seizures, dizziness, lightheadedness, psychotic symptoms, insomnia, paresthesia, asthenia
Gastrointestinal: Constipation (more of a problem in elderly), nausea, abdominal discomfort, diarrhea, dry mouth
Hepatic: Increase in hepatic enzymes
Ocular: Blurred vision
Respiratory: May precipitate insufficiency of respiratory muscle function in Duchenne muscular dystrophy
Miscellaneous: Peripheral edema

Overdosage Symptoms of overdose include hypotension, peripheral vasodilation
Toxicology Ipecac-induced emesis can hypothetically worsen calcium antagonist toxicity, since it can produce vagal stimulation. The potential for seizures precipitously following acute ingestion of large doses of a calcium antagonist may also contraindicate the use of ipecac. Supportive and symptomatic treatment, including I.V. fluids and Trendelenburg positioning, should be initiated as intoxication may cause hypotension. Although calcium (calcium chloride I.V. 1-2 g over 5-10 minutes with repeats as needed) has been used as an "antidote" for acute intoxications, there is limited experience to support its routine use and should be reserved for those cases where definite signs of myocardial depression are evident. Heart block may respond to isoproterenol, glucagon, atropine and/or calcium although a temporary pacemaker may be required.

Drug Interactions
Beta-blockers increased cardiac and A-V conduction depression
Fentanyl increased volume requirements and hypotension; although this drug is new, other drug interactions not reported to the same degree as older agents; however, should be suspect of any drug interaction reported with other calcium channel blockers

Mechanism of Action Nimodipine is a calcium channel blocker; animal studies indicate that nimodipine has a greater effect on cerebral arterials than other arterials; this increased specificity may be due to the drug's increased lipophilicity and cerebral distribution as compared to nifedipine; inhibits calcium ion from entering the "slow channels" or select voltage sensitive areas of vascular smooth muscle and myocardium during depolarization

Pharmacokinetics
Protein binding: >95%
Metabolism: Extensive in the liver
Bioavailability: 13% absolute
Half-life: 3 hours, increases with reduced renal function
Time to peak: Oral: Peak serum levels occur within 1 hour
Elimination: In feces (32%) and in urine (50% within 4 days)
Usual Dosage Geriatrics and Adults: Oral: 60 mg every 4 hours for 21 days; if capsule

(Continued)
503

Nimodipine *(Continued)*

cannot be swallowed, extract capsule contents with 18-gauge needle and empty into NG tube; flush with 30 mL normal saline

Monitoring Parameters CNS response, heart rate, blood pressure, signs and symptoms of CHF

Reference Range No data

Patient Information Do not crush or chew capsule; notify physician if you experience irregular heartbeat, shortness of breath, swelling, constipation, nausea, hypotension, or dizziness; do not stop or interrupt therapy without advice of physician

Nursing Implications If capsules cannot be swallowed, the liquid may be removed by making a hole in each end of the capsule with an 18-gauge needle and extracting the contents into a syringe; if given via NG tube, follow with a flush of 30 mL NS

Special Geriatric Considerations Elderly may experience a greater hypotensive response; constipation may be more of a problem in elderly; studies in the treatment of Alzheimer's disease have not demonstrated clear clinical effect

Dosage Forms Capsule, liquid: 30 mg

Nimotop® *see Nimodipine on previous page*

Nipride® *see Nitroprusside Sodium on page 507*

Nitro-Bid® *see Nitroglycerin on next page*

Nitrocap® TD *see Nitroglycerin on next page*

Nitrocine® *see Nitroglycerin on next page*

Nitrodisc® *see Nitroglycerin on next page*

Nitro-Dur® *see Nitroglycerin on next page*

Nitrofurantoin *(nye troe fyoor an' toyn)*

Related Information

Antacid Drug Interactions *on page 764*

Brand Names Furadantin®; Furalan®; Furan®; Furanite®; Macrodantin®

Generic Available Yes: Tablet and suspension

Therapeutic Class Antibiotic, Miscellaneous

Use Prevention and treatment of urinary tract infections caused by susceptible gram-negative and some gram-positive organisms; *Pseudomonas*, *Serratia*, and most species of *Proteus* are generally resistant to nitrofurantoin

Contraindications Hypersensitivity to nitrofurantoin or any component; renal impairment

Warnings Therapeutic concentrations of nitrofurantoin are not attained in the urine of patients with Cl_{cr} <40 mL/minute

Precautions Use with caution in patients with G-6-PD deficiency, patients with anemia, vitamin B deficiency, diabetes mellitus or electrolyte abnormalities; superinfection

Adverse Reactions

Cardiovascular: Chest pains

Central nervous system: Dizziness, headache, fever, chills, drowsiness

Dermatologic: Rash, exfoliative dermatitis, urticaria

Gastrointestinal: Nausea, vomiting, anorexia, pancreatitis, sore throat

Hematologic: Hemolytic anemia

Hepatic: Hepatotoxicity

Neuromuscular & skeletal: Peripheral neuropathy, arthralgia

Respiratory: Interstitial pneumonitis and/or fibrosis, asthma, cough

Overdosage Symptoms of overdose include vomiting

Drug Interactions

Probenecid decreased renal excretion of nitrofurantoin, antacids decreased absorption of nitrofurantoin

Anticholinergic drugs and food increased absorption of nitrofurantoin

Magnesium trisilicate delays or decreases absorption

Mechanism of Action Inhibits several bacterial enzyme systems including acetyl coenzyme A

Pharmacokinetics

Absorption: Well from the GI tract; the macrocrystalline form is absorbed more slowly due to slower dissolution, but causes less GI distress

Distribution: V_d: 0.8 L/kg

Protein binding: ~40%

Metabolism: 60% of the drug is metabolized by body tissues throughout the body, with the exception of plasma, to inactive metabolites

Bioavailability: Presence of food increases bioavailability

Half-life: 20-60 minutes and is prolonged with renal impairment

Elimination: As metabolites and unchanged drug (40%) in urine and small amounts in bile; renal excretion is via glomerular filtration and tubular secretion

Usual Dosage Geriatrics and Adults: Oral: 50-100 mg every 6 hours

Prophylaxis: 50-100 mg/dose at bedtime; see Special Geriatric Considerations

Administration Higher peak serum levels may cause increased GI upset; give with meals to slow the rate of absorption and thus decrease adverse effects; give around-the-clock rather than 4 times/day, 3 times/day, etc (ie, 12-6-12-6, not 9-1-5-9) to promote less variation in peak and trough serum levels

Monitoring Parameters Signs of pulmonary reaction, signs of numbness or tingling of the extremities; periodic liver function tests; signs and symptoms of infection

Test Interactions Causes false-positive urine glucose with Clinitest®

Patient Information Take with food or milk; may discolor urine to a dark yellow or brown color; complete full course of therapy; notify physician or pharmacist if diarrhea, tingling in extremities, skin rash, or difficulty breathing occurs

Nursing Implications See Administration

Special Geriatric Considerations Because of nitrofurantoin's decreased efficacy in patients with a Cl$_{cr}$ <40 mL/minute and its side effect profile, it is not an antibiotic of choice for acute or prophylactic treatment of urinary tract infections in the elderly.

Dosage Forms
Capsule: 50 mg, 100 mg
Capsule:
Extended release: 100 mg
Macrocrystal: 25 mg, 50 mg, 100 mg
Macrocrystal/monohydrate: 100 mg
Suspension, oral: 25 mg/5 mL (470 mL)

Nitrogard® see Nitroglycerin *on this page*

Nitroglycerin (nye troe gli' ser in)
Brand Names Deponit®; Minitran®; Nitro-Bid®; Nitrocap® TD; Nitrocine®; Nitrodisc®; Nitro-Dur®; Nitrogard®; Nitroglyn®; Nitrol®; Nitrolingual®; Nitrong®; Nitrospan®; Nitrostat®; Transdermal-NTG®; Transderm-Nitro®; Tridil®

Synonyms Glyceryl Trinitrate; Nitroglycerol; NTG

Generic Available Yes

Therapeutic Class Antianginal Agent; Nitrate; Vasodilator, Coronary

Use Angina pectoris; I.V. for congestive heart failure (especially when associated with acute myocardial infarction); pulmonary hypertension; hypertensive emergencies occurring perioperatively (especially during cardiovascular surgery)

Contraindications Hypersensitivity to nitroglycerin or any component; closed-angle glaucoma; severe anemia, postural hypotension, early myocardial infarction, head trauma, cerebral hemorrhage, allergy to adhesive (transdermal), uncorrected hypovolemia (I.V.), inadequate cerebral circulation, increased intracranial pressure, constrictive pericarditis, pericardial tamponade; transdermal NTG is not effective for immediate relief of angina

Warnings Do not chew or swallow sublingual dosage form.

Precautions Do not use extended release preparations in patients with GI hypermotility or malabsorptive syndrome; use with caution in patients with hypovolemia, constrictive pericarditis, hypertension, and hypotension; use with caution in patients with increased intracranial pressure; do not abruptly withdraw therapy for treatment of angina

Adverse Reactions
Cardiovascular: Flushing, headache, hypotension, reflex tachycardia, severe hypotension and bradycardia have been described; abrupt withdrawal may result in acute coronary vascular insufficiency
Central nervous system: Dizziness, restlessness
Dermatologic: Allergic contact dermatitis may be seen with ointment and patches
Gastrointestinal: Nausea, vomiting
Miscellaneous: Perspiration and collapse, pallor

Overdosage Symptoms of overdose include hypotension, throbbing headache, palpitations, bloody diarrhea, bradycardia, cyanosis, tissue hypoxia, metabolic acidosis, clonic convulsions, circulatory collapse

Toxicology If ingested, perform gastric lavage or induce emesis followed by charcoal administration; keep patient warm and in recumbent position to prevent shock; administer oxygen and artificial ventilation if needed. Monitor methemoglobin levels if indicated; if severely hypotensive, elevate legs; administer I.V. fluids, consider alpha-adrenergics; treat methemoglobinemia if present

Drug Interactions I.V. nitroglycerin may antagonize the anticoagulant effect of heparin, monitor closely, may need to decrease heparin dosage when nitroglycerin is discontinued; alcohol, beta-blockers, calcium channel blockers may enhance nitroglycerin's hypotensive effect

Stability I.V. infusion solution in NS or D$_5$W, is stable for 48 hours at room temperature, mixed and stored in glass containers; maximum concentration not to exceed 400 mcg/mL; do not mix with other drugs; store sublingual tablets and ointment in tightly closed container; store at 15°C to 30°C

Mechanism of Action Relax vascular smooth muscle via stimulation of intracellular cyclic GMP production which stimulates a cyclic GMP-dependent protein kinases that

(Continued)

Nitroglycerin (Continued)

alters phosphorylation of the smooth muscle myosin resulting in relaxation of the muscle; venous dilation is predominate action causing peripheral pooling which decreases venous return to heart and, therefore, workload, central venous pressure, and pulmonary capillary wedge pressure; reduction in pulmonary vascular resistance occurs secondary to pulmonary arterial dilation; reduces cardiac oxygen demand by decreasing left ventricular pressure and systemic vascular resistance; dilates coronary arteries and improves collateral flow to ischemic regions

Pharmacodynamics Onset and duration of action is dependent upon dosage form administered; see table.

Dosage Form	Onset of Effect	Peak Effect	Duration
Sublingual tablet	1–3 min	4–8 min	30–60 min
Lingual spray	2 min	4–10 min	30–60 min
Buccal tablet	2–5 min	4–10 min	2 h
Sustained release	20–45 min	45–120 min	4–8 h
Topical	15–60 min	30–120 min	2–12 h
Transdermal	40–60 min	60–180 min	18–24 h
I.V. drip	Immediate	Immediate	3–5 min

Pharmacokinetics
Protein binding: 60%
Metabolism: Extensive first-pass
Half-life: 1-4 minutes
Elimination: Excretion of inactive metabolites in urine

Usual Dosage Geriatrics and Adults:
Buccal: Initial: 1 mg every 5 hours while awake (3 times/day); titrate dosage upward if angina occurs with tablet in place
Oral: 2.5-9 mg every 8-12 hours
I.V.: 5 mcg/minute, increase by 5 mcg/minute every 3-5 minutes to 20 mcg/minute then increase by 10 mcg/minute every 3-5 minutes, up to 200 mcg/minute
Lingual: 1-2 sprays into mouth under tongue every 3-5 minutes for maximum of 3 doses in 15 minutes
Ointment: 1" to 2" every 8 hours
Patch, transdermal: 2.5-15 mg/24 hours (recommended to remove patch at bedtime for a drug-free period of 10-12 hours)
Sublingual: 0.2-0.6 mg every 5 minutes for maximum of 3 doses in 15 minutes

Monitoring Parameters Orthostatic blood pressure, blood pressure, heart rate; therapeutic dose may be determined by observing for a decrease in systolic blood pressure by 15 mm Hg, diastolic reduction of 10 mm Hg or an increase in heart rate of 10 bpm

Test Interactions Increased catecholamines (U)

Patient Information Go to hospital or call 911 if no relief after 3 sublingual doses; do not swallow or chew sublingual form; keep in original container and tightly closed; remove and do not reinsert cotton plug; for the sublingual tablets, it is best to get a fresh bottle 3-6 months after opening. Get instructions on proper use of transdermal patches or ointment.

Nursing Implications I.V. must be prepared in glass bottles and use special sets intended for nitroglycerin; transdermal patches labeled as mg/hour; do not crush sublingual drug product

Additional Information I.V. preparations contain alcohol and/or propylene glycol; may need to use nitrate-free internal (10-12 hours/day) to avoid tolerance development; tolerance may possibly be reversed with acetylcysteine; gradually decrease dose in patients receiving NTG for prolonged period to avoid withdrawal reaction

Special Geriatric Considerations Caution should be used when using nitrate therapy in elderly due to hypotension; hypotension is enhanced in elderly due to decreased baroreceptor response, decreased venous tone, and often hypovolemia (dehydration) or other hypotensive drugs

Dosage Forms
Capsule, sustained release: 2.5 mg, 6.5 mg, 9 mg
Injection: 0.5 mg/mL (10 mL); 0.8 mg/mL (10 mL); 5 mg/mL (1 mL, 5 mL, 10 mL, 20 mL); 10 mg/mL (5 mL, 10 mL)
Ointment, topical (Nitrol®): 2% (30 g, 60 g)
Patch, transdermal: Systems designed to deliver 2.5 mg, 5 mg, 7.5 mg, 10 mg, or 15 mg NTG over 24 hours. See table.
Spray, translingual: 0.4 mg/metered spray (13.8 g)
Tablet:
Buccal, controlled release: 1 mg, 2 mg, 3 mg
Sublingual (Nitrostat®): 0.15 mg, 0.3 mg, 0.4 mg, 0.6 mg
Sustained release: 2.6 mg, 6.5 mg, 9 mg

Nitroglycerin

Product	Release Rate		Surface Area (cm²)	Total Content (mg)
	mg/h	mg/24 h		
Deponit®				
5	0.2	5	16	16
10	0.42	10	32	32
Minitran®				
2.5	0.1	2.5	3.3	9
5	0.2	5	6.7	18
10	0.42	10	13.3	36
15	0.625	15	20	54
Nitrocine®				
5	0.2	5	10	62.5
10	0.42	10	20	125
15	0.625	15	30	187.5
Nitrodisc®				
5	0.2	5	8	6
7.5	0.312	7.5	12	24
10	0.42	10	16	32
Nitro–Dur®				
2.5	0.1	2.5	5	20
5	0.2	5	10	40
7.5	0.312	7.5	15	60
10	0.42	10	20	80
15	0.625	15	30	120
Transderm–Nitro®				
2.5	0.1	2.5	5	12.5
5	0.2	5	10	25
10	0.42	10	20	50
15	0.625	15	30	75

References
Elkayam U, "Tolerance to Organic Nitrates: Evidence, Mechanisms, Clinical Relevance, and Strategies for Prevention," *Ann Intern Med*, 1991, 114(8):667-77.

◀Nitroglycerol *see* Nitroglycerin *on page 505*

◀Nitroglyn® *see* Nitroglycerin *on page 505*

◀Nitrol® *see* Nitroglycerin *on page 505*

◀Nitrolingual® *see* Nitroglycerin *on page 505*

◀Nitrong® *see* Nitroglycerin *on page 505*

◀Nitropress® *see* Nitroprusside Sodium *on this page*

◀Nitroprusside Sodium (nye troe pruss' ide)

Brand Names Nipride®; Nitropress®
Synonyms Sodium Nitroferricyanide; Sodium Nitroprusside
Generic Available Yes
Therapeutic Class Vasodilator
Use Management of hypertensive crises; congestive heart failure; used for controlled hypotension to reduce bleeding during surgery
Contraindications Hypersensitivity to nitroprusside or components; decreased cerebral perfusion; arteriovenous shunt or coarctation of the aorta (ie, compensatory hypertension)
Warnings Use only as an infusion with 5% dextrose in water; continuously monitor patient's blood pressure; excessive amounts of nitroprusside can cause cyanide toxicity (usually in patients with decreased liver function) or thiocyanate toxicity (usually in patients with decreased renal function, or in patients with normal renal function but prolonged nitroprusside use)
Precautions Use with caution in patients with increased intracranial pressure (head trauma, cerebral hemorrhage); severe renal impairment, hepatic failure, hypothyroidism, hyponatremia
Adverse Reactions
Cardiovascular: Excessive hypotensive response, palpitations
Central nervous system: Restlessness, disorientation, psychosis, headache, increased intracranial pressure
Endocrine & metabolic: Thyroid suppression, thiocyanate toxicity
Gastrointestinal: Nausea, vomiting
(Continued)

507

Nitroprusside Sodium *(Continued)*

    Neuromuscular & skeletal: Muscle spasm, weakness
    Otic: Tinnitus
    Respiratory: Substernal distress, hypoxia
    Miscellaneous: Sweating

Overdosage Symptoms of overdose include hypotension, vomiting, hyperventilation, tachycardia, muscular twitching, hypothyroidism, cyanide or thiocyanate toxicity

Toxicology Thiocyanate toxicity includes psychosis, hyperreflexia, confusion, weakness, tinnitus, seizures, and coma; cyanide toxicity includes acidosis (decreased HCO_3, decreased pH, increased lactate), increase in mixed venous blood oxygen tension, tachycardia, altered consciousness, coma, convulsions, and almond smell on breath. Nitroprusside has been shown to release cyanide *in vivo* with hemoglobin. Cyanide toxicity does not usually occur because of the rapid uptake of cyanide by erythrocytes and its eventual incorporation into cyanocobalamin. However, prolonged administration of nitroprusside or its reduced elimination can lead to cyanide intoxication. In these situations, airway support with oxygen therapy is germane, followed closely with antidotal therapy of amyl nitrate perles, sodium nitrate 300 mg I.V. and sodium thiosulfate 12.5 g I.V.

Stability Discard solution 24 hours after reconstitution and dilution in D_5W; promptly wrap in aluminum foil or other opaque material to protect from light; reconstituted solution should be very faint brown, discard if highly colored (blue, green or red); store powder in carton until ready to use

Mechanism of Action Causes peripheral vasodilation by direct action on venous and arteriolar smooth muscle, thus reducing peripheral resistance; will increase cardiac output by decreasing afterload; reduces aortal and left ventricular impedance

Pharmacodynamics
    Onset of action: Hypotensive effects occur in <2 minutes
    Duration: Following discontinuation of therapy, effects cease within 1-10 minutes

Pharmacokinetics
    Metabolism: Converted to cyanide by erythrocyte and tissue sulfhydryl group interactions; cyanide is converted in the liver by rhodanese to thiocyanate
    Half-life: <10 minutes; half-life (thiocyanate): 2.7-7 days
    Elimination: In urine

Usual Dosage Geriatrics and Adults: I.V.: Continuous infusion: Start 0.5 mcg/kg/minute, titrate to effect; usual dose: 3 mcg/kg/minute, rarely need >4 mcg/kg/minute; maximum: 10 mcg/kg/minute

Monitoring Parameters Blood pressure, cardiac status, thiocyanate levels

Reference Range Monitor thiocyanate levels if requiring prolonged infusion (>4 days) or ≥4 μg/kg/minute; Therapeutic: 6-29 μg/mL (SI: 103-499 μmol/L)

Nursing Implications I.V. infusion only, not for direct injection; protect from light; brownish solution is usable, discard if bluish in color

Additional Information Nitroprusside is converted to cyanide ions in the bloodstream; decomposes to prussic acid which in the presence of sulfur donor is converted to thiocyanate (liver and kidney rhodanase systems); thiocyanate is then renally eliminated

Special Geriatric Considerations Elderly patients may have an increased sensitivity to nitroprusside possibly due to a decreased baroreceptor reflex, altered sensitivity to vasodilating effects or a resistance of cardiac adrenergic receptors to stimulation by catecholamines

Dosage Forms Injection: 10 mg/mL (5 mL); 25 mg/mL (2 mL)

Nitrospan® *see* Nitroglycerin *on page 505*
Nitrostat® *see* Nitroglycerin *on page 505*
Nix™ *see* Permethrin *on page 548*

Nizatidine (ni za' ti deen)

Brand Names Axid®
Generic Available No
Therapeutic Class Histamine-2 Antagonist
Use Treatment and maintenance of duodenal ulcer, benign gastric ulcer, GERD
Contraindications Hypersensitivity to nizatidine or any component; hypersensitivity to other H_2 blockers since a cross-sensitivity has been observed in this class of drugs
Warnings Adjust dosages in renal/hepatic impairment; elderly due to renal decline with age
Precautions Modify dosage in patients with renal and/or hepatic impairment; gastric malignancy may be masked, gynecomastia; cardiac arrhythmias and hypotension; CNS side effects (confusion, depression, psychosis, hallucinations, anxiety)
Adverse Reactions
    Cardiovascular: Ventricular (asymptomatic) tachycardia
    Central nervous system: Somnolence, headache, fatigue, dizziness, hallucinations, insomnia, fever

Dermatologic: Urticaria, exfoliative dermatitis, rash, pruritus
Endocrine & metabolic: Gynecomastia, hyperuricemia
Gastrointestinal: Nausea, vomiting, abdominal pain, diarrhea, constipation
Genitourinary: Impotence, loss of libido
Hematologic: Eosinophilia, thrombocytopenia
Hepatic: Cholestatic and hepatocellular damage
Miscellaneous: Sweating

Overdosage No experience with intentional overdose; reported ingestions of 20 g have had transient side effects seen with recommended doses; animal data have shown respiratory failure, tachycardia, muscle tremors, vomiting, restlessness, hypotension, salivation, emesis, and diarrhea (LD$_{50}$ ~80 mg/kg)

Toxicology Treatment is primarily symptomatic and supportive

Drug Interactions Does not bind to cytochrome P-450 *in vitro*; antacids may decrease absorption (~10%); aspirin (increased levels) with high doses (3.9 g/day), diazepam; food may increase absorption

Mechanism of Action Nizatidine is an H$_2$ receptor antagonist. In healthy volunteers, nizatidine has been effective in suppressing gastric acid secretion induced by pentagastrin infusion or food. Nizatidine reduces gastric acid secretion by 29.4% to 78.4%. This compares with a 60.3% reduction by cimetidine. Nizatidine 100 mg is reported to provide equivalent acid suppression as cimetidine 300 mg.

Pharmacokinetics
Bioavailability: >90% (rapidly absorbed)
Protein binding: ~35%
Time to peak serum concentration: 0.5-3 hours
Elimination:
  Renal: Unchanged, 60%
  Hepatic: <18%

Usual Dosage Geriatrics and Adults: Oral: 300 mg at bedtime or 150 mg twice daily; maintenance: 150 mg once daily (bedtime); GERD 150 mg twice daily

Dosing interval in renal impairment:
  Cl$_{cr}$ 20-50 mL/minute: Administer 150 mg/day for duodenal ulcer; 150 mg every other day for maintenance therapy
  Cl$_{cr}$ <20 mL/minute: Administer 150 mg every other day; 150 mg every 3rd day for maintenance therapy

Monitoring Parameters Signs and symptoms of peptic ulcer disease, occult blood with GI bleeding, gastric pH where necessary; monitor renal function to correct dose; monitor for side effects

Test Interactions False-positive tests for urobilinogen

Patient Information May take several days before relief of stomach pain occurs; take with or immediately after meals; inform pharmacist and physician (nurse practitioner) of any concomitant drug therapy; stagger doses with antacids with this medication by taking antacids 30-60 minutes before or after taking nizatidine

Nursing Implications Giving a dose at 6 PM may more effectively suppress nocturnal acid secretion than giving a dose at 10 PM; See Warnings, Precautions, Monitoring Parameters, and Special Geriatric Considerations

Special Geriatric Considerations H$_2$ blockers are the preferred drugs for treating PUD in elderly due to cost and ease of administration. These agents are no less or more effective than any other therapy. The preferred agents (due to side effects and drug interaction profile and pharmacokinetics) are ranitidine, famotidine, and nizatidine. Treatment for PUD in elderly is recommended for 12 weeks since their lesions are larger, and therefore, take longer to heal; always adjust dose based upon creatinine clearance.

Dosage Forms Capsule: 150 mg, 300 mg

References
Fennerty MD and Higbee M, "Drug Therapy of Gastrointestinal Disease," *Geriatric Pharmacology*, Bressler R and Katz MD, eds, New York, NY: McGraw-Hill, 1993, 585-608.

Nizoral® *see* Ketoconazole *on page 389*

Nostrilla® [OTC] *see* Oxymetazoline Hydrochloride *on page 530*

NaSal™ [OTC] *see* Sodium Chloride *on page 648*

Noctec® *see* Chloral Hydrate *on page 146*

Nolvadex® *see* Tamoxifen Citrate *on page 669*

Norcet® *see* Hydrocodone and Acetaminophen *on page 350*

Nordeoxyguanosine *see* Ganciclovir *on page 318*

Nordryl® *see* Diphenhydramine Hydrochloride *on page 228*

Nor-Feran® *see* Iron Dextran Complex *on page 377*

Norflex™ *see* Orphenadrine Citrate *on page 520*

Norfloxacin (nor flox' a sin)
Brand Names Noroxin®
Generic Available No
Therapeutic Class Antibiotic, Quinolone
(Continued)

509

Norfloxacin *(Continued)*

Use Complicated and uncomplicated urinary tract infections caused by susceptible gram-negative and gram-positive bacteria; ophthalmic solution for conjunctivitis

Contraindications Known hypersensitivity to quinolones including cinoxacin and nalidixic acid

Warnings Convulsion in persons with CNS disorders (seizure disorder, increased intracranial pressure, and toxic psychosis); CNS stimulation, tremor, headache, pseudomembranous colitis

Precautions Superinfection, crystalluria, phototoxicity

Adverse Reactions
Central nervous system: Headache, dizziness, fatigue, hallucinations, confusion
Dermatologic: Erythema multiforme
Gastrointestinal: Nausea, dry mouth, flatulence, abdominal pain, vomiting, heartburn, diarrhea
Hematologic: Leukopenia
Hepatic: Increased liver function tests, hepatitis
Neuromuscular & skeletal: Tremors
Renal: Acute renal failure, increased creatinine and BUN

Drug Interactions
Antacids, iron salts, sucralfate, zinc salts may reduce absorption by up to 98% if given at the same time
Antineoplastic agents may decrease norfloxacin levels
Cimetidine may increase levels
Nitrofurantoin may antagonize norfloxacin's effects
Probenecid may decrease urinary excretion
Norfloxacin may increase the effects of anticoagulants, increase nephrotoxicity of cyclosporine, and decrease clearance (increase levels) of theophylline and caffeine, hence, monitor appropriately

Mechanism of Action Exerts a broad spectrum antimicrobial effect. The primary target of the fluoroquinolones is DNA gyrase (topoisomerase II), an essential bacterial enzyme that maintains the superhelical structure of DNA. DNA gyrase is required for DNA replication and transcription, DNA repair, recombination, and transposition.

Pharmacokinetics
Absorption: Oral: Rapid, up to 40%
Protein binding: 15%
Metabolism: In the liver
Half-life: 4.8 hours (can be higher with reduced glomerular filtration rates)
Time to peak: Peak serum levels occur within 1-2 hours
Elimination: In urine and feces (30%); increased area under the curve (AUC), a 30% to 40% decrease in renal clearance without a significant change in half-life has been reported in elderly

Usual Dosage Geriatrics and Adults:
Oral: 400 mg twice daily for 7-21 days depending on infection; do not give as single or 3-day course of therapy
Ophthalmic: Instill 1-2 drops in affected eye(s) 4 times/day for up to 7 days
Dosing interval in renal impairment: Oral: Cl_{cr} ≤30 mL/minute/1.73 m^2: Administer 400 mg once daily for appropriate duration

Administration Hold antacids and sucralfate for 2-4 hours before and after giving dose

Monitoring Parameters Signs and symptoms of infection, WBC, mental status, culture, and sensitivity

Patient Information Take 1 hour before or 2 hours after meals; do not take with antacids, dairy products, iron, or zinc products; may cause dizziness, headache, or stimulation; avoid excess natural or artificial sunlight exposure; complete full course of therapy

Nursing Implications See Administration

Special Geriatric Considerations See Pharmacokinetics and Usual Dosage; assess ability to self-administer eye drops; adjust dose for renal function

Dosage Forms
Solution, ophthalmic: 0.3% [3 mg/mL] (5 mL)
Tablet: 400 mg

References
Nilsson-Ehle I and Ljungberg B, "Quinolone Disposition in the Elderly: Practical Implications," *Drugs Aging*, 1991, 1(4):279-88.

Norpace® *see* Disopyramide Phosphate *on page 234*

Norpace® CR *see* Disopyramide Phosphate *on page 234*

Norpramin® *see* Desipramine Hydrochloride *on page 205*

Nor-Pred S® *see* Prednisolone *on page 584*

Nor-Pred T.B.A.® *see* Prednisolone *on page 584*

Nor-tet® *see* Tetracycline *on page 678*

Nortriptyline Hydrochloride (nor trip' ti leen)
Related Information
Antidepressant Agents Comparison *on page 800*
Drug Levels Commonly Monitored Guidelines *on page 771-772*
Brand Names Aventyl® Hydrochloride; Pamelor®
Therapeutic Class Antidepressant, Tricyclic
Use Treatment of various forms of depression, often in conjunction with psychotherapy
Contraindications Narrow-angle glaucoma
Precautions Use with caution in patients with cardiac conduction disturbances, history of hyperthyroidism, bipolar illness; renal or hepatic impairment; nortriptyline should not be abruptly discontinued in patients receiving high doses for prolonged periods; to avoid cholinergic crisis; an EKG prior to initiating therapy is advised
Adverse Reactions
Cardiovascular: Postural hypotension, arrhythmias, tachycardia, sudden death
Central nervous system: Sedation, fatigue, anxiety, impaired cognitive function, seizures have occurred occasionally, delirium, headache
Gastrointestinal: Dry mouth, constipation, increased appetite
Genitourinary: Urinary retention
Hematologic: Rarely agranulocytosis, eosinophilia
Hepatic: Jaundice
Neuromuscular & skeletal: Tremors, weakness
Ocular: Blurred vision, increased intraocular pressure
Miscellaneous: Allergic reactions
Overdosage Symptoms of overdose include agitation, confusion, hallucinations, urinary retention, hypothermia, hypotension, tachycardia
Toxicology Following initiation of essential overdose management, toxic symptoms should be treated. Ventricular arrhythmias often respond to phenytoin 15-20 mg/kg with concurrent systemic alkalinization (sodium bicarbonate 0.5-2 mEq/kg I.V.). Arrhythmias unresponsive to this therapy may respond to lidocaine 1 mg/kg I.V. followed by a titrated infusion. Physostigmine (1-2 mg I.V. slowly) may be indicated in reversing cardiac arrhythmias that are due to vagal blockade or for anticholinergic effects. Seizures usually respond to diazepam I.V. boluses (5-10 mg, up to 30 mg). If seizures are unresponsive or recur, phenytoin or phenobarbital may be required.
Drug Interactions
Nortriptyline blocks the uptake of guanethidine and thus prevents the hypotensive effect of guanethidine; nortriptyline may be additive with or may potentiate the action of other CNS depressants, anticholinergic agents, dicumarol; nortriptyline potentiates the pressor and cardiac effects of sympathomimetic agents such as isoproterenol, epinephrine, etc; cimetidine, fluoxetine, methylphenidate, and haloperidol may decrease the metabolism and/or elevate TCA levels; phenobarbital may increase TCA metabolism; disulfiram may increase bioavailability
With MAO inhibitors, hyperpyrexia, hypertension, tachycardia, confusion, seizures, and death have been reported
Additive anticholinergic effects seen with other anticholinergic agents
Clonidine used concurrently has been reported to cause hypertensive crisis and increase blood pressure
Stability Protect from light
Mechanism of Action Traditionally believed to increase the synaptic concentration of serotonin and/or norepinephrine in the central nervous system by inhibition of their reuptake by the presynaptic neuronal membrane. However, additional receptor effects have been found including desensitization of adenyl cyclase, down regulation of beta-adrenergic receptors, and down regulation of serotonin receptors.
Pharmacodynamics Onset of therapeutic effects: Takes 1-3 weeks before effects are seen; NE >>5-HT
Pharmacokinetics
Distribution: V_d: 21 L/kg
Protein binding: 93% to 95%
Metabolism: Undergoes significant first-pass metabolism
Half-life: 28-31 hours
Time to peak: Oral: Peak serum levels occur within 7-8.5 hours
Elimination: Primarily detoxified in the liver and excreted as metabolites and small amounts of unchanged drug in the urine; small amounts of biliary elimination occurs.
(Continued)

Nortriptyline Hydrochloride *(Continued)*

Geriatric: Single-dose pharmacokinetic studies have found the mean half-life to range from 37-45 hours in older subjects; the mean metabolic clearance was significantly lower compared to younger subjects, 20 vs 54 L/hour

Usual Dosage Oral:

Geriatrics: Initial: 10-25 mg at bedtime; dosage can be increased by 25 mg every 3 days for inpatients and weekly for outpatients if tolerated; usual maintenance dose: 75 mg as a single bedtime dose, however, lower or higher doses may be required to stay within the therapeutic window

Adults: 25 mg 3-4 times/day up to 150 mg/day

Monitoring Parameters Blood pressure and pulse; serum levels, target symptoms

Reference Range Therapeutic: 50-150 ng/mL (SI: 190-570 nmol/L); Toxic: >500 ng/mL (SI: >1900 nmol/L)

Test Interactions Elevated glucose

Patient Information Do not stop abruptly, rise slowly to avoid dizziness; may cause dry mouth, constipation, blurred vision; use sugarless hard candy for dry mouth

Nursing Implications Offer patient sugarless hard candy for dry mouth, monitor for orthostatic changes, weight gain, decreased appetite

Additional Information Maximum antidepressant effect may not be seen for 2 or more weeks after initiation of therapy

Special Geriatric Considerations Since it is the least likely of the TCAs to cause orthostatic hypotension and one of the least anticholinergic and sedating TCAs, it is a preferred agent when a TCA is indicated

Dosage Forms

Capsule: 10 mg, 25 mg, 50 mg, 75 mg

Solution: 10 mg/5 mL

References

Dawling S, Crome P, and Braithwaite R, "Pharmacokinetics of Single Oral Doses of Nortriptyline in Depressed Elderly Hospital Patients and Young Healthy Volunteers," *Clin Pharmacokinet*, 1980, 5(4):394-401.

Schneider LS, Cooper TB, Staples FR, et al, "Prediction of Individual Dosage of Nortriptyline in Depressed Elderly Outpatients," *J Clin Psychopharmacol*, 1987, 7(5):311-4.

Turbott J, Norman TR, Burrows GD, et al, "Pharmacokinetics of Nortriptyline in Elderly Volunteers," *Commun Psychopharmacol*, 1980, 4(3):225-31.

Nortussin® [OTC] *see* Guaifenesin *on page 331*

Norvasc® *see* Amlodipine *on page 45*

Nostril® Nasal Solution [OTC] *see* Phenylephrine Hydrochloride *on page 557*

Novafed® *see* Pseudoephedrine *on page 609*

Novolin® 70/30 *see* Insulin Preparations *on page 372*

Novolin® L *see* Insulin Preparations *on page 372*

Novolin® N *see* Insulin Preparations *on page 372*

Novolin® R *see* Insulin Preparations *on page 372*

Novolin® R Penfill *see* Insulin Preparations *on page 372*

NP-27® [OTC] *see* Tolnaftate *on page 705*

NPH *see* Insulin Preparations *on page 372*

NPH Iletin®I *see* Insulin Preparations *on page 372*

NPH Insulin (Beef) *see* Insulin Preparations *on page 372*

NPH Purified Pork *see* Insulin Preparations *on page 372*

NTG *see* Nitroglycerin *on page 505*

NTZ® Long Acting Nasal Solution [OTC] *see* Oxymetazoline Hydrochloride *on page 530*

Nubain® *see* Nalbuphine Hydrochloride *on page 488*

Nuprin® [OTC] *see* Ibuprofen *on page 360*

Nutracort® *see* Hydrocortisone *on page 351*

Nydrazid® *see* Isoniazid *on page 379*

Nylidrin Hydrochloride *(nye' li drin)*

Brand Names Adrin®; Arlidin®

Generic Available Yes

Therapeutic Class Vasodilator, Peripheral

Use Considered "possibly effective" for increasing blood supply to treat peripheral disease (arteriosclerosis obliterans, diabetic vascular disease, nocturnal leg cramps, Raynaud's disease, frost bite, ischemic ulcer, thrombophlebitis) and circulatory disturbances of the inner ear (cochlear ischemia, macular or ampullar ischemia, etc)

Contraindications Paroxysmal tachycardia, acute myocardial infarction, progressive angina pectoris, thyrotoxicosis

Warnings Use with caution in patients with tachyarrhythmias, uncompensated CHF

Precautions See Warnings

Adverse Reactions
Cardiovascular: Postural hypotension, palpitations
Central nervous system: Dizziness
Gastrointestinal: Nausea, vomiting
Neuromuscular & skeletal: Trembling, weakness

Overdosage Symptoms of overdose include tremors, hypotension

Toxicology Hypotension can be treated by fluids and alpha-adrenergic pressors if needed

Drug Interactions May enhance action of drugs causing vasodilation/hypotension; use with caution in elderly

Mechanism of Action Nylidrin is a peripheral vasodilator. This results from direct relaxation of vascular smooth muscle and beta agonist action. Nylidrin does not appear to affect cutaneous blood flow. It reportedly increases heart rate and cardiac output. Cutaneous blood flow is not enhanced to any appreciable extent.

Pharmacodynamics
Onset of action: ~10 minutes
Peak effect: 30 minutes
Duration: ~2 hours

Pharmacokinetics Absorption: Well absorbed from GI tract

Usual Dosage Geriatrics and Adults: Oral: 3-12 mg 3-4 times/day; best to start with lower dose in elderly due to hypotensive effect

Monitoring Parameters Monitor orthostatic blood pressure

Patient Information May cause dizziness, arise slowly from prolonged sitting or lying; may impair judgment and coordination

Nursing Implications See Monitoring Parameters

Special Geriatric Considerations Vasodilators have been used to treat dementia upon the premise that dementia is secondary to a cerebral blood flow insufficiency. The hypothesis is that if blood flow could be increased, cognitive function would be increased. This hypothesis is no longer valid. The use of vasodilators for cognitive dysfunction is not recommended or proven by appropriate scientific study.

Dosage Forms Tablet: 6 mg, 12 mg

References
Erwin WG, "Senile Dementia of the Alzheimer Type," *Clin Pharm*, 1984, 3:497-504.
Higbee MD, "Noncholinergic Approaches to Treating Senile Dementia of the Alzheimer's Type," *Consult Pharm*, 1992, 7(6):635-41.
Waters C, "Cognitive Enhancing Agents: Current Status in the Treatment of Alzheimer's Disease," *Can J Neurol Sci*, 1988, 15:249-56.
Yesavage JA, Tinklenberg JR, Hollister LE, et al, "Vasodilators in Senile Dementias: A Review of the Literature," *Arch Gen Psychiatry*, 1979, 36:220-3.

Nystatin (nye stat' in)

Brand Names Mycostatin®; Mykinac®; Nilstat®; Nystat-Rx®; Nystex®; O-V Staticin®

Generic Available Yes

Therapeutic Class Antifungal Agent, Oral Nonabsorbed; Antifungal Agent, Topical; Antifungal Agent, Vaginal

Use Treatment of susceptible cutaneous, mucocutaneous, and oral cavity fungal infections normally caused by the *Candida* species

Contraindications Hypersensitivity to nystatin or any component

Adverse Reactions
Dermatologic: Contact dermatitis
Gastrointestinal: Nausea, vomiting, diarrhea, stomach pain
Local: Irritation
Miscellaneous: Hypersensitivity reactions

Overdosage Symptoms of overdose include nausea, vomiting, diarrhea

Stability Keep vaginal inserts in refrigerator; protect from temperature extremes, moisture and light

Mechanism of Action Binds to sterols in fungal cell membrane, changing the cell wall permeability allowing for leakage of cellular contents

Pharmacokinetics
Absorption: Not absorbed through mucous membranes or intact skin; poorly absorbed from the GI tract
Elimination: In feces as unchanged drug

Usual Dosage Geriatrics and Adults:
Intestinal infections: Oral: 500,000-1,000,000 units every 8 hours

Oral candidiasis: 400,000-600,000 units 4 times/day; pastilles: 200,000-400,000 units 4-5 times/day

Cutaneous and mucocutaneous infections: Topical: Apply 2-3 times/day

Vaginal infections: Vaginal tablets: Insert 1-2 tablets/day at bedtime for 2 weeks

(Continued)

Nystatin *(Continued)*

Patient Information The oral suspension should be swished about the mouth and retained in the mouth for as long as possible (several minutes) before swallowing. Troches must be allowed to dissolve slowly and should not be chewed or swallowed whole. *Candida* infections should be treated for 48 hours after symptoms have disappeared. Avoid contact with the eyes.

Nursing Implications Give around-the-clock rather than 4 times/day, 3 times/day, etc (ie, 12-6-12-6, not 9-1-5-9) to promote less variation in peak and trough serum levels

Additional Information Very moist topical lesions are treated best with powder

Special Geriatric Considerations See Usual Dosage; for oral infections, patients who wear dentures must have them removed and cleaned in order to eliminate source of reinfection

Dosage Forms
Cream: 100,000 units/g (15 g, 30 g)
Ointment, topical: 100,000 units/g (15 g, 30 g)
Powder:
For preparation of oral suspension: 50 million units, 1 billion units, 2 billion units, 5 billion units
Topical: 100,000 units/g (15 g)
Suspension, oral: 100,000 units/mL (5 mL 60 mL, 480 mL)
Tablet:
Oral: 500,000 units
Vaginal: 100,000 units (15 and 30/box with applicator)
Troches: 200,000 units

References
Dismukes WE, Wade JS, Lee JY, et al, "A Randomized, Double-Blind Trial of Nystatin Therapy for the Candidiasis Hypersensitivity Syndrome," *N Engl J Med*, 1990, 323(25):1717-23.

Nystatin and Triamcinolone *(nye stat' in)*

Related Information
Nystatin *on previous page*
Triamcinolone *on page 710*

Brand Names Dermacomb® Topical; Mycogen II Topical; Mycolog®-II Topical; Myconel® Topical; Mytrex® F Topical; NGT® Topical; Nyst-Olone® II Topical; Tri-Statin® II Topical

Synonyms Triamcinolone and Nystatin

Generic Available Yes

Therapeutic Class Antifungal Agent, Topical; Corticosteroid, Topical (Medium Potency)

Use Treatment of cutaneous candidiasis

Contraindications Known hypersensitivity to nystatin or triamcinolone

Warnings Avoid use of occlusive dressings; limit therapy to least amount necessary for effective therapy

Adverse Reactions
Dermatologic: Dryness, folliculitis, hypertrichosis, acne, hypopigmentation, allergic dermatitis, maceration of the skin, skin atrophy
Local: Burning, itching, irritation
Miscellaneous: Increased incidence of secondary infection

Mechanism of Action Binds to sterols in fungal cell membrane, changing the cell wall permeability allowing for leakage of cellular contents; decreases inflammation by suppression of migration of polymorphonuclear leukocytes and reversal of increased capillary permeability; suppresses the immune system by reducing activity and volume of the lymphatic system suppresses adrenal function at high doses

Usual Dosage Geriatrics and Adults: Topical: Apply sparingly 2-4 times/day

Administration External use only; do not use on open wounds; apply sparingly to occlusive dressings; should not be used in the presence of open or weeping lesions

Patient Information Before applying, gently wash area to reduce risk of infection; apply a thin film to cleansed area and rub in gently and thoroughly until medication vanishes; avoid exposure to sunlight, severe sunburn may occur

Nursing Implications See Administration

Special Geriatric Considerations No specific dose adjustment or use consideration necessary in the elderly

Dosage Forms
Cream: Nystatin 100,000 units and triamcinolone acetonide 0.1% (15 g, 30 g, 45 g, 60 g, 240 g)
Ointment, topical: Nystatin 100,000 units and triamcinolone acetonide 0.1% (15 g, 30 g, 60 g, 120 g)

Nystat-Rx® *see Nystatin on previous page*
Nystex® *see Nystatin on previous page*
Nyst-Olone® II Topical *see Nystatin and Triamcinolone on this page*

Nytilax® [OTC] *see* Senna *on page 641*

Nytol® [OTC] *see* Diphenhydramine Hydrochloride *on page 228*

Ocean Nasal Mist [OTC] *see* Sodium Chloride *on page 648*

Octamide® PFS *see* Metoclopramide *on page 462*

Octocaine® *see* Lidocaine Hydrochloride *on page 406*

Ocu-Carpine® *see* Pilocarpine *on page 563*

Ocu-Chlor® *see* Chloramphenicol *on page 148*

OcuClear® Ophthalmic [OTC] *see* Oxymetazoline Hydrochloride *on page 530*

Ocu-Dex® *see* Dexamethasone *on page 207*

Ocu-Drop® [OTC] *see* Tetrahydrozoline Hydrochloride *on page 680*

Ocufen® *see* Flurbiprofen Sodium *on page 306*

Ocugestrin® Ophthalmic Solution *see* Phenylephrine Hydrochloride *on page 557*

Ocular Lubricant
Brand Names AKWA Tears™ [OTC]; Dey-Lube®; Duolube® [OTC]; Duratears® [OTC]; HypoTears® [OTC]; Lacri-Lube® [OTC]
Therapeutic Class Ophthalmic Agent, Miscellaneous
Use Ocular lubricant
Contraindications Known hypersensitivity to any of the components
Warnings Discontinue if eye pain, vision change, redness or eye irritation occurs or if condition worsens or persists for more than 72 hours
Precautions Do not use with contact lenses
Adverse Reactions Local: Temporary blurring of vision
Stability Store away from heat
Usual Dosage Geriatrics and Adults: Ointment: Instill $\frac{1}{4}$" of ointment to the inside of the lower lid as needed
Patient Information If condition worsens or persists more than 72 hours, discontinue use and consult a physician; do not touch tube tip to any surface to avoid contamination; do not use with contact lenses
Additional Information Contains petrolatum and mineral oil
Special Geriatric Considerations Ointment is useful at bedtime; make sure patient is able to apply correctly
Dosage Forms Ointment, ophthalmic: 3.5 g

Ocumycin® *see* Gentamicin Sulfate *on page 320*

Ocu-Phrin® Ophthalmic Solution *see* Phenylephrine Hydrochloride *on page 557*

Ocu-Pred® *see* Prednisolone *on page 584*

Ocupress® *see* Carteolol Hydrochloride *on page 122*

Ocusert® Pilo *see* Pilocarpine *on page 563*

Ocu-Trol® Ophthalmic *see* Neomycin, Polymyxin B, and Dexamethasone *on page 495*

Ocu-Tropine® *see* Atropine Sulfate *on page 65*

Ocu-Zoline® *see* Naphazoline Hydrochloride *on page 492*

Ofloxacin (oh floks' a sin)
Brand Names Floxin®
Generic Available No
Therapeutic Class Antibiotic, Quinolone
Use Quinolone antibiotic for skin and skin structure, lower respiratory and urinary tract infections and sexually transmitted diseases, bacterial conjunctivitis caused by susceptible organisms
Contraindications Known hypersensitivity to quinolones including cinoxacin and nalidixic acid
Warnings Convulsion in persons with CNS disorders (seizure disorder, increased intracranial pressure, and toxic psychosis); CNS stimulation, tremor, headache, pseudomembranous colitis; use with caution in patients with renal impairment; failure to respond to an ophthalmic antibiotic after 2-3 days may indicate the presence of resistant organisms or another causative agent (ie, viral or allergy)
Precautions Superinfection, crystalluria, phototoxicity
Adverse Reactions
Central nervous system: Headache, dizziness, fatigue, drowsiness, insomnia, seizures, nervousness

(Continued)

ALPHABETICAL LISTING OF DRUGS

Ofloxacin *(Continued)*

Dermatologic: Rash, pruritus
Gastrointestinal: Nausea, diarrhea, flatulence, dysgeusia, dry mouth
Genitourinary: Vaginitis, external genital pruritus in women
Hematologic: Eosinophilia
Neuromuscular & skeletal: Tremors
Ocular: Visual disturbance, photophobia

Drug Interactions
Antacids, iron and zinc salts, sucralfate may reduce absorption by up to 98% if given at the same time
Antineoplastic agents may decrease absorption; cimetidine may increase levels
Probenecid may decrease urinary excretion
Ofloxacin may increase effects of anticoagulant, increased nephrotoxicity of cyclosporine, and decrease clearance (increased levels) of theophylline, hence, monitor appropriately

Food/Drug Interactions Food causes alteration in absorption; best to avoid concomitant administration

Mechanism of Action Ofloxacin, a fluorinated quinolone, is a pyridone carboxylic acid derivative which exerts a broad spectrum antimicrobial effect. Ofloxacin is related to the older quinolone derivatives, nalidixic acid, and oxolinic acid, and to the newer quinolone derivatives, norfloxacin and ciprofloxacin. The primary target of the fluoroquinolones is DNA gyrase (topoisomerase II), an essential bacterial enzyme that maintains the superhelical structure of DNA. DNA gyrase is required for DNA replication and transcription, DNA repair, recombination, and transposition.

Pharmacokinetics
Absorption: Fraction absorbed increases proportionately with the dose; age does not affect absorption
Half-life:
Young adults: 5 hours
Older adults with normal renal function: 6-8 hours
Sick, older, hospitalized adults: Between 9-13 hours
Time to peak serum concentration: Within 1-2 hours
Elimination: Primarily renal with ~5% excreted in feces

Usual Dosage Oral, I.V.:
Geriatrics: 200-400 mg every 12-24 hours (based on estimated renal function) for 7 days to 6 weeks depending on indication.
Adults: 200-400 mg every 12 hours for 3 days to 6 weeks; single 400 mg dose for acute uncomplicated gonorrhea.

Dosing interval in renal impairment:
Cl_{cr} 10-50 mL/minute: Administer recommended dose every 24 hours
Cl_{cr} <10 mL/minute: Administer half of recommended dose every 24 hours

Monitoring Parameters Signs and symptoms of infection; WBC, mental status

Patient Information Do not take antacids or multivitamins with minerals within 6 hours before or 2 hours after taking drug; take 1 hour before or 2 hours after meals; do not take with dairy products, iron, or zinc products; may cause dizziness, headache, or stimulation; avoid excess natural or artificial sunlight exposure; complete full course of therapy

Nursing Implications Hold antacids for 2-4 hours before and after giving dose

Special Geriatric Considerations See Pharmacokinetics and Usual Dosage; must adjust dose for renal function

Dosage Forms
Injection: 200 mg (50 mL); 400 mg (10 mL, 20 mL, 100 mL)
Tablet: 200 mg, 300 mg, 400 mg

References
Nilsson-Ehle I and Ljungberg B, "Quinolone Disposition in the Elderly: Practical Implications," *Drugs Aging,* 1991, 1(4):279-88.

Oleum Ricini *see* Castor Oil *on page 124*

Olsalazine Sodium *(ole sal' a zeen)*

Brand Names Dipentum®
Generic Available No
Therapeutic Class 5-Aminosalicylic Acid Derivative; Anti-inflammatory Agent
Use Maintenance of remission of ulcerative colitis in patients intolerant to sulfasalazine
Contraindications Hypersensitivity to salicylates
Warnings Bladder tumors in rats receiving 10-100 times the equivalent dose for man have been found in studies; liver tumors have also been reported in mice. No evidence exists for such problems in people receiving recommended doses.
Precautions Diarrhea appears to be dose related, but is difficult to distinguish from underlying disease symptoms; diarrhea occurs in up to 33% of patients
Adverse Reactions
Dermatologic: Rash, pruritus

Gastrointestinal: Diarrhea, abdominal pain/cramps, nausea, anorexia, dyspepsia

Miscellaneous: Depression, arthralgia, fever, hepatitis, blood dyscrasias (<1%)

Overdosage Symptoms of overdose include decreased motor activity, diarrhea

Toxicology Supportive care and discontinuation of drug may be initiated at a decreased dose after symptoms clear

Mechanism of Action Olsalazine is converted to two molecules of 5-ASA (mesalamine) by colonic bacteria. Mechanism of action is unknown but appears action is topical rather than systemic and decreases inflammation by inhibiting cyclooxygenase production of prostaglandins. Other actions may contribute to the antiinflammatory action such as inhibition of polymorphonuclear cell migration and inhibition of leukotriene production.

Pharmacokinetics

Absorption: 2% to 4%

Protein binding: 98%

Metabolism: 98% to 99% is converted to 5-aminosalicylic acid

Half-life: 0.9 hours; olsalazine-0-sulfate (olsalazine-S) accounts for 0.1% of the dose and has a half-life of 7 days

Time to peak serum concentration: Within 1 hour

Elimination: Primarily in feces

Usual Dosage Geriatrics and Adults: Oral: 1 g twice daily

Monitoring Parameters Stool frequency

Reference Range Olsalazine: 0-4.3 mmol/L; olsalazine sodium: 3.3-12.4 mmol/L. These are not therapeutic guideline levels. These are reported levels after administration that have been observed on study. No correlation to response is known at this time.

Test Interactions Increases in ALT/AST reported

Patient Information Take with food in evenly divided doses; contact physician if rash or diarrhea occur

Nursing Implications Monitor stool frequency

Special Geriatric Considerations No specific data on elderly to suggest the drug needs alterations in dose. Since so little is absorbed, dosing should not be changed for reasons of age. Diarrhea may pose a serious problem for elderly in that it may cause dehydration, electrolyte imbalance, hypotension, and confusion.

Dosage Forms Capsule: 250 mg

Omeprazole (oh me' pray zol)

Brand Names Prilosec™

Generic Available No

Formerly Known As Losec®

Therapeutic Class Gastric Acid Secretion Inhibitor

Use Short-term (4-8 weeks) treatment of duodenal ulcer and severe erosive esophagitis (grade 2 or above), diagnosed by endoscopy and short-term treatment of symptomatic gastroesophageal reflux disease (GERD) poorly responsive to customary medical treatment; pathological hypersecretory conditions

Unlabeled use: Gastric ulcer therapy and healing NSAID-induced ulcers

Contraindications Known hypersensitivity to omeprazole

Warnings In long-term (2-year) studies in rats, omeprazole produced a dose-related increase in gastric carcinoid tumors (doses were in excess of what is recommended in humans). While available endoscopic evaluations and histologic examinations of biopsy specimens from human stomachs have not detected a risk from short-term exposure to omeprazole, further human data on the effect of sustained hypochlorhydria and hypergastrinemia are needed to rule out the possibility of an increased risk for the development of tumors in humans receiving long-term therapy with omeprazole. Omeprazole should be prescribed only for the conditions, dosage and duration described. Bioavailability may be increased in elderly patients.

Precautions Symptomatic response to omeprazole does not preclude gastric malignancy

Adverse Reactions

Cardiovascular: Headache (most frequent at 7%), angina, tachycardia, bradycardia, edema

Central nervous system: Dizziness, fever, fatigue, malaise, apathy, somnolence, nervousness, anxiety

Dermatologic: Rash, urticaria, pruritus, dry skin

Endocrine & metabolic: Hypoglycemia

Gastrointestinal: Diarrhea, nausea, abdominal pain, vomiting, constipation, abdominal swelling, anorexia, irritable colon, fecal discoloration, esophageal candidiasis, dry mouth, taste alterations

Genitourinary: Urinary frequency, testicular pain

Renal: Pyuria, proteinuria, hematuria, glycosuria

Hematologic: Thrombocytopenia, pancytopenia, leukocytosis

Hepatic: Hepatitis, elevated AST/ALT/GGT/alkaline phosphatase, jaundice, increases in serum creatinine

Neuromuscular & skeletal: Back pain, asthenia occurred in more frequently than 1% of patients, muscle cramps, myalgia, joint pain, leg pain

(Continued)

Omeprazole *(Continued)*

Otic: Tinnitus
Respiratory: Cough

Overdosage Symptoms of overdose include hypothermia, sedation, convulsions, decreased respiratory rate (animal data)

Toxicology Symptomatic and general supportive care; not dialyzable

Drug Interactions Diazepam → ↑ half-life with increased CNS effects (toxicity), phenytoin, warfarin, ketoconazole (decreased absorption), nifedipine

Mechanism of Action Suppresses gastric acid secretion by inhibiting the parietal cell H+/K+ ATP pump

Pharmacodynamics
Onset of antisecretory action: Oral: Within 1 hour
Maximum effect: 2 hours
Duration: 72 hours

Pharmacokinetics
Protein binding: 95%
Metabolism: Extensive in the liver
Half-life: 30-90 minutes

Usual Dosage Geriatrics and Adults: Oral:
Duodenal ulcer: 20 mg/day for 4-8 weeks

GERD or severe erosive esophagitis: 20 mg/day for 4-8 weeks

Pathological hypersecretory conditions: 60 mg once daily initially; doses up to 120 mg 3 times/day have been administered; administer daily doses >80 mg in divided doses; patients with Zollinger-Ellison syndrome have been treated continuously for over 5 years

Dosing adjustment in renal impairment: No adjustment for dose is necessary for patients with renal or hepatic impairment or for elderly

Monitoring Parameters Monitor symptoms, occult blood; use of gastroscopy is preferred

Patient Information Take before eating; do not chew, crush, or open capsule; if need to open capsule for ease of administration, place contents in acid juice (orange juice, tomato juice, etc); may take with antacids concomitantly

Nursing Implications Capsule should be swallowed whole, not chewed, crushed, or opened

Special Geriatric Considerations The incidence of side effects in elderly is no different than that of younger adults (≤65 years of age) despite slight decrease in elimination and increase in bioavailability. Bioavailability may be increased in elderly (≥65 years of age), however, dosage adjustments are not necessary.

Dosage Forms Capsule, sustained release: 20 mg

Omnipen® see Ampicillin *on page 51*

OMS® see Morphine Sulfate *on page 481*

Ondansetron *(on dan' se tron)*

Brand Names Zofran®
Generic Available No
Therapeutic Class Antiemetic

Use May be prescribed for patients who are refractory to or have severe adverse reactions to standard antiemetic therapy. Ondansetron may be prescribed for young patients (ie, <45 years of age who are more likely to develop extrapyramidal reactions to high-dose metoclopramide) who are to receive highly emetogenic chemotherapeutic agents as listed:

Agents with high emetogenic potential (>90%) (dose/m²):
Carmustine ≥200 mg
Cisplatin ≥75 mg
Cyclophosphamide ≥1000 mg
Cytarabine ≥1000 mg
Dacarbazine ≥500 mg
Ifosfamide ≥1000 mg
Lomustine ≥60 mg
Mechlorethamine
Pentostatin
Streptozocin

or two agents classified as having high or moderately high emetogenic potential as listed:

Agents with moderately high emetogenic potential (60% to 90%) (dose/m²):
Carmustine <200 mg
Cisplatin <75 mg
Cyclophosphamide 1000 mg
Cytarabine 250-1000 mg
Dacarbazine <500 mg
Doxorubicin ≥75 mg

Ifosfamide
Lomustine <60 mg
Methotrexate ≥250 mg
Mitomycin
Mitoxantrone
Procarbazine

Ondansetron should not be prescribed for chemotherapeutic agents with a low emetogenic potential (eg, bleomycin, busulfan, cyclophosphamide <1000 mg, etoposide, 5-fluorouracil, vinblastine, vincristine)

Contraindications Hypersensitivity to ondansetron or any component

Warnings Ondansetron should be used on a scheduled basis, not as an "as needed" (PRN) basis, since data supports the use of this drug in the prevention of nausea and vomiting and not in the rescue of nausea and vomiting. Ondansetron should only be used in the first 24-48 hours of receiving chemotherapy. Data does not support any increased efficacy of ondansetron in delayed nausea and vomiting

Adverse Reactions
Cardiovascular: Headache, tachycardia, angina
Central nervous system: Lightheadedness, seizures
Dermatologic: Rash
Endocrine & metabolic: Hypokalemia
Gastrointestinal: Constipation, diarrhea
Hepatic: Transient elevations in serum levels of aminotransferases and bilirubin
Respiratory: Rarely bronchospasm
Miscellaneous: There have been 2 cases of EPS reaction

Overdosage In a few reported cases, the following symptoms have been noted: sudden blindness for 2-3 minutes, severe constipation, syncope, hypotension, transient vasovagal response

Toxicology No antidote; manage with general supportive care; doses 10 times greater than recommended have not shown significant adverse effects

Drug Interactions Metabolized by the hepatic cytochrome P-450 enzymes; therefore, the drug's clearance and half-life may be changed with concomitant use of cytochrome P-450 inducers (eg, barbiturates, carbamazepine, rifampin, phenytoin, and phenylbutazone) or inhibitors (eg, cimetidine, allopurinol, and disulfiram). Carmustine, etoposide, and cisplatin do not affect the pharmacokinetics of ondansetron in humans.

Stability Currently available only by the injectable route, as the oral form is still under investigation. The injection may be stored between 36°F and 86°F. Ondansetron is stable when mixed in 5% dextrose or 0.9% sodium chloride for 48 hours at room temperature and does not need protection from light.

Ondansetron is physically compatible with the following drugs for Y-site administration: amikacin, aztreonam, bleomycin, carboplatin, cefazolin, ceftazidime, ceftizoxime, cefuroxime, chlorpromazine, doxorubicin, doxycycline, droperidol, etoposide, floxuridine, fluconazole, gentamicin, haloperidol, hydrocortisone, ifosfamide, imipenem-cilastatin, magnesium sulfate, mannitol, mechlorethamine, mesna, methotrexate, miconazole, mitomycin, mitoxantrone, pentostatin, potassium chloride, streptozocin, tetracycline, ranitidine, ticarcillin/clavulanate, vancomycin, vinblastine, and vincristine.

Ondansetron is incompatible with the following drugs: acyclovir, aminophylline, amphotericin B, ampicillin, ampicillin/sulbactam, amsacrine, fluorouracil, furosemide, ganciclovir, lorazepam, methylprednisolone, mezlocillin, and piperacillin.

Mechanism of Action Selective 5-HT$_3$ receptor antagonist, blocking serotonin, both peripherally on vagal nerve terminals and centrally in the chemoreceptor trigger zone

Pharmacokinetics
Protein binding: Plasma 70% to 76%
Metabolism: Extensive by hydroxylation, followed by glucuronide or sulfate conjugation; elderly >75 years of age have a decreased hepatic clearance
Half-life: Geriatric patients <75 years of age and Adults: 4 hours
Elimination: In urine and feces; <10% of the parent drug is recovered unchanged in urine

Usual Dosage Geriatrics and Adults:
Oral: 8 mg 3 times/day; first dose 30 minutes prior to chemotherapy; administer for 1-2 days after completion of each chemotherapy treatment
I.V.: 0.15 mg/kg/dose or a single dose 32 mg over 15 minutes, infused 30 minutes before the start of emetogenic chemotherapy, with subsequent doses administered 4 and 8 hours after the first dose; decreased effectiveness has been reported when administered for prolonged therapy (eg, more than 3 doses); dilute in 50 mL D$_5$W or sodium chloride 0.9% for injection; elderly may need dosage adjustment if >75 years of age; however, no dosage adjustment is recommended

Dosing in hepatic impairment: Oral, I.V.: Do not exceed 8 mg/day dose

Postoperative nausea/vomiting: I.V.: 4 mg undiluted over 2-5 minutes; may give before anesthesia and after procedure

(Continued)

Ondansetron (Continued)

Administration See Stability; if injected undiluted, administer over a 2- to 5-minute period

Monitoring Parameters Emetic episodes, diarrhea, headache

Patient Information May cause diarrhea and headache

Nursing Implications First dose should be given 30 minutes prior to starting chemotherapy treatment

Additional Information The I.V. product has been used orally successfully

Special Geriatric Considerations Elderly have a slightly decreased hepatic clearance rate; this does not, however, require a dose adjustment

Dosage Forms
Tablet: 4 mg, 8 mg
Injection: 2 mg/mL (20 mL)

References

Marty M, Pouillart P, Scholl S, et al, "Comparison of the 5-hydroxytryptamine 3 (Serotonin) Antagonist Ondansetron (GR 38032F) With High-Dose Metoclopramide in the Control of Cisplatin-Induced Emesis," N Engl J Med, 1990, 322(12):816-21.

Pinkerton CR, Williams D, Wootton C, et al, "5-HT₃ Antagonist Ondansetron – An Effective Outpatient Antiemetic in Cancer Treatment," Arch Dis Child, 1990, 65(8):822-5.

Opcon® see Naphazoline Hydrochloride on page 492

Ophthalgan® see Glycerin on page 325

Ophthochlor® see Chloramphenicol on page 148

Opticrom® see Cromolyn Sodium on page 190

Optigene® [OTC] see Tetrahydrozoline Hydrochloride on page 680

Optimine® see Azatadine Maleate on page 69

OPV see Poliovirus Vaccine, Live, Trivalent on page 575

Orabase® HCA see Hydrocortisone on page 351

Oracit® see Sodium Citrate and Citric Acid on page 649

Orajel® Brace-Aid Rinse [OTC] see Carbamide Peroxide on page 119

Oraminic® II see Brompheniramine Maleate on page 95

Orap™ see Pimozide on page 565

Orasone® see Prednisone on page 586

Orazinc® [OTC] see Zinc Sulfate on page 742

Orciprenaline Sulfate see Metaproterenol Sulfate on page 449

Oretic® see Hydrochlorothiazide on page 347

Orex® [OTC] see Saliva Substitute on page 636

Original Doan's® [OTC] see Salicylates (Various Salts) on page 633

Orimune® see Poliovirus Vaccine, Live, Trivalent on page 575

Orinase® see Tolbutamide on page 702

Ormazine see Chlorpromazine Hydrochloride on page 153

Orphenadrine Citrate (or fen' a dreen)

Brand Names Norflex™

Generic Available Yes

Therapeutic Class Skeletal Muscle Relaxant

Use Treatment of muscle spasm associated with acute painful musculoskeletal conditions

Unlabeled use: Orphenadrine 100 mg at bedtime may be useful in the treatment of quinine-resistant leg cramps

Contraindications Glaucoma, GI obstruction, prostatic hypertrophy or GU obstruction, cardiospasm, myasthenia gravis, hypersensitivity to orphenadrine or any component

Warnings Use with caution in patients with CHF or cardiac arrhythmias; some products contain sulfites

Precautions Safety of continuous long-term therapy has not been established

Adverse Reactions Adverse effects are mainly due to its anticholinergic effects
Cardiovascular: Tachycardia, palpitations
Central nervous system: Dizziness, drowsiness, confusion in the elderly, hallucinations, agitation
Gastrointestinal: Dry mouth, nausea, constipation
Genitourinary: Urinary hesitancy and retention
Neuromuscular & skeletal: Tremors
Ocular: Blurred vision, dilated pupils

Overdosage Symptoms of overdose include blurred vision, tachycardia, confusion, seizures, respiratory arrest, dysrhythmias

Toxicology There is no specific treatment; however, most of its clinical toxicity is due to anticholinergic effects. Anticholinesterase inhibitors may be useful by reducing acetylcholinesterase. Anticholinesterase inhibitors include physostigmine, neostigmine, pyridostigmine and edrophonium. For anticholinergic overdose with severe life-threatening symptoms, physostigmine 1-2 mg I.V., slowly may be given to reverse these effects. Lethal dose is 2-3 g

Drug Interactions
Decreased effect of phenothiazines, haloperidol, tacrine
Increased toxicity with amantadine (anticholinergic effects)

Mechanism of Action Has not been identified, may be related to its analgesic properties; acts centrally at the brain stem

Pharmacodynamics
Peak effect: Oral: Within 2-4 hours
Duration: 4-6 hours

Pharmacokinetics
Protein binding: 20%
Metabolism: Extensive
Half-life: 14-16 hours
Elimination: Urine (8% as unchanged drug)

Usual Dosage
Geriatrics: See Special Geriatric Considerations
Adults:
Oral: 100 mg twice daily
I.M., I.V.: 60 mg every 12 hours

Monitoring Parameters Relief of symptoms, mental status, anticholinergic effects

Patient Information May cause drowsiness, dizziness, blurred vision, or fainting; do not crush or chew sustained release product; avoid alcohol, may impair coordination and judgment

Nursing Implications Do not crush sustained release drug product; raise bed rails, institute safety measures, assist with ambulation

Special Geriatric Considerations Because of its anticholinergic side effects, orphenadrine is not a drug of choice in the elderly

Dosage Forms
Injection: 30 mg/mL (2 mL, 10 mL)
Tablet: 100 mg
Tablet, sustained release: 100 mg

Or-tyl® see Dicyclomine Hydrochloride on page 215

Orudis® see Ketoprofen on page 390

Os-Cal® 500 [OTC] see Calcium Salts (Oral) on page 111

Osmoglyn® see Glycerin on page 325

O-V Staticin® see Nystatin on page 513

Oxacillin Sodium (ox a sill' in)
Brand Names Bactocill®; Prostaphlin®
Synonyms Isoxazolyl Penicillin; Methylphenyl
Generic Available Yes
Therapeutic Class Antibiotic, Penicillin
Use Treatment of susceptible bacterial infections such as osteomyelitis, septicemia, endocarditis, and CNS infections due to penicillinase-producing strains of *Staphylococcus* (except methicillin resistant)
Contraindications Hypersensitivity to oxacillin or other penicillins or any component
Precautions Use with caution in patients with severe renal impairment; use with caution in patients with cephalosporin allergy
Adverse Reactions
Cardiovascular: Thrombophlebitis
Central nervous system: Fever
Dermatologic: Rash
Gastrointestinal: Diarrhea, nausea, vomiting
Hematologic: Mild leukopenia, agranulocytosis, thrombocytopenia
Hepatic: Elevated AST, hepatotoxicity
Renal: Acute interstitial nephritis, hematuria
Miscellaneous: Allergy, serum sickness-like reactions
Overdosage Symptoms of overdose include neuromuscular hypersensitivity, seizure
Toxicology Many beta-lactam-containing antibiotics have the potential to cause neuromuscular hyperirritability or convulsive seizures. Hemodialysis may be helpful to aid in the removal of the drug from the blood, otherwise most treatment is supportive or symptom directed.
Drug Interactions Increased effect with probenecid
Food/Drug Interactions Food decreases bioavailability
(Continued)

Oxacillin Sodium *(Continued)*

Stability Reconstituted parenteral solution is stable for 3 days at room temperature and 7 days when refrigerated; for I.V. infusion in NS or D_5W, solution is stable for 6 hours at room temperature

Mechanism of Action Interferes with bacterial cell wall synthesis during active multiplication causing cell death and resultant bactericidal activity against susceptible bacteria

Pharmacokinetics

Absorption: Oral: ~35% to 67%

Distribution: Penetrates the blood-brain barrier only when meninges are inflamed

Protein binding: 90% to 95%

Metabolism: In the liver to active metabolites

Half-life: 23-60 minutes (prolonged with reduced renal function)

Time to peak:

Oral: Peak serum levels occur within 120 minutes

I.M.: Peak serum levels occur 30-60 minutes

Elimination: By the kidneys and to small degree the bile as parent drug and metabolites

Usual Dosage Geriatrics and Adults:

Oral: 500-1000 mg every 4-6 hours

I.M., I.V.: 250 mg to 2 g/dose every 4-6 hours

Dosing interval in renal impairment: Cl_{cr} <10 mL/minute: Use lower range of the usual dosage

Not dialyzable (0% to 5%)

Administration Give around-the-clock rather than 4 times/day, 3 times/day, etc (ie, 12-6-12-6, not 9-1-5-9) to promote less variation in peak and trough serum levels; I.M. injections should be given deep into a large muscle mass such as the gluteus maximus

Monitoring Parameters Monitor signs and symptoms of infection, WBC, mental status

Test Interactions False-positive urinary and serum proteins

Patient Information Take on an empty stomach 1 hour before meals or 2 hours after meals; complete full course of therapy; call your physician or pharmacist if diarrhea, cramping, or skin rash occur

Nursing Implications See Administration

Additional Information Sodium content of 1 g: 2.5 mEq

Special Geriatric Considerations Oxacillin has not been studied in the elderly; dosing adjustments are not necessary except in renal failure (ie, Cl_{cr} <10 mL/minute)

Dosage Forms

Capsule: 250 mg, 500 mg

Injection: 250 mg, 500 mg, 1 g, 2 g, 4 g, 10 g

Solution: 250 mg/5 mL (100 mL)

References

Yoshikawa TT, "Antimicrobial Therapy for the Elderly Patient," *J Am Geriatr Soc*, 1990, 38(12):1353-72.

Oxaprozin *(ox a proe' zin)*

Brand Names Daypro™

Therapeutic Class Nonsteroidal Anti-inflammatory Agent (NSAID), Oral

Use Acute and long-term use in the management of signs and symptoms of osteoarthritis and rheumatoid arthritis

Unlabeled use: Mild to moderate pain, acute painful shoulder

Contraindications Hypersensitivity to oxaprozin or other NSAIDs; due to the potential cross-sensitivity, use extreme caution when a history of allergy exists to aspirin, iodides, or other NSAIDs; hypersensitivity has caused symptoms of rhinitis, urticaria, asthma, nasal polyps, bronchospasm, angioedema, and anaphylaxis

Warnings GI toxicity (bleeding, ulceration, perforation); CNS effects may occur (headaches, confusion, depression); hypersensitivity, anaphylactoid reactions (intermittent tolmetin use more often); renal function decline, acute renal insufficiency, interstitial nephritis, dysuria, cystitis, hematuria, nephrotic syndrome, hyperkalemia in acute renal insufficiency, hyponatremia, papillary necrosis, hepatic function impairment; elderly have increased risk for adverse reactions to NSAIDs; see Special Geriatric Considerations

Precautions Use with caution in patients with congestive heart failure, hypertension, decreased renal or hepatic function, history of GI disease (bleeding or ulcers), or those receiving anticoagulants; perform ophthalmologic evaluation for those who develop eye complaints during therapy (blurred vision, diminished vision, changes in color vision, retinal changes); NSAIDs may mask signs/symptoms of infections; photosensitivity reported

Adverse Reactions

Cardiovascular: Congestive heart failure, angina, hypertension, hypotension, fluid retention, arrhythmias, edema

Central nervous system: Headache, drowsiness, vertigo, dizziness, fatigue, hallucinations, confusion, depression, emotional lability, psychotic behavior, asthenia

Dermatologic: Rash, urticaria, angioedema, Stevens-Johnson syndrome, exfoliative dermatitis, ecchymosis, petechiae, purpura, bruising

Endocrine & metabolic: Hyperglycemia, hypoglycemia, hyperkalemia, gynecomastia, hyponatremia

Gastrointestinal: Dyspepsia, heartburn, nausea, diarrhea, constipation, flatulence, stomatitis, vomiting, abdominal pain, peptic ulcer, GI bleeding, GI perforation, gingival ulcers, pancreatitis, proctitis, paralytic ulcers, colitis, anorexia, weight loss

Genitourinary: Impotence, azotemia

Hematologic: Neutropenia, anemia, agranulocytosis, bone marrow suppression, hemolytic anemia, hemorrhage, inhibition of platelet aggregation

Hepatic: Hepatitis, elevated LFTs, cholestatic jaundice

Neuromuscular & skeletal: Involuntary muscle movements, muscle weakness, tremors

Ocular: Vision changes

Otic: Tinnitus

Renal: Dysuria, polyuria, pyuria, oliguria, anuria, acute renal failure

Respiratory: Exacerbation of asthma, dyspnea

Miscellaneous: Dry mucous membranes, thirst, pyrexia, sweating

Overdosage Symptoms include drowsiness, lethargy, disorientation, confusion, dizziness, numbness, paresthesia, nausea, vomiting, gastric irritation, abdominal pain, headache, tinnitus, sweating, blurred vision, muscle twitching, seizures, coma, acute renal failure, increased BUN and serum creatinine, hypotension, tachycardia, and metabolic acidosis

Toxicology Management of a nonsteroidal anti-inflammatory agent (NSAID) intoxication is primarily supportive and symptomatic. Fluid therapy is commonly effective in managing the hypotension that may occur following an acute NSAID overdose, except when this is due to an acute blood loss. Seizures tend to be very short-lived and often do not require drug treatment although recurrent seizures should be treated with I.V. diazepam. Since many of the NSAIDs undergo enterohepatic cycling, multiple doses of charcoal may be needed to reduce the potential for delayed toxicities. NSAIDs are highly bound to plasma proteins, therefore hemodialysis and peritoneal dialysis are not useful.

Drug Interactions
May increase digoxin, methotrexate, and lithium serum concentrations

Aspirin may decrease NSAID serum concentrations

Other NSAIDs may increase adverse GI effects

Increased prothrombin time with anticoagulants

Decrease antihypertensive effects of ACE inhibitors, beta-blockers, and thiazide diuretics

Increased response to sympathomimetics

Probenecid may increase toxicity of NSAIDs by increase in serum concentrations

Diuretics may increase risk of acute renal function

Azotemia may be enhanced in elderly receiving loop diuretics

Mechanism of Action Inhibits prostaglandin synthesis, acts on the hypothalamus heat-regulating center to reduce fever, blocks prostaglandin synthetase action which prevents formation of the platelet-aggregating substance thromboxane A_2; decreases pain receptor sensitivity. Other proposed mechanisms of action are lysosomal stabilization, kinin and leukotriene production, alteration of chemotactic factors, and inhibition of neutrophil activation. This latter mechanism may be the most significant pharmacologic action to reduce inflammation.

Pharmacodynamics Onset of anti-inflammatory action: Up to 7 days

Pharmacokinetics
Absorption: Almost completely

Protein binding: >99%

Half-life: 40-50 hours; with continued dosing, half-life decreases to ~40 hours

Time to peak: 3-5 hours

Elimination: Has a dual pathway, hepatic and renal; with continued dosing, this dual pathway explains the lower half-life of chronic dosing vs single dose half-life

Usual Dosage Geriatrics and Adults: Oral (individualize dosage to lowest effective dose to minimize adverse effects):

Osteoarthritis: 600-1200 mg once daily

Rheumatoid arthritis: 1200 mg once daily

Maximum dose: 1800 mg/day or 26 mg/kg (whichever is lower) in divided doses
See Additional Information

Monitoring Parameters Monitor response (pain, range of motion, grip strength, mobility, ADL function), inflammation; observe for weight gain, edema; monitor renal function; observe for bleeding, bruising; evaluate gastrointestinal effects (abdominal pain, bleeding, dyspepsia); mental confusion, disorientation, CBC, serum, creatinine, BUN, liver function tests

Test Interactions Increased chloride (S), increased sodium (S)

Patient Information Serious gastrointestinal bleeding can occur as well as ulceration and perforation. Pain may or may not be present. Avoid aspirin and aspirin-containing

(Continued)

Oxaprozin *(Continued)*

products while taking this medication. If gastric upset occurs, take with food, milk, or antacid. If gastric adverse effects persist, contact physician. May cause drowsiness, dizziness, blurred vision, and confusion. Use caution when performing tasks which require alertness (eg, driving). Do not take for more than 3 days for fever or 10 days for pain without physician's advice.

Nursing Implications See Patient Information, Overdosage, Monitoring Parameters, and Special Geriatric Considerations

Additional Information There are no clinical guidelines to predict which NSAID will give response in a particular patient; trials with each must be initiated until response determined; consider dose, patient convenience, and cost

Special Geriatric Considerations Elderly are a high-risk population for adverse effects from nonsteroidal anti-inflammatory agents. As much as 60% of elderly can develop peptic ulceration and/or hemorrhage asymptomatically. The concomitant use of H_2 blockers, omeprazole, and sucralfate is not generally effective as prophylaxis. Misoprostol is the only prophylactic agent proven effective. Also, concomitant disease and drug use contribute to the risk for GI adverse effects. Use lowest effective dose for shortest period possible. Consider renal function decline with age. Use of NSAIDs can compromise existing renal function especially when Cl_{cr} is ≤ 30 mL/minute. Tinnitus may be a difficult and unreliable indication of toxicity due to age-related hearing loss or eighth cranial nerve damage. CNS adverse effects such as confusion, agitation, and hallucination are generally seen in overdose or high dose situations, but elderly may demonstrate these adverse effects at lower doses than younger adults.

Dosage Forms Tablet: 600 mg

References

Brooks PM, Day RO, "Nonsteroidal Anti-inflammatory Drugs – Differences and Similarities," *N Engl J Med*, 1991, 324(24):1716-25.

Clinch D, Banerjee AK, Ostick G, "Absence of Abdominal Pain in Elderly Patients With Peptic Ulcer," *Age Ageing*, 1984, 13(2):120-3.

Clive DM, Stoff JS, "Renal Syndromes Associated With Nonsteroidal Anti-inflammatory Drugs," *N Engl J Med*, 1984, 310(9):563-72.

Graham DY, "Prevention of Gastroduodenal Injury Induced by Chronic Nonsteroidal Anti-inflammatory Drug Therapy," *Gastroenterology*, 1989, 96(2 Pt 2 Suppl):675-81.

Gurwitz JH, Avarn J, Ross-Degan D, et al, "Nonsteroidal Anti-Inflammatory Drug-Associated Azotemia in the Very Old," *JAMA*, 1990, 264(4):471-5.

Knodel LC, "Preventing NSAID-Induced Ulcers: The Role of Misoprostol," *Consult Pharm*, 1989, 4:37-41.

Pounder R, "Silent Peptic Ulceration: Deadly Silence or Golden Silence?" *Gastroenterology*, 1989, 96:(2 Pt 2 Suppl)626-31.

Oxazepam *(ox a' ze pam)*

Related Information

Antacid Drug Interactions *on page 764*

Anxiolytic/Hypnotic Use in Long-Term Care Facilities *on page 755-756*

Benzodiazepines Comparison *on page 802-803*

Brand Names Serax®

Generic Available Yes

Therapeutic Class Benzodiazepine

Use Treatment of anxiety and management of alcohol withdrawal

Restrictions C-IV

Contraindications Hypersensitivity to oxazepam or any component, cross-sensitivity with other benzodiazepines may exist; avoid using in patients with pre-existing CNS depression, severe uncontrolled pain, or narrow-angle glaucoma

Precautions Use with caution in patients with a history of drug dependence

Adverse Reactions

Central nervous system: Drowsiness, confusion, dizziness, ataxia, amnesia, slurred speech, paradoxical excitement or rage

Gastrointestinal: Constipation, dry mouth, diarrhea, nausea, vomiting

Neuromuscular & skeletal: Impaired coordination

Ocular: Blurred vision, diplopia

Respiratory: Decrease in respiratory rate, apnea, laryngospasm

Miscellaneous: Physical and psychological dependence with prolonged use

Overdosage Symptoms of overdose include somnolence, confusion, coma, and diminished reflexes

Toxicology Treatment for benzodiazepine overdose is supportive; rarely is mechanical ventilation required

Flumazenil has been shown to selectively block the binding of benzodiazepines to CNS receptors, resulting in a reversal of benzodiazepine-induced sedation; however, its use may not alter the course of overdose

Drug Interactions Increased toxicity: CNS depressants, alcohol

Mechanism of Action Benzodiazepines appear to potentiate the effects of GABA and other inhibitory neurotransmitters by binding to specific benzodiazepine-receptor sites in various areas of the CNS

Pharmacodynamics Studies have shown that the elderly are more sensitive to the effects of benzodiazepines as compared to younger adults

Pharmacokinetics No significant changes in pharmacokinetics are seen in the elderly

Absorption: Oral: Almost completely
Protein binding: 86% to 99%
Metabolism: In the liver to inactive compounds (primarily as glucuronides)
Half-life: 5-20 hours
Time to peak serum concentration: Within 2-4 hours
Elimination: Urinary excretion of unchanged drug (50%) and metabolites; excreted without need for liver metabolism

Usual Dosage Oral:
Geriatrics: Anxiety: 10 mg 2-3 times/day; increase gradually as needed to a total of 30-45 mg/day

Adults:
Anxiety: 10-15 mg 3-4 times/day
Alcohol withdrawal: 15-30 mg 3-4 times/day

Not dialyzable (0% to 5%)

Monitoring Parameters Respiratory, cardiovascular and mental status, symptoms of anxiety

Reference Range Therapeutic: 0.2-1.4 μg/mL (SI: 0.7-4.9 μmol/L)

Patient Information Avoid alcohol and other CNS depressants; may cause drowsiness; avoid activities needing good psychomotor coordination until CNS effects are known; may cause physical or psychological dependence; avoid abrupt discontinuation after prolonged use

Nursing Implications Assist patient with ambulation, monitor for alertness

Special Geriatric Considerations Because of its relatively short half-life and its lack of active metabolites, oxazepam is recommended for use in the elderly when a benzodiazepine is indicated; see Pharmacodynamics

Dosage Forms Capsule: 10 mg, 15 mg, 30 mg

References
Hicks R, Dysken MW, Davis JM, et al, "The Pharmacokinetics of Psychotropic Medication in the Elderly: A Review," *J Clin Psychiatry*, 1981, 42(10)374-85.

Oxilapine Succinate see Loxapine on page 421
Oxpentifylline see Pentoxifylline on page 547

Oxtriphylline (ox trye' fi lin)

Brand Names Choledyl®
Synonyms Choline Theophyllinate
Generic Available Yes
Therapeutic Class Antiasthmatic; Bronchodilator; Theophylline Derivative
Use Bronchodilator in symptomatic treatment of asthma and reversible bronchospasm
Contraindications Uncontrolled arrhythmias, peptic ulcer, hyperthyroidism, uncontrolled seizure disorders; hypersensitivity to oxtriphylline, other xanthines, or any component
Warnings May precipitate or worsen existing arrhythmias
Precautions Use with caution in patients with peptic ulcer, hyperthyroidism, hypertension, and patients with compromised cardiac function; hepatic function, esophageal reflux disease, alcoholism, and elderly
Adverse Reactions Adverse reactions are uncommon at serum theophylline concentrations <20 μg/mL

Cardiovascular: Palpitation, sinus tachycardia, extrasystoles, hypotension, ventricular arrhythmias, flushing
Central nervous system: Irritability, restlessness, fever, headache, insomnia, seizures
Endocrine & metabolic: Hyperglycemia
Gastrointestinal: Nausea, vomiting, esophageal reflux, diarrhea, hematemesis, rectal bleeding, epigastric pain
Genitourinary: Diuresis
Neuromuscular & skeletal: Tremors, muscle twitching
Renal: Proteinuria
Respiratory: Tachypnea, respiratory arrest

Overdosage Symptoms of overdose include tachycardia, extrasystoles, nausea, vomiting, anorexia, tonic-clonic seizures, insomnia, circulatory failure; agitation, irritability, headache

Toxicology If seizures have not occurred, induce vomiting; ipecac syrup is preferred. Do not induce emesis in the presence of impaired consciousness. Repeated doses of charcoal have been shown to be effective in enhancing the total body clearance of theophylline. Do not repeat charcoal doses if an ileus is present. Charcoal hemoperfusion may be considered if the serum theophylline level exceeds 40 mcg/mL, the patient is unable to tolerate repeat oral charcoal administrations, or if severe toxic symptoms are present. Clearance with hemoperfusion is better than clearance from hemodialysis. Administer a cathartic, especially if sustained release agents were used. Phenobarbital administered prophylactically may prevent seizures.

(Continued)

Oxtriphylline *(Continued)*

Drug Interactions

Changes in diet may affect the elimination of theophylline; theophylline may decrease the effects of phenytoin, lithium, and neuromuscular blocking agents

Theophylline increases the excretion of lithium; theophylline may have synergistic toxicity with sympathomimetics

Cimetidine, ranitidine, allopurinol, beta-blockers (nonspecific), erythromycin, influenza virus vaccine, corticosteroids, ephedrine, quinolones, thyroid hormones, oral contraceptives, amiodarone, troleandomycin, clindamycin, carbamazepine, isoniazid, loop diuretics, and lincomycin may increase theophylline concentrations

Cigarette and marijuana smoking, rifampin, barbiturates, hydantoins, ketoconazole, sulfinpyrazone, sympathomimetics, isoniazid, loop diuretics, carbamazepine, and aminoglutethimide may decrease theophylline concentrations

Tetracyclines enhance toxicity and may antagonize benzodiazepine's action

Mechanism of Action Causes bronchodilatation, diuresis, CNS and cardiac stimulation, and gastric acid secretion by blocking phosphodiesterase which increases tissue concentrations of cyclic adenine monophosphate (cAMP), which in turn promotes catecholamine stimulation of lipolysis, glycogenolysis, and gluconeogenesis and induces release of epinephrine from adrenal medulla cells. Other proposed mechanisms include inhibition of extracellular adenosine, stimulation of endogenous catecholamines, antagonism of PGE_2 and $PGE_{2\alpha}$, mobilization of intracellular calcium, and increased sensitivity of beta-adrenergic receptors in reactive airways.

Pharmacokinetics

Absorption: Oral: Up to 100% of dose is absorbed depending upon the formulation used; contains 64% theophylline, the active form

Distribution: V_d: 0.45 L/kg

Metabolism: In the liver by demethylation

Half-life: Varies from 3-15 hours in healthy adults (nonsmokers); 4-5 hours in smokers (1-2 packs/day); see table.

Half–life (h)	Patient Population
7–9	Normal healthy geriatrics/adults
18–24	Severe congestive heart failure
29	Cirrhosis

Time to peak: Peak plasma concentrations are reached in 1-2 hours, 4 hours for sustained release

Elimination: In urine; adults excrete 10% in urine as unchanged drug

Usual Dosage Geriatrics and Adults:

Oral: 4-7 mg/kg every 6-8 hours; see Additional Information

Sustained release: Initiate therapy with 400 mg every 12 hours

Monitoring Parameters Heart rate, CNS effects (insomnia, irritability); respiratory rate (COPD patients often have resting controlled respiratory rates in the low 20's)

Reference Range

Sample size: 0.5-1 mL serum (red top tube)

Therapeutic: 10-20 µg/mL; Toxic: >20 µg/mL; some patients may have adequate clinical response with serum levels from 5-10 µg/mL

Timing of serum samples: If toxicity is suspected, draw a level any time during a continuous I.V. infusion, or 2 hours after an oral dose; if lack of therapeutic is effected, draw a trough immediately before the next oral dose or intermittent I.V. dose

Test Interactions May elevate uric acid tests

Patient Information Oral preparations should be taken with a full glass of water; avoid drinking or eating large quantities of caffeine-containing beverages or food; take at regular intervals; take with food if GI upset occurs; notify physician if nausea, vomiting, insomnia, nervousness, irritability, palpitations, seizures occur; do not change from one brand to another without consulting physician and pharmacist; do not change doses without consulting your physician

Nursing Implications Give oral administration around-the-clock rather than 4 times/day, 3 times/day, etc (ie, 12-6-12-6, not 9-1-5-9) to promote less variation in peak and trough serum levels; do not crush sustained release drug products; monitor vital signs, serum concentrations, and CNS effects (insomnia, irritability); encourage patient to drink adequate fluids (2 L/day) to decrease mucous viscosity in airways

Additional Information When dosing with oxtriphylline, assure equivalent doses are used especially when switching from theophylline or aminophylline products to oxtriphylline, as the theophylline content is much lower for oxtriphylline agents (eg, 156 mg oxtriphylline = 100 mg theophylline)

Special Geriatric Considerations Although there is a great intersubject variability for half-lives of methylxanthines (2-10 hours), elderly as a group have slower hepatic clearance. Therefore, use lower initial doses and monitor closely for response and adverse reactions. Additionally, elderly are at greater risk for toxicity due to concomitant disease (eg, CHF, arrhythmias), and drug use (eg, cimetidine, ciprofloxacin, etc); there exists no therapeutic benefit using this product instead of less expensive theophylline products; see Precautions and Drug Interactions

Dosage Forms
Elixir: 100 mg/5 mL
Syrup: 50 mg/5 mL
Tablet: 100 mg, 200 mg
Tablet, sustained release: 400 mg, 600 mg

References
Kearney TE, Manoguerra AS, Curtis GP, et al, "Theophylline Toxicity and the Beta-Adrenergic System," *Ann Intern Med*, 1985, 102(6):766-9.
Mahler DA, Barlow PB, and Matthay RA, "Chronic Obstructive Pulmonary Disease," *Clin Geriatr Med*, 1986, 2(2):285-312.
Upton RA, "Pharmacokinetic Interactions Between Theophylline and Other Medication (Part II)," *Clin Pharmacokinet*, 1991, 20(2):135-50.

Oxybutynin Chloride (ox i byoo' ti nin)

Brand Names Ditropan®
Generic Available Yes
Therapeutic Class Antispasmodic Agent, Urinary
Use Antispasmodic for bladder (urgency, frequency, urge incontinence) and uninhibited bladder
Contraindications Glaucoma, myasthenia gravis, partial or complete GI obstruction, GU obstruction, ulcerative colitis; patients hypersensitive to the drug; intestinal atony, megacolon, toxic megacolon
Precautions Use with caution in patients with hepatic or renal disease, heart disease, hyperthyroidism, reflux esophagitis; use with caution in elderly, autonomic neuropathy, ulcerative colitis (may cause ileus and toxic megacolon), hypertension, hiatal hernia, and prostatic hypertrophy; use caution in patients with heat prostration, diarrhea (may be early sign of intestinal obstruction)
Adverse Reactions
Cardiovascular: Tachycardia, palpitations
Central nervous system: Drowsiness, fever, dizziness, insomnia, hallucinations, restlessness
Dermatologic: Rash
Endocrine & metabolic: Hot flashes
Gastrointestinal: Dry mouth, nausea, vomiting, constipation, decreased GI motility
Genitourinary: Urinary hesitancy or retention, impotence
Neuromuscular & skeletal: Weakness
Ocular: Blurred vision, mydriasis, amblyopia
Miscellaneous: Decreased sweating
Overdosage Symptoms of overdose include hypotension, circulatory failure, psychotic behavior, flushing, respiratory failure, paralysis, restlessness, tremor, irritability, seizures, delirium, hallucinations, coma
Toxicology Symptomatic and supportive; induce emesis or perform gastric lavage followed by charcoal and a cathartic; physostigmine may be required; treat hyperpyrexia with cooling techniques (ice bags, cold applications, alcohol sponges)
Drug Interactions
Oxybutynin may increase serum concentrations of digoxin
May decrease serum concentrations of haloperidol
May enhance development of tardive dyskinesia; may enhance anticholinergic effect of drugs exhibiting anticholinergic pharmacologic action
Mechanism of Action Direct antispasmodic effect on smooth muscle, also inhibits the action of acetylcholine on smooth muscle (exhibits $\frac{1}{5}$ the anticholinergic activity of atropine, but is 4-10 times the antispasmodic activity); does not block effects at skeletal muscle or at autonomic ganglia; increases bladder capacity, decreases uninhibited contractions, and delays desire to void; therefore, decreases urgency and frequency
Pharmacodynamics
Onset of action: Oral: 30-60 minutes
Peak effects: 3-6 hours
Duration: 6-10 hours
Pharmacokinetics
Absorption: Oral: Rapid
Metabolism: In the liver
Half-life: 1-2.3 hours
Time to peak: Peak serum levels occur within 60 minutes
Elimination: In urine
Usual Dosage Oral (see Additional Information):
Geriatrics: 2.5-5 mg twice daily; increase by 2.5 mg increments every 1-2 days
Adults: 5 mg 2-3 times/day up to 5 mg 4 times/day maximum
Monitoring Parameters Monitor incontinence episodes, post void residual (PVR)
Patient Information May impair ability to perform activities requiring mental alertness or physical coordination; alcohol or other sedating drugs may enhance drowsiness
(Continued)

Oxybutynin Chloride *(Continued)*

Nursing Implications See Adverse Reactions, Precautions, Monitoring Parameters, and Special Geriatric Considerations

Additional Information Should be discontinued periodically to determine whether the patient can manage without the drug and to minimize resistance to the drug

Special Geriatric Considerations Caution should be used in elderly due to anticholinergic activity (eg, confusion, constipation, blurred vision, and tachycardia)

Dosage Forms
Syrup: 5 mg/5 mL (473 mL)
Tablet: 5 mg

Oxycodone and Acetaminophen
(ox i koe' done & a seet a min' oh fen)

Related Information
Acetaminophen *on page 13*
Oxycodone Hydrochloride *on next page*
Pharmacokinetics of Narcotic Agonist Analgesics *on page 812*

Brand Names Percocet®; Roxicet®; Tylox®

Synonyms Acetaminophen and Oxycodone

Generic Available Yes

Therapeutic Class Analgesic, Narcotic

Use Management of moderate to severe pain

Restrictions C-II

Contraindications Hypersensitivity to oxycodone, acetaminophen or any component; severe respiratory depression, severe liver or renal insufficiency

Warnings Some preparations may contain bisulfites which may cause allergies

Precautions Use with caution in patients with hypersensitivity to other phenanthrene derivative opioid agonists (morphine, codeine, hydrocodone, hydromorphone, oxymorphone, levorphanol)

Adverse Reactions
Cardiovascular: Palpitations, hypotension, bradycardia, peripheral vasodilation
Central nervous system: CNS depression, increased intracranial pressure
Dermatologic: Pruritus
Endocrine & metabolic: Antidiuretic hormone release
Gastrointestinal: Nausea, vomiting, constipation
Ocular: Miosis
Respiratory: Respiratory depression
Miscellaneous: Physical and psychological dependence, biliary or urinary tract spasm, histamine release

Overdosage Symptoms of overdose include hepatic necrosis, transient azotemia, renal tubular necrosis with acute toxicity, anemia, renal damage, and GI disturbances with chronic toxicity

Toxicology Treatment of an overdose includes support of the patient's airway, establishment of an I.V. line and administration of naloxone 2 mg I.V. with repeat administration as necessary. Mucomyst® (acetylcysteine) 140 mg/kg orally (loading) followed by 70 mg/kg (maintenance) every 4 hours for 17 doses. Therapy should be initiated based upon laboratory analysis suggesting high probability of hepatotoxic potential.

Drug Interactions
Decreased effect with phenothiazines
Increased effect/toxicity with CNS depressants, TCAs, dextroamphetamine

Usual Dosage Oral (doses should be titrated to appropriate analgesic effects):
Geriatrics: 1 tablet or capsule every 6 hours as needed; do not exceed 4 g/day of acetaminophen
Adults: 1-2 tablets every 4-6 hours as needed for pain

Monitoring Parameters Pain relief, respiratory and mental status, blood pressure

Patient Information May cause drowsiness, avoid alcoholic beverages; do not exceed recommended dose

Nursing Implications Monitor for pain relief, excessive sedation, confusion, and constipation

Special Geriatric Considerations Enhanced analgesia has been seen in elderly patients on therapeutic doses of narcotics; duration of action may be increased in the elderly; the elderly may be particularly susceptible to the CNS depressant and constipating effects of narcotics; if one tablet/dose is used, it may be useful to add an additional 325 mg of acetaminophen to maximize analgesic effect

Dosage Forms
Capsule: Oxycodone hydrochloride 5 mg and acetaminophen 500 mg
Solution: Oxycodone hydrochloride 5 mg and acetaminophen 325 mg per 5 mL (5 mL, 500 mL)
Tablet: Oxycodone hydrochloride 5 mg and acetaminophen 325 mg

Oxycodone and Aspirin (ox i koe' done and as' pir in)

Related Information
  Aspirin *on page 58*
  Oxycodone Hydrochloride *on this page*
  Pharmacokinetics of Narcotic Agonist Analgesics *on page 812*
Brand Names Codoxy®; Percodan®; Percodan®-Demi; Roxiprin®
Synonyms Aspirin and Oxycodone
Generic Available Yes
Therapeutic Class Analgesic, Narcotic
Use Relief of moderate to moderately severe pain
Restrictions C-II
Contraindications Known hypersensitivity to oxycodone or aspirin; severe respiratory depression, severe liver or renal insufficiency
Precautions Use with caution in patients with hypersensitivity to other phenanthrene derivative opioid agonists (morphine, codeine, hydrocodone, hydromorphone, oxymorphone, levorphanol)
Adverse Reactions
  Cardiovascular: Palpitations, hypotension, bradycardia, peripheral vasodilation
  Central nervous system: CNS depression, increased intracranial pressure
  Dermatologic: Pruritus
  Endocrine & metabolic: Antidiuretic hormone release
  Gastrointestinal: Nausea, vomiting, constipation
  Ocular: Miosis
  Respiratory: Respiratory depression
  Miscellaneous: Physical and psychological dependence, biliary or urinary tract spasm, histamine release
Overdosage Symptoms of overdose include CNS and respiratory depression, gastrointestinal cramping, constipation, tinnitus, headache, dizziness, confusion, metabolic acidosis, hyperpyrexia
Toxicology Naloxone 2 mg I.V. with repeat administration as necessary up to a total of 10 mg; see also Aspirin toxicology
Drug Interactions
  Decreased effect with phenothiazines
  Increased effect/toxicity with CNS depressants, TCAs, dextroamphetamine
Usual Dosage Geriatrics and Adults: Oral (based on oxycodone combined salts): Percodan®: 1 tablet every 6 hours as needed for pain or Percodan®-Demi: 1-2 tablets every 6 hours as needed for pain
Monitoring Parameters Pain relief, respiratory and mental status, blood pressure
Patient Information May cause drowsiness, avoid alcoholic beverages; do not exceed recommended dose
Nursing Implications Monitor for pain relief, excessive sedation, confusion, and constipation
Special Geriatric Considerations Enhanced analgesia has been seen in elderly patients on therapeutic doses of narcotics; duration of action may be increased; the elderly may be particularly susceptible to the CNS depressant and constipating effects of narcotics; if one tablet/dose is used, it may be useful to add an additional 325 mg of acetaminophen to maximize analgesic effect
Dosage Forms Tablet: Oxycodone hydrochloride 4.5 mg, oxycodone terephthalate 0.38 mg, and aspirin 325 mg; oxycodone hydrochloride 2.25 mg, oxycodone terephthalate 0.19 mg, and aspirin 325 mg

Oxycodone Hydrochloride (ox i koe' done)

Related Information
  Narcotic Agonist Comparative Pharmacology *on page 811*
  Pharmacokinetics of Narcotic Agonist Analgesics *on page 812*
Brand Names Roxicodone™
Synonyms Dihydrohydroxycodeinone
Generic Available No
Therapeutic Class Analgesic, Narcotic
Use Management of moderate to severe pain, normally used in combination with non-narcotic analgesics
Restrictions C-II
Contraindications Hypersensitivity to oxycodone or any component
Warnings Use with caution in patients with hypersensitivity reactions to other phenanthrene derivative opioid agonists (morphine, hydrocodone, hydromorphone, levorphanol, oxycodone, oxymorphone); respiratory diseases including asthma, emphysema, COPD, or severe liver or renal insufficiency; some preparations contain sulfites which may cause allergic reactions
Adverse Reactions
  Cardiovascular: Palpitations, hypotension, bradycardia, peripheral vasodilation
  Central nervous system: CNS depression, increased intracranial pressure
  Dermatologic: Pruritus
  Endocrine & metabolic: Antidiuretic hormone release
(Continued)

Oxycodone Hydrochloride *(Continued)*

Gastrointestinal: Nausea, vomiting, constipation
Ocular: Miosis
Respiratory: Respiratory depression
Miscellaneous: Physical and psychological dependence, histamine release, biliary or urinary tract spasm

Overdosage Symptoms of overdose include CNS depression, respiratory depression, miosis

Toxicology Treatment of an overdose includes support of the patient's airway, establishment of an I.V. line and administration of naloxone 2 mg I.V. with repeat administration as necessary up to a total of 10 mg.

Drug Interactions
Decreased effect with phenothiazines
Increased effect/toxicity with CNS depressants, TCAs, dextroamphetamine

Mechanism of Action Binds to opiate receptors in the CNS, causing inhibition of ascending pain pathways, altering the perception of and response to pain; produces generalized CNS depression

Pharmacodynamics
Onset of action: Oral: Pain relief occurs within 10-15 minutes
Peak effects: 30-60 minutes
Duration: 4-5 hours; enhanced analgesia has been seen in elderly patients on therapeutic doses of narcotics; duration of action may be increased in the elderly

Pharmacokinetics
Metabolism: In the liver
Elimination: In urine

Usual Dosage Oral:
Geriatrics: 2.5-5 mg every 6 hours as needed
Adults: 5 mg every 6 hours as needed

Monitoring Parameters Pain relief, respiratory and mental status, blood pressure

Patient Information May cause drowsiness, avoid alcoholic beverages; do not exceed recommended dose

Nursing Implications Monitor patient for pain relief, excessive sedation, confusion, and constipation

Additional Information
Oxycodone: Roxicodone™
Oxycodone and acetaminophen: Oxycet®, Percocet®, Roxicet®, Tylox®
Oxycodone and aspirin: Percodan®, Percodan®-Demi, Codoxy®, Roxiprin®

Special Geriatric Considerations See Pharmacodynamics; the elderly may be particularly susceptible to the CNS depressant and constipating effects of narcotics

Dosage Forms
Liquid: 5 mg/5 mL
Tablet: 5 mg

Oxymetazoline Hydrochloride *(ox i met az' oh leen)*

Brand Names Afrin® Nasal Solution [OTC]; Allerest® 12 Hour Nasal Solution [OTC]; Chlorphed®-LA Nasal Solution [OTC]; Dristan® Long Lasting Nasal Solution [OTC]; Duration® Nasal Solution [OTC]; Genasal® Nasal Solution [OTC]; Nasal Relief® [OTC]; Neo-Synephrine® 12 Hour Nasal Solution [OTC]; Nõstrilla® [OTC]; NTZ® Long Acting Nasal Solution [OTC]; OcuClear® Ophthalmic [OTC]; Sinarest® 12 Hour Nasal Solution; Twice-A-Day® Nasal Solution [OTC]; Vicks Sinex® Long-Acting Nasal Solution [OTC]; Visine® L.R. Ophthalmic [OTC]; 4-Way® Long Acting Nasal Solution [OTC]

Generic Available Yes

Therapeutic Class Adrenergic Agonist Agent; Decongestant, Nasal; Vasoconstrictor, Nasal; Vasoconstrictor, Ophthalmic

Use Symptomatic relief of nasal mucosal congestion and adjunctive therapy of middle ear infections, associated with acute or chronic rhinitis, the common cold, sinusitis, hay fever, or other allergies
Ophthalmic: Relief of redness of eye due to minor eye irritations

Contraindications Hypersensitivity to oxymetazoline or any component

Warnings Rebound congestion may occur with extended use (>3 days); use with caution in the presence of hypertension, diabetes, hyperthyroidism, heart disease, coronary artery disease, cerebral arteriosclerosis, or long-standing bronchial asthma

Adverse Reactions
Cardiovascular: Hypertension, palpitations, reflex bradycardia
Central nervous system: Nervousness, dizziness, insomnia, headache
Gastrointestinal: Nausea
Local: Transient burning, stinging, dryness of nasal mucosa, rebound congestion with prolonged use
Respiratory: Sneezing

Overdosage Symptoms of overdose include CNS depression, hypothermia, bradycardia, cardiovascular collapse, coma, apnea

Toxicology Following initiation of essential overdose management, toxic symptoms should be treated. The patient should be kept warm and monitored for alterations in vital functions. Seizures commonly respond to diazepam (5-10 mg I.V. bolus in adults every 15 minutes if needed up to a total of 30 mg) or to phenytoin or phenobarbital; hypotension should be treated with fluids.

Drug Interactions Increased toxicity: MAO inhibitors

Mechanism of Action Stimulates alpha-adrenergic receptors in the arterioles of the nasal mucosa to produce vasoconstriction

Pharmacodynamics
Onset of effect: Intranasal: Within 5-10 minutes
Duration: 5-6 hours

Pharmacokinetics Metabolism: Metabolic fate is unknown

Usual Dosage Geriatrics and Adults (therapy should not exceed 3-5 days):
Intranasal: 0.05% solution: Instill 2-3 drops or 2-3 sprays into each nostril twice daily

Ophthalmic: Instill 1-2 drops into affected eye(s) every 6 hours

Monitoring Parameters Blood pressure in hypertensives

Patient Information Should not be used for self-medication for longer than 3 days, if symptoms persist, drug should be discontinued and a physician consulted; notify physician of insomnia, tremor, or irregular heartbeat; burning, stinging, or drying of the nasal mucosa may occur

Special Geriatric Considerations Evaluate the patient's ability to self-administer; use with caution in patients with cardiovascular disease

Dosage Forms
Nasal solution:
Drops: Afrin®, NTZ® Long Acting Nasal Solution: 0.05% (15 mL, 20 mL)
Spray: Afrin®, Allerest® 12 Hours, Chlorphed®-LA, Dristan® Long Lasting, Duration®, 4-Way® Long Acting, Genasal®, Nasal Relief®, Neo-Synephrine® 12 Hour, Nostrilla®, NTZ® Long Acting Nasal Solution, Sinex® Long-Acting, Twice-A-Day®: 0.05% (15 mL, 30 mL)
Ophthalmic solution (OcuClear®, Visine® L.R.): 0.025% (15 mL, 30 mL)

Oxytetracycline Hydrochloride (ox i tet ra sye' kleen)

Brand Names Terramycin® IV; Uri-Tet®

Therapeutic Class Antibiotic, Tetracycline Derivative

Use Treatment of susceptible bacterial infections; both gram-positive and gram-negative, as well as *Rickettsia* and *Mycoplasma* organisms

Contraindications Hypersensitivity to tetracycline or any component

Precautions Photosensitivity can occur with oxytetracycline

Adverse Reactions
Cardiovascular: Thrombophlebitis
Central nervous system: Pseudotumor cerebri
Dermatologic: Photosensitivity
Gastrointestinal: Nausea, vomiting, diarrhea, antibiotic-associated pseudomembranous colitis, staphylococcal enterocolitis
Hepatic: Hepatotoxicity
Neuromuscular & skeletal: Injury to growing bones and teeth
Renal: Renal damage
Miscellaneous: Candidal superinfection, discoloration of teeth and enamel hypoplasia, hypersensitivity reactions

Drug Interactions
Antacids, milk, iron, calcium, methoxyflurane, zinc, penicillins, cimetidine, food (particularly dairy products) may decrease absorption
May increase the effects of anticoagulants, digoxin; may increase or decrease lithium level

Food/Drug Interactions Food, particularly dairy products, may decrease absorption

Mechanism of Action Inhibits bacterial protein synthesis by binding with the 30S and possibly the 50S ribosomal subunit(s) of susceptible bacteria, cell wall synthesis is not affected

Pharmacokinetics
Absorption:
Oral: Adequately, ~75%
I.M.: Poor
Metabolism: Small amounts metabolized in the liver
Half-life: 8.5-9.6 hours (increases with renal impairment)
Time to peak: Peak serum levels occur within 2-4 hours
Elimination: In urine, while much higher amounts can be found in bile

Usual Dosage Geriatrics and Adults: I.V.: 250-500 mg every 12 hours

Administration Injection for intramuscular use only; do not administer with food or antacids

Monitoring Parameters Signs and symptoms of infection, WBC, mental status

Test Interactions Increased catecholamines (U), increased uric acid (S); decreased urea nitrogen (B)

Patient Information Complete full course of therapy; take on an empty stomach 1 hour before or 2 hours after meals; do not take with antacids or vitamins or iron; avoid excessive exposure to natural or artificial sunlight

(Continued)

Oxytetracycline Hydrochloride *(Continued)*

Nursing Implications Reduce dose in renal insufficiency; see Administration
Special Geriatric Considerations Oxytetracycline has not been studied in the elderly, however, dose reduction for renal function is not necessary
Dosage Forms
Capsule: 250 mg
Injection: 250 mg/2 mL
Ointment, ophthalmic: 5 mg and polymyxin B sulfate 10,000 units (3.5 g)
Powder for injection: 250 mg, 500 mg

Oyst-Cal 500 [OTC] *see* Calcium Salts (Oral) *on page 111*

Oystercal® 500 *see* Calcium Salts (Oral) *on page 111*

P₁E₁,® *see* Pilocarpine and Epinephrine *on page 565*

P₂E₁,® *see* Pilocarpine and Epinephrine *on page 565*

P₄E₁,® *see* Pilocarpine and Epinephrine *on page 565*

P₆E₁,® *see* Pilocarpine and Epinephrine *on page 565*

Pamelor® *see* Nortriptyline Hydrochloride *on page 511*

Pamidronate Disodium *(pa mi droe' nate)*

Brand Names Aredia™
Synonyms Aminohydroxypropylidine Diphosphonate
Generic Available No
Therapeutic Class Antidote, Hypercalcemia; Biphosphonate Derivative
Use Hypercalcemia associated with malignancy with or without bone metastases

Unlabeled use: Symptomatic treatment of Paget's disease, postmenopausal osteoporosis; reduce severe bone pain in malignancy; prevent steroid-induced osteoporosis
Contraindications Hypersensitivity to biphosphonates
Warnings Has not been tested in patients with serum creatinine >5 mg/dL; renal dysfunction when used to treat hypercalcemia secondary to malignancy
Precautions Patients should maintain adequate intake of calcium and vitamin D; use with caution in patients with pre-existing fractures, for uninterrupted periods of >6 months, and in patients with renal dysfunction (serum creatinine: >5 mg/dL)
Adverse Reactions
Cardiovascular: Fluid overload, hypertension, syncope, tachycardia, atrial fibrillation
Central nervous system: Fatigue, somnolence, insomnia, self-limiting pyrexia (within the first 72 hours)
Endocrine & metabolic: Hypokalemia, hypomagnesemia, hypophosphatemia, hypothyroidism, hypocalcemia
Gastrointestinal: Abdominal pain, nausea, anorexia, constipation, GI bleeding
Genitourinary: Urinary tract infections
Hematologic: Anemia
Hepatic: Elevated liver function tests
Local: Soft tissue erythema, swelling or induration, pain on palpation at site of injection
Neuromuscular & skeletal: Generalized pain, bone pain
Ocular: Uveitis, abnormal vision
Miscellaneous: Transient elevation of body temperature (1°C) at initiation of therapy, moniliasis, rhinitis
Overdosage Symptoms of overdose include hypocalcemia, EKG changes, seizures, bleeding, paresthesia, carpopedal spasm, fever
Toxicology Treat hypocalcemia with I.V. calcium gluconate; general supportive care; fever and hypotension can be treated with corticosteroids
Drug Interactions Calcium (see Additional Information)
Stability Reconstitute with 10 mL of sterile water for injection, USP; resulting solution has a pH of 6-7.4; infusion is stable for 24 hours at room temperature; solution should be diluted with ½ normal or normal saline USP or 5% dextrose injection, USP. Reconstituted with sterile water for injection may be stored in refrigerator at temperatures of 36°F to 46°F (2°C to 8°C) for 24 hours. Do not use calcium-containing solutions such as Ringer's solution as a diluent.
Mechanism of Action Inhibits normal and abnormal bone resorption; this action is achieved without inhibiting bone formation and mineralization; the exact mechanism is not known, but may be due to inhibition of hydroxyapatite crystal dissolution or its action on osteoclasts; decreased phosphate serum levels due to release from bone and increase in parathyroid hormone levels (suppressed during hypercalcemia)
Pharmacokinetics Data in humans is limited
Half-life:
Alpha (distribution): 1.6 hours
Urinary (elimination): 2.5 hours

Bone: 300 days

Elimination, biphasic: ~50% excreted unchanged in urine within 72 hours

Usual Dosage Geriatrics and Adults (dose is dependent on the severity and symptoms of hypercalcemia): I.V.:

Moderate hypercalcemia (corrected serum calcium 12-13.5 mg/dL): 60-90 mg given as a slow infusion over 24 hours

Severe hypercalcemia (corrected serum calcium >13.5 mg/dL): 90 mg given as a slow infusion over 24 hours

Consider retreatment if needed; allow at least 7 days before retreatment; see Additional Information

Monitoring Parameters Serum calcium, electrolytes, phosphate, magnesium, potassium, serum creatinine, CBC with differential

Reference Range Calcium (total): Adults: 9.0-11.0 mg/dL (2.05-2.54 mmol/L), may slightly decrease with aging; phosphorus: 2.5-4.5 mg/dL (0.81-1.45 mmol/L)

Patient Information Maintain adequate intake of calcium and vitamin D; report any fever, sore throat, or unusual bleeding to your physician

Nursing Implications Patient should be adequately hydrated while receiving this medication; see Additional Information and Special Geriatric Considerations

Additional Information Do not mix with calcium containing solutions (ie, lactated Ringer's solution); reconstitute in 10 mL sterile water for injection USP for each vial (results in 30 mg/10 mL); dilute in 0.45% NS, 0.9% NS, or D_5W to administer

Special Geriatric Considerations Has not been studied exclusively in the elderly; monitor serum electrolytes periodically since elderly are often receiving diuretics which can result in decreases in serum calcium, potassium, and magnesium

Dosage Forms Injection, lyophilized: 30 mg, 60 mg, 90 mg

References

Drug Facts and Comparisons, St Louis, MO: JB Lippincott Co, 1992, 134f-134m.

Kellihan MJ and Mangino PD, "Pamidronate," *Ann Pharmacother*, 1992, 26(10):1262-9.

Pamisyl® see Aminosalicylic Acid on page 41

Pamprin IB® [OTC] see Ibuprofen on page 360

Panadol® [OTC] see Acetaminophen on page 13

Panmycin® see Tetracycline on page 678

Panwarfin® see Warfarin Sodium on page 739

Papaverine Hydrochloride (pa pav' er een)

Brand Names Cerespan®; Genabid®; Pavabid® Plateau Caps®; Pavagen®; Pavarine® Spancaps®; Pavaspan®; Pavasule®; Pavatine® Pavased®; Pavatym®; Paverolan®

Generic Available Yes

Therapeutic Class Vasodilator

Use Papaverine has been used for many conditions where vasodilatation is felt to be of some benefit; however, to date, insufficient scientific evidence exists for any therapeutic value to its use except in testing for impotence

Oral: Relief of peripheral and cerebral ischemia associated with arterial spasm; smooth muscle relaxant

Parenteral: Various vascular spasms associated with muscle spasms as in myocardial infarction, angina, peripheral and pulmonary embolism, peripheral vascular disease, angiospastic states, and visceral spasm (ureteral, biliary, and GI colic); testing for impotence

Contraindications Complete atrioventricular block; Parkinson's disease

Warnings May, in large doses, depress cardiac conduction (eg, A-V node) leading to arrhythmias; may interfere with levodopa therapy of Parkinson's disease

Precautions Use with caution in patients with glaucoma; administer I.V. cautiously since apnea and arrhythmias may result; hepatic hypersensitivity noted with jaundice, eosinophilia, and abnormal LFTs

Adverse Reactions

Cardiovascular: Flushing of the face, tachycardia, hypotension, arrhythmias with rapid I.V. use

Central nervous system: Depression, dizziness, vertigo, drowsiness, sedation, lethargy, headache

Dermatologic: Pruritus

Gastrointestinal: Dry mouth, nausea, constipation

Hepatic: Hepatic hypersensitivity

Local: Thrombosis at the I.V. administration site

Respiratory: Apnea with rapid I.V. use

Miscellaneous: Sweating

Overdosage Symptoms of overdose include constipation, diplopia, weakness, drowsiness, liver damage, nystagmus, respiratory depression, anxiety, ataxia, gastric upset, urticaria, macular eruptions

Toxicology

Acute overdose: Gastric lavage or emesis, then follow with catharsis; with coma and respiratory depression, give general supportive care and respiratory support

(Continued)

Papaverine Hydrochloride *(Continued)*

Chronic overdose: Discontinue medication; give supportive care

Parenteral overdose: Give general supportive care, monitor vital signs, blood gases, and blood chemistry

Treat convulsions with diazepam, phenytoin, or phenobarbital; refractory seizures may be treated with general anesthesia (thiopental, halothane) and muscular paralysis with neuromuscular blocking agents; treat hypotension with I.V. fluids, elevation of legs, and vasopressor agents (dopamine/norepinephrine); cardiovascular effects may be treated with calcium gluconate; monitor EKG and serum calcium; dialysis (peritoneal or charcoal hemoperfusion) does not show any benefit

Drug Interactions

Additive effects with CNS depressants or morphine

Papaverine decreases the effects of levodopa

May enhance hypotensive action of drugs causing hypotension; use with caution in elderly

Stability Protect from heat or freezing; refrigerate injection at 2°C to 8°C (35°F to 46°F); solutions should be clear to pale yellow; precipitates with lactated Ringer's

Mechanism of Action Smooth muscle spasmolytic producing a generalized smooth muscle relaxation including: vasodilatation, gastrointestinal sphincter relaxation, bronchiolar muscle relaxation, and potentially a depressed myocardium; muscle relaxation may occur due to inhibition or cyclic nucleotide phosphodiesterase, increasing cyclic AMP; muscle relaxation is unrelated to nerve innervation; papaverine increases cerebral blood flow in normal subjects; oxygen uptake is unaltered; atrioventricular conduction and intraventricular conduction are depressed with large doses

Pharmacodynamics Peak levels: 1-2 hours

Pharmacokinetics

Absorption: Sustained preparations erratically absorbed

Protein binding: 90%

Metabolism: Rapidly in the liver

Bioavailability: Oral: ~54%

Half-life: 30-120 minutes

Elimination: Primarily as metabolites in urine

Usual Dosage Geriatrics and Adults:

Oral: 100-300 mg 3-5 times/day (start with lowest dose in elderly due to hypotensive potential)

Oral, sustained release: 150-300 mg every 12 hours; may increase to 150 mg every 8 hours or 300 mg every 12 hours

I.M., I.V.: 30-120 mg every 3 hours as needed

Cardiac extrasystoles: 2 doses 10 minutes apart; I.V. should be given over 1-2 minutes

Monitoring Parameters Monitor blood pressure

Patient Information Inform patient about potential for dizziness, hypotension, drowsiness; alcohol may enhance these effects; may cause flushing, sweating, headache, tiredness, jaundice, skin rash, nausea, anorexia, abdominal discomfort, constipation, or diarrhea

Nursing Implications Rapid I.V. administration may result in arrhythmias and fatal apnea

Additional Information Therapeutic value is lacking

Special Geriatric Considerations Vasodilators have been used to treat dementia upon the premise that dementia is secondary to a cerebral blood flow insufficiency. The hypothesis is that if blood flow could be increased, cognitive function would be increased. This hypothesis is no longer valid. The use of vasodilators for cognitive dysfunction is not recommended or proven by appropriate scientific study.

Dosage Forms

Capsule, sustained release: 150 mg

Injection: 30 mg/mL (2 mL, 10 mL)

Tablet: 30 mg, 60 mg, 100 mg, 150 mg, 200 mg, 300 mg

Tablet, timed release: 200 mg

References

Erwin WG, "Senile Dementia of the Alzheimer Type," *Clin Pharm*, 1984, 3:497-504.

Higbee MD, "Noncholinergic Approaches to Treating Senile Dementia of the Alzheimer's Type," *Consult Pharm*, 1992, 7(6):635-41.

Waters C, "Cognitive Enhancing Agents: Current Status in the Treatment of Alzheimer's Disease," *Can J Neurol Sci*, 1988, 15:249-56.

Yesavage JA, Tinklenberg JR, Hollister LE, et al, "Vasodilators in Senile Dementias: A Review of the Literature," *Arch Gen Psychiatry*, 1979, 36:220-3.

Parabromdylamine *see* Brompheniramine Maleate *on page 95*

Paracetamol *see* Acetaminophen *on page 13*

Paracort® *see* Prednisone *on page 586*

Paraflex® *see* Chlorzoxazone *on page 160*

Parafon Forte™ DSC *see* Chlorzoxazone *on page 160*

Parepectolin® *see* Kaolin and Pectin With Opium *on page 388*

Parlodel® *see* Bromocriptine Mesylate *on page 93*

Parnate® *see* Tranylcypromine Sulfate *on page 707*

Paroxetine (pa rox' e teen)
Related Information
Antidepressant Agents Comparison *on page 800*
Brand Names Paxil™
Therapeutic Class Antidepressant; Serotonin Antagonist

Use Treatment of depression; presently being investigated for obsessive-compulsive disorder

Contraindications Hypersensitivity to paroxetine or any component; do not use within 14 days of MAO inhibitors

Warnings Use cautiously in patients with a history of seizures, mania, renal disease, cardiac disease, suicidal patients; avoid ECT

Adverse Reactions
Cardiovascular: Bradycardia, hypotension, palpitations, tachycardia, vasodilation, postural hypotension

Central nervous system: Headache, asthenia, nervousness, anxiety, somnolence, dizziness, insomnia, paresthesia, migraine, seizures

Dermatologic: Alopecia

Fluid & electrolytes: Hyponatremia possibly due to SIADH

Gastrointestinal: Constipation, diarrhea, nausea, dry mouth, anorexia, flatulence, vomiting, gastritis, thirst

Genitourinary: Ejaculatory disturbances, decreased libido

Hematologic: Anemia, leukopenia

Hepatic: Increased LFTs

Neuromuscular & skeletal: Akinesia, arthritis, tremors

Ocular: Eye pain

Otic: Ear pain

Respiratory: Asthma

Miscellaneous: Bruxism, sweating

Overdosage Symptoms of overdose include nausea, vomiting, drowsiness, sinus tachycardia, and dilated pupils

Toxicology There are no specific antidotes, following attempts at decontamination, treatment is supportive and symptomatic; forced diuresis, dialysis, and hemoperfusion are unlikely to be beneficial

Drug Interactions
Decreased effect with phenobarbital, phenytoin (also decreased phenytoin effects)

Increased effect/toxicity with alcohol, cimetidine, MAO inhibitors (hyperpyrexic crisis); increased effect/toxicity of TCAs, fluoxetine, sertraline, phenothiazines, class 1C antiarrhythmics, warfarin

Mechanism of Action Selectively inhibits the CNS neuronal reuptake of serotonin, thereby enhancing serotonergic activity and inhibiting adrenergic activity in the locus ceruleus; minimal or no effect on reuptake of norepinephrine, dopamine, or cholinergic receptors; no effects on the regulation of beta receptors

Pharmacodynamics Maximum antidepressant effect usually seen after 4 weeks

Pharmacokinetics
Metabolism: Extensive following absorption by cytochrome P-450 enzymes

Half-life: 21 hours

Elimination: Metabolites are excreted in bile and urine

Elderly: Half-life and steady-state concentration increase disproportionately to dose with single and multiple dosing; see table.

Paroxetine

	Median Half-life (h)	Css (ng/mL)
Elderly 20 mg	30	46
Elderly 30 mg	38	80

Usual Dosage Oral:
Geriatrics: Initial: 10 mg once daily, preferably in the morning; usual dose: 20-30 mg/day; maximum: 40 mg/day

Adults: 20 mg once daily (maximum: 50 mg/day), preferably in the morning

Administration Best given in the morning unless too sedating; then give as divided dose or at bedtime

Monitoring Parameters Improvement of depression symptoms, anxiety, sleep disturbance, weight and appetite, hepatic and renal function tests, blood pressure, heart rate

(Continued)

Paroxetine *(Continued)*

Reference Range Not established

Test Interactions Elevated LFTs

Patient Information If currently on another antidepressant, notify physician; refrain from alcohol; if taking warfarin, anticonvulsants, or other drugs with CNS effects, notify physician

Nursing Implications See Administration and Monitoring Parameters

Special Geriatric Considerations Paroxetine's favorable side effect profile make it a useful alternative to the traditional tricyclic antidepressants; paroxetine is the most sedating of the currently available selective serotonin reuptake inhibitors; see Usual Dosage and Pharmacokinetics

Dosage Forms Tablet: 20 mg, 30 mg

References

Grimsley SR and Jann MW, "Paroxetine, Sertraline, and Fluvoxamine: New Selective Serotonin Reuptake Inhibitors," *Clin Pharm*, 1992, 11(11):930-57.

Hebenstreit GF, Fellerer K, Zochling R, et al, "A Pharmacokinetic Dose Titration Study in Adult and Elderly Depressed Patients," *Acta Psychiatr Scand Suppl*, 1989, 350:81-4.

Lundmark J, Scheel Thomsen I, Fjord-Larsen T, et al, "Paroxetine: Pharmacokinetic and Antidepressant Effect in the Elderly," *Acta Psychiatr Scand Suppl*, 1989, 350:76-80.

Schone W and Ludwig M, "A Double-Blind Study of Paroxetine Compared With Fluoxetine in Geriatric Patients With Major Depression," *J Clin Psychopharmacol*, 1993, 13(6 Suppl 2):34S-9S.

Parsidol® *see* Ethopropazine Hydrochloride *on page 274*

PAS *see* Aminosalicylic Acid *on page 41*

Pathocil® *see* Dicloxacillin Sodium *on page 214*

Pavabid® Plateau Caps® *see* Papaverine Hydrochloride *on page 533*

Pavagen® *see* Papaverine Hydrochloride *on page 533*

Pavarine® Spancaps® *see* Papaverine Hydrochloride *on page 533*

Pavaspan® *see* Papaverine Hydrochloride *on page 533*

Pavasule® *see* Papaverine Hydrochloride *on page 533*

Pavatine® Pavased® *see* Papaverine Hydrochloride *on page 533*

Pavatym® *see* Papaverine Hydrochloride *on page 533*

Paverolan® *see* Papaverine Hydrochloride *on page 533*

Paxil™ *see* Paroxetine *on previous page*

Paxipam® *see* Halazepam *on page 336*

PCE® *see* Erythromycin *on page 263*

Pectin and Kaolin *see* Kaolin and Pectin *on page 388*

Penamp® *see* Ampicillin *on page 51*

Penbutolol Sulfate

Related Information

Beta-Blockers Comparison *on page 804-805*

Brand Names Levatol®

Generic Available No

Therapeutic Class Beta-Adrenergic Blocker

Use Treatment of mild to moderate arterial hypertension

Contraindications Uncompensated congestive heart failure, cardiogenic shock, bradycardia or heart block, bronchial asthma, bronchospasms, hypersensitivity to beta-blocking agents, diabetes mellitus

Warnings Abrupt withdrawal of beta-blockers may result in an exaggerated cardiac beta-adrenergic responsiveness. Symptomatology has included reports of tachycardia, hypertension, ischemia, angina, myocardial infarction, and sudden death. It is recommended that patients be tapered gradually off of beta-blockers over a 2-week period rather than via abrupt discontinuation.

Precautions Increase dosing interval in patients with renal dysfunction; administer with caution to patients with bronchospastic disease, diabetes mellitus, hyperthyroidism, myasthenia gravis, and renal function decline and severe peripheral vascular disease; abrupt withdrawal of the drug should be avoided, drug should be discontinued over 2 weeks

Adverse Reactions Other adverse effects similar to other beta-blockers

Cardiovascular: Persistent bradycardia, hypotension, chest pain, edema, heart failure, Raynaud's phenomena

Central nervous system: Depression, confusion, dizziness, nightmares, fatigue, insomnia, lethargy, headache

Gastrointestinal: Constipation, diarrhea, nausea

Genitourinary: Impotence

Respiratory: Chest pain

Miscellaneous: Cold extremities

Overdosage Symptoms of overdose include bradycardia, congestive heart failure, hypotension, bronchospasm, hypoglycemia; see Toxicology

Toxicology Sympathomimetics (eg, epinephrine or dopamine), glucagon, or a pacemaker can be used to treat the toxic bradycardia, asystole, and/or hypotension; initially fluids may be the best treatment for toxic hypotension; patients should remain supine; serum glucose and potassium should be measured; use supportive measures: lavage, syrup of ipecac. I.V. glucose should be administered for hypoglycemia; seizures may be treated with phenytoin or diazepam intravenously; continuous monitoring of blood pressure and EKG is necessary. If PVCs occur, treat with lidocaine or phenytoin; avoid quinidine, procainamide, and disopyramide since these agents further depress myocardial function; bronchospasm can be treated with theophylline or beta$_2$ agonists (epinephrine).

Drug Interactions

Other hypotensive agents, diuretics and phenothiazines may increase hypotensive effects of penbutolol

Penbutolol may enhance neuromuscular blocking agents and will antagonize beta-sympathomimetic drugs; other drug interactions similar to propranolol may occur

Mechanism of Action Blocks both beta$_1$- and beta$_2$-receptors and has mild intrinsic sympathomimetic activity; has negative inotropic and chronotropic effects and can significantly slow A-V nodal conduction; lipid solubility is high which may result in CNS side effects

Pharmacokinetics

Absorption: Well absorbed, ~100%

Protein binding: 80% to 98%

Metabolism: Extensive in the liver (oxidation and conjugation)

Bioavailability: Oral: ~100%

Half-life: 5 hours

Elimination: Hepatic oxidation and conjugation with metabolites; excreted renally

Usual Dosage Oral:

Geriatrics: Initial: 10 mg once daily

Adults: Initial: 20 mg once daily, full effect of a 20 or 40 mg dose is seen by the end of a 2-week period, full effect not seen for 4-6 weeks; doses of 40-80 mg have been tolerated but have shown little additional antihypertensive effects

Monitoring Parameters Blood pressure, orthostatic hypotension, heart rate, CNS effects

Patient Information Do not discontinue medication abruptly, sudden stopping of medication may precipitate or cause angina; consult pharmacist or physician before taking with other adrenergic drugs (eg, cold medications); notify physician if any of the following symptoms occur: difficult breathing, night cough, swelling of extremities, slow pulse, dizziness, lightheadedness, confusion, depression, skin rash, fever, sore throat, unusual bleeding or bruising; may produce drowsiness, dizziness, lightheadedness, blurred vision, confusion; use with caution while driving or performing tasks requiring alertness; may mask signs of hypoglycemia in diabetics; may be taken without regard to meals

Nursing Implications Advise against abrupt withdrawal; monitor orthostatic blood pressures, apical and peripheral pulse and mental status changes (ie, confusion, depression)

Special Geriatric Considerations Due to alterations in the beta-adrenergic autonomic nervous system, beta-adrenergic blockade may result in less hemodynamic response than seen in younger adults. Studies indicate that despite decreased sensitivity to the chronotropic effects of beta blockade with age, there appears to be an increased myocardial sensitivity to the negative inotropic effect during stress (ie, exercise). Controlled trials have shown the overall response rate for propranolol to be only 20% to 50% in elderly populations. Therefore, all beta-adrenergic blocking drugs may result in a decreased response as compared to younger adults.

Dosage Forms Tablet: 20 mg

Penecort® see Hydrocortisone *on page 351*

Penetrex™ see Enoxacin *on page 253*

Penicillamine (pen i sill' a meen)

Related Information

Antacid Drug Interactions *on page 764*

Brand Names Cuprimine®; Depen®

Synonyms D-3-Mercaptovaline; β,β-Dimethylcysteine; D-Penicillamine

Generic Available No

Therapeutic Class Antidote, Copper Toxicity; Antidote, Lead Toxicity; Chelating Agent, Oral

Use Treatment of Wilson's disease, cystinuria, adjunct in the treatment of rheumatoid arthritis; lead poisoning, primary biliary cirrhosis

(Continued)

Penicillamine *(Continued)*

Contraindications Hypersensitivity to penicillamine and possibly penicillin; rheumatoid arthritis patients with renal insufficiency; patients with previous penicillamine-related aplastic anemia or agranulocytosis

Warnings Leukopenia, thrombocytopenia, proteinuria, hematuria, nephrotic syndrome, autoimmune syndrome, polymyositis, diffuse alveolitis, dermatomyositis, Goodpasture's syndrome, obliterative bronchiolitis, myasthenia gravis, and pemphigoid-like reaction; lupus erythematosus reaction

Precautions Patients on penicillamine should receive pyridoxine supplementation 25 mg/day; drug fever, skin rash, pemphigoid rash, oral ulcerations, hypogeusia, hypoglycemia, cross-sensitivity with penicillin may exist; delayed wound healing

Adverse Reactions

Central nervous system: Fever

Dermatologic: Rash, pruritus, pemphigus, increased friability of the skin, alopecia, lichen planus, TEN, increased skin irritability, excessive wrinkling in skin

Endocrine & metabolic: Iron deficiency, mammary hyperplasia

Gastrointestinal: Oral lesions, nausea, vomiting, loss of taste, epigastric pain, diarrhea, reactivate peptic ulcers, pancreatitis, cholestasis

Hematologic: Leukopenia, thrombocytopenia, eosinophilia, aplastic anemia, bone marrow depression

Hepatic: Hepatic dysfunction, increased alkaline phosphatase, and LDH

Neuromuscular & skeletal: Arthralgia

Ocular: Optic neuritis

Otic: Tinnitus

Renal: Nephrotic syndrome, proteinuria, membranous glomerulopathy

Miscellaneous: Allergic reactions, hyperpyrexia, lymphadenopathy, SLE-like syndrome

High evidence of adverse effects (>50%), medical supervision essential

Overdosage Symptoms of overdose include proteinuria, leukopenia, thrombocytopenia, skin rashes, bruising, nausea, vomiting, dysgeusia, diarrhea

Toxicology Toxic effects will reverse upon discontinuation of drug therapy; general supportive care; renal effects may take one year to reverse

Drug Interactions

Concomitant use of gold therapy, antimalarials, or cytotoxic agents should not be used due to similar toxic/adverse effects

Penicillamine has decreased absorption when taken with food (50% to 60%), antacids (65%), and iron compounds (35%)

Digoxin blood levels decreased by penicillamine

Stability Store in tight, well-closed containers

Mechanism of Action Chelates with lead, copper, mercury, iron, and other heavy metals to form stable, soluble complexes that are excreted in the urine; depresses circulating IgM rheumatoid factor, depresses T-cell but not B-cell activity; combines with cystine to form a compound which is more soluble, thus cystine calculi is prevented

Pharmacokinetics

Absorption: Oral: 40% to 70%

Protein binding: 80% bound to albumin

Half-life: 1.7-3.2 hours

Time to peak: Peak serum levels within 1 hour

Elimination: Primarily (30% to 60%) in urine as unchanged drug with small amounts of hepatic metabolism

Usual Dosage Geriatrics and Adults: Oral:

Rheumatoid arthritis: 125-250 mg/day, may increase dose at 1- to 3-month intervals up to 1-1.5 g/day (750 mg maximum daily dose for elderly)

Wilson's disease: 1 g/day in 4 divided doses, doses titrated to maintain urinary copper excretion >1 mg/day (750 mg maximum daily dose for elderly)

Cystinuria: 1-4 g/day divided every 6 hours

Lead poisoning: 250 mg/dose divided every 8-12 hours

Primary biliary cirrhosis: 250 mg/day to start, increase by 250 mg every 2 weeks up to a maintenance dose of 1 g/day, usually given 250 mg 4 times/day (750 mg maximum daily dose for elderly)

Monitoring Parameters CBC: WBC <3500/mm^2, neutrophils <2000/mm^2 or monocytes >500/mm^2 indicate need to stop therapy immediately; quantitative 24-hour urine protein at 1- to 2-week intervals initially (first 2-3 months); urinalysis, LFTs occasionally; platelet counts <100,000/mm^3 indicate need to stop therapy until numbers of platelets increase

Patient Information Take at least 1 hour before a meal; loss of taste may occur; probable severe allergic reaction if patient allergic to penicillin; report any signs of toxicity to physician; patients with cystinuria should drink copious amounts of water; report any unusual bleeding, bruising, persistent fever, fatigue, sore throat, shortness of breath

Nursing Implications For patients who cannot swallow, content of capsules may be administered in 15-30 mL of chilled puréed fruit or fruit juice; patients should be warned to report promptly any symptoms suggesting toxicity; see Monitoring Parameters

Additional Information Approximately 33% of patients will experience an allergic reaction

Special Geriatric Considerations Close monitoring of elderly is necessary; since steady-state serum/tissue concentrations rise slowly, "go slow" with dose increase intervals; steady-state concentrations decline slowly after discontinuation suggesting extensive tissue distribution. Skin rashes and taste abnormalities occur more frequently in elderly than in young adults; leukopenia, thrombocytopenia, and proteinuria occur with equal frequency in both younger adults and elderly. Since toxicity may be dose related, it is recommended not to exceed 750 mg/day in elderly.

Dosage Forms
Capsule: 125 mg, 250 mg
Tablet: 250 mg

References
Stein HB, Patterson AC, Offer RC, et al, "Adverse Effects of D-Penicillamine in Rheumatoid Arthritis," *Ann Intern Med*, 1980, 92:24-9.

Penicillin G Benzathine and Procaine Combined

Brand Names Bicillin® C-R; Bicillin® C-R 900/300
Synonyms Penicillin G Procaine and Benzathine Combined
Therapeutic Class Antibiotic, Penicillin
Use Active against most gram-positive organisms; some gram-negative such as *Neisseria gonorrhoeae* and some anaerobes and spirochetes
Contraindications Known hypersensitivity to penicillin or any component
Precautions Use with caution in patients with impaired renal function, impaired cardiac function, seizure disorder, or history of cephalosporin allergy
Adverse Reactions
Cardiovascular: Thrombophlebitis
Central nervous system: Convulsions, confusion, drowsiness, fever
Dermatologic: Rash
Endocrine & metabolic: Electrolyte imbalance
Hematologic: Hemolytic anemia, positive Coombs' reaction
Neuromuscular & skeletal: Myoclonus
Renal: Acute interstitial nephritis
Miscellaneous: Jarisch-Herxheimer reaction, hypersensitivity reactions, anaphylaxis
Overdosage Symptoms of overdose include neuromuscular hypersensitivity, seizure
Drug Interactions Probenecid, tetracyclines, aminoglycosides
Stability Store in the refrigerator
Mechanism of Action Interferes with bacterial cell wall synthesis during active multiplication causing cell death and resultant bactericidal activity against susceptible bacteria
Usual Dosage Geriatrics and Adults: I.M.: 2.4 million units in a single dose
Administration Administer by deep I.M. injection in the upper outer quadrant of the buttock do **not** administer I.V., intravascularly, or intra-arterially
Test Interactions Positive Coombs' [direct], increased protein
Nursing Implications See Administration
Special Geriatric Considerations See Usual Dosage; no adjustment for renal function or age is necessary
Dosage Forms
Injection: 300,000 units = 150,000 units each of penicillin G benzathine and penicillin G procaine (10 mL); 600,000 units = 300,000 units each penicillin G benzathine and penicillin G procaine (1 mL); 1,200,000 units = 600,000 units each penicillin G benzathine and penicillin G procaine (2 mL); 2,400,000 units = 1,200,000 units each penicillin G benzathine and penicillin G procaine (4 mL)
Injection: Penicillin G benzathine 900,000 units and penicillin G procaine/dose 300,000 units (2 mL)

Penicillin G Benzathine, Parenteral

Brand Names Bicillin®; Bicillin® L-A; Megacillin®; Permapen®
Synonyms Benzathine Benzylpenicillin; Benzathine Penicillin G; Benzylpenicillin Benzathine
Therapeutic Class Antibiotic, Penicillin
Use Active against most gram-positive organisms; some gram-negative organisms such as *Neisseria gonorrhoeae* and some anaerobes and spirochetes; used only for the treatment of mild to moderately severe infections caused by organisms susceptible to low concentrations of penicillin G, or for prophylaxis of infections caused by these organisms
Contraindications Known hypersensitivity to penicillin or any component
Precautions Use with caution in patients with impaired renal function, impaired cardiac function, or seizure disorder; history of cephalosporin allergy

(Continued)

539

Penicillin G Benzathine, Parenteral *(Continued)*

Adverse Reactions
Cardiovascular: Thrombophlebitis
Central nervous system: Convulsions, confusion, drowsiness, fever
Dermatologic: Rash
Endocrine & metabolic: Electrolyte imbalance
Hematologic: Hemolytic anemia, positive Coombs' reaction
Local: Pain at injection site
Neuromuscular & skeletal: Myoclonus
Renal: Acute interstitial nephritis
Miscellaneous: Jarisch-Herxheimer reaction, hypersensitivity reactions, anaphylaxis

Overdosage Symptoms of overdose include neuromuscular hypersensitivity, seizure

Toxicology Many beta-lactam-containing antibiotics have the potential to cause neuromuscular hyperirritability or convulsive seizures. Hemodialysis may be helpful to aid in the removal of the drug from the blood, otherwise most treatment is supportive or symptom directed.

Drug Interactions Probenecid, tetracyclines, aminoglycosides, anticoagulants (I.M. administration only)

Stability Store in the refrigerator

Mechanism of Action Interferes with bacterial cell wall synthesis during active multiplication causing cell death and resultant bactericidal activity against susceptible bacteria

Pharmacokinetics
Absorption: I.M.: Slow
Time to peak: Peak serum levels attained within 12-24 hours; serum levels are usually detectable for 1-4 weeks depending on the dose; larger doses result in more sustained levels rather than higher levels; following equal, simple I.M. injections, the elderly have serum penicillin concentrations approximately twice that of younger adults 48, 96, and 144 hours postadministration

Usual Dosage Dosage frequency depends on infection being treated

Geriatrics and Adults: I.M.:
Group A streptococcal upper respiratory infection: 1.2 million units as a single dose
Prophylaxis of recurrent rheumatic fever: 1.2 million units every 3-4 weeks or 600,000 units twice monthly
Early syphilis: 2.4 million units as a single dose
Syphilis >1 year duration: 2.4 million units once weekly for 3 doses

Administration Administer by deep I.M. injection in the upper outer quadrant of the buttock do **not** give I.V., intra-arterially, or S.C.

Monitoring Parameters Signs and symptoms of infection

Test Interactions Positive Coombs' [direct], false-positive urinary and/or serum proteins

Nursing Implications See Administration

Additional Information A single dose of 600,000 to 1,2000,000 units is effective in the prevention of rheumatic fever secondary to streptococcal pharyngitis; used when patient cannot be kept in a hospital environment and neurosyphilis has been ruled out

Special Geriatric Considerations See Pharmacokinetics. Not indicated as single drug therapy for neurosyphilis, but may be given 1 time/week for 3 weeks following I.V. treatment (see Penicillin G for dosing); no adjustment for renal function or age is necessary

Dosage Forms Injection: 300,000 units/mL (10 mL); 600,000 units/mL (1 mL, 2 mL, 4 mL)

References
Collart P, Poitevin M, Milovanovic A, et al, "Kinetic Study of Serum Penicillin Concentrations After Single Doses of Benzathine and Benethamine Penicillins in Young and Old People," *Br J Vener Dis,* 1980, 56(6):355-62.
WHO Study Group, "Rheumatic Fever and Rheumatic Heart Disease," *WHO Tech Rep Ser,* 1988, 764:1-58.

Penicillin G, Parenteral
Brand Names Pfizerpen®

Synonyms Benzylpenicillin Potassium; Benzylpenicillin Sodium; Crystalline Penicillin; Penicillin G Potassium; Penicillin G Sodium

Generic Available Yes

Therapeutic Class Antibiotic, Penicillin

Use Active against most gram-positive organisms except *Staphylococcus aureus;* some gram-negative such as *Neisseria gonorrhoeae* and some anaerobes and spirochetes; although ceftriaxone is now the drug of choice for lyme disease and gonorrhea

Contraindications Known hypersensitivity to penicillin or any component

Warnings Contains ~2 mEq sodium/one million units

Precautions Avoid I.V., intravascular or intra-arterial administration or injection into or near major peripheral nerves or blood vessels since such injections may cause severe and/or permanent neurovascular damage; use with caution in patients with severe renal impairment; use with caution in patients with cephalosporin allergy

Adverse Reactions
Cardiovascular: Thrombophlebitis
Central nervous system: Convulsions, confusion, drowsiness, fever
Dermatologic: Rash
Endocrine & metabolic: Electrolyte imbalance
Hematologic: Hemolytic anemia, positive Coombs' reaction
Neuromuscular & skeletal: Myoclonus
Renal: Acute interstitial nephritis
Miscellaneous: Jarisch-Herxheimer reaction, hypersensitivity reactions, anaphylaxis

Overdosage Symptoms of overdose include neuromuscular hypersensitivity, seizure

Toxicology Many beta-lactam-containing antibiotics have the potential to cause neuromuscular hyperirritability or convulsive seizures. Hemodialysis may be helpful to aid in the removal of the drug from the blood, otherwise most treatment is supportive or symptom directed.

Drug Interactions Probenecid (increased levels), tetracyclines, aminoglycosides, anticoagulants (I.M. administration only)

Stability Reconstituted parenteral solution is stable for 7 days when refrigerated; for I.V. infusion in NS or D_5W, solution is stable for 24 hours at room temperature

Mechanism of Action Interferes with bacterial cell wall synthesis during active multiplication causing cell death and resultant bactericidal activity against susceptible bacteria

Pharmacokinetics
Distribution: Penetration across the blood-brain barrier is poor, despite inflamed meninges
Protein binding: 65%
Metabolism: In the liver (30%) to penicilloic acid
Half-life: 20-50 minutes; prolonged half-life reported in some elderly (~1 hour) compared to younger subjects presumably due to decreased renal function
Time to peak: I.V.: Peak serum levels occur within 1 hour
Elimination: In urine

Usual Dosage
Geriatrics and Adults:
I.V.: 3-5 million units every 4-6 hours; higher doses and/or more frequent administration may be necessary for some infections such as meningitis
Neurosyphilis: 2-4 million units every 4 hours for 10-14 days

Dosing interval in renal impairment:
Cl_{cr} 10-30 mL/minute: Administer every 8-12 hours
Cl_{cr} <10 mL/minute: Administer every 12-18 hours
Moderately dialyzable (20% to 50%)

Monitoring Parameters Fever, mental status, WBC count, appetite

Test Interactions Positive Coombs' [direct], increased protein

Patient Information Complete full course of treatment; notify physician if rash, itching, hives, diarrhea, or any other unusual finding

Nursing Implications Dosage modification required in patients with renal insufficiency; give around-the-clock rather than 4 times/day to avoid variations in peak and trough concentrations

Special Geriatric Considerations Despite a reported prolonged half-life, it is usually not necessary to adjust the dose of penicillin G or VK in the elderly to account for renal function changes with age, however, it is advised to calculate an estimated creatinine clearance and adjust dose accordingly; see Usual Dosage

Dosage Forms
Injection, as potassium: 200,000 units, 500,000 units, 1 million units, 5 million units, 10 million units, 20 million units
Injection, as sodium: 5 million units

References
Hansen JM, Kampmann J, and Laursen H, "Renal Excretion of Drugs in the Elderly," *Lancet*, 1970, 1(657):1170.
Leikola E and Vartia KO, "On Penicillin Levels in Young and Geriatric Subjects," *J Gerontol*, 1957, 12:48-52.
Yoshikawa TT, "Antimicrobial Therapy for the Elderly Patient," *J Am Geriatr Soc*, 1990, 38(12):1353-72.

Penicillin G Potassium *see* Penicillin G, Parenteral *on previous page*

Penicillin G Procaine and Benzathine Combined *see* Penicillin G Benzathine and Procaine Combined *on page 539*

Penicillin G Procaine, Aqueous
Brand Names Crysticillin® A.S.; Duracillin® A.S.; Pfizerpen®-AS; Wycillin®
Synonyms APPG; Aqueous Procaine Penicillin G; Procaine Benzylpenicillin; Procaine Penicillin G
(Continued)

Penicillin G Procaine, Aqueous *(Continued)*

Generic Available Yes

Therapeutic Class Antibiotic, Penicillin

Use Moderately severe infections due to *Neisseria gonorrhoeae*, *Treponema pallidum* and other penicillin G-sensitive microorganisms that are susceptible to low but prolonged serum penicillin concentrations

Contraindications Known hypersensitivity to penicillin or any component; also contraindicated in patients hypersensitive to procaine

Precautions Modify dosage in patients with severe renal impairment; use with caution in patients with cephalosporin allergy

Adverse Reactions
Cardiovascular: Myocardial depression, vasodilation, conduction disturbances
Central nervous system: Confusion, drowsiness, CNS stimulation, seizures
Hematologic: Hemolytic anemia, positive Coombs' reaction
Local: Sterile abscess at injection site, pain at injection site
Neuromuscular & skeletal: Myoclonus
Renal: Interstitial nephritis
Miscellaneous: Pseudoanaphylactic reactions, Jarisch-Herxheimer reaction, hypersensitivity reactions

Overdosage Symptoms of overdose include neuromuscular hypersensitivity, seizure

Toxicology Many beta-lactam-containing antibiotics have the potential to cause neuromuscular hyperirritability or convulsive seizures. Hemodialysis may be helpful to aid in the removal of the drug from the blood, otherwise most treatment is supportive and symptom directed.

Drug Interactions Probenecid, tetracycline, aminoglycosides, anticoagulants (I.M. administration)

Stability Store in refrigerator

Mechanism of Action Interferes with bacterial cell wall synthesis during active multiplication causing cell death and resultant bactericidal activity against susceptible bacteria

Pharmacokinetics
Absorption: I.M.: Slow
Distribution: Penetration across the blood-brain barrier is poor, despite inflamed meninges
Protein binding: 65%
Half-life: 20-50 minutes
Time to peak: Peak serum levels occur within 1-4 hours and can persist within the therapeutic range for 15-24 hours
Elimination: 60% to 90% of drug is excreted unchanged via renal tubular excretion; ~30% of dose inactivated in the liver
Renal clearance is delayed in patients with impaired renal function

Usual Dosage Geriatrics and Adults: I.M.: 0.6-2.4 million units every 6-12 hours
Uncomplicated gonorrhea: 1 g probenecid orally, then 4.8 million units procaine penicillin divided into 2 injection sites 30 minutes later. When used in conjunction with an aminoglycoside for the treatment of endocarditis caused by susceptible *S. viridans*: 1.2 million units every 6 hours for 2-4 weeks

Neurosyphilis: I.M.: 2-4 million units/day with 500 mg probenecid by mouth 4 times/day for 10-14 days; penicillin G aqueous I.V. is the preferred agent

Dosing interval in renal impairment:
Cl_{cr} 10-30 mL/minute: Administer every 8-12 hours
Cl_{cr} <10 mL/minute: Administer every 12-18 hours
Moderately dialyzable (20% to 50%)

Administration Procaine suspension for deep I.M. injection only; give around-the-clock rather than 4 times/day, 3 times/day, etc (ie, 12-6-12-6, not 9-1-5-9) to promote less variation in peak and trough serum levels; when doses are repeated, rotate the injection site; avoid I.V., intravascular, or intra-arterial administration of penicillin G procaine since severe and/or permanent neurovascular damage may occur; renal and hematologic systems should be evaluated periodically during prolonged therapy

Monitoring Parameters Fever, mental status, WBC count, appetite

Test Interactions Positive Coombs' [direct], false-positive urinary and/or serum proteins

Patient Information Notify physician if skin rash, itching, hives or severe diarrhea occurs; complete full course of therapy

Nursing Implications See Administration

Special Geriatric Considerations Dosage does not usually need to be adjusted in the elderly, however, if multiple doses are to be given, adjust dose for renal function; see Usual Dosage

Dosage Forms Injection: 300,000 units/mL (10 mL); 500,000 units/mL (12 mL); 600,000 units (1 mL, 2 mL, 4 mL); 1,200,000 units (2 mL); 2,400,000 units (4 mL)

References
Yoshikawa TT, "Antimicrobial Therapy for the Elderly Patient," *J Am Geriatr Soc*, 1990, 38(12):1353-72.

Penicillin G Sodium *see* Penicillin G, Parenteral *on page 540*

Penicillin V Potassium

Brand Names Beepen-VK®; Betapen®-VK; Ledercillin® VK; Pen.Vee® K; Robicillin® VK; V-Cillin K®; Veetids®; Wincillin®-VK

Synonyms Phenoxymethyl Penicillin

Generic Available Yes

Therapeutic Class Antibiotic, Penicillin

Use Treatment of moderate to severe susceptible bacterial infections; no longer recommended for dental procedure prophylaxis; prophylaxis in rheumatic fever; infections caused by susceptible organisms involving the respiratory tract, otitis media, sinusitis, skin, and urinary tract;

Contraindications Known hypersensitivity to penicillin or any component

Precautions Use with caution in patients with renal impairment, dosage adjustment may be necessary; use with caution in patients with cephalosporin allergy

Adverse Reactions
Central nervous system: Convulsions, fever
Dermatologic: Rash
Gastrointestinal: nausea, diarrhea, vomiting, oral candidiasis
Hematologic: Hemolytic anemia, positive Coombs' reaction
Renal: Acute interstitial nephritis
Miscellaneous: Hypersensitivity reactions, anaphylaxis

Overdosage Symptoms of overdose include neuromuscular hypersensitivity, seizure

Toxicology Many beta-lactam-containing antibiotics have the potential to cause neuromuscular hyperirritability or convulsive seizures. Hemodialysis may be helpful to aid in the removal of the drug from the blood, otherwise most treatment is supportive or symptom directed.

Drug Interactions Probenecid, tetracycline, aminoglycosides (synergism)

Stability Refrigerate suspension after reconstitution; discard after 14 days

Mechanism of Action Interferes with bacterial cell wall synthesis during active multiplication causing cell death and resultant bactericidal activity against susceptible bacteria

Pharmacokinetics
Absorption: Oral: 60% to 73% from GI tract
Protein binding: 80%
Half-life: 30 minutes, prolonged in patients with renal impairment
Time to peak: Oral: Peak serum levels occur within 30-60 minutes
Elimination: Penicillin V and its metabolites are excreted in urine mainly by tubular secretion

Usual Dosage Geriatrics and Adults: 125-500 mg every 6 hours
Dosing adjustment in renal impairment: Do not exceed 250 mg every 6 hours

Administration Give on an empty stomach (ie, 1 hour prior to, or 2 hours after meals) to increase total absorption; give around-the-clock rather than 4 times/day, 3 times/day, etc (ie, 12-6-12-6, not 9-1-5-9) to promote less variation in peak and trough serum levels

Monitoring Parameters Fever, WBC count, mental status, appetite

Test Interactions False-positive or negative urinary glucose determination using Clinitest®; positive Coombs' [direct]; false-positive urinary and/or serum proteins

Patient Information Take on an empty stomach 1 hour before or 2 hours after meals; complete full course of therapy, do not skip doses

Nursing Implications See Administration

Additional Information 0.7 mEq of potassium per 250 mg penicillin V; 250 mg equals 400,000 units of penicillin; each gram contains 2.6 mEq of potassium

Special Geriatric Considerations Dosage adjustment in the elderly is usually not necessary; see Usual Dosage

Dosage Forms
Liquid, oral: 125 mg/5 mL (3 mL, 100 mL, 150 mL, 200 mL); 250 mg/5 mL (100 mL, 150 mL, 200 mL)
Tablet: 125 mg, 250 mg, 500 mg

Pentaerythritol Tetranitrate (pen ta er ith' ri tole)

Brand Names Duotrate®; Duotrate® 45; Pentylan®; Peritrate®; Peritrate® SA

Synonyms PETN

Generic Available Yes

Therapeutic Class Antianginal Agent; Nitrate; Vasodilator, Coronary

Use Possibly effective for the prophylactic long-term management of angina pectoris.
Note: Not indicated to abort acute anginal episodes

Contraindications Known hypersensitivity to pentaerythritol tetranitrate or other nitrates; severe anemia, closed-angle glaucoma, postural hypotension, cerebral hemorrhage, head trauma

Warnings Do not crush or chew sustained release preparations; use with caution in patients with hypovolemia, glaucoma, increased intracranial pressure or hypotension

(Continued)

Pentaerythritol Tetranitrate *(Continued)*

Precautions Do not use sustained-release products in patients with GI hypermotility or malabsorption syndrome; do not stop use abruptly to avoid withdrawal reactions (angina); must gradually reduce daily doses to withdraw; tolerance to vascular effects of nitrates has been demonstrated; see Dosage for recommendation to minimize development of tolerance

Adverse Reactions
Cardiovascular: Orthostatic hypotension, tachycardia, cutaneous flushing of head, neck, and clavicular area
Central nervous system: Dizziness, headache, vertigo
Dermatologic: Rash
Gastrointestinal: Dry mouth, nausea, GI upset
Ocular: Blurred vision

Overdosage Symptoms of overdose include hypotension, throbbing headache, palpitations, visual disturbances, flushing, perspiring skin, vertigo, diaphoresis, dizziness, syncope, nausea, vomiting, anorexia, dyspnea, heart block, confusion, fever, paralysis

Toxicology Formation of methemoglobinemia is dose-related and unusual in normal doses; high levels can cause signs and symptoms of hypoxemia; treatment consists of placing patient in recumbent position and administer fluids; alpha-adrenergic vasopressors may be required; treat methemoglobinemia with oxygen and methylene blue at a dose of 1-2 mg/kg I.V. slowly

Drug Interactions
May antagonize the anticoagulant effect of heparin; alcohol (increased hypotension)
Aspirin (increases serum nitrate concentration)
Calcium channel blockers (increases hypotension)

Mechanism of Action Stimulation of intracellular cyclic-GMP results in vascular smooth muscle relaxation of both arterial and venous vasculature. Increased venous pooling decreases left ventricular pressure (preload) and arterial dilatation decreases arterial resistance (afterload). Therefore, this reduces cardiac oxygen demand by decreasing left ventricular pressure and systemic vascular resistance by dilating arteries. Additionally, coronary artery dilation improves collateral flow to ischemic regions; esophageal smooth muscle is relaxed via the same mechanism.

Pharmacodynamics
Onset of action: Oral: Within 20-60 minutes; 30 minutes with sustained release
Duration: 4-5 hours, or up to 12 hours with the sustained release formulations

Pharmacokinetics
Metabolism: In the liver
Half-life: 10 minutes
Elimination: In urine and to a smaller degree in bile

Usual Dosage Geriatrics and Adults: Oral: 10-20 mg 4 times/day up to 40 mg 4 times/day before or after meals and at bedtime; sustained release preparation 80 mg twice daily; use lowest recommended doses in elderly initially; titrations up to 100 mg/day are tolerated, however, headache may occur with increasing doses; should headache occur, reduce dose for a few days; if headache returns or is persistent, an analgesic can be used to treat symptoms

Monitoring Parameters Monitor anginal episodes, orthostatic blood pressures; a decrease of 15 mm Hg pressure systolic and/or 10 mm Hg diastolic or an increase in heart rate of 10 beats/minute from baseline (no drug) indicates approximate maximal cardiodynamic effects to nitrates and end point for dosing

Test Interactions Decreased cholesterol (S)

Patient Information Dispense drug in easy-to-open container; do not chew or crush sustained-release dosage form; do not change brands without consulting your pharmacist or physician; any angina that persists for more than 20 minutes should be evaluated by a physician immediately

Nursing Implications Do not crush sustained release drug product; monitor blood pressure reduction for maximal effect and orthostatic hypotension

Special Geriatric Considerations The first dose of nitrates should be taken in a physician's office to observe for maximal cardiovascular dynamic effects (see Monitoring Parameters) and adverse effects (orthostatic blood pressure drop, headache). The use of nitrates for angina may occasionally promote reflux esophagitis. This may require dose adjustments or changing therapeutic agents to correct this adverse effect; the use of this agent does not demonstrate any benefit over other forms of nitrate therapy.

Dosage Forms
Tablet: 10 mg, 20 mg, 40 mg
Tablet, sustained release: 30 mg, 45 mg, 80 mg

Pentam-300® *see* Pentamidine Isethionate *on this page*

Pentamidine Isethionate *(pen tam' i deen)*
Brand Names NebuPent™; Pentam-300®
Generic Available No
Therapeutic Class Antibiotic, Miscellaneous

Use Treatment and prevention of pneumonia caused by *Pneumocystis carinii*

Unlabeled use: Treatment of trypanosomiasis

Contraindications Hypersensitivity to pentamidine isethionate or any component (inhalation and injection)

Precautions Use with caution in patients with diabetes mellitus, renal or hepatic dysfunction; hypertension or hypotension

Adverse Reactions

Cardiovascular: Hypotension, tachycardia

Central nervous system: Dizziness, fever, fatigue

Dermatologic: Rash

Endocrine & metabolic: Hypoglycemia, hyperglycemia, hypocalcemia, hyperkalemia

Gastrointestinal: Vomiting, metallic taste in mouth, pancreatitis

Hematologic: Megaloblastic anemia, granulocytopenia, leukopenia, thrombocytopenia

Local: Pain at injection site

Renal/Hepatic: Mild renal or hepatic injury

Respiratory: Irritation of the airway, cough, bronchospasm, dyspnea, chest pain/congestion, pharyngitis

Miscellaneous: Jarisch-Herxheimer-like reaction,

Stability Reconstituted solution is stable for 24 hours at room temperature; do not refrigerate due to the possibility of crystallization; do not use NS as a diluent, NS is **incompatible** with pentamidine

Mechanism of Action It is proposed to interfere with RNA/DNA, phospholipids, and protein synthesis through inhibition of oxidative phosphorylation and/or interference with incorporation of nucleotides and nucleic acids into RNA and DNA, in protozoa

Pharmacokinetics

Absorption: I.M.: Well absorbed; systemic accumulation of pentamidine does not appear to occur following inhalation therapy

Half-life, terminal: 6.4-9.4 hours; may be prolonged in patients with severe renal impairment

Elimination: 33% to 66% excreted in urine as unchanged drug

Usual Dosage Geriatrics and Adults:

Treatment: I.M., I.V. (I.V. preferred): 4 mg/kg/day once daily for 14 days

Prevention: Inhalation: 300 mg every 4 weeks via Respirgard® II nebulizer

Dosing interval in renal impairment:

Cl_{cr} 10-50 mL/minute: Administer every 24-36 hours

Cl_{cr} <10 mL/minute: Administer every 48 hours

Administration Infuse I.V. slowly over a period of at least 60 minutes or administer deep I.M.; patients receiving I.V. or I.M. pentamidine should be lying down and blood pressure should be monitored closely during administration of drug and several times thereafter until it is stable; see Stability

Monitoring Parameters Inhaler technique, BUN, serum creatinine, blood glucose, CBC, platelet count, LFTs, serum calcium should be monitored before, during, and after acute treatment, EKG

Test Interactions Decreased glucose

Patient Information Get instructions on how to use inhaler

Nursing Implications See Administration and Stability

Special Geriatric Considerations 10% of acquired immune syndrome (AIDS) cases are in the elderly and this figure is expected to increase; pentamidine has not as yet been studied exclusively in this population; adjust dose for renal function

Dosage Forms

Inhalation: 300 mg

Injection: 300 mg

Pentazocine (pen taz' oh seen)

Related Information

Pharmacokinetics of Narcotic Agonist Analgesics *on page 812*

Brand Names Talwin®; Talwin® NX

Synonyms Pentazocine Hydrochloride; Pentazocine Lactate

Therapeutic Class Analgesic, Narcotic

Use Relief of moderate to severe pain; has also been used as a sedative prior to surgery and as a supplement to surgical anesthesia

Restrictions C-IV

Contraindications Hypersensitivity to pentazocine or any component, increased intracranial pressure (unless the patient is mechanically ventilated)

Warnings Pentazocine may precipitate opiate withdrawal symptoms in patients who have been receiving opiates regularly; injection contains sulfites which may cause allergic reaction

Precautions Use with caution in seizure-prone patients, acute MI, patients undergoing biliary tract surgery, patients with renal and hepatic dysfunction, and patients with a history of prior opioid dependence or abuse

(Continued)

Pentazocine *(Continued)*

Adverse Reactions

Cardiovascular: Palpitations, hypotension, bradycardia, peripheral vasodilation

Central nervous system: CNS depression, sedation, dizziness, euphoria, lightheadedness, hallucinations, confusion, disorientation, increased intracranial pressure, seizures may occur in seizure-prone patients

Dermatologic: Pruritus, rash

Endocrine & metabolic: Antidiuretic hormone release

Gastrointestinal: Nausea, vomiting, constipation, biliary spasm

Genitourinary: Urinary tract spasm

Local: Tissue damage and irritation with I.M./S.C. use

Ocular: Miosis

Respiratory: Respiratory depression

Miscellaneous: Physical and psychological dependence, histamine release

Overdosage Symptoms of overdose include drowsiness, sedation, respiratory depression, coma

Toxicology Treatment of an overdose includes support of the patient's airway, establishment of an I.V. line and administration of naloxone 2 mg I.V. with repeat administration as necessary up to a total of 10 mg.

Drug Interactions

May potentiate or reduce analgesic effect of opiate agonist (eg, morphine) depending on patients tolerance to opiates can precipitate withdrawal in narcotic addicts

Increased effect/toxicity with tripelennamine (can be lethal), CNS depressants (phenothiazines, tranquilizers, anxiolytics, sedatives, hypnotics, or alcohol)

Stability Store at room temperature, protect from heat and from freezing

Mechanism of Action Binds to opiate receptors in the CNS, causing inhibition of ascending pain pathways, altering the perception of and response to pain; produces generalized CNS depression; partial agonist-antagonist

Pharmacodynamics

Onset of action:

Oral, I.M., S.C.: Within 15-30 minutes

I.V.: Within 2-3 minutes

Duration:

Parenteral: 2-3 hours

Oral: 4-5 hours

Pharmacokinetics

Protein binding: 60%

Bioavailability: Oral: ~20% due to large first-pass effect; increased oral bioavailability to 60% to 70% in patients with cirrhosis

Metabolism: In liver via oxidative and glucuronide conjugation pathways

Half-life: 2-3 hours, increased half-life with decreased hepatic function

Elimination: Excreted unchanged in urine

Usual Dosage

Geriatrics:

Oral: 50 mg every 4 hours

I.M.: 30 mg every 4 hours

Adults:

Oral: 50-100 mg every 3-4 hours

I.M., S.C.: 30-60 mg every 3-4 hours

I.V.: 30 mg every 3-4 hours

Dosing adjustment in renal impairment:

Cl_{cr} 10-50 mL/minute: Administer 75% of normal dose

Cl_{cr} <10 mL/minute: Administer 50% of normal dose

Dosing adjustment in hepatic impairment: Reduce dose or avoid use in patients with liver disease

Monitoring Parameters Relief of pain, respiratory and mental status, blood pressure

Patient Information May cause drowsiness; avoid alcohol and CNS depressants; may be addicting if used for prolonged periods; will cause withdrawal in patients currently dependent on narcotics

Nursing Implications Rotate injection site for I.M., S.C. use; avoid intra-arterial injection; observe patient for excessive sedation, respiratory depression, implement safety measures, assist with ambulation; observe for narcotic withdrawal

Additional Information

Pentazocine hydrochloride: Talwin® NX tablet (with naloxone); naloxone is used to prevent abuse by dissolving tablets in water and using as injection

Pentazocine lactate: Talwin® injection

Special Geriatric Considerations See Warnings and Precautions; pentazocine is not recommended for use in the elderly because of its propensity to cause delirium and agitation; adjust dose for renal function

Dosage Forms

Injection, as lactate: 30 mg/mL (1 mL, 1.5 mL, 2 mL, 10 mL)

Tablet: Pentazocine hydrochloride 50 mg and naloxone hydrochloride 0.5 mg

Pentazocine Hydrochloride *see* Pentazocine *on page 545*

Pentazocine Lactate *see* Pentazocine *on page 545*

Pentobarbital (pen toe bar' bi tal)
Related Information
Anxiolytic/Hypnotic Use in Long-Term Care Facilities *on page 755-756*
Brand Names Nembutal®
Synonyms Pentobarbital Sodium
Therapeutic Class Barbiturate; Sedative
Special Geriatric Considerations Use of this agent as a hypnotic in the elderly is not recommended due to its long half-life and addiction potential

Pentobarbital Sodium *see* Pentobarbital *on this page*

Pentoxifylline (pen tox i' fi leen)
Brand Names Trental®
Synonyms Oxpentifylline
Generic Available No
Therapeutic Class Blood Viscosity Reducer Agent
Use Symptomatic management of peripheral vascular disease, mainly intermittent claudication
Contraindications Hypersensitivity to pentoxifylline or any component and other xanthine derivatives (caffeine, theophylline)
Precautions Dose may need adjustment in patients with impaired renal function and in the elderly
Adverse Reactions
Cardiovascular: Mild hypotension, angina, arrhythmias
Central nervous system: Agitation, dizziness, headache
Gastrointestinal: Nausea, dyspepsia, vomiting
Ocular: Blurred vision
Otic: Earache
Overdosage Symptoms of overdose include hypotension, flushing, convulsions, deep sleep, agitation, tremors, bradycardia with first or second degree A-V block
Toxicology Gastric lavage and activated charcoal; symptomatic treatment for cardiovascular, respiratory, and neurologic events
Drug Interactions Warfarin's effects may be enhanced
Mechanism of Action Mechanism of action remains unclear; is thought to reduce blood viscosity and improve blood flow by altering the rheology of red blood cells
Pharmacokinetics
Absorption: Oral: Well absorbed
Half-life: 24-48 minutes (metabolites half-life: 60-96 minutes)
Time to peak: Peak serum levels occur within 1 hour
Metabolism: Undergoes first-pass metabolism; metabolized in the liver and excreted mainly in the urine
Usual Dosage Geriatrics and Adults: Oral: 400 mg 3 times/day with meals; may reduce to 400 mg twice daily if GI or CNS side effects occur
Monitoring Parameters PT, PTT if used in conjunction with other agents that may affect coagulation or platelet aggregation
Test Interactions Decrease calcium (S), decreased magnesium (S), false-positive theophylline levels
Patient Information Take with food or meals; if GI or CNS side effects continue, contact physician; while effects may be seen in 2-4 weeks, continue treatment for at least 8 weeks
Special Geriatric Considerations See Usual Dosage and Monitoring Parameters
Dosage Forms Tablet, controlled release: 400 mg

Pentylan® *see* Pentaerythritol Tetranitrate *on page 543*

Pen.Vee® K *see* Penicillin V Potassium *on page 543*

Pepcid® *see* Famotidine *on page 280*

Pepto-Bismol® [OTC] *see* Bismuth *on page 88*

Percocet® *see* Oxycodone and Acetaminophen *on page 528*

Percodan® *see* Oxycodone and Aspirin *on page 529*

Percodan®-Demi *see* Oxycodone and Aspirin *on page 529*

Perdiem® Plain [OTC] *see* Psyllium *on page 610*

Pergolide Mesylate (per' go lide)
Brand Names Permax®
Generic Available No
Therapeutic Class Anti-Parkinson's Agent; Ergot Alkaloid
(Continued)

Pergolide Mesylate *(Continued)*

Use Adjunctive treatment to levodopa/carbidopa in the management of Parkinson's Disease

Contraindications Known hypersensitivity to pergolide mesylate or other ergot derivatives

Precautions High incidence of syncope and orthostatic hypotension upon initiation of therapy; use with caution in patients prone to cardiac dysrhythmias and in patients with a history of confusion or hallucinations

Adverse Reactions
Cardiovascular: Myocardial infarction, postural hypotension, syncope, arrhythmias
Central nervous system: Dizziness, somnolence, insomnia, confusion, hallucinations, anxiety
Gastrointestinal: Nausea, constipation
Neuromuscular & skeletal: Dyskinesias
Respiratory: Rhinitis
Miscellaneous: Peripheral edema

Overdosage Symptoms of overdose include vomiting, hypotension, agitation, hallucinations, ventricular extrasystoles, possible seizures; data on overdose are limited

Toxicology Treatment is supportive and may require antiarrhythmias and/or neuroleptics for agitation; hypotension, when unresponsive to I.V. fluids or Trendelenburg positioning, often responds to norepinephrine infusions started at 0.1-0.2 mcg/kg/minute followed by a titrated infusion. If signs of CNS stimulation are present, a neuroleptic may be indicated; antiarrhythmics may be indicated, monitor EKG; activated charcoal is useful to prevent further absorption and to hasten elimination.

Drug Interactions
Decreased effect: Dopamine antagonists, metoclopramide
Increased toxicity: Highly plasma protein bound drugs

Mechanism of Action Pergolide is a semisynthetic ergot alkaloid similar to bromocriptine but stated to be more potent and longer acting; it is a centrally-active dopamine agonist stimulating both D_1 and D_2 receptors

Pharmacokinetics
Absorption: Oral: Well absorbed
Metabolism: Extensive in the liver (on first-pass)
Elimination: ~50% in urine and 50% in feces

Usual Dosage Geriatrics and Adults: Oral: Start with 0.05 mg/day for 2 days, then increase dosage by 0.1 or 0.15 mg/day every 3 days over next 12 days, increase dose by 0.25 mg/day every 3 days until optimal therapeutic dose is achieved; usual dosage range: 2-3 mg/day in 3 divided doses

Monitoring Parameters Blood pressure, both standing and sitting/supine, symptoms of parkinsonism, dyskinesias, mental status

Patient Information Take with food or milk; rise slowly from sitting or lying down; report any confusion or change in mental status

Nursing Implications Raise bed rails and institute safety measures, aid patient with ambulation; may cause postural hypotension and drowsiness

Additional Information When adding pergolide to levodopa/carbidopa, the dose of the latter can usually and should be decreased. Patients no longer responsive to bromocriptine may benefit by being switched to pergolide.

Special Geriatric Considerations See Precautions and Adverse Reactions

Dosage Forms Tablet: 0.05 mg, 0.25 mg, 1 mg

References
Collier DS, Berg MJ, and Fincham RW, "Parkinsonism Treatment: Part III
Koller WC, Silver DE, and Lieberman A, "An Algorithm for the Management of Parkinson's Disease," *Neurology*, 1994, 44(12):S1-52. - Update," *Ann Pharmacother*, 1992, 26(2):227-33.

Periactin® *see* Cyproheptadine Hydrochloride *on page 200*

Peri-Colace® [OTC] *see* Docusate and Casanthranol *on page 237*

Peridex® *see* Chlorhexidine Gluconate *on page 151*

Peri-DOS® [OTC] *see* Docusate and Casanthranol *on page 237*

Peritrate® *see* Pentaerythritol Tetranitrate *on page 543*

Peritrate® SA *see* Pentaerythritol Tetranitrate *on page 543*

Permapen® *see* Penicillin G Benzathine, Parenteral *on page 539*

Permax® *see* Pergolide Mesylate *on previous page*

Permethrin *(per meth' rin)*

Brand Names Elimite™; Nix™

Therapeutic Class Antiparasitic Agent, Topical; Scabicidal Agent

Use Single application treatment of infestation with *Pediculus humanus capitis* (head louse) and its nits, or *Sarcoptes scabiei* (scabies)

Contraindications Known hypersensitivity to pyrethyroid, pyrethrin or to chrysanthemums

Precautions Treatment with Nix™ may temporarily exacerbate the symptoms of itching, redness, swelling; for external use only

Adverse Reactions
Cardiovascular: Edema
Dermatologic: Pruritus, numbness or scalp discomfort, erythema, rash of the scalp
Local: Burning, stinging, tingling

Mechanism of Action Inhibits sodium ion influx through nerve cell membrane channels in parasites resulting in delayed repolarization and thus paralysis of the pest

Pharmacokinetics
Absorption: Topical: Minimal, <2%
Metabolism: In the liver
Elimination: In urine

Usual Dosage Geriatrics and Adults: Topical:
Head lice: After hair has been washed with shampoo, rinsed with water and towel dried, apply a sufficient volume to saturate the hair and scalp. Leave on hair for 10 minutes before rinsing off with water; remove remaining nits; may repeat in 1 week if lice or nits still present

Scabies: Apply cream from head to toe; leave on for 8-14 hours before washing off with water, a single application is usually adequate; may repeat in 1 week

Administration Because scabies and lice are so contagious, use caution to avoid spreading or infecting oneself; wear gloves when applying; see Usual Dosage

Patient Information Avoid contact with eyes during application; shake well before using; notify physician if irritation persists; clothing and bedding should be washed in hot water or dry cleaned to kill the scabies mite

Nursing Implications See Administration

Special Geriatric Considerations Because of its minimal absorption, permethrin is a drug of choice and is preferred over lindane

Dosage Forms
Cream: 5% (60 g)
Liquid: 1% (60 mL)

Perphenazine (per fen' a zeen)
Related Information
Antacid Drug Interactions *on page 764*
Antipsychotic Agents Comparison *on page 801*
Antipsychotic Medication Guidelines *on page 754*

Brand Names Trilafon®

Generic Available Yes

Therapeutic Class Antiemetic; Antipsychotic Agent; Phenothiazine Derivative

Use Management of manifestations of psychotic disorders; depressive neurosis; alcohol withdrawal; nausea and vomiting; nonpsychotic symptoms associated with dementia in elderly; Tourette's syndrome; Huntington's chorea; spasmodic torticollis and Reye's syndrome; see Special Geriatric Considerations

Contraindications Hypersensitivity to perphenazine or any component, cross-sensitivity with other phenothiazines may exist; avoid use in patients with narrow-angle glaucoma, bone marrow depression, severe liver or cardiac disease; subcortical brain damage; circulatory collapse; severe hypotension or hypertension

Warnings
Tardive dyskinesia: Prevalence rate may be 40% in elderly; elderly women especially at risk; embarrassment from dyskinesias may lead to greater social isolation; development of the syndrome and the irreversible nature are proportional to duration and total cumulative dose over time. May be reversible if diagnosed early in therapy; intermittent use of antipsychotics (not proven use) helps decrease total cumulative dose.

EPS: Extrapyramidal reactions are more common in elderly with up to 50% developing these reactions after age 60. These reactions may be more common in dementia patients. Drug-induced **Parkinson's syndrome** occurs often. Discontinuation usually resolves symptoms but may take weeks to months (12+) to clear. **Akathisia** is the most common EPS reaction in elderly. The symptoms of motor restlessness are difficult to diagnose in demented elderly; increased nervousness, assertiveness, restlessness with constant movement may indicate this adverse event. Consider decreasing dose if antipsychotic to treat as well as diagnose problem; usually see this reaction within 2-3 months of initiating antipsychotic drug.

Anticholinergic effects: These side effects most common with low potency antipsychotics (eg, thioridazine, chlorpromazine). CNS toxicity occurs more frequently and severely in elderly; increased confusion, memory loss, psychotic behavior, and agitation frequently occur as a consequence of anticholinergic effects to antipsychotic agents. Peripheral anticholinergic action troublesome to elderly; most peripheral anticholinergic effects last only 2-3 weeks; see Adverse Reactions.

Orthostatic hypotension: More common with low potency agents (eg, thioridazine, chlorpromazine, and clozapine) but of concern with all antipsychotic agents;

(Continued)

549

Perphenazine *(Continued)*

orthostasis due to alpha-receptor blockade by antipsychotic agents. Elderly present many risk factors for orthostatic hypotension: blunted baroreceptor reflexes, decreased vascular tone, decreased vascular volume, and possible presence of cardiac diseases which result in decreased cardiac output.

Sedation: Common side effect with antipsychotic therapy; should not be used as a hypnotic unless insomnia is associated with target behavior symptoms treated with antipsychotic medications; see Special Geriatric Considerations. Anecdotal reports suggesting antipsychotic sedation in nonpsychotic patients is extremely unpleasant due to feelings of depersonalization, derealization, and dysphoria. Due to the long duration of action with antipsychotic drugs, these reactions may last up to 24 hours and result in decreased daytime function.

Cardiac toxicity: Life-threatening arrhythmias have occurred at therapeutic doses of antipsychotics. Thioridazine more commonly demonstrates EKG changes than other antipsychotics; suggested to use high potency antipsychotic agents (ie, haloperidol) in patients with cardiac conduction defects.

Precautions Use with caution in patients with cardiovascular disease, seizures, and Parkinson's disease; benefits of therapy must be weighed against risks

Adverse Reactions Sedation and anticholinergic effects are more pronounced than extrapyramidal effects

Cardiovascular: EKG changes, hypotension (especially orthostatic), tachycardia, arrhythmias, abnormal T waves with prolonged ventricular repolarization
Central nervous system: Drowsiness, restlessness, anxiety, extrapyramidal reactions, dystonic reactions, pseudoparkinsonian signs and symptoms, tardive dyskinesia, neuroleptic malignant syndrome, seizures, altered central temperature regulation
Dermatologic: Hyperpigmentation, pruritus, rash, contact dermatitis, photosensitivity (rare)
Endocrine & metabolic: Amenorrhea, galactorrhea, gynecomastia
Gastrointestinal: Dry mouth (problem for denture user), constipation, adynamic ileus, GI upset, weight gain
Genitourinary: Overflow incontinence, urinary retention, priapism, sexual dysfunction (up to 60%)
Hematologic: Agranulocytosis, leukopenia
Hepatic: Cholestatic jaundice
Ocular: Retinal pigmentation (more common than with chlorpromazine), blurred vision, decreased visual acuity (may be irreversible)

Overdosage Symptoms of overdose include deep sleep, coma, extrapyramidal symptoms, abnormal involuntary muscle movements, hypotension or hypertension; agitation, restlessness, fever, hypothermia or hyperthermia, seizures, cardiac arrhythmias, EKG changes

Toxicology Following initiation of essential overdose management, toxic symptom treatment and supportive treatment should be initiated. Hypotension usually responds to I.V. fluids or Trendelenburg positioning. If unresponsive to these measures the use of a parenteral inotrope may be required (eg, norepinephrine 0.1-0.2 mcg/kg/minute titrated to response). Seizures commonly respond to diazepam (I.V. 5-10 mg bolus every 15 minutes if needed up to a total of 30 mg) or to phenytoin or phenobarbital. Also critical cardiac arrhythmias often respond to I.V. phenytoin (15 mg/kg up to 1 g), while other antiarrhythmics can be used. Neuroleptics often cause extrapyramidal symptoms (eg, dystonic reactions) requiring management with diphenhydramine 1-2 mg/kg up to a maximum of 50 mg I.M. or I.V. slow push followed by a maintenance dose for 48-72 hours. When these reactions are unresponsive to diphenhydramine, benztropine mesylate I.V. 1-2 mg may be effective. These agents are generally effective within 2-5 minutes.

Drug Interactions
Alcohol may increase CNS sedation
Anticholinergic agents may decrease pharmacologic effects; increase anticholinergic side effects; may enhance tardive dyskinesia
Aluminum salts may decrease absorption of phenothiazines
Barbiturates may decrease phenothiazine serum concentrations
Bromocriptine may have decreased efficacy when administered with phenothiazines
Guanethidine's hypotensive effect is decreased by phenothiazines
Lithium administration with phenothiazines may increase disorientation
Meperidine and phenothiazine coadministration increases sedation and hypotension
Methyldopa administration with phenothiazine (trifluoperazine) may significantly increase blood pressure
Norepinephrine, epinephrine have decreased pressor effect when administered with chlorpromazine; therefore, be aware of possible decreased effectiveness or when any phenothiazine is used
Phenytoin serum concentrations may increase or decrease with phenothiazines; tricyclic antidepressants may have increased serum concentrations with concomitant administration with phenothiazines
Propranolol administered with phenothiazines may increase serum concentrations of both drugs

Valproic acid may have increased half-life when administered with phenothiazines (chlorpromazine)

Stability Do not mix with beverages containing caffeine (coffee, cola), tannins (tea), or pectinates (apple juice) since physical incompatibility exists; use ~60 mL diluent for each 5 mL of concentrate; protect all dosage forms from light, clear or slightly yellow solutions may be used; should be dispensed in amber or opaque vials/bottles. Solutions may be diluted or mixed with fruit juices or other liquids but must be administered immediately after mixing; do not prepare bulk dilutions or store bulk dilutions.

Mechanism of Action Blocks postsynaptic mesolimbic dopaminergic D_1 and D_2 receptors in the brain; exhibits a strong alpha-adrenergic blocking and anticholinergic effect; depresses the release of hypothalamic and hypophyseal hormones; believed to depress the reticular activating system thus affecting basal metabolism, body temperature, wakefulness, vasomotor tone, and emesis

Pharmacokinetics

Absorption: Oral: Well absorbed; absorption may be affected by the inherent anticholinergic action on the gastrointestinal tissue causing variable absorption. Absorption from tablets is erratic with less variation seen with solutions. These agents are widely distributed in tissues with CNS concentrations exceeding that of plasma due to their lipophilic characteristics.

Protein binding: Antipsychotic agents are bound 90% to 99% to plasma or proteins; highly bound to brain and lung tissue and other tissues with a high blood perfusion

Metabolism: Metabolized in the liver

Time to peak: Peak serum levels occur within 4-8 hours; peak concentrations between 2-4 hours

Elimination: Excreted in urine and bile; excretion occurs through hepatic metabolism (oxidation) where numerous active metabolites are produced; active metabolites excreted in urine; elimination half-lives of antipsychotics ranges from 20-40 hours which may be extended in elderly due to decline in oxidative hepatic reactions (phase I) with age.

The biologic effect of a single dose persists for 24 hours. When the patient has accommodated to initial side effects (sedation), once daily dosing is possible due to the long half-life of antipsychotics.

Steady-state plasma levels are achieved in 4-7 days; therefore, if possible, do not make dose adjustments more than once in a 7-day period. Due to the long half-lives of antipsychotics, as needed (PRN) use is ineffective since repeated doses are necessary to achieve therapeutic tissue concentrations in the CNS.

Usual Dosage Oral:

Geriatrics (nonpsychotic patient; dementia behavior): Initial: 2-4 mg 1-2 times/day; increase at 4- to 7-day intervals by 2-4 mg/day. Increase dose intervals (bid, tid, etc) as necessary to control behavior response or side effects. Maximum daily dose: 32 mg; gradual increase (titration) may prevent some side effects or decrease their severity

Adults:

Psychoses: 4-16 mg 2-4 times/day; I.M.: 5 mg every 6 hours

Nausea/vomiting: 8-16 mg/day in divided doses

I.M.: 5-10 mg

I.V. (severe): 1 mg at 1- to 2-minute intervals up to a total of 5 mg

Not dialyzable (0% to 5%)

Monitoring Parameters Orthostatic blood pressures; tremors; gait changes, abnormal movement in trunk, neck, buccal area or extremities; monitor target behaviors for which the agent is given

Reference Range 0.8-1.2 ng/mL; serum concentrations are controversial and dosing to response is recommended

Test Interactions Increased cholesterol (S), increased glucose; decreased uric acid (S)

Patient Information Oral concentrate must be diluted in 2-4 oz of liquid (water, fruit juice, carbonated drinks, milk, or pudding); do not take antacid within 1 hour of taking drug; avoid alcohol; avoid excess sun exposure (use sun block); may cause drowsiness, rise slowly from recumbent position; use of supportive stockings may help prevent orthostatic hypotension

Nursing Implications Monitor for hypotension when administering I.M. or I.V.; dilute oral concentration to at least 2 oz with water, juice, or milk; for I.V. use, injection should be diluted to at least 0.5 mg/mL with NS and given at a rate of 1 mg/minute. Monitor for orthostatic hypotension 3-5 days after initiation of therapy or a dose increase; observe for tremor and abnormal movement or posturing.

Special Geriatric Considerations See Warnings

Many elderly patients receive antipsychotic medications for inappropriate nonpsychotic behavior. Before initiating antipsychotic medication, the clinician should investigate any possible reversible cause; any stress or stress from any disease can cause acute "confusion" or worsening of baseline nonpsychotic behavior. Most commonly acute changes in behavior are due to increases in drug dose or addition of new drug to regimen; fluid electrolyte loss; infections; and changes in environment.

(Continued)

Perphenazine *(Continued)*
Any changes in disease status in any organ system can result in behavior changes.
Dosage Forms
Concentrate: 16 mg/5 mL (118 mL)
Injection: 5 mg/mL (1 mL)
Tablet: 2 mg, 4 mg, 8 mg, 16 mg

Perphenazine and Amitriptyline *see* Amitriptyline and Perphenazine
on page 43

Persantine® *see* Dipyridamole *on page 233*

Pertofrane® *see* Desipramine Hydrochloride *on page 205*

Pethadol® *see* Meperidine Hydrochloride *on page 441*

Pethidine Hydrochloride *see* Meperidine Hydrochloride *on page 441*

PETN *see* Pentaerythritol Tetranitrate *on page 543*

Pfizerpen® *see* Penicillin G, Parenteral *on page 540*

Pfizerpen®-AS *see* Penicillin G Procaine, Aqueous *on page 541*

Pharmacokinetics of Narcotic Agonist Analgesics *see page 812*

Phazyme®-25 [OTC] *see* Simethicone *on page 645*

Phazyme®-95 [OTC] *see* Simethicone *on page 645*

Phazyme® [OTC] *see* Simethicone *on page 645*

Phenantoin *see* Mephenytoin *on page 442*

Phenaphen® With Codeine *see* Acetaminophen and Codeine
on page 14

Phenazine® *see* Promethazine Hydrochloride *on page 599*

Phenazopyridine Hydrochloride *(fen az oh peer' i deen)*
Brand Names Azo-Standard®; Geridium®; Phenzodine®; Pyridiate®; Pyridium®; Uro-dine®
Synonyms Phenylazo Diamino Pyridine Hydrochloride
Generic Available Yes
Therapeutic Class Analgesic, Urinary; Local Anesthetic, Urinary
Use Symptomatic relief of urinary burning, itching, frequency and urgency in association with urinary tract infection or following urologic procedures
Contraindications Hypersensitivity to phenazopyridine or any component; kidney or liver disease
Warnings Long-term administration has induced neoplasia in rats and mice
Precautions Yellowish tinge of the skin or sclera may indicate accumulation due to impaired renal function. If this occurs, discontinue therapy; phenazopyridine should only be given for 2 days when used with an antibiotic for the treatment of a urinary tract infection. Do not use in patients with Cl_{cr} <50 mL/minute.
Adverse Reactions
Central nervous system: Vertigo, headache
Dermatologic: Skin pigmentation, rash
Hematologic: Methemoglobinemia, hemolytic anemia
Hepatic: Hepatitis
Renal: Acute renal failure
Overdosage Symptoms of overdose include methemoglobinemia, hemolytic anemia, skin pigmentation, renal and hepatic impairment
Toxicology Antidote: Methylene blue 1-2 mg/kg I.V. or 100-200 g ascorbic acid orally
Mechanism of Action Exerts local anesthetic or analgesic action on urinary tract mucosa through an unknown mechanism
Pharmacokinetics
Metabolism: In the liver and other tissues
Elimination: In urine (where it exerts its action); renal excretion (as unchanged drug) is rapid and accounts for 65% of the drug's elimination
Usual Dosage Geriatrics and Adults: Oral: 100-200 mg 3-4 times/day after meals for 2 days
Monitoring Parameters Relief of urinary discomfort
Test Interactions Phenazopyridine may cause delayed reactions with glucose oxidase reagents (Clinistix®, Tes-Tape®); occasional false-positive tests occur with Tes-Tape®; cupric sulfate tests (Clinitest®) are not affected; interference may also occur with urine ketone tests (Acetest®, Ketostix®) and urinary protein tests; tests for urinary steroids and porphyrins may also occur
Patient Information Take by mouth after meals; tablets may color the urine orange or red and may stain clothing. This medication treats the painful symptoms of a urinary tract infection but does not cure the infection.
Nursing Implications Colors urine orange or red; stains clothing and is difficult to remove; give after meals

Special Geriatric Considerations Use of this agent in the elderly is limited since accumulation of phenazopyridine can occur in patients with renal insufficiency; it should not be used in patients with a Cl$_{cr}$ <50 mL/minute

Dosage Forms Tablet: 100 mg, 200 mg

Phencen® *see* Promethazine Hydrochloride *on page 599*

Phenelzine Sulfate (fen' el zeen)
Brand Names Nardil®
Therapeutic Class Antidepressant, Monoamine Oxidase Inhibitor
Use Symptomatic treatment of depressed patients refractory to or intolerant to other antidepressants or electroconvulsive therapy
Contraindications Pheochromocytoma, hepatic or renal disease, cerebrovascular defect, cardiovascular disease, hypersensitivity to phenelzine or any component
Warnings Hypertensive crisis within several hours of ingestion of a contraindicated substance (such as tyramine-containing foods)
Adverse Reactions
Cardiovascular: Hypotension, edema, tachycardia
Central nervous system: Drowsiness, paresthesias, nervousness
Dermatologic: Skin rash
Gastrointestinal: Dry mouth, constipation, anorexia
Genitourinary: Urinary retention, impotence
Hematologic: Leukopenia
Hepatic: Hepatocellular (hepatitis-like) damage
Neuromuscular & skeletal: Peripheral neuropathy, trembling
Ocular: Blurred vision
Overdosage Symptoms of overdose include tachycardia, palpitations, muscle twitching, seizures
Toxicology Competent supportive care is the most important treatment for an overdose with a monoamine oxidase (MAO) inhibitor. Both hypertension or hypotension can occur with intoxication. Hypotension may respond to I.V. fluids or vasopressors and hypertension usually responds to an alpha-adrenergic blocker. While treating the hypertension, care is warranted to avoid sudden drops in blood pressure, since this may worsen the MAO inhibitor toxicity. Muscle irritability and seizures often respond to diazepam, while hyperthermia is best treated antipyretics and cooling blankets. Cardiac arrhythmias are best treated with phenytoin or procainamide.
Drug Interactions
Increased effect/toxicity of barbiturates, psychotropics, rauwolfia alkaloids, CNS depressants
Increased toxicity with disulfiram (seizures), fluoxetine and other serotonin active agents (increased cardiac effect), tricyclic antidepressants (increased cardiovascular instability), meperidine (increased cardiovascular instability), phenothiazine (hypertensive crisis), sympathomimetics (hypertensive crisis), levodopa (hypertensive crisis), dextroamphetamine
Note: Many of these interactions can occur weeks after the MAO inhibitor has been stopped; in patients undergoing general anesthesia, discontinue the MAO inhibitors several weeks before to avoid cardiovascular effects
Food/Drug Interactions Avoid tyramine-containing foods (may increase blood pressure)
Stability Protect from light
Mechanism of Action Inhibits the enzymes monoamine oxidase A and B which is responsible for the intraneuronal metabolism of norepinephrine and serotonin, and dopamine and phenylethylamine, respectively. Also involved in the down regulation of beta$_2$- and alpha$_2$-nonadrenergic receptors and serotonin alpha-receptos
Pharmacodynamics
Onset of action: Expect to see some clinical response in 2-4 weeks, provided that the dosing is adequate
Duration of action: May continue to have a therapeutic effect and interactions 2 weeks after discontinuing therapy
Geriatric patients receiving an average of 55 mg/day developed a mean platelet MAO activity inhibition of about 85%
Pharmacokinetics
Absorption: Oral: Well absorbed; undergoes acetylation in the liver
Older patients have been reported to have higher blood concentrations than younger adults after 2 weeks of continuous treatment
Elimination: In urine primarily as metabolites and unchanged drug
Usual Dosage Oral:
Geriatrics: Initial: 7.5 mg/day, increase by 7.5-15 mg/day every 3-4 days as tolerated; usual therapeutic dose: 15-60 mg/day in 3-4 divided doses

Adults: 15 mg 3 times/day; may increase to 60-90 mg/day
Monitoring Parameters Blood pressure, heart rate; diet; weight; mood if depressive symptoms
(Continued)

Phenelzine Sulfate *(Continued)*

Reference Range Inhibition of platelet monoamine oxidase (≥80%) correlates with clinical response

Test Interactions Decreased glucose

Patient Information Avoid tyramine-containing foods: red wine, aged cheese (except cottage, ricotta, and cream), smoked or pickled fish, beef or chicken liver, dried sausage, fava or broad bean pods, yeast, vitamin supplements. Report severe headaches, irregular heartbeats, skin rash, insomnia, sedation, changes in strength, sensations of pain, burning, touch, or vibration, or any other unusual symptoms to your physician; avoid alcohol; get up slowly from chair or bed.

Nursing Implications Watch for postural hypotension; monitor blood pressure carefully, especially at therapy onset or if other CNS drugs or cardiovascular drugs are added; check for dietary and drug restriction

Special Geriatric Considerations The MAO inhibitors are effective and generally well tolerated by older patients. It is their potential interactions with tyramine or tryptophan-containing foods (see Warnings) and other drugs (see Drug Interactions), and their effects on blood pressure that have limited their use. The MAO inhibitors are usually reserved for patients who do not tolerate or respond to the traditional "cyclic" or "second generation" antidepressants. The brain activity of monoamine oxidase increases with age and even more so in patients with Alzheimer's disease. Therefore, the MAO inhibitors may have an increased role in patients with Alzheimer's disease who are depressed. Phenelzine is less stimulating than tranylcypromine; see Pharmacokinetics and Pharmacodynamics.

Dosage Forms Tablet: 15 mg

References

Alexopoulos GS, "Treatment of Depression," *Clinical Geriatric Psychopharmacology*, 2nd ed, 137-74, Salzman C, ed, Baltimore, MD: Williams & Wilkins, 1992.

Georgotas A, Friedman E, McCarthy M, et al, "Resistant Geriatric Depression and Therapeutic Response to Monoamine-Oxidase Inhibitors," *Biol Psychiatry*, 1983, 18:195-205.

Goff DC and Jenike MA, "Treatment-Resistant Depression in the Elderly," *J Am Geriatr Soc*, 1986, 34(1):63-70.

Jenike MA, "MAO Inhibitors as Treatment for Depressed Patients With Primary Degenerative Dementia (Alzheimer's Disease)," *Am J Psychiatry*, 1985, 142:763.

Phenergan® *see* Promethazine Hydrochloride *on page 599*

Phenetron® *see* Chlorpheniramine Maleate *on page 152*

Pheniramine and Naphazoline *see* Naphazoline and Pheniramine *on page 491*

Phenobarbital *(fee noe bar' bi tal)*

Related Information

Drug Levels Commonly Monitored Guidelines *on page 771-772*

Brand Names Barbita®; Luminal®; Solfoton®

Synonyms Phenobarbital Sodium; Phenobarbitone; Phenylethylmalonylurea

Generic Available Yes

Therapeutic Class Anticonvulsant, Barbiturate; Barbiturate; Hypnotic; Sedative

Use Management of generalized tonic-clonic (grand mal) and partial seizures; sedation; hypnosis; lowering of bilirubin in chronic cholestasis

Restrictions C-IV

Contraindications Hypersensitivity to phenobarbital or any component; pre-existing CNS depression, severe uncontrolled pain, porphyria, severe respiratory disease with dyspnea or obstruction

Warnings Abrupt withdrawal may precipitate status epilepticus

Precautions Use with caution in patients with renal or hepatic impairment; abrupt withdrawal in patients with epilepsy may precipitate status epilepticus

Adverse Reactions

Cardiovascular: Hypotension, cardiac arrhythmias, bradycardia, hypotension, circulatory collapse, thrombophlebitis with I.V. use, arterial spasm, and gangrene with inadvertent intra-arterial injection

Central nervous system: Drowsiness, lethargy, CNS excitation or depression, impaired judgment, paradoxical excitement, cognitive impairment, defects in general comprehension, short-term memory deficits, decreased attention span, ataxia

Dermatologic: Rash, skin eruptions, exfoliative dermatitis

Gastrointestinal: Nausea, vomiting

Hematologic: Megaloblastic anemia

Hepatic: Hepatitis

Neuromuscular & skeletal: Osteomalacia, hyperkinetic activity

Renal: Oliguria

Respiratory: Respiratory depression, apnea (especially with rapid I.V. use)

Miscellaneous: Hypothermia

Overdosage Symptoms of overdose include CNS depression, respiratory depression, hypotension, tachycardia, areflexia

Toxicology Treatment is mainly supportive; emesis may be induced if the patient is conscious and has not lost his/her gag reflex; activated charcoal may be administered; if renal function is normal, forced diuresis is helpful. Alkalinization of the urine with I.V. sodium bicarbonate helps enhance elimination; hemodialysis and hemoperfusion may be used in severe barbiturate intoxications.

Drug Interactions

Decreased effect of phenothiazines, haloperidol, quinidine, cyclosporine, TCAs, corticosteroids, theophylline, ethosuximide, warfarin, oral contraceptives, chloramphenicol, griseofulvin, doxycycline, beta-blockers

Increased effect/toxicity of phenobarbital with propoxyphene, benzodiazepines, CNS depressants, valproic acid, methylphenidate, chloramphenicol

Stability Protect elixir from light; not stable in aqueous solutions; use only clear solutions; do not add to acidic solutions, precipitation may occur

Mechanism of Action Interferes with transmission of impulses from the thalamus to the cortex of the brain resulting in an imbalance in central inhibitory and facilitatory mechanisms

Pharmacodynamics

Hypnosis after oral dose:
Onset of action: Within 20-60 minutes
Duration: 6-10 hours
I.V.:
Onset: Within 5 minutes with peak effect within 30 minutes
Duration: 4-10 hours; the elderly may be more sensitive to the sedative effects of phenobarbital

Pharmacokinetics

Absorption: Oral: 70% to 90%
Protein binding: 20% to 45%
Metabolism: In liver via hydroxylation and glucuronide conjugation
Half-life: 53-140 hours; half-life may be increased in elderly; clearance can be increased with alkalinization of urine or with oral multiple dose activated charcoal
Time to peak: Oral: Peak serum levels occur within 1-6 hours
Elimination: 20% to 50% excreted unchanged in urine

Usual Dosage

Geriatrics and Adults:
Anticonvulsant: 2-4 mg/kg/day at bedtime or in divided doses; adjust dose until serum concentration is therapeutic; in status epilepticus, load with 15 mg/kg I.V. given over 10-15 minutes
Status epilepticus: I.V.: 15-20 mg/kg; may possibly be increased to up to 25 mg/kg at a rate not to exceed 100 mg/minute

Adults:
Sedation: Oral, I.M.: 30-120 mg/day in 2-3 divided doses
Hypnotic: Oral, I.M., I.V., S.C.: 100-320 mg at bedtime
Hyperbilirubinemia: Oral: 90-180 mg/day in 2-3 divided doses
Preoperative sedation: I.M.: 100-200 mg 1-1.5 hours before procedure

Moderately dialyzable (20% to 50%)

Monitoring Parameters Phenobarbital serum concentrations, mental status, CBC, LFTs, seizure activity

Reference Range Adults: Therapeutic: 15-40 μg/mL (SI: 65-172 μmol/L); Toxic: >40 μg/mL (SI: >172 μmol/L)

Test Interactions Increased alkaline phosphatase (S), increased ammonia (B); decreased bilirubin (S), decreased calcium (S)

Patient Information May cause drowsiness, avoid alcohol and other CNS depressants

Nursing Implications Observe patient for excessive sedation, respiratory depression

Additional Information Sodium content of injection (65 mg, 1 mL): 6 mg (0.3 mEq)
Phenobarbital: Barbita®, Solfoton®
Phenobarbital sodium: Luminal®

Special Geriatric Considerations Due to its long half-life and risk of dependence, phenobarbital is not recommended as a sedative or hypnotic in the elderly; interpretive guidelines from the Health Care Financing Administration discourage the use of this agent as a sedative/hypnotic in long-term care residents

Dosage Forms

Capsule: 16 mg
Elixir: 20 mg/5 mL (3.75 mL, 5 mL, 7.5 mL, 120 mL, 473 mL, 946 mL, 4000 mL)
Injection, as sodium: 30 mg/mL (1 mL), 60 mg/mL (1 mL), 65 mg/mL (1 mL); 130 mg/mL (1 mL)
Powder for injection: 120 mg
Tablet: 8 mg, 15 mg, 16 mg, 30 mg, 32 mg, 60 mg, 65 mg, 100 mg

Phenobarbital Sodium see Phenobarbital on previous page

Phenobarbitone see Phenobarbital on previous page

Phenolax® [OTC] *see* Phenolphthalein *on this page*

Phenolphthalein (fee nole thay' leen)

Brand Names Alophen Pills® [OTC]; Evac-U-Gen® [OTC]; Evac-U-Lax® [OTC]; Ex-Lax® [OTC]; Feen-A-Mint® [OTC]; Lax-Pills® [OTC]; Medilax® [OTC]; Modane® [OTC]; Modane® Mild [OTC]; Phenolax® [OTC]; Prulet® [OTC]

Synonyms Phenolphthalein, White; Phenolphthalein, Yellow

Generic Available Yes

Therapeutic Class Laxative, Stimulant

Use Stimulant laxative

Contraindications Do not use in patients with abdominal pain, obstruction, nausea or vomiting; appendicitis, acute surgical abdomen

Warnings Excessive use may lead to fluid and electrolyte balance

Precautions Drug is habit-forming and may result in laxative dependence and loss of normal bowel function with prolonged use; rectal bleeding and failure to respond to therapy may require further evaluation; discoloration of urine may occur

Adverse Reactions

Endocrine & metabolic: Electrolyte imbalance

Gastrointestinal: Abdominal cramps, nausea, griping, vomiting, rectal burning, irritation and sensation of burning on rectal mucosa and mild proctitis, bloating, flatulence

Miscellaneous: Sweating

Overdosage Symptoms of overdose include abdominal pain, diarrhea, hypotension, fatigue, lethargy, nausea, vomiting

Mechanism of Action Stimulates peristalsis by directly irritating the smooth muscle of the intestine, possibly the colonic intramural plexus and causes secretion of water and electrolyte into intestine; bile must be present for phenolphthalein to produce its effects; see Additional Information

Pharmacodynamics Onset of action: Within 6-10 hours

Pharmacokinetics Elimination: In feces and skin, with up to 15% excreted in urine as the conjugate; enterohepatically recycled

Usual Dosage Geriatrics and Adults: Oral: 60-200 mg preferably at bedtime; elderly may respond with lower doses; yellow phenolphthalein is 2-3 times more potent than white phenolphthalein

Monitoring Parameters Monitor stools daily or weekly; fluid/electrolyte status

Test Interactions Decreased calcium (S), decreased potassium (S)

Patient Information Do not exceed recommended doses; swallow tablet whole, do not crush or chew; may discolor urine (pink, red)

Nursing Implications See Contraindications, Adverse Reactions, and Special Geriatric Considerations

Additional Information

Phenolphthalein, white: Alophen Pills® [OTC], Medilax® [OTC], Modane® [OTC], Modane® Mild [OTC], Phenolax® [OTC], Prulet® [OTC]

Phenolphthalein, yellow: Evac-U-Gen® [OTC], Evac-U-Lax® [OTC], Ex-Lax® [OTC], Feen-A-Mint® [OTC], Lax-Pills® [OTC] yellow is 2-3 times more potent than white

Special Geriatric Considerations The chronic use of stimulant cathartics is inappropriate and should be avoided; although constipation is a common complaint from elderly, such complaints require evaluation; short term use of stimulants is best; if prophylaxis is desired, this can be accomplished with bulk agents (psyllium), stool softeners, and hyperosmotic agents (sorbitol 70%); stool softeners are unnecessary if stools are well hydrated, soft, or "mushy"

Dosage Forms Tablet: 60 mg

Phenolphthalein, White *see* Phenolphthalein *on this page*

Phenolphthalein, Yellow *see* Phenolphthalein *on this page*

Phenoxybenzamine Hydrochloride (fen ox ee ben' za meen)

Brand Names Dibenzyline®

Generic Available No

Therapeutic Class Alpha-Adrenergic Blocking Agent, Oral; Antihypertensive; Vasodilator, Coronary

Use Symptomatic management of pheochromocytoma; treatment of hypertensive crisis caused by sympathomimetic amines

Unlabeled use: Micturition problems associated with neurogenic bladder, functional outlet obstruction, and partial prostatic obstruction

Contraindications Shock and other conditions where a fall in blood pressure would be undesirable

Warnings Do not give with drugs that stimulate beta-adrenergic receptors as this may cause hypotension and tachycardia

Precautions Use with caution in patients with renal damage, congestive heart failure, or cerebral or coronary arteriosclerosis; can exacerbate symptoms of respiratory tract infections

Adverse Reactions
  Cardiovascular: Postural hypotension, tachycardia, syncope, shock
  Central nervous system: Lethargy, headache
  Gastrointestinal: Vomiting, nausea, diarrhea, dry mouth
  Genitourinary: Inhibition of ejaculation
  Neuromuscular & skeletal: Weakness
  Respiratory: Nasal congestion

Overdosage Symptoms of overdose include hypotension, tachycardia, lethargy, dizziness, shock

Toxicology Place patient in Trendelenburg's position; norepinephrine may be used in severe hypotension; do not use epinephrine; keep patient flat for 24 hours or more as phenoxybenzamine's effect is prolonged

Drug Interactions
  Decreased effect with alpha agonists
  Increased toxicity with beta-blockers, epinephrine (hypotension, tachycardia)

Mechanism of Action Irreversible noncompetitive alpha-adrenergic blockade of postganglionic synapses in exocrine glands and smooth muscle; relaxes the urethra and increases the opening of the bladder

Pharmacodynamics
  Onset of action: Oral: Within 2 hours
  Peak effects: Within 4-6 hours
  Duration: 4 or more days

Pharmacokinetics
  Half-life: 24 hours
  Elimination: Primarily in urine and feces

Usual Dosage Geriatrics and Adults: Oral:
  Initial: 10 mg twice daily, increase by 10 mg every other day until optimum dose is achieved. Usual range: 20-40 mg 2-3 times/day

  Urinary incontinence: 10 mg 1-3 times/day

Monitoring Parameters Blood pressure, pulse, urine output

Patient Information Avoid alcoholic beverages; if dizziness occurs, avoid sudden changes in posture; may cause nasal congestion and constricted pupils; may inhibit ejaculation; avoid cough, cold or allergy medications containing sympathomimetics

Nursing Implications Monitor vital signs

Special Geriatric Considerations Because of the risk of adverse effects, avoid the use of this medication in the elderly if possible

Dosage Forms Capsule: 10 mg

Phenoxymethyl Penicillin *see* Penicillin V Potassium *on page 543*

Phenylazo Diamino Pyridine Hydrochloride *see* Phenazopyridine Hydrochloride *on page 552*

Phenylephrine Hydrochloride (fen ill ef' rin)

Brand Names AK-Dilate® Ophthalmic Solution; AK-Nefrin® Ophthalmic Solution; Alconefrin® Nasal Solution [OTC]; Dilatair® Ophthalmic Solution; Doktors® Nasal Solution [OTC]; I-Phrine® Ophthalmic Solution; Isopto® Frin Ophthalmic Solution; I-White® Ophthalmic Solution; Mydfrin® Ophthalmic Solution; Neo-Synephrine® Nasal Solution [OTC]; Neo-Synephrine® Ophthalmic Solution; Nostril® Nasal Solution [OTC]; Ocugestrin® Ophthalmic Solution; Ocu-Phrin® Ophthalmic Solution; Prefrin™ Ophthalmic Solution; Relief® Ophthalmic Solution; Rhinall® Nasal Solution [OTC]; Sinarest® Nasal Solution [OTC]; St. Joseph® Measured Dose Nasal Solution [OTC]; Vicks® Sinex® Nasal Solution [OTC]

Generic Available Yes

Therapeutic Class Adrenergic Agonist Agent; Adrenergic Agonist Agent, Ophthalmic; Alpha-Adrenergic Blocking Agent, Ophthalmic; Nasal Agent, Vasoconstrictor; Ophthalmic Agent, Mydriatic

Use Treatment of hypotension, vascular failure in shock; as a vasoconstrictor in regional analgesia; symptomatic relief of nasal and nasopharyngeal mucosal congestion; as a mydriatic in ophthalmic procedures and treatment of wide-angle glaucoma

Contraindications Pheochromocytoma, severe hypertension, tachyarrhythmias; hypersensitivity to phenylephrine or any component

Warnings Injection may contain sulfites which may cause allergic reactions in some patients; do not use if solution turns brown or contains a precipitate. Administer all dosage forms with caution to patients with hypertension, hyperthyroidism, diabetes mellitus, cardiovascular disease, ischemic heart disease, increased intraocular pressure, or prostatic hypertrophy. Elderly patients are more likely to experience adverse reactions to sympathomimetics. Overdosage may cause hallucinations, seizures, CNS depression, and death.

Precautions Topical phenylephrine should only be used for 3-5 days. Rebound congestion may occur after the effects of the topical application subside.

Adverse Reactions
  Cardiovascular: Hypertension, angina, reflex bradycardia, arrhythmias, palpitations
  Central nervous system: Headache, restlessness, anxiety, excitability

(Continued)

Phenylephrine Hydrochloride *(Continued)*

Genitourinary: Difficult urination
Neuromuscular & skeletal: Tremors (with systemic use)
Miscellaneous: Rebound nasal stuffiness

Overdosage Symptoms of overdose include vomiting, hypertension, palpitations, paresthesia, ventricular extrasystoles

Toxicology Treatment is supportive; in extreme cases, I.V. phentolamine may be used

Drug Interactions
Decreased effect with alpha-blockers, beta-blockers
Increased effect/toxicity with oxytocic drugs, sympathomimetics (tachycardia, arrhythmias), MAO inhibitors

Stability Stable for 48 hours in 5% dextrose in water at pH 3.5-7.5; do not use brown colored solutions

Mechanism of Action Potent, direct-acting, alpha-adrenergic stimulator with weak beta-adrenergic activity; causes vasoconstriction of the arterioles of the nasal mucosa and conjunctiva; activates the dilator muscle of the pupil to cause contraction; produces vasoconstriction of arterioles in the body

Pharmacodynamics
Onset of action: Parenteral injection: Effects occur immediately
Duration:
I.M., S.C.: 45-60 minutes
I.V.: 20-30 minutes

Pharmacokinetics
Half-life: 2.5 hours
Metabolism: To phenolic conjugates
Elimination: Urine (90%)

Usual Dosage
Ophthalmic preparations for pupil dilation:
Geriatrics: Instill 1 drop of 2.5% solution, may repeat in 1 hour if necessary
Adults: Instill 1 drop of 2.5% or 10% solution, may repeat in 10-60 minutes as needed

Nasal decongestant:
Geriatrics: Administer 2-3 drops or 1-2 sprays every 4 hours of 0.125% to 0.25% solution as needed; do not use more than 3 days
Adults: Administer 2-3 drops or 1-2 sprays every 4 hours of 0.25% solution as needed; the 0.5% or 1% solution may be used in cases of extreme nasal congestion; do not use nasal solutions more than 3 days

Ophthalmic decongestant: Instill 1-2 drops of 0.12% solution 2-4 times/day

Hypotension/shock: Geriatrics and Adults:
I.M., S.C.: 2-5 mg/dose every 1-2 hours as needed (initial dose should not exceed 5 mg)
I.V. bolus: 0.1-0.5 mg/dose every 10-15 minutes as needed (initial dose should not exceed 0.5 mg)
I.V. infusion: 10 mg in 250 mL D_5W or NS (1:25,000 dilution) (40 mcg/mL); start at 100-180 mcg/minute (2-5 mL/minute; 50-90 drops/minute) initially. When blood pressure is stabilized, maintenance rate: 40-60 mcg/minute (20-30 drops/minute).

Paroxysmal supraventricular tachycardia: Geriatrics and Adults: I.V.: 0.25-0.5 mg/dose over 20-30 seconds

Monitoring Parameters Blood pressure, pulse, EKG (systemic), relief of symptoms (topical)

Patient Information Nasal decongestant should not be used for >3 days in a row, hereby reducing problems of rebound congestion. Consult physician or pharmacist before using. Notify physician of insomnia, weakness, dizziness, tremor, or irregular heartbeat.

Nursing Implications May cause necrosis or sloughing tissue if extravasation occurs during I.V. administration or S.C. administration; monitor elderly patients closely while on phenylephrine

Special Geriatric Considerations Phenylephrine I.V. should be used with extreme caution in the elderly. The 10% ophthalmic solution has caused increased blood pressure in elderly patients and its use should, therefore, be avoided. Since topical decongestants can be obtained over-the-counter, elderly patients should be counseled about their proper use and in what disease states they should be avoided; see Warnings

Dosage Forms
Jelly: 0.5% (18.75 g)
Injection: 10 mg/mL (1 mL)
Solution:
Nasal:
Drops: 0.125% (15 mL, 30 mL); 0.16% (30 mL); 0.2% (30 mL); 0.25% (15 mL, 30 mL, 473 mL)
Spray: 0.25% (15 mL, 30 mL); 0.5% (15 mL, 30 mL); 1% (15 mL)
Ophthalmic: 0.12% (15 mL); 2.5% (2 mL, 3 mL, 5 mL, 15 mL); 10% (1 mL, 2 mL, 5 mL)

Phenylethylmalonylurea *see* Phenobarbital *on page 554*

Phenylpropanolamine Hydrochloride (fen ill proe pa nole' a meen)
Brand Names Control® [OTC]; Dex-A-Diet® [OTC]; Dexatrim® [OTC]; Maigret-50®; Precision Release® [OTC]; Prolamine® [OTC]; Propadrine; Propagest® [OTC]; Rhindecon®; Stay Trim® Diet Gum [OTC]; Westrim® LA [OTC]

Synonyms *dl*-Norephedrine Hydrochloride; PPA

Generic Available Yes

Therapeutic Class Adrenergic Agonist Agent; Anorexiant; Decongestant; Nasal Agent, Vasoconstrictor

Use Anorexiant and nasal decongestant

Unlabeled use: Urinary incontinence, stress type

Contraindications Known hypersensitivity to phenylpropanolamine

Warnings Administer with caution to patients with hypertension, hyperthyroidism, diabetes mellitus, cardiovascular disease, ischemic heart disease, increased intraocular pressure, or prostatic hypertrophy. Elderly patients are more likely to experience adverse reactions to sympathomimetics; overdosage may cause hallucinations, seizures, CNS depression, and death.

Adverse Reactions
Cardiovascular: Palpitations, reflex bradycardia, arrhythmias, hypertension, angina, stimulating sympathomimetic agents
Central nervous system: Anxiety, nervousness, restlessness, headache
Gastrointestinal: Dry mouth, nausea
Genitourinary: Difficult urination

Overdosage Symptoms of overdose include vomiting, hypertension, palpitations, paresthesias, excitation, seizures

Toxicology Treatment is supportive; in extreme cases, I.V. phentolamine may be used

Drug Interactions
Decreased effect of antihypertensives
Increased effect/toxicity with tricyclic antidepressants, MAO inhibitors, increased effect of caffeine

Mechanism of Action Releases tissue stores of epinephrine and thereby produces an alpha- and beta-adrenergic stimulation; this causes vasoconstriction and nasal mucosa blanching; also appears to depress central appetite centers; increases urethral resistance to prevent urine leakage during times of increased intra-abdominal pressure

Pharmacokinetics
Absorption: Oral: Well absorbed
Bioavailability: Close to 100%
Half-life: 4.6-6.6 hours
Metabolism: In the liver to norephedrine
Elimination: In urine primarily as unchanged drug (80% to 90%)

Usual Dosage Oral:
Geriatrics:
Decongestant: 25 mg every 4-6 hours as needed
Urinary incontinence: 75 mg twice daily

Adults: Decongestant: 25 mg every 4 hours or 50 mg every 8 hours as needed, not to exceed 150 mg/day; sustained release: 75 mg every 12 hours

Monitoring Parameters Blood pressure, pulse, relief of symptoms, episodes of urinary incontinence

Patient Information Do not exceed recommended doses; consult physician or pharmacist before using; notify physician of insomnia, weakness, dizziness, tremor, or irregular heartbeat

Additional Information Phenylpropanolamine is found is many combination cough and cold products

Special Geriatric Considerations Not recommended for use an as anorexiant in the elderly. Phenylpropanolamine is ~75% effective in controlling mild to moderate stress incontinence. Elderly patients should be counseled about the proper use of over-the-counter cough and cold preparations; see Warnings.

Dosage Forms
Capsules, timed release: 75 mg
Tablets: 25 mg, 50 mg

References
Romanowski GL, Shimp LA, Balson AB, et al, "Urinary Incontinence in the Elderly: Etiology and Treatment," *Drug Intell Clin Pharm*, 1988, 22(7-8):525-33.

Phenytoin (fen' i toyn)
Related Information
Antacid Drug Interactions *on page 764*
Drug Levels Commonly Monitored Guidelines *on page 771-772*

Brand Names Dilantin®; Diphenylan Sodium®

Synonyms Diphenylhydantoin; DPH; Phenytoin Sodium, Extended; Phenytoin Sodium, Prompt

(Continued)

Phenytoin *(Continued)*

Generic Available Yes

Therapeutic Class Antiarrhythmic Agent, Class IB; Anticonvulsant, Hydantoin

Use Management of generalized tonic-clonic (grand mal), simple partial and complex partial seizures; prevention of seizures following head trauma/neurosurgery; ventricular arrhythmias, including those associated with digitalis intoxication, also used for epidermolysis bullosa; trigeminal neuralgia

Contraindications Hypersensitivity to phenytoin or any component; heart block, sinus bradycardia

Warnings Do not withdraw abruptly in seizure patients; elderly and patients with hepatic disease may accumulate and cause toxicity; discontinue in hepatic failure; patients with a low serum albumin or Cl_{cr} <10 mL/minute, may have an increase unbound (free) concentration

Precautions May increase frequency of petit mal seizures; I.V. form may cause hypotension, skin necrosis at I.V. site; avoid I.V. administration in small veins; use with caution in patients with porphyria; discontinue if rash or lymphadenopathy occurs

Adverse Reactions

Dose-related:

Central nervous system: Ataxia, slurred speech, dizziness, drowsiness, lethargy, confusion, fever, mood changes, coma

Dermatologic: Rash, hirsutism, coarsening of facial features

Endocrine & metabolic: Folic acid depletion, hyperglycemia

Gastrointestinal: Nausea, vomiting, gingival hyperplasia

Neuromuscular & skeletal: Peripheral neuropathy, tenderness, osteomalacia

Ocular: Nystagmus, blurred vision, diplopia

I.V.:

Cardiovascular: Hypotension, bradycardia, cardiac arrhythmias, thrombophlebitis

Local: Venous irritation and pain

Rarely:

Dermatologic: Stevens-Johnson syndrome

Hematologic: Blood dyscrasias, pseudolymphoma, lymphoma

Hepatic: Hepatitis

Neuromuscular & skeletal: Dyskinesias

Miscellaneous: SLE-like syndrome, lymphadenopathy

Overdosage Symptoms of overdose include unsteady gait, slurred speech, confusion, nausea, hypothermia, fever, hypotension, respiratory depression, coma

Drug Interactions

Phenytoin may decrease the serum concentration or effectiveness of valproic acid, ethosuximide, primidone, warfarin, corticosteroids, cyclosporin, theophylline, chloramphenicol, rifampin, doxycycline, quinidine, mexiletine, disopyramide, dopamine, or nondepolarizing skeletal muscle relaxants

Protein binding of phenytoin can be affected by valproic acid or salicylates

Serum phenytoin concentrations may be increased by cimetidine, chloramphenicol, INH, trimethoprim, or sulfonamides and decreased by rifampin, cisplatin, vinblastine, bleomycin, folic acid, or continuous NG feeds; do not use extended release capsules for enteral feeding (NG)

Stability Parenteral solution may be used as long as there is no precipitate and it is not hazy; slightly yellowed solution may be used; refrigeration may cause precipitate, sometimes the precipitate is resolved by allowing the solution to reach room temperature again; drug may precipitate with pH ≤11.5; do not mix with other medications; may dilute with normal saline for I.V. infusion, but must be diluted to concentration <6 mg/mL

Mechanism of Action Stabilizes neuronal membranes and decreases seizure activity by increasing efflux or decreasing influx of sodium ions across cell membranes in the motor cortex during generation of nerve impulses; prolongs effective refractory period and suppresses ventricular pacemaker automaticity, shortens action potential in the heart

Pharmacokinetics

Absorption: Oral: Slow

Distribution: V_d: 0.6-0.7 L/kg

Protein binding: 90% to 95%

Bioavailability and peak serum levels are dependent upon formulation administered

Time to peak: Oral:

Extended release capsule: Within 4-12 hours

Immediate release preparation: Within 2-3 hours

Elimination: <5% excreted unchanged in urine

Highly variable clearance, dependent upon intrinsic hepatic function and dose administered; major metabolite (via oxidation) HPPA undergoes enterohepatic recycling and elimination in urine as glucuronides

Increased clearance and decreased serum concentrations with febrile illness

ALPHABETICAL LISTING OF DRUGS

Usual Dosage Geriatrics and Adults:

Status epilepticus: I.V.:

Loading dose: 15-18 mg/kg in a single or divided dose at a rate of 25 mg/minute; maintenance, anticonvulsant: usual: 300 mg/day or 5-6 mg/kg/day in 3 divided doses or 1-2 divided doses using extended release; do not exceed 25-50 mg/minute infusion rate with I.V. use; recommended to initiate status epilepticus loading with 25 mg/minute, especially if elderly have any cardiovascular disease, to avoid adverse effects

Anticonvulsant: Oral:

Loading dose: 15-20 mg/kg; based on phenytoin serum concentrations and recent dosing history; administer oral loading dose in 3 divided doses given every 2-4 hours to decrease GI adverse effects and to ensure complete oral absorption; maintenance dose: same as I.V.; doses >400 mg should be divided to avoid possible gastric irritation and reduced absorption

Arrhythmias:

Loading dose: I.V.: 1.25 mg/kg IVP every 5 minutes may repeat up to total loading dose: 15 mg/kg; do not exceed 25-50 mg/minute infusion rate with I.V. use
Maintenance dose: Oral: 250 mg 4 times/day for 1 day, 250 mg twice daily for 2 days, then maintenance at 300-400 mg/day in divided doses 1-4 times/day

See tables.

Adjustment of Serum Concentration in Patients With Low Serum Albumin

Measured Total Phenytoin Concentration (μg/mL)	Patient's Serum Albumin (g/dL)			
	3.5	3	2.5	2
	Adjusted Total Phenytoin Concentration (μg/mL)*			
5	6	7	8	10
10	13	14	17	20
15	19	21	25	30

*Adjusted concentration = measured total concentration ÷ [(0.2 x albumin) + 0.1].

Adjustment of Serum Concentration in Patients With Renal Failure (Cl_cr ≤10 mL/min)
(Product Information from Parke–Davis)

Measured Total Phenytoin Concentration (μg/mL)	Patient's Serum Albumin (g/dL)				
	4	3.5	3	2.5	2
	Adjusted Total Phenytoin Concentration (μg/mL)*				
5	10	11	13	14	17
10	20	22	25	29	33
15	30	33	38	43	50

*Adjusted concentration = measured total concentration ÷ [(0.1 x albumin) + 0.1].

Monitoring Parameters Monitor serum concentration, gait, CNS effects, speech; free concentrations for patients with low serum albumin

Reference Range

Therapeutic: 10-20 μg/mL (SI: 40-79 μmol/L); for status epilepticus, initial serum concentrations should be between 20-25 μg/mL with later serum concentrations (24 hours) in the 10-20 μg/mL range; some recommend the therapeutic range be extended to 5-20 μg/mL; free serum concentration: 0.5-2 μg/mL

Toxicity is measured clinically, and some patients require levels outside the suggested therapeutic range; Toxic: 30-50 μg/mL (SI: 120-200 μmol/L)

Lethal: >100 μg/mL (SI: >400 μmol/L)

Do not obtain serum for analysis 8-12 hours after administration; spurious elevations will be seen due to slow distribution of phenytoin

Test Interactions Increased glucose, alkaline phosphatase (S); decreased thyroxine (S), calcium (S)

Patient Information Shake oral suspension well prior to each dose; do not change brand or dosage form without consulting physician; may cause drowsiness; report

(Continued)

Phenytoin *(Continued)*

any incoordination, blurred vision; good oral hygiene may help prevent gingival tissue hyperplasia

Nursing Implications I.V. injections should be followed by normal saline flushes through the same needle or I.V. catheter to avoid local irritation of the vein; must be diluted to concentrations <6 mg/mL, in normal saline, for I.V. infusion; patients with enteral feeding tubes should have feeding stopped 2 hours before and after dosing with suspension

Additional Information Not recommended to be given I.M. unless no other route exists due to erratic absorption; best to not switch brands once stabilized

Special Geriatric Considerations Elderly may have reduced hepatic clearance due to age decline in phase I metabolism; elderly may have low albumin which will increase free fraction and, therefore, pharmacologic response; monitor closely in those who are hypoalbuminemic; free fraction measurements advised, also elderly may display a higher incidence of adverse effects (cardiovascular) when using the I.V. loading regimen; therefore, recommended to decrease loading I.V. dose to 25 mg/minute; see Warnings

Dosage Forms
Capsule, as sodium, extended: 30 mg, 100 mg
Capsule, as sodium, prompt: 30 mg, 100 mg
Injection, as sodium: 50 mg/mL (2 mL, 5 mL)
Suspension, oral: 30 mg/5 mL (5 mL, 240 mL); 125 mg/5 mL (5 mL, 240 mL)
Tablet, chewable: 50 mg

Phenytoin Sodium, Extended *see* Phenytoin *on page 559*

Phenytoin Sodium, Prompt *see* Phenytoin *on page 559*

Phenzodine® *see* Phenazopyridine Hydrochloride *on page 552*

Phillips® LaxCaps® [OTC] *see* Docusate and Phenolphthalein *on page 238*

Phillips'® Milk of Magnesia [OTC] *see* Magnesium Hydroxide *on page 427*

Phos-Ex® *see* Calcium Acetate *on page 107*

Phos-Flur® *see* Fluoride *on page 299*

PhosLo® *see* Calcium Acetate *on page 107*

Phosphaljel® [OTC] *see* Aluminum Phosphate *on page 33*

Phosphate, Potassium *see* Potassium Phosphate *on page 579*

Phospholine Iodide® *see* Echothiophate Iodide *on page 248*

p-Hydroxyampicillin *see* Amoxicillin Trihydrate *on page 49*

Phyllocontin® *see* Aminophylline *on page 39*

Phylloquinone *see* Vitamin K and Menadiol *on page 738*

Physostigmine *(fye zoe stig' meen)*

Related Information
Glaucoma Drug Therapy Comparison *on page 810*

Brand Names Antilirium®; Isopto® Eserine

Synonyms Eserine Salicylate

Generic Available Yes: Ophthalmic

Therapeutic Class Antidote, Anticholinergic Agent; Cholinergic Agent; Cholinergic Agent, Ophthalmic

Use Reverse toxic CNS effects caused by anticholinergic drugs; used as miotic in treatment of glaucoma

Unlabeled use: Alzheimer's disease

Contraindications Hypersensitivity to physostigmine or any component; GI or GU obstruction, asthma, diabetes, gangrene, cardiovascular disease

Precautions Use with caution in patients with epilepsy, bradycardia. Discontinue if excessive salivation or emesis, frequent urination or diarrhea occur. Reduce dosage if excessive sweating or nausea occur. Administer I.V. slowly or at a controlled rate not faster than 1 mg/minute. Due to the possibility of hypersensitivity or overdose/cholinergic crisis, atropine should be readily available.

Adverse Reactions
Cardiovascular: Palpitations, bradycardia
Central nervous system: Restlessness, hallucinations, seizures
Gastrointestinal: Nausea, vomiting, salivation
Genitourinary: Frequent urge to urinate
Local: Topical stinging, burning, lacrimation
Neuromuscular & skeletal: Muscle twitching, weakness
Ocular: Miosis, blurred vision, eye pain

Respiratory: Dyspnea, bronchospasm, respiratory paralysis, pulmonary edema
Miscellaneous: Sweating

Overdose Symptoms of overdose include muscle weakness, blurred vision, excessive sweating, tearing and salivation, nausea, vomiting, bronchospasm, seizures

Toxicology Physostigmine has proven useful in the treatment of central nervous system effects caused by anticholinergic agents. However, physostigmine has been associated with intoxications as well. If physostigmine is used in excess or in the absence of an anticholinergic overdose, patients may manifest signs of cholinergic toxicity. At this point an anticholinergic agent (eg, atropine 0.015-0.05 mg/kg) may be necessary.

Drug Interactions Increased toxicity with bethanechol, methacholine, succinylcholine

Mechanism of Action Inhibits destruction of acetylcholine by acetylcholinesterase which facilitates transmission of impulses across myoneural junction

Pharmacodynamics
Onset of action:
Ophthalmic: Within 2 minutes
Parenteral: Within 5 minutes

Pharmacokinetics
Absorption: I.M., S.C., ophthalmic: Readily absorbed
Distribution: Crosses the blood-brain barrier readily and reverses both central and peripheral anticholinergic effects
Half-life: 1-2 hours
Metabolism: In the liver

Usual Dosage Geriatrics and Adults:
I.M., I.V., S.C.: 0.5-2 mg to start, repeat every 20 minutes until response occurs or adverse effect occurs; maximum I.V. rate: 1 mg/minute
I.M., I.V. to reverse the anticholinergic effects of atropine or scopolamine given as preanesthetic medications: Give twice the dose, on a weight basis of the anticholinergic drug
Ointment, ophthalmic: Administer ¼" up to 3 times/day
Solution, ophthalmic: Instill 1-2 drops up to 4 times/day

Monitoring Parameters Blood pressure, pulse, intraocular pressure

Test Interactions Increased aminotransferase [ALT (SGPT)/AST (SGOT)] (S), increased amylase (S)

Nursing Implications Too rapid administration (I.V. rate not to exceed 1 mg/minute) can cause bradycardia, hypersalivation leading to respiratory difficulties and seizures

Special Geriatric Considerations Studies on the use of physostigmine in Alzheimer's disease have reported variable results. Doses generally were in the range of 2-4 mg 4 times/day. Limitations to the use of physostigmine include a short half-life requiring frequent dosing, variable absorption from the GI tract, and no commercially available oral product; therefore, not recommended for treatment of Alzheimer's disease

Dosage Forms
Injection, as salicylate: 1 mg/mL (2 mL)
Ointment, ophthalmic: 0.25% (3.5 g, 3.7 g)
Solution, ophthalmic: 0.25% (15 mL); 0.5% (2 mL, 15 mL)

References
Jenike MA, Albert MS, Heller H, et al, "Oral Physostigmine Treatment for Patients With Presenile and Senile Dementia of the Alzheimer's Type: A Double-Blind Placebo-Controlled Trial," *J Clin Psychiatry*, 1990, 51(1):3-7.
Theesen KA, Boyd JA, "Dementia of the Alzheimer's Type: An Update," *Consult Pharm*, 1990, 5:535-40.

Phytomenadione *see* Vitamin K and Menadiol *on page 738*

Phytonadione *see* Vitamin K and Menadiol *on page 738*

Pilagan® *see* Pilocarpine *on this page*

Pilocar® *see* Pilocarpine *on this page*

Pilocarpine (pye loe kar' peen)
Related Information
Glaucoma Drug Therapy Comparison *on page 810*

Brand Names Adsorbocarpine®; Akarpine®; I-Pilocarpine®; Isopto® Carpine; Ocu-Carpine®; Ocusert® Pilo; Pilagan®; Pilocar®; Pilopine HS®; Piloptic®; Pilostat®

Generic Available Yes: Solution

Therapeutic Class Cholinergic Agent, Ophthalmic; Ophthalmic Agent, Miotic

Use Management of chronic simple glaucoma, chronic and acute angle-closure glaucoma; counter effects of cycloplegics; treat xerostomia

Contraindications Hypersensitivity to pilocarpine or any component; acute inflammatory disease of anterior chamber

Precautions Use with caution in patients with corneal abrasion; narrow-angle glaucoma (may promote acute-angle closure)

(Continued)

Pilocarpine (Continued)

Adverse Reactions
Cardiovascular: Hypertension, tachycardia
Central nervous system: Headache, browache
Gastrointestinal: Salivation, nausea, vomiting, diarrhea
Genitourinary: Urination
Local: Stinging, burning, lacrimation
Ocular: Miosis, ciliary spasm, blurred vision, retinal detachment, photophobia, acute iritis, conjunctival and ciliary congestion early in therapy, decreased night vision
Miscellaneous: Sweating, hypersensitivity reactions

Overdosage Symptoms of overdose include bronchospasm, bradycardia, involuntary urination, vomiting, hypotension, tremors

Toxicology Atropine is the treatment of choice for intoxications manifesting with significant muscarinic symptoms. Atropine I.V. 2-4 mg every 3-60 minutes should be repeated to control symptoms and then continued as needed for 1-2 days following the acute ingestion. Epinephrine 0.1-1 mg S.C. may be useful in reversing severe cardiovascular or pulmonary sequel.

Stability Refrigerate gel

Mechanism of Action Directly stimulates cholinergic receptors in the eye causing miosis (by contraction of the iris sphincter), loss of accommodation (by constriction of ciliary muscle), and lowering of intraocular pressure (with decreased resistance to aqueous humor outflow)

Pharmacodynamics
Ophthalmic:
  Onset of action: Miosis occurs within 10-30 minutes
  Duration: 4-8 hours
Intraocular pressure reduction requires an hour to begin and persists for 4-12 hours
Ocusert® Pilo application:
  Onset of action: 90-120 minutes; miosis occurs within 10-30 minutes
  Peak effect: Within 30-40 minutes
  Duration: 4-8 hours; reduced intraocular pressure is detectable within 60 minutes and lasts 4-14 hours, depending on concentration

Usual Dosage Geriatrics and Adults: Ophthalmic:
Nitrate solution: Shake well before using; instill 1-2 drops 2-4 times/day
Hydrochloride solution:
  Instill 1-2 drops up to 6 times/day; adjust the concentration and frequency as required to control elevated intraocular pressure
  To counteract the mydriatic effects of sympathomimetic agents: Instill 1 drop of a 1% solution in the affected eye
Gel: Instill ½" ribbon into lower conjunctival sac once daily at bedtime
Ocular systems: Systems are labeled in terms of mean rate of release of pilocarpine over 7 days; begin with 20 μg/hour at night and adjust based on response

Monitoring Parameters Intraocular pressure, fundoscopic exam, visual field testing

Patient Information May sting on instillation, do not touch dropper to eye; visual acuity may be decreased after administration; night vision may be decreased; distance vision may be altered. Do not leave damaged Ocusert® system in the eye; read package instructions for insertion; after topical instillation, finger pressure should be applied to lacrimal sac to decrease drainage into the nose and throat and minimize possible systemic absorption

Dosage Form	Strength %	1 mL	2 mL	15 mL	30 mL	3.5 g
Gel	4					x
Solution as hydrochloride	0.25			x		
	0.5			x	x	
	1	x	x	x	x	
	2		x	x	x	
	3			x	x	
	4	x	x	x	x	
	6			x	x	
	8		x			
	10			x		
Solution as nitrate	1			x		
	2			x		
	4			x		
Ocusert® Pilo–20: Releases 20 mcg/hour for 1 week						
Ocusert® Pilo–40: Releases 40 mcg/hour for 1 week						

Nursing Implications Usually causes difficulty in dark adaptation; advise patients to use caution while night driving or performing hazardous tasks in poor illumination; after topical instillation, finger pressure should be applied to lacrimal sac to decrease drainage into the nose and throat and minimize possible systemic absorption

Special Geriatric Considerations Assure the patient or a caregiver can adequately administer ophthalmic medication dosage form

Dosage Forms See table.

Pilocarpine and Epinephrine (pye loe kar' peen & ep i nef' rin)
Related Information
Epinephrine *on page 256*
Pilocarpine *on previous page*
Brand Names P$_1$E$_1$®; P$_2$E$_1$®; P$_4$E$_1$®; P$_6$E$_1$®
Therapeutic Class Ophthalmic Agent, Miotic
Use Treatment of glaucoma; counter effect of cycloplegics
Contraindications Hypersensitivity to pilocarpine, epinephrine or any component; acute inflammatory disease of anterior chamber
Precautions Use with caution in patients with corneal abrasion and narrow-angle glaucoma
Adverse Reactions
Cardiovascular: Tachycardia, hypertension
Central nervous system: Headache, brow ache
Gastrointestinal: Salivation
Local: Stinging, itching
Ocular: Miosis, ciliary spasm, blurred vision, retinal detachment vitreous hemorrhages, photophobia, acute iritis, lacrimation
Miscellaneous: Hypersensitivity reactions
Pharmacodynamics
Onset of action: Miosis occurs within 10-30 minutes
Peak effect: Within 30-40 minutes
Duration: 4-8 hours; reduced intraocular pressure is detectable within 60 minutes and lasts 4-14 hours, depending on concentration
Usual Dosage Geriatrics and Adults: Instill 1-2 drops up to 6 times/day
Monitoring Parameters Intraocular pressure, fundiscopic exam, visual field testing
Patient Information May sting on instillation, do not touch dropper to eye
Nursing Implications Usually causes difficulty in dark adaptation; advise patients to use caution while night driving or performing hazardous tasks in poor illumination
Special Geriatric Considerations Assess patient's ability to self-administer ophthalmic drops; use with caution in patients with cardiovascular disease
Dosage Forms Solution, ophthalmic: Epinephrine bitartrate 1% and pilocarpine hydrochloride 1%, 2%, 4%, 6% (15 mL)

Pilopine HS® *see* Pilocarpine *on page 563*
Piloptic® *see* Pilocarpine *on page 563*
Pilostat® *see* Pilocarpine *on page 563*

Pimozide (pi' moe zide)
Related Information
Antipsychotic Agents Comparison *on page 801*
Brand Names Orap™
Generic Available No
Therapeutic Class Neuroleptic Agent
Use Suppression of severe motor and phonic tics in patients with Tourette's disorder who have failed to respond to other standard treatment
Contraindications Simple tics other than Tourette's, phonic tics and drug-induced motor tics (eg, amphetamines, methylphenidate, pemoline), history of cardiac dysrhythmias, administration with other medications is known to prolong Q-T interval, known hypersensitivity to pimozide, use with caution in patients with hypersensitivity to other neuroleptics; do not use in patients with severe CNS depression or comatose patients
Warnings Tardive dyskinesia may develop, especially in elderly females taking high doses; prolongation of Q-T intervals with sudden death has occurred in patients receiving doses of approximately 1 mg/kg; sudden death and grand mal seizures have occurred at doses >20 mg/kg; prolongation of Q-T interval may be responsible for sudden deaths since this may predispose patient to ventricular arrhythmias; recommend baseline EKG and EKG with dosage increases to observe for serious adverse effects; carcinogenic potential suggested in mice studies, however, no clinical significance known in man; neuroleptic malignant syndrome can occur with the use of neuroleptics
(Continued)

Pimozide (Continued)

Precautions Hypokalemia is associated with ventricular arrhythmias, therefore correct any existing deficiency before starting pimozide; use with caution in elderly as anticholinergic side effects are caused by pimozide; use with caution in patients with renal/hepatic impairment; may caused decreased alertness

Adverse Reactions

Cardiovascular: Ventricular dysrhythmias, sudden death, Q-T interval increase, hypertension, hypotension, postural hypotension, chest pain, palpitations, tachycardia, syncope

Central nervous system: Extrapyramidal effects (usually in first few days of treatment), tardive dyskinesia, motor restlessness, akathisia, dystonias, opisthotonos, oculogyric crisis, neuroleptic malignant syndrome, seizures, headache, sedation, drowsiness, insomnia, speech difficulties, akinesia, dizziness, nervousness, anxiety, Parkinson's syndrome, depression, hyperpyrexia

Dermatologic: Rash

Gastrointestinal: Diarrhea, constipation, thirst, dry mouth, belching, salivation, anorexia, nausea, vomiting, GI distress

Genitourinary: Nocturia, urinary frequency, impotence

Neuromuscular & skeletal: Tremors, hyperreflexia

Ocular: Visual disturbances, light sensitivity, spots before eyes

Respiratory: Respiratory failure

Miscellaneous: Taste changes, sweating

Overdosage Symptoms of overdose include hypotension, coma, respiratory depression, EKG abnormalities, extrapyramidal symptoms

Toxicology Following attempts at decontamination, treatment is supportive and symptomatic. Seizures can be treated with diazepam, phenytoin, or phenobarbital; monitor EKG until normal EKG is achieved; use I.V. fluids for hypotension/circulating collapse, plasma, vasopressors (norepinephrine) **do not use epinephrine**; observe patient for 4 days

Drug Interactions Pimozide lowers seizures threshold, therefore may interfere with anticonvulsant therapy; Q-T interval may be increased when pimozide is used with tricyclic antidepressants, phenothiazines, or other antiarrhythmics; pimozide will increase sedation associated with CNS depressant drugs

Mechanism of Action A potent centrally acting dopamine receptor antagonist resulting in its characteristic neuroleptic effects

Pharmacokinetics

Absorption: Oral: 50%

Protein binding: 99%

Metabolism: In the liver with significant first-pass decay

Half-life: 50 hours

Time to peak serum concentration: Within 6-8 hours

Elimination: Metabolites excreted in urine

Usual Dosage

Geriatrics: Recommend initial dose of 1 mg/day; periodically attempt gradual reduction of dose to determine if tic persists; follow up for 1-2 weeks before concluding the tic is a persistent disease phenomenon and not a manifestation of drug withdrawal

Adults: **Note:** Recommend obtaining a baseline EKG and done periodically, especially with dose increases or addition of drugs which may interact. Oral: Initial: 1-2 mg/day, increase dosage as needed every other day; maximum dose: 10 mg

Dosing adjustment in hepatic impairment: Reduction of dose is necessary in patients with liver disease

Monitoring Parameters Monitor EKG, blood pressure, and CNS side effects

Test Interactions Increased prolactin (S)

Patient Information May cause drowsiness; use caution when driving or performing tasks which require alertness; do not stop medication without physician advice

Nursing Implications Must obtain baseline EKG and an EKG with dose increases; see Adverse Reactions and Monitoring Parameters

Additional Information Treatment with pimozide exposes the patient to serious risks; a decision to use pimozide chronically in Tourette's disorder is one that deserves full consideration by the patient (or patient's family) as well as by the treating physician. Because the goal of treatment is symptomatic improvement, the patient's view of the need for treatment and assessment of response are critical in evaluating the impact of therapy and weighing its benefits against the risks.

Special Geriatric Considerations No specific clinical studies in the use of this drug in elderly; use with extreme caution in elderly due to cardiovascular effects; consider cardiovascular effects of drugs the elderly patient may be receiving

Dosage Forms Tablet: 2 mg

Pindolol (pin' doe lole)

Related Information

Beta-Blockers Comparison on page 804-805

Brand Names Visken®
Generic Available No
Therapeutic Class Beta-Adrenergic Blocker
Use Management of hypertension

Unlabeled use: Ventricular arrhythmias/tachycardia, antipsychotic-induced akathisia, situational anxiety; aggressive behavior associated with dementia

Contraindications Uncompensated congestive heart failure, cardiogenic shock, bradycardia or heart block, asthma, bronchospasm, COPD

Warnings Use with caution in patients with inadequate myocardial function; acute withdrawal may exacerbate symptoms; use with caution in patients undergoing anesthesia, bronchospastic disease, hyperthyroidism, impaired hepatic function, diabetes mellitus, hyperthyroidism. Abrupt withdrawal of the drug should be avoided, drug should be discontinued over 1-2 weeks; may potentiate hypoglycemia in a diabetic patient and mask signs and symptoms; sweating will continue

Adverse Reactions
Cardiovascular: A-V block, edema, hypotension, impaired myocardial contractility
Central nervous system: Dizziness, fatigue, insomnia, depression
Gastrointestinal: Ischemic colitis, nausea, vomiting, diarrhea, GI distress
Genitourinary: Decreased sexual ability
Neuromuscular & skeletal: Muscle pain, cold extremities
Respiratory: Bronchospasm

Overdosage Symptoms of overdose include severe hypotension, bradycardia, heart failure, and bronchospasm

Toxicology Sympathomimetics (eg, epinephrine or dopamine), glucagon or a pacemaker can be used to treat the toxic bradycardia, asystole, and/or hypotension; initially fluids may be the best treatment for toxic hypotension.

Drug Interactions
Decreased effect with NSAIDs, sympathomimetics
Increased effect with diuretics, other antihypertensives

Mechanism of Action Blocks both beta$_1$- and beta$_2$-receptors and has mild intrinsic sympathomimetic activity; pindolol has negative inotropic and chronotropic effects and can significantly slow A-V nodal conduction

Pharmacodynamics One study found that beta blockade lasted longer in elderly patients as compared to younger patients

Pharmacokinetics
Absorption: Oral: Rapid, 50% to 95%
Protein binding: 50%
Metabolism: In the liver (60% to 65%) to conjugates
Half-life: 2.5-4 hours (increased with renal insufficiency, and cirrhosis); half-life is not significantly prolonged in the elderly, though some accumulation of drug may occur (related to renal function)
Time to peak: Within 1-2 hours
Elimination: In urine (35% to 50% unchanged drug)

Usual Dosage
Geriatrics: Initial: 5 mg once daily, increase as necessary by 5 mg/day every 3-4 weeks

Adults: Initial: 5 mg twice daily, increase as necessary by 10 mg/day every 3-4 weeks; maximum daily dose: 60 mg

Monitoring Parameters Blood pressure, standing and sitting/supine, pulse, respiratory function, signs of congestive heart failure

Test Interactions Increased cholesterol (S), decreased glucose; decreased bilirubin (S)

Patient Information Do not discontinue medication abruptly; consult pharmacist or physician before taking over-the-counter cold preparations

Nursing Implications Do not discontinue abruptly; see Monitoring Parameters

Special Geriatric Considerations Due to alterations in the beta-adrenergic autonomic nervous system, beta-adrenergic blockade may result in less hemodynamic response than seen in younger adults. Studies indicate that despite decreased sensitivity to the chronotropic effects of beta blockade with age, there appears to be an increased myocardial sensitivity to the negative inotropic effect during stress (ie, exercise). Controlled trials have shown the overall response rate for propranolol to be only 20% to 50% in elderly populations. Therefore, all beta-adrenergic blocking drugs may result in a decreased response as compared to younger adults; see Pharmacodynamics and Pharmacokinetics.

Dosage Forms Tablet: 5 mg, 10 mg

References
Gretzer I, Alvan G, Duner H, et al, "Beta-Blocking Effect and Pharmacokinetics of Pindolol in Young and Elderly Hypertensive Patients," *Eur J Clin Pharmacol*, 1986, 31(4):415-8.

Pink Bismuth® [OTC] *see* Bismuth *on page 88*

Piperacillin Sodium (pi per' a sill in)

Brand Names Pipracil®

Generic Available No

Therapeutic Class Antibiotic, Penicillin

Use Treatment of *Pseudomonas aeruginosa* infections in combination with an aminoglycoside which are susceptible to piperacillin; also effective against other gram-negative microorganisms and nonpenicillinase-producing anaerobes (including *B. fragilis*) and gram-positive organisms; normally used with other antibiotics (ie, aminoglycosides)

Contraindications Hypersensitivity to piperacillin or any component or penicillins

Precautions Dosage modification required in patients with impaired renal function; use with caution in patients with cephalosporin allergy

Adverse Reactions
Cardiovascular: Thrombophlebitis
Central nervous system: Convulsions, confusion, drowsiness, seizures, fever
Dermatologic: Rash, exfoliative dermatitis
Endocrine & metabolic: Electrolyte imbalance, hypokalemia
Gastrointestinal: Diarrhea
Hematologic: Hemolytic anemia, eosinophilia, neutropenia, prolonged bleeding time
Hepatic: Positive Coombs' reaction, elevated liver enzymes
Neuromuscular & skeletal: Myoclonus
Renal: Acute interstitial nephritis
Miscellaneous: Hypersensitivity reactions, anaphylaxis, serum sickness-like reaction

Overdosage Symptoms of overdose include neuromuscular hypersensitivity, seizure

Toxicology Many beta-lactam-containing antibiotics have the potential to cause neuromuscular hyperirritability or convulsive seizures. Hemodialysis may be helpful to aid in the removal of the drug from the blood, otherwise most treatment is supportive or symptom directed.

Drug Interactions
Decreased effect if administration is within 1 hour prior to or 4 hours after aminoglycosides in patients with renal impairment
Increased levels with probenecid

Stability Reconstituted solution is stable (I.V. infusion) in NS or D$_5$W for 24 hours at room temperature, 7 days when refrigerated or 4 weeks when frozen; after freezing, thawed solution is stable for 24 hours at room temperature or 48 hours when refrigerated; 40 g bulk vial should NOT be frozen after reconstitution; incompatible with aminoglycosides

Mechanism of Action Interferes with bacterial cell wall synthesis during active multiplication causing cell death and resultant bactericidal activity against susceptible bacteria

Pharmacodynamics Bactericidal

Pharmacokinetics
Absorption: I.M.: 70% to 80%
Protein binding: 22%
Half-life: Adults: 36-80 minutes (dose-dependent), prolonged with moderately severe renal or hepatic impairment
Time to peak: Peak serum levels occur within 30-50 minutes
Elimination: Principally in urine and partially in feces (via bile)

Usual Dosage
Geriatrics:
I.M.: 1-2 g every 8-12 hours
I.V.: 2-4 g every 6-8 hours
Adults: I.M., I.V.: 2-4 g/dose every 4-8 hours

Dosing interval in renal impairment:
Cl$_{cr}$ 20-40 mL/minute: Administer every 8 hours
Cl$_{cr}$ <20 mL/minute: Administer every 12 hours
Moderately dialyzable (20% to 50%)

Monitoring Parameters Temperature, WBC count, mental status, appetite

Test Interactions False-positive urinary and serum proteins, positive Coombs' test [direct]

Nursing Implications Administer 1 hour apart from aminoglycosides; extended spectrum includes *Pseudomonas aeruginosa*; dosage modification required in patients with impaired renal function

Additional Information Sodium content of 1 g: 1.85 mEq

Special Geriatric Considerations Antipseudomonal penicillins should not be used alone and are often combined with an aminoglycoside as empiric therapy for lower respiratory infections and sepsis in which gram-negative (including *Pseudomonal sp.*) and/or anaerobes are of a high probability; because of piperacillin's lower sodium content, it is preferred over ticarcillin in patients with a history of heart failure and/or renal or hepatic disease; adjust dose for renal function

Dosage Forms Injection: 2 g, 3 g, 4 g, 40 g

References
Donowitz GR and Mandell GL, "Beta-Lactam Antibiotics," *N Engl J Med*, 1988, 318(7):419-26 and 318(8):490-500.

Yoshikawa TT, "Antimicrobial Therapy for the Elderly Patient," *J Am Geriatr Soc*, 1990, 38(12):1353-72.

Piperacillin Sodium and Tazobactam Sodium
Related Information
Piperacillin Sodium *on previous page*
Brand Names Zosyn™
Therapeutic Class Antibiotic, Penicillin
Use Treatment of infections of lower respiratory tract, urinary tract, skin and skin structures, gynecologic, bone and joint infections, and septicemia caused by susceptible organisms. Tazobactam expands activity of piperacillin to include beta-lactamase producing strains of *S. aureus, H. influenzae, Enterobacteriaceae, Pseudomonas, Klebsiella, Citrobacter, Serratia, Bacteroides,* and other gram-negative anaerobes.
Contraindications Hypersensitivity to piperacillin, tazobactam, other penicillins, or any component
Warnings Use with caution in patients with known hypersensitivity to cephalosporins or other beta-lactamase inhibitors; use with caution in patients with a history of seizures and in patients with renal function impairment
Adverse Reactions
Cardiovascular: Hypertension, hypotension, edema
Central nervous system: Insomnia, headache, dizziness, agitation, confusion
Dermatologic: Rash
Gastrointestinal: Diarrhea, constipation, nausea, vomiting, dyspepsia, pseudomembranous colitis
Hematologic: Leukopenia
Respiratory: Bronchospasm
Overdosage Symptoms of overdose include neuromuscular hypersensitivity, seizures
Toxicology Many beta-lactam-containing antibiotics have the potential to cause neuromuscular hyperirritability or convulsive seizures. Hemodialysis may be helpful to aid in the removal of the drug from the blood, otherwise most treatment is supportive or symptom directed.
Drug Interactions
Increased duration of neuromuscular blockers
Increased/prolonged levels with probenecid
Stability Store at controlled room temperature; after reconstitution, stable for 24 hours at room temperature and 1 week when refrigerated; unused portions should be discarded after 24 hours at room temperature and 48 hours when refrigerated; not compatible with lactated Ringer's solution
Mechanism of Action Piperacillin interferes with bacterial cell wall synthesis during active multiplication, causing cell wall death and resultant bactericidal activity against susceptible bacteria; tazobactam prevents degradation of piperacillin by binding to the active side on beta-lactamase
Pharmacokinetics Both AUC and peak concentrations are dose proportional
Distribution: Distributes well into lungs, intestinal mucosa, skin, muscle, uterus, ovary, prostate, gallbladder, and bile; penetration into CSF is low in subject with noninflamed meninges
Metabolism:
Piperacillin: 6% to 9%
Tazobactam: ~26%
Protein binding:
Piperacillin: ~26% to 33%
Tazobactam: 31% to 32%
Half-life:
Piperacillin: 1 hour
Metabolite: 1-1.5 hours
Tazobactam: 0.7-0.9 hour
Elimination: Both piperacillin and tazobactam are directly proportional to renal function
Piperacillin: 50% to 70% eliminated unchanged in urine, 10% to 20% excreted in bile
Tazobactam: Found in urine at 24 hours, with 26% as the inactive metabolite
Hemodialysis removes 30% to 40% of piperacillin and tazobactam; peritoneal dialysis removes 11% to 21% of tazobactam and 6% of piperacillin; hepatic impairment does not affect the kinetics of piperacillin or tazobactam significantly
Usual Dosage Geriatrics and Adults: I.V.: 3.375 g (3 g piperacillin/0.375 g tazobactam) every 6 hours

Dosing interval in renal impairment:
Cl_{cr} >40 mL/minute: No change
Cl_{cr} 20-40 mL/minute: Administer 2.25 g every 6 hours
Cl_{cr} <20 mL/minute: Administer 2.25 g every 8 hours
Hemodialysis: Administer 2.25 g every 8 hours with an additional dose of 0.75 g after each dialysis
Administration See Stability
Monitoring Parameters Signs and symptoms of infection, mental status, WBC
(Continued)

Piperacillin Sodium and Tazobactam Sodium *(Continued)*

Test Interactions Positive Coombs' [direct] test 3.8%, increased ALT, increased AST

Nursing Implications Administer 1 hour apart from aminoglycosides; give around-the-clock (ie, 6-12-6-12); see Stability

Special Geriatric Considerations Has not been studied exclusively in the elderly; see Usual Dosage; adjust dose for renal function

Dosage Forms Injection: Piperacillin sodium 2 g and tazobactam sodium 0.25 g; piperacillin sodium 3 g and tazobactam sodium 0.375 g; piperacillin sodium 4 g and tazobactam sodium 0.5 g (vials at an 8:1 ratio of piperacillin sodium to tazobactam sodium)

Piperazine Citrate (pi' per a zeen)

Brand Names Vermizine®

Generic Available Yes

Therapeutic Class Anthelmintic

Use Treatment of pinworm and roundworm infections (used as an alternative to first-line agents, mebendazole, or pyrantel pamoate)

Contraindications Seizure disorders, liver or kidney impairment, hypersensitivity to piperazine or any component

Precautions Use with caution in patients with anemia or malnutrition

Adverse Reactions
Central nervous system: Dizziness, vertigo, seizures, EEG changes, headache
Gastrointestinal: Nausea, vomiting, diarrhea
Hematologic: Hemolytic anemia
Neuromuscular & skeletal: Weakness
Ocular: Visual impairment
Respiratory: Bronchospasm
Miscellaneous: Hypersensitivity reactions

Drug Interactions Pyrantel pamoate (antagonistic mode of action)

Mechanism of Action Causes muscle paralysis of the roundworm by blocking the effects of acetylcholine at the neuromuscular junction

Pharmacokinetics
Absorption: Well absorbed from GI tract
Time to peak: Peak plasma levels at 1 hour
Elimination: In urine as metabolites and unchanged drug

Usual Dosage Geriatrics and Adults: Oral:
Pinworms: 65 mg/kg/day as a single daily dose for 7 days, in severe infections, repeat course after a 1-week interval; not to exceed 2.5 g/day

Roundworms: 3.5 g/day for 2 days (in severe infections, repeat course, after a 1-week interval)

Monitoring Parameters Stool exam for worms and ova

Patient Information Take on an empty stomach; contact physician if headache, dizziness, poor coordination, muscle weakness, seizures, nausea, vomiting, diarrhea, or rash occur; wash bed clothes, towels, night clothes, and maintain good hygiene to prevent spread or reinfection

Nursing Implications Cure rates may be decreased with massive infections or in patients with hypermotility of the GI tract; give on an empty stomach

Special Geriatric Considerations Not a drug of choice; see Adverse Reactions and monitor closely in the elderly

Dosage Forms
Syrup: 500 mg/5 mL (473 mL, 4000 mL)
Tablet: 250 mg

Pipracil® *see* Piperacillin Sodium *on page 568*

Pirbuterol Acetate (peer byoo' ter ole)

Brand Names Maxair™

Synonyms Pyrbuterol

Generic Available No

Therapeutic Class Beta-2-Adrenergic Agonist Agent; Bronchodilator

Use Prevention and treatment of reversible bronchospasm including asthma

Contraindications Hypersensitivity to pirbuterol, adrenergic amines, or any ingredient

Warnings Administer with caution to individuals with unstable vasomotor systems, diabetes, hyperthyroidism, prostatic hypertrophy, or a history of seizures. Also administer with caution to elderly patients, psychoneurotic individuals, and to patients with long-standing bronchial asthma and emphysema who have developed degenerative heart disease

Precautions Excessive use may result in tolerance; deaths have been reported after excessive use; though the exact cause is unknown, cardiac arrest after a severe asthmatic crisis is suspected

Adverse Reactions
Cardiovascular: Tachycardia, palpitations, elevation or depression of blood pressure
Central nervous system: Nervousness, CNS stimulation, hyperactivity, insomnia

Gastrointestinal: GI upset

Neuromuscular: Tremors (may be more common in the elderly)

Overdosage Symptoms of overdose include hypertension, tachycardia, seizures, angina, hypokalemia, and tachyarrhythmias

Toxicology In cases of overdose, supportive therapy should be instituted, and prudent use of a cardioselective beta-adrenergic blocker (eg, atenolol or metoprolol) should be considered, keeping in mind the potential for induction of bronchoconstriction in an asthmatic individual. Dialysis has not been shown to be of value in the treatment of an overdose with this agent.

Drug Interactions

Decreased therapeutic effect: Beta-adrenergic blockers (eg, propranolol)

Increased therapeutic effect: Inhaled ipratropium → ↑ duration of bronchodilation, nifedipine → ↑ FEV-1

Increased toxicity (cardiovascular): MAO inhibitors, tricyclic antidepressants, sympathomimetic agents (eg, amphetamine, dopamine, dobutamine), inhaled anesthetics (eg, enflurane)

Mechanism of Action Relaxes bronchial smooth muscle by action on $beta_2$-receptors with little effect on heart rate (minor $beta_1$ activity)

Pharmacodynamics

Onset of action: Within 5 minutes

Peak effect: 30-60 minutes

Duration of action: 3-5 hours

Pharmacokinetics

Metabolism: In the liver

Elimination: Urine as unchanged drug and metabolites

Usual Dosage Geriatrics and Adults: 2 inhalations (puffs) every 4-6 hours; some patients may be controlled on 1 puff every 4 hours; do not exceed 12 puffs/day

Monitoring Parameters Pulmonary function, blood pressure, pulse

Patient Information Patient instructions are available with product. Do not exceed recommended dosage; rinse mouth with water following each inhalation to help with dry throat and mouth. May cause nervousness, restlessness, insomnia – if these effects continue after dosage reduction, notify physician. Also notify physician if palpitations, tachycardia, chest pain, muscle tremors, dizziness, headache, flushing or if breathing difficulty persists.

Nursing Implications Before using, the inhaler must be shaken well; assess lung sounds, pulse, and blood pressure before administration and during peak of medication; observe patient for wheezing after administration, if this occurs, call physician

Special Geriatric Considerations Elderly patients may find it useful to utilize a spacer device when using a metered dose inhaler. Difficulty in using the inhaler often limits its effectiveness.

Dosage Forms Aerosol, oral: 0.2 mg/actuation (25.6 g) (~300 inhalations)

Piroxicam (peer ox' i kam)

Brand Names Feldene®

Generic Available No

Therapeutic Class Analgesic, Non-narcotic; Anti-inflammatory Agent; Nonsteroidal Anti-inflammatory Agent (NSAID), Oral

Use Management of inflammatory disorders; symptomatic treatment of acute and chronic rheumatoid arthritis, osteoarthritis, and sunburn

Contraindications Hypersensitivity to piroxicam, any component, aspirin or other non-steroidal anti-inflammatory drugs (NSAIDs); active GI bleeding

Warnings GI toxicity (bleeding, ulceration, perforation); CNS effects may occur (headaches, confusion, depression); hypersensitivity, anaphylactoid reactions (intermittent tolmetin use more often); renal function decline, acute renal insufficiency, interstitial nephritis, dysuria, cystitis, hematuria, nephrotic syndrome, hyperkalemia in acute renal insufficiency, hyponatremia, papillary necrosis, hepatic function impairment; elderly have increased risk for adverse reactions to NSAIDs; see Special Geriatric Considerations

Precautions Use with caution in patients with congestive heart failure, hypertension, decreased renal or hepatic function, history of GI disease (bleeding or ulcers), or those receiving anticoagulants; perform ophthalmologic evaluation for those who develop eye complaints during therapy (blurred vision, diminished vision, changes in color vision, retinal changes); NSAIDs may mask signs/symptoms of infections; photosensitivity reported

Adverse Reactions

Cardiovascular: Congestive heart failure, angina, hypertension, hypotension, fluid retention, arrhythmias, edema

Central nervous system: Headache, drowsiness, vertigo, dizziness, fatigue, hallucinations, confusion, depression, emotional lability, psychotic behavior, asthenia

Dermatologic: Rash, urticaria, angioedema, Stevens-Johnson syndrome, exfoliative dermatitis, ecchymosis, petechiae, purpura, bruising

Endocrine & metabolic: Hyperglycemia, hypoglycemia, hyperkalemia, gynecomastia, hyponatremia

(Continued)

Piroxicam *(Continued)*

Gastrointestinal: Dyspepsia, heartburn, nausea, diarrhea, constipation, flatulence, stomatitis, vomiting, abdominal pain, peptic ulcer, GI bleeding, GI perforation, gingival ulcers, pancreatitis, proctitis, paralytic ulcers, colitis, anorexia, weight loss

Genitourinary: Impotence, azotemia

Hematologic: Neutropenia, anemia, agranulocytosis, bone marrow suppression, hemolytic anemia, hemorrhage, inhibition of platelet aggregation

Hepatic: Hepatitis, elevated LFTs, cholestatic jaundice

Neuromuscular & skeletal: Involuntary muscle movements, muscle weakness, tremors

Ocular: Vision changes

Otic: Tinnitus

Renal: Dysuria, polyuria, pyuria, oliguria, anuria, acute renal failure

Respiratory: Exacerbation of asthma, dyspnea

Miscellaneous: Dry mucous membranes, thirst, pyrexia, sweating

Overdosage Symptoms include drowsiness, lethargy, disorientation, confusion, dizziness, numbness, paresthesia, nausea, vomiting, gastric irritation, abdominal pain, headache, tinnitus, sweating, blurred vision, muscle twitching, seizures, coma, acute renal failure, increased BUN and serum creatinine, hypotension, tachycardia, and metabolic acidosis

Toxicology Management of a nonsteroidal anti-inflammatory agent (NSAID) intoxication is primarily supportive and symptomatic. Fluid therapy is commonly effective in managing the hypotension that may occur following an acute NSAID overdose, except when this is due to an acute blood loss. Seizures tend to be very short-lived and often do not require drug treatment although recurrent seizures should be treated with I.V. diazepam. Since many of the NSAIDs undergo enterohepatic cycling, multiple doses of charcoal may be needed to reduce the potential for delayed toxicities.

Drug Interactions

May increase digoxin, methotrexate, and lithium serum concentrations

Aspirin or other salicylates may decrease NSAID serum concentrations

Other NSAIDs may increase adverse GI effects

Increased prothrombin time with anticoagulants

Decreased antihypertensive effects of ACE inhibitors, beta-blockers, and thiazide diuretics

Effects of loop diuretics may decrease

Increased response to sympathomimetics

Probenecid may increase toxicity of NSAIDs by increase in serum concentrations

Diuretics may increase risk of acute renal insufficiency

Azotemia may be enhanced in elderly receiving loop diuretics

Mechanism of Action Inhibits prostaglandin synthesis, acts on the hypothalamus heat-regulating center to reduce fever, blocks prostaglandin synthetase action which prevents formation of the platelet-aggregating substance thromboxane A_2; decreases pain receptor sensitivity. Other proposed mechanisms of action are lysosomal stabilization, kinin and leukotriene production, alteration of chemotactic factors, and inhibition of neutrophil activation. This latter mechanism may be the most significant pharmacologic action to reduce inflammation.

Pharmacodynamics

Onset of analgesia: Oral: Within 1 hour

Duration: 2-3 days

Onset of anti-inflammatory effect: 7-12 days

Peak effect: 2-3 weeks

Pharmacokinetics

Protein binding: 99%

Metabolism: In the liver

Half-life: 45-50 hours

Time to peak: Peak levels achieved 3-5 hours after ingestion

Elimination: Excreted as unchanged drug (5%) and metabolites primarily in urine and to a small degree in feces

Usual Dosage Geriatrics and Adults: Oral: 10-20 mg/day once daily; although associated with increase in GI adverse effects, doses >20 mg/day have been used (ie, 30-40 mg/day); maximum recommended dose: 20 mg/day; assess therapeutic effect after 2 weeks of therapy before increasing doses

Note: Some clinicians have used 10 mg every other day to initiate therapy in elderly to help avoid side effects and produce effect at minimal dose

Monitoring Parameters Monitor response (pain, range of motion, grip strength, mobility, ADL function), inflammation; observe for weight gain, edema; monitor renal function; observe for bleeding, bruising; evaluate gastrointestinal effects (abdominal pain, bleeding, dyspepsia); mental confusion, disorientation, CBC, serum, creatinine, BUN, liver function tests

Test Interactions Increased chloride (S), increased sodium (S)

Patient Information Serious gastrointestinal bleeding can occur as well as ulceration and perforation. Pain may or may not be present. Avoid aspirin and aspirin-containing products while taking this medication. If gastric upset occurs, take with food, milk, or antacid. If gastric adverse effects persist, contact physician. May cause drowsiness, dizziness, blurred vision, and confusion. Use caution when performing tasks which require alertness (eg, driving). Do not take for more than 3 days for fever or 10 days for pain without physician's advice.

Nursing Implications Administer with food to decrease GI adverse effect; monitor CBC, BUN, serum creatinine, liver enzymes; periodic ophthalmologic exams with chronic use

Additional Information Because of its long half-life, may be dosed once daily. There are no clinical guidelines to predict which NSAID will give response in a particular patient. Trials with each must be initiated until response determined. Consider dose, patient convenience, and cost.

Special Geriatric Considerations Elderly are a high-risk population for adverse effects from nonsteroidal anti-inflammatory agents. As much as 60% of elderly can develop peptic ulceration and/or hemorrhage asymptomatically. The concomitant use of H_2 blockers, omeprazole, and sucralfate is not generally effective as prophylaxis. Misoprostol is the only prophylactic agent proven effective. Also, concomitant disease and drug use contribute to the risk for GI adverse effects. Use lowest effective dose for shortest period possible. Consider renal function decline with age. Use of NSAIDs can compromise existing renal function especially when Cl_{cr} is ≤ 30 mL/minute. Tinnitus may be a difficult and unreliable indication of toxicity due to age-related hearing loss or eighth cranial nerve damage. CNS adverse effects such as confusion, agitation, and hallucination are generally seen in overdose or high dose situations, but elderly may demonstrate these adverse effects at lower doses than younger adults.

Dosage Forms Capsule: 10 mg, 20 mg

References

Brooks PM, Day RO, "Nonsteroidal Anti-inflammatory Drugs – Differences and Similarities," *N Engl J Med*, 1991, 324(24):1716-25.

Clinch D, Banerjee AK, Ostick G, "Absence of Abdominal Pain in Elderly Patients With Peptic Ulcer," *Age Ageing*, 1984, 13:120-3.

Clive DM, Stoff JS, "Renal Syndromes Associated With Nonsteroidal Anti-inflammatory Drugs," *N Engl J Med*, 1984, 310(9):563-72.

Graham DY, "Prevention of Gastroduodenal Injury Induced by Chronic Nonsteroidal Anti-inflammatory Drug Therapy," *Gastroenterology*, 1989, 96(2 Pt 2 Suppl):675-81.

Gurwitz JH, Avarn J, Ross-Degan D, et al, "Nonsteroidal Anti-Inflammatory Drug-Associated Azotemia in the Very Old," *JAMA*, 1990, 264(4):471-5.

Knodel LC, "Preventing NSAID-Induced Ulcers: The Role of Misoprostol," *Consult Pharm*, 1989, 4:37-41.

Pounder R, "Silent Peptic Ulceration: Deadly Silence or Golden Silence?" *Gastroenterology*, 1989, 96(2 Pt 2 Suppl):626-31.

***p*-Isobutylhydratropic Acid** *see Ibuprofen on page 360*

Pitressin® *see Vasopressin on page 732*

Pitressin® Tannate in Oil *see Vasopressin on page 732*

Plantago Seed *see Psyllium on page 610*

Plantain Seed *see Psyllium on page 610*

Plaquenil® *see Hydroxychloroquine Sulfate on page 354*

Plendil® *see Felodipine on page 281*

Pneumococcal Vaccine, Polyvalent

Related Information

Immunization Guidelines *on page 759-762*

Brand Names Pneumovax® 23; Pnu-Imune® 23

Therapeutic Class Vaccine, Inactivated Bacteria

Use Immunity to pneumococcal lobar pneumonia and bacteremia in individuals ≥ 2 years of age who are at high risk of morbidity and mortality from pneumococcal infection; patients with a chronic disease which predisposes them to pneumococcal pneumonia (pulmonary, cardiovascular disease, diabetes, alcoholism, liver disease); patients with immunodeficiency due to drugs and/or disease; persons whose living environments place them at risk (nursing homes, hospitals, community epidemics)

Contraindications Active infections, immunosuppressive therapy, Hodgkin's disease patients, hypersensitivity to pneumococcal vaccine or any component

Warnings Hypersensitivity reactions (have epinephrine 1:1000 available); limited effectiveness in preventing infections in patients with skull fractures, external communication with CSF, immune deficiency diseases, certain myeloproliferative diseases, immunosuppressive drugs, splenectomy (vaccination should still be administered)

Precautions Should be administered with caution in individuals who have had episodes of pneumococcal infection within the preceding 3 years – pre-existing pneumococcal antibodies may result in increased reactions to the vaccine; may cause relapse in patients with stable idiopathic thrombocytopenia purpura; patients with cardiac and/or pulmonary disease whom adverse effects to vaccine may be undesirable; revaccination may result in an arthus reaction or other systemic reactions which may be

(Continued)

573

Pneumococcal Vaccine, Polyvalent (Continued)

more frequent and severe; those who received the 14 valent vaccine may benefit from 23 valent vaccine only if at high risk for pneumococcal pneumonia; those at less risk do not have significant benefit

Adverse Reactions Booster doses are associated with an increase in adverse reactions and are currently not recommended

Central nervous system: Fever, paresthesia
Dermatologic: Rash
Local: Erythema, induration, and soreness at the injection site (2-3 days)
Neuromuscular & skeletal: Myalgia, arthralgia
Miscellaneous: Anaphylaxis (rare), Guillain-Barré syndrome

Drug Interactions Immunosuppressive agents

Stability Refrigerate at 2°C to 8°C (36°F to 46°F); at room temperature (25°C) Pnu-Imune® 23 is stable for several days; Pneumovax® 23 is stable for 1 month at temperatures 15°C to 30°C (59°F to 86°F)

Usual Dosage Geriatrics and Adults: I.M., S.C.: 0.5 mL as a one time only dose; recent studies indicate that high-risk patients (ie, severe COPD, immunosuppressed patients) should have this vaccine administered every 6 years

Patient Information Be aware of adverse effects

Nursing Implications Do not inject I.V., avoid intradermal, administer S.C. or I.M. (deltoid muscle or lateral midthigh); no dilution or reconstitution necessary

Additional Information Federal law requires that the date of administration, the vaccine manufacturer, lot number of vaccine, and the administering person's name, title and address be entered into the patient's permanent medical record; inactivated bacteria vaccine

Special Geriatric Considerations Elderly have ~3 times the incidence of pneumococcal pneumonia than younger adults and 30% of all pneumococcal meningitis occurs in persons >50 years of age with a 20% mortality; limited data on elderly; however, the elderly, compared to young adults, develop slightly lower antibody titers; provides 60% to 70% protection for bacterial pneumonia; 90% protection for pneumococcal pneumonia strains; 20% of elderly with pneumococcal pneumonia have an associated bacteremia with a 17% to 40% fatality

Dosage Forms Injection: 25 mcg each of 23 polysaccharide isolates/0.5 mL dose (1 mL, 5 mL)

References

Davidson M, Bulkow LR, Grabman J, et al, "Immunogenicity of Pneumococcal Revaccination in Patients With Chronic Disease," *Arch Intern Med*, 1994, 154(19):2209-14.

Gardner P and Schaffner W, "Immunization of Adults," *N Engl J Med*, 1993, 328(17):1252-8.

Pneumovax® 23 see Pneumococcal Vaccine, Polyvalent on previous page

Pnu-Imune® 23 see Pneumococcal Vaccine, Polyvalent on previous page

Poliomyelitis Vaccine see Poliovirus Vaccine, Inactivated on this page

Poliovax® see Poliovirus Vaccine, Inactivated on this page

Poliovirus Vaccine, Inactivated (poe lee oh vye' russ)

Related Information
Immunization Guidelines on page 759-762

Brand Names IPOL®; Poliovax®

Synonyms IPV; Poliomyelitis Vaccine; Salk

Therapeutic Class Vaccine, Live Virus and Inactivated Virus

Use Active immunization for prevention of poliomyelitis from types 1, 2, and 3; routine primary polio vaccination of adults who reside in the U.S. is not recommended unless patient is at increased risk due to contact or travel

Contraindications Acute febrile illness, including respiratory infections; allergy to streptomycin, polymyxin B, or neomycin; immunodeficiency conditions

Warnings Hypersensitivity reactions, have epinephrine 1:1000 available

Precautions Review patient history and allergy status; HIV infection

Adverse Reactions
Cardiovascular: Fever
Central nervous system: Drowsiness
Gastrointestinal: Decreased appetite
Local: Erythema, induration, pain at injection site
Miscellaneous: Guillain-Barré syndrome

Drug Interactions Immunosuppressive drugs and therapy may blunt response to vaccine

Stability Refrigerate at 2°C to 8°C (36°F to 46°F); do not freeze

Usual Dosage Geriatrics and Adults: S.C.: 3 doses of 0.5 mL; the first 2 doses should be administered at an interval of 1-2 months; the third dose should be given at least 6 months and preferably 12 months after the second dose; see Additional Information

Reference Range >1:8 titer

Patient Information Be aware of adverse reactions

Nursing Implications Do not give I.V.

Additional Information If <3 months exists for series, give 3 doses at 1-month intervals; if <1 month available, it is recommended to give OPV single dose or IPV single dose; for adults incompletely vaccinated, give remainder of doses needed to complete series

Special Geriatric Considerations For elderly who cannot document a primary immunization series or at risk to contact or travel, give the initial series; boosters may be necessary for travel since antibody titers may diminish with age

Dosage Forms Injection: Suspension of three types of poliovirus (Types 1, 2 and 3) grown in human diploid cell cultures (0.5 mL)

References
Gardner P and Schaffner W, "Immunization of Adults," *N Engl J Med*, 1993, 328(17):1252-8.

Poliovirus Vaccine, Live, Trivalent (poe lee oh vye' russ)

Brand Names Orimune®

Synonyms OPV; Sabin; TOPV

Therapeutic Class Vaccine, Live Virus

Use Poliovirus immunization to prevent poliomyelitis types 1, 2, and 3

Contraindications Persistent vomiting or diarrhea, patients allergic to sorbitol, streptomycin, or neomycin, known hypersensitivity to poliovirus vaccine; defer administration in presence of any acute illness; patients with any immunodeficiency condition (drug induced or disease)

Precautions The vaccine will not modify or prevent cases of existing or incubating poliomyelitis; do not administer TOPV after ISG administration; if given a short time after ISG, repeat dose of TOPV in 3 months

Adverse Reactions Central nervous system: Paralytic poliomyelitis

Drug Interactions May temporarily suppress tuberculin skin test sensitivity (4-6 weeks), immunosuppressive agents, immune globulin

Stability Keep in freezer; vaccine must remain frozen to retain potency; thawed dose must be refrigerated at 2°C to 8°C (36°F to 46°F) and used within 30 days

Usual Dosage Geriatrics and Adults: Oral: Two 0.5 mL doses 8 weeks apart; third dose of 0.5 mL 6-12 months after second dose

Booster dose: If an individual is at increased risk due to contact, travel, or occupation and has completed a primary series of immunization, a single booster dose (0.5 mL) orally is suggested

Reference Range >1:8 titer

Nursing Implications Do not administer parenterally; administer directly or dilute with distilled water, simple syrup USP, or milk; may be administered on bread or sugar cubes

Additional Information Federal law requires that the date of administration, the vaccine manufacturer, lot number of vaccine, and the administering person's name, title and address be entered into the patient's permanent medical record

Special Geriatric Considerations For elderly who cannot document a primary immunization series or at risk due to contact or travel, give the initial series; boosters may be necessary for travel since antibody titers may diminish with age

Dosage Forms Oral: Mixture of type 1, 2, and 3 viruses in monkey kidney tissue (0.5 mL)

References
Gardner P and Schaffner W, "Immunization of Adults," *N Engl J Med*, 1993, 328(17):1252-8.

Polycillin® *see* Ampicillin *on page 51*

Polycitra® *see* Sodium Citrate and Potassium Citrate Mixture *on page 649*

Polymox® *see* Amoxicillin Trihydrate *on page 49*

Ponstel® *see* Mefenamic Acid *on page 437*

Pork NPH Iletin® II *see* Insulin Preparations *on page 372*

Pork Regular Iletin® II *see* Insulin Preparations *on page 372*

Posture® [OTC] *see* Calcium Salts (Oral) *on page 111*

Potago® *see* Potassium Chloride *on next page*

Potasalan® *see* Potassium Chloride *on next page*

Potassium Acid Phosphate

Brand Names K-Phos® Original

Generic Available No

Therapeutic Class Electrolyte Supplement, Oral; Potassium Salt; Urinary Acidifying Agent

Use Acidifies urine and lowers urinary calcium concentration; reduces odor and rash caused by ammoniacal urine; to increase the antibacterial activity of methenamine

Contraindications Severe renal impairment, hyperkalemia, hyperphosphatemia, and infected magnesium ammonium phosphate stones

(Continued)

Potassium Acid Phosphate *(Continued)*

Warnings Use with caution in patients receiving other potassium supplementation and in patients with renal insufficiency, or severe tissue breakdown as seen in chemotherapy or hemodialysis

Precautions Use cautiously, serum potassium needs regulation; use caution in patients receiving digitalis products, Addison's disease, dehydrated patients, renal insufficiency, hepatic disease, peripheral or pulmonary edema, hypertension, hypernatremia, hypoparathyroidism, acute pancreatitis, osteomalacia

Adverse Reactions
Cardiovascular: Irregular heartbeat
Central nervous system: Tetany, dizziness, tiredness, tingling or numbness of lips
Endocrine & metabolic: Hyperphosphatemia, hyperkalemia, hypocalcemia
Gastrointestinal: Nausea; vomiting; diarrhea; abdominal discomfort; a mild laxative effect may occur, but resolves with dose reduction; weight gain
Genitourinary: Decreased urine output
Neuromuscular & skeletal: Pain/weakness of extremities, bone/joint pain
Respiratory: Shortness of breath
Miscellaneous: Thirst, edema

Overdosage Symptoms of overdose include muscle weakness, paralysis, peaked T waves, flattened P waves, prolongation of QRS complex, ventricular arrhythmias

Toxicology Removal of potassium can be accomplished by various means; removal through the GI tract with Kayexalate® administration; by way of the kidney through diuresis, mineralocorticoid administration or increased sodium intake; by hemodialysis or peritoneal dialysis; or by shifting potassium back into the cells by insulin and glucose infusion or sodium bicarbonate; calcium chloride will reverse cardiac effects.

Drug Interactions
Antacids containing magnesium, calcium or aluminum binds phosphate and decreased absorption
Potassium or potassium-sparing diuretics may increase chance of hyperkalemia
Salicylates have increased serum concentrations
Angiotensin-converting enzyme inhibitors may increase serum potassium

Mechanism of Action The principal intracellular cation; involved in transmission of nerve impulses, muscle contractions, enzyme activity, and glucose utilization

Pharmacokinetics
Absorption: Absorbed well from upper GI tract
Distribution: Enters cells via active transport from extracellular fluid
Elimination: Largely by the kidneys, but also small amount via the skin and feces, with most intestinal potassium being reabsorbed

Usual Dosage Geriatrics and Adults: Oral: 1000 mg dissolved in 6-8 oz of water 4 times/day with meals and at bedtime; for best results, soak tablets in water for 2-5 minutes, then stir and swallow

Monitoring Parameters Serum potassium, sodium, phosphate, calcium; serum salicylates (if taking salicylates); signs of muscle weakness, cramps

Test Interactions Decreased ammonia (B)

Patient Information Dissolve tablets completely before drinking; avoid taking magnesium, calcium, or aluminum antacids at the same time; patients may pass old kidney stones when starting therapy; notify physician if experiencing nausea, vomiting, or abdominal pain, muscle weakness, or cramps

Special Geriatric Considerations A complete drug history should be taken to rule out potential drug interactions since elderly frequently may be taking potassium and potassium-sparing diuretics or salicylates as antacids

Dosage Forms Tablet, sodium free: 500 mg [potassium 3.67 mEq]

Potassium Chloride

Brand Names Cena-K®; Gen-K®; Kaochlor® S-F; Kaon-CL®; Kato®; K-Dur® 20; K-Lor™; Klor-con®; Klorvess®; Klotrix®; K-Lyte/CL®; K-Tab®; Micro-K®; Potago®; Potasalan®; Rum-K®; Slow-K® K⁺8®

Synonyms KCl

Generic Available Yes

Therapeutic Class Electrolyte Supplement, Oral; Electrolyte Supplement, Parenteral; Potassium Salt

Use Treatment or prevention of hypokalemia

Unlabeled use: Treatment of hypertension

Contraindications Severe renal impairment, untreated Addison's disease, acute dehydration, heat cramps, hyperkalemia, severe tissue trauma; liquid potassium preparation should be used in patients with esophageal compression or delayed gastric emptying time

Warnings Potassium injections should be administered only in patients with adequate urine flow; patients with impaired potassium excretion (renal failure) can develop hyperkalemia and cardiac arrhythmias or arrest; potassium tablets have been reported to produce stenotic or ulcerative lesions in gastrointestinal tract

Precautions Use with caution in patients with cardiac disease, patients receiving potassium-sparing drugs; patients must be on a cardiac monitor during intermittent infusions

Adverse Reactions
Cardiovascular: Cardiac arrhythmias, heart block, hypotension
Central nervous system: Parethesias, mental confusion
Endocrine & metabolic: Hyperkalemia
Gastrointestinal: Nausea, vomiting, diarrhea, abdominal pain, GI lesions
Local: Pain at the site of injection, phlebitis
Neuromuscular & skeletal: Muscle weakness

Overdosage See Adverse Reactions

Toxicology Removal of potassium can be accomplished by various means; removal through the GI tract with Kayexalate® administration; by way of the kidney through diuresis, mineralocorticoid administration or increased sodium intake; by hemodialysis or peritoneal dialysis; or by shifting potassium back into the cells by insulin and glucose infusion.

Drug Interactions Potassium-sparing diuretics, salt substitutes, digitalis, angiotensin-converting enzyme inhibitors

Stability Store at room temperature, protect from freezing; use only clear solutions; use admixtures within 24 hours

Mechanism of Action Needed for the conduction of nerve impulses in heart, brain, and skeletal muscle; contraction of cardiac, skeletal and smooth muscles; maintenance of normal renal function

Pharmacokinetics
Absorption: Well from upper GI tract; enters cells via active transport from extracellular fluid
Elimination: Largely by the kidneys, but also small amount via skin and feces, with most intestinal potassium being reabsorbed

Usual Dosage I.V. doses should be incorporated into the patient's maintenance I.V. fluids, intermittent I.V. potassium administration should be reserved for severe depletion situations in patients undergoing EKG monitoring.

Geriatrics and Adults:
Normal daily requirement: Oral, I.V.: 30-80 mEq/day
Prevention during diuretic therapy: Oral: 10-40 mEq/day in 1-2 divided doses
Treatment: Oral, I.V.: 20-100 mEq/day
I.V. intermittent infusion: 10-20 mEq/hour, not to exceed 40 mEq/hour and 150 mEq/day. See table.

Potassium Dosage/Rate of Infusion Guidelines

Serum K^+	Maximum Infusion Rate	Maximum Concentration	Maximum 24-Hour Dose
>2.5 mEq/L	10 mEq/h	40 mEq/L	200 mEq
<2.5 mEq/L	40 mEq/h	80 mEq/L	400 mEq

Monitoring Parameters Serum potassium, blood pressure, pulse, EKG (as needed), signs of muscle weakness, cramps

Reference Range 3.5-5.0 mEq/L (3.5-5.0 mmol/L)

Test Interactions Decreased ammonia (B)

Patient Information Swallow tablets whole, do not crush or chew; take with food, water, or juice

Nursing Implications Maximum concentration (peripheral line): 80 mEq/L; usual rate: 10 mEq/hour; maximum concentration (central line): 30 mEq/100 mL; may not be given I.V. push or I.V. retrograde; oral liquid potassium supplements should be diluted (2-6 parts diluent) with water or fruit juice during administration; wax matrix tablets must be swallowed and not allowed to dissolve in mouth

Special Geriatric Considerations Elderly may require less potassium than younger adults due to decreased renal function; for elderly who do not respond to replacement therapy, check serum magnesium; due to long-term diuretic use, elderly may be hypomagnesemic

Dosage Forms
Capsule, controlled release, micro encapsulated (Micro-K®): 600 mg [8 mEq]; 750 mg [10 mEq]
Injection: 1.5 mEq/mL, 2 mEq/mL, 3 mEq/mL
Liquid, oral: 10 mEq/15 mL, 15 mEq/15 mL, 20 mEq/15 mL, 30 mEq/15 mL, 40 mEq/15 mL, 45 mEq/15 mL
Powder, oral: 15 mEq, 20 mEq, 25 mEq packet
Tablet:
Effervescent, as potassium chloride: 25 mEq
Effervescent, as potassium bicarbonate: 20 mEq, 25 mEq, 50 mEq

(Continued)

Potassium Chloride *(Continued)*

Extended release (K⁺8®): 8 mEq
Sustained release, microcrystalloids (K-Dur®): 750 mg [10 mEq]; 1500 mg [20 mEq]
Wax matrix:
Kaon-Cl®: 500 mg [6.7 mEq]
Slow-K®: 600 mg [8 mEq]; 750 mg [10 mEq]

Potassium Gluconate

Brand Names Glu-K®; Kaon®; Kaylixir®
Generic Available Yes
Therapeutic Class Electrolyte Supplement, Oral; Potassium Salt
Use Treatment of potassium deficiency (hypokalemia) or prevention of hypokalemia

Unlabeled use: Treatment of hypertension

Contraindications Severe renal impairment, untreated Addison's disease, acute dehydration, heat cramps, hyperkalemia, severe tissue trauma; liquid potassium preparation should be used in patients with esophageal compression or delayed gastric emptying time

Warnings Patients with impaired potassium excretion (renal failure) can develop hyperkalemia and cardiac arrhythmias or arrest; potassium tablets have been reported to produce stenotic or ulcerative lesions in gastrointestinal tract

Precautions Use with caution in patients with cardiac disease, patients receiving potassium-sparing drugs; patients must be on a cardiac monitor during intermittent infusions

Adverse Reactions
Cardiovascular: Cardiac arrhythmias, heart block, hypotension
Central nervous system: Parethesias, mental confusion
Endocrine & metabolic: Hyperkalemia
Gastrointestinal: Nausea, vomiting, diarrhea, abdominal pain, GI lesions
Local: Phlebitis
Neuromuscular & skeletal: Muscle weakness

Overdosage See Adverse Reactions

Toxicology Removal of potassium can be accomplished by various means; removal through the GI tract with Kayexalate® administration; by way of the kidney through diuresis, mineralocorticoid administration or increased sodium intake; by hemodialysis or peritoneal dialysis; or by shifting potassium back into the cells by insulin and glucose infusion

Drug Interactions Potassium-sparing diuretics, salt substitutes, digitalis, angiotensin-converting enzyme inhibitors

Stability Store at room temperature, protect from freezing; use only clear solutions; use admixtures within 24 hours

Mechanism of Action Needed for the conduction of nerve impulses in heart, brain, and skeletal muscle; contraction of cardiac, skeletal and smooth muscles; maintenance of normal renal function

Pharmacokinetics
Absorption: Well from upper GI tract
Distribution: Enters cells via active transport from extracellular fluid
Elimination: Largely by the kidneys, but also small amount via skin and feces, with most intestinal potassium being reabsorbed

Usual Dosage Geriatrics and Adults: Oral:
Normal daily requirement: 40-80 mEq/day
Prevention during diuretic therapy: 10-40 mEq/kg/day in 1-2 divided doses
Treatment of hypokalemia: 20-100 mEq/day in 2-4 divided doses

Monitoring Parameters Serum potassium, blood pressure, pulse, EKG (as needed), signs of muscle weakness, cramps

Reference Range 3.5-5 mEq/L (3.5-5 mmol/L)

Test Interactions Decreased ammonia (B)

Patient Information Take with food, water, or fruit juice; swallow tablets whole; do not crush or chew

Nursing Implications Maximum concentration (peripheral line): 80 mEq/L; maximum concentration (central line): 30 mEq/100 mL; oral liquid potassium supplements should be diluted (2-6 parts diluent) with water or fruit juice during administration; wax matrix tablets must be swallowed and not chewed

Additional Information 9.4 g potassium gluconate is approximately equal to 40 mEq potassium (4.3 mEq potassium/g salt)

Special Geriatric Considerations Elderly may require less potassium than younger adults due to decreased renal function; for elderly who do not respond to replacement therapy, check serum magnesium; long-term use of diuretics may result in hypomagnesemia

Dosage Forms
Elixir: 20 mEq/15 mL (5 mL, 15 mL, 118 mL, 473 mL, 946 mL, 4000 mL)
Tablet: 500 mg, 595 mg

Potassium Phosphate

Brand Names Neutra-Phos®-K

Synonyms Phosphate, Potassium

Generic Available Yes

Therapeutic Class Electrolyte Supplement, Oral; Electrolyte Supplement, Parenteral; Phosphate Salt; Potassium Salt

Use Source of potassium and phosphorus in parenteral nutrition and large volume I.V. fluids; treatment of conditions associated with excessive renal phosphate and potassium loss, inadequate GI absorption of these electrolytes, or inadequate phosphate and potassium in the diet

Contraindications Hyperphosphatemia, hyperkalemia, low calcium levels, severe renal impairment

Warnings Use with caution in patients with renal insufficiency, cardiac disease, metabolic alkalosis; admixture of phosphate and calcium in I.V. fluids can result in calcium phosphate precipitation; cases where severe tissue breakdown occurs (eg, hemolysis, chemotherapy)

Precautions Use cautiously, serum potassium needs regulation; use caution in patients receiving digitalis products, Addison's disease, dehydrated patients, renal insufficiency, hepatic disease, peripheral or pulmonary edema, hypertension, hypernatremia, hypoparathyroidism, acute pancreatitis, osteomalacia

Adverse Reactions

Cardiovascular: Irregular heartbeat

Central nervous system: Tetany, dizziness, tiredness, tingling or numbness of lips

Endocrine & metabolic: Hyperphosphatemia, hyperkalemia, hypocalcemia

Gastrointestinal: Nausea; vomiting; diarrhea; abdominal discomfort; a mild laxative effect may occur, but resolves with dose reduction; weight gain

Genitourinary: Decreased urine output

Neuromuscular & skeletal: Pain/weakness of extremities, bone/joint pain

Respiratory: Shortness of breath

Miscellaneous: Thirst, edema

Overdosage Symptoms of overdose include muscle weakness, paralysis, peaked T waves, flattened P waves, prolongation of QRS complex, ventricular arrhythmias, tetany, calcium-phosphate precipitation

Toxicology Removal of potassium can be accomplished by various means; removal through the GI tract with Kayexalate® administration; by way of the kidney through diuresis, mineralocorticoid administration or increased sodium intake; by hemodialysis or peritoneal dialysis; or by shifting potassium back into the cells by insulin, glucose infusion, or sodium bicarbonate; calcium chloride reverses cardiac effects.

Drug Interactions

Decreased effect/levels with aluminum- and magnesium-containing antacids or sucralfate which can act as phosphate binders

Increased effect/levels with potassium-sparing diuretics or ACE-inhibitors

Stability Store at room temperature, protect from freezing; use only clear solutions; up to 10-15 mEq of calcium may be added per liter before precipitate may occur

Stability of parenteral admixture at room temperature (25°C): 24 hours

Usual Dosage I.V. doses should be incorporated into the patient's maintenance I.V. fluids; intermittent I.V. infusion should be reserved for severe depletion situations in patients undergoing continuous EKG monitoring. It is difficult to determine total body phosphorus deficit; the following dosages are empiric guidelines:

Geriatrics and Adults: Normal requirements elemental phosphorus: Oral: 1200 mg/day

Treatment: It is difficult to provide concrete guidelines for the treatment of severe hypophosphatemia because the extent of total body deficits and response to therapy are difficult to predict. Aggressive doses of phosphate may result in a transient serum elevation followed by redistribution into intracellular compartments or bone tissue. It is recommended that repletion of severe hypophosphatemia (<1 mg/dL) be done I.V. because large doses of oral phosphate may cause diarrhea and intestinal absorption may be unreliable

Geriatrics and Adults: I.V. phosphate repletion:

Initial dose: 0.08 mmol/kg if recent uncomplicated hypophosphatemia

Initial dose: 0.16 mmol/kg if prolonged hypophosphatemia with presumed total body deficits; increase dose by 25% to 50% if patient symptomatic with severe hypophosphatemia

Do not exceed 0.24 mmol/kg/day; administer over 6 hours by I.V. infusion

With orders for I.V. phosphate, there is considerable confusion associated with the use of millimoles (mmol) versus milliequivalents (mEq) to express the phosphate requirement. Because inorganic phosphate exists as monobasic and dibasic anions, with the mixture of valences dependent on pH, ordering by mEq amounts is unreliable and may lead to large dosing errors. In addition, I.V. phosphate is available in the sodium and potassium salt; therefore, the content of these cations must be considered when ordering phosphate. The most reliable method of ordering I.V. phosphate is by millimoles, then specifying the potassium or sodium

(Continued)

579

Potassium Phosphate *(Continued)*

salt. For example, an order for 15 mmol of phosphate as potassium phosphate in one liter of normal saline would also provide 22 mEq of potassium.

Phosphate maintenance electrolyte requirement in parenteral nutrition: Geriatrics and Adults: 2 mmol/kg/24 hours or 35 mmol/kcal/24 hours; maximum: 15-30 mmol/24 hours

Maintenance: Geriatrics and Adults:
I.V. solutions: 15-30 mmol/24 hours I.V. or 50-150 mmol/24 hours in divided doses
Oral: 1-2 capsules (250-500 mg phosphorus/8-16 mmol) 4 times/day; dilute as instructed

Fleet® Phospho®-Soda: Laxative: Oral: Single dose: 20-30 mL mixed with 120 mL cold water

Administration For intermittent infusion, if peripheral line, dilute to a maximum concentration of 0.05 mmol/mL; if central line, dilute to a maximum concentration of 0.12 mmol/mL; maximum rate of infusion: 0.06 mmol/kg/hour; do **not** infuse with calcium containing IV. fluids (ie, TPN)

Monitoring Parameters Serum potassium, phosphate, calcium, EKG, salicylate serum levels if patient is taking salicylates; signs of muscle weakness, cramps

Reference Range Geriatrics and Adults: 2.5-5 mg/dL

Test Interactions Decreased ammonia (B)

Patient Information Do not swallow the capsule; empty contents of capsule into 75 mL (2.5 oz) of water before taking; take with food to reduce the risk of diarrhea

Nursing Implications Injection must be diluted in appropriate I.V. solution and volume prior to administration and administered over a minimum of 4 hours; capsule must be emptied into 3-4 oz of water before administration

Special Geriatric Considerations A complete drug history should be taken to rule out potential drug interactions since elderly frequently may be taking potassium and potassium-sparing diuretics or salicylates as antacids

Dosage Forms
Injection: Potassium 4.4 mEq and phosphate 3 mmol per mL (15 mL)
Powder packet (Neutra-Phos®-K): Potassium 556 mg [14.25 mEq] and phosphorus 250 mg [8 mmol] per packet

Potassium Phosphate and Sodium Phosphate

Brand Names K-Phos® MF; K-Phos® Neutral; K-Phos® No. 2; Neutra-Phos®; Uro-KP-Neutral®

Synonyms Sodium Phosphate and Potassium Phosphate

Generic Available Yes

Therapeutic Class Electrolyte Supplement, Oral; Phosphate Salt; Potassium Salt

Use Treatment of conditions associated with excessive renal phosphate loss or inadequate GI absorption of phosphate; to acidify the urine to lower calcium concentrations; to increase the antibacterial activity of methenamine; reduce odor and rash caused by ammonia in urine

Contraindications Severe renal impairment, hyperkalemia, hyperphosphatemia, and infected magnesium ammonium phosphate stones

Warnings Use with caution in patients with renal disease, hyperkalemia, cardiac disease, Addison's disease, hyperkalemia, infected urolithiasis or struvite stone formation, patients with severely impaired renal function

Precautions Use cautiously in sodium-restricted patients; serum potassium needs regulation; use caution in patients receiving digitalis products, Addison's disease, dehydrated patients, renal insufficiency, hepatic disease, peripheral or pulmonary edema, hypertension, hypernatremia, hypoparathyroidism, acute pancreatitis, osteomalacia

Adverse Reactions
Cardiovascular: Irregular heartbeat
Central nervous system: Tetany, dizziness, tiredness, tingling or numbness of lips
Endocrine & metabolic: Hyperphosphatemia, hyperkalemia, hypocalcemia
Gastrointestinal: Nausea; vomiting; diarrhea; abdominal discomfort; a mild laxative effect may occur, but resolves with dose reduction; weight gain
Genitourinary: Decreased urine output
Neuromuscular & skeletal: Pain/weakness of extremities, bone/joint pain
Respiratory: Shortness of breath
Miscellaneous: Thirst, edema

Overdosage Symptoms of overdose include muscle weakness, paralysis, peaked T waves, flattened P waves, prolongation of QRS complex, ventricular arrhythmias, tetany, calcium phosphate precipitation

Toxicology Removal of potassium can be accomplished by various means; removal through the GI tract with Kayexalate® administration; by way of the kidney through diuresis, mineralocorticoid administration or increased sodium intake; by hemodialysis or peritoneal dialysis; or by shifting potassium back into the cells by insulin and glucose infusion; calcium chloride reverses cardiac effects.

Drug Interactions
Decreased effect/levels with aluminum- and magnesium-containing antacids or sucralfate which can act as phosphate binders

Increased effect/levels with potassium-sparing diuretics or ACE-inhibitors

Salicylates may have increased serum concentrations

Usual Dosage All dosage forms to be mixed in 6-8 oz of water prior to administration

Geriatrics and Adults: 1-2 capsules (250-500 mg phosphorus/8-16 mmol) 4 times/day after meals and at bedtime; do not exceed 8 doses in 24 hours; if urine is difficult to acidify, give 1 dose (tablet/capsule/powder) every 2 hours, not to exceed 8 doses in 24 hours

Monitoring Parameters Serum potassium, sodium, calcium, phosphate, EKG; signs of muscle weakness, cramps

Patient Information Do not swallow, open capsule and dissolve in 6-8 oz of water; powder packets are to be mixed in 6-8 oz of water; tablets should be crushed and mixed in 6-8 oz of water

Nursing Implications Tablets may be crushed and stirred vigorously to speed dissolution

Special Geriatric Considerations A complete drug history should be taken to rule out potential drug interactions since elderly frequently may be taking potassium and potassium-sparing diuretics or salicylates as antacids

Dosage Forms
Capsule: Phosphate 8 mmol, sodium 7.125 mEq, and potassium 7.125 mEq (250 mg of phosphorus)

Powder, concentrate: Phosphate 8 mmol, sodium 7.125 mEq, and potassium 7.125 mEq per 75 mL when reconstituted

Tablet: Phosphate 8 mmol, sodium 13 mEq, and potassium 1.1 mEq (114 mg of phosphorus)

PPA *see* Phenylpropanolamine Hydrochloride *on page 559*

PPD *see* Tuberculin Purified Protein Derivative *on page 725*

Prazepam (pra' ze pam)
Related Information
Antacid Drug Interactions *on page 764*

Anxiolytic/Hypnotic Use in Long-Term Care Facilities *on page 755-756*

Benzodiazepines Comparison *on page 802-803*

Brand Names Centrax®

Generic Available No

Therapeutic Class Antianxiety Agent; Anticonvulsant, Benzodiazepine; Benzodiazepine

Use Treatment of anxiety and management of alcohol withdrawal

Restrictions C-IV

Contraindications Hypersensitivity to prazepam or any component, cross-sensitivity with other benzodiazepines may exist; avoid using in patients with pre-existing CNS depression, severe uncontrolled pain, or narrow-angle glaucoma

Warnings May cause drug dependency; avoid abrupt discontinuance in patients with prolonged therapy or seizure disorders

Precautions Use with caution in patients with a history of drug dependence

Adverse Reactions
Central nervous system: Drowsiness, dizziness, confusion, sedation, ataxia, headache

Gastrointestinal: Dry mouth, constipation, diarrhea, nausea, vomiting

Neuromuscular & skeletal: Impaired coordination

Ocular: Blurred vision

Respiratory: Decreased respiratory rate, apnea, laryngospasm

Miscellaneous: Physical and psychological dependence with prolonged use

Overdosage Symptoms of overdose include somnolence, confusion, coma, and diminished reflexes

Toxicology Treatment for benzodiazepine overdose is supportive; rarely is mechanical ventilation required

Flumazenil has been shown to selectively block the binding of benzodiazepines to CNS receptors, resulting in a reversal of benzodiazepine-induced sedation; however, its use may not alter the course of overdose

Drug Interactions Benzodiazepines may increase digoxin concentrations and may decrease the effect of levodopa

Decreased metabolism: Cimetidine, fluoxetine

Increased metabolism: Rifampin

Increased toxicity: CNS depressants, alcohol

Mechanism of Action Benzodiazepines appear to potentiate the effects of GABA and other inhibitory neurotransmitters by binding to specific benzodiazepine-receptor sites in various areas of the CNS

(Continued)

Prazepam (Continued)

Pharmacodynamics
Peak effects: Within 6 hours

Duration: 48 hours; studies have shown that the elderly are more sensitive to the effects of benzodiazepines as compared to younger adults

Pharmacokinetics
Distribution: V_d is increased in elderly

Half-life:

Parent: 78 minutes

Desmethyldiazepam: 30-100 hours; significantly prolonged in elderly men (127.8 hours) as compared to young men (61.8 hours) and older women (75.4 hours)

Metabolism: Prazepam, itself, is pharmacologically inactive; first-pass hepatic metabolism

Elimination: Renal excretion of unchanged drug and primarily N-desmethyldiazepam (active)

Usual Dosage Oral:
Geriatrics: Initial: 5 mg 2-3 times/day

Adults: 30 mg/day in divided doses; may increase gradually to 60 mg/day

Monitoring Parameters Respiratory, cardiovascular and mental status, symptoms of anxiety

Patient Information Avoid alcohol and other CNS depressants; may cause drowsiness; avoid activities needing good psychomotor coordination until CNS effects are known; may cause physical or psychological dependence; avoid abrupt discontinuation after prolonged use

Nursing Implications Assist patient with ambulation, monitor for alertness

Additional Information Prazepam offers no significant advantage over other benzodiazepines

Special Geriatric Considerations See Pharmacokinetics and Pharmacodynamics; because of its long-acting metabolite, prazepam is not considered a drug of choice in the elderly; long-acting benzodiazepines have been associated with falls in the elderly; interpretive guidelines from the Health Care Financing Administration (HCFA) discourage the use of this agent in residents of long-term care facilities

Dosage Forms
Capsule: 5 mg, 10 mg, 20 mg

Tablet: 10 mg

References
Allen MD, Greenblatt DJ, Harmatz JS, et al, "Desmethyldiazepam Kinetics in the Elderly After Oral Prazepam," Clin Pharmacol Ther, 1986, 28:196-202.

Prazosin Hydrochloride (pra' zoe sin)

Brand Names Minipress®

Synonyms Furazosin

Generic Available Yes

Therapeutic Class Alpha-Adrenergic Blocking Agent, Oral; Antihypertensive; Vasodilator, Coronary

Use Hypertension

Unlabeled use: Severe congestive heart failure (in conjunction with diuretics and cardiac glycosides), overflow incontinence secondary to prostatic obstruction

Contraindications Hypersensitivity to prazosin or any component

Warnings Can cause marked hypotension and syncope with sudden loss of consciousness with the first few doses. Anticipate a similar effect if therapy is interrupted for a few days, if dosage is increased rapidly, or if another antihypertensive drug is introduced.

Precautions Marked orthostatic hypotension, syncope, and loss of consciousness may occur with first dose ("first-dose phenomenon"). This reaction is more likely to occur in patients receiving beta-blockers, diuretics, low sodium diets or larger first doses (ie, >1 mg/dose in adults); avoid rapid increase in dose; use with caution in patients with renal impairment.

Adverse Reactions
Cardiovascular: Orthostatic hypotension, syncope, palpitations, tachycardia, edema

Central nervous system: Dizziness, lightheadedness, nightmares, drowsiness, headache

Dermatologic: Rash

Endocrine & metabolic: Fluid retention

Gastrointestinal: Nausea, dry mouth

Genitourinary: Urinary frequency, priapism, sexual dysfunction

Neuromuscular & skeletal: Weakness

Respiratory: Nasal congestion

Miscellaneous: Hypothermia

Overdosage Symptoms of overdose include hypotension and drowsiness

Toxicology Hypotension usually responds to I.V. fluids or Trendelenburg positioning. If unresponsive to these measures the use of a parenteral vasoconstrictor may be required (eg, norepinephrine 0.1-0.2 mcg/kg/minute titrated to response). Treatment is primarily supportive and symptomatic.

Drug Interactions Increased effect (hypotensive) with diuretics and antihypertensive medications (especially beta-blockers)

Mechanism of Action Competitively inhibits postsynaptic alpha$_1$-adrenergic receptors which results in vasodilation of veins and arterioles and a decrease in total peripheral resistance and blood pressure

Pharmacodynamics
Onset of hypotensive effect: Within 2 hours; maximum decrease: 2-4 hours
Duration: 10-24 hours

Pharmacokinetics
Distribution: V_d: 0.5 L/kg (hypertensive adults)
Protein binding: 92% to 97%
Metabolism: Extensive in the liver; metabolites may be active
Bioavailability: Oral: 43% to 82%
Half-life: 2-4 hours; increased half-life with congestive heart failure
Elimination: 6% to 10% excreted renally as unchanged drug
In the elderly, half-life and volume of distribution may be increased and the oral absorption decreased, though the clinical significance is unknown

Usual Dosage Oral (first dose given at bedtime):
Geriatrics: Initial: 1 mg 1-2 times/day
Adults: Initial: 1 mg/dose 2-3 times/day; usual maintenance dose: 3-15 mg/day in divided doses 2-4 times/day; maximum daily dose: 20 mg

Monitoring Parameters Blood pressure, standing and sitting/supine

Patient Information Rise from sitting/lying carefully, may cause dizziness; take first dose at bedtime

Nursing Implications Syncope may occur usually within 90 minutes of the initial dose; give initial dose at bedtime; see Monitoring Parameters

Special Geriatric Considerations See Warnings and Pharmacokinetics; adverse effects such as dry mouth and urinary problems can be particularly bothersome in the elderly

Dosage Forms Capsule: 1 mg, 2 mg, 5 mg

References
Rubin PC, Scott PJ, and Reid JL, "Prazosin Disposition in Young and Elderly Subjects," *Br J Clin Pharmacol*, 1981, 12(3):401-4.

Precision Release® [OTC] *see* Phenylpropanolamine Hydrochloride *on page 559*

Predair® *see* Prednisolone *on next page*

Predaject® *see* Prednisolone *on next page*

Predalone T.B.A.® *see* Prednisolone *on next page*

Predate® S *see* Prednisolone *on next page*

Predate® TBA *see* Prednisolone *on next page*

Predcor® *see* Prednisolone *on next page*

Predcor-TBA® *see* Prednisolone *on next page*

Pred Forte® *see* Prednisolone *on next page*

Pred-G® *see* Prednisolone and Gentamicin *on page 585*

Pred Mild® *see* Prednisolone *on next page*

Prednicarbate

Brand Names Dermatop®

Therapeutic Class Corticosteroid, Topical (Medium Potency)

Use Relief of the inflammatory and pruritic manifestations of corticosteroid-responsive dermatoses

Contraindications Hypersensitivity to prednicarbate or any component; fungal, viral, or tubercular skin lesions, herpes simplex or zoster

Precautions Systemic absorption of topical corticosteroids has produced reversible HPA axis suppression. This is more likely to occur when the preparation is used on large surface or denuded areas for prolonged periods of time or with an occlusive dressing.

Adverse Reactions
Dermatologic: Acne, hypopigmentation, allergic dermatitis, maceration of the skin, skin atrophy
Endocrine & metabolic: HPA suppression, Cushing's syndrome, growth retardation
Local: Burning, itching, irritation, dryness, folliculitis, hypertrichosis
Miscellaneous: Secondary infection

Mechanism of Action Topical corticosteroids have anti-inflammatory, antipruritic, vasoconstrictive, and antiproliferative actions

Usual Dosage Geriatrics and Adults: Topical: Apply a thin film to affected area twice daily

(Continued)

Prednicarbate *(Continued)*

Monitoring Parameters Relief of symptoms

Patient Information Use only as prescribed and for no longer than the period prescribed; apply sparingly in a thin film and rub in lightly; avoid contact with eyes; notify physician if condition persists or worsens

Nursing Implications Use sparingly

Additional Information Considered a moderate-potency steroid; has been shown that the atrophic activity of prednicarbate is many times less than agents with similar clinical potency, nevertheless, avoid prolonged use on the face

Special Geriatric Considerations See Precautions; due to age-related changes in skin, limit use of topical corticosteroids

Dosage Forms Cream: 0.1% (15 g, 60 g)

References
Rumbaugh MM, "High Potency Topical Corticosteroids," *US Pharmacist*, 1993, 18(6):30-41.

Prednicen-M® *see Prednisone on page 586*

Prednisolone *(pred niss' oh lone)*

Related Information

Antacid Drug Interactions *on page 764*

Corticosteroids Comparison, Systemic *on page 808*

Brand Names AK-Pred®; AK-Tate®; Cortalone®; Delta-Cortef®; Econopred®; Econopred® Plus; Hydeltrasol®; Hydeltra-T.B.A.®; Inflamase®; Inflamase® Mild; I-Pred®; Key-Pred®; Key-Pred-SP®; Metreton®; Nor-Pred S®; Nor-Pred T.B.A.®; Ocu-Pred®; Pre-dair®; Predaject®; Predalone T.B.A.®; Predate® S; Predate® TBA; Predcor®; Predcor-TBA®; Pred Forte®; Pred Mild®; Prelone®

Synonyms Deltahydrocortisone; Metacortandralone; Prednisolone Acetate; Prednisolone Acetate, Ophthalmic; Prednisolone Sodium Phosphate; Prednisolone Sodium Phosphate, Ophthalmic; Prednisolone Tebutate

Generic Available Yes

Therapeutic Class Adrenal Corticosteroid; Anti-inflammatory Agent; Anti-inflammatory Agent, Ophthalmic; Corticosteroid, Ophthalmic; Corticosteroid, Systemic

Use Treatment of palpebral and bulbar conjunctivitis; corneal injury from chemical, radiation, thermal burns, or foreign body penetration; endocrine disorders, rheumatic disorders, collagen diseases, dermatologic diseases, allergic states, ophthalmic diseases, respiratory diseases, hematologic disorders, neoplastic diseases, edematous states, and gastrointestinal diseases; useful in patients unable to activate prednisone (ie, liver disease)

Contraindications Acute superficial herpes simplex keratitis; systemic fungal infections; varicella; hypersensitivity to prednisolone or any component

Precautions Use with caution in patients with hypothyroidism, cirrhosis, hypertension, congestive heart failure, nonspecific ulcerative colitis, thromboembolic disorders and in patients at increased risk for peptic ulcer disease; gradually taper dose to withdraw therapy

Adverse Reactions

Cardiovascular: Hypertension, edema, accelerated atherogenesis

Central nervous system: Euphoria, mental changes, headache, vertigo, seizures, psychoses, pseudotumor cerebri

Dermatologic: Folliculitis, hypertrichosis, acneiform eruption dermatitis, maceration, skin atrophy, acne, impaired wound healing, hirsutism

Endocrine & metabolic: Growth suppression, Cushing's syndrome, pituitary-adrenal axis suppression, alkalosis, glucose intolerance, hypokalemia, postmenopausal bleeding, hot flashes

Gastrointestinal: Peptic ulcer, nausea, vomiting, pancreatitis

Local: Burning, irritation

Neuromuscular & skeletal: Muscle weakness, osteoporosis, fractures, aseptic necrosis of femoral and humeral heads, steroid myopathy

Ocular: Cataracts, glaucoma

Miscellaneous: Increased susceptibility to infection

Toxicology When consumed in excessive quantities for prolonged periods, systemic hypercorticism and adrenal suppression may occur; in those cases, discontinuation and withdrawal of the corticosteroid should be done judiciously

Drug Interactions

Steroids decrease the effect of anticholinesterases, isoniazid, salicylates, insulin, oral hypoglycemics

Decreased effect: Barbiturates, phenytoin, rifampin

Increased effect (hypokalemia) of potassium-depleting diuretics

Increased risk of digoxin toxicity (due to hypokalemia)

Increased effect: Estrogens, ketoconazole

Mechanism of Action Decreases inflammation by suppression of migration of polymorphonuclear leukocytes and reversal of increased capillary permeability; suppresses the immune system by reducing activity and volume of the lymphatic system

Pharmacokinetics
Half-life: 3.6 hours; biologic: 18-36 hours
Protein binding: 65% to 91% (concentration dependent)
Metabolism: Primarily in the liver, but also metabolized in most tissues, to inactive compounds
Elimination: In urine principally as glucuronides, sulfates and unconjugated metabolites

Usual Dosage Dose depends upon condition being treated and response of patient; alternate day dosing may be attempted in some disease states

Geriatrics: Use the lowest effective dose
Adults:
Oral, I.M.: 5-60 mg/day
Rheumatoid arthritis: Oral: Initial: 5-7.5 mg/day; adjust dose as necessary
Ophthalmic suspension: Instill 1-2 drops into conjunctival sac every hour during day, every 2 hours at night until favorable response is obtained, then use 1 drop every 4 hours

Monitoring Parameters Blood pressure, blood glucose, electrolytes, symptoms of fluid retention

Test Interactions Increased amylase (S), chloride (S), increased cholesterol (S), increased glucose, increased protein, increased sodium (S); decreased calcium (S), decreased chloride (S), decreased potassium (S), decreased thyroxine (S)

Patient Information Take oral form after meals or with food or milk; do not abruptly discontinue if on long-term therapy; notify physician of any signs of infection

Nursing Implications Give with food or milk; parenteral product is not for I.V. use – only give I.M., intralesional, intra-articular, or soft tissue injections

Additional Information
Prednisolone: Cortalone®, Delta-Cortef®, Prelone®
Prednisolone acetate: Key-Pred®, Predaject®, Predate®, Predcor®
Prednisolone acetate, ophthalmic: AK-Tate®, Econopred®, Econopred® Plus, Ocu-Pred®, Pred Forte®, Pred Mild®
Prednisolone sodium phosphate: Hydeltrasol®, Key-Pred-SP®, Nor-Pred S®, Predate® S
Prednisolone sodium phosphate, ophthalmic: AK-Pred®, Inflamase®, Inflamase® Mild, I-Pred®, Predair®
Prednisolone tebutate: Hydeltra-T.B.A.®, Nor-Pred T.B.A.®, Predalone T.B.A.®, Predate® TBA, Predcor-TBA®

Special Geriatric Considerations Useful in patients with inability to activate prednisone (liver disease). Because of the risk of adverse effects, systemic corticosteroids should be used cautiously in the elderly, in the smallest possible dose, and for the shortest possible time.

Dosage Forms
Injection, as acetate: 25 mg/mL (10 mL, 30 mL); 50 mg/mL (10 mL, 30 mL); 100 mg/mL (10 mL)
Injection, as sodium phosphate: 20 mg/mL (2 mL, 5 mL, 10 mL)
Injection, as tebutate: 20 mg/mL (1 mL, 5 mL, 10 mL)
Liquid, oral, as sodium phosphate: 5 mg/5 mL (120 mL)
Solution, ophthalmic, as sodium phosphate: 0.125% (5 mL, 10 mL, 15 mL); 0.5% (5 mL)
Suspension, ophthalmic, as acetate: 0.12% (5 mL, 10 mL); 0.125% (5 mL, 10 mL); 1% (1 mL, 5 mL, 10 mL, 15 mL)
Syrup: 15 mg/5 mL (240 mL)
Tablet: 5 mg

Prednisolone Acetate see Prednisolone on previous page

Prednisolone Acetate, Ophthalmic see Prednisolone on previous page

Prednisolone and Gentamicin (pred niss' oh lone)

Related Information
Prednisolone on previous page

Brand Names Pred-G®

Synonyms Gentamicin and Prednisolone

Therapeutic Class Antibiotic, Ophthalmic; Corticosteroid, Ophthalmic

Use Treatment of steroid responsive inflammatory conditions and superficial ocular infections due to strains of microorganisms susceptible to gentamicin

Contraindications Known hypersensitivity to a drug component, dendritic keratitis, fungal diseases, vaccinia, varicella and most other viral infections, mycobacterial infection of the eye. The product's use is contraindicated after uncomplicated removal of a corneal foreign body.

Warnings Prolonged use may result in glaucoma, damage to the optic nerve, defects in visual acuity, posterior subcapsular cataract formation, and secondary ocular infections

(Continued)

Prednisolone and Gentamicin (Continued)

Adverse Reactions
Local: Burning, stinging

Ocular: Elevation of intraocular pressure, glaucoma, infrequent optic nerve damage, posterior subcapsular cataract formation, superficial punctate keratitis

Miscellaneous: Delayed wound healing, development of secondary infection, allergic sensitization

Usual Dosage Geriatrics and Adults: Ophthalmic: Instill 1 drop 2-4 times/day; during the initial 24-48 hours, the dosing frequency may be increased if necessary

Monitoring Parameters With use >10 days, monitor intraocular pressure

Nursing Implications Shake well before using

Special Geriatric Considerations No specific recommendations for use in elderly necessary

Dosage Forms
Ointment, ophthalmic: Prednisolone acetate 0.6% and gentamicin sulfate 0.3% (3.5 g)

Suspension, ophthalmic: Prednisolone acetate 1% and gentamicin sulfate 0.3% (5 mL)

Prednisolone Sodium Phosphate see Prednisolone on page 584

Prednisolone Sodium Phosphate, Ophthalmic see Prednisolone on page 584

Prednisolone Tebutate see Prednisolone on page 584

Prednisone (pred' ni sone)

Related Information
Antacid Drug Interactions on page 764

Corticosteroids Comparison, Systemic on page 808

Brand Names Cortan®; Deltasone®; Liquid Pred®; Meticorten®; Orasone®; Paracort®; Prednicen-M®; Sterapred®

Synonyms Deltacortisone; Deltadehydrocortisone

Generic Available Yes

Therapeutic Class Adrenal Corticosteroid; Anti-inflammatory Agent; Corticosteroid, Systemic

Use Treatment of a variety of diseases including adrenocortical insufficiency, hypercalcemia, rheumatic and collagen disorders, dermatologic, ocular, respiratory, gastrointestinal and neoplastic diseases, organ transplantation and a variety of diseases including those of hematologic, allergic, inflammatory, and autoimmune in origin

Contraindications Serious infections, except septic shock or tuberculous meningitis; systemic fungal infections; hypersensitivity to prednisone or any component; varicella

Precautions Use with caution in patients with hypothyroidism, cirrhosis, hypertension, congestive heart failure, nonspecific ulcerative colitis, thromboembolic disorders, and patients at increased risk for peptic ulcer disease; gradually taper dose to withdraw therapy

Adverse Reactions
Cardiovascular: Hypertension, edema, accelerated atherogenesis

Central nervous system: Euphoria, mental changes, headache, vertigo, seizures, psychoses, pseudotumor cerebri

Dermatologic: Folliculitis, hypertrichosis, acneiform eruption dermatitis, maceration, skin atrophy, acne, impaired wound healing, hirsutism

Endocrine & metabolic: Growth suppression, Cushing's syndrome, pituitary-adrenal axis suppression, alkalosis, glucose intolerance, hypokalemia, postmenopausal bleeding, hot flashes

Gastrointestinal: Peptic ulcer, nausea, vomiting, pancreatitis

Neuromuscular & skeletal: Muscle weakness, osteoporosis, fractures, aseptic necrosis of femoral and humeral heads, steroid myopathy

Ocular: Cataracts, glaucoma

Miscellaneous: Increased susceptibility to infection

Toxicology When consumed in excessive quantities for prolonged periods, systemic hypercorticism and adrenal suppression may occur; in those cases, discontinuation and withdrawal of the corticosteroid should be done judiciously

Drug Interactions
Steroids decrease the effect of anticholinesterases, isoniazid, salicylates, insulin, oral hypoglycemics

Decreased effect: Barbiturates, phenytoin, rifampin

Increased effect (hypokalemia) of potassium-depleting diuretics

Increased risk of digoxin toxicity (due to hypokalemia)

Increased effect: Estrogens, ketoconazole

Mechanism of Action Decreases inflammation by suppression of migration of polymorphonuclear leukocytes and reversal of increased capillary permeability; suppresses the immune system by reducing activity and volume of the lymphatic system; suppresses adrenal function at high doses

Pharmacokinetics Converted rapidly to prednisolone in the liver (active); see Prednisolone for full kinetic information

Usual Dosage Oral (dose depends upon condition being treated and response of patient; alternate day dosing may be attempted):

Geriatrics: Use the lowest effective dose

Adults: 5-60 mg/day in divided doses 1-4 times/day

Monitoring Parameters Blood pressure, blood glucose, electrolytes, symptoms of fluid retention

Test Interactions Increased amylase (S), chloride (S), increased cholesterol (S), increased glucose, increased protein, increased sodium (S); decreased calcium (S), decreased chloride (S), decreased potassium (S), decreased thyroxine (S)

Patient Information Take with food or milk or after meals; do not discontinue or decrease the drug without contacting your physician; carry an identification card or bracelet advising that you are on steroids; notify physician if signs of infection occur

Nursing Implications Give with meals to decrease GI upset; withdraw therapy with gradual tapering of dose

Additional Information Not available in injectable form, prednisolone must be used

Special Geriatric Considerations Because of the risk of adverse effects, systemic corticosteroids should be used cautiously in the elderly, in the smallest possible dose, and for the shortest possible time

Dosage Forms
Solution:
Concentrate: 5 mg/mL (5 mL, 30 mL)
Oral: 5 mg/5 mL (10 mL, 20 mL, 500 mL)
Syrup: 5 mg/5 mL (120 mL, 240 mL)
Tablet: 1 mg, 2.5 mg, 5 mg, 10 mg, 20 mg, 50 mg

Prefrin™ Ophthalmic Solution see Phenylephrine Hydrochloride on page 557

Pregnenedione see Progesterone on page 596

Prelone® see Prednisolone on page 584

Premarin® see Estrogens, Conjugated on page 270

Pretz® [OTC] see Sodium Chloride on page 648

Prevident® see Fluoride on page 299

Prilosec™ see Omeprazole on page 517

Primaclone see Primidone on this page

Primatene® Mist [OTC] see Epinephrine on page 256

Primaxin® see Imipenem/Cilastatin on page 363

Primidone (pri' mi done)
Related Information
Drug Levels Commonly Monitored Guidelines on page 771-772

Brand Names Mysoline®; Neurosyn®

Synonyms Desoxyphenobarbital; Primaclone

Generic Available Yes: Tablet

Therapeutic Class Anticonvulsant, Barbiturate

Use Management of grand mal, complex partial, and psychomotor or focal seizures

Unlabeled use: Benign familial tremor (essential tremor)

Contraindications Hypersensitivity to primidone, phenobarbital, or any component; porphyria

Warnings Do not abruptly withdraw therapy

Precautions Use with caution in patients with renal or hepatic impairment, pulmonary insufficiency; monitor for hematologic effects every 6 months; drowsiness may occur, therefore, patients should exercise caution when performing hazardous tasks

Adverse Reactions
Central nervous system: Drowsiness, vertigo, ataxia, lethargy, behavior change (mood changes with paranoia)
Dermatologic: Rash
Gastrointestinal: Nausea, vomiting
Genitourinary: Impotence
Hematologic: Leukopenia, malignant lymphoma-like syndrome, megaloblastic anemia
Ocular: Diplopia, nystagmus
Miscellaneous: Systemic lupus-like syndrome

Overdosage Symptoms of overdose include unsteady gait, slurred speech, confusion, jaundice, hypothermia, fever, hypotension

Toxicology Repeated oral doses of activated charcoal significantly reduces the half-life of primidone resulting from an enhancement of nonrenal elimination. The usual dose is 30-60 g every 4-6 hours for 3-4 days unless the patient has no bowel move-

(Continued)

Primidone *(Continued)*

ment causing the charcoal to remain in the GI tract. Assure adequate hydration and renal function. Urinary alkalinization with I.V. sodium bicarbonate also helps to enhance elimination. Hemodialysis or hemoperfusion is of uncertain value. Patients in stage IV coma due to high serum drug levels may require charcoal hemoperfusion.

Drug Interactions

Primidone may decrease serum concentrations of ethosuximide, valproic acid, griseofulvin

Succinimides may also decrease primidone and phenobarbital serum concentrations

Methylphenidate, nicotinamide, and isoniazid may increase primidone serum concentrations

Phenytoin (hydantoins) may increase primidone serum concentrations

Valproic acid may increase phenobarbital concentrations derived from primidone

Acetazolamide decrease primidone concentrations

Primidone and carbamazepine concomitantly given together may influence each others serum concentration (decrease or increased)

Stability Protect from light

Mechanism of Action Decreases neuron excitability, raises seizure threshold similar to phenobarbital; primidone has two active metabolites, phenobarbital and phenylethylmalonamide (PEMA); PEMA may enhance the activity of phenobarbital

Pharmacokinetics

Distribution: V_d: 2-3L/kg (adults)

Protein binding: 99%

Metabolism: In the liver to phenobarbital (active) and phenylethylmalonamide (PEMA)

Bioavailability: 60% to 80%

Half-life:

Primidone: 10-12 hours

PEMA: 16 hours

Phenobarbital: 52-118 hours (age-dependent with elderly generally having the longer half-life)

Time to peak: Oral: Peak concentration: Within 4 hours

Elimination: Urinary excretion of both active metabolites and unchanged primidone (15% to 25%)

Usual Dosage Geriatrics and Adults: Oral:

Initial: 125-250 mg/day at bedtime; increase by 125-250 mg/day every 3-7 days

Usual dose: 750-1500 mg/day in divided doses 3-4 times/day with maximum dosage of 2 g/day

Essential tremor: 750 mg early in divided doses; see Additional Information

Dosing interval in renal impairment:

Cl_{cr} 50-80 mL/minute: Administer every 8 hours

Cl_{cr} 10-50 mL/minute: Administer every 8-12 hours

Cl_{cr} <10 mL/minute: Administer every 12-24 hours

Moderately dialyzable (20% to 50%)

Monitoring Parameters Monitor CBC, serum concentrations of primidone, and if applicable, other anticonvulsants when given concomitantly

Reference Range

Therapeutic: Adults: 5-12 µg/mL (SI: 23-55 µmol/L); Toxic effects rarely present with levels <10 µg/mL (SI: 46 µmol/L) if phenobarbital concentrations are low

Dosage of primidone is adjusted with reference mostly to the phenobarbital level

Toxic: >15 µg/mL (SI: >69 µmol/L)

Test Interactions Increased alkaline phosphatase (S); decreased calcium (S)

Patient Information May cause drowsiness; if stomach upset occurs, take with food; do not stop therapy without consulting physician

Nursing Implications Observe patient for excessive sedation; see Monitoring Parameters and Reference Range

Additional Information Bioequivalence problems have been noted with primidone from one manufacturer to another, therefore, brand interchange is not recommended

Special Geriatric Considerations Due to CNS effects, monitor closely when initiating drug in elderly; see Adverse Reactions. Monitor CBC at 6-month intervals to compare with baseline obtained at start of therapy. Since elderly metabolize phenobarbital at a slower rate than younger adults, it is suggested to measure both primidone and phenobarbital levels together. Adjust dose for renal function in elderly when initiating or changing dose.

Dosage Forms

Suspension, oral: 250 mg/5 mL (240 mL)

Tablet: 50 mg, 250 mg

Principen® *see* Ampicillin *on page 51*

Prinivil® *see* Lisinopril *on page 412*

Privine® [OTC] *see* Naphazoline Hydrochloride *on page 492*

Probalan® *see* Probenecid *on next page*

Pro-Banthine® *see* Propantheline Bromide *on page 602*

Probenecid (proe ben' e sid)
Brand Names Benemid®; Probalan®
Therapeutic Class Adjuvant Therapy, Penicillin Level Prolongation; Uric Acid Lowering Agent
Use Prevention of gouty arthritis; hyperuricemia; prolong serum levels of penicillin/cephalosporin
Contraindications Hypersensitivity to probenecid or any component; high dose aspirin therapy; moderate to severe renal impairment
Precautions Rapid lowering of uric acid may precipitate acute gout; use with caution in patients with peptic ulcer; use extreme caution in the use of probenecid with penicillin in patients with renal insufficiency; probenecid may not be effective in patients with a Cl_{cr} <50 mL/minute
Adverse Reactions
Cardiovascular: Flushing
Central nervous system: Dizziness, headache
Dermatologic: Rash
Gastrointestinal: Anorexia, nausea, vomiting
Genitourinary: Urinary frequency, uric acid stones
Hematologic: Anemia, leukopenia
Hepatic: Hepatic necrosis
Renal: Nephrotic syndrome
Overdosage Symptoms of overdose include nausea, vomiting, tonic-clonic seizures, coma
Toxicology Activated charcoal is especially effective at binding probenecid
Drug Interactions
Decreased effect with high-dose salicylates
Increased effect/toxicity of acyclovir, thiopental, benzodiazepines, dapsone, methotrexate, sulfonylureas, zidovudine, penicillins, and cephalosporins
Mechanism of Action Competitively inhibits the reabsorption of uric acid at the proximal convoluted tubule, thereby promoting its excretion and reducing serum uric acid levels; increases plasma levels of weak organic acids (penicillins, cephalosporins or other beta-lactam antibiotics) by competitively inhibiting their renal tubular secretion
Pharmacodynamics Onset of action: Effect on penicillin levels is reached in about 2 hours
Pharmacokinetics
Absorption: Rapid and complete from GI tract
Metabolism: In the liver
Half-life: 6-12 hours (dose dependent)
Time to peak: Within 2-4 hours
Elimination: In urine
Usual Dosage Geriatrics and Adults: Oral:
Hyperuricemia: 250 mg twice daily for one week; increase by 250-500 mg/day until uric acid normalizes; maximum: 2-3 g/day

Prolongation of penicillin serum levels: 500 mg 4 times/day

Dosing adjustment in renal impairment: Cl_{cr} <50 mL/minute: Avoid use
Monitoring Parameters Uric acid, renal function, CBC
Test Interactions False-positive glucosuria with Clinitest®
Patient Information Take with food or antacids; drink plenty of fluids to reduce the risk of uric acid stones; the frequency of acute gouty attacks may increase during the first 6-12 months of therapy; avoid taking large doses of aspirin or other salicylates
Nursing Implications Give with food or antacids
Special Geriatric Considerations Since probenecid loses its effectiveness when the Cl_{cr} is <50 mL/minute, its usefulness in the elderly is limited
Dosage Forms Tablet: 500 mg

Probenecid and Colchicine *see* Colchicine and Probenecid
on page 186

Pro-Bionate® [OTC] *see* Lactobacillus acidophilus *and* Lactobacillus
bulgaricus *on page 397*

Probucol (proe' byoo kole)
Brand Names Lorelco®
Synonyms Biphenabid
Generic Available No
Therapeutic Class Antilipemic Agent
Use Adjunct to dietary therapy to decrease elevated serum total and LDL cholesterol concentrations in primary hypercholesterolemia
Contraindications Ventricular arrhythmias, hypersensitivity to probucol or any component
(Continued)

Probucol *(Continued)*

Warnings Hypokalemia, hypomagnesemia, severe bradycardia due to intrinsic heart disease, recent or AMI, ischemia or inflammation, and those receiving other cardioactive drugs that prolong the Q-T interval; serious cardiovascular toxicity and arrhythmias associated with abnormally long Q-T intervals have been reported; the manufacturer recommends that an EKG be performed before therapy is initiated and at appropriate intervals during therapy; use with caution in patients with prolonged Q-T intervals

Adverse Reactions
Cardiovascular: Q-T prolongation, serious arrhythmias
Central nervous system: Dizziness, paresthesia, headache
Dermatologic: Rash, pruritus
Gastrointestinal: Diarrhea, abdominal pain, nausea, GI bleeding, and decreased taste and smell, bloating, vomiting
Hematologic: Thrombocytopenia, anemia
Hepatic: Increase in liver function tests
Ocular: Blurred vision
Otic: Tinnitus

Overdosage Symptoms of overdose include diarrhea, flatulence

Drug Interactions Concomitant use of drugs that prolong the Q-T interval (eg, tricyclic antidepressants, some antiarrhythmic agents, phenothiazines) or with drugs that affect the atrial rate (eg, beta-adrenergic blocking agents) or that can cause A-V block (eg, digoxin) should be avoided; see Additional Information

Mechanism of Action Increases the fecal loss of bile acid-bound low density lipoprotein cholesterol, decreases the synthesis of cholesterol and inhibits enteral cholesterol absorption; decreased HDL

Pharmacokinetics
Absorption: Very slowly and poorly absorbed
Half-life: 20 days (elimination)
Time to peak: Peak serum levels require ~3 months of continuous oral administration
Elimination: Primarily via bile in feces

Usual Dosage Geriatrics and Adults: Oral: 500 mg twice daily administered with the morning and evening meals

Monitoring Parameters Fractionated serum cholesterol; EKG before starting therapy and monthly every 3 months

Patient Information Take with meals; may cause diarrhea, flatulence, abdominal pain, nausea, or vomiting

Nursing Implications Give with meals

Additional Information Concurrent use with clofibrate is not recommended since it does not provide additional lowering of LDL or total cholesterol, and may lower HDLs

Special Geriatric Considerations The definition of and, therefore, when to treat hyperlipidemia in the elderly is a controversial issue. The National Cholesterol Education Program recommends that all adults 20 years of age and older maintain a plasma cholesterol of <200 mg/dL. By this definition, 60% of all elderly would be considered to have a borderline high (200-239 mg/dL) or high (≥240 mg/dL) blood cholesterol. However, plasma cholesterol has been shown to be a less reliable predictor of coronary heart disease in the elderly. Therefore, it is the authors' belief that pharmacologic treatment be reserved for those who are unable to obtain a desirable plasma cholesterol level by diet alone and for whom the benefits of treatment are believed to outweigh the potential adverse effects, drug interactions, and cost of treatment.

Dosage Forms Tablet: 250 mg

References
"Summary of the Second Report of the National Cholesterol Education Program (NCEP) Expert Panel on Detection, Evaluation, and Treatment of High Blood Cholesterol in Adults," *JAMA,* 1993, 269(23):3015-23.

Procainamide Hydrochloride *(proe kane a' mide)*

Related Information
Drug Levels Commonly Monitored Guidelines *on page 771-772*
Brand Names Procan® SR; Promine®; Pronestyl®; Rhythmin®
Synonyms Procaine Amide Hydrochloride
Generic Available Yes
Therapeutic Class Antiarrhythmic Agent, Class IA
Use Ventricular tachycardia, premature ventricular contractions considered life-threatening, paroxysmal atrial tachycardia, and atrial fibrillation; to prevent recurrence of ventricular tachycardia, paroxysmal supraventricular tachycardia, atrial fibrillation or flutter
Contraindications Complete heart block; second or third degree heart block without pacemaker; "torsade de pointes" (twisting of the points) an unusual ventricular tachycardia; prolonged Q-T syndrome; hypokalemia; hypersensitivity to the drug or procaine, or related drugs; myasthenia gravis; SLE
Warnings Long-term administration leads to the development of a positive antinuclear antibody test in 50% of patients which may lead to a lupus erythematosus-like syn-

drome (in 20% to 30% of patients); assess relative benefits and risks if ANA titer becomes positive and consider alternative agent; discontinue PCA with SLE symptoms and change to alternative agent; serious blood dyscrasias have been reported; neutropenia and granulocytosis induced on rare occasions and associated more commonly with sustained release products; proarrhythmic potential is low

Precautions Marked A-V conduction disturbances, bundle-branch block or severe cardiac glycoside intoxication, ventricular arrhythmias in patients with organic heart disease or coronary occlusion, supraventricular tachyarrhythmias unless digitalis levels adequate to prevent marked increases in ventricular rates; drug may accumulate in patients with renal or hepatic dysfunction; some tablets contain tartrazine; injection may contain bisulfite

Adverse Reactions

Cardiovascular: Pericarditis, flushing, hypotension, tachycardia, arrhythmias, A-V block, Q-T prolongation, widening QRS complex

Central nervous system: Lightheadedness, fever, clouded sensorium, inability to concentrate, confusion, disorientation, depression, psychosis, hallucination, fatigue

Dermatologic: Rash, urticaria, pruritus

Gastrointestinal: Nausea, vomiting, GI complaints, anorexia, diarrhea, abdominal pain, bitter taste

Hematologic: Agranulocytosis, neutropenia, thrombocytopenia, positive ANA titer in 70% or more of patients

Hepatic: Positive Coombs' test

Neuromuscular & skeletal: Arthralgia, myalgia

Respiratory: Pleural effusion

Miscellaneous: Drug fever, systemic lupus erythematosus

Overdosage Symptoms of overdose include hypotension, widening of QRS complex, junctional tachycardia, intraventricular conduction delay, oliguria, lethargy, confusion

Toxicology Hypotension usually responds to I.V. fluids or Trendelenburg positioning. If unresponsive to these measures the use of a parenteral inotrope may be required (eg, norepinephrine 0.1-0.2 mcg/kg/minute titrated to response). Concurrent sodium bicarbonate and sodium lactate infusions have been effective in reversing the drug-induced cardiac toxicity.

Drug Interactions

Cimetidine, ranitidine, trimethoprim, and amiodarone may increase plasma PCA and NAPA concentrations, PCA dosage adjustment may be required

PCA may potentiate skeletal muscle relaxants and anticholinergic drugs may have enhanced effects

Propranolol may increase PCA levels

PCA may enhance neuromuscular blockade of succinylcholine

May enhance quinidine and lidocaine cardiac response (depression)

Stability Use only clear or slightly yellow solutions; stability of parenteral admixture at room temperature (25°C) and refrigeration (4°C): 24 hours

Mechanism of Action Decreases myocardial excitability and conduction velocity and depresses myocardial contractility, by increasing the electrical stimulation threshold of ventricle, HIS-Purkinje system and through direct cardiac effects

Pharmacodynamics Onset of action: I.M.: 10-30 minutes

Pharmacokinetics

Protein binding: 15% to 20%

Distribution: V_d: 2 L/kg, decreased V_d with congestive heart failure or shock

Metabolism: By acetylation in the liver to produce N-acetyl procainamide (NAPA) (active metabolite)

Bioavailability: 75% to 95% orally

Half-life (PCA):

Adults with normal renal function: 2.5-4.7 hours; half-life dependent upon hepatic acetylator phenotype, cardiac function, and renal function

NAPA (adults with normal renal function): 6-8 hours

Anephric half-life (procainamide): 11 hours

NAPA: 42 hours; half-life for procainamide and NAPA increases with age; clearance is 4.3 L/minute/kg for patients >60 years and whereas those younger have a clearance of procainamide of 7.7 mL/minute/kg

Time to peak:

Capsule: Within 45 minutes to 2.5 hours

I.M.: 15-60 minutes

Elimination: Urinary excretion (25% as NAPA)

Usual Dosage Geriatrics and Adults: Must be titrated to patient's response

Oral: 250-500 mg/dose every 3-6 hours or 500 mg to 1 g every 6 hours sustained release; usual dose: 50 mg/kg/24 hours or 2-4 g/24 hours; must individualize dose; if possible, start with lowest doses in elderly

I.V.: Load: 50-100 mg/dose, repeated every 5-10 minutes until patient controlled; or load with 15-18 mg/kg, maximum loading dose: 1-1.5 g; maintenance: 2-6 mg/minute continuous I.V. infusion, usual maintenance: 3-4 mg/minute; use lowest recommended doses for elderly

Patients with chronic hepatic disease have a reduced urinary clearance of PCA, therefore, reduce dose 50%

(Continued)

591

Procainamide Hydrochloride *(Continued)*

Dosing interval in renal impairment:
Cl$_{cr}$ 10-50 mL/minute: Administer every 6-12 hours
Cl$_{cr}$ <10 mL/minute: Administer every 8-24 hours
Moderately dialyzable (20% to 50%)

Monitoring Parameters Blood pressure, apical pulse, pulse, EKG; monitor for SLE, obtain CBC to monitor WBC every 2 weeks for first 3 months of treatment

Reference Range
Therapeutic: 4.9-12 μg/mL (SI: 15-37 μmol/L) for procainamide, <30 μg/mL (SI: <127 μmol/L) for sum of procainamide and NAPA. Optimal ranges must be ascertained for individual patients, with EKG monitoring; Toxic: >10-12 μg/mL (SI: >42-51 μmol/L).

Patient Information Do not discontinue therapy unless instructed by physician; notify physician or pharmacist if soreness of mouth, throat or gums, unexplained fever, symptoms of upper respiratory tract infection. Do not break or chew sustained release tablets. Sustained release tablets contain a wax core that slowly releases the drug. When this process is complete, the empty, nonabsorbable wax core is eliminated.

Nursing Implications Dilute I.V. with D$_5$W; maximum rate: 25-50 mg/minute

Special Geriatric Considerations Monitor closely since clearance is reduced in those >60 years of age; if clinically possible, start doses at lowest recommended dose; also, elderly frequently have drug therapy which may interfere with the use of procainamide; adjust dose for renal function in elderly; see Drug Interactions, Pharmacokinetics, and Usual Dosage

Dosage Forms
Capsule: 250 mg, 375 mg, 500 mg
Injection: 100 mg/mL (10 mL); 500 mg/mL (2 mL)
Tablet: 250 mg, 375 mg, 500 mg
Tablet, sustained release: 250 mg, 500 mg, 750 mg, 1000 mg

References
Fenster PE and Nolan PE, "Antiarrhythmic Drugs," *Geriatric Pharmacology,* Bressler R and Katz MD, eds, New York, NY: McGraw-Hill, 1993, 6:105-49.

Procaine Amide Hydrochloride *see* Procainamide Hydrochloride *on page 590*

Procaine Benzylpenicillin *see* Penicillin G Procaine, Aqueous *on page 541*

Procaine Penicillin G *see* Penicillin G Procaine, Aqueous *on page 541*

Procan® SR *see* Procainamide Hydrochloride *on page 590*

Procardia® *see* Nifedipine *on page 501*

Procardia XL® *see* Nifedipine *on page 501*

Prochlorperazine *(proe klor per' a zeen)*

Related Information
Antacid Drug Interactions *on page 764*
Antipsychotic Medication Guidelines *on page 754*

Brand Names Compazine®

Synonyms Prochlorperazine Edisylate; Prochlorperazine Maleate

Generic Available Yes: Injection and tablet

Therapeutic Class Antiemetic; Antipsychotic Agent; Phenothiazine Derivative

Use Management of nausea and vomiting; acute and chronic psychosis; nonpsychotic symptoms associated with dementia (not commonly used); see Special Geriatric Considerations

Contraindications Hypersensitivity to prochlorperazine or any component; cross-sensitivity with other phenothiazines may exist; avoid use in patients with narrow-angle glaucoma; bone marrow depression; severe liver or cardiac disease; subcortical brain damage; severe hypotension or hypertension

Warnings High incidence of extrapyramidal reactions occurs; injection contains sulfites which may cause allergic reactions; hypotension with parenteral use

Tardive dyskinesia: Prevalence rate may be 40% in elderly; elderly women especially at risk; embarrassment from dyskinesias may lead to greater social isolation; development of the syndrome and the irreversible nature are proportional to duration and total cumulative dose over time. May be reversible if diagnosed early in therapy; intermittent use of antipsychotics (not proven use) helps decrease total cumulative dose.

EPS: Extrapyramidal reactions are more common in elderly with up to 50% developing these reactions after age 60. These reactions may be more common in dementia patients. Drug-induced **Parkinson's syndrome** occurs often. Discontinuation usually resolves symptoms but may take weeks to months (12+) to clear. **Akathisia** is the most common EPS reaction in elderly. The symptoms of motor restlessness are difficult to diagnose in demented elderly; increased nervousness, assertiveness, restlessness with constant movement may indicate this adverse event. Consider decreasing dose if antipsychotic to treat as well as diagnose problem; usually see this reaction within 2-3 months of initiating antipsychotic drug.

Anticholinergic effects: These side effects most common with low potency antipsychotics (eg, thioridazine, chlorpromazine). CNS toxicity occurs more frequently and severely in elderly; increased confusion, memory loss, psychotic behavior, and agitation frequently occur as a consequence of anticholinergic effects to antipsychotic agents. Peripheral anticholinergic action troublesome to elderly; most peripheral anticholinergic effects last only 2-3 weeks; see Adverse Reactions.

Orthostatic hypotension: More common with low potency agents (eg, thioridazine, chlorpromazine, and clozapine) but of concern with all antipsychotic agents; orthostasis due to alpha-receptor blockade by antipsychotic agents. Elderly present many risk factors for orthostatic hypotension: blunted baroreceptor reflexes, decreased vascular tone, decreased vascular volume, and possible presence of cardiac diseases which result in decreased cardiac output.

Sedation: Common side effect with antipsychotic therapy; should not be used as a hypnotic unless insomnia is associated with target behavior symptoms treated with antipsychotic medications; see Special Geriatric Considerations. Anecdotal reports suggesting antipsychotic sedation in nonpsychotic patients is extremely unpleasant due to feelings of depersonalization, derealization, and dysphoria. Due to the long duration of action with antipsychotic drugs, these reactions may last up to 24 hours and result in decreased daytime function.

Cardiac toxicity: Life-threatening arrhythmias have occurred at therapeutic doses of antipsychotics. Thioridazine more commonly demonstrates EKG changes than other antipsychotics; suggested to use high potency antipsychotic agents (ie, haloperidol) in patients with cardiac conduction defects.

Precautions Extrapyramidal reactions associated with prochlorperazine are relatively high; use with caution in patients with severe cardiovascular disorder, seizures, and Parkinson's disease; benefits of therapy must be weighed against risks

Adverse Reactions
Cardiovascular: Hypotension (especially with I.V. use), orthostatic hypotension, tachycardia, arrhythmias, abnormal T waves with prolonged ventricular repolarization

Central nervous system: Sedation, drowsiness, restlessness, anxiety, extrapyramidal reactions, pseudoparkinsonian signs and symptoms, tardive dyskinesia, neuroleptic malignant syndrome, seizures, altered central temperature regulation

Dermatologic: Hyperpigmentation, pruritus, rash, photosensitivity

Endocrine & metabolic: Amenorrhea, galactorrhea, gynecomastia

Gastrointestinal: GI upset, dry mouth (problem for denture users), constipation, adynamic ileus, weight gain

Genitourinary: Urinary retention, overflow incontinence, priapism, sexual dysfunction (up to 60%), impotence

Hematologic: Agranulocytosis, leukopenia (usually in patients with large doses for prolonged periods), thrombocytopenia, hemolytic anemia, eosinophilia

Hepatic: Cholestatic jaundice (rare)

Ocular: Retinal pigmentation, blurred vision

Miscellaneous: Anaphylactoid reactions

Incidence of extrapyramidal reactions are higher with prochlorperazine than chlorpromazine

Overdosage Symptoms of overdose include deep sleep, coma, extrapyramidal symptoms, abnormal involuntary muscle movements, hypotension or hypertension; agitation, restlessness, fever, hypothermia or hyperthermia, seizures, cardiac arrhythmias, EKG changes

Toxicology Following initiation of essential overdose management, toxic symptom treatment and supportive treatment should be initiated. Hypotension usually responds to I.V. fluids or Trendelenburg positioning. If unresponsive to these measures the use of a parenteral inotrope may be required (eg, norepinephrine 0.1-0.2 mcg/kg/minute titrated to response). Do not use epinephrine. Seizures commonly respond to diazepam (I.V. 5-10 mg bolus in adults every 15 minutes if needed up to a total of 30 mg) or to phenytoin or phenobarbital. Also critical cardiac arrhythmias often respond to I.V. phenytoin (15 mg/kg up to 1 g), while other antiarrhythmics can be used. Neuroleptics often cause extrapyramidal symptoms (eg, dystonic reactions) requiring management with diphenhydramine 1-2 mg/kg up to a maximum of 50 mg I.M. or I.V. slow push followed by a maintenance dose for 48-72 hours. When these reactions are unresponsive to diphenhydramine, benztropine mesylate I.V. 1-2 mg may be effective. These agents are generally effective within 2-5 minutes.

Drug Interactions
Alcohol may increase CNS sedation
Anticholinergic agents may decrease pharmacologic effects; increase anticholinergic side effects; may enhance tardive dyskinesia

(Continued)

593

Prochlorperazine (Continued)

Aluminum salts may decrease absorption of phenothiazines

Barbiturates may decrease phenothiazine serum concentrations

Bromocriptine may have decreased efficacy when administered with phenothiazines

Guanethidine's hypotensive effect is decreased by phenothiazines

Lithium administration with phenothiazines may increase disorientation

Meperidine and phenothiazine coadministration increases sedation and hypotension

Methyldopa administration with phenothiazine (trifluoperazine) may significantly increase blood pressure

Norepinephrine, epinephrine have decreased pressor effect when administered with chlorpromazine; therefore, be aware of possible decreased effectiveness or when any phenothiazine is used

Phenytoin serum concentrations may increase or decrease with phenothiazines; tricyclic antidepressants may have increased serum concentrations with concomitant administration with phenothiazines

Propranolol administered with phenothiazines may increase serum concentrations of both drugs

Valproic acid may have increased half-life when administered with phenothiazines (chlorpromazine)

Stability Protect all dosage forms from light, clear or slightly yellow solutions may be used; should be dispensed in amber or opaque vials/bottles. Solutions may be diluted or mixed with fruit juices or other liquids but must be administered immediately after mixing; do not prepare bulk dilutions or store bulk dilutions.

Mechanism of Action Blocks postsynaptic mesolimbic dopaminergic D_1 and D_2 receptors in the brain, including the medullary chemoreceptor trigger zone; exhibits a strong alpha-adrenergic and anticholinergic blocking effect and depresses the release of hypothalamic and hypophyseal hormones; believed to depress the reticular activating system, thus affecting basal metabolism, body temperature, wakefulness, vasomotor tone and emesis

Pharmacodynamics

Onset of action:
Oral: Within 30-40 minutes
I.M.: Within 10-20 minutes
Rectal: Within 60 minutes

Duration: Effect persists longest with I.M. and oral extended release doses (12 hours) and shortest following rectal and immediate release oral administration (3-4 hours)

Pharmacokinetics

Half-life: 23 hours

Elimination: Primarily by hepatic metabolism

Usual Dosage

Geriatrics (nonpsychotic patient; dementia behavior): Initial: 2.5-5 mg 1-2 times/day; increase dose at 4- to 7-day intervals by 2.5-5 mg/day; increase dosing intervals (bid, tid, etc) as necessary to control response or side effects; maximum daily dose should probably not exceed 75 mg in elderly; gradual increases (titration) may prevent some side effects or decrease their severity

Adults, antiemetic:
Oral: 5-10 mg 3-4 times/day; usual maximum: 40 mg/day; doses up to 150 mg/day may be required in some patients
I.M.: 5-10 mg every 3-4 hours; usual maximum: 40 mg/day; doses up to 10-20 mg every 4-6 hours may be required in some patients; do not dilute with any diluent containing parabens; see Nursing Implications
I.V.: 2.5-10 mg; maximum 10 mg/dose or 40 mg/day; may repeat dose every 3-4 hours as needed; do not dilute with any diluent containing parabens
Rectal: 25 mg twice daily

Not dialyzable (0% to 5%)

Monitoring Parameters Orthostatic blood pressures; tremors, gait changes, abnormal movement in trunk, neck, buccal area or extremities; monitor target behaviors for which the agent is given

Test Interactions False-positives for phenylketonuria, urinary amylase, uroporphyrins, urobilinogen

Patient Information Do not take antacid within 1 hour of taking drug; avoid alcohol; avoid excess sun exposure (use sunblock); may cause drowsiness, rise slowly from recumbent position; use of supportive stockings may help prevent orthostatic hypotension

Nursing Implications Avoid skin contact with oral suspension or solution; may cause contact dermatitis; monitor orthostatic blood pressures 3-5 days after initiation of therapy or a dose increase; observe for tremor and abnormal movement or posturing (extrapyramidal symptoms)

Special Geriatric Considerations Due to side effect profile (dystonias, EPs) this is not a preferred drug in elderly for antiemetic therapy; see Warnings

Many elderly patients receive antipsychotic medications for inappropriate nonpsychotic behavior. Before initiating antipsychotic medication, the clinician should investigate any possible reversible cause; any stress or stress from any disease can cause acute "confusion" or worsening of baseline nonpsychotic behavior. Most commonly acute changes in behavior are due to increases in drug dose or addition of new drug to regimen, fluid electrolyte loss, infections, and changes in environment. Any changes in disease status in any organ system can result in behavior changes.

Dosage Forms
Capsule, sustained action, as maleate: 10 mg, 15 mg, 30 mg
Injection, as edisylate: 5 mg/mL (2 mL, 10 mL)
Suppository, rectal: 2.5 mg, 5 mg, 25 mg
Syrup, as edisylate: 5 mg/5 mL (120 mL)
Tablet, as maleate: 5 mg, 10 mg, 25 mg

Prochlorperazine Edisylate *see* Prochlorperazine *on page 592*

Prochlorperazine Maleate *see* Prochlorperazine *on page 592*

Procrit® *see* Epoetin Alfa *on page 258*

Proctocort™ *see* Hydrocortisone *on page 351*

Procyclidine Hydrochloride (proe sye' kli deen)
Brand Names Kemadrin®
Generic Available No
Therapeutic Class Anticholinergic Agent; Anti-Parkinson's Agent
Use Relieve symptoms of parkinsonian syndrome and drug-induced extrapyramidal symptoms
Contraindications Patients with narrow-angle glaucoma; hypersensitivity to any component; pyloric or duodenal obstruction, stenosing peptic ulcers; bladder neck obstructions; achalasia; myasthenia gravis
Precautions Use with caution in hot weather or during exercise. Elderly patients frequently develop increased sensitivity and require strict dosage regulation; side effects may be more severe in elderly patients with atherosclerotic changes. Use with caution in patients with tachycardia, cardiac arrhythmias, hypertension, hypotension, prostatic hypertrophy (especially in the elderly) or any tendency toward urinary retention, liver or kidney disorders and obstructive disease of the GI or GU tract. May exacerbate mental symptoms and precipitate a toxic psychosis when used to treat extrapyramidal reactions resulting from phenothiazines. When given in large doses or to susceptible patients, may cause weakness and inability to move particular muscle groups. Anticholinergic agents can aggravate tardive dyskinesia caused by neuroleptic agents.
Adverse Reactions
Cardiovascular: Tachycardia, hypotension
Central nervous system: Lightheadedness, hallucinations, memory loss, drowsiness, nervousness, coma **(elderly may be at increased risk for confusion and hallucinations)**
Gastrointestinal: Dry mouth, nausea, vomiting, constipation
Genitourinary: Urinary hesitancy or retention
Neuromuscular & skeletal: Muscle weakness
Ocular: Blurred vision, mydriasis
Miscellaneous: Heat intolerance
Overdosage Symptoms of overdose include CNS depression, confusion, nervousness, hallucinations, dizziness, blurred vision, nausea, vomiting, hyperthermia
Toxicology Anticholinergic toxicity is caused by strong binding of the drug to cholinergic receptors. Anticholinesterase inhibitors reduce acetylcholinesterase, the enzyme that breaks down acetylcholine and thereby allows acetylcholine to accumulate and compete for receptor binding with the offending anticholinergic. For anticholinergic overdose with severe life-threatening symptoms, physostigmine 1-2 mg S.C. or I.V., slowly may be given to reverse these effects.
Drug Interactions
Decreased effect of levodopa (decreased absorption); decreased effect with tacrine
Increased toxicity (central anticholinergic syndrome): Narcotic analgesics, phenothiazines, and other antipsychotics, tricyclic antidepressants, some antihistamines, quinidine, disopyramide
Mechanism of Action Thought to act by blocking excess acetylcholine at cerebral synapses; many of its effects are due to its pharmacologic similarities with atropine
Pharmacodynamics
Onset of action: Oral: Within 30-40 minutes
Duration: 4-6 hours; effects may still be seen at 12 hours after the dose
Pharmacokinetics
Half-life: 12 hours
Metabolism: In the liver
Elimination: In urine
Usual Dosage Oral:
Geriatrics: Initial: 2.5 mg once or twice daily, gradually increasing as necessary
(Continued)

Procyclidine Hydrochloride *(Continued)*

Adults:
 Parkinsonism: 2.5 mg 3 times/day; gradually increase to 5 mg 3-4 times/day
 Drug-induced extrapyramidal symptoms: 2.5 mg 3 times/day; increase as necessary by 2.5 mg/day; most patients require 10-20 mg/day

Monitoring Parameters Symptoms of EPS or Parkinson's, pulse, anticholinergic effects (ie, CNS< bowel and bladder function)

Patient Information Take after meals or with food if GI upset occurs; do not discontinue drug abruptly; notify physician if adverse GI effects, rapid or pounding heartbeat, confusion, eye pain, rash, fever or heat intolerance occurs. Observe caution when performing hazardous tasks or those that require alertness such as driving, as may cause drowsiness. Avoid alcohol and other CNS depressants. May cause dry mouth – adequate fluid intake or hard sugar-free candy may relieve. Difficult urination or constipation may occur – notify physician if effects persist; may increase susceptibility to heat stroke.

Nursing Implications Do not discontinue drug abruptly

Special Geriatric Considerations Anticholinergic agents are generally not well tolerated in the elderly and their use should be avoided when possible. See Precautions, Adverse Reactions. In the elderly, anticholinergic agents should not be used as prophylaxis against extrapyramidal symptoms.

Dosage Forms Tablet: 5 mg

References
Feinberg M, "The Problems of Anticholinergic Adverse Effects in Older Patients," *Drugs Aging*, 1993, 3(4):335-48.

Profenal® *see* Suprofen *on page 667*

Proferdex® *see* Iron Dextran Complex *on page 377*

Progestaject® *see* Progesterone *on this page*

Progesterone *(proe jess' ter one)*

Brand Names Gesterol®; Progestaject®

Synonyms Pregnenedione; Progestin

Generic Available Yes

Therapeutic Class Progestin

Use Endometrial carcinoma or renal carcinoma as well as secondary amenorrhea or abnormal uterine bleeding due to hormonal imbalance

Contraindications Thrombophlebitis, cerebral apoplexy, undiagnosed vaginal bleeding, hypersensitivity to progesterone or any component; carcinoma of the breast

Precautions Use with caution in patients with impaired liver function

Adverse Reactions
 Cardiovascular: Edema, thrombophlebitis, central thrombosis and embolism
 Dermatologic: Allergic rash or pruritus
 Endocrine & metabolic: Breakthrough bleeding or spotting, breast tenderness
 Gastrointestinal: Secretions, weight gain or loss, anorexia
 Hepatic: Cholestatic jaundice
 Local: Pain at injection site
 Respiratory: Pulmonary embolism

Toxicology Toxicity is unlikely following single exposures of excessive doses, and supportive treatment is adequate in most cases

Stability Refrigerate suppositories

Mechanism of Action Natural steroid hormone that induces secretory changes in the endometrium, promotes mammary gland development, relaxes uterine smooth muscle, blocks follicular maturation and ovulation and maintains pregnancy

Pharmacodynamics Duration of action: 24 hours

Pharmacokinetics
 Absorption: Inactivated by liver when taken orally, absorbed rapidly after injection
 Half-life: 5 minutes
 Elimination: In urine

Usual Dosage Geriatrics and Adults: I.M.: 5-10 mg/day for 6-8 days

Monitoring Parameters Before starting therapy, a physical exam including the breasts and pelvis are recommended, also a PAP smear; signs or symptoms of depression, glucose in diabetics

Test Interactions Liver function tests, coagulation tests, thyroid, metyrapone test, and endocrine function tests

Patient Information Diabetics should monitor their blood glucose closely

Nursing Implications Patients should receive a copy of the patient labeling for the drug; administer deep I.M. only

Additional Information May be used to prepare suppositories

Special Geriatric Considerations Not a progestin of choice in the elderly for hormonal cycling; see Adverse Reactions

Dosage Forms
 Injection: 50 mg/mL in oil (10 mL vials)
 Powder for prescription compounding

Progestin *see* Progesterone *on previous page*

Prolamine® [OTC] *see* Phenylpropanolamine Hydrochloride *on page 559*

Prolixin® *see* Fluphenazine *on page 302*

Prolixin Decanoate® *see* Fluphenazine *on page 302*

Prolixin Enanthate® *see* Fluphenazine *on page 302*

Proloid® *see* Thyroglobulin *on page 690*

Proloprim® *see* Trimethoprim *on page 721*

Promazine Hydrochloride (proe' ma zeen)

Related Information
 Antacid Drug Interactions *on page 764*
 Antipsychotic Agents Comparison *on page 801*
 Antipsychotic Medication Guidelines *on page 754*
Brand Names Sparine®
Generic Available Yes: Injection only
Therapeutic Class Antipsychotic Agent; Phenothiazine Derivative
Use Management of manifestations of psychotic disorders; depressive neurosis; alcohol withdrawal; nausea and vomiting; nonpsychotic symptoms associated with dementia in elderly, Tourette's syndrome; Huntington's chorea; spasmodic torticollis and Reye's syndrome; see Special Geriatric Considerations
Contraindications Hypersensitivity to promazine or any component; severe CNS depression, cross-sensitivity to other phenothiazines may exist; avoid use in patients with narrow-angle glaucoma, blood dyscrasias, severe liver or cardiac disease; subcortical brain damage; circulatory collapse; severe hypotension or hypertension
Warnings
 Tardive dyskinesia: Prevalence rate may be 40% in elderly; elderly women especially at risk; embarrassment from dyskinesias may lead to greater social isolation; development of the syndrome and the irreversible nature are proportional to duration and total cumulative dose over time. May be reversible if diagnosed early in therapy; intermittent use of antipsychotics (not proven use) helps decrease total cumulative dose.

 EPS: Extrapyramidal reactions are more common in elderly with up to 50% developing these reactions after age 60. These reactions may be more common in dementia patients. Drug-induced **Parkinson's syndrome** occurs often. Discontinuation usually resolves symptoms but may take weeks to months (12+) to clear. **Akathisia** is the most common EPS reaction in elderly. The symptoms of motor restlessness are difficult to diagnose in demented elderly; increased nervousness, assertiveness, restlessness with constant movement may indicate this adverse event. Consider decreasing dose if antipsychotic to treat as well as diagnose problem; usually see this reaction within 2-3 months of initiating antipsychotic drug.

 Anticholinergic effects: These side effects most common with low potency antipsychotics (eg, thioridazine, chlorpromazine). CNS toxicity occurs more frequently and severely in elderly; increased confusion, memory loss, psychotic behavior, and agitation frequently occur as a consequence of anticholinergic effects to antipsychotic agents. Peripheral anticholinergic action troublesome to elderly; most peripheral anticholinergic effects last only 2-3 weeks; see Adverse Reactions.

 Orthostatic hypotension: More common with low potency agents (eg, thioridazine, chlorpromazine, and clozapine) but of concern with all antipsychotic agents; orthostasis due to alpha-receptor blockade by antipsychotic agents. Elderly present many risk factors for orthostatic hypotension: blunted baroreceptor reflexes, decreased vascular tone, decreased vascular volume, and possible presence of cardiac diseases which result in decreased cardiac output.

 Sedation: Common side effect with antipsychotic therapy; should not be used as a hypnotic unless insomnia is associated with target behavior symptoms treated with antipsychotic medications; see Special Geriatric Considerations. Anecdotal reports suggesting antipsychotic sedation in nonpsychotic patients is extremely unpleasant due to feelings of depersonalization, derealization, and dysphoria. Due to the long duration of action with antipsychotic drugs, these reactions may last up to 24 hours and result in decreased daytime function.

 Cardiac toxicity: Life-threatening arrhythmias have occurred at therapeutic doses of antipsychotics. Thioridazine more commonly demonstrates EKG changes than other antipsychotics; suggested to use high potency antipsychotic agents (ie, haloperidol) in patients with cardiac conduction defects.
Precautions Use with caution in patients with severe cardiovascular disorder, seizures, and Parkinson's disease; benefits of therapy must be weighed against risks
Adverse Reactions
 Cardiovascular: Hypotension (especially with I.V. use), orthostatic hypotension, tachycardia, arrhythmias, abnormal T waves with prolonged ventricular repolarization

(Continued)

Promazine Hydrochloride *(Continued)*

Central nervous system: Sedation, drowsiness, restlessness, anxiety, extrapyramidal reactions, pseudoparkinsonian signs and symptoms, tardive dyskinesia, neuroleptic malignant syndrome, seizures, altered central temperature regulation

Dermatologic: Hyperpigmentation, pruritus, rash, photosensitivity

Endocrine & metabolic: Amenorrhea, galactorrhea, gynecomastia

Gastrointestinal: GI upset, dry mouth (problem for denture users), constipation, adynamic ileus, weight gain

Genitourinary: Urinary retention, overflow incontinence, priapism, sexual dysfunction (up to 60%), impotence

Hematologic: Agranulocytosis, leukopenia (usually in patients with large doses for prolonged periods), thrombocytopenia, hemolytic anemia, eosinophilia

Hepatic: Cholestatic jaundice (rare)

Ocular: Retinal pigmentation, blurred vision

Miscellaneous: Anaphylactoid reactions

Anticholinergic effects are more pronounced than extrapyramidal effects

Toxicology Following initiation of essential overdose management, toxic symptom treatment and supportive treatment should be initiated. Hypotension usually responds to I.V. fluids or Trendelenburg positioning. If unresponsive to these measures the use of a parenteral inotrope may be required (eg, norepinephrine 0.1-0.2 mcg/kg/minute titrated to response). Do not use epinephrine. Seizures commonly respond to diazepam (I.V. 5-10 mg bolus in adults every 15 minutes if needed up to a total of 30 mg) or to phenytoin or phenobarbital. Also critical cardiac arrhythmias often respond to I.V. phenytoin (15 mg/kg up to 1 g), while other antiarrhythmics can be used. Neuroleptics often cause extrapyramidal symptoms (eg, dystonic reactions) requiring management with diphenhydramine 1-2 mg/kg up to a maximum of 50 mg I.M. or I.V. slow push followed by a maintenance dose for 48-72 hours. When these reactions are unresponsive to diphenhydramine, benztropine mesylate I.V. 1-2 mg may be effective. These agents are generally effective within 2-5 minutes.

Drug Interactions

Alcohol may increase CNS sedation

Anticholinergic agents may decrease pharmacologic effects; increase anticholinergic side effects; may enhance tardive dyskinesia

Aluminum salts may decrease absorption of phenothiazines

Barbiturates may decrease phenothiazine serum concentrations

Bromocriptine may have decreased efficacy when administered with phenothiazines

Guanethidine's hypotensive effect is decreased by phenothiazines

Lithium administration with phenothiazines may increase disorientation

Meperidine and phenothiazine coadministration increases sedation and hypotension

Methyldopa administration with phenothiazine (trifluoperazine) may significantly increase blood pressure

Norepinephrine, epinephrine have decreased pressor effect when administered with chlorpromazine; therefore, be aware of possible decreased effectiveness or when any phenothiazine is used

Phenytoin serum concentrations may increase or decrease with phenothiazines; tricyclic antidepressants may have increased serum concentrations with concomitant administration with phenothiazines

Propranolol administered with phenothiazines may increase serum concentrations of both drugs

Valproic acid may have increased half-life when administered with phenothiazines (chlorpromazine)

Stability Protect all dosage forms from light, clear or slightly yellow solutions may be used; should be dispensed in amber or opaque vials/bottles. Solutions may be diluted or mixed with fruit juices or other liquids but must be administered immediately after mixing; do not prepare bulk dilutions or store bulk dilutions.

Mechanism of Action Blocks postsynaptic mesolimbic dopaminergic D_1 and D_2 receptors in the brain; exhibits a strong alpha-adrenergic blocking and anticholinergic effect, depresses the release of hypothalamic and hypophyseal hormones; believed to depress the reticular activating system thus affecting basal metabolism, body temperature, wakefulness, vasomotor tone, and emesis

Pharmacokinetics

Absorption: May be affected by the inherent anticholinergic action on the gastrointestinal tissue causing variable absorption. Absorption from tablets is erratic with less variation seen with solutions. These agents are widely distributed in tissues with CNS concentrations exceeding that of plasma due to their lipophilic characteristics.

Protein binding: Antipsychotic agents are bound 90% to 99% to plasma proteins; highly bound to brain and lung tissue and other tissues with a high blood perfusion

Time to peak: Oral absorption results in peak concentrations between 2-4 hours

Elimination: Excretion occurs through hepatic metabolism (oxidation) where numerous active metabolites are produced; active metabolites excreted in urine; elimination half-lives of antipsychotics ranges from 20-40 hours which may be extended in elderly due to decline in oxidative hepatic reactions (phase I) with age.

The biologic effect of a single dose persists for 24 hours. When the patient has accommodated to initial side effects (sedation), once daily dosing is possible due to the long half-life of antipsychotics.

Steady-state plasma levels are achieved in 4-7 days; therefore, if possible, do not make dose adjustments more than once in a 7-day period. Due to the long half-lives of antipsychotics, as needed (PRN) use is ineffective since repeated doses are necessary to achieve therapeutic tissue concentrations in the CNS.

Usual Dosage

Geriatrics (nonpsychotic patients; dementia behavior): Initial: 25 mg 1-2 times/day; increase dose at 4- to 7-day intervals by 25 mg/day; increase dose intervals (bid, tid, etc) as necessary to control response or side effects; maximum daily dose: 500 mg; gradual increases (titration) may prevent some side effects or decrease their severity

Adults: Oral, I.M.: 10-200 mg every 4-6 hours; I.M. injection preferred, I.V. not recommended

Not dialyzable (0% to 5%)

Test Interactions Increased cholesterol (S), increased glucose; decreased uric acid (S)

Patient Information Do not take antacid within 1 hour of taking drug; avoid alcohol; avoid excess sun exposure (use sun block); may cause drowsiness, rise slowly from recumbent position; use of supportive stockings may help prevent orthostatic hypotension

Nursing Implications I.M. injections should be deep injections; if giving I.V., dilute to at least 25 mg/mL and give slowly; watch for hypotension; protect injection from light; monitor orthostatic blood pressures 3-5 days after initiation of therapy or a dose increase; observe for tremor and abnormal movement or posturing (extrapyramidal symptoms)

Special Geriatric Considerations See Warnings

Many elderly patients receive antipsychotic medications for inappropriate nonpsychotic behavior. Before initiating antipsychotic medication, the clinician should investigate any possible reversible cause; any stress or stress from any disease can cause acute "confusion" or worsening of baseline nonpsychotic behavior. Most commonly acute changes in behavior are due to increases in drug dose or addition of new drug to regimen; fluid electrolyte loss; infections; and changes in environment.

Any changes in disease status in any organ system can result in behavior changes.

Dosage Forms

Injection: 25 mg/mL, 50 mg/mL

Tablet: 25 mg, 50 mg, 100 mg

Prometa® *see* Metaproterenol Sulfate *on page 449*

Prometh® *see* Promethazine Hydrochloride *on this page*

Promethazine Hydrochloride (proe meth' a zeen)

Related Information

Antacid Drug Interactions *on page 764*

Brand Names Anergan®; Phenazine®; Phencen®; Phenergan®; Prometh®; Prorex®; V-Gan®

Generic Available Yes

Therapeutic Class Antiemetic; Antihistamine; Phenothiazine Derivative; Sedative

Use Symptomatic treatment of various allergic conditions, antiemetic, motion sickness, and as a sedative

Contraindications Hypersensitivity to promethazine or any component; narrow-angle glaucoma

Warnings Do not give S.C. or intra-arterially, necrotic lesions may occur; injection may contain sulfites which may cause allergic reactions in some patients. Antihistamines are more likely to cause dizziness, excessive sedation, syncope, toxic confusion states, and hypotension in the elderly. Phenothiazine-type side effects (especially EPS) are more prone to develop in the elderly.

Precautions Use with caution in patients with cardiovascular disease, impaired liver function, asthma, sleep apnea, seizures, hypertensive crisis; avoid in patients with Reye's syndrome

Adverse Reactions

Cardiovascular: Tachycardia, bradycardia with I.V. administration

Central nervous system: Sedation (pronounced), confusion, fatigue, excitation, extrapyramidal reactions with high doses, dystonia, faintness with I.V. administration

Dermatologic: Photosensitivity

Gastrointestinal: Dry mouth, abdominal pain, nausea, diarrhea

Genitourinary: Urinary retention

Hematologic: Thrombocytopenia

Hepatic: Jaundice

Ocular: Blurred vision

(Continued)

Promethazine Hydrochloride *(Continued)*

Respiratory: Irregular respiration, bronchospasm

Miscellaneous: Allergic reactions

Overdosage Symptoms of overdose include CNS depression, respiratory depression, possible CNS stimulation, dry mouth, fixed and dilated pupils, hypotension

Toxicology Following initiation of essential overdose management, toxic symptom treatment and supportive treatment should be initiated. Hypotension usually responds to I.V. fluids or Trendelenburg positioning. If unresponsive to these measures the use of a parenteral vasopressor may be required (eg, norepinephrine 0.1-0.2 mcg/kg/minute titrated to response). Seizures commonly respond to diazepam (I.V. 5-10 mg bolus every 15 minutes if needed up to a total of 30 mg); or to phenytoin or phenobarbital. Also critical cardiac arrhythmias often respond to I.V. phenytoin (15 mg/kg up to 1 g), while other antiarrhythmics can be used. Neuroleptics often cause extrapyramidal symptoms (eg, dystonic reactions) requiring management with diphenhydramine 1-2 mg/kg up to a maximum of 50 mg I.M. or I.V. slow push followed by a maintenance dose for 48-72 hours. When these reactions are unresponsive to diphenhydramine, benztropine mesylate I.V. 1-2 mg may be effective. These agents are generally effective within 2-5 minutes. Anticholinesterase inhibitors including physostigmine, neostigmine, pyridostigmine and edrophonium may be useful in treating life-threatening anticholinergic symptoms. Physostigmine 1-2 mg I.V., slowly may be given to reverse these effects.

Drug Interactions Increased toxicity with epinephrine (increased blood pressure), CNS depressants, alcohol

Stability Protect from light and from freezing

Mechanism of Action Blocks postsynaptic mesolimbic dopaminergic receptors in the brain; exhibits a strong alpha-adrenergic blocking effect and depresses the release of hypothalamic and hypophyseal hormones; competes with histamine for the H_1-receptor; reduces stimuli to the brainstem reticular system

Pharmacodynamics

Onset of action: Within 20 minutes (3-5 minutes with I.V. injection)

Duration: 4-6 hours

Pharmacokinetics

Metabolism: In the liver

Elimination: Principally as inactive metabolites in urine and feces

Usual Dosage Geriatrics and Adults:

Antihistamine:

Oral: 25 mg at bedtime or 12.5 mg 3 times/day

I.M., I.V., rectal: 25 mg, may repeat in 2 hours

Antiemetic: Oral, I.M., I.V., rectal: 12.5-25 mg every 4 hours as needed

Motion sickness: Oral: 25 mg 30 minutes to 1 hour before departure, then every 12 hours as needed

Sedation: Oral, I.M., I.V., rectal: 25-50 mg/dose

Not dialyzable (0% to 5%)

Administration When administering IVP, do not give any faster than 25 mg/minute

Monitoring Parameters Relief of symptoms, mental status

Test Interactions Alters the flare response in intradermal allergen tests

Patient Information May cause drowsiness; avoid the use of alcohol and other CNS depressants; may cause photosensitivity

Nursing Implications Rapid I.V. administration may produce a transient fall in blood pressure, rate of administration should not exceed 25 mg/minute; slow I.V. administration may produce a slightly elevated blood pressure; avoid extravasation since tissue necrosis has occurred with extravasation; monitor patient's mental status, monitor for EPS

Additional Information Promethazine is available in various combinations. These include codeine; phenylephrine; phenylephrine and codeine.

Special Geriatric Considerations Because promethazine is a phenothiazine (and can, therefore, cause side effects such as extrapyramidal symptoms), it is not considered an antihistamine of choice in the elderly; see Warnings

Dosage Forms

Injection: 25 mg/mL (1 mL, 10 mL); 50 mg/mL (1 mL, 10 mL)

Suppository, rectal: 12.5 mg, 25 mg, 50 mg

Syrup: 6.25 mg/5 mL (5 mL, 120 mL, 240 mL, 480 mL, 4000 mL)

Tablet: 12.5 mg, 25 mg, 50 mg

Promine® *see* Procainamide Hydrochloride *on page 590*

Pronestyl® *see* Procainamide Hydrochloride *on page 590*

Propacet® *see* Propoxyphene and Acetaminophen *on page 604*

Propadrine *see* Phenylpropanolamine Hydrochloride *on page 559*

Propafenone Hydrochloride *(proe pa feen' one)*

Brand Names Rythmol®

Therapeutic Class Antiarrhythmic Agent, Class IC

Use Life-threatening ventricular arrhythmias

Unlabeled use: Supraventricular tachycardias, including those patients with Wolff-Parkinson-White syndrome

Contraindications Hypersensitivity to propafenone or any component; patients with uncontrolled congestive heart failure or bronchospastic disorders; cardiogenic shock, conduction disorders (A-V block, sick sinus syndrome), bradycardia

Warnings The CAST study issues warnings for increased mortality for any class IC antiarrhythmic agent; may be proarrhythmia, nonallergic bronchospasm, worsening or induction of CHF, decreased A-V conduction including A-V block; alterations of pacemaker thresholds; use cautiously in patients with hepatic and renal impairment; elderly may be at risk for toxicity due to decreased renal and hepatic function with age

Precautions Propafenone may cause elevation of ANA titers; both renal and hepatic tissue changes (interstitial nephritis, fatty degeneration respectively) reported in animal studies at doses above those recommended in humans; agranulocytosis has been reported

Adverse Reactions

Cardiovascular: New or worsened arrhythmias (proarrhythmic effect); prolonged A-V conduction; aggravated existing A-V block; first degree A-V block; CHF; ventricular tachycardia, palpitations, and proarrhythmia in high doses

Central nervous system: Dizziness, headache, loss of balance, fatigue, numbness, paresthesias, abnormal speech, bad dreams; occasionally: depression, confusion, memory loss, psychosis, vertigo

Gastrointestinal: Bitter or metallic taste sensation, dyspepsia, nausea, vomiting, flatulence, anorexia, abdominal pain, and constipation

Hematologic: Leukopenia, thrombocytopenia, agranulocytosis

Neuromuscular & skeletal: Weakness

Ocular: Blurred vision

Otic: Tinnitus

Majority of adverse reactions are noncardiac; for other less frequent (rare) side effects, refer to product information circular

Overdosage Most severe 3 hours after ingestion; symptoms of overdose include hypotension, bradycardia, atrial and ventricular conduction disturbances, somnolence, possibly seizures

Toxicology Symptoms of overdose include hypotension, somnolence, bradycardia, conduction disturbances, convulsions, ventricular arrhythmias; treatment is supportive; I.V. fluids and the Trendelenburg position are employed for hypotension; bradycardia can be treated with atropine but may require a pacemaker; ventricular arrhythmias are often resistant to conventional therapy; however, lidocaine 1.5 mg/kg bolus followed by 1-2 mg/minute may be effective; magnesium may be helpful in wide complex tachycardia; however, defibrillation, or isoproterenol may be needed; not dialyzable

Drug Interactions Increases effect of levels of local anesthetics, cimetidine, quinidine, anticoagulants, beta-blockers, cyclosporine, digoxin (reduce dose of digoxin 25%); rifampin increases propafenone clearance (decreases serum concentration)

Mechanism of Action Direct myocardial membrane stabilization; decreased velocity of phase O (upstroke), decreased velocity in Purkinje fibers; increased diastolic excitability threshold; prolonged effective refractory period; reduced spontaneous automaticity; exhibits beta-blockade activity

Pharmacokinetics

Absorption: Well absorbed

Metabolism: Two genetically determined metabolism groups exist: fast or slow metabolizers; 10% of Caucasians are slow metabolizers

Half-life after a single dose (100-300 mg): 2-8 hours; half-life after chronic dosing ranges from 10-32 hours

Time to peak: Peak levels occur in 2 hours with a 150 mg dose and 3 hours after a 300 mg dose; this agent exhibits nonlinear pharmacokinetics; when dose is increased from 300 mg to 900 mg/day, serum concentrations increase tenfold; this nonlinearity is thought to be due to saturable first-pass hepatic enzyme metabolism

Usual Dosage Geriatrics and Adults: Oral: 150 mg every 8 hours, increase dose at 3- to 4-day intervals; increase to 225 mg every 8 hours; increase up to 300 mg every 8 hours (maximum dose); patients who exhibit significant widening of QRS complex or second or third degree A-V block may need dose reduction

Dosing adjustment in hepatic impairment: Dose reduction is necessary

Monitoring Parameters EKG, blood pressure, pulse (particularly at initiation of therapy), signs and symptoms of CHF; titrate dose according to response and tolerance

Patient Information Take dose the same way each day, either with or without food; very important to take drug correctly, do not double the next dose if present dose is missed; report any palpitations, chest pain, difficult breathing, blurred vision, fever, sore throat, bleeding, bruising, or drowsiness; may impair coordination and judgment

Nursing Implications Watch for signs of infection; monitor heart sounds and pulses for rate, rhythm and quality

(Continued)

Propafenone Hydrochloride *(Continued)*

Additional Information An oral sodium channel blocker similar to encainide and flecainide; in clinical trials was used effectively to treat atrial flutter, atrial fibrillation, and other arrhythmias, but are not labeled indications; can worsen or even cause new ventricular arrhythmias (proarrhythmic effect)

Special Geriatric Considerations Elderly may have age-related decreases in hepatic phase I metabolism; propafenone is dependent upon liver metabolism, therefore, monitor closely in elderly and dose more gradually during initial treatment. See Warnings. No differences in clearance noted with impaired renal function and, therefore, no adjustment for renal function in elderly is necessary.

Dosage Forms Tablet: 150 mg, 300 mg

References

Fenster PE and Nolan PE, "Antiarrhythmic Drugs," *Geriatric Pharmacology*, Bressler R and Katz MD, eds, New York, NY: McGraw-Hill, 1993, 6:105-49.

Propagest® [OTC] *see* Phenylpropanolamine Hydrochloride *on page 559*

Propantheline Bromide (proe pan' the leen)

Brand Names Pro-Banthine®

Generic Available Yes: 15 mg tablet

Therapeutic Class Antispasmodic Agent, Gastrointestinal

Use Adjunctive treatment of peptic ulcer, irritable bowel syndrome, pancreatitis, ureteral and urinary bladder spasm; to reduce duodenal motility during diagnostic radiologic procedures

Contraindications Narrow-angle glaucoma, known hypersensitivity to propantheline; ulcerative colitis; toxic megacolon; obstructive disease of the GI or urinary tract

Precautions Use with caution in febrile patients, patients with hyperthyroidism, hepatic, cardiac, or renal disease, hypertension, GI infections

Adverse Reactions

Cardiovascular: Tachycardia, palpitations, flushing, orthostatic hypotension

Central nervous system: Insomnia, drowsiness, dizziness, nervousness

Dermatologic: Rash

Gastrointestinal: Dry mouth, nausea, vomiting, constipation

Genitourinary: Urinary retention, impotence

Ocular: Mydriasis, blurred vision

Miscellaneous: Diaphoresis

Overdosage Symptoms of overdose include CNS disturbances, flushing, respiratory failure, paralysis, coma, urinary retention, hyperthermia

Toxicology Anticholinergic toxicity is caused by strong binding of the drug to cholinergic receptors; for anticholinergic overdose with severe life-threatening symptoms, physostigmine 1-2 mg S.C. or I.V., slowly may be given to reverse these effects

Drug Interactions

Decreased effect with antacids (decreased absorption), tacrine; decreased effect of sustained release dosage forms (decreased absorption)

Increased effect/toxicity with anticholinergics, disopyramide, narcotic analgesics, bretylium, type I antiarrhythmics, antihistamines, phenothiazines, TCAs, corticosteroids (increased IOP), CNS depressants (sedation), adenosine, amiodarone, betablockers, amoxapine

Mechanism of Action Competitively blocks the action of acetylcholine at postganglionic parasympathetic receptor sites

Pharmacodynamics

Onset of action: Oral: Within 30-45 minutes

Duration: 4-6 hours

Pharmacokinetics

Metabolism: In the liver and GI tract

Elimination: In urine, bile, and other body fluids

Usual Dosage Oral:

Geriatrics: 7.5 mg 2-3 times/day increasing as necessary to a maximum of 30 mg 3 times/day

Adults: 15 mg 3 times/day before meals or food and 30 mg at bedtime

Monitoring Parameters Anticholinergic effects, blood pressure, pulse, urinary output, postvoid residual, GI symptoms

Patient Information Take 30 minutes before meals and at bedtime. Maintain good oral hygiene habits, because lack of saliva may increase chance of cavities. Observe caution while driving or performing other tasks requiring alertness, as may cause drowsiness, dizziness, or blurred vision. Notify physician if skin rash, flushing or eye pain occurs; or if difficulty in urinating, constipation or sensitivity to light becomes severe or persists.

Nursing Implications Give 30 minutes before meals so that the drug's peak effect occurs at the proper time; monitor for anticholinergic effects, orthostatic changes

Additional Information Because propantheline is a quaternary ammonium compound, it does not cross the blood-brain barrier and is less likely to cause CNS effects as compared to atropine

Special Geriatric Considerations The primary use of propantheline in the geriatric population is for treatment of urinary incontinence due to detrusor instability. Even though it does not cross the blood-brain barrier, CNS effects have been reported. Orthostatic hypotension may also occur, therefore, avoid long-term use in the elderly.

Dosage Forms Tablet: 7.5 mg, 15 mg

Propine® *see* Dipivefrin *on page 232*

Propoxyphene (proe pox' i feen)
Related Information
Narcotic Agonist Comparative Pharmacology *on page 811*
Pharmacokinetics of Narcotic Agonist Analgesics *on page 812*

Brand Names Darvon®; Darvon-N®

Synonyms Dextropropoxyphene; Propoxyphene Hydrochloride; Propoxyphene Napsylate

Generic Available Yes: Capsule

Therapeutic Class Analgesic, Narcotic

Use Management of mild to moderate pain

Restrictions C-IV

Contraindications Hypersensitivity to propoxyphene or any component

Warnings Give with caution in patients dependent on opiates, substitution may result in acute opiate withdrawal symptoms, use with caution in patients with severe renal or hepatic dysfunction; when given in excessive doses, either alone or in combination with other CNS depressants, propoxyphene is a major cause of drug-related deaths; do not exceed recommended dosage

Adverse Reactions
Central nervous system: Dizziness, lightheadedness, sedation, paradoxical excitement and insomnia, headache
Dermatologic: Rashes
Gastrointestinal: GI upset, nausea, vomiting, constipation
Hepatic: Increased liver enzymes
Neuromuscular & skeletal: Weakness
Miscellaneous: Psychologic and physical dependence with prolonged use

Overdosage Symptoms of overdose include CNS, respiratory, depression, hypotension, pulmonary edema, seizures

Toxicology Treatment of an overdose includes support of the patient's airway, establishment of an I.V. line and administration of naloxone 2 mg I.V. with repeat administration as necessary up to a total of 10 mg.

Drug Interactions
Decreased effect with charcoal, cigarette smoking
Increased effect/toxicity of carbamazepine, warfarin, tricyclic antidepressants, propranolol, metoprolol
Increased toxicity with CNS depressants

Mechanism of Action Binds to opiate receptors in the CNS, causing inhibition of ascending pain pathways, altering the perception of and response to pain; produces generalized CNS depression

Pharmacodynamics
Onset of effect: Oral: Within 30-60 minutes
Duration: 4-6 hours

Pharmacokinetics
Bioavailability: Oral: 30% to 70% due to first-pass effect
Half-life: 8-24 hours (mean: ~15 hours)
Metabolism: In the liver to an active metabolite (norpropoxyphene) and inactive metabolites; metabolism is decreased in the elderly and hepatic dysfunction; propoxyphene and norpropoxyphene accumulate in renal failure
Half-life: Norpropoxyphene: 34 hours

Usual Dosage Oral:
Geriatrics:
Hydrochloride: 65 mg every 4-6 hours as needed for pain
Napsylate: 100 mg every 4-6 hours as needed for pain

Adults:
Hydrochloride: 65 mg every 3-4 hours as needed for pain; maximum: 390 mg/day
Napsylate: 100 mg every 4 hours as needed for pain; maximum: 600 mg/day

Monitoring Parameters Pain relief, respiratory and mental status, blood pressure

Reference Range Therapeutic: 0.1-0.4 μg/mL (SI: 0.3-1.2 μmol/L) (therapeutic ranges published vary between laboratories and may not correlate with clinical effect); Toxic: >0.5 μg/mL (SI: >1.5 μmol/L)

Patient Information May cause drowsiness, dizziness, or blurring of vision; avoid alcohol and other sedatives; may take with food

(Continued)

Propoxyphene *(Continued)*

Nursing Implications Monitor for excessive sedation

Additional Information Some studies have found no significant difference in pain relief between propoxyphene and aspirin or acetaminophen

Propoxyphene hydrochloride: Darvon®

Propoxyphene napsylate: Darvon-N®

Special Geriatric Considerations The elderly may be particularly susceptible to the CNS depressant and constipating effects of narcotics; see Pharmacokinetics, Usual Dosage, and Additional Information

Dosage Forms

Capsule, as hydrochloride: 32 mg, 65 mg

Suspension, as napsylate: 50 mg/5 mL (480 mL)

Tablet, as napsylate: 100 mg

References

Ferrell BA, "Pain Management in Elderly People," *J Am Geriatr Soc*, 1991, 39(1):64-73.

Propoxyphene and Acetaminophen

(proe pox' i feen & a seet a min' oh fen)

Related Information

Acetaminophen *on page 13*

Pharmacokinetics of Narcotic Agonist Analgesics *on page 812*

Propoxyphene *on previous page*

Brand Names Darvocet-N®; Dolene® AP-65; Genagesic®; Propacet®; Wygesic®

Synonyms Propoxyphene Hydrochloride and Acetaminophen; Propoxyphene Napsylate and Acetaminophen

Generic Available Yes

Therapeutic Class Analgesic, Narcotic

Use Management of mild to moderate pain

Restrictions C-IV

Contraindications Hypersensitivity to propoxyphene, acetaminophen or any component

Warnings Give with caution in patients dependent on opiates, substitution may result in acute opiate withdrawal symptoms, use with caution in patients with severe renal or hepatic dysfunction; when given in excessive doses, either alone or in combination with other CNS depressants, propoxyphene is a major cause of drug-related deaths; do not exceed recommended dosage

Precautions Give with caution in patients dependent on opiates, substitution may result in acute opiate withdrawal symptoms

Adverse Reactions

Central nervous system: Dizziness, lightheadedness, sedation, paradoxical excitement and insomnia, headache

Dermatologic: Rashes

Gastrointestinal: GI upset, nausea, vomiting, constipation

Hepatic: Increased liver enzymes

Neuromuscular & skeletal: Weakness

Miscellaneous: Psychologic and physical dependence with prolonged use

Toxicology Treatment of an overdose includes support of the patient's airway, establishment of an I.V. line and administration of naloxone 2 mg I.V. with repeat administration as necessary up to a total of 10 mg. Mucomyst® (acetylcysteine) 140 mg/kg orally (loading) followed by 70 mg/kg (maintenance) every 4 hours for 17 doses. Therapy should be initiated based upon laboratory analysis suggesting high probability of acetaminophen hepatotoxic potential.

Drug Interactions

Decreased effect with charcoal, cigarette smoking

Increased effect/toxicity of carbamazepine, warfarin, tricyclic antidepressants, propranolol, metoprolol

Increased toxicity with CNS depressants

Usual Dosage Geriatrics and Adults:

Darvocet-N® 50: 1-2 tablets every 4 hours as needed; maximum: 600 mg propoxyphene napsylate/day

Darvocet-N® 100: 1 tablet every 4 hours as needed; maximum: 600 mg propoxyphene napsylate/day

Dolene® AP-65: 1 tablet every 4 hours as needed

Monitoring Parameters Pain relief, respiratory and mental status, blood pressure

Patient Information Do not exceed recommended dose; may cause drowsiness, avoid alcoholic beverages

Nursing Implications Monitor for excessive sedation

Additional Information Some studies have found no significant difference in pain relief between propoxyphene and aspirin or acetaminophen

Propoxyphene hydrochloride and acetaminophen: Dolene® AP-65, Wygesic®, Genagesic®

Propoxyphene napsylate and acetaminophen: Darvocet-N®, Darvocet-N® 100; Propacet®

Propoxyphene napsylate 100 mg and propoxyphene hydrochloride contain same amount of propoxyphene

Special Geriatric Considerations Elderly may be particularly susceptible to the CNS depressant and constipating effects of narcotics; do not exceed 4 g/day of acetaminophen; see Warnings

Dosage Forms Tablet: Propoxyphene napsylate 50 mg and acetaminophen 325 mg; propoxyphene napsylate 100 mg and acetaminophen 650 mg; propoxyphene hydrochloride 65 mg and acetaminophen 650 mg

Propoxyphene Hydrochloride see Propoxyphene on page 603

Propoxyphene Hydrochloride and Acetaminophen see Propoxyphene and Acetaminophen on previous page

Propoxyphene Napsylate see Propoxyphene on page 603

Propoxyphene Napsylate and Acetaminophen see Propoxyphene and Acetaminophen on previous page

Propranolol and Hydrochlorothiazide
Related Information
Hydrochlorothiazide on page 347
Propranolol Hydrochloride on this page
Brand Names Inderide®
Generic Available Yes: Immediate release
Therapeutic Class Antihypertensive, Combination
Use Management of hypertension
Special Geriatric Considerations Combination products are not recommended for first-line therapy and divided doses of diuretics may increase the incidence of nocturia in the elderly
Dosage Forms
Capsule, long acting (Inderide® LA):
80/50 Propranolol hydrochloride 80 mg and hydrochlorothiazide 50 mg
120/50 Propranolol hydrochloride 120 mg and hydrochlorothiazide 50 mg
160/50 Propranolol hydrochloride 160 mg and hydrochlorothiazide 50 mg
Tablet (Inderide®):
40/25 Propranolol hydrochloride 40 mg and hydrochlorothiazide 25 mg
80/25 Propranolol hydrochloride 80 mg and hydrochlorothiazide 25 mg

Propranolol Hydrochloride (proe pran' oh lole)
Related Information
Beta-Blockers Comparison on page 804-805
Brand Names Inderal®; Inderal® LA; Ipran®
Generic Available Yes
Therapeutic Class Antianginal Agent; Antiarrhythmic Agent, Class IB; Antiarrhythmic Agent, Class II; Beta-Adrenergic Blocker
Use Management of hypertension, angina pectoris, pheochromocytoma, essential tremor, and arrhythmias (such as atrial fibrillation, PVCs, and flutter, A-V nodal re-entrant tachycardias, and catecholamine-induced arrhythmias); prevention of myocardial infarction, migraine headache; symptomatic treatment of hypertrophic subaortic stenosis, digitalis-induced arrhythmias, resistant tachyarrhythmias, migraine prophylaxis
Unlabeled use: Tremor due to Parkinson's disease, alcohol withdrawal, aggressive behavior, antipsychotic-induced akathisia, esophageal varices bleeding, anxiety, schizophrenia, acute panic, and gastric bleeding in portal hypertension
Contraindications Uncompensated congestive heart failure, cardiogenic shock, bradycardia or heart block, asthma, hyperactive airway disease, chronic obstructive lung disease, Raynaud's syndrome, diabetes mellitus, and those with hypersensitivity to beta-blocking agents
Warnings In patients with angina pectoris, exacerbation of angina and, in some cases, myocardial infarction, occurred following abrupt discontinuance of therapy abrupt withdrawal of the drug should be avoided; drug should be discontinued over 2 weeks
Precautions Use with caution in patients with renal or hepatic impairment administer to CHF patients with caution; administer with caution to patients with bronchospastic disease, diabetes mellitus, hyperthyroidism, myasthenia gravis, renal function decline, and severe peripheral vascular disease; abrupt withdrawal of the drug should be avoided, drug should be discontinued over 2 weeks.
Adverse Reactions
Cardiovascular: Hypotension, impaired myocardial contractility, congestive heart failure, bradycardia, worsening of A-V conduction disturbances
Central nervous system: Lightheadedness, insomnia, vivid dreams, lethargy, depression
Endocrine & metabolic: Hypoglycemia, hyperglycemia
Gastrointestinal: Nausea, vomiting, diarrhea, GI distress, constipation
Hematologic: Agranulocytosis
(Continued)

Propranolol Hydrochloride *(Continued)*

Neuromuscular & skeletal: Weakness
Respiratory: Bronchospasm
Miscellaneous: Cold extremities

Overdosage Symptoms of overdose include severe hypotension, bradycardia, heart failure and bronchospasm; isoproterenol may be used to counteract; see Toxicology

Toxicology Sympathomimetics (eg, epinephrine or dopamine), glucagon or a pacemaker can be used to treat the toxic bradycardia, asystole, and/or hypotension. Initially, fluids may be the best treatment for toxic hypotension. Patients should remain supine; serum glucose and potassium should be measured; use supportive measures: lavage, syrup of ipecac; propranolol not significantly removed by hemodialysis; I.V. glucose should be administered for hypoglycemia. Seizures may be treated with phenytoin or diazepam intravenously; continuous monitoring of blood pressure and EKG is necessary. If PVCs occur, treat with lidocaine or phenytoin; avoid quinidine, procainamide, and disopyramide since these agents further depress myocardial function; bronchospasm can be treated with theophylline or beta$_2$ agonists (epinephrine).

Drug Interactions

Phenobarbital, rifampin may increase propranolol clearance and may decrease its activity

Cimetidine may reduce propranolol clearance and may increase its effects

Aluminum-containing antacid may reduce GI absorption of propranolol; nonsteroidal anti-inflammatory agents, salicylates, sympathomimetics, thyroid hormones, insulins, lidocaine, calcium channel blockers, nifedipine, catecholamine depleting drugs, clonidine, disopyramide, prazosin, theophylline

Stability Compatible in saline, incompatible with HCO_3^-; protect injection from light

Mechanism of Action Competitively blocks response to beta$_1$- and beta$_2$-adrenergic stimulation; demonstrates high membrane stabilization activity but has no intrinsic sympathomimetic activity; highly lipid soluble, therefore, penetrates the blood-brain barrier

Pharmacodynamics

Onset of action: Oral: Beta blockade occurs within 1-2 hours
Duration: ~6 hours

Pharmacokinetics Extensive first-pass effect

Distribution: V_d: 3.9 L/kg
Protein binding: 93%
Metabolism: In the liver to active and inactive compounds
Bioavailability: 30% to 40%
Half-life: 4-6 hours
Elimination: Primarily in urine (96% to 99%)

Usual Dosage

Arrhythmias:

Adults:
Oral: 10-80 mg/dose every 6-8 hours
I.V.: 1 mg/dose slow IVP; repeat every 5 minutes up to a total of 5 mg
Geriatrics: Initial: 10 mg twice daily or 60 mg once daily as sustained release capsules; increase dosage every 3-7 days; usual dose range: 10-320 mg given 1-2 times/day

Hypertension: Geriatrics and Adults: Oral: Initial: 40 mg twice daily or 60-80 mg once daily as sustained release capsules; increase dosage every 3-7 days; usual dose: ≤320 mg divided in 2-3 doses/day or once daily as sustained release; maximum daily dose: 640 mg

Migraine headache prophylaxis: Geriatrics and Adults: Oral: Initial: 80 mg/day divided every 6-8 hours; increase by 20-40 mg/dose every 3-4 weeks to a maximum of 160-240 mg/day given in divided doses every 6-8 hours

Thyrotoxicosis: Geriatrics and Adults:
Oral: 10-40 mg/dose every 6 hours
I.V.: 1-3 mg/dose slow IVP as a single dose

Not dialyzable (0% to 5%)

Monitoring Parameters Blood pressure, orthostatic hypotension, heart rate, CNS effects

Reference Range Therapeutic: 50-100 ng/mL (SI: 190-390 nmol/L) at end of dose interval

Test Interactions Increased thyroxine (S), cholesterol (S), glucose, triglycerides, potassium, uric acid; decreased HDL

Patient Information Do not discontinue abruptly, sudden stopping of medication may precipitate or cause angina; consult pharmacist or physician before taking with other adrenergic drugs (eg, cold medications); notify physician if any of the following symptoms occur: difficult breathing, night cough, swelling of extremities, slow pulse, dizziness, lightheadedness, confusion, depression, skin rash, fever, sore throat, unusual bleeding, or bruising; may produce drowsiness, dizziness, lightheadedness, blurred vision, confusion; use with caution while driving or performing tasks requiring alertness; take at the same time each day, may be taken without regard to meals; may mask signs of hypoglycemia in diabetes

Nursing Implications I.V. dose much smaller than oral dose; I.V. administration should not exceed 1 mg/minute; monitor EKG and CVP; patient's therapeutic response may be evaluated by looking at blood pressure, apical and radial pulses, fluid I & O, daily weight, respirations, and circulation in extremities before and during therapy; modify dosage in patients with renal insufficiency

Special Geriatric Considerations Since bioavailability increased in elderly about twofold, geriatric patients may require lower maintenance doses, therefore, as serum and tissue concentrations increase beta$_1$ selectivity diminishes; due to alterations in the beta-adrenergic autonomic nervous system, beta-adrenergic blockade may result in less hemodynamic response than seen in younger adults. Studies indicate that despite decreased sensitivity to the chronotropic effects of beta blockade with age, there appears to be an increased myocardial sensitivity to the negative inotropic effect during stress (ie, exercise). Controlled trials have shown the overall response rate for propranolol to be only 20% to 50% in elderly populations. Therefore, all beta-adrenergic blocking drugs may result in a decreased response as compared to younger adults. Due to propranolol's CNS penetration and nonselective action, it may not be the beta-blocker of choice for use in elderly.

Dosage Forms
Capsule, sustained action: 60 mg, 80 mg, 120 mg, 160 mg
Injection: 1 mg/mL (1 mL)
Solution, oral: 4 mg/mL (5 mL, 500 mL); 8 mg/mL (5 mL, 500 mL)
Solution, oral, concentrate: 80 mg/mL (30 mL)
Tablet: 10 mg, 20 mg, 40 mg, 60 mg, 80 mg, 90 mg

References
Aagaard GN, "Treatment of Hypertension in The Elderly," *Drug Treatment in the Elderly*, Vestal RE, ed, Boston, MA: ADIS Health Science Press, 1984, 77.

Propulsid® see Cisapride *on page 169*

2-Propylpentanoic Acid see Valproic Acid and Derivatives *on page 728*

Propylthiouracil (proe pill thye oh yoor' a sill)

Synonyms PTU
Generic Available Yes
Therapeutic Class Antithyroid Agent
Use Palliative treatment of hyperthyroidism as an adjunct to ameliorate hyperthyroidism in preparation for surgical treatment or radioactive iodine therapy and in the management of thyrotoxic crisis
Contraindications Hypersensitivity to propylthiouracil or any component
Warnings Use of antithyroid drugs may cause agranulocytosis, thyroid, hyperplasia, thyroid carcinoma (PTU for longer than 1 year)
Precautions Use with caution in patients >40 years of age because PTU may cause hypoprothrombinemia and bleeding, monitor prothrombin time during therapy; use with extreme caution in patients receiving other drugs known to cause agranulocytosis; monitor thyroid function tests periodically (T$_4$, TSH)

Adverse Reactions
Cardiovascular: Edema, cutaneous vasculitis, periarteritis
Central nervous system: Headache, drowsiness, paresthesia, CNS stimulation, depression, neuritis, vertigo
Dermatologic: Rash, urticaria, pruritus, exfoliative dermatitis
Gastrointestinal: Nausea, vomiting, loss of taste
Hematologic: Aplastic anemia, agranulocytosis, thrombocytopenia, bleeding
Hepatic: Jaundice, hepatitis
Neuromuscular & skeletal: Arthralgia
Renal: Nephritis
Miscellaneous: Drug fever, lupus-like syndrome

Overdosage Symptoms of overdose include nausea, vomiting, arthralgia, pancytopenia, epigastric distress, and signs of hypothyroidism
Toxicology General supportive care; monitor bone marrow response, forced diuresis, peritoneal and hemodialysis as well as charcoal hemoperfusion **have not** been helpful in overdose situation
Drug Interactions Activity of oral anticoagulants may be increased by the antivitamin K activity of PTU
Mechanism of Action Inhibits the synthesis of thyroid hormones by blocking the oxidation of iodine in the thyroid gland; blocks synthesis of thyroxine and triiodothyronine; does not inactivate circulatory T$_4$ and T$_3$
Pharmacodynamics For significant therapeutic effects, 24-36 hours are required and remissions of hyperthyroidism do not usually occur before 4 months of continued therapy

Pharmacokinetics
Protein binding: 75% to 80%
(Continued)

Propylthiouracil *(Continued)*

Metabolism: Hepatic

Half-life: 1-2 hours

Time to peak: Oral: Peak serum levels occur within 1 hour and persist for 2-3 hours

Elimination: 35% in urine

Usual Dosage Oral:

Geriatrics: Initial: 150-300 mg/day in divided doses every 8 hours

Adults: Initial: 300-450 mg/day in divided doses every 8 hours

Geriatrics and Adults: Maintenance: 100-150 mg/day in divided doses every 8-12 hours

Monitoring Parameters Monitor signs of hypo- and hyperthyroidism, T_4, T_3, TSH, CBC

Test Interactions Increased prothrombin time (S)

Patient Information Do not exceed prescribed dosage; take at regular intervals around-the-clock; notify physician or pharmacist if fever, sore throat, unusual bleeding or bruising, headache, or general malaise occurs

Nursing Implications See Warnings, Precautions, Monitoring Parameters, and Special Geriatric Considerations

Additional Information Periodic blood counts are recommended with chronic therapy; see Warnings

Special Geriatric Considerations The use of antithyroid thioamides is as effective in elderly as they are in younger adults; however, the expense, potential adverse effects, and inconvenience (compliance, monitoring) make them undesirable. The use of radioiodine, due to ease of administration and less concern for long-term side effects and reproduction problems, makes it a more appropriate therapy

Dosage Forms Tablet: 50 mg

References

Johnson DG and Campbell S, "Hormonal and Metabolic Agents," *Geriatric Pharmacology*, Bressler R and Katz MD, eds, New York, NY: McGraw-Hill, 1993, 427-50.

Raby C, Lagorce JF, Jambut-Absil AC, et al, "The Mechanism of Action of Synthetic Antithyroid Drugs: Iodine Complexation During Oxidation of Iodide," *Endocrinology*, 1990, 126(3):1683-91.

2-Propylvaleric Acid *see* Valproic Acid and Derivatives *on page 728*

Prorex® *see* Promethazine Hydrochloride *on page 599*

Proscar® *see* Finasteride *on page 292*

ProSom™ *see* Estazolam *on page 268*

Prostaphlin® *see* Oxacillin Sodium *on page 521*

Protostat® *see* Metronidazole *on page 467*

Protriptyline Hydrochloride *(proe trip' ti leen)*

Related Information

Antidepressant Agents Comparison *on page 800*

Brand Names Vivactil®

Therapeutic Class Antidepressant, Tricyclic

Use Treatment of various forms of depression, often in conjunction with psychotherapy

Contraindications Narrow-angle glaucoma, hypersensitivity to protriptyline or any component

Precautions Use with caution in patients with cardiac conduction disturbances, history of hyperthyroid; protriptyline should not be abruptly discontinued in patients receiving high doses for prolonged periods to avoid cholinergic crisis; an EKG prior to initiation of therapy is advised

Adverse Reactions

Cardiovascular: Postural hypotension, arrhythmias, tachycardia, sudden death

Central nervous system: Sedation, dizziness, fatigue, anxiety, confusion, insomnia, impaired cognitive function, delirium, seizures; extrapyramidal symptoms are possible

Dermatologic: Photosensitivity

Endocrine & metabolic: SIADH

Gastrointestinal: Dry mouth, increased appetite and weight gain, constipation, decreased lower esophageal sphincter tone may cause GE reflux, unpleasant taste

Genitourinary: Urinary retention, sexual dysfunction

Hematologic: Rarely agranulocytosis, leukopenia, eosinophilia

Hepatic: Jaundice, cholestatic jaundice

Neuromuscular & skeletal: Tremors, weakness

Ocular: Blurred vision, increased intraocular pressure

Miscellaneous: Allergic reactions

Overdosage Symptoms of overdose include agitation, confusion, hallucinations, urinary retention, hypothermia, hypotension, tachycardia

Toxicology Following initiation of essential overdose management, toxic symptoms should be treated. Ventricular arrhythmias often respond to phenytoin 15-20 mg/kg with concurrent systemic alkalinization (sodium bicarbonate 0.5-2 mEq/kg I.V.). Arrhythmias unresponsive to this therapy may respond to lidocaine 1 mg/kg I.V. followed by a titrated infusion. Physostigmine (1-2 mg I.V. slowly) may be indicated in reversing cardiac arrhythmias that are due to vagal blockade or for anticholinergic effects. Seizures usually respond to diazepam I.V. boluses (5-10 mg, up to 30 mg). If seizures are unresponsive or recur, phenytoin or phenobarbital may be required.

Drug Interactions
May decrease effects of guanethidine and clonidine
May increase effects of CNS depressants, adrenergic agents, dicumarol, anticholinergic agents
With MAO inhibitors, hyperpyrexia, tachycardia, hypertension, seizures, and death may occur; interactions similar to other tricyclics may occur
Cimetidine, fluoxetine, methylphenidate, and haloperidol may decrease the metabolism and/or increase TCA levels
Phenobarbital may increase TCA metabolism; use with clonidine may result in hypertensive crisis

Mechanism of Action Traditionally believed to increase the synaptic concentration of serotonin and/or norepinephrine in the central nervous system by inhibition of their reuptake by the presynaptic neuronal membrane. However, additional receptor effects have been found including desensitization of adenyl cyclase, down regulation of beta-adrenergic receptors, and down regulation of serotonin receptors.

Pharmacodynamics Onset of therapeutic effects: Takes 1-3 weeks before effects are seen; NE >>5-HT

Pharmacokinetics
Protein binding: 92%
Metabolism: Undergoes first-pass metabolism (10% to 25%); extensively metabolized in the liver by N-oxidation, hydroxylation and glucuronidation
Half-life: 54-92 hours, averaging 74 hours
Time to peak: Oral: Peak serum levels occur within 24-30 hours
Elimination: In urine

Usual Dosage Oral:
Geriatrics: Initial dose: 5-10 mg/day; increase every 3-7 days by 5-10 mg; usual dose: 15-20 mg/day

Adults: 15-60 mg in 3-4 divided doses

Monitoring Parameters Blood pressure, pulse, target symptoms, mental status
Reference Range Therapeutic: 70-250 ng/mL (SI: 266-950 nmol/L); Toxic: >500 ng/mL (SI: >1900 nmol/L)
Test Interactions Elevated glucose
Patient Information Do not drink alcoholic beverages, may cause dry mouth, constipation, blurred vision, dizziness, avoid sudden changes in position
Nursing Implications Offer patient sugarless hard candy for dry mouth; monitor sitting and standing blood pressure and pulse
Special Geriatric Considerations Little data on its use in the elderly; strong anticholinergic properties which may limit its use; more often stimulating rather than sedating
Dosage Forms Tablet: 5 mg, 10 mg

Proventil® see Albuterol on page 24
Provera® see Medroxyprogesterone Acetate on page 437
Proxigel® Oral [OTC] see Carbamide Peroxide on page 119
Prozac® see Fluoxetine Hydrochloride on page 301
Prulet® [OTC] see Phenolphthalein on page 556

Pseudoephedrine (soo doe e fed' rin)
Brand Names Afrinol® [OTC]; Cenafed® [OTC]; Decofed® Syrup [OTC]; Neofed® [OTC]; Novafed®; Sudafed® [OTC]; Sudafed® 12 Hour [OTC]; Sufedrin® [OTC]
Synonyms d-Isoephedrine Hydrochloride; Pseudoephedrine Hydrochloride; Pseudoephedrine Sulfate
Generic Available Yes
Therapeutic Class Adrenergic Agonist Agent; Decongestant
Use Temporary symptomatic relief of nasal congestion due to common cold, upper respiratory allergies, and sinusitis; also promotes nasal or sinus drainage

Unlabeled use: Urinary incontinence (stress type) due to urethral sphincter weakness
Contraindications Hypersensitivity to pseudoephedrine or any component; MAO inhibitor therapy
Warnings Administer with caution to patients with hypertension, hyperthyroidism, diabetes mellitus, cardiovascular disease, ischemic heart disease, increased intraocular pressure, or prostatic hypertrophy. Elderly patients are more likely to experience adverse reactions to sympathomimetics. Overdosage may cause hallucinations, seizures, CNS depression, and death.
Adverse Reactions
Cardiovascular: Tachycardia, palpitations, arrhythmias
(Continued)

Pseudoephedrine *(Continued)*

Central nervous system: Nervousness, excitability, dizziness, insomnia, drowsiness, headache

Gastrointestinal: Nausea, vomiting

Genitourinary: Difficult urination

Neuromuscular & skeletal: Tremors

Overdosage Symptoms of overdose include seizures, nausea, vomiting, cardiac arrhythmias, hypertension, agitation

Toxicology There is no specific antidote for pseudoephedrine intoxication and the bulk of the treatment is supportive. Hyperactivity and agitation usually respond to reduced sensory input, however with extreme agitation haloperidol may be required. Hyperthermia is best treated with external cooling measures, or when severe or unresponsive, muscle paralysis with pancuronium may be needed. Hypertension is usually transient and generally does not require treatment unless severe. For diastolic blood pressures >110 mm Hg, a nitroprusside infusion should be initiated. Seizures usually respond to diazepam I.V. and/or phenytoin maintenance regimens.

Drug Interactions

Decreased effect: Beta-blockers, methyldopa

Increased toxicity/effect: Tricyclic antidepressants, MAO inhibitors (increased blood pressure), sympathomimetics

Mechanism of Action Stimulates alpha-adrenergic receptors of the vascular smooth muscle, thus constricting dilated arterioles within the nasal mucosa and reducing blood flow to the engaged area; increases urethral sphincter tone due to alpha-adrenergic actions

Pharmacodynamics

Onset of action: Oral: Decongestant effects occur within 15-30 minutes

Duration: 4-6 hours (up to 12 hours with extended release formulation administration)

Pharmacokinetics

Half-life: 9-16 hours

Metabolism: Partially in liver

Elimination: 70% to 90% of dose excreted in urine as unchanged drug and 1% to 6% as norpseudoephedrine (active); renal elimination is dependent on urine pH and flow rate; alkaline urine decreases renal elimination of pseudoephedrine

Usual Dosage

Nasal congestion:

Geriatrics: 30-60 mg every 6 hours as needed

Adults: 60 mg every 4-6 hours; maximum: 240 mg/24 hours; sustained release: 120 mg every 12 hours

Urinary incontinence: Geriatrics and Adults: 15-30 mg 3 times/day

Monitoring Parameters Blood pressure, pulse, relief of symptoms, urinary output, episodes of incontinence

Patient Information Do not crush sustained release products; consult pharmacist or physician before using; do not exceed recommended dose; notify physician of insomnia, weakness, dizziness, tremor, or irregular heartbeat

Additional Information Pseudoephedrine is found in many combination cough and cold products

Pseudoephedrine hydrochloride: Cenafed® syrup [OTC], Decofed® syrup [OTC], Neofed® [OTC], Novafed®, Sudafed® [OTC], Sudafed® 12 Hour [OTC], Sudafed® tablet [OTC], Sufedrin® [OTC]

Pseudoephedrine sulfate: Afrinol® [OTC]

Special Geriatric Considerations Elderly patients should be counseled about the proper use of over-the-counter cough and cold preparations; see Warnings

Dosage Forms

Capsule, timed release, as hydrochloride: 120 mg

Liquid, as hydrochloride: 15 mg/5 mL (120 mL); 30 mg/5 mL (120 mL, 240 mL, 473 mL)

Tablet: 30 mg, 60 mg

Tablet, repeat action: 120 mg

Pseudoephedrine and Triprolidine *see* Triprolidine and Pseudoephedrine *on page 723*

Pseudoephedrine Hydrochloride *see* Pseudoephedrine *on previous page*

Pseudoephedrine Sulfate *see* Pseudoephedrine *on previous page*

Pseudomonic Acid A *see* Mupirocin *on page 482*

Psyllium *(sill' i yum)*

Brand Names Effer-Syllium® [OTC]; Fiberall® [OTC]; Hydrocil® [OTC]; Konsyl® [OTC]; Konsyl-D® [OTC]; Metamucil® [OTC]; Metamucil® Instant Mix [OTC]; Modane® Bulk [OTC]; Naturacil® [OTC]; Perdiem® Plain [OTC]; Reguloid® [OTC]; Serutan® [OTC]; Siblin® [OTC]; Syllact® [OTC]; V-Lax® [OTC]

Synonyms Plantago Seed; Plantain Seed; Psyllium Hydrophilic Mucilloid

Generic Available Yes

Therapeutic Class Laxative, Bulk-Producing

Use Treatment of chronic atonic or spastic constipation and in constipation associated with rectal disorders; treatment of diverticulosis and diverticulitis; management of irritable bowel syndrome; nonspecific acute diarrhea

Contraindications Fecal impaction, GI obstruction; hypersensitivity to psyllium

Warnings May contribute to fecal impaction if insufficient fluid intake exists or other predisposing causes

Precautions Some products contain aspartame which is metabolized in the GI tract to phenylalanine; rectal bleeding may indicate a more serious medical condition which may require further evaluation; impaction and obstruction may occur in diseases which inhibit passage through the gastrointestinal tract (eg, strictures, ileus); use caution in patients with intestinal ulceration, bowel adhesions, or stenosis; not to be used for acute constipation

Adverse Reactions
Gastrointestinal: Esophageal or bowel obstruction, bloating, flatulence, abdominal cramps
Ocular: Rhinoconjunctivitis
Respiratory: Bronchospasm
Miscellaneous: Anaphylaxis upon inhalation in susceptible (hypersensitive) individuals

Overdosage Symptoms of overdose include abdominal pain, diarrhea, flatulence, possible impaction

Drug Interactions Digitalis, nitrofurantoin, salicylates may have their absorption decreased by psyllium

Mechanism of Action Absorbs water in the intestine to form a viscous liquid which promotes peristalsis and reduces transit time through mechanical distention; fiber decreases intraluminal pressures in the colon and rectum which is beneficial in treatment of diverticular disease and irritable bowel syndrome

Pharmacodynamics Onset of action: 12-24 hours, but full effect may take 2-3 days; considered the safest and most physiologic laxative agent

Pharmacokinetics Absorption: Oral: Generally not absorbed, small amounts of grain extracts present in the preparation have been reportedly absorbed following colonic hydrolysis

Usual Dosage Geriatrics and Adults: Oral: 1-2 rounded teaspoonfuls (5-11 g) or 1-2 packets 1-3 times/day in water or fruit juice; see Additional Information

Monitoring Parameters Monitor for diarrhea, abdominal pain, bowel obstruction, or impaction

Patient Information Must be mixed in a glass of water or juice; drink a full glass of liquid with each dose; must drink fluids throughout the day to be effective and avoid impaction; report bleeding or failure to respond to physician, pharmacist, or nurse; do not use for acute constipation

Nursing Implications Inhalation of psyllium dust may cause sensitivity to psyllium (runny nose, watery eyes, wheezing); fiber therapy increases stool frequency; do not use for acute constipation; see Monitoring Parameters

Additional Information 3.4 g psyllium hydrophilic mucilloid per 7 g powder is equivalent to a rounded teaspoonful or one packet; fiber therapy results in increased frequency of defecation. Diabetic patients may need or prefer sugar-free products; psyllium using aspartame is available for diabetic patients.

Special Geriatric Considerations Elderly may have insufficient fluid intake which may predispose them to fecal impaction and bowel obstruction. Patients should have a 1 month trial, with at least 14 g/day, before effects in bowel function are determined. Bloating and flatulence are mostly a problem in first 4 weeks of therapy.

Dosage Forms
Chewable pieces: 3.4 g
Granules: 4.03 g per rounded teaspoon (100 g, 250 g); 2.5 g per rounded teaspoon
Powder, effervescent: 3 g per dose (270 g, 480 g); 3.4 g per dose (single dose packets)
Powder: Psyllium 50% and dextrose 50% (6.5 g, 325 g, 420 g, 480 g, 500 g); psyllium hydrophilic: 3.4 g per rounded teaspoon (210 g, 300 g, 420 g, 630 g)
Wafer: 3.4 g

Psyllium Hydrophilic Mucilloid see Psyllium on previous page

Pteroylglutamic Acid see Folic Acid on page 310

PTU see Propylthiouracil on page 607

Purge® [OTC] see Castor Oil on page 124

Purinethol® see Mercaptopurine on page 444

Pyopen® see Carbenicillin on page 120

Pyrazinamide (peer a zin' a mide)

Synonyms Pyrazinoic Acid Amide

Therapeutic Class Antitubercular Agent

Use Adjunctive treatment of tuberculosis when primary and secondary agents cannot be used or have failed

(Continued)

Pyrazinamide *(Continued)*

Contraindications Severe hepatic damage; hypersensitivity to pyrazinamide or any component, acute gout

Precautions Use with caution in patients with renal failure, gout or diabetes mellitus

Adverse Reactions
Central nervous system: Malaise, fever
Dermatologic: Urticaria, rash, photosensitivity
Endocrine & metabolic: Gout, hyperuricemia
Gastrointestinal: Nausea, vomiting, anorexia
Hepatic: Hepatotoxicity, jaundice
Neuromuscular & skeletal: Arthralgia

Overdosage Symptoms of overdose include gout, gastric upset, hepatic damage

Drug Interactions Isoniazid (decreased INH serum levels)

Mechanism of Action Converted to pyrazinoic acid in susceptible strains of *Mycobacterium* which lowers the pH of the environment

Pharmacodynamics Bacteriostatic or bactericidal depending on the drug's concentration at the site of infection

Pharmacokinetics
Absorption: Oral: Well absorbed
Distribution: Widely distributed into body tissues and fluids including the liver, lung, and CSF
Protein binding: 50%
Metabolism: In the liver
Half-life: 9-10 hours, increased with reduced renal or hepatic function
Time to peak: Peak serum levels appear within 2 hours
Elimination: In urine (4% as unchanged drug)

Usual Dosage Oral:
Geriatrics: Start with a lower daily dose (15 mg/kg) and increase as tolerated

Adults: 15-30 mg/kg/day in 3-4 divided doses; maximum daily dose: 2 g/day
Alternative dose: A dosing regimen of 50-70 mg/kg twice weekly (based upon lean body weight) has been recommended to improve patient compliance

Monitoring Parameters Periodic liver function tests, serum uric acid, sputum culture, chest x-ray 2-3 months into treatment and at completion

Test Interactions May interfere with Acetest® and Ketostix® urine tests to produce a pink-brown color

Patient Information Compliance must be stressed; inform physician if fever, malaise, weakness, nausea or vomiting, darkened urine, skin or eye discoloration (yellow), or swollen or painful joints develop

Special Geriatric Considerations Pyrazinamide is used in the 2-month intensive treatment phase of a 6-month treatment plan. Most elderly acquired their *Mycobacterium tuberculosis* infection before effective chemotherapy was available; however, older persons with new infections (not reactivation), or who are from areas where drug-resistant *M. tuberculosis* is endemic, or who are HIV-infected should receive 3-4 drug therapies including pyrazinamide.

Dosage Forms Tablet: 500 mg

References
Bass JB Jr, Farer LS, Hopewell PC, et al, "Treatment of Tuberculosis and Tuberculosis Infection in Adults and Children," *Am J Respir Crit Care Med*, 1994, 149(5):1359-74.
Van Scoy RE and Wilkowske CJ, "Antituberculous Agents: Isoniazid, Rifampin, Streptomycin, Ethambutol, and Pyrazinamide," *Mayo Clin Proc*, 1983, 58(4):233-40.
Yoshikawa TT, "Tuberculosis in Aging Adults," *J Am Geriatr Soc*, 1992, 40(2):178-87.

Pyrazinoic Acid Amide *see Pyrazinamide on previous page*

Pyrbuterol *see Pirbuterol Acetate on page 570*

Pyridiate® *see Phenazopyridine Hydrochloride on page 552*

Pyridium® *see Phenazopyridine Hydrochloride on page 552*

Pyridostigmine Bromide *(peer id oh stig' meen)*

Brand Names Mestinon®; Regonol®

Generic Available No

Therapeutic Class Antidote, Neuromuscular Blocking Agent; Cholinergic Agent

Use Symptomatic treatment of myasthenia gravis; also used as an antidote for nondepolarizing neuromuscular blockers

Contraindications Hypersensitivity to pyridostigmine, bromides, or any component; GI or GU obstruction

Precautions Use with caution in patients with epilepsy, asthma, bradycardia, hyperthyroidism, arrhythmias, or peptic ulcer

Adverse Reactions
Cardiovascular: Bradycardia, A-V block
Central nervous system: Headache, seizures, drowsiness
Dermatologic: Rash

Gastrointestinal: Nausea, vomiting, diarrhea, salivation

Genitourinary: Urge to urinate

Neuromuscular & skeletal: Muscle cramps, weakness

Ocular: Miosis

Respiratory: Increased bronchial secretions, bronchospasm

Miscellaneous: Sweating

Overdosage Symptoms of overdose include muscle weakness, blurred vision, excessive sweating, tearing and salivation, nausea, vomiting, diarrhea, hypertension, bradycardia, paralysis

Toxicology Atropine is the treatment of choice for intoxications manifesting with significant muscarinic symptoms. Atropine I.V. 2-4 mg every 3-60 minutes should be repeated to control symptoms and then continued as needed for 1-2 days following the acute ingestion.

Drug Interactions

Decreased effect with corticosteroids, magnesium, antiarrhythmics

Increased effect of depolarizing neuromuscular relaxants (succinylcholine) effect

Increased effect/toxicity with edrophonium, aminoglycosides

Stability Protect from light

Mechanism of Action Inhibits destruction of acetylcholine by acetylcholinesterase which facilitates transmission of impulses across myoneural junction

Pharmacodynamics

Onset of action:

Oral, I.M.: Within 15-30

I.V.: Within 2-5 minutes

Duration:

Oral: 3-6 hours

I.M., I.V.: 2-4 hours

Pharmacokinetics

Absorption: Oral: Very poor (10% to 20%) from GI tract

Metabolism: In the liver

Usual Dosage Geriatrics and Adults:

Myasthenia gravis:

Oral: Initial: 60 mg 3 times/day with maintenance dose ranging from 60 mg to 1.5 g/day; sustained release: 180-540 mg once or twice daily

I.M., I.V.: 2 mg every 2-3 hours or 1/30th of oral dose

Reversal of nondepolarizing neuromuscular blocker: I.V.: 10-20 mg preceded by atropine (I.V. 0.6-1.2 mg)

Monitoring Parameters Symptoms of myasthenia gravis, blood pressure, pulse

Test Interactions Increased aminotransferase [ALT (SGPT)/AST (SGOT)] (S), increased amylase (S)

Patient Information Take drug as ordered; take with food; report adverse reactions to physician promptly; do not chew or crush sustained release tablets

Nursing Implications Do not crush sustained release drug product; observe patient closely for cholinergic symptoms especially if I.V. dose is used

Additional Information Not a cure; patient may develop resistance to the drug; normally, sustained release dosage form is used at bedtime for patients who complain of morning weakness

Special Geriatric Considerations See Precautions and Adverse Reactions

Dosage Forms

Injection: 5 mg/mL (2 mL, 5 mL)

Syrup: 60 mg/5 mL (480 mL)

Tablet: 60 mg

Tablet, sustained release: 180 mg

Pyridoxine Hydrochloride (peer i dox' een)

Brand Names Nestrex®

Synonyms Vitamin B$_6$

Generic Available Yes

Therapeutic Class Antidote, Cycloserine Toxicity; Antidote, Hydralazine Toxicity; Antidote, Isoniazid Toxicity; Vitamin, Water Soluble

Use Prevents and treats vitamin B$_6$ deficiency, adjunct to treatment of acute toxicity from isoniazid, cycloserine, or hydralazine overdose

Contraindications Hypersensitivity to pyridoxine or any component

Warnings Dependence and withdrawal may occur with doses >200 mg/day

Adverse Reactions

Central nervous system: Paresthesia, sensory neuropathy, seizures

Miscellaneous: Following I.V. administration of very large doses, headache, nausea, decreased serum folic acid secretions (especially in patients with homocystinuria), increased AST, allergic reactions

Overdosage Signs and symptoms of overdose include ataxia, sensory neuropathy with doses of 50 mg to 2 g daily over prolonged periods

(Continued)

Pyridoxine Hydrochloride *(Continued)*

Drug Interactions Decreased serum levels of levodopa, phenobarbital, and phenytoin (patients taking levodopa should avoid supplemental vitamin B₆ >5 mg/day; includes many multivitamin preparations)

Stability Protect from light

Mechanism of Action Precursor to pyridoxal, which functions in the metabolism of proteins, carbohydrates, and fats; pyridoxal also aids in the release of liver and muscle stored glycogen

Pharmacokinetics

Absorption: Enteral, parenteral: Well absorbed

Metabolism: In 4-pyridoxic acid, and other metabolites

Half-life: 2-3 weeks

Elimination: Urinary excretion

Usual Dosage Geriatrics and Adults:

Dietary deficiency: Oral: 10-20 mg/day for 3 weeks

Drug-induced neuritis (eg, isoniazid, hydralazine, penicillamine, cycloserine): Oral treatment: 100-200 mg/24 hours; prophylaxis: 10-100 mg/24 hours

For the treatment of seizures and/or coma from acute isoniazid toxicity, a dose of pyridoxine hydrochloride equal to the amount of INH ingested can be given I.M./I.V. in divided doses together with other anticonvulsants

For the treatment of acute hydralazine toxicity, a pyridoxine dose of 25 mg/kg in divided doses I.M./I.V. has been used

Administration Give slow I.V.

Monitoring Parameters When administering large I.V. doses, monitor respiratory rate, heart rate, and blood pressure

Reference Range >50 ng/mL (SI: 243 nmol/L) (varies considerably with method). A broad range is ~25-80 ng/mL (SI: 122-389 nmol/L). HPLC method for pyridoxal phosphate has normal range of 3.5-18 ng/mL (SI: 17-88 nmol/L).

Test Interactions Urobilinogen

Patient Information Dietary sources of pyridoxine include red meats, bananas, potatoes, yeast, lima beans, whole grain cereals; do not exceed recommended doses

Nursing Implications Burning may occur at the injection site after I.M. or S.C. administration; seizures have occurred following I.V. administration of very large doses

Additional Information

For the treatment of seizures and/or coma from acute isoniazid toxicity, a dose of pyridoxine hydrochloride equal to the amount of INH ingested can be given I.M./I.V. in divided doses together with other anticonvulsants

For the treatment of acute hydrazine toxicity, pyridoxine 25 mg/kg/dose I.M./I.V. has been used

Dosage Forms

Injection: 100 mg/mL (10 mL, 30 mL)

Tablet: 25 mg, 50 mg, 100 mg

Tablet, extended release: 100 mg

Quazepam *(kway' ze pam)*

Related Information

Antacid Drug Interactions *on page 764*

Anxiolytic/Hypnotic Use in Long-Term Care Facilities *on page 755-756*

Benzodiazepines Comparison *on page 802-803*

Brand Names Doral®

Generic Available No

Therapeutic Class Benzodiazepine; Hypnotic; Sedative

Use Short-term treatment of insomnia

Restrictions C-IV

Contraindications Narrow-angle glaucoma, known hypersensitivity to quazepam, cross-sensitivity with other benzodiazepines may occur; severe uncontrolled pain, sleep apnea

Warnings Abrupt discontinuance may precipitate withdrawal or rebound insomnia

Precautions Has potential for drug dependence and abuse, use with caution in patients with a history of drug dependence

Adverse Reactions

Central nervous system: Daytime sedation, ataxia, amnesia, confusion, dizziness, hallucinations, headache

Gastrointestinal: Dry mouth, nausea, vomiting

Hepatic: Cholestatic jaundice

Miscellaneous: Physical and psychological dependence may occur with prolonged use

Overdosage Symptoms of overdose include somnolence, confusion, coma, and diminished reflexes

Toxicology Treatment for benzodiazepine overdose is supportive; rarely is mechanical ventilation required

Flumazenil has been shown to selectively block the binding of benzodiazepines to CNS receptors, resulting in a reversal of benzodiazepine-induced sedation; however, its use may not alter the course of overdose

Drug Interactions Benzodiazepines may increase digoxin concentrations and may decrease the effect of levodopa

Decreased metabolism: Cimetidine, fluoxetine

Increased metabolism: Rifampin

Increased toxicity: CNS depressants, alcohol

Mechanism of Action Benzodiazepines appear to potentiate the effects of GABA and other inhibitory neurotransmitters by binding to specific benzodiazepine-receptor sites in various areas of the CNS

Pharmacodynamics Studies have shown that the elderly are more sensitive to the effects of benzodiazepines as compared to younger adults

Pharmacokinetics

Absorption: Oral: Rapidly absorbed

Half-life:

Geriatrics:

Parent: 53 hours

Active metabolite: 190 hours

Adults:

Parent: 25-41 hours

Active metabolite: 40-114 hours

Metabolism: In the liver to at least one active compound

Protein binding: 95%.

Usual Dosage Oral:

Geriatrics: Initial: 7.5-15 mg at bedtime, if giving 15 mg initially, decrease to 7.5 mg on the second or third night

Adults: Initial: 15 mg at bedtime, in some patients the dose may be reduced to 7.5 mg after a few nights

Monitoring Parameters Respiratory, cardiovascular and mental status

Patient Information Avoid alcohol and other CNS depressants; may cause drowsiness; avoid activities needing good psychomotor coordination until CNS effects are known; may cause physical or psychological dependence; avoid abrupt discontinuation after prolonged use; may cause "hangover" effect

Nursing Implications Provide safety measures (ie, side rails, night light, call button); remove smoking materials from area; supervise ambulation

Additional Information More likely than short-acting benzodiazepine to cause daytime sedation and fatigue; is classified as a long-acting benzodiazepine hypnotic (like flurazepam - Dalmane®), this long duration of action may prevent withdrawal symptoms when therapy is discontinued.

Special Geriatric Considerations See Pharmacodynamics; two short-term placebo controlled studies found minimal daytime drowsiness or other side effects with quazepam in elderly patients; there is little clinical experience with this drug in the elderly, but because of its long duration of action, it is probably not a drug of choice; long-acting benzodiazepines have been associated with falls in the elderly; interpretive guidelines from the Health Care Financing Administration (HCFA) discourage the use of this agent in residents of long-term care facilities

Dosage Forms Tablet: 7.5 mg, 15 mg

References

Martinez HT and Serna CT, "Short-Term Treatment With Quazepam in Insomnia in Geriatric Patients," *Clin Ther*, 1982, 5(2):174-8.

Winsauer HJ and O'Hair DE, "Quazepam: Short-Term Treatment of Insomnia in Geriatric Outpatients," *Curr Ther Res*, 1984, 35(2):228-34.

Queltuss® [OTC] see Guaifenesin and Dextromethorphan on page 332

Questran® see Cholestyramine Resin on page 163

Quibron®-T see Theophylline on page 681

Quibron®-T/SR see Theophylline on page 681

Quiess® see Hydroxyzine on page 356

Quinacrine Hydrochloride (kwin' a kreen)

Brand Names Atabrine®

Synonyms Mepacrine Hydrochloride

Therapeutic Class Anthelmintic; Antimalarial Agent

Use Treatment of giardiasis and cestodiasis (tapeworm); reserve agent for suppression and chemoprophylaxis of malaria

Contraindications Hypersensitivity to quinacrine or any component; patients receiving primaquine

Precautions Use with caution in patients with renal, cardiac, hepatic disease, G-6-PD deficiency, porphyria reported to cause psychosis in persons >60 years or who have a history of psychosis

(Continued)

Quinacrine Hydrochloride (Continued)

Adverse Reactions

Central nervous system: Dizziness, psychosis, restlessness, confusion, seizures, headache

Dermatologic: Urticaria, yellow discoloration of skin, black skin and nail pigmentation, exfoliative dermatitis, lichen planus-like eruptions

Gastrointestinal: Nausea, vomiting, diarrhea, abdominal cramps

Hematologic: Blood dyscrasias

Hepatic: Hepatitis

Ocular: Retinopathy, corneal deposits

Renal: Yellow discoloration of urine

Overdosage Symptoms of overdose include CNS excitation with restlessness, insomnia, psychic stimulation, seizures, nausea, vomiting, abdominal cramps, diarrhea, hypotension, cardiac arrhythmias or arrest, yellow skin pigmentation

Toxicology No specific therapy is indicated after GI decontamination; therapy is supportive in nature. Diazepam 0.1 mg/kg for seizures, I.V. fluids/Trendelenburg position for hypotension; norepinephrine or dopamine may be required; lidocaine for cardiac arrhythmias.

Drug Interactions Primaquine increased serum concentrations, alcohol (disulfiram-like reaction)

Mechanism of Action Binds to parasite's DNA by intercalation between adjacent base pairs inhibiting replication and protein synthesis

Pharmacokinetics

Absorption: Oral: Well absorbed

Protein binding: 90%

Metabolism: Concentrates in the liver where it is slowly metabolized

Half-life: 120 hours

Time to peak: Peak serum levels occur within 1-3 hours

Elimination: Principally in urine with secondary elimination in saliva, bile, sweat; 11% of dose excreted unchanged in urine

Usual Dosage Geriatrics and Adults: Oral:

Dwarf tapeworm: 900 mg in 3 portions 20 minutes apart, then 100 mg 3 times/day for 3 days

Tapeworm (beef, pork, or fish): 200 mg every 10 minutes for 4 doses

Giardiasis: 100 mg 3 times/day for 5-7 days

Suppression of malaria: 100 mg/day, continue for 1-3 months; for endemic areas, drug therapy should be started 2 weeks before arrival and continued for 3-4 weeks after departure

Administration For tapeworms use cathartic 1-2 hours after quinacrine administered in order to expel the worms for examination; collect and examine all stool for 48 hours after treatment for worm's attachment organ (stained yellow)

Monitoring Parameters CBC, periodic ophthalmic exams with prolonged therapy

Patient Information May discolor urine and skin yellow; give after meals; report to physician any visual disturbances, skin rash, or mental aberrations during therapy

Nursing Implications See Administration

Additional Information See Administration

Special Geriatric Considerations Due to side effect profile, this agent is not a drug of choice for giardiasis or tapeworm treatment in elderly; see Precautions and Adverse Reactions

Dosage Forms

Tablet: 100 mg

Tablet, as sulfate: 100 mg, 200 mg, 300 mg

Quinaglute® Dura-Tabs® see Quinidine on page 618

Quinalan® see Quinidine on page 618

Quinalbarbitone Sodium see Secobarbital Sodium on page 640

Quin-Amino® see Quinine Sulfate on page 620

Quinaminoph® see Quinine Sulfate on page 620

Quinamm® see Quinine Sulfate on page 620

Quinapril Hydrochloride

Brand Names Accupril®

Generic Available No

Therapeutic Class Angiotensin-Converting Enzyme (ACE) Inhibitors

Use Management of hypertension and treatment of congestive heart failure; increase circulation in Raynaud's phenomenon; idiopathic edema

Unlabeled use: Hypertensive crisis, diabetic nephropathy, rheumatoid arthritis, diagnosis of anatomic renal artery stenosis, hypertension secondary to scleroderma renal crisis, diagnosis of aldosteronism, idiopathic edema, Bartter's syndrome, postmyocardial infarction for prevention of ventricular failure

Contraindications Hypersensitivity to captopril or any component or any ACE inhibitor

Warnings Neutropenia, agranulocytosis, angioedema, decreased renal function (hypertension, renal artery stenosis, CHF), hepatic dysfunction (elimination, activation), proteinuria, first-dose hypotension (hypovolemia, CHF, dehydrated patients at risk, eg, diuretic use, elderly), elderly (due to renal function changes)

Precautions Use with caution and modify dosage in patients with renal impairment; use with caution in patients with collagen vascular disease, CHF, hypovolemia, valvular stenosis, hyperkalemia (>5.7 mEq/L), anesthesia

Adverse Reactions

Cardiovascular: Arrhythmias, orthostatic blood pressure changes, CVA, myocardial infarction, angina, palpitations, chest pain, hypotension, tachycardia, syncope, cardiogenic shock, heart failure

Central nervous system: Nervousness, depression, confusion, somnolence, fatigue, dizziness, headache, paresthesia, insomnia, malaise, vertigo

Dermatologic: Rash, exfoliative dermatitis, photosensitivity, pruritus, dermatopolymyositis, angioedema

Endocrine & metabolic: Hyperkalemia

Gastrointestinal: Loss of taste perception, pancreatitis, dry mouth, constipation, anorexia, nausea, vomiting, abdominal pain, dry mouth, pancreatitis, GI hemorrhage

Genitourinary: Impotence

Hematologic: Neutropenia, agranulocytosis, thrombocytopenia (0.5% to 1%)

Hepatic: Hepatitis

Neuromuscular & skeletal: Myalgia, arthralgia

Ocular: Blurred vision

Renal: Increased BUN, serum creatinine, proteinuria, oliguria, worsening of renal failure

Respiratory: Chronic cough (nonproductive, persistent; more often in women and seen in 15% to 30% of patients), asthma, bronchospasm

Miscellaneous: Sweating

Overdosage Symptoms of overdose include hypotension

Toxicology Following initiation of essential overdose management, toxic symptom treatment and supportive treatment should be initiated. Hypotension usually responds to I.V. fluids or Trendelenburg positioning. If unresponsive to these measures, the use of a parenteral inotrope may be required (eg, norepinephrine 0.1-0.2 mcg/kg/minute titrated to response). Seizures commonly respond to diazepam (I.V. 5-10 mg bolus in adults every 15 minutes if needed up to a total of 30 mg) or to phenytoin or phenobarbital.

Drug Interactions

ACE inhibitors (quinapril) and potassium-sparing diuretics → additive hyperkalemic effect

ACE inhibitors (quinapril) and indomethacin or nonsteroidal anti-inflammatory agents → reduced antihypertensive response to ACE inhibitors (quinapril)

Allopurinol and quinapril → neutropenia

Antacids and ACE inhibitors → ↓ absorption of ACE inhibitors

Phenothiazines and ACE inhibitors → ↑ ACE inhibitor effect

Probenecid and ACE inhibitors (quinapril) → ↑ ACE inhibitors (quinapril) levels

Rifampin and ACE inhibitors (enalapril) → ↓ ACE inhibitor effect

Digoxin and ACE inhibitors → ↑ serum digoxin levels

Lithium and ACE inhibitors → ↑ lithium serum levels

Tetracycline and ACE inhibitors (quinapril) → ↓ tetracycline absorption (up to 37%)

Food decreases quinapril absorption; rate, but not extent, of ramipril and fosinopril is reduced by concomitant administration with food; food does not reduce absorption of enalapril, lisinopril or benazepril; quinapril has a decreased rate and extent (25% to 30%) of absorption when taken with a high fat meal

Stability Unstable in aqueous solutions; to prepare solution for oral administration, mix prior to administration and use within 10 minutes

Mechanism of Action Competitive inhibitor of angiotensin-converting enzyme (ACE); prevents conversion of angiotensin I to angiotensin II, a potent vasoconstrictor; results in lower levels of angiotensin II which causes an increase in plasma renin activity and a reduction in aldosterone secretion; a CNS mechanism may also be involved in hypotensive effect as angiotensin II increases adrenergic outflow from CNS; vasoactive kallikreins may be decreased in conversion to active hormones by ACE inhibitors, thus reducing blood pressure

Pharmacodynamics

Onset of action: Within 1 hour

Duration: 24 hours

Pharmacokinetics

Absorption: Oral: 60%

Metabolism: To some degree in liver; active metabolite quinaprilat

Half-life (quinaprilat): 2 hours; prolonged with renal impairment, see Usual Dosage

Elimination: As metabolites in urine and feces

(Continued)

Quinapril Hydrochloride *(Continued)*

Usual Dosage Oral:

Geriatrics: Initial: 2.5-5 mg/day; increase dosage at increments of 2.5-5 mg at 1- to 2-week intervals; see following creatinine clearance recommendations; see Additional Information

Adults: Initial: 10 mg once daily, adjust at 1- to 2-week intervals according to blood pressure response at peak and trough blood levels; in general, the normal dosage range is 40-80 mg/day

Dosing adjustment in renal impairment (daily initial dose):

Cl_{cr} >60 mL/minute: Administer 10 mg; elderly: 5 mg

Cl_{cr} 30-60 mL/minute: Administer 5 mg; elderly: 2.5

Cl_{cr} 10-30 mL/minute: Administer 2.5 mg

Monitoring Parameters Serum calcium levels, BUN, serum creatinine, renal function, WBC, and potassium

Test Interactions Increased potassium (S)

Patient Information Do not discontinue medication without advice of physician; notify physician if sore throat, swelling, palpitations, cough, chest pains, difficulty swallowing, swelling of face, eyes, tongue, lips, hoarseness, sweating, vomiting, or diarrhea occurs; may cause dizziness, lightheadedness during first few days; may also cause changes in taste perception; do not use salt substitutes containing potassium without consulting a physician

Nursing Implications May cause depression in some patients; discontinue if angioedema of the face, extremities, lips, tongue, or glottis occurs; watch for hypotensive effects within 1-3 hours of first dose or new higher dose; see Precautions and Special Geriatric Considerations

Additional Information Patients taking diuretics are at risk for developing hypotension on initial dosing; to prevent this, discontinue diuretics 2-3 days prior to initiating quinapril; may restart diuretics if blood pressure is not controlled by quinapril alone

Special Geriatric Considerations Due to frequent decreases in glomerular filtration (also creatinine clearance) with aging, elderly patients may have exaggerated responses to ACE inhibitors; differences in clinical response due to hepatic changes are not observed. ACE inhibitors may be preferred agents in elderly patients with CHF and diabetes mellitus. Diabetic proteinuria is reduced and insulin sensitivity is enhanced. In general, the side effect profile is favorable in elderly and causes little or no CNS confusion; use lowest dose recommendations initially.

Dosage Forms Tablet: 5 mg, 10 mg, 20 mg, 40 mg

References

McAreavey D and Robertson JIS, "Angiotensin Converting Enzyme Inhibitors and Moderate Hypertension," *Drugs*, 1990, 40(3):326-45.

Quinatime® *see* Quinidine *on this page*

Quindan® *see* Quinine Sulfate *on page 620*

Quine® [OTC] *see* Quinine Sulfate *on page 620*

Quinidex® Extentabs® *see* Quinidine *on this page*

Quinidine *(kwin' i deen)*

Related Information

Antacid Drug Interactions *on page 764*

Drug Levels Commonly Monitored Guidelines *on page 771-772*

Brand Names Cardioquin®; Cin-Quin®; Duraquin®; Quinaglute® Dura-Tabs®; Quinalan®; Quinatime®; Quinidex® Extentabs®; Quinora®

Synonyms Quinidine Gluconate; Quinidine Polygalacturonate; Quinidine Sulfate

Generic Available Yes

Therapeutic Class Antiarrhythmic Agent, Class IA

Use Prophylaxis after cardioversion of atrial fibrillation and/or flutter to maintain normal sinus rhythm; also used to prevent reoccurrence of paroxysmal supraventricular tachycardia, paroxysmal A-V junctional rhythm, paroxysmal ventricular tachycardia, paroxysmal atrial fibrillation, and atrial or ventricular premature contractions; also has activity against *Plasmodium falciparum* malaria

Contraindications Patients with complete A-V block with an A-V junctional or idioventricular pacemaker; patients with intraventricular conduction defects (marked widening of QRS complex); patients with cardiac glycoside-induced A-V conduction disorders; myasthenia gravis; thrombocytopenia associated with quinidine administration; digitalis intoxication, aberrant ectopic rhythms, history of drug-induced torsade de pointes, history of long Q-T syndrome, hypersensitivity to the drug or cinchona derivatives

Warnings May cause syncope, most likely due to ventricular tachycardia or fibrillation; syncope may subside spontaneously, but occasionally may be fatal; discontinue quinidine if syncope occurs; hepatotoxicity, atrial flutter/fibrillation or conversion to sinus rhythm, cardiotoxicity, hypersensitivity; use caution in renal/hepatic impairment or patients with cardiac insufficiency

Precautions Myocardial depression, sick sinus syndrome, incomplete A-V block, cardiac glycoside intoxication, hepatic and/or renal insufficiency, myasthenia gravis; hemolysis may occur in patients with G-6-PD (glucose-6-phosphate dehydrogenase) deficiency; quinidine-induced hepatotoxicity, including granulomatous hepatitis, increased serum AST and alkaline phosphatase concentrations, and jaundice may occur

Adverse Reactions

Cardiovascular: Hypotension, tachycardia, heart block, torsade de pointes, syncope, vascular collapse, ventricular fibrillation, severe hypotension with rapid I.V. administration

Central nervous system: Headache, fever, vertigo, confusion, delirium, dementia

Dermatologic: Angioedema, rash

Gastrointestinal: GI disturbances, nausea, vomiting, abdominal pain, cramps

Hematologic: Blood dyscrasias, thrombotic thrombocytopenic

Hepatic: Purpura

Ocular: Impaired vision

Otic: Tinnitus, impaired hearing

Respiratory: Respiratory depression

Overdosage Symptoms of overdose include ataxia, lethargy, respiratory distress, apnea, severe hypotension, anuria, absence of P waves, broadening QRS complex, PR and Q-T intervals, ventricular arrhythmias, hallucinations, and seizures.

Toxicology Electrolyte balance should be monitored and treated, especially when refractory arrhythmias develop. Sodium bicarbonate 1-2 mEq/kg I.V. may decrease drug toxicity. Phenytoin or lidocaine are often effective at controlling drug-induced arrhythmias, while phenytoin is preferred due to its beneficial effects on A-V conduction velocity.

Drug Interactions

Quinidine potentiates nondepolarizing and depolarizing muscle relaxants

Verapamil, amiodarone, alkalinizing agents, and cimetidine may increase quinidine serum concentrations

Phenobarbital, phenytoin, and rifampin may decrease quinidine serum concentrations

Quinidine may increase plasma concentration of digoxin, closely monitor digoxin concentrations, digoxin dosage may need to be reduced (by one-half) when quinidine is initiated, new steady-state digoxin plasma concentrations occur in 5-7 days; beta-blockers + quinidine → ↑ bradycardia

Quinidine may enhance coumarin anticoagulants

Quinidine alters pharmacokinetics of encainide, flecainide, propafenone, and metoprolol

Stability Do not use discolored parenteral solution

Mechanism of Action Depresses phase O (upstroke) of the action potential; decreases myocardial excitability and conduction velocity, and myocardial contractility by decreasing sodium influx during depolarization and potassium efflux in repolarization; also reduces calcium transport across cell membrane

Pharmacokinetics

Distribution: V_d: 2-3.5 L/kg, decreased V_d with congestive heart failure, malaria; increased V_d with cirrhosis; V_d is not significantly changed with age

Protein binding: 80% to 90% (younger adults); decreased protein binding with cyanotic congenital heart disease, cirrhosis, or acute myocardial infarction.

Metabolism: Extensive in the liver (50% to 90%) to inactive compounds

Bioavailability: 80% (sulfate), 70% (gluconate); 87% (elderly)

Half-life, plasma: 6-8 hours (average 5.7 hours) in young adults, increased half-life with elderly (average 9.7 hours), cirrhosis and congestive heart failure

Elimination: In urine (15% to 25% as unchanged drug)

Usual Dosage Note: Dosage expressed in terms of the salt: 267 mg of quinidine gluconate = 275 mg of quinidine polygalacturonate = 200 mg of quinidine sulfate

Geriatrics and Adults: Test dose: 200 mg (sulfate or its equivalent) administered several hours before full dosage (to determine possibility of idiosyncratic reaction)

Oral:

Sulfate: 100-600 mg/dose every 4-6 hours; begin at 200 mg/dose and titrate to desired effect

Gluconate: 324-972 mg every 8-12 hours

Polygalacturonate: 275 mg every 8-12 hours

I.M.: 400 mg/dose every 4-6 hours

I.V.: 200-400 mg/dose diluted and given at a rate ≤10 mg/minute

Slightly dialyzable (5% to 20%)

Monitoring Parameters EKG, apical pulse, heart rate, blood levels; monitor for syncope initially, diarrhea, periodic CBC, renal and liver function tests

Reference Range Therapeutic: 2-5 μg/mL (SI: 6.2-15.4 μmol/L). Patient dependent therapeutic response occurs at levels of 3-6 μg/mL (SI: 9.2-18.5 μmol/L). Optimal therapeutic level is method dependent; >6 μg/mL (SI: >18 μmol/L).

Test Interactions Increased prothrombin time (S)

Patient Information Patients should notify their physician if rash, fever, diarrhea, unusual bleeding or bruising, ringing in the ears or visual disturbances occur. Complete blood counts, liver and renal function tests should be routinely performed during long-term administration; do not chew or crush sustained release dose forms

(Continued)

Quinidine (Continued)

Nursing Implications When injecting I.M., aspirate carefully to avoid injection into a vessel; give around-the-clock rather than 4 times/day, 3 times/day, etc (ie, 12-6-12-6, not 9-1-5-9) to promote less variation in peak and trough serum levels; do not crush sustained release drug product

Additional Information Sulfate form is the standard dosage preparation

Special Geriatric Considerations Clearance may be decreased with a resultant increased half-life; must individualize dose; bioavailability and half-life are increased in elderly due to decreases in both renal and hepatic function with age

Dosage Forms
Capsule, as sulfate: 200 mg, 300 mg
Injection, as gluconate: 80 mg/mL (10 mL)
Injection, as sulfate: 200 mg/mL (1 mL)
Tablet, as polygalacturonate: 275 mg
Tablet:
Sustained action, as sulfate: 300 mg
Sustained release, as gluconate: 324 mg, 330 mg

References
Fenster PE and Nolan PE, "Antiarrhythmic Drugs," *Geriatric Pharmacology*, Bressler R and Katz MD, eds, New York, NY: McGraw-Hill, 1993, 6:105-49.

Quinidine Gluconate *see* Quinidine *on page 618*

Quinidine Polygalacturonate *see* Quinidine *on page 618*

Quinidine Sulfate *see* Quinidine *on page 618*

Quinine Sulfate (kwye' nine)

Brand Names Legatrin® [OTC]; Quin-Amino®; Quinaminoph®; Quinamm®; Quindan®; Quine® [OTC]; Quiphile®

Generic Available Yes

Therapeutic Class Antimalarial Agent; Skeletal Muscle Relaxant

Use Suppression or treatment of chloroquine-resistant *P. falciparum* malaria; treatment of *Babesia microti* infection
Unlabeled use: Prevention and treatment of nocturnal recumbency leg muscle cramps

Contraindications Tinnitus, optic neuritis, G-6-PD deficiency, hypersensitivity to quinine or any component, history of black water fever, and thrombocytopenia with quinine or quinidine

Precautions Use with caution in patients with cardiac arrhythmias (quinine has quinidine-like activity) and in patients with myasthenia gravis

Adverse Reactions
Cardiovascular: Flushing of the skin, anginal symptoms
Central nervous system: Fever, headache
Dermatologic: Rash, pruritus
Endocrine & metabolic: Hypoglycemia
Gastrointestinal: Nausea, vomiting, epigastric pain, diarrhea
Hematologic: Hemolysis, thrombocytopenia
Hepatic: Hepatitis
Ocular: Nightblindness, diplopia, optic atrophy, blurred vision
Otic: Tinnitus, impaired hearing
Miscellaneous: Hypersensitivity reactions

Overdosage Symptoms of overdose include cinchonism (tinnitus, headache, nausea, abdominal pain, visual disturbance) blood dyscrasias, photosensitivity, cardiac arrhythmias, hypotension, renal injury, hemolysis, hypoprothrombinemia

Drug Interactions
Decreased serum concentrations with phenobarbital, phenytoin, and rifampin
Increased effect of nondepolarizing/depolarizing muscle relaxants and coumarin anticoagulants
Increased serum concentrations with verapamil, amiodarone, alkalinizing agents, and cimetidine
Increased plasma concentration of digoxin, closely monitor digoxin concentrations, digoxin dosage may need to be reduced (by one-half) when quinine is initiated, new steady-state digoxin plasma concentrations occur in 5-7 days

Stability Protect from light

Mechanism of Action Depresses oxygen uptake and carbohydrate metabolism; intercalates into DNA, disrupting the parasite's replication and transcription; affects calcium distribution within muscle fibers and decreases the excitability of the motor end-plate region

Pharmacokinetics
Absorption: Oral: Readily absorbed, mainly from the upper small intestine
Protein binding: 70% to 95%
Metabolism: Primarily in the liver

Half-life (adults): 8-14 hours

Time to peak: Peak serum levels occur within 1-3 hours after dose

Elimination: In bile and saliva with <5% excreted unchanged in urine

Not effectively removed by peritoneal dialysis, removed by hemodialysis

Usual Dosage Geriatrics and Adults: Oral:

Chloroquine-resistant malaria: 650 mg every 8 hours for 5-7 days in conjunction with another agent

Babesiosis: 650 mg every 6-8 hours for 7 days

Leg cramps: 250-300 mg at bedtime

Reference Range Toxic: >10 μg/mL

Test Interactions Positive Coombs' [direct], increased prothrombin time (S)

Patient Information Avoid use of aluminum-containing antacids because of drug absorption problems; swallow dose whole to avoid bitter taste; take with food; notify physician if diarrhea, nausea, and other GI complaints or blurred vision, vertigo, confusion or dizziness occurs

Nursing Implications Administer by slow I.V. infusion

Additional Information Parenteral dosage form may be obtained from Centers for Disease Control if needed

Special Geriatric Considerations Efficacy in nocturnal leg cramps is not well supported in the medical and pharmacy literature, however, some patients do respond; nonresponders should be evaluated for other possible etiologies

Dosage Forms

Capsule: 65 mg, 200 mg, 300 mg, 325 mg

Tablet: 162.5 mg, 250 mg, 325 mg

Quinora® see Quinidine on page 618

Quiphile® see Quinine Sulfate on previous page

Racemic Epinephrine see Epinephrine on page 256

Ramipril (ra mi' prill)

Brand Names Altace™

Generic Available No

Therapeutic Class Angiotensin-Converting Enzyme (ACE) Inhibitors

Use Treatment of hypertension, alone or in combination with thiazide diuretics

Unlabeled use: Congestive heart failure

Contraindications Hypersensitivity to ramipril or ramiprilat, or any other angiotensin-converting enzyme inhibitors

Warnings Neutropenia, agranulocytosis, angioedema, decreased renal function (hypertension, renal artery stenosis, CHF), hepatic dysfunction (elimination, activation), proteinuria, first-dose hypotension (hypovolemia, CHF, dehydrated patients at risk, eg, diuretic use, elderly), elderly (due to renal function changes)

Precautions Use with caution and modify dosage in patients with renal impairment (decrease dosage) (especially renal artery stenosis), severe congestive heart failure or with coadministered diuretic therapy. Severe hypotension may occur in patients who are sodium and/or volume depleted, initiate lower doses and monitor closely when starting therapy in these patients; may cause hyperkalemia.

Adverse Reactions

Cardiovascular: Arrhythmias, orthostatic blood pressure changes, angina, palpitations, chest pain, hypotension, tachycardia, syncope, myocardial infarction

Central nervous system: Nervousness, depression, confusion, somnolence, fatigue, dizziness, headache, paresthesias, asthenia, insomnia, malaise, vertigo, anxiety

Dermatologic: Rash, photosensitivity, pruritus, purpura, angioedema

Endocrine & metabolic: Hyperkalemia

Gastrointestinal: Loss of taste perception, pancreatitis, dry mouth, constipation, anorexia, nausea, vomiting, diarrhea, dysphagia, gastroenteritis, increased salivation, abdominal pain, dysgeusia, dyspepsia

Genitourinary: Impotence

Hematologic: Eosinophilia, leukopenia

Hepatic: Hepatitis

Neuromuscular & skeletal: Myalgia, arthralgia, muscle cramps, arthritis

Ocular: Blurred vision

Otic: Tinnitus

Renal: Proteinuria, increased BUN, serum creatinine, oliguria

Respiratory: Chronic cough (nonproductive, persistent; more often in women and seen in 15% to 30% of patients), asthma, bronchospasm, dyspnea, upper respiratory infections

Miscellaneous: Sweating

Overdosage Severe hypotension

Toxicology Following initiation of essential overdose management, toxic symptom treatment and supportive treatment should be initiated. Hypotension usually responds to I.V. fluids or Trendelenburg positioning. If unresponsive to these measures,

(Continued)

621

Ramipril *(Continued)*

the use of a parenteral inotrope may be required (eg, norepinephrine 0.1-0.2 mcg/kg/minute titrated to response). Seizures commonly respond to diazepam (I.V. 5-10 mg bolus in adults every 15 minutes if needed up to a total of 30 mg) or to phenytoin or phenobarbital.

Drug Interactions

ACE inhibitors (ramipril) and potassium-sparing diuretics → additive hyperkalemic effect

ACE inhibitors (ramipril) and indomethacin or nonsteroidal anti-inflammatory agents → reduced antihypertensive response to ACE inhibitors (ramipril)

Allopurinol and ACE inhibitors (ramipril) → neutropenia

Antacids and ACE inhibitors → ↓ absorption of ACE inhibitors

Phenothiazines and ACE inhibitors → ↑ ACE inhibitor effect

Probenecid and ACE inhibitors (ramipril) → ↑ ACE inhibitor (ramipril) levels

Rifampin and ACE inhibitors (enalapril) → ↓ ACE inhibitor effect

Digoxin and ACE inhibitors → ↑ serum digoxin levels

Lithium and ACE inhibitors → ↑ lithium serum levels

Tetracycline and ACE inhibitors (quinapril) → ↓ tetracycline absorption (up to 37%)

Food decreases ramipril absorption, see Additional Information; rate, but not extent, of ramipril and fosinopril is reduced by concomitant administration with food; food does not reduce absorption of enalapril, lisinopril, or benazepril

Mechanism of Action Ramipril is an angiotensin-converting enzyme (ACE) inhibitor which prevents the formation of angiotensin II from angiotensin I and exhibits pharmacologic effects that are similar to captopril. Ramipril must undergo enzymatic saponification by esterases in the liver to its biologically active metabolite, ramiprilat. The pharmacodynamic effects of ramipril result from the high-affinity, competitive, reversible binding of ramiprilat to angiotensin-converting enzyme thus preventing the formation of the potent vasoconstrictor angiotensin II. This isomerized enzyme-inhibitor complex has a slow rate of dissociation, which results in high potency and a long duration of action; a CNS mechanism may also be involved in the hypotensive effect as angiotensin II increases adrenergic outflow from CNS; vasoactive kallikreins may be decreased in conversion to active hormones by ACE inhibitors, thus reducing blood pressure

Pharmacodynamics

Onset of action: Reduction of blood pressure occurs in 2 hours

Duration: 24 hours

Pharmacokinetics

Absorption: Well absorbed from GI tract (50% to 60%)

Distribution: Plasma levels decline in a triphasic fashion; rapid decline is a distribution phase to peripheral compartment, plasma protein and tissue ACE (half-life 2-4 hours); 2nd phase is an apparent elimination phase representing the clearance of free ramiprilat (half-life: 9-18 hours); and final phase is the terminal elimination phase representing the equilibrium phase between tissue binding and dissociation (half-life: >50 hours)

Metabolism: Hepatic to the active form, ramiprilat

Half-life: Ramiprilat: >50 hours

Time to peak serum concentration: ~1 hour

Elimination: Ramipril and its metabolites are eliminated primarily through the kidneys (60%) and feces (40%)

Usual Dosage Geriatrics and Adults: Oral: 2.5-5 mg once daily, maximum: 20 mg/day; see Special Geriatric Considerations; must adjust dose for renal function for elderly since glomerular filtration rates are decreased; may see exaggerated hypotensive effects if renal clearance is not considered; see Additional Information

Dosing adjustment in renal impairment: Cl_{cr} <40 mL/minute: Initial: 1.25 mg/day, titrate upward to 5 mg/day maximum

Monitoring Parameters Serum calcium levels, BUN, serum creatinine, renal function, WBC, and potassium

Test Interactions Increases BUN, creatinine, potassium, positive Coombs' [direct]; decreases cholesterol (S); may cause false-positive results in urine acetone determinations using sodium nitroprusside reagent

Patient Information Notify physician if vomiting, diarrhea, excessive perspiration, or dehydration should occur; also if swelling of face, lips, tongue, or difficulty in breathing occurs or if persistent cough develops; do not stop therapy or use potassium salt substitutes without physician's advice; may be taken with food

Nursing Implications May cause depression in some patients; discontinue if angioedema of the face, extremities, lips, tongue, or glottis occurs; watch for hypotensive effects within 1-3 hours of first dose or new higher dose; see Warnings, Precautions, Monitoring Parameters, and Special Geriatric Considerations

Additional Information Some patients may have a decreased hypotensive effect between 12 and 16 hours; consider dividing total daily dose into 2 doses 12 hours apart; if patient is receiving a diuretic, a potential for first-dose hypotension is increased; to decrease this potential, stop diuretic for 2-3 days prior to initiating ramipril; continue diuretic if needed to control blood pressure

Special Geriatric Considerations Due to frequent decreases in glomerular filtration (also creatinine clearance) with aging, elderly patients may have exaggerated responses to ACE inhibitors; differences in clinical response due to hepatic changes are not observed. ACE inhibitors may be preferred agents in elderly patients with CHF and diabetes mellitus. Diabetic proteinuria is reduced and insulin sensitivity is enhanced. In general, the side effect profile is favorable in elderly and causes little or no CNS confusion; use lowest dose recommendations initially.

Dosage Forms Capsule: 1.25 mg, 2.5 mg, 5 mg, 10 mg

References
McAreavey D and Robertson JIS, "Angiotensin Converting Enzyme Inhibitors and Moderate Hypertension," *Drugs*, 1990, 40(3):326-45.

Ranitidine Hydrochloride (ra nye' te deen)

Related Information
Antacid Drug Interactions *on page 764*

Brand Names Zantac®

Generic Available No

Therapeutic Class Histamine-2 Antagonist

Use Short-term treatment of active duodenal ulcers and benign gastric ulcers; long-term prophylaxis of duodenal ulcer and gastric hypersecretory states, gastroesophageal reflux, erosive esophagitis

Unlabeled use: Upper GI bleeding, prevention of acid-aspiration pneumonias, prevention of stress-induced ulcers, and prevention of duodenal NSAID ulcers

Contraindications Hypersensitivity to ranitidine or any component

Warnings Use with caution in people (elderly) with reduced renal function, liver disease may impair clearance

Precautions Modify dosage in patients with renal and/or hepatic impairment; gastric malignancy may be masked, gynecomastia; cardiac arrhythmias and hypotension (I.V.); CNS side effects (confusion, depression, psychosis, hallucinations, anxiety)

Adverse Reactions
Cardiovascular: Bradycardia or tachycardia, arrhythmias, edema
Central nervous system: Headache, dizziness, sedation, hallucinations, agitation, anxiety, depression, vertigo, insomnia, malaise, mental confusion
Dermatologic: Alopecia, erythema multiforme
Endocrine & metabolic: Gynecomastia
Gastrointestinal: Constipation, nausea, vomiting, rash, diarrhea, pancreatitis
Genitourinary: Impotence, loss of libido
Hematologic: Agranulocytosis, granulocytopenia, thrombocytopenia, hemolytic anemia, reversible leukopenia, pancytopenia
Hepatic: Hepatitis, increase in serum creatinine
Neuromuscular & skeletal: Arthralgias
Ocular: Blurred vision

Overdosage Symptoms of overdose include muscular tremors, vomiting, rapid respiration

Toxicology LD$_{50}$ ~80 mg/kg; treatment is primarily symptomatic and supportive.

Drug Interactions
Binds weakly to cytochrome P-450 and, therefore, does not cause significant inhibition of drug metabolism
Antacids may decrease absorption; decreased absorption of diazepam may occur (ranitidine)
Increased serum levels of procainamide (ranitidine)
Increased hypoglycemic effects observed with sulfonylureas
Serum concentrations may be increased (case reports with ranitidine)
May decrease warfarin clearance and increase anticoagulant effect (ranitidine) but data are conflicting

Stability Solution for I.V. infusion in NS or D$_5$W is stable for 48 hours at room temperature or 30 days when frozen; is stable for 24 hours in TPN solutions; is stable only for 12 hours in total nutrient admixtures (TPN) when lipids are added

Mechanism of Action Competitive inhibition of histamine at H$_2$ receptors of the gastric parietal cells, which inhibits gastric acid secretion; gastric volume and hydrogen ion concentration reduced

Pharmacodynamics
Efficacy of healing rate: 63% to 77% at 4 weeks; 82% to 95% at 8 weeks
Duration of effect: Oral: 12 hours; I.V.: 6-8 hours

Pharmacokinetics
Absorption: Oral: ~50% to 60%
Protein binding: 15%
Metabolism: In the liver (<10%)
Half-life: 2-2.5 hours; minimally penetrates the blood-brain barrier
Time to peak: Peak serum levels occur within 1-3 hours and persist for 8 hours, 15 minutes for I.M.
Elimination: Primarily in urine (35% as unchanged drug) and feces

(Continued)

Ranitidine Hydrochloride (Continued)

Usual Dosage Geriatrics and Adults:

Short-term treatment of ulceration: 150 mg/dose twice daily or 300 mg at bedtime (100 mg orally twice daily has been found as effective as 150 mg twice daily)

Prophylaxis of recurrent duodenal ulcer: 150 mg at bedtime

Gastric hypersecretory conditions: Oral: 150 mg twice daily, more frequent doses may be necessary up to 6 g/day

GERD: Oral: 150 mg twice daily

Erosive esophagitis: Oral: 150 mg 4 times/day

I.M., I.V.: 50 mg/dose every 6-8 hours (dose not to exceed 400 mg/day)

Dosing interval in renal impairment:
Oral: Cl_{cr} <50 mL/minute: Administer each dose every 24 hours
I.V.: Cl_{cr} <50 mL/minute: Administer each dose every 18-24 hours
Slightly dialyzable (5% to 20%)

Monitoring Parameters Signs and symptoms of peptic ulcer disease, occult blood with GI bleeding, gastric pH where necessary; monitor renal function to correct dose; monitor for side effects

Test Interactions False-positive urine protein using Multistix® (test with sulfasalicylic acid), gastric acid secretion test, skin tests allergen extracts, serum creatinine and serum transaminase concentrations, urine protein test

Patient Information It may take several days before this medicine begins to relieve stomach pain; antacids may be taken with ranitidine unless your physician has told you not to use them; wait 30-60 minutes between taking the antacid and ranitidine; inform prescribers of any concomitant medications

Nursing Implications I.M. solution does not need to be diluted before use; monitor creatinine clearance for renal impairment; giving dose at 6 PM may be better than 10 PM bedtime, the highest acid production usually starts at approximately 7 PM, thus giving at 6 PM controls acid secretion better; observe caution in patients with renal function impairment and hepatic function impairment

Additional Information Giving dose at 6 PM may be better than 10 PM bedtime, the highest acid production usually starts at approximately 7 PM, thus giving at 6 PM controls acid secretion better; give I.V. administration over a 30 minute period to avoid bradycardia; causes fewer adverse reactions and interactions than cimetidine; most patient's ulcers have healed within 4 weeks, however, elderly require 12 weeks of therapy; long-term therapy may cause vitamin B_{12} deficiency

Special Geriatric Considerations H_2 blockers are the preferred drugs for treating PUD in elderly due to cost and ease of administration. These agents are no less or more effective than any other therapy. The preferred agents, due to side effects and drug interaction profile and pharmacokinetics are ranitidine, famotidine, and nizatidine. Treatment for PUD in elderly is recommended for 12 weeks since their lesions are larger; therefore, take longer to heal. Always adjust dose based upon creatinine clearance.

Dosage Forms
Infusion: 0.5 mg/mL in $^1/_2$ NS (50 mL)
Injection: 25 mg/mL (2 mL, 10 mL, 40 mL)
Syrup: 15 mg/mL (473 mL)
Tablet: 150 mg, 300 mg

References
Fennerty MD and Higbee M, "Drug Therapy of Gastrointestinal Disease," *Geriatric Pharmacology*, Bressler R and Katz MD, eds, New York, NY: McGraw-Hill, 1993, 585-608.
Morris DL, Markham SJ, Beechey A, et al, "Ranitidine--Bolus or Infusion Prophylaxis for Stress Ulcer," *Crit Care Med*, 1988, 16(3):229-32.
Roberts CJ, "Clinical Pharmacokinetics of Ranitidine," *Clin Pharmacokinet*, 1984, 9(3):211-21.

Recombivax HB® *see* Hepatitis B Vaccine *on page 342*

Redisol® *see* Cyanocobalamin *on page 192*

Reglan® *see* Metoclopramide *on page 462*

Regonol® *see* Pyridostigmine Bromide *on page 612*

Regular Iletin® I *see* Insulin Preparations *on page 372*

Regular Insulin (Pork) *see* Insulin Preparations *on page 372*

Regular Purified Pork *see* Insulin Preparations *on page 372*

Reguloid® [OTC] *see* Psyllium *on page 610*

Rela® *see* Carisoprodol *on page 121*

Relafen® *see* Nabumetone *on page 483*

Relaxadon® *see* Hyoscyamine, Atropine, Scopolamine and Phenobarbital *on page 357*

Relief® Ophthalmic Solution *see* Phenylephrine Hydrochloride *on page 557*

Reserpine (re ser' peen)

Brand Names Serpalan®; Serpasil®
Generic Available Yes
Therapeutic Class Rauwolfia Alkaloid
Use Management of mild to moderate hypertension

Unlabeled use: Management of tardive dyskinesia

Contraindications Any ulcerative condition, gallstones, mental depression, electroshock therapy, hypersensitivity to reserpine or any component

Precautions Electroshock therapy: discontinue reserpine 7 days before electroshock therapy; may increase GI motility and secretions; acute hypersensitivity reactions may occur; some products may contain tartrazine; use cautiously in patients with renal insufficiency

Adverse Reactions

Cardiovascular: Hypotension, bradycardia

Central nervous system: Drowsiness, fatigue, mental depression, parkinsonism

Endocrine & metabolic: Sodium and water retention

Gastrointestinal: Abdominal cramps, nausea, vomiting, increased gastric acid secretion, diarrhea

Genitourinary: Impotence, urination difficulty

Respiratory: Nasal congestion

Overdosage Symptoms of overdose include hypotension, bradycardia, CNS depression, sedation, coma, hypothermia, vomiting, diarrhea, miosis, tremors

Toxicology Hypotension usually responds to I.V. fluids or Trendelenburg positioning. If unresponsive to these measures the use of a parenteral vasopressor may be required (eg, norepinephrine 0.1-0.2 mcg/kg/minute titrated to response). Anticholinergic agents may be useful in reducing the parkinsonian effects; avoid the use of digoxin in these patients. Since reserpine is long-acting, observe the patient for at least 72 hours.

Drug Interactions

Decreased effect of indirect-acting sympathomimetics, levodopa

Increased effect/toxicity of other antihypertensives, digoxin, quinidine, general anesthesia, MAO inhibitors, direct-acting sympathomimetics

Stability Protect oral dosage forms from light

Mechanism of Action Reduces blood pressure via depletion of sympathetic biogenic amines (norepinephrine and dopamine); this also commonly results in sedative effects

Pharmacodynamics

Onset of action: Within 3-6 days

Duration: 2-6 weeks

Pharmacokinetics

Absorption: Oral: ~40%

Protein binding: 96%

Metabolism: Extensive in the liver (>90%)

Half-life: 50-100 hours

Elimination: Principal excretion in feces (30% to 60%) and small amounts in urine (10%)

Usual Dosage Oral:

Geriatrics: Initial: 0.05 mg once daily increasing by 0.05 mg every week as necessary

Adults: 0.5 mg/day for 1-2 weeks, then decrease to 0.1-0.25 mg once daily

Monitoring Parameters Blood pressure, standing and sitting/supine, symptoms of depression

Test Interactions Decreased catecholamines (U)

Patient Information Take with food or milk; impotency is reversible; notify physician if a weight gain of more than 5 pounds has taken place during therapy; may cause drowsiness

Nursing Implications Observe for mental depression and alert family members to report any symptoms

Additional Information Full antihypertensive effects may take as long as 3 weeks; at high doses, mental depression is possible and might lead to suicide

Special Geriatric Considerations Some studies advocate the use of reserpine because of its low cost, long half-life, and efficacy, but it is generally not considered a first-line drug. If it is to be used, doses should not exceed 0.25 mg and the patient should be monitored for depressed mood.

Dosage Forms

Injection: 2.5 mg/mL (2 mL)

Tablet: 0.1 mg, 0.25 mg, 1 mg

References

Adelman AM, Daly MP, and Michocki RJ, "Alternate Drugs," *Clin Geriatr Med*, 1990, 6(2):423-44.

Reserpine and Hydrochlorothiazide see Hydrochlorothiazide and Reserpine on page 348

Respbid® *see* Theophylline *on page 681*

Restoril® *see* Temazepam *on page 671*

Retrovir® *see* Zidovudine *on page 741*

Rev-Eyes™ *see* Dapiprazole Hydrochloride *on page 202*

Rexolate® *see* Salicylates (Various Salts) *on page 633*

Rheaban® [OTC] *see* Attapulgite *on page 66*

Rheumatrex® *see* Methotrexate *on page 455*

Rhinall® Nasal Solution [OTC] *see* Phenylephrine Hydrochloride
on page 557

Rhindecon® *see* Phenylpropanolamine Hydrochloride *on page 559*

Rhythmin® *see* Procainamide Hydrochloride *on page 590*

Ribavirin (rye ba vye' rin)
Brand Names Virazole® Aerosol
Synonyms RTCA; Tribavirin
Generic Available No
Therapeutic Class Antiviral Agent, Inhalation Therapy
Use Treatment of patients with respiratory syncytial virus (RSV) infections; may also be used in other viral infections including influenza A and B and adenovirus; specially indicated for treatment of severe lower respiratory tract RSV infections in patients with an underlying compromising condition (prematurity, bronchopulmonary dysplasia, congenital heart disease, immunodeficiency, and immunosuppression)
Warnings Use with caution in patients requiring assisted ventilation because precipitation of the drug in the respiratory equipment may interfere with safe and effective patient ventilation; also monitor carefully in patients with COPD and asthma for deterioration of respiratory function. Ribavirin is potentially mutagenic, tumor-promoting, and gonadotoxic; there is evidence that ribavirin is teratogenic in small animals. Health care workers who are pregnant or may become pregnant should be advised of the potential risks of exposure and counseled about risk reduction strategies including alternate job responsibilities; virus resistance does not appear to develop; incubation period for RSV is 4-8 days.
Adverse Reactions
　Cardiovascular: Hypotension, cardiac arrest
　Dermatologic: Rash, skin irritation
　Hematologic: Anemia
　Ocular: Conjunctivitis
　Respiratory: Mild bronchospasm, worsening of respiratory function, bacterial pneumonia, pneumothorax, apnea, ventilator dependence
Drug Interactions Decreased effect of zidovudine
Stability Do not use any water containing an antimicrobial agent to reconstitute drug; reconstituted solution is stable for 24 hours at room temperature
Mechanism of Action Inhibits replication of RNA and DNA viruses; inhibits influenza virus RNA polymerase activity and inhibits the initiation and elongation of RNA fragments resulting in inhibition of viral protein synthesis
Pharmacokinetics
　Absorption: Systemically from the respiratory tract following nasal and oral inhalation; absorption is dependent upon respiratory factors and method of drug delivery; maximal absorption occurs with the use of the aerosol generator via an endotracheal tube; highest concentrations are found in the respiratory tract and erythrocytes
　Metabolism: Occurs intracellularly and may be necessary for drug action
　Plasma half-life: Adults: 24 hours, much longer in the erythrocyte (16-40 days), which can be used as a marker for intracellular metabolism
　Time to peak serum concentration: Inhalation: Within 60-90 minutes
　Elimination: Hepatic metabolism is major route of elimination with 40% of the drug cleared renally as unchanged drug and metabolites
Usual Dosage Geriatrics and Adults:
　Aerosol inhalation: Use with Viratek® small particle aerosol generator (SPAG-2) at a concentration of 20 mg/mL (6 g reconstituted with 300 mL of sterile water without preservatives)
　Aerosol only: 12-18 hours/day for 3 days, up to 7 days in length
Administration Read the Viratek Small Particle Aerosol Generator (SPAG) Model SPAG-2 Operator's Manual before use
Monitoring Parameters Respiratory function
Nursing Implications Keep accurate I & O record, discard solutions placed in the SPAG-2 unit at least every 24 hours and before adding additional fluid; see Administration
Additional Information RSV season is usually December to April; viral shedding period for RSV is usually 3-8 days
Special Geriatric Considerations No specific recommendations are necessary in elderly; see Usual Dosage and Adverse Reactions
Dosage Forms Powder for aerosol: 6 g (100 mL)

Ridaura® *see* Auranofin *on page 67*

Rifabutin (rif a bu' tin)
Brand Names Mycobutin® Oral
Synonyms Ansamycin
Therapeutic Class Antibiotic, Miscellaneous; Antitubercular Agent
Use Prevention of disseminated *Mycobacterium avium* complex (MAC) in patients with advanced HIV infection; also utilized in multiple drug regimens for treatment of MAC
Contraindications Hypersensitivity to rifabutin or any other rifamycins; rifabutin is contraindicated in patients with a WBC <1000/mm³ or a platelet count <50,000/mm³
Warnings Rifabutin as a single agent must not be administered to patients with active tuberculosis since its use may lead to the development of tuberculosis that is resistant to both rifabutin and rifampin; rifabutin should be discontinued in patients with AST >500 IU/L or if total bilirubin is >3 mg/dL. Use with caution in patients with liver impairment; modification of dosage should be considered in patients with renal impairment.
Adverse Reactions
  Cardiovascular: Chest pain
  Central nervous system: Fever, headache, seizures, confusion, insomnia
  Dermatologic: Rash
  Gastrointestinal: Abdominal pain, diarrhea, dyspepsia, nausea, vomiting, taste perversion, anorexia, flatulence, eructation
  Hematologic: Thrombocytopenia, anemia, leukopenia, neutropenia
  Hepatic: Elevated liver enzymes
  Neuromuscular & skeletal: Arthralgia, myalgia
  Ocular: Uveitis
  Miscellaneous: Discolored urine
Overdosage Symptoms of overdose include nausea, vomiting, hepatotoxicity, lethargy, CNS depression
Toxicology Treatment is supportive; lavage with activated charcoal is preferred to ipecac as emesis is frequently present with overdose; hemodialysis will remove rifabutin, its effect on outcome is unknown
Drug Interactions Decreased plasma concentration (because of induced liver enzymes) of verapamil, methadone, digoxin, cyclosporine, corticosteroids, oral anticoagulants, theophylline, barbiturates, chloramphenicol, ketoconazole, oral contraceptives, quinidine, halothane
Mechanism of Action Inhibits DNA-dependent RNA polymerase at the beta subunit which prevents chain initiation
Pharmacokinetics
  Absorption: Oral: Readily absorbed 53%
  Distribution: V_d: 9.32 L/kg; distributes to body tissues including the lungs, liver, spleen, eyes, and kidneys
  Protein binding: 85%
  Metabolism: To active and inactive metabolites
  Bioavailability: Absolute, 20% in HIV patients
  Half-life, terminal: 45 hours (range: 16-69 hours)
  Peak serum level: Within 2-4 hours
  Elimination: Renal and biliary clearance of unchanged drugs is 10%; 30% excreted in feces; 53% in urine unchanged
Usual Dosage Geriatrics and Adults: Oral: 300 mg once daily; for patients who experience gastrointestinal upset, rifabutin can be administered 150 mg twice daily with food
Administration May be mixed with food (ie, applesauce)
Monitoring Parameters Periodic liver function tests, CBC with differential, platelet count, hemoglobin, hematocrit
Patient Information May discolor urine, tears, sweat, or other body fluids to a red-orange color; soft contact lenses may be permanently stained; report to physician any severe or persistent flu-like symptoms, nausea, vomiting, dark urine or pale stools, or unusual bleeding or bruising; can be taken with meals or sprinkled on applesauce
Nursing Implications Administer with meals
Special Geriatric Considerations No specific recommendations for elderly
Dosage Forms Capsule: 150 mg
Extemporaneous Preparation(s) Rifabutin is insoluble in water and ethanol; prepare powder packets or compound with a suspending agent and shake well before using

Rifadin® *see* Rifampin *on this page*

Rifampicin *see* Rifampin *on this page*

Rifampin (rif' am pin)
Brand Names Rifadin®; Rimactane®
Synonyms Rifampicin
Therapeutic Class Antibiotic, Miscellaneous; Antitubercular Agent
(Continued)

Rifampin *(Continued)*

Use Management of active tuberculosis; eliminate meningococci from asymptomatic carriers; prophylaxis of *Haemophilus influenzae* type B infection

Contraindications Hypersensitivity to rifampin or any component

Precautions Use with caution in patients with liver impairment; modification of dosage should be considered in patients with severe liver impairment; monitor closely if intermittent therapy is used; hypersensitivity reactions and thrombocytopenia occur more frequently in this setting

Adverse Reactions

Central nervous system: Drowsiness, fatigue, ataxia, confusion, fever, headache

Dermatologic: Rash, pruritus

Gastrointestinal: Nausea, vomiting, diarrhea, stomatitis, abdominal cramps

Hematologic: Eosinophilia, blood dyscrasias (leukopenia, thrombocytopenia)

Hepatic: Hepatitis

Local: Irritation at the I.V. site

Renal: Renal failure

Miscellaneous: Discoloration of urine, feces, saliva, sputum, sweat, and tears (reddish orange), flu-like syndrome

Overdosage Symptoms of overdose include nausea, vomiting, hepatotoxicity

Toxicology Asymptomatic increases in liver enzymes occur in 10% to 20% of patients; most often these increases occur in the first 6 months of treatment and are transient. If AST or ALT increases to 5 times baseline or signs of hepatitis are present, rifampin (and isoniazid) should be stopped; therapy can be reinitiated with close monitoring once symptoms have resolved and/or liver enzymes have returned to normal.

Drug Interactions Rifampin induces liver enzymes which may decrease the plasma concentration of the following drugs: acetaminophen, benzodiazepines (only those that undergo oxidation), beta-blockers, clofibrate, digitoxin, disopyramide, estrogens, phenytoin, and other hydantoins, mexiletine, sulfones, sulfonylureas, enalapril (decreased blood pressure control), verapamil, methadone, digoxin, cyclosporine, corticosteroids, oral anticoagulants, theophylline, barbiturates, chloramphenicol, ketoconazole, oral contraceptives, quinidine; halothane

Stability Reconstituted I.V. solution is stable for 24 hours at room temperature; rifampin oral suspension can be compounded with simple syrup or wild cherry syrup at a concentration of 10 mg/mL; the suspension is stable for 4 weeks at room temperature or in a refrigerator when stored in a glass amber prescription bottle

Mechanism of Action Inhibits bacterial RNA synthesis by binding to the beta subunit of DNA-dependent RNA polymerase, blocking RNA transcription

Pharmacodynamics

Peak serum levels: Within 2-4 hours

Duration: Up to 24 hours

Pharmacokinetics

Absorption: Oral: Well absorbed

Half-life: 3-4 hours, prolonged with hepatic impairment

Protein binding: 80%

Metabolism: In the liver

Highly lipophilic; crosses the blood-brain barrier well, undergoes enterohepatic recycling

Time to peak: Peak serum levels occur within 2-4 hours; food may delay or slightly reduce peak serum level

Elimination: Principally in feces (60% to 65%) and urine (~30%)

Plasma rifampin concentrations are not significantly affected by hemodialysis or peritoneal dialysis

In a small (n=6) single-dose study, rifampin's pharmacokinetic parameters in elderly subjects were not significantly different compared to values of younger subjects reported in the literature

Usual Dosage Geriatrics and Adults: I.V. infusion dose is the same as for the oral route; Adults:

Tuberculosis: Oral: 10 mg/kg/day; maximum: 600 mg/day

American Thoracic Society and CDC currently recommend twice weekly therapy as part of a short-course regimen which follows 1-2 months of daily treatment of uncomplicated pulmonary tuberculosis in the compliant patient. Adults: 10 mg/kg (up to 600 mg) twice weekly

H. influenza prophylaxis: 600 mg every 24 hours for 4 days

Meningococcal prophylaxis: 600 mg every 12 hours for 2 days

Nasal carriers of *Staphylococcus aureus*: 600 mg/day for 5-10 days in combination with other antibiotics

Administration Give on an empty stomach (ie, 1 hour prior to, or 2 hours after meals) to increase total absorption

Monitoring Parameters Liver function tests (ALT and AST) at baseline and 1, 3, and 6 months; sputum culture; chest x-ray 2-3 months into treatment and at completion

Test Interactions Increased bilirubin (S), positive Coombs' [direct]; inhibit standard assay's ability to measure serum folate and B_{12}

Patient Information May discolor urine, tears, sweat, or other body fluids to a red-orange color; take 1 hour before or 2 hours after a meal on an empty stomach; soft contact lenses may be permanently stained

Nursing Implications Evaluate hepatic status and mental status; see Administration

Additional Information Since resistant strains occur rapidly, is normally used with other anti-TB drugs

Special Geriatric Considerations Rifampin, in combination with isoniazid, is the foundation of tuberculosis treatment; since most older patients acquired their *Mycobacterium tuberculosis* infection before effective chemotherapy was available, either a 9-month regimen of isoniazid and rifampin or a 6-month regimen of isoniazid and rifampin with pyrazinamide (the first 2 months) should be effective

Dosage Forms
Capsule: 150 mg, 300 mg
Injection: 600 mg

References
Advenier C, Gobert C, Houin G, et al, "Pharmacokinetic Studies of Rifampicin in the Elderly," *Ther Drug Monit*, 1983, 5(1):61-5.
Bass JB Jr, Farer LS, Hopewell PC, et al, "Treatment of Tuberculosis and Tuberculosis Infection in Adults and Children," *Am J Respir Crit Care Med*, 1994, 149(5):1359-74.
Van Scoy RE & Wilkowske CJ, "Antituberculous Agents: Isoniazid, Rifampin, Streptomycin, Ethambutol, and Pyrazinamide," *Mayo Clin Proc*, 1983, 58(4):233-40.
Yoshikawa TT, "Tuberculosis in Aging Adults," *J Am Geriatr Soc*, 1992, 40(2):178-87.

Rimactane® *see* Rifampin *on page 627*

Rimantadine Hydrochloride (ri man' to deen)

Brand Names Flumadine® Oral

Therapeutic Class Antiviral Agent, Oral

Use Prophylaxis and treatment of influenza A viral infection

Contraindications Hypersensitivity to drugs of the adamantine class (rimantadine or amantadine)

Warnings Use with caution in patients with liver disease, a history of recurrent and eczematoid dermatitis, uncontrolled psychosis or severe psychoneurosis, seizures in those receiving CNS stimulant drugs

Adverse Reactions
Cardiovascular: Hypertension, tachycardia, heart block, orthostatic hypotension, syncope
Central nervous system: Insomnia, dizziness, headache, nervousness, fatigue, impaired concentration, ataxia, confusion, irritability, hallucinations
Gastrointestinal: Nausea, vomiting, anorexia, dry mouth, abdominal pain, diarrhea, dyspepsia, constipation, dysgeusia
Genitourinary: Urinary retention
Neuromuscular & skeletal: Tremors
Ocular: Eye pain
Otic: Tinnitus
Respiratory: Dyspnea, bronchospasm, cough

Overdosage Symptoms of overdose include agitation, hallucinations, cardiac arrhythmias, and death

Toxicology I.V. physostigmine, 1-2 mg repeated as needed up to 2 mg/hour may be beneficial; supportive therapy

Drug Interactions Acetaminophen and aspirin decrease rimantadine plasma concentration and AUC 10% to 11%; cimetidine reduced rimantadine clearance

Mechanism of Action Believed to inhibit early viral replication, perhaps by inhibiting viral uncoating

Pharmacokinetics
Absorption: Tablet and syrup essentially completely absorbed
Distribution: 40% bound to plasma protein
Metabolism: 90%
Half-life:
Adults: Mean: 25.4 hours
Elderly (healthy): Mean: 32 hours

At steady-state, AUC, plasma concentration, and half-life are 20% to 30% greater in persons >60 years of age; elderly nursing home residents were found to have steady-state plasma concentrations 2-4 times greater than elderly by community residents

Usual Dosage Oral:
Prophylaxis:
Geriatrics: 100 mg/day
Adults: 100 mg twice daily

Treatment:
Geriatrics: 100 mg/day
Adults: 100 mg twice daily

Dosing adjustment in renal/hepatic impairment: Cl_{cr} 10 mL/minute: Dosage should be reduced to 100 mg/day

(Continued)

Rimantadine Hydrochloride *(Continued)*

Monitoring Parameters Signs and symptoms of toxicity, especially CNS

Reference Range No relationship between plasma concentration and antiviral effects has been established

Nursing Implications See Monitoring Parameters

Special Geriatric Considerations Dosing must be individualized (100 mg 1-2 times/day); it is recommended that nursing home patients receive 100 mg/day; see Pharmacokinetics

Dosage Forms

Syrup: 50 mg/5 mL (60 mL, 240 mL, 480 mL)

Tablet: 100 mg

References

Douglas RG Jr, "Prophylaxis and Treatment of Influenza," *N Engl J Med,* 1990, 322(7):443-50.

Guay DR, "Amantadine and Rimantadine Prophylaxis of Infuenza A in Nursing Homes," *Drugs Aging,* 1994, 5(1):8-19.

Patriarca PA, Kater NA, Kendal AP, et al, "Safety of Prolonged Administration of Rimantadine Hydrochloride in the Prophylaxis of Influenza A Virus Infections in Nursing Homes," *Antimicrob Agents Chemother,* 1984, 26:101-3.

Riopan Extra Strength® [OTC] *see* Magaldrate *on page 424*

Riopan Plus® [OTC] *see* Magaldrate and Simethicone *on page 425*

Riopan® [OTC] *see* Magaldrate *on page 424*

Risperdal® *see* Risperidone *on this page*

Risperidone *(ris per' i done)*

Related Information

Antipsychotic Agents Comparison *on page 801*

Brand Names Risperdal®

Therapeutic Class Antipsychotic Agent

Use Management of psychotic disorders (eg, schizophrenia); nonpsychotic symptoms associated with dementia in elderly

Contraindications Known hypersensitivity to risperidone or any component of the product

Warnings Long-term use (>8 weeks) not evaluated; neuroleptic malignant syndrome has been reported with antipsychotics

Tardive dyskinesia: Prevalence rate may be 40% in elderly; elderly women especially at risk; embarrassment from dyskinesias may lead to greater social isolation; development of the syndrome and the irreversible nature are proportional to duration and total cumulative dose over time. May be reversible if diagnosed early in therapy; intermittent use of antipsychotics (not proven use) helps decrease total cumulative dose.

EPS: Extrapyramidal reactions are more common in elderly with up to 50% developing these reactions after 60 years of age. These reactions may be more common in dementia patients. Drug-induced **Parkinson's syndrome** occurs often. Discontinuation usually resolves symptoms but may take weeks to months (12+) to clear. **Akathisia** is the most common EPS reaction in elderly. The symptoms of motor restlessness are difficult to diagnose in demented elderly; increased nervousness, assertiveness, restlessness with constant movement may indicate this adverse event. Consider decreasing dose if antipsychotic to treat as well as diagnose problem; usually see this reaction within 2-3 months of initiating antipsychotic drug.

Anticholinergic effects: These side effects most common with low potency antipsychotics (eg, thioridazine, chlorpromazine). CNS toxicity occurs more frequently and severely in elderly; increased confusion, memory loss, psychotic behavior, and agitation frequently occur as a consequence of anticholinergic effects to antipsychotic agents. Peripheral anticholinergic action troublesome to elderly; most peripheral anticholinergic effects last only 2-3 weeks; see Adverse Reactions.

Orthostatic hypotension: More common with low potency agents (eg, thioridazine, chlorpromazine, and clozapine) but of concern with all antipsychotic agents; orthostasis due to alpha-receptor blockade by antipsychotic agents. Elderly present many risk factors for orthostatic hypotension: blunted baroreceptor reflexes, decreased vascular tone, decreased vascular volume, and possible presence of cardiac diseases which result in decreased cardiac output.

Sedation: Common side effect with antipsychotic therapy; should not be used as a hypnotic unless insomnia is associated with target behavior symptoms treated with antipsychotic medications; see Special Geriatric Considerations. Anecdotal reports suggesting antipsychotic sedation in nonpsychotic patients is extremely unpleasant due to feelings of depersonalization, derealization, and dysphoria. Due to the long duration of action with antipsychotic drugs, these reactions may last up to 24 hours and result in decreased daytime function.

Cardiac toxicity: Life-threatening arrhythmias have occurred at therapeutic doses of antipsychotics. Thioridazine more commonly demonstrates EKG changes than other antipsychotics; suggested to use high potency antipsychotic agents (ie, haloperidol) in patients with cardiac conduction defects.

Precautions Use with caution in patients with cardiovascular disease, seizures, and Parkinson's disease; benefits of therapy must be weighed against risks of therapy

Adverse Reactions

Anticholinergic: Dry mouth (problem for denture user), urinary retention, constipation, adynamic ileus, overflow incontinence, blurred vision

Cardiovascular: Hypotension (especially orthostatic), tachycardia, arrhythmias, abnormal T waves with prolonged ventricular repolarization, EKG changes

Central nervous system: Sedation, drowsiness, restlessness, anxiety, extrapyramidal reactions, dystonic reactions, pseudoparkinsonian signs and symptoms, tardive dyskinesia, neuroleptic malignant syndrome, seizures, altered central temperature regulation

Dermatologic: Photosensitivity (rare)

Endocrine & metabolic: Amenorrhea, galactorrhea, gynecomastia

Gastrointestinal: Constipation, adynamic ileus, GI upset, dry mouth (problem for denture user), weight gain

Genitourinary: Urinary retention, overflow incontinence, priapism, sexual dysfunction (up to 60%)

Hematologic: Agranulocytosis, leukopenia (usually in patients with large doses for prolonged periods)

Hepatic: Cholestatic jaundice

Ocular: Blurred vision, retinal pigmentation, decreased visual acuity (may be irreversible)

Overdosage In reports of doses ranging from 20-30 mg, no fatalities have occurred; symptoms of overdose include drowsiness, sedation, hypotension, tachycardia, extrapyramidal symptoms, seizures

Toxicology Following initiation of essential overdose management, toxic symptom treatment and supportive treatment should be initiated. Hypotension usually responds to I.V. fluids or Trendelenburg positioning. If unresponsive to these measures the use of a parenteral inotrope may be required (eg, norepinephrine 0.1-0.2 mcg/kg/ minute titrated to response). Do not use epinephrine. Seizures commonly respond to diazepam (I.V. 5-10 mg bolus in adults every 15 minutes if needed up to a total of 30 mg) or to phenytoin or phenobarbital. Also critical cardiac arrhythmias often respond to I.V. phenytoin (15 mg/kg up to 1 g), while other antiarrhythmics can be used. Neuroleptics often cause extrapyramidal symptoms (eg, dystonic reactions) requiring management with diphenhydramine 1-2 mg/kg up to a maximum of 50 mg I.M. or I.V. slow push followed by a maintenance dose for 48-72 hours. When these reactions are unresponsive to diphenhydramine, benztropine mesylate I.V. 1-2 mg may be effective. These agents are generally effective within 2-5 minutes.

Drug Interactions

May antagonize effects of levodopa

Carbamazepine decreased risperidone serum concentrations

Clozapine decreases clearance of risperidone

Mechanism of Action Risperidone is a benzisoxazole derivative, mixed serotonin-dopamine antagonist; binds to $5\text{-}HT_2$ receptors in the CNS and in the periphery with a very high affinity; binds to dopamine D_2 receptors with less affinity. The binding affinity to the dopamine D_2 receptor is 20 times lower than the $5\text{-}HT_2$ affinity. The addition of serotonin antagonism to dopamine antagonism (classic neuroleptic mechanism) is thought to improve negative symptoms of psychoses and reduce the incidence of extrapyramidal side effects.

Pharmacokinetics

Absorption: Oral: Rapid

Metabolism: Extensively by cytochrome P-450IID_6

Protein binding: Plasma: 90%

Half-life: 24 hours (risperidone and its active metabolite)

Time to peak: Peak plasma concentrations within 1 hour

Usual Dosage

Geriatrics: **Dosing adjustment in renal, hepatic impairment, and elderly:** Starting dose of 0.5 mg twice daily is advisable; dosages >6 mg/day increase incidence of side effects; increase dose at 0.5 mg twice daily at weekly intervals if possible

Adults: Recommended starting dose: 1 mg twice daily; slowly increase to the optimum range of 4-8 mg/day; daily dosages >5 mg do not appear to confer any additional benefit, and the incidence of extrapyramidal reactions is higher than with lower doses; maximum dose: 16 mg/day

Monitoring Parameters Orthostatic blood pressures; tremors, gait changes, abnormal movement in trunk, neck, buccal area or extremities; monitor target behaviors for which the agent is given

Patient Information Explain to patients that orthostatic hypotension may occur at initiation of therapy; may cause impairment of alertness and judgment; enhanced sedation will occur with the ingestion of alcohol; photosensitivity may occur; use sunscreen or avoid exposure to sunlight and ultraviolet light

Nursing Implications Monitor and observe for extrapyramidal effects, orthostatic blood pressure changes for 3-5 days after starting or increasing dose

(Continued)

Risperidone *(Continued)*

Special Geriatric Considerations See Warnings

Many elderly patients receive antipsychotic medications for inappropriate nonpsychotic behavior. Before initiating antipsychotic medication, the clinician should investigate any possible reversible cause; any stress or stress from any disease can cause acute "confusion" or worsening of baseline nonpsychotic behavior. Most commonly acute changes in behavior are due to increases in drug dose or addition of new drug to regimen; fluid electrolyte loss; infections; and changes in environment.

Any changes in disease status in any organ system can result in behavior changes.

Dosage Forms Tablet: 1 mg, 2 mg, 3 mg, 4 mg

References

Cohen LJ, "Risperidone," *Pharmacotherapy*, 1994, 14(3):253-65.

Ritalin® *see* Methylphenidate Hydrochloride *on page 459*

Ritalin-SR® *see* Methylphenidate Hydrochloride *on page 459*

rIFN-b *see* Interferon Beta-1b *on page 374*

RMS® *see* Morphine Sulfate *on page 481*

Robafen® [OTC] *see* Guaifenesin *on page 331*

Robaxin® *see* Methocarbamol *on page 454*

Robicillin® VK *see* Penicillin V Potassium *on page 543*

Robinul® *see* Glycopyrrolate *on page 326*

Robitet® *see* Tetracycline *on page 678*

Robitussin® A-C *see* Guaifenesin and Codeine *on page 332*

Robitussin-DM® [OTC] *see* Guaifenesin and Dextromethorphan *on page 332*

Robitussin® [OTC] *see* Guaifenesin *on page 331*

Robomol® *see* Methocarbamol *on page 454*

Rocaltrol® *see* Calcitriol *on page 105*

Ro-Ceph® *see* Cephradine *on page 145*

Rocephin® *see* Ceftriaxone Sodium *on page 139*

Rogaine® *see* Minoxidil *on page 474*

Rolaids® Calcium Rich [OTC] *see* Calcium Salts (Oral) *on page 111*

Ronase® *see* Tolazamide *on page 702*

Rowasa® *see* Mesalamine *on page 445*

Roxanol™ *see* Morphine Sulfate *on page 481*

Roxanol SR™ *see* Morphine Sulfate *on page 481*

Roxicet® *see* Oxycodone and Acetaminophen *on page 528*

Roxicodone™ *see* Oxycodone Hydrochloride *on page 529*

Roxiprin® *see* Oxycodone and Aspirin *on page 529*

RTCA *see* Ribavirin *on page 626*

Rubella Virus Vaccine, Live (rue bell' a)

Related Information

Immunization Guidelines *on page 759-762*

Brand Names Meruvax® II

Synonyms German Measles Vaccine

Generic Available No

Therapeutic Class Vaccine, Live Virus

Use Provide vaccine-induced immunity to rubella

Contraindications Hypersensitivity to neomycin, patients receiving ACTH, corticosteroids, irradiation; patients with respiratory infections; active tuberculosis; immunosuppressed patients (drug induced or disease)

Precautions Hypersensitivity, allergic reactions to the vaccine; do not administer with other live vaccines; do not vaccinate for at least 3 months following patient receiving blood transfusion and immune serum globulin; may temporarily depress tuberculin skin testing

Adverse Reactions

Central nervous system: Malaise, fever, headache, rarely encephalitis, polyneuritis

Dermatologic: Urticaria, rash

Hematologic: Thrombocytopenia

Local: Local tenderness and erythema

Neuromuscular & skeletal: Arthralgias

Respiratory: Sore throat

Miscellaneous: Lymphadenopathy, hypersensitivity, allergic reactions to the vaccine

Drug Interactions Whole blood, immune globulin

Stability Refrigerate, discard reconstituted vaccine after 8 hours; store at 2°C to 8°C (36°F to 46°F); ship vaccine at 10°C; may use dry ice

Mechanism of Action Antibody titers after immunization last 6 years without significant decline; 90% of those vaccinated have protection for at least 15 years

Usual Dosage S.C.: 1000 $TCID_{50}$ of rubella (entire single-dose vial) into outer aspect of upper arm; do not give I.V.

Monitoring Parameters See Adverse Reactions

Patient Information Patient may experience burning or stinging at the injection site; joint pain usually occurs 1-10 weeks after vaccination and persists 1-3 days

Nursing Implications Reconstituted vaccine should be used within 8 hours; S.C. injection only; federal law requires that the date of administration, the vaccine manufacturer, lot number of vaccine, and the administering person's name, title, and address be entered into the patient's permanent record

Special Geriatric Considerations Not a vaccine necessary for most adults and elderly adults; however, necessary to protect persons without immunity traveling into endemic or epidemic countries; may need to test for rubella immunity if no record of disease of vaccination is available

Dosage Forms Injection: 1000 $TCID_{50}$ (Wistar RA 27/3 Strain) single dose

Rubeola vaccine see Measles Virus Vaccine, Live, Attenuated on page 433

Rubramin-PC® see Cyanocobalamin on page 192

Ru-Est-Span® see Estradiol on page 269

Rufen® see Ibuprofen on page 360

Rum-K® see Potassium Chloride on page 576

Ru-Vert-M® see Meclizine Hydrochloride on page 434

Rythmol® see Propafenone Hydrochloride on page 600

Sabin see Poliovirus Vaccine, Live, Trivalent on page 575

Salbutamol see Albuterol on page 24

Saleto-200® [OTC] see Ibuprofen on page 360

Saleto-400® see Ibuprofen on page 360

Salflex® see Salsalate on page 637

Salgesic® see Salsalate on page 637

Salicylates (Various Salts)
Related Information
Antacid Drug Interactions on page 764

Brand Names Arthropan®; Asproject®; Extra Strength Doan's® [OTC]; Magan®; Mobidin®; Original Doan's® [OTC]; Rexolate®; Tusal®

Synonyms Choline Salicylate; Magnesium Salicylate; Sodium Salicylate; Sodium Thiosalicylate

Generic Available Yes

Therapeutic Class Analgesic, Non-narcotic

Use Treatment of mild to moderate pain, inflammation, and fever; management of rheumatic fever, rheumatoid arthritis, osteoarthritis, and gout

Contraindications Bleeding disorders (factor VII or IX deficiencies), hypersensitivity to salicylates or other nonsteroidal anti-inflammatory drugs (NSAIDs); tartrazine dye and asthma

Warnings Tinnitus or impaired hearing may indicate toxicity; discontinue use 1 week prior to surgical procedures

Precautions Use with caution in patients with platelet and bleeding disorders, renal dysfunction, hepatic disease, history of salicylate-induced gastric irritation, peptic ulcer disease, erosive gastritis, bleeding disorders, hypoprothrombinemia, and vitamin K deficiency; use cautiously in asthmatics, especially those with aspirin intolerance and nasal polyps

Adverse Reactions
Central nervous system: Fever, dizziness, mental confusion, CNS depression, headache, lassitude
Dermatologic: Rash, urticaria, angioedema
Gastrointestinal: Nausea, vomiting, GI distress, bleeding, ulcers
Hematologic: Leukopenia, thrombocytopenia
Hepatic: Hepatotoxicity (high dose)
Otic: Tinnitus
Respiratory: Bronchospasm, hyperventilation
Miscellaneous: Thirst, sweating

Overdosage 10-30 g; symptoms of overdose include tinnitus, headache, dizziness, confusion, metabolic acidosis, hyperpyrexia, hyperpnea, tachypnea, nausea, vomiting, irritability, disorientation, hallucinations, lethargy, stupor, dehydration, hyperven-

(Continued)

Salicylates (Various Salts) *(Continued)*

tilation, hyperthermia, hyperactivity, depression leading to coma, respiratory failure, and collapse; laboratory abnormalities include hypokalemia, hypoglycemia or hyperglycemia with alterations in pH

Toxicology The "Done" nomogram is very helpful for estimating the severity of aspirin poisoning and directing treatment using serum salicylate levels. Treatment can also be based upon symptomatology; see table.

Aspirin or Other Salicylate Toxicity

Toxic Symptoms	Treatment
Overdose	Induce emesis with ipecac, and/or lavage with saline, followed with activated charcoal
Dehydration	I.V. fluids with KCl (no D_5W only)
Metabolic acidosis (must be treated)	Sodium bicarbonate
Hyperthermia	Cooling blankets or sponge baths
Coagulopathy/hemorrhage	Vitamin K I.V.
Hypoglycemia (with coma, seizures or change in mental status)	Dextrose 25 g I.V.
Seizures	Diazepam 5-10 mg I.V.

Drug Interactions

May increase nephrotoxicity of cyclosporin; diclofenac + K^+ sparing diuretics → ↑ serum K^+

Concomitant insulin or oral hypoglycemic agents → ↑ or ↓ serum glucose

May increase digoxin, methotrexate, and lithium serum concentrations

Aspirin or other salicylates may decrease NSAID serum concentrations

Other NSAIDs may increase adverse GI effects

Increased prothrombin time with anticoagulants

Decreased antihypertensive effects of ACE inhibitors, beta-blockers, and thiazide diuretics

Increased response to sympathomimetics

Probenecid may increase toxicity of NSAIDs by increase in serum concentrations

Effects of loop diuretics may decrease; concomitant use with loop diuretics may enhance azotemia in elderly

Mechanism of Action Inhibits prostaglandin synthesis, acts on the hypothalamus heat-regulating center to reduce fever; decreases pain receptor sensitivity. Other proposed mechanisms of action for salicylate anti-inflammatory action are lysosomal stabilization, kinin and leukotriene production, alteration of chemotactic factors, and inhibition of neutrophil activation. This latter mechanism may be the most significant pharmacologic action to reduce inflammation.

Pharmacokinetics

Absorption: From the stomach and small intestine

Distribution: Readily into most body fluids and tissues

Aspirin is hydrolyzed to salicylate (active) by esterases in the GI mucosa, red blood cells, synovial fluid and blood

Metabolism: Metabolism of salicylate occurs primarily by hepatic microsomal enzymes

Half-life, aspirin: 15-20 minutes; metabolic pathways are saturable such that salicylates half-life is dose-dependent ranging from 3 hours at lower doses (300-600 mg), 5-6 hours (after 1 g) and 15-30 hours with higher doses; in therapeutic anti-inflammatory doses, half-lives generally range from 6-12 hours

Time to peak: Peak plasma levels appear in about 1-2 hours

Usual Dosage Geriatrics and Adults:

Sodium salicylate: Oral: 325-650 mg every 4 hours

Sodium thiosalicylate: I.M.:
Acute gout: 100 mg every 3-4 hours for 2 days, then 100 mg/day until resolved
Rheumatic fever: 100-150 mg every 4-8 hours for 3 days, then 100 mg twice/day until asymptomatic
Musculoskeletal pain: 50-100 mg/day or every other day

Magnesium salicylate: Oral: 650 mg every 4 hours or 1090 mg 3 times/day; may increase dose to 3.6-4.8 g/day in divided dose (3-4 doses); use caution in patients with renal failure and reduced renal function (ie, elderly – magnesium accumulation); see Additional Information

Monitoring Parameters Serum concentrations, renal function; hearing changes or tinnitus; monitor for response (ie, pain, inflammation, range of motion, grip strength); observe for abnormal bleeding, bruising, weight gain

Reference Range

Sample size: 1.5-2 mL blood (purple top tube)

Timing of serum samples: Peak levels usually occur 2 hours after ingestion; the half-life increases with the dosage (eg, the half-life after 300 mg is 3 hours, and after 1 g is 5-6 hours, and after 8-10 g is 10-15 hours).

Salicylate serum concentrations correlate with the pharmacological actions and adverse effects observed. Anti-inflammatory therapeutic serum concentrations 15-30 mg/dL. See table.

Serum Salicylate: Clinical Correlations

Serum Salicylate Concentration (mg/dL)	Desired Effects	Adverse Effects/ Intoxication
~10	Antiplatelet Antipyresis Analgesia	GI intolerance and bleeding, hypersensitivity, hemostatic defects
15–30	Anti–inflammatory	Mild salicylism
25–40	Treatment of rheumatic fever	Nausea/vomiting, hyperventilation, salicylism, flushing, sweating, thirst, headache, diarrhea and tachycardia
>40–50		Respiratory alkalosis, hemorrhage, excitement, confusion, asterixis, pulmonary edema, convulsions, tetany, metabolic acidosis, fever, coma, cardiovascular collapse, renal and respiratory failure

Test Interactions False-negative results for glucose oxidase urinary glucose tests (Clinistix®); false-positives using the cupric sulfate method (Clinitest®); also, interferes with Gerhardt test (urinary ketone analysis), VMA determination; 5-HIAA, xylose tolerance test, and T_3 and T_4; increased PBI; increased uric acid

Patient Information Watch for any signs of bleeding (stool); take with food to minimize GI distress; report ringing in ears, persistent GI pain to physician or pharmacist

Nursing Implications See Monitoring Parameters, Reference Range, and Special Geriatric Considerations

Additional Information Liquid dosage form may be useful for those who have difficulty swallowing tablets or caplets. These agents do not appear to inhibit platelet aggregation. Nonacetylated salicylates have less GI toxicity and renal effects than aspirin and other NSAIDs. They also do not cause reactions in aspirin sensitive patients.

Choline salicylate: Arthropan®

Sodium thiosalicylate: Asproject®; Rexolate®; Tusal®

Magnesium salicylate: Extra Strength Doan's® [OTC]; Magan®; Mobidin®; Original Doan's® [OTC]

Special Geriatric Considerations Elderly are a high-risk population for adverse effects from nonsteroidal anti-inflammatory agents. As much as 60% of elderly can develop peptic ulceration and/or hemorrhage asymptomatically. The concomitant use of H_2-blockers, omeprazole, and sucralfate is not effective as prophylaxis. Misoprostol is the only prophylactic agent proven effective. Also, concomitant disease and drug use contribute to the risk for GI adverse effects. Use lowest effective dose for shortest period possible. Consider renal function decline with age. Use of NSAIDs can compromise existing renal function especially when Cl_{cr} is ≤30 mL/minute. Tinnitus may be a difficult and unreliable indication of toxicity due to age-related hearing loss or eighth cranial nerve damage. CNS adverse effects such as confusion, agitation, and hallucination are generally seen in overdose or high dose situations, but elderly may demonstrate these adverse effects at lower doses than younger adults.

Dosage Forms

Injection: 50 mg/mL

Liquid: 870 mg/mL (choline salicylate)

Tablet, enteric coated: 325 mg, 545 mg, 600 mg, 650 mg

References

Gurwitz JH, Avarn J, Ross-Degan D, et al, "Nonsteroidal Anti-Inflammatory Drug-Associated Azotemia in the Very Old," *JAMA*, 1990, 264(4):471-5.

Weissmann G, "Aspirin," *Sci Am*, 1991, 264(1):84-90.

Salicylazosulfapyridine *see* Sulfasalazine *on page 661*

Salicylsalicylic Acid *see* Salsalate *on page 637*

Saline® [OTC] *see* Sodium Chloride *on page 648*

Salivart® [OTC] *see* Saliva Substitute *on next page*

Saliva Substitute
Brand Names Moi-Stir® [OTC]; Orex® [OTC]; Salivart® [OTC]; Xero-Lube® [OTC]

Therapeutic Class Gastrointestinal Agent, Miscellaneous

Use Relief of dry mouth and throat in xerostomia

Usual Dosage Geriatrics and Adults: Use as needed

Special Geriatric Considerations Saliva production has not been shown to change with aging, however, many drugs used by the elderly can cause dry mouth; these patients may benefit from a saliva substitute

Dosage Forms

Solution: 60 mL, 75 mL, 120 mL, 180 mL

Swabstix: 300s

Salk *see* Poliovirus Vaccine, Inactivated *on page 574*

Salmeterol Xinafoate
Brand Names Serevent®

Therapeutic Class Adrenergic Agonist Agent; Beta-2-Adrenergic Agonist Agent; Bronchodilator

Use Bronchodilator in reversible airway obstruction due to asthma or COPD; prevention of exercise-induced bronchospasm

Contraindications Hypersensitivity to salmeterol, adrenergic amines or any ingredients

Warnings Not to be used for the treatment of acute symptoms; if patient has an increased need for short-acting, "as needed" beta-agonists, medical evaluation should be obtained; patients should be warned not to exceed recommended dose; use with caution in patients with unstable vasomotor symptoms, diabetes, hyperthyroidism, prostatic hypertrophy, or a history of seizures; also use caution in the elderly and those patients with cardiovascular disorders such as coronary artery disease, arrhythmias and hypertension

Precautions Excessive use may result in tolerance; deaths have been reported after excessive use; though the exact cause is unknown, cardiac arrest after a severe asthmatic crisis is suspected

Adverse Reactions

Cardiovascular: Tachycardia, palpitations, elevation or depression of blood pressure

Central nervous system: Nervousness, CNS stimulation, hyperactivity, insomnia

Gastrointestinal: GI upset

Neuromuscular & skeletal: Tremors (may be more common in the elderly)

Overdosage Symptoms of overdose include hypertension, tachycardia, seizures, angina, hypokalemia, and tachyarrhythmias

Toxicology Prudent use of a cardioselective beta-adrenergic blocker (eg, atenolol or metoprolol); keep in mind the potential for induction of bronchoconstriction in an asthmatic. Dialysis has not been shown to be of value in the treatment of an overdose with this agent.

Drug Interactions

Decreased therapeutic effect: Beta-adrenergic blockers (eg, propranolol)

Increased toxicity (cardiovascular): MAO inhibitors, tricyclic antidepressants

Mechanism of Action Relaxes bronchial smooth muscle by action on beta$_2$-receptors with little effect on heart rate

Pharmacodynamics

Onset of effective bronchodilation: 10-20 minutes

Peak effect: Within 3 hours

Duration: 12 hours

Pharmacokinetics

Protein binding: 94% to 98%

Metabolism: Extensive by hydroxylation in the liver; systemic levels are low or undetectable

Usual Dosage Geriatrics and Adults:

Inhalation: 42 mcg (2 puffs) every 12 hours

Prevention of exercise-induced bronchospasm: 2 puffs 30-60 minutes before exercise; do not repeat dose for 12 hours

Monitoring Parameters Pulmonary function tests, blood pressure, pulse

Patient Information Not to be used for the relief of acute attacks; do not exceed recommended dosage; rinse mouth with water following each inhalation to help with dry throat and mouth; follow specific instructions accompanying inhaler; if more than one inhalation is necessary, wait at least 1 full minute between inhalations. May cause nervousness, restlessness, insomnia – if these effects continue after dosage reduction, notify physician; also notify physician if palpitations, tachycardia, chest pain, muscle tremors, dizziness, headache, flushing or if breathing difficulty persists

Nursing Implications Not to be used for the relief of acute attacks; monitor lung sounds, pulse, blood pressure

Special Geriatric Considerations Geriatric patients were included in four clinical studies of salmeterol; no apparent differences in efficacy and safety were noted in geriatric patients compared to younger adults. Because salmeterol is only to be used for prevention of bronchospasm, patients also need a short-acting beta-agonist to treat acute attacks. Elderly patients should be carefully counseled about which inhaler to use and the proper scheduling of doses; a spacer device may be utilized to maximize effectiveness.

Dosage Forms Inhaler: 21 mcg/metered inhalation (60 & 120 doses)

Salsalate (sal' sa late)

Brand Names Anigesic®; Argesic®-SA; Artha-G®; Disalcid®; Mono-Gesic®; Salflex®; Salgesic®; Salsitab®

Synonyms Disalicylic Acid; Salicylsalicylic Acid

Generic Available Yes

Therapeutic Class Analgesic, Non-narcotic; Anti-inflammatory Agent; Antipyretic; Nonsteroidal Anti-inflammatory Agent (NSAID), Oral; Salicylate

Use Treatment of mild to moderate pain, inflammation and fever; management of rheumatic fever, rheumatoid arthritis, osteoarthritis, and gout

Contraindications Known hypersensitivity to salsalate; bleeding disorders (factor VII or IX deficiencies), hypersensitivity to salicylates or other nonsteroidal anti-inflammatory drugs (NSAIDs); tartrazine dye and asthma

Warnings Tinnitus or impaired hearing may indicate toxicity; discontinue use 1 week prior to surgical procedures

Precautions Use with caution in patients with platelet and bleeding disorders, renal dysfunction, hepatic disease, history of salicylate-induced gastric irritation, peptic ulcer disease, erosive gastritis, bleeding disorders, hypoprothrombinemia, and vitamin K deficiency; use cautiously in asthmatics, especially those with aspirin intolerance and nasal polyps

Adverse Reactions
Central nervous system: Fever, dizziness, mental confusion, CNS depression, lassitude, headache
Dermatologic: Rash, urticaria, angioedema
Gastrointestinal: Nausea, vomiting, GI distress, bleeding, ulcers, thirst
Hematologic: Leukopenia, thrombocytopenia
Hepatic: Hepatotoxicity (high dose)
Otic: Tinnitus
Respiratory: Hyperventilation, bronchospasm
Miscellaneous: Sweating

Overdosage 10-30 g; symptoms of overdose include tinnitus, headache, dizziness, confusion, metabolic acidosis, hyperpyrexia, hyperpnea, tachypnea, nausea, vomiting, irritability, disorientation, hallucinations, lethargy, stupor, dehydration, hyperventilation, hyperthermia, hyperactivity, depression leading to coma, respiratory failure, and collapse; laboratory abnormalities include hypokalemia, hypoglycemia or hyperglycemia with alterations in pH

Toxicology The "Done" nomogram is very helpful for estimating the severity of aspirin poisoning and directing treatment using serum salicylate levels. Treatment can also be based upon symptomatology; see table.

Aspirin or Other Salicylate Toxicity

Toxic Symptoms	Treatment
Overdose	Induce emesis with ipecac, and/or lavage with saline, followed with activated charcoal
Dehydration	I.V. fluids with KCl (no D_5W only)
Metabolic acidosis (must be treated)	Sodium bicarbonate
Hyperthermia	Cooling blankets or sponge baths
Coagulopathy/hemorrhage	Vitamin K I.V.
Hypoglycemia (with coma, seizures or change in mental status)	Dextrose 25 g I.V.
Seizures	Diazepam 5–10 mg I.V.

Drug Interactions
May increase nephrotoxicity of cyclosporin
Diclofenac + K^+ sparing diuretics → ↑ serum K^+
Concomitant insulin or oral hypoglycemic agents → ↑ or ↓ serum glucose
May increase digoxin, methotrexate, and lithium serum concentrations
Aspirin or other salicylates may decrease NSAID serum concentrations
Other NSAIDs may increase adverse GI effects
Increased prothrombin time with anticoagulants
(Continued)

ALPHABETICAL LISTING OF DRUGS

Salsalate *(Continued)*

Decreased antihypertensive effects of ACE inhibitors, beta-blockers, and thiazide diuretics

Increased response to sympathomimetics

Probenecid may increase toxicity of NSAIDs by increase in serum concentrations

Effects of loop diuretics may decrease

Concomitant use with loop diuretics may enhance azotemia in elderly

Mechanism of Action Inhibits prostaglandin synthesis, acts on the hypothalamus heat-regulating center to reduce fever; decreases pain receptor sensitivity. Other proposed mechanisms of action for salicylate anti-inflammatory action are lysosomal stabilization, kinin and leukotriene production, alteration of chemotactic factors, and inhibition of neutrophil activation. This latter mechanism may be the most significant pharmacologic action to reduce inflammation.

Pharmacodynamics Onset of action: Within 3-4 days of continuous dosing

Pharmacokinetics

Absorption: Oral: Completely from the small intestine; insoluble in gastric acid secretions and, therefore, is not absorbed until it reaches the small intestine

Protein binding: 90%

Half-life: 7-8 hours; half-life increases with dose, 15-30 hours with higher doses hydrolyzed in the liver to 2 moles of salicylic acid (active)

Elimination: Almost totally excreted renally

Usual Dosage Geriatrics and Adults: Oral: 500-1000 mg 2-4 times/day

Monitoring Parameters Serum concentrations, renal function; hearing changes or tinnitus; monitor for response (ie, pain, inflammation, range of motion, grip strength); observe for abnormal bleeding, bruising, weight gain

Reference Range

Sample size: 1.5-2 mL blood (purple top tube)

Timing of serum samples: Peak levels usually occur 2 hours after ingestion; the half-life increases with the dosage (eg, the half-life after 300 mg is 3 hours, and after 1 g is 5-6 hours, and after 8-10 g is 10-15 hours).

Salicylate serum concentrations correlate with the pharmacological actions and adverse effects observed. Anti-inflammatory therapeutic serum concentrations 15-30 mg/dL. See table.

Serum Salicylate: Clinical Correlations

Serum Salicylate Concentration (mg/dL)	Desired Effects	Adverse Effects/ Intoxication
~10	Antiplatelet Antipyresis Analgesia	GI intolerance and bleeding, hypersensitivity, hemostatic defects
15-30	Anti-inflammatory	Mild salicylism
25-40	Treatment of rheumatic fever	Nausea/vomiting, hyperventilation, salicylism, flushing, sweating, thirst, headache, diarrhea and tachycardia
>40-50		Respiratory alkalosis, hemorrhage, excitement, confusion, asterixis, pulmonary edema, convulsions, tetany, metabolic acidosis, fever, coma, cardiovascular collapse, renal and respiratory failure

Test Interactions False-negative results for glucose oxidase urinary glucose tests (Clinistix®); false-positives using the cupric sulfate method (Clinitest®); also, interferes with Gerhardt test (urinary ketone analysis), VMA determination; 5-HIAA, xylose tolerance test, and T_3 and T_4; increased PBI; increased uric acid

Patient Information Avoid alcohol; do not self-medicate with other drug products containing aspirin; use antacids to relieve upset stomach; watch for any signs of bleeding (stool); take with food to minimize GI distress; report ringing in ears, persistent GI pain to physician or pharmacist

Nursing Implications See Monitoring Parameters, Reference Range, and Special Geriatric Considerations

Additional Information Does not appear to inhibit platelet aggregation; salsalate causes less GI and renal toxicity than aspirin and other NSAIDs.

Special Geriatric Considerations Elderly are a high-risk population for adverse effects from nonsteroidal anti-inflammatory agents. As much as 60% of elderly can develop peptic ulceration and/or hemorrhage asymptomatically. The concomitant use of H_2-blockers, omeprazole, and sucralfate is not effective as prophylaxis. Misoprostol is the only prophylactic agent proven effective. Also, concomitant disease and drug use contribute to the risk for GI adverse effects. Use lowest effective dose for shortest period possible. Consider renal function decline with age. Use of NSAIDs can compromise existing renal function especially when Cl_{cr} is ≤ 30 mL/minute. Tinnitus may be a difficult and unreliable indication of toxicity due to age-related hearing loss or eighth cranial nerve damage. CNS adverse effects such as confusion, agitation, and hallucinations are generally seen in overdose or high dose situations, but elderly may demonstrate these adverse effects at lower doses than younger adults. See Additional Information

Dosage Forms
Capsule: 500 mg
Tablet: 500 mg, 750 mg

References
Gurwitz JH, Avarn J, Ross-Degan D, et al, "Nonsteroidal Anti-Inflammatory Drug-Associated Azotemia in the Very Old," *JAMA*, 1990, 264(4):471-5.
Weissmann G, "Aspirin," *Sci Am*, 1991, 264(1):84-90.

Salsitab® *see* Salsalate *on page 637*

Salt *see* Sodium Chloride *on page 648*

Sandimmune® *see* Cyclosporine *on page 199*

Sandoglobulin® *see* Immune Globulin *on page 366*

Sani-Supp® [OTC] *see* Glycerin *on page 325*

Santyl® *see* Collagenase *on page 187*

Scabene® *see* Lindane *on page 407*

Sclavo-PPD® Solution *see* Tuberculin Purified Protein Derivative *on page 725*

Sclavo-Test-PPD® *see* Tuberculin Purified Protein Derivative *on page 725*

Scopolamine (skoe pol' a meen)

Brand Names Isopto® Hyoscine; Transderm Scop®
Synonyms Hyoscine; Scopolamine Hydrobromide
Generic Available Yes
Therapeutic Class Anticholinergic Agent; Anticholinergic Agent, Ophthalmic; Anticholinergic Agent, Transdermal; Ophthalmic Agent, Mydriatic
Use Preoperative medication to produce amnesia and decrease salivation and respiratory secretions; ophthalmic: to produce cycloplegia and mydriasis prior to refraction; treatment of iridocyclitis; patch: prevention of nausea and vomiting by motion
Contraindications Hypersensitivity to scopolamine or any component; narrow-angle glaucoma; acute hemorrhage
Precautions Use with caution in the elderly or in individuals with hepatic or renal impairment since adverse CNS effects occur more often in these patients; use with caution in patients with pyloric obstruction, urinary bladder neck obstruction or intestinal obstruction, cardiovascular disease, hypertension
Adverse Reactions
Cardiovascular: Tachycardia, palpitations
Central nervous system: Disorientation, drowsiness, hallucinations, confusion, psychosis, delirium **(the elderly are at increased risk for confusion and hallucinations)**
Gastrointestinal: Dry mouth, constipation
Genitourinary: Urinary retention
Ocular: Blurred vision, cycloplegia, mydriasis, photophobia, increased intraocular pressure, local irritation
Miscellaneous: Anaphylaxis, allergic reactions **Note:** Systemic adverse effects have been reported with both the transdermal and ophthalmic preparations. Drug withdrawal has occurred in patients using the transdermal system for longer than 3 days; symptoms include dizziness, nausea, vomiting, headache, and equilibrium disturbance.
Overdosage Symptoms of overdose include dilated pupils, flushed skin, tachycardia, hypertension, EKG abnormalities, CNS manifestations resembling acute psychosis; CNS depression, circulatory collapse, respiratory failure
Toxicology Pure scopolamine intoxication is extremely rare. However, for a scopolamine overdose with severe life-threatening symptoms, physostigmine 1-2 mg S.C. or I.V. slowly should be given to reverse the toxic effects.
Drug Interactions
Decreased effect due to impaired absorption of acetaminophen, levodopa, ketoconazole, digoxin, riboflavin, potassium chloride in wax matrix preparations
Increased effect/toxicity with anticholinergic agents
Stability Avoid acid solutions, because hydrolysis occurs at pH <3
Mechanism of Action Blocks the action of acetylcholine at parasympathetic sites in smooth muscle, secretory glands and the CNS; increases cardiac output, dries secretions, antagonizes histamine and serotonin
Pharmacodynamics Peak effects: 20-60 minutes; may take 3-7 days for full recovery
Pharmacokinetics Absorption: Well absorbed by all routes of administration

(Continued)

Scopolamine *(Continued)*

Usual Dosage Geriatrics and Adults:
Preoperatively and Antiemetic: I.M., I.V., S.C.: 0.3-0.65 mg

Motion sickness: Apply 1 patch behind the ear at least 4 hours before the antiemetic effect is required; if therapy is required for longer than 3 days, remove the first patch and apply a new one behind the other ear

Ophthalmic:
Refraction: Instill 1-2 drops of 0.25% to eye(s) 1 hour before procedure
Iridocyclitis: Instill 1-2 drops of 0.25% to eye(s) up to 3 times/day

Monitoring Parameters Blood pressure, pulse, anticholinergic effects

Patient Information Report any changes of vision; wait 5 minutes after instilling ophthalmic preparation before using any other drops; do not blink excessively; after instilling ophthalmic preparation, apply pressure to the side of the nose near the eye to minimize systemic absorption; put patch on at least 4 hours before traveling; once applied, do not remove the patch for 3 full days. May cause dry mouth, drowsiness, blurred vision. If eye pain, blurred vision, dizziness, or rapid pulse occurs, remove patch and consult physician. Wash hands thoroughly after handling the patch.

Nursing Implications Disc (patch) is programmed to deliver *in vivo* 0.5 mg over 3 days; wash hands before and after applying the disc to avoid drug contact with eyes; after instilling ophthalmic preparation, apply pressure to the side of the nose near the eye to minimize systemic absorption

Additional Information Produces more CNS depression, mydriasis, and cycloplegia but less effective in preventing reflex bradycardia and affecting the intestines than atropine

Scopolamine: Transderm Scop®
Scopolamine hydrobromide: Isopto® hyoscine

Special Geriatric Considerations Because of its long duration of action as a mydriatic agent, it should be avoided in elderly patients. Anticholinergic agents are not well tolerated in the elderly and their use should be avoided when possible; see Precautions, Adverse Reactions

Dosage Forms
Disc, transdermal: 1.5 mg/disc (4's)
Injection, as hydrobromide: 0.3 mg/mL (1 mL); 0.4 mg/mL (0.5 mL, 1 mL); 0.86 mg/mL (0.5 mL); 1 mg/mL (1 mL)
Solution, ophthalmic, as hydrobromide: 0.25% (5 mL, 15 mL)

References
Feinberg M, "The Problems of Anticholinergic Adverse Effects in Older Patients," *Drugs Aging*, 1993, 3(4):335-48.

Scopolamine Hydrobromide *see* Scopolamine *on previous page*

Sebaquin® [OTC] *see* Iodoquinol *on page 375*

Secobarbital and Amobarbital *see* Amobarbital and Secobarbital *on page 46*

Secobarbital Sodium *(see koe bar' bi tal)*

Related Information
Anxiolytic/Hypnotic Use in Long-Term Care Facilities *on page 755-756*
Brand Names Seconal™
Synonyms Quinalbarbitone Sodium
Therapeutic Class Barbiturate; Hypnotic; Sedative
Special Geriatric Considerations Use of this agent in the elderly is not recommended due to its long half-life and addiction potential

Seconal™ *see* Secobarbital Sodium *on this page*

Sectral® *see* Acebutolol Hydrochloride *on page 12*

Seldane® *see* Terfenadine *on page 674*

Selegiline Hydrochloride *(seh ledge' ah leen)*

Brand Names Eldepryl®
Synonyms Deprenyl; L-Deprenyl
Generic Available No
Therapeutic Class Anti-Parkinson's Agent
Use Adjunct in the management of parkinsonian patients in which levodopa/carbidopa therapy is deteriorating.

Unlabeled use: Early Parkinson's disease
Investigational use: Alzheimer's disease
Contraindications Known hypersensitivity to selegiline
Warnings Do not use at daily doses exceeding 10 mg/day because of the risks associated with nonselective inhibition of MAO

Precautions At doses ≤10 mg/day patients can safely consume tyramine-containing foods without the risk of uncontrolled hypertension

Adverse Reactions
Cardiovascular: Orthostatic hypotension, arrhythmias, hypertension
Central nervous system: Hallucinations, confusion, depression, insomnia, agitation, loss of balance
Gastrointestinal: Nausea, vomiting, dry mouth
Neuromuscular & skeletal: Increased involuntary movements, bradykinesia

Overdosage Symptoms of overdose include tachycardia, palpitations, muscle twitching, seizures

Toxicology Competent supportive care is the most important treatment; both hypertension or hypotension can occur with intoxication. Hypotension may respond to I.V. fluids or vasopressors, and hypertension usually responds to an alpha-adrenergic blocker. While treating the hypertension, care is warranted to avoid sudden drops in blood pressure, since this may worsen the MAO inhibitor toxicity. Muscle irritability and seizures often respond to diazepam, while hyperthermia is best treated antipyretics and cooling blankets. Cardiac arrhythmias are best treated with phenytoin or procainamide.

Drug Interactions Increased toxicity: Meperidine in combination with selegiline has caused agitation, delirium, and death; it may be prudent to avoid other opioids as well; fluoxetine increased pressor effects

Mechanism of Action Potent monoamine oxidase (MAO) type-B inhibitor; MAO-B plays a major role in the metabolism of dopamine; selegiline may also increase dopaminergic activity by interfering with dopamine reuptake at the synapse

Pharmacodynamics
Onset of action: Oral: Within 60 minutes
Duration: 24-72 hours

Pharmacokinetics
Half-life: 9 minutes
Metabolism: To amphetamine and methamphetamine in the liver

Usual Dosage Oral:
Geriatrics: Initial: 5 mg in the morning; may increase to a total of 10 mg/day
Adults: 5 mg twice daily with breakfast and lunch or 10 mg in the morning

Monitoring Parameters Blood pressure, symptoms of parkinsonism

Patient Information Do not take more than the prescribed dose; explain the tyramine reaction to patients and tell them to report severe headaches or other unusual symptoms to physician

Nursing Implications Selegiline is a monoamine oxidase inhibitor type "B"; there should **not** be a problem with tyramine-containing products as long as the typical doses are employed

Additional Information When adding selegiline to levodopa/carbidopa the dose of the latter can usually (and should) be decreased. Studies are investigating the use of selegiline in early Parkinson's disease to slow the progression of the disease.

Special Geriatric Considerations Selegiline is also being studied in Alzheimer's disease; small studies have shown some improvement in behavioral and cognitive performance in patients, however, further study is needed; see Warnings and Adverse Reactions

Dosage Forms Tablet: 5 mg

References
Collier DS, Berg MJ, and Fincham RW, "Parkinsonism Treatment: Part III - Update," *Ann Pharmacother*, 1992, 26(2):227-33.
Koller WC, Silver DE, and Lieberman A, "An Algorithm for the Management of Parkinson's Disease," *Neurology*, 1994, 44(12):S1-52.
Schneider LS, Pollock VE, Zemansky MF, et al, "A Pilot Study of Low-Dose L-Deprenyl in Alzheimer's Disease," *J Geriatr Psychiatry Neurol*, 1991, 4(3):143-8.
The Parkinson Study Group, "Effect of Deprenyl on the Progression of Disability in Early Parkinson's Disease," *N Engl J Med*, 1989, 321(20):1364-71.
The Parkinson Study Group, "Effects of Tocopherol and Deprenyl on the Progression of Disability in Early Parkinson's Disease," *N Engl J Med*, 1993, 328(3):176-83.

Selestoject® *see* Betamethasone *on page 82*

Semilente *see* Insulin Preparations *on page 372*

Semilente® Iletin®I *see* Insulin Preparations *on page 372*

Semilente® Insulin (Beef) *see* Insulin Preparations *on page 372*

Semilente® Purified Pork Human *see* Insulin Preparations *on page 372*

Senexon® [OTC] *see* Senna *on this page*

Senna

Brand Names Black Draught® [OTC]; Dr Caldwell Senna Laxative® [OTC]; Ex-Lax® Gentle Nature® [OTC]; Fletcher's Castoria® [OTC]; Gentlax® [OTC]; Gentle Nature® [OTC]; Nytilax® [OTC]; Senexon® [OTC]; Senna-Gen® [OTC]; Senokot® [OTC]; Senolax® [OTC]; X-Prep® Liquid [OTC]

(Continued)

Senna *(Continued)*

Synonyms Sennosides

Therapeutic Class Laxative, Stimulant

Use Short-term treatment of constipation; evacuate the colon for bowel or rectal examinations

Contraindications Hypersensitivity to senna or any component; nausea and vomiting; undiagnosed abdominal pain, appendicitis, intestinal obstruction or perforation

Warnings Laxatives used excessively may lead to fluid/electrolyte imbalance; stimulant cathartics may lead to abuse or dependency with chronic use (laxative abuse syndrome); cathartic colon, which may present as ulcerative colitis, occurs with chronic use of stimulant cathartics; melanosis coli is a dark pigmentation of the colonic mucosa from chronic use of anthraquinone derivatives

Precautions Habit-forming and may result in laxative dependence and loss of normal bowel function with prolonged use; rectal bleeding or failure to respond requires further evaluation for possibly serious medical problems

Adverse Reactions
Cardiovascular: Palpitations
Central nervous system: Dizziness, fainting
Endocrine & metabolic: Fluid and electrolyte loss
Gastrointestinal: Nausea, vomiting, diarrhea, abdominal cramps, bloating, flatulence, perianal irritation
Neuromuscular & skeletal: Weakness
Miscellaneous: Sweating

Overdosage Symptoms of overdose include hypokalemia, hypocalcemia, metabolic acidosis or alkalosis, abdominal pain, diarrhea, malabsorption, weight loss and protein-losing enteropathy

Drug Interactions MAO inhibitors, disulfiram, metronidazole, procarbazine

Mechanism of Action Active metabolite (aglycone) acts as a local irritant on the colon, stimulates Auerbach's plexus to produce peristalsis; alters water and electrolyte secretion

Pharmacodynamics Onset of action: Oral: Within 6-10 hours

Pharmacokinetics
Metabolism: In the liver
Elimination: In feces (via bile) and urine

Usual Dosage Geriatrics and Adults:
Granules: 1 teaspoonful at bedtime, not to exceed 2 teaspoonfuls twice daily
Syrup: 2-3 teaspoonfuls at bedtime, not to exceed 3 teaspoonfuls twice daily
Tablet: 2 tablets at bedtime, not to exceed 4 tablets twice daily (8 tablets total)

Monitoring Parameters Monitor stools daily for consistency, occult or gross blood; also with chronic use, monitor serum electrolytes; monitor for dehydration and hypotension

Test Interactions Decreased calcium (S), decreased potassium (S)

Patient Information May discolor urine or feces (yellow-brown); do not use in presence of nausea, vomiting, or abdominal pain; stimulant laxative use should be limited; notify physician if unrelieved by laxative, rectal bleeding occurs, or signs of electrolyte imbalance develop (dizziness, weakness, muscle cramps); take with a full glass of water

Nursing Implications May discolor urine or feces; liquid syrups contain 7% alcohol; liquids 3.5% to 4.9% alcohol; see Monitoring Parameters and Special Geriatric Considerations

Additional Information Long term, chronic use should be avoided; patients should be encouraged to increase fluid intake, fiber intake, and exercise

Special Geriatric Considerations Elderly are often predisposed to constipation due to disease, immobility, drugs, and a decreased "thirst reflex" with age. Avoid stimulant cathartic use on a chronic basis if possible. Use osmotic, lubricant, stool softeners, and bulk agents as prophylaxis. Patients should be instructed for proper dietary fiber and fluid intake as well as regular exercise. Monitor closely for fluid/electrolyte imbalance, CNS signs of fluid/electrolyte loss, and hypotension.

Dosage Forms
Granules: 326 mg/teaspoonful
Liquid: 33.3 mg/mL (75 mL, 150 mL, 360 mL)
Suppository: 652 mg
Syrup: 218 mg/5 mL (60 mL, 240 mL)
Tablet: 187 mg, 217 mg, 600 mg

Senna-Gen® [OTC] *see* Senna *on previous page*

Sennosides *see* Senna *on previous page*

Senokot® [OTC] *see* Senna *on previous page*

Senolax® [OTC] *see* Senna *on previous page*

Septra® *see* Co-trimoxazole *on page 189*

Septra® DS *see* Co-trimoxazole *on page 189*

Ser-Ap-Es® *see* Hydralazine, Hydrochlorothiazide, and Reserpine *on page 346*

Serax® *see* Oxazepam *on page 524*

Serentil® *see* Mesoridazine Besylate *on page 446*

Serevent® *see* Salmeterol Xinafoate *on page 636*

Seromycin® Pulvules® *see* Cycloserine *on page 198*

Serpalan® *see* Reserpine *on page 625*

Serpasil® *see* Reserpine *on page 625*

Serpasil®-Apresoline® *see* Hydralazine and Reserpine *on page 345*

Sertraline Hydrochloride
Related Information
Antidepressant Agents Comparison *on page 800*
Brand Names Zoloft™
Generic Available No
Therapeutic Class Antidepressant; Serotonin Antagonist
Use Treatment of major depression

Unlabeled use: Obsessive-compulsive disorder
Contraindications Hypersensitivity to sertraline or any component; patients receiving MAO inhibitors currently or in the past 2 weeks
Warnings Do not use in combination with monoamine oxidase inhibitor or within 14 days of discontinuing treatment or initiating treatment with a monoamine oxidase inhibitor due to the risk of serotonin syndrome; use with caution in patients with pre-existing seizure disorders, patients in whom weight loss is undesirable, patients with recent myocardial infarction, unstable heart disease, hepatic or renal impairment, patients taking other psychotropic medications, agitated or hyperactive patients as drug may produce or activate mania or hypomania; because the risk of suicide is inherent in depression, patient should be closely monitored until depressive symptoms remit and prescriptions should be written for minimum quantities to reduce the risk of overdose. A weak uricosuric effect has been noted; its significance is unknown.
Adverse Reactions In clinical trials, dizziness and nausea were two most frequent side effects that led to discontinuation of therapy in the elderly

Cardiovascular: Palpitations
Central nervous system: Insomnia, agitation, dizziness, headache, somnolence, nervousness, fatigue
Dermatologic: Dermatological reactions
Gastrointestinal: Dry mouth, diarrhea or loose stools, nausea, constipation, vomiting
Genitourinary: Sexual dysfunction in men, micturition disorders, hyponatremia
Neuromuscular & skeletal: Pain, tremors
Ocular: Visual difficulty
Otic: Tinnitus
Miscellaneous: Sweating
Toxicology Establish and maintain an airway, ensure adequate oxygenation and ventilation. Activated charcoal with 70% sorbitol may be as or more effective than emesis or lavage. Monitoring of cardiac and vital signs is recommended along with general symptomatic and supportive measures. There is no specific antidote for sertraline. Forced diuresis, dialysis, hemoperfusion and exchange transfusion are unlikely to enhance elimination due to sertraline's large volume of distribution.
Drug Interactions MAO inhibitors, see Warnings; alcohol, diazepam, tolbutamide (decreased clearance), warfarin (increased PT); desipramine (slight increase in desipramine concentration)
Mechanism of Action Selectively inhibits the CNS neuronal reuptake of serotonin, thereby enhancing serotonergic activity and inhibiting adrenergic activity in the locus ceruleus. Minimal or no effect on reuptake of norepinephrine or dopamine and does not significantly bind to alpha-adrenergic, histamine, or cholinergic receptors; as a result, it may be useful in patients at risk for sedation, hypotension, and anticholinergic effects of tricyclic antidepressants.
Pharmacodynamics Maximum antidepressant effects usually seen after 4 weeks
Pharmacokinetics Peak plasma concentrations were achieved 4.5-8.4 hours after single daily doses of 50-200 mg for 14 days. Food appears to increase both the area under the curve and peak plasma concentrations, while decreasing time to peak plasma concentration. Sertraline is subject to extensive first-pass metabolism. Its principle metabolite, N-desmethylsertraline is 8 times less active as a serotonin reuptake inhibitor and 4 times less active in its inhibition of norepinephrine and dopamine, and is considered to have little or no clinical Both sertraline and N-desmethylsertraline undergo activity. The mean elimination half-life of sertraline is 26 hours. It is further metabolized via hydroxylation, reduction, and glucuronide conjugation. highly protein bound (87%); <15% is eliminated unchanged in feces. In the elderly, sertraline's clearance has been found to be reduced by 40%
(Continued)

Sertraline Hydrochloride *(Continued)*

Usual Dosage Oral:

Geriatrics: Start treatment with 25 mg/day in the morning and increase by 25 mg/day increments every 2-3 days if tolerated to 75-100 mg/day; additional increases may be necessary; maximum dose: 200 mg/day

Adults: Start with 50 mg/day in the morning and increase by 50 mg/day increments every 2-3 days if tolerated to 100 mg/day; additional increases may be necessary; maximum dose: 200 mg/day. If somnolence is noted, give at bedtime.

Monitoring Parameters Improvement of depressive symptoms, anxiety, sleep disturbance, weight, and appetite

Patient Information If currently on another antidepressant drug, patients should notify their physician. Although sertraline has not been shown to increase the effects of alcohol, it is recommended to refrain from drinking while on this medication. May experience some weight loss, but it is usually minimal. If on warfarin, digoxin, an oral hypoglycemic drug, or a drug having an effect on the central nervous system, such as a medication for insomnia or anxiety, patients should notify physician. There are no known interactions between sertraline and over-the-counter medications; however, these should be used with caution and the directions for their use should be followed carefully.

Nursing Implications Monitor nutritional intake and weight; if patient becomes anxious or overstimulated, notify physician; if somnolent, give dose at bedtime; see Monitoring Parameters and Usual Dosage. Offer hard, sugarless candy or ice chips for dry mouth.

Special Geriatric Considerations Sertraline's favorable side effect profile makes it a useful alternative to the traditional tricyclic antidepressants; its potential stimulation effect and anorexia may be bothersome. Has the shortest half-life of the currently marketed serotonin-reuptake inhibitors.

Dosage Forms Tablet: 50 mg, 100 mg

References

Cohn CK, Shrivastava R, Mendels J, et al, "Double-Blind, Multicenter Comparison of Sertraline and Amitriptyline in Elderly Depressed Patients," *J Clin Psychiatry*, 1990, 51(Suppl B):28-33.

Drug Facts and Comparisons, St Louis, MO: JB Lippincott Co, 1992, 263r-4a.

Grimsley SR and Jann MW, "Paroxetine, Sertraline, and Fluvoxamine: New Selective Serotonin Reuptake Inhibitors," *Clin Pharm*, 1992, 11(11):930-57.

Reimherr FW, Chouinard G, Cohn CK, et al, "Antidepressant Efficacy of Sertraline: A Double-Blind Placebo- and Amitriptyline-Controlled, Multicenter Comparison Study in Outpatients With Major Depression," *J Clin Psychiatry*, 1990, 51(Suppl B):18-27.

Serutan® [OTC] *see* Psyllium *on page 610*

Siblin® [OTC] *see* Psyllium *on page 610*

Silain® [OTC] *see* Simethicone *on next page*

Silvadene® *see* Silver Sulfadiazine *on this page*

Silver Sulfadiazine *(sul fa dye' a zeen)*

Brand Names Flint SSD®; Silvadene®; Thermazene®

Therapeutic Class Antibacterial, Topical

Use Adjunct in the prevention and treatment of infection in second and third degree burns

Contraindications Hypersensitivity to silver sulfadiazine or any component

Precautions Use with caution in patients with G-6-PD deficiency and renal impairment; sulfadiazine may accumulate in patients with impaired hepatic or renal function; systemic absorption is significant and adverse reactions may be due to the sulfa component

Adverse Reactions

Dermatologic: Itching, rash, erythema multiforme, skin discoloration, photosensitivity

Hematologic: Hemolytic anemia, leukopenia, agranulocytosis, aplastic anemia

Hepatic: Hepatitis

Local: Pain, burning

Renal: Interstitial nephritis

Drug Interactions Silver may inactivate topical proteolytic enzymes

Stability Discard if cream is darkened (reacts with heavy metals resulting in release of silver)

Mechanism of Action Acts upon the bacterial cell wall and cell membrane and is bactericidal

Pharmacokinetics

Absorption: Significant percutaneous absorption of sulfadiazine can occur especially when applied to extensive burns

Half-life: 10 hours, prolonged in patients with renal insufficiency

Time to peak: Peak serum levels occur within 3-11 days of continuous therapy

Elimination: ~50% excreted unchanged in urine

Usual Dosage Geriatrics and Adults: Topical: Apply once or twice daily with a sterile gloved hand; apply to a thickness of $1/16$; burned area should be covered with cream at all times

Administration See Patient Information

Patient Information Bathe daily to aid in debridement (if not contraindicated); apply liberally to burned areas; for external use only; notify physician if condition persists or worsens

Nursing Implications Evaluate the development of granulation

Additional Information Contains methylparaben and propylene glycol; use of analgesic might be needed before application

Special Geriatric Considerations See Usual Dosage; no specific recommendations for use in the elderly

Dosage Forms Cream, topical: 10 mg/g (20 g, 50 g, 400 g, 100 g)

Simethicone (sye meth' i kone)

Brand Names Gas-X® [OTC]; Mylicon® [OTC]; Mylicon®-80 [OTC]; Phazyme® [OTC]; Phazyme®-25 [OTC]; Phazyme®-95 [OTC]; Silain® [OTC]

Synonyms Activated Dimethicone; Activated Methylpolysiloxane

Generic Available Yes: Tablet

Therapeutic Class Antiflatulent

Use Relieve flatulence and functional gastric bloating, and postoperative gas pains; painful distention due to air swallowing, peptic ulcer, diverticulitis, irritable (spastic) colon, and functional dyspepsia

Contraindications Hypersensitivity to drug or components

Mechanism of Action Decreases the surface tension of gas bubbles thereby dispersing and preventing gas pockets in the GI system

Pharmacokinetics Elimination: In feces

Usual Dosage Geriatrics and Adults:
Oral: 40-120 mg after meals and at bedtime as needed, not to exceed 500 mg/day
Drops: 40 mg after meals and at bedtime

Monitoring Parameters Monitor for feelings of relief, decreased pain, bloating

Patient Information Chew tablets thoroughly before swallowing; shake drops well before using

Nursing Implications Shake drops before using; mix with water or other liquids; monitor for decrease in pain, bloating, cramping

Additional Information Drops have small amount of saccharin calcium and sodium benzoate

Special Geriatric Considerations Before treating excess gas or pain due to gas accumulation, a thorough evaluation must be made to determine cause since many bowel diseases may present with flatulence and bloating.

Dosage Forms
Capsule: 125 mg
Drops: 40 mg/0.6 mL (30 mL)
Tablet: 50 mg, 60 mg, 95 mg
Tablet, chewable: 40 mg, 80 mg, 125 mg

Simethicone and Magaldrate *see* Magaldrate and Simethicone
on page 425

Simvastatin

Brand Names Zocor™

Generic Available No

Therapeutic Class Antilipemic Agent; HMG-CoA Reductase Inhibitor

Use Adjunct to dietary therapy to decrease elevated serum total and LDL cholesterol concentrations in primary hypercholesterolemia

Contraindications Active liver disease or unexplained persistent elevations of LFTs, hypersensitivity to simvastatin or other HMG-CoA reductase inhibitors

Warnings Musculoskeletal effects include myopathy (myalgia and/or muscle weakness accompanied by markedly elevated CK concentrations), rash and/or pruritus; hepatocellular carcinomas have been found in mice taking in excess of 300 times the recommended dose based on body weight

Precautions May elevate aminotransferases; LFTs should be performed before and every 4-6 weeks during the first 12-15 months of therapy and periodically thereafter; serum cholesterol and triglyceride concentrations should be determined prior to and regularly during therapy; use with caution in patients who consume large quantities of alcohol

Adverse Reactions
Central nervous system: Headache, dizziness
Dermatologic: Rash
Gastrointestinal: Flatulence, dyspepsia, abdominal pain and/or cramps diarrhea and/or constipation, nausea
Neuromuscular & skeletal: Myalgia, muscle cramps, myopathy
Ocular: Blurred vision

Overdosage Few cases have been reported; no patients were symptomatic and all recovered without adverse effects

(Continued)

Simvastatin (Continued)

Drug Interactions Increased anticoagulant effect of warfarin, niacin, gemfibrozil, erythromycin, and cyclosporine (rhabdomyolysis or myopathy)

Mechanism of Action Simvastatin is a methylated derivative of lovastatin that acts by competitively inhibiting 3-hydroxy-3-methylglutaryl-coenzyme A reductase (HMG-CoA reductase), the enzyme that catalyzes the rate-limiting step in cholesterol biosynthesis

Pharmacokinetics

Absorption: Oral: Although 85% is absorbed following administration, <5% reaches the general circulation due to an extensive first-pass effect

Time to peak concentrations: 1.3-2.4 hours

Protein binding: ~95%

Elimination: 13% excreted in urine and 60% in feces; the elimination half-life is unknown

In patients with severe renal insufficiency, high systemic levels may occur

Usual Dosage Oral:

Geriatrics: Start at 5 mg/day as a single evening dose; increase as needed every 4 weeks by 5-10 mg; maximum LDL lowering may be achieved with ≤20 mg/day

Adults: Start with 5-10 mg/day as a single bedtime dose; if LDL is ≤90 mg/dL start with 5 mg; if LDL >100 mg/dL, start with 10 mg/day; increase every 4 weeks as needed; maximum dose: 40 mg/day

Monitoring Parameters Serum cholesterol (total and fractionated), CPK levels; reduce dose if indicated; see Precautions

Test Interactions Increased ALT, AST, CPK, alkaline phosphatase, bilirubin; altered thyroid function tests

Patient Information Promptly report any unexplained muscle pain, tenderness or weakness, especially if accompanied by malaise or fever; follow prescribed diet; take with meals

Special Geriatric Considerations Effective and well tolerated in the elderly. The definition of and, therefore, when to treat hyperlipidemia in the elderly is a controversial issue. The National Cholesterol Education Program recommends that all adults 20 years of age and older maintain a plasma cholesterol of <200 mg/dL. By this definition, 60% of all elderly would be considered to have a borderline high (200-239 mg/dL) or high blood (≥240 mg/dL) cholesterol. However, plasma cholesterol has been shown to be a less reliable predictor of coronary heart disease in the elderly. Therefore, it is the authors' belief that pharmacologic treatment be reserved for those who are unable to obtain a desirable plasma cholesterol level by diet alone and for whom the benefits of treatment are believed to outweigh the potential adverse effects, drug interactions, and cost of treatment.

Dosage Forms Tablet: 5 mg, 10 mg, 20 mg, 40 mg

References

Bach LA, Cooper ME, O'Brien RC, et al, "The Use of Simvastatin, an HMG-CoA Reductase Inhibitor, in Older Patients With Hypercholesterolemia and Atherosclerosis," *J Am Geriatr Soc*, 1990, 38(1):10-4.

Lintott CJ and Scott RS, "HMG-CoA Reductase Inhibitor Use in the Aged: A Review of Clinical Experience," *Drugs Aging*, 1992, 2(6):518-29.

"Summary of the Second Report of the National Cholesterol Education Program (NCEP) Expert Panel on Detection, Evaluation, and Treatment of High Blood Cholesterol in Adults," *JAMA*, 1993, 269(23):3015-23.

Sinarest® 12 Hour Nasal Solution see Oxymetazoline Hydrochloride on page 530

Sinarest® Nasal Solution [OTC] see Phenylephrine Hydrochloride on page 557

Sinemet® see Levodopa and Carbidopa on page 402

Sinequan® see Doxepin Hydrochloride on page 242

Sinusol-B® see Brompheniramine Maleate on page 95

Sleep-eze 3® [OTC] see Diphenhydramine Hydrochloride on page 228

Slo-bid™ see Theophylline on page 681

Slo-Niacin® [OTC] see Niacin on page 498

Slo-Phyllin® see Theophylline on page 681

Slo-Salt® [OTC] see Sodium Chloride on page 648

Slow-K® K+8® see Potassium Chloride on page 576

Slow-Mag® [OTC] see Magnesium Salts (Various Salts) on page 430

SMX-TMP see Co-trimoxazole on page 189

Sodium Acid Carbonate see Sodium Bicarbonate on this page

Sodium Bicarbonate

Brand Names Neut®

Synonyms Baking Soda; NaHCO₃; Sodium Acid Carbonate; Sodium Hydrogen Carbonate

Therapeutic Class Alkalinizing Agent, Oral; Alkalinizing Agent, Parenteral; Antacid; Electrolyte Supplement, Oral; Electrolyte Supplement, Parenteral; Sodium Salt

Use Management of metabolic acidosis; antacid; alkalinize urine

Contraindications Alkalosis, hypocalcemia; unknown abdominal pain, inadequate ventilation during cardiopulmonary resuscitation

Warnings Use of I.V. NaHCO$_3$ should be reserved for documented metabolic acidosis and for hyperkalemia-induced cardiac arrest. Routine use in cardiac arrest is not recommended. Avoid extravasation, tissue necrosis can occur due to the hypertonicity of NaHCO$_3$. May cause sodium retention especially if renal function is impaired; not to be used in treatment of peptic ulcer; use with caution in patients with CHF, edema, cirrhosis, or renal failure; attenuation of effects of hyperkalemia

Adverse Reactions
Cardiovascular: Edema, cerebral hemorrhage
Endocrine & metabolic: Metabolic alkalosis, hypernatremia, hypokalemia, hypocalcemia, intracranial acidosis, increased affinity of hemoglobin for oxygen-reduced pH in myocardia
Gastrointestinal: Gastric distention, flatulence
Local: Tissue necrosis when extravasated

Overdosage Symptoms of overdose include hypocalcemia, hypokalemia, hypernatremia, seizures

Drug Interactions
Decreased effect/levels of lithium, chlorpropamide, salicylates due to urinary alkalinization
Increased toxicity/levels of amphetamines, ephedrine, pseudoephedrine, flecainide, quinidine, quinine due to urinary alkalinization

Stability Store injection at room temperature; protect from heat and from freezing; use only clear solutions; incompatible with acids, acidic salts, alkaloid salts, calcium salts, catecholamines, atropine

Mechanism of Action Dissociates to provide bicarbonate ion which neutralizes hydrogen ion concentration and raises blood and urinary pH

Pharmacodynamics
Oral:
Onset of action: Rapid
Duration: of 8-10 minutes

I.V.:
Onset of action: 15 minutes
Duration: 1-2 hours

Pharmacokinetics
Absorption: Oral: Well absorbed
Elimination: Reabsorbed by kidney and <1% excreted by urine

Usual Dosage Geriatrics and Adults:
Cardiac arrest: See Precautions. Patient should be adequately ventilated before administering NaHCO$_3$
HCO$_3$-(mEq) = 0.3 x weight (kg) x base deficit (mEq/L); **routine use of NaHCO$_3$ is not recommended and should be given only after adequate alveolar ventilation has been established and effective cardiac compressions are provided**
I.V.: Initial: 1 mEq/kg/dose one time; maintenance: 0.5 mEq/kg/dose every 10 minutes or as indicated by arterial blood gases

Metabolic acidosis: I.V.: 2-5 mEq/kg/dose over 4-8 hours infusion or calculate dose based on base deficit (re-evaluate acid-base status) mEq NaHCO$_3$ = 0.3 x body weight (kg) x base deficit (mEq/L); give up to 1 mEq/kg/dose over several minutes or dilute larger doses in maintenance fluids for slow infusion; re-evaluate acid-base status frequently
Maximum daily dose: 200 mEq in adults <60 years and 100 mEq in adults >60 years
Maintenance electrolyte requirements of sodium: Daily requirements: 3-4 mEq/kg/24 hours or 25-40 mEq/1000 kcal/24 hours

Chronic renal failure: Oral: Initiate when plasma HCO$_3$ <15 mEq/L; start with 20-36 mEq/day in divided doses, titrate to bicarbonate level of 18-20 mEq/L

Reference Range Therapeutic (sodium): 135-145 mmol/L (SI: 135-145 mmol/L)

Patient Information Avoid chronic use as an antacid (<2 weeks)

Nursing Implications Advise patient of milk-alkali syndrome if use is long-term; observe for extravasation when giving I.V.

Additional Information May cause sodium retention especially if renal function is impaired; not to be used in treatment of peptic ulcer

Sodium content of injection 50 mL, 8.4%: 1150 mg (50 mEq); each 6 mg of NaHCO$_3$ contains 12 mEq sodium; 1 mEq NaHCO$_3$ = 84 mg; 1 mEq NaHCO$_3$ = 0.3 x body weight (kg) x base deficit (mEq/L)
Each 84 mg of sodium bicarbonate provides 1 mEq of sodium and bicarbonate ions; each gram of sodium bicarbonate provides 12 mEq of sodium and bicarbonate ions

(Continued)

Sodium Bicarbonate *(Continued)*

Special Geriatric Considerations Not the antacid of choice for the elderly because of sodium content and potential for systemic alkalosis

Dosage Forms
Injection: 4% (5 mL, 10 mL); 4.2% (1 mL, 5 mL, 10 mL); 5% (500 mL); 7.5% (50 mL); 8.4% (10 mL, 50 mL)
Powder: 120 g, 480 g
Tablet: 300 mg, 324 mg, 600 mg, 648 mg

Sodium Chloride

Brand Names Adsorbonac® [OTC] Ophthalmic; Ayr® [OTC]; HuMIST® [OTC]; Muro 128® Ophthalmic [OTC]; NaSal™ [OTC]; Ocean Nasal Mist [OTC]; Pretz® [OTC]; Saline® [OTC]; Slo-Salt® [OTC]

Synonyms NaCl; Normal Saline; Salt

Generic Available Yes

Therapeutic Class Electrolyte Supplement, Oral; Electrolyte Supplement, Parenteral; Lubricant, Ocular; Sodium Salt

Use Prevention of muscle cramps and heat prostration; restoration of sodium ion in hyponatremia; restore moisture to nasal membranes; GU irrigant; reduction of corneal edema; source of electrolytes and water for expansion of the extracellular fluid compartment

Contraindications Hypersensitivity to sodium chloride or any component; hypernatremia, fluid retention

Warnings Sodium toxicity is almost exclusively related to how fast a sodium deficit is corrected; both rate and magnitude are extremely important

Precautions Use with caution in patients with congestive heart failure, renal insufficiency, liver cirrhosis, hypertension

Adverse Reactions
Cardiovascular: Congestive conditions
Endocrine & metabolic: Extravasation, hypervolemia, hypernatremia, dilution of serum electrolytes, overhydration, hypokalemia
Local: Thrombosis, phlebitis, extravasation
Respiratory: Pulmonary edema

Overdosage Symptoms of overdose include nausea, vomiting, diarrhea, abdominal cramps, hypocalcemia, hypokalemia, hypernatremia

Toxicology Hypernatremia is resolved through the use of diuretics and free water replacement

Drug Interactions Decreased levels of lithium

Stability Store injection at room temperature; protect from heat and from freezing; use only clear solutions

Mechanism of Action Principal extracellular cation; functions in fluid and electrolyte balance, osmotic pressure control and water distribution

Pharmacokinetics
Absorption: Oral, I.V.: Rapid
Distribution: Widely distributed
Elimination: Mainly in urine but also in sweat, tears, and saliva

Usual Dosage Geriatrics and Adults:
Heat cramps: Oral: 0.5-1 g with full glass of water, up to 4.8 g/day

Replacement: Determined by laboratory determinations

Nasal: Use as often as needed

Ophthalmic:
Ointment: Apply once daily or more often
Solution: 1-2 drops in affected eye(s) every 3-4 hours

To correct acute, serious hyponatremia: mEq sodium = (desired sodium (mEq/L) - actual sodium (mEq/L) x 0.6 x wt (kg)); for acute correction use 125 mEq/L as the desired serum sodium; acutely correct serum sodium in 5 mEq/L/dose increments; more gradual correction in increments of 10 mEq/L/day is indicated in the asymptomatic patient

Monitoring Parameters I & O, weight, presence or worsening of rales and degree of peripheral edema with infusions, electrolyte levels

Reference Range Serum/plasma levels: 135-145 mEq/L

Patient Information Blurred vision is common with ophthalmic ointment; may sting eyes when first applied

Nursing Implications I.V. infusion of 3% or 5% sodium chloride should not exceed 100 mL/hour and should be administered via a central line only

Special Geriatric Considerations See Contraindications and Precautions

Dosage Forms
Injection: 0.45% (500 mL, 1000 mL); 0.9% (10 mL, 20 mL, 50 mL, 100 mL, 150 mL, 250 mL, 500 mL, 1000 mL); 3% (500 mL); 5% (500 mL); 20% (250 mL); 23.4% (30 mL, 100 mL)

Injection:
   Admixtures: 50 mEq, 100 mEq, 625 mEq
   Bacteriostatic: 0.9% (30 mL)
Ointment, ophthalmic: 5% (3.5 g)
Solution:
   Irrigation: 0.45% (500 mL, 1000 mL, 1500 mL); 0.9% (150 mL, 250 mL, 500 mL, 1000 mL, 1500 mL, 2000 mL, 4000 mL)
   Ophthalmic: 2% (15 mL); 5% (15 mL, 30 mL)
Tablet: 650 mg, 1 g, 2.25 g
Tablet:
   Enteric coated: 1 g
   Slow release: 600 mg

Sodium Citrate and Citric Acid

Brand Names Bicitra®; Oracit®

Synonyms Modified Shohl's Solution

Therapeutic Class Alkalinizing Agent, Oral

Use Treatment of metabolic acidosis; alkalinizing agent in conditions where long-term maintenance of an alkaline urine is desirable

Contraindications Severe renal insufficiency, sodium-restricted diet

Warnings Conversion to bicarbonate may be impaired in patients with hepatic failure or in shock

Precautions Use with caution in patients with congestive heart failure, hypertension, pulmonary edema; severe renal impairment

Adverse Reactions
  Endocrine & metabolic: Metabolic alkalosis, hyperkalemia
  Gastrointestinal: Diarrhea, nausea, vomiting, laxative effect
  Genitourinary: Urolithiasis
  Neuromuscular & skeletal: Tetany

Overdosage Symptoms of overdose include diarrhea, nausea, vomiting, excessive mental activity

Drug Interactions Other alkylating agents; acts as a urinary alkalinizer which may increase urinary excretion and decrease serum levels of chlorpropamide, lithium, methenamine, methotrexate, salicylates, tetracyclines; the converse is true (decreased urinary excretion, increased serum levels) for flecainide, mecamylamine, quinidine, and sympathomimetics

Usual Dosage Geriatrics and Adults: Oral: 15-30 mL with water after meals and at bedtime

Monitoring Parameters Blood gas for pH and bicarbonate; serum bicarbonate

Patient Information Palatability is improved by chilling solution, dilute each dose with 1-3 oz of water and follow with additional water (will also minimize laxative effect); take after meals to prevent saline laxative effect

Nursing Implications May be ordered as modified Shohl's solution; dilute with 30-90 mL of chilled water to enhance taste; 1 mL Bicitra® contains 1 mEq sodium and bicarbonate; take after meals

Additional Information 1 mL of Bicitra® contains 1 mEq of sodium and is metabolized to form the equivalent of 1 mEq of bicarbonate/mL

Special Geriatric Considerations See Precautions, Usual Dosage, and Additional Information

Dosage Forms Solution, oral: Sodium citrate 500 mg and citric acid 334 mg per 5 mL (15 mL 30 mL, 120 mL, 473 mL, 4000 mL)

Sodium Citrate and Potassium Citrate Mixture

Brand Names Polycitra®

Therapeutic Class Alkalinizing Agent, Oral

Use Conditions where long-term maintenance of an alkaline urine is desirable as in control and dissolution of uric acid and cystine calculi of the urinary tract

Contraindications Oliguria, azotemia, untreated Addison's disease

Warnings Citrate is converted to bicarbonate in the liver; this conversion may be blocked in patients who are severely ill, in shock, or in hepatic failure

Precautions Use caution in patients with congestive heart failure, hypertension, edema or any condition sensitive to sodium or potassium intake

Adverse Reactions
  Cardiovascular: Cardiac abnormalities
  Endocrine & metabolic: Metabolic alkalosis, calcium levels, hyperkalemia, hypernatremia
  Gastrointestinal: Diarrhea
  Neuromuscular & skeletal: Tetany

Toxicology Treat hyperkalemia

Drug Interactions Potassium-sparing diuretics; will alkalinize the urine which may increase the urinary excretion and decrease serum levels of chlorpropamide, lithium, methenamine, methotrexate, salicylate, tetracycline; the converse is true (decreased

(Continued)

Sodium Citrate and Potassium Citrate Mixture (Continued)

urinary excretion, increased serum levels) for flecainide, mecamylamine, quinidine, and sympathomimetics

Usual Dosage Geriatrics and Adults: Oral: 15-30 mL diluted in water after meals and at bedtime

Monitoring Parameters Blood gas (pH and bicarbonate); serum bicarbonate

Patient Information Palatability is improved by chilling solution, dilute each dose with 1-3 oz of water and follow with additional water; take after meals to prevent saline laxative effect

Nursing Implications Dilute each dose in 30-90 mL of water prior to administration; give after meals to prevent laxative effect

Special Geriatric Considerations See Precautions, Adverse Reactions, and Usual Dosage

Dosage Forms Syrup: Potassium citrate 550 mg, sodium citrate 500 mg, citric acid 334 mg/5 mL (1 mEq sodium, 1 mEq potassium, 2 mEq bicarbonate/mL)

Sodium Etidronate see Etidronate Disodium on page 276

Sodium Fluoride see Fluoride on page 299

Sodium Hydrogen Carbonate see Sodium Bicarbonate on page 646

Sodium L-Tri-iodothyronine see Liothyronine Sodium on page 408

Sodium Methicillin see Methicillin Sodium on page 453

Sodium Nafcillin see Nafcillin Sodium on page 487

Sodium Nitroferricyanide see Nitroprusside Sodium on page 507

Sodium Nitroprusside see Nitroprusside Sodium on page 507

Sodium Phosphate and Potassium Phosphate see Potassium Phosphate and Sodium Phosphate on page 580

Sodium Polystyrene Sulfonate (pol ee stye' reen)

Related Information
  Antacid Drug Interactions on page 764
Brand Names Kayexalate®; SPS®
Synonyms SPS
Generic Available Yes
Therapeutic Class Antidote, Hyperkalemia; Antidote, Potassium
Use Treatment of hyperkalemia
Contraindications Hypernatremia
Warnings Enema may be prepared with powder and diluted with sorbitol 10% solution or oral solution with 25% sorbitol solution. Enema will reduce the serum potassium faster than oral administration, but the oral route will result in a greater reduction over several hours. In severe hyperkalemia, consider treatment concomitantly with I.V. calcium, sodium bicarbonate, or glucose and insulin; hypokalemia may be precipitated by this agent. Measure serum potassium frequently; loss of magnesium and calcium occurs with polystyrene sulfonate

Precautions Use with caution in patients with severe congestive heart failure, hypertension, or edema

Adverse Reactions
  Endocrine & metabolic: Hypokalemia, hypocalcemia, hypomagnesemia, sodium retention
  Gastrointestinal: Anorexia, nausea, vomiting, constipation, intestinal necrosis, gastric irritation, occasionally diarrhea

Overdosage Symptoms of overdose include hypokalemia including cardiac dysrhythmias, confusion, irritability, EKG changes, muscle weakness; irritable confusion may be first sign of hypokalemia

Drug Interactions Cation-donating antacids (eg, magnesium, calcium, aluminum) and saline cathartics should be avoided

Stability Store prepared suspensions at 15°C to 30°C (59°F to 86°F); store repackaged product in refrigerator and use within 14 days; freshly prepared suspensions should be used within 24 hours; do not heat resin suspension

Mechanism of Action Removes potassium by exchanging sodium ions for potassium ions in the intestine before the resin is passed from the body

Pharmacodynamics
  Onset of action: Within 2-12 hours
  Exchange capacity is ~1 mEq/g in vivo; in vitro capacity is 3.1 mEq/g; therefore, a wide range of exchange capacity exists such that close monitoring of serum electrolytes is necessary

Pharmacokinetics Remains in the GI tract to be completely excreted in the feces (primarily as potassium polystyrene sulfonate)

Usual Dosage Geriatrics and Adults:
  Oral: 15 g 1-4 times/day

Powder formula: Prepare suspension in a ratio of liquid vehicle to powder of 3-4 mL/g of resin; water, syrup, or sorbitol may be used; sorbitol helps prevent constipation
Rectal: 30-50 g every 6 hours; retention time 30 minutes minimum

Monitoring Parameters Monitor serum electrolytes (potassium, sodium) frequently/ 24 hours; occasional serum calcium and magnesium is recommended; monitor for constipation and bowel obstruction; EKG monitoring for hypokalemia

Nursing Implications Administer oral (or NG) as ~25% sorbitol solution, never mix in orange juice; enema route is less effective than oral administration; retain enema in colon for at least 30-60 minutes and for several hours, if possible

Additional Information 1 gram of resin binds ~1 mEq of potassium; chilling the oral mixture will increase palatability
Sodium content of 1 g: 31 mg (1.3 mEq)

Special Geriatric Considerations Large doses in elderly may cause fecal impaction and intestinal obstruction; best to administer using sorbitol 70% as vehicle

Dosage Forms
Powder for suspension, oral or rectal: 454 g
Suspension, oral or rectal: 1.25 g/5 mL (60 mL, 120 mL, 200 mL, 480 mL, 500 mL)

Sodium Salicylate see Salicylates (Various Salts) on page 633

Sodium Sulamyd® see Sodium Sulfacetamide on this page

Sodium Sulfacetamide (sul fa see' ta mide)

Brand Names AK-Sulf®; Bleph®-10; Cetamide®; Isopid®; I-Sulfacet®; Sodium Sulamyd®; Sulfair®

Synonyms Sulfacetamide Sodium

Generic Available Yes

Therapeutic Class Antibiotic, Ophthalmic

Use Treatment and prophylaxis of conjunctivitis due to susceptible organisms; corneal ulcers; adjunctive treatment with systemic sulfonamides for therapy of trachoma

Contraindications Hypersensitivity to sulfacetamide or any component, sulfonamides

Warnings Inactivated by purulent exudates containing PABA; use with caution in patients with severe dry eye; ointment may retard corneal wound healing

Precautions Inactivated by purulent exudates containing PABA; use with caution in severe dry eye; ointment may retard corneal epithelial healing; sulfite in some products may cause hypersensitivity reactions

Adverse Reactions
Central nervous system: Headache, brow ache
Dermatologic: Stevens-Johnson syndrome, exfoliative dermatitis, toxic epidermal necrolysis
Local: Irritation, stinging, burning
Ocular: Blurred vision
Miscellaneous: Hypersensitivity reactions

Drug Interactions Silver, gentamicin (antagonism)

Stability Protect from light; discolored solution should not be used; incompatible with silver and zinc sulfate; sulfacetamide is inactivated by blood or purulent exudates

Mechanism of Action Interferes with bacterial growth by inhibiting bacterial folic acid synthesis through competitive antagonism of PABA

Pharmacokinetics Unknown

Usual Dosage Geriatrics and Adults: Ophthalmic:
Ointment: Apply to lower conjunctival sac 1-4 times/day and at bedtime
Solution: Instill 1-2 drops every 2-3 hours in the lower conjunctival sac during the waking hours and less frequently at night

Monitoring Parameters Response to therapy

Patient Information Eye drops will burn upon instillation; wait at least 10 minutes before using another eye preparation; ointment may sting eyes when first applied and blur vision; do not touch dropper to eye to maintain sterility

Nursing Implications Eye drops will burn upon instillation (especially 30% solution); wait at least 10 minutes before administering another eye preparation

Special Geriatric Considerations Assess whether patient can adequately instill drops or ointment

Dosage Forms Ophthalmic:
Ointment: 10% (3.5 g)
Solution: 10% (1 mL, 2 mL, 3.75 mL, 5 mL, 15 mL); 15% (2 mL, 15 mL); 30% (5 mL, 15 mL)

Sodium Sulfacetamide and Phenylephrine

Related Information
Phenylephrine Hydrochloride on page 557
Sodium Sulfacetamide on this page

Brand Names Vasosulf®

Therapeutic Class Antibiotic, Ophthalmic; Ophthalmic Agent, Vasoconstrictor

(Continued)

ALPHABETICAL LISTING OF DRUGS

Sodium Sulfacetamide and Phenylephrine *(Continued)*

Stability Keep tightly closed; protect from light

Usual Dosage Geriatrics and Adults: Instill 1 or 2 drops into the lower conjunctival sac(s) every 2 or 3 hours during the day, less often at night

Dosage Forms Solution, ophthalmic: Sodium sulfacetamide 15% and phenylephrine hydrochloride 0.125% (5 mL, 15 mL)

Sodium Sulfacetamide and Prednisolone Acetate

Related Information

Prednisolone *on page 584*

Sodium Sulfacetamide *on previous page*

Brand Names Blephamide®; Cetapred®; Metimyd®; Vasocidin®

Therapeutic Class Antibiotic, Ophthalmic; Corticosteroid, Ophthalmic

Use Steroid-responsive inflammatory ocular conditions where infection is present or there is a risk of infection

Contraindications Mycobacteria infections, fungal infections, hypersensitivity to sulfacetamide, prednisolone or any component

Precautions Inactivated by purulent exudates containing PABA; use with caution in severe dry eyes; ointment may retard corneal epithelial healing; sulfite in some products may cause hypersensitivity reactions

Adverse Reactions

Central nervous system: Vertigo, headache

Dermatologic: Stevens-Johnson syndrome, skin atrophy

Endocrine & metabolic: Cushing's syndrome, pituitary-adrenal axis suppression

Local: Irritation, stinging, burning

Ocular: Cataracts, glaucoma

Drug Interactions Silver, gentamicin, vaccines, toxoids

Usual Dosage Geriatrics and Adults:

Ointment: Apply to lower conjunctival sac 1-4 times/day

Solution: 1-3 drops every 2-3 hours

Patient Information Shake ophthalmic solution before using; eye drops will burn upon instillation; wait at least 10 minutes before using another eye preparation; ointment may sting eyes when first applied and blur vision; do not touch dropper to eye

Nursing Implications Shake ophthalmic suspension before using

Additional Information The ophthalmic suspension may be used as an otic preparation

Special Geriatric Considerations Assess whether patient can adequately instill drops or ointment

Dosage Forms Ophthalmic:

Ointment:

Blephamide®: Sodium sulfacetamide 10% and prednisolone acetate 0.2% (3.5 g)

Cetapred®: Sodium sulfacetamide 10% and prednisolone acetate 0.25% (3.5 g)

Metimyd®: Sodium sulfacetamide 10% and prednisolone acetate 0.5% (3.5 g)

Suspension:

Blephamide®: Sodium sulfacetamide 10% and prednisolone acetate 0.2% (2.5 mL, 5 mL, 10 mL)

Isopto® Cetapred®: Sodium sulfacetamide 10% and prednisolone acetate 0.25% (5 mL, 15 mL)

Optimyd®: Sodium sulfacetamide 10% and prednisolone sodium phosphate 0.5% (5 mL)

Vasocidin®: Sodium sulfacetamide 10% and prednisolone acetate 0.25% (5 mL, 10 mL)

Sodium Thiosalicylate *see* Salicylates (Various Salts) *on page 633*

Sodol® *see* Carisoprodol *on page 121*

Sofarin® *see* Warfarin Sodium *on page 739*

Solfoton® *see* Phenobarbital *on page 554*

Solganal® *see* Aurothioglucose *on page 68*

Solu-Cortef® *see* Hydrocortisone *on page 351*

Solu-Medrol® *see* Methylprednisolone *on page 461*

Solurex L.A.® *see* Dexamethasone *on page 207*

Soma® *see* Carisoprodol *on page 121*

Soma® Compound *see* Carisoprodol *on page 121*

Sominex® [OTC] *see* Diphenhydramine Hydrochloride *on page 228*

Somnos® *see* Chloral Hydrate *on page 146*

Somophyllin® *see* Aminophylline *on page 39*

Somophyllin®-CRT *see* Theophylline *on page 681*

Somophyllin®-DF *see* Aminophylline *on page 39*

Somophyllin®-T *see* Theophylline *on page 681*

Soothe® [OTC] *see* Tetrahydrozoline Hydrochloride *on page 680*

Soprodol® *see* Carisoprodol *on page 121*

Sorbitol (sor' bi tole)

Generic Available Yes

Therapeutic Class Genitourinary Irrigant

Use Genitourinary irrigant in transurethral prostatic resection or other transurethral resection or other transurethral surgical procedures; diuretic; humectant; sweetening agent; hyperosmotic laxative; facilitate the passage of sodium polystyrene sulfonate through the intestinal tract

Contraindications Anuria

Warnings When used for TURP irrigation, large volumes of fluid may enter systemic circulation. The osmotic diuresis it may induce can affect renal, pulmonary, and cardiac status. Use in diabetics may cause hyperglycemia when absorbed systemically from urethral irrigation.

Precautions Systemic absorption may cause a shift of intracellular fluid to the extracellular space, thus causing or aggravating existing hyponatremia. Systemic absorption may cause significant diuresis to cause or aggravate existing hypovolemia and dehydration.

Adverse Reactions

I.V. infusion:
Cardiovascular: Edema, hypotension, tachycardia, angina, thrombophlebitis
Central nervous system: Seizures, vertigo, chills
Dermatologic: Urticaria
Endocrine & metabolic: Acidosis, electrolyte loss, dehydration
Gastrointestinal: Dry mouth, thirst, nausea, vomiting, diarrhea
Genitourinary: Urinary retention, marked diuresis
Ocular: Blurred vision

Oral:
Cardiovascular: Hypotension
Endocrine & metabolic: Dehydration, fluid and electrolyte loss
Gastrointestinal: Diarrhea, flatulence, abdominal cramps, unpleasant sweet taste for some patients

Overdosage Symptoms of overdose include diarrhea, hypotension, dehydration, lethargy

Stability Protect from freezing; avoid storage in temperatures >150°F

Mechanism of Action A polyalcoholic sugar (monosaccharide) with osmotic cathartic actions

Pharmacodynamics Onset of action: ~15-60 minutes

Pharmacokinetics
Absorption: Oral, rectal: Poor
Metabolism: Mainly in the liver to carbon dioxide (70%) and dextrose (30%)
Elimination: In kidneys

Usual Dosage Hyperosmotic laxative (as single dose, at infrequent intervals): Geriatrics and Adults:
Oral: 30-150 mL (as 70% solution)
Rectal enema: 120 mL as 25% to 30% solution

Adjunct to sodium polystyrene sulfonate: 15 mL as 70% solution orally until diarrhea occurs (10-20 mL/2 hours) or 20-100 mL as an oral vehicle for the sodium polystyrene sulfonate resin

When administered with charcoal: Oral: 4.3 mL/kg of 70% sorbitol with 1 g/kg of activated charcoal

Monitoring Parameters Blood pressure, serum electrolytes, number of stools per day; when used as an irrigant in TURP, see Warnings and Precautions

Patient Information Take with a full glass of water. When used as a cathartic, report failure of laxative effect, dizziness, weakness, and dehydration to physician, pharmacist, or nurse. Contact physician if more than 3-5 stools per day are produced.

Nursing Implications Do not use unless solution is clear; see Monitoring Parameters

Special Geriatric Considerations Causes for constipation must be evaluated prior to initiating treatment. Nonpharmacological dietary treatment should be initiated before laxative use. Sorbitol is as effective as lactulose but is much less expensive.

Dosage Forms Solution: 3% (1500 mL, 3000 mL); 3.3% (2000 mL)

References
Lederle FA, Busch DL, Mattox KM, et al, "Cost-Effective Treatment of Constipation in the Elderly: A Randomized Double-Blend Comparison of Sorbitol and Lactulose," *Am J Med*, 1990, 89(5):597-601.

Sorbitrate® *see* Isosorbide Dinitrate *on page 382*

Soridol® *see* Carisoprodol *on page 121*

Sotalol Hydrochloride (soe' ta lole)
Related Information
Beta-Blockers Comparison *on page 804-805*
Brand Names Betapace®
Therapeutic Class Antiarrhythmic Agent, Class II; Antiarrhythmic Agent, Class III
Use Treatment of ventricular arrhythmias, prevention of life-threatening arrhythmias, and sudden death postmyocardial infarction

Contraindications Uncompensated congestive heart failure, cardiogenic shock, bradycardia or heart block, pulmonary edema, asthma

Warnings Use with caution in patients with congestive heart failure, peripheral vascular disease, hypokalemia, hypomagnesemia, renal dysfunction, sick sinus syndrome; abrupt withdrawal may result in return of life-threatening arrhythmias; sotalol can provoke new or worsening ventricular arrhythmias

Adverse Reactions
Cardiovascular: Hypotension (especially with higher doses), bradycardia, Raynaud's phenomena

Central nervous system: Dizziness, somnolence, confusion, lethargy, depression, headache

Gastrointestinal: Nausea, vomiting

Local: Skin necrosis after extravasation, phlebitis

Miscellaneous: Cold extremities, diaphoresis

Overdosage Symptoms of overdose include severe hypotension, bradycardia, heart failure and bronchospasm, hypoglycemia

Toxicology Sympathomimetics (eg, epinephrine or dopamine), glucagon or a pacemaker can be used to treat the toxic bradycardia, asystole, and/or hypotension. Initially, fluids may be the best treatment for toxic hypotension. Following GI decontamination, treatment is supportive. Lidocaine should be used for torsade de pointes or other ventricular arrhythmias; magnesium may be helpful; may require isoproterenol or cardioversion.

Drug Interactions Decreased effect/levels with coadministration of aluminum and/or magnesium-containing antacids

Mechanism of Action Has both beta$_1$- and beta$_2$-receptor blocking activity; also passes some type III antiarrhythmic activity

Pharmacokinetics
Onset of action: Rapid, 1-2 hours

Peak effect: 3-4 hours

Absorption: Decreased 20% to 30% by meals

Distribution: Low lipid solubility

Protein binding: Not protein bound

Bioavailability: 90% to 100%

Half-life: 12 hours

Elimination: Unchanged through kidney

Usual Dosage Geriatrics and Adults: Oral: Initial: 80 mg twice daily; may be increased to 240-320 mg/day and up to 480-640 mg/day in patients with life-threatening refractory ventricular arrhythmias; adjust dose every 2-3 days; due to half-life twice daily dosing is all that is necessary; see Additional Information

Dosing adjustment in renal impairment:
Cl_{cr} >60 mL/minute: Administer every 12 hours
Cl_{cr} 30-60 mL/minute: Administer every 24 hours
Cl_{cr} 10-30 mL/minute: Administer every 36-48 hours
Cl_{cr} <10 mL/minute: Individualize dose

Monitoring Parameters Serum magnesium, potassium, EKG, pulse

Patient Information Seek emergency help if palpitations occur; do not discontinue abruptly or change dose without notifying physician; take on an empty stomach

Nursing Implications Initiation of therapy and dose escalation should be done in a hospital with cardiac monitoring; lidocaine and other resuscitative measures should be available

Additional Information If patients are receiving another antiarrhythmic, must generally withdraw agent, with careful monitoring, for at least 2-3 half-lives of the previous agent if clinical condition allows; treatment with sotalol has been initiated in some with patients receiving I.V. lidocaine without problems; if patients are receiving amiodarone, **do not** start sotalol until Q-T interval is normal

Special Geriatric Considerations Since elderly frequently have Cl_{cr} <60 mL/minute, attention to dose, creatinine clearance, and monitoring is important; make dosage adjustments at 3-day intervals or after 5-6 doses at any dosage

Dosage Forms Tablet: 80 mg, 160 mg, 240 mg

Sparine® *see* Promazine Hydrochloride *on page 597*

Spasmolin *see* Hyoscyamine, Atropine, Scopolamine and Phenobarbital *on page 357*

Spasquid® see Hyoscyamine, Atropine, Scopolamine and Phenobarbital
   on page 357

Spectrobid® see Bacampicillin Hydrochloride on page 73

Spectro-Chlor® see Chloramphenicol on page 148

Spironolactone (speer on oh lak' tone)

Brand Names Aldactone®

Generic Available Yes

Therapeutic Class Diuretic, Potassium Sparing

Use Management of edema associated with excessive aldosterone excretion; hypertension; primary hyperaldosteronism; hypokalemia; cirrhosis of the liver accompanied by edema or ascites

Unlabeled use: Treatment of hirsutism

Contraindications Renal insufficiency, hypersensitivity to spironolactone or any component, hyperkalemia, patients receiving other potassium-sparing diuretics or potassium supplements

Warnings Spironolactone has been shown to be tumorigenic in toxicity studies using rats at 25-250 times the usual human dose

Precautions Use with caution in patients with dehydration, hepatic disease, hyponatremia; potassium excretion may be decreased in the elderly, increasing the risk of hyperkalemia with the use of spironolactone

Adverse Reactions

Central nervous system: Lethargy, headache, confusion, ataxia

Dermatologic: Rash

Endocrine & metabolic: Hyperkalemia, dehydration, hyponatremia, gynecomastia, hyperchloremic metabolic acidosis, postmenopausal bleeding

Gastrointestinal: Anorexia, nausea, vomiting, diarrhea, cramping, gastric bleeding, ulceration, gastritis

Genitourinary: Inability to achieve or maintain an erection

Overdosage Symptoms of overdose include drowsiness, confusion, clinical signs of dehydration, and electrolyte imbalance

Toxicology Ingestion of large amounts of potassium-sparing diuretics, may result in life-threatening hyperkalemia. This can be treated with I.V. glucose (dextrose 25% in water), with concurrent I.V. sodium bicarbonate (1 mEq/kg up to 44 mEq/dose). If needed, Kayexalate® oral or rectal solutions in sorbitol may also be used.

Drug Interactions Increased serum potassium levels with potassium, potassium-sparing diuretics, indomethacin, angiotensin-converting enzymes inhibitors

Food/Drug Interactions Administration of spironolactone with food increases its absorption

Stability Protect from light

Mechanism of Action Competes with aldosterone for receptor sites in the distal renal tubules, increasing sodium, chloride and water excretion while conserving potassium and hydrogen ions; may block the effect of aldosterone on arteriolar smooth muscle as well

Pharmacokinetics

Protein binding: 91% to 98%

Metabolism: In the liver to multiple metabolites, including canrenone (active)

Half-life: 78-84 minutes

Time to peak: Oral: Peak serum levels occur within 1-3 hours (primarily as the active metabolite)

Elimination: Urinary and biliary

In the elderly, levels of the metabolites were found to be twice as high as in younger patients

Usual Dosage Oral:

Geriatrics: Initial: 25-50 mg/day in 1-2 divided doses increasing by 25-50 mg every 5 days as needed

Adults:

Edema, hypertension, hypokalemia: 25-200 mg/day in 1-2 divided doses

Diagnosis of primary aldosteronism: 100-400 mg/day in 1-2 divided doses

Monitoring Parameters Blood pressure, serum electrolytes, renal function, weight, I & O

Test Interactions May cause false elevation in serum digoxin concentrations measured by RIA

Patient Information Avoid hazardous activity such as driving, until response to drug is known (may cause lethargy or confusion); take with meals or milk; avoid excessive ingestion of foods high in potassium or use of salt substitutes. Take in the morning; take the last dose of multiple doses no later than 6 PM unless instructed otherwise.

Nursing Implications Diuretic effect may be delayed 2-3 days and maximum hypertensive may be delayed 2-3 weeks

Additional Information To reduce delay in onset of effect, a loading dose of 2 or 3 times the daily dose may be administered on the first day of therapy; it is recommend-

(Continued)

Spironolactone *(Continued)*

ed the drug be discontinued several days prior to adrenal vein catheterization; adverse reactions are dose related and usually disappear upon drug withdrawal, except possibly gynecomastia

Special Geriatric Considerations See Precautions and Pharmacokinetics; monitor serum potassium

Dosage Forms Tablet: 25 mg, 50 mg, 100 mg

Spironolactone and Hydrochlorothiazide *see* Hydrochlorothiazide and Spironolactone *on page 348*

Sporanox® Oral *see* Itraconazole *on page 386*

SPS *see* Sodium Polystyrene Sulfonate *on page 650*

SPS® *see* Sodium Polystyrene Sulfonate *on page 650*

S-P-T *see* Thyroid *on page 691*

Stadol® *see* Butorphanol Tartrate *on page 101*

Stadol® NS *see* Butorphanol Tartrate *on page 101*

Stannous Fluoride *see* Fluoride *on page 299*

Staphcillin® *see* Methicillin Sodium *on page 453*

Staticin® *see* Erythromycin, Topical *on page 266*

Stay Trim® Diet Gum [OTC] *see* Phenylpropanolamine Hydrochloride *on page 559*

Stelazine® *see* Trifluoperazine Hydrochloride *on page 714*

Stemetic® *see* Trimethobenzamide Hydrochloride *on page 720*

Sterapred® *see* Prednisone *on page 586*

Stilbestrol *see* Diethylstilbestrol *on page 217*

Stilphostrol® *see* Diethylstilbestrol *on page 217*

Stimate™ *see* Desmopressin Acetate *on page 206*

St. Joseph® Measured Dose Nasal Solution [OTC] *see* Phenylephrine Hydrochloride *on page 557*

Streptase® *see* Streptokinase *on this page*

Streptokinase *(strep toe kye' nase)*

Brand Names Kabikinase®; Streptase®

Therapeutic Class Thrombolytic Agent

Use Thrombolytic agent used in treatment of recent severe or massive deep vein thrombosis, pulmonary emboli, myocardial infarction, and occluded arteriovenous cannulas

Contraindications Hypersensitivity to streptokinase or any component; recent strep infection; active internal bleeding, recent CVA (within 2 months), or intracranial or intraspinal surgery, major surgery within the last 10 days, GI bleeding, recent trauma severe hypertension

Warnings Avoid I.M. injections

Adverse Reactions
Cardiovascular: Hypotension, arrhythmias, noncardiac pulmonary edema, flushing
Central nervous system: Fever
Dermatologic: Itching, urticaria, angionecrotic edema
Hematologic: Surface bleeding, internal bleeding, cerebral hemorrhage
Neuromuscular & skeletal: Musculoskeletal pain
Respiratory: Bronchospasm

Overdosage Symptoms of overdose include epistaxis, bleeding gums, hematoma spontaneous ecchymoses, oozing at catheter site

Drug Interactions Increased effect of anticoagulants (discontinue heparin before giving streptokinase), and antiplatelet agents; decreased effect with antifibrinolytic agents (aminocaproic acid)

Stability Keep in refrigerator, use reconstituted solutions within 24 hours; store unopened vials at room temperature

Mechanism of Action Activates the conversion of plasminogen to plasmin by forming a complex exposing plasminogen-activating site and clearing a peptide bond that converts plasminogen to plasmin; plasmin being capable of thrombolysis, by degrading fibrin, fibrinogen and other procoagulant proteins into soluble fragments; effective both outside and within the formed thrombus/embolus

Pharmacodynamics
Onset of effect: Following injection, activation of plasminogen occurs almost immediately
Duration: Fibrinolytic effects last only a few hours, while anticoagulant effects can persist for 12-24 hours

Pharmacokinetics
Half-life: 83 minutes
Elimination: By circulating antibodies and via the reticuloendothelial system

Usual Dosage Geriatrics and Adults: I.V. (best results are realized if used within 5-6 hours of myocardial infarction; antibodies to streptokinase remain for 3-6 months after initial dose; use another thrombolytic enzyme (ie, urokinase), if thrombolytic therapy is indicated):

Guidelines for acute myocardial infarction (AMI):
1.5 million units infused over 60 minutes. Monitor for the first few hours for signs of anaphylaxis or allergic reaction. **Infusion should be slowed if blood pressure is lowered by 25 mm Hg or if asthmatic symptoms appear.** Begin heparin 5000-10,000 unit bolus followed by 1000 units/hour approximately 3-4 hours after completion of streptokinase infusion or when PTT is <100 seconds.

Guidelines for acute pulmonary embolism (APE):
3 million unit dose; administer 250,000 units over 30 minutes followed by 100,000 units/hour for 24 hours. Monitor for the first few hours for signs of anaphylaxis or allergic reaction. **Infusion should be slowed if blood pressure is lowered by 25 mm Hg or if asthmatic symptoms appear**. Begin heparin 1000 units/hour approximately 3-4 hours after completion of streptokinase infusion or when PTT is <100 seconds.

Thromboses: 250,000 units to start, then 100,000 units/hour for 24-72 hours depending on location

Cannula occlusion: 250,000 units into cannula, clamp for 2 hours, then aspirate contents and flush with normal saline

Monitoring Parameters Before therapy, hematocrit, platelet count, PT, APTT, thrombin time (TT), fibrinogen concentration; check PT, APTT, TT, or fibrinogen level every 4 hours after starting therapy

Test Interactions I.V. and intracoronary administration will increase thrombin time, APTT, PT, and decrease fibrinogen and plasminogen levels

Nursing Implications For I.V. or intracoronary use only; monitor for bleeding every 15 minutes for the first hour of therapy; avoid I.M. injections

Special Geriatric Considerations Investigators applied analysis to data for patients ≥75 years of age from two large trials studying the impact of streptokinase on patient outcome after acute myocardial infarction; their conclusion was that age alone is not a contraindication to the use of streptokinase and that thrombolytic therapy is cost-effective and is beneficial toward the survival of elderly patients. Additional studies are needed to determine if a weight-adjusted dose will maintain efficacy but decrease adverse events such as stroke

Dosage Forms Injection: 250,000 units (5 mL, 6.5 mL); 600,000 units (5 mL); 750,000 units (6 mL, 6.5 mL); 1,500,000 units (6.5 mL, 50 mL)

References
Krumholz HM, Pasternak RC, Weinstein MC, et al, "Cost Effectiveness of Thrombolytic Therapy With Streptokinase in Elderly Patients With Suspected Acute Myocardial Infarction," *N Engl J Med*, 1992, 327:7-13.

Streptomycin Sulfate (strep toe mye' sin)
Generic Available Yes

Therapeutic Class Antibiotic, Aminoglycoside; Antitubercular Agent

Use Combination therapy of active tuberculosis; used in combination with other agents for treatment of streptococcal or enterococcal endocarditis, mycobacterial infections, plague, tularemia, and brucellosis

Contraindications Hypersensitivity to streptomycin or any component

Warnings Aminoglycosides are associated with significant nephrotoxicity or ototoxicity; the ototoxicity is directly proportional to the amount of drug given and the duration of treatment; tinnitus or vertigo are indications of vestibular injury and impending bilateral irreversible damage; renal damage is usually reversible

Precautions Use with caution in patients with pre-existing vertigo, tinnitus, hearing loss, neuromuscular disorders, or renal impairment; modify dosage in patients with renal impairment

Adverse Reactions
Cardiovascular: Myocarditis, cardiovascular collapse
Central nervous system: Dizziness, vertigo, ataxia, neuromuscular blockade, headache
Dermatologic: Toxic epidermal necrolysis
Gastrointestinal: Vomiting
Otic: Ototoxicity
Renal: Nephrotoxicity
Miscellaneous: Serum sickness

Overdosage Symptoms of overdose include ototoxicity, nephrotoxicity, and neuromuscular toxicity

Toxicology The treatment of choice following a single acute overdose appears to be the maintenance of good urine output of at least 3 mL/kg/hour. Dialysis is of question-

(Continued)

Streptomycin Sulfate *(Continued)*

able value in the enhancement of aminoglycoside elimination. If required, hemodialysis is preferred over peritoneal dialysis in patients with normal renal function. Careful hydration may be all that is required to promote diuresis and therefore the enhancement of the drug's elimination.

Drug Interactions
Increased/prolonged effect: Depolarizing and nondepolarizing neuromuscular blocking agents
Increased toxicity: Concurrent use of amphotericin may increase nephrotoxicity

Stability Depending upon manufacturer reconstituted solution remains stable for 2-4 weeks when refrigerated; exposure to light causes darkening of solution without apparent loss of potency

Mechanism of Action Inhibits bacterial protein synthesis by binding directly to the 30S ribosomal subunits causing faulty peptide sequence to form in the protein chain

Pharmacodynamics Bactericidal at an alkaline pH

Pharmacokinetics
Protein binding: 34%; CNS penetration is fair
Half-life: 2-4.7 hours and is prolonged with renal impairment (up to 100 hours)
Time to peak: I.M.: Peak serum levels occur within 1 hour
Elimination: Almost completely (90%) as unchanged drug in urine, with small amounts (1%) excreted in bile, saliva, sweat, and tears

Usual Dosage
Geriatrics: 10 mg/kg/day not to exceed 750 mg/day; dosing interval should be adjusted for renal function; some authors suggest not to give more than 5 days/week or give as 20-25 mg/kg/dose twice weekly

Adults: I.M.:
Tuberculosis: 15 mg/kg/day in divided doses every 12 hours, not to exceed 2 g/day
Enterococcal endocarditis: 1 g every 12 hours for 2 weeks, 500 mg every 12 hours for 4 weeks in combination with penicillin
Streptococcal endocarditis: 1 g every 12 hours for 1 week, 500 mg every 12 hours for 1 week
Tularemia: 1-2 g/day in divided doses for 7-10 days or until patient is afebrile for 5-7 days
Plague: 2-4 g/day in divided doses until the patient is afebrile for at least 3 days

Monitoring Parameters BUN and serum creatinine, hearing (if appropriate); in tuberculosis patients, monitor sputum culture and chest x-ray 2-3 months into treatment and at its completion

Reference Range
Therapeutic: Peak: 20-30 μg/mL; trough: <5 μg/mL
Toxic: Peak: >50 μg/mL; trough: >10 μg/mL

Test Interactions False-positive urine glucose with Benedict's solution

Patient Information Report any unusual symptom

Nursing Implications Inject deep I.M. into large muscle mass; I.V. administration is not recommended. Modify dosage in patients with renal insufficiency.

Additional Information Eighth cranial nerve damage is usually preceded by high-pitched tinnitus, roaring noises, sense of fullness in ears, or impaired hearing and may persist for weeks after drug is discontinued

Special Geriatric Considerations Streptomycin is indicated for persons from endemic areas of drug-resistant *Mycobacterium tuberculosis* or who are HIV infected; since most older patients acquired the *M. tuberculosis* infection prior to the availability of effective chemotherapy, isoniazid and rifampin are usually effective unless resistant organisms are suspected or the patient is HIV infected

Dosage Forms
Injection: 400 mg/mL (12.5 mL)
Powder for injection: 1 g, 5 g

References
Bass JB Jr, Farer LS, Hopewell PC, et al, "Treatment of Tuberculosis and Tuberculosis Infection in Adults and Children," *Am J Respir Crit Care Med*, 1994, 149(5):1359-74.
Stead WW and Dutt AK, "Tuberculosis: A Special Problem in the Elderly," *Principles of Geriatric Medicine and Gerontology*, 2nd ed, 1990, 522.
Yoshikawa TT, "Tuberculosis in Aging Adults," *J Am Geriatr Soc*, 1992, 40(2):178-87.

Strifon® Forte DSC *see* Chlorzoxazone *on page 160*

Sublimaze® *see* Fentanyl *on page 284*

Sucralfate *(soo kral' fate)*
Brand Names Carafate®
Synonyms Aluminum Sucrose Sulfate, Basic
Generic Available No
Therapeutic Class Gastrointestinal Agent, Miscellaneous
Use Short-term management of duodenal ulcers

Unlabeled uses: Gastric ulcers; maintenance of duodenal ulcers; suspension may be used topically for treatment of stomatitis due to cancer chemotherapy and other causes of esophageal and gastric erosions; GERD, esophagitis, treatment of NSAID mucosal damage, prevention of stress ulcers

Contraindications Hypersensitivity to sucralfate or any component

Warnings Use caution with chronic renal failure, dialysis (aluminum accumulation)

Precautions Successful therapy with sucralfate should not be expected to alter the posthealing frequency of recurrence or the severity of duodenal ulceration

Adverse Reactions

Central nervous system: Dizziness, sleepiness, vertigo, headache

Dermatologic: Rash, pruritus

Gastrointestinal: Constipation, diarrhea, nausea, gastric discomfort, indigestion, dry mouth

Neuromuscular & skeletal: Back pain

Overdosage Risk appears minimal

Toxicology Deferoxamine, traditionally used as an iron chelator, has been shown to increase urinary aluminum output. Deferoxamine chelation of aluminum has resulted in improvements of clinical symptoms and bone histology. Deferoxamine, however, remains an experimental treatment for aluminum poisoning and has a significant potential for adverse effects.

Drug Interactions Cimetidine, digoxin, phenytoin (hydantoins), warfarin, ketoconazole, quinidine, ciprofloxacin, norfloxacin (quinolones), ranitidine, tetracycline, theophylline; because of the potential for sucralfate to alter the absorption of some drugs, separate administration (2 hours before or after) should be considered when alterations in bioavailability are believed to be critical; do not give antacids within 30 minutes of administration

Note: When given with aluminum-containing antacids, may increase serum/body aluminum concentrations; see Warnings

Mechanism of Action Forms a complex by binding with positively charged proteins in exudates, forming a viscous paste-like, adhesive substance, when combined with gastric acid adheres to the damaged mucosal area. This selectively forms a protective coating that protects the lining against peptic acid, pepsin, and bile salts.

Pharmacodynamics

Onset of paste formation and ulcer adhesion: within 1-2 hours

Duration of action: Up to 6 hours

Pharmacokinetics

Absorption: Oral: <5% of dose

Metabolism: Not metabolized

Protein binding: Unbound in GI tract to aluminum and sucrose octasulfate

Elimination: Small amounts that are absorbed are excreted in urine as unchanged compounds

Usual Dosage Geriatrics and Adults: Oral: 1 g 4 times/day, 1 hour before meals or food and at bedtime, or alternatively 2 g twice daily; adult treatment is recommended for 4-8 weeks; elderly will often require 12 weeks

Prophylaxis (maintenance): 1 g twice daily (tablets only)

Stomatitis: 2.5-5 mL, swish and spit or swish and swallow 4 times/day

Monitoring Parameters Monitor signs and symptoms of disease process and adverse effects; evaluate by endoscopic examination or x-ray

Patient Information Take 1 hour before meals or on an empty stomach; may allow tablet to disintegrate in ~1 oz of room temperature water and drink the resulting suspension, if unable to swallow tablets whole; do not take within 30 minutes of antacids (before or after)

Nursing Implications Monitor for constipation; give 2 hours before or after administration of other oral drugs; tablets may be disintegrated in water before administering

Additional Information May decrease gastric emptying; many trials have demonstrated sucralfate is equivalent in efficacy to antacids and H_2-blockers; equivalence of sucralfate suspension to sucralfate tablets has not been established in studies

Special Geriatric Considerations Caution should be used in elderly due to reduced renal function; patients with Cl_{cr} <30 mL/minute may be at risk for aluminum intoxication; due to low side effect profile, this may be an agent of choice in elderly with PUD

Dosage Forms

Suspension: 1 g/10 mL (420 mL)

Tablet: 1 g

Sudafed® 12 Hour [OTC] *see* Pseudoephedrine *on page 609*

Sudafed® [OTC] *see* Pseudoephedrine *on page 609*

Sudahist® [OTC] *see* Triprolidine and Pseudoephedrine *on page 723*

Sufedrin® [OTC] *see* Pseudoephedrine *on page 609*

Sulbactam and Ampicillin *see* Ampicillin Sodium and Sulbactam Sodium *on page 52*

Sulfacetamide Sodium *see* Sodium Sulfacetamide *on page 651*

ALPHABETICAL LISTING OF DRUGS

Sulfair® see Sodium Sulfacetamide *on page 651*

Sulfamethoprim® see Co-trimoxazole *on page 189*

Sulfamethoxazole (sul fa meth ox' a zole)

Brand Names Gantanol®

Generic Available Yes: Tablet

Therapeutic Class Antibiotic, Sulfonamide Derivative

Use Treatment of urinary tract infections, nocardiosis, toxoplasmosis, acute otitis media, and acute exacerbations of chronic bronchitis due to susceptible organisms

Contraindications Porphyria; known hypersensitivity to sulfa drug or any component

Warnings Should not be used for group A beta-hemolytic streptococcal infections

Precautions Maintain adequate fluid intake to prevent crystalluria; use with caution in patients with renal or hepatic impairment, and patients with G-6-PD deficiency

Adverse Reactions

Central nervous system: Dizziness, fever, headache

Dermatologic: Rash, exfoliative dermatitis, Stevens-Johnson syndrome, photosensitivity

Endocrine & metabolic: Folic acid deficiency (rare)

Gastrointestinal: Nausea, vomiting

Hematologic: Granulocytopenia, leukopenia, thrombocytopenia, aplastic anemia, hemolytic anemia

Hepatic: Jaundice

Renal: Acute nephropathy

Miscellaneous: Serum sickness-like reactions

Overdosage Symptoms of overdose include drowsiness, dizziness, anorexia, abdominal pain, nausea, vomiting, hemolytic anemia, acidosis, jaundice

Drug Interactions

Decreased effect with PABA or PABA metabolites of drugs (ie, procaine, proparacaine, tetracaine)

Increased effect of oral anticoagulants and oral hypoglycemic agents

Stability Protect from light

Mechanism of Action Interferes with bacterial growth by inhibiting bacterial folic acid synthesis through competitive antagonism of PABA

Pharmacokinetics

Absorption: Oral: 90%

Protein binding: 70%

Metabolism: Primarily in the liver, with 10% to 20% as the N-acetylated form in the plasma

Half-life: 9-12 hours, prolonged with renal impairment; in elderly, half-life has been reported to be increased while total and renal clearances are decreased

Time to peak: Peak serum levels occur within 3-4 hours

Elimination: Unchanged drug (20%) and its metabolites are excreted in urine

Usual Dosage Oral:

Geriatrics: Same as adults unless Cl_{cr} <30 mL/minute; see below. Single dose or 3-day dosing has not been shown to be reliable for treating urinary tract infections in the elderly

Adults: 2 g stat, 1 g 2-3 times/day; maximum: 3 g/24 hours

Dosing interval in renal impairment: Cl_{cr} <30 mL/minute: Decrease dose by 50%

Moderately dialyzable (20% to 50%)

Monitoring Parameters Temperature, WBC, urine analysis and culture, appetite, mental status

Reference Range Therapeutic: Peak: 100-500 mg/L; Trough: 75-120 mg/L (not routinely monitored)

Test Interactions Increased cholesterol (S), increased protein, increased uric acid (S)

Patient Information Report sore throat, mouth sores, unusual bleeding or fever; drink plenty of fluid; avoid aspirin and vitamin C products; complete full course of therapy; wear sunscreen if going out in the sun

Nursing Implications Shake suspension before administering; watch for signs of adverse reactions

Special Geriatric Considerations Sulfamethoxazole is an effective anti-infective agent; most prescribers prefer the combination of sulfamethoxazole and trimethoprim for its dual mechanism of action; trimethoprim penetrates the prostate; adjust dose for renal function; see Usual Dosage and Pharmacokinetics

Dosage Forms

Suspension, oral: 500 mg/5 mL (480 mL)

Tablet: 500 mg

References

Ljungberg B and Nilsson-Ehle I, "Pharmacokinetics of Antimicrobial Agents in the Elderly," *Rev Infect Dis*, 1987, 9(2):250-64.

Varoquaux O, Lajoie D, Gobert C, et al, "Pharmacokinetics of the Trimethoprim-Sulfamethoxazole Combination in the Elderly," *Br J Clin Pharmacol*, 1985, 20:575-81.

Sulfamethoxazole and Trimethoprim *see Co-trimoxazole on page 189*

Sulfasalazine (sul fa sal' a zeen)
Brand Names Azulfidine®; Azulfidine® EN-tabs®
Synonyms Salicylazosulfapyridine
Generic Available Yes
Therapeutic Class 5-Aminosalicylic Acid Derivative; Anti-inflammatory Agent
Use Management of ulcerative colitis
Contraindications Hypersensitivity to sulfasalazine, sulfa drugs, or any component; porphyria, GI or GU obstruction; hypersensitivity to salicylates
Precautions Use with caution in patients with renal impairment; impaired hepatic function or urinary obstruction, blood dyscrasias, severe allergies or asthma, or G-6-PD deficiency
Adverse Reactions
Cardiovascular: Vasculitis
Central nervous system: Headache, fever, dizziness
Dermatologic: Rash, toxic epidermal necrolysis, itching, photosensitivity, Stevens-Johnson syndrome
Endocrine & metabolic: Folic acid deficiency, thyroid function disturbance
Gastrointestinal: Nausea, vomiting, diarrhea, anorexia
Genitourinary: Crystalluria
Hematologic: Hemolytic anemia, agranulocytosis, aplastic anemia, granulocytopenia, leukopenia
Hepatic: Hepatitis, jaundice
Renal: Hematuria, interstitial nephritis
Respiratory: Fibrosing alveolitis
Miscellaneous: Orange-yellow discoloration of urine and skin (rare), serum sickness-like reaction
Overdosage Symptoms of overdose include drowsiness, dizziness, anorexia, abdominal pain, nausea, vomiting, hemolytic anemia, acidosis, jaundice
Toxicology Doses of as little as 2-5 g/day may produce toxicity; the aniline radical is responsible for hematologic toxicity; high volume diuresis may aid in elimination and prevention of renal failure
Drug Interactions
Folic acid decreased absorption, digoxin decreased serum levels
Iron decreased sulfasalazine absorption
Decreased effect with PABA or PABA metabolites of drugs (ie, procaine, proparacaine, tetracaine); decreased effect of oral anticoagulants and oral hypoglycemic agents
Stability Protect from light; shake suspension well
Mechanism of Action Acts locally in the colon to decrease the inflammatory response and interferes with secretion by inhibiting prostaglandin synthesis
Pharmacokinetics
Absorption: Oral: Up to 33% as unchanged drug from the small intestine
Metabolism: Following absorption, both components are metabolized in the liver
Half-life: 5.7-10 hours; upon administration, the drug is split into sulfapyridine and 5-aminosalicylic acid (5-ASA) in the colon
Time to peak: Peak serum 5-aminosalicylic acid (active metabolite) levels appear within 1.5-6 hours and serum sulfapyridine (active metabolite) levels peak in 6-24 hours
Elimination: Primary excretion in urine (as unchanged drug, components, and acetylated metabolites)
Usual Dosage Geriatrics and Adults: Oral: 1 g 3-4 times/day, 2 g/day maintenance in divided doses; not to exceed 6 g/day; individualize dose based upon patient's response; start with lower dose, 1-2 g/day, to avoid GI intolerance

Dosing interval in renal impairment:
Cl$_{cr}$ 10-30 mL/minute: Administer twice daily
Cl$_{cr}$ <10 mL/minute: Administer once daily
Dosing adjustment in hepatic impairment: Avoid use
Monitoring Parameters Response to therapy, GI complaints
Patient Information Maintain adequate fluid intake; may cause orange-yellow discoloration of urine and skin; take after meals or with food; do not take with antacids; may permanently stain soft contact lenses yellow; avoid prolonged exposure to sunlight (wear sunscreen)
Nursing Implications Shake suspension well; GI intolerance is common during the first few days of therapy; drug commonly imparts an orange-yellow discoloration to urine and skin; see Administration
Additional Information This drug should be administered after food to reduce GI irritation
Special Geriatric Considerations See Usual Dosage; adjust dose for renal function
Dosage Forms
Suspension, oral: 250 mg/5 mL (473 mL)
Tablet: 500 mg
Tablet, enteric coated: 500 mg

Sulfatrim® see Co-trimoxazole on page 189
Sulfatrim® DS see Co-trimoxazole on page 189
Sulfimycin® see Erythromycin and Sulfisoxazole on page 265

Sulfinpyrazone (sul fin peer' a zone)
Brand Names Anturane®
Generic Available Yes
Therapeutic Class Uric Acid Lowering Agent
Use Treatment of chronic gouty arthritis and intermittent gouty arthritis

Unlabeled use: To decrease the incidence of sudden death postmyocardial infarction
Contraindications Active peptic ulcers, GI inflammation, blood dyscrasias, hypersensitivity to sulfinpyrazone or any component
Precautions Avoid in patients with a Cl_{cr} <50 mL/minute (sulfinpyrazone loses its effectiveness and may cause acute renal failure); administer with caution to patients with healed peptic ulcers
Adverse Reactions
Cardiovascular: Flushing
Central nervous system: Dizziness, headache
Dermatologic: Rash
Gastrointestinal: Anorexia, nausea, vomiting
Hematologic: Anemia, leukopenia, increased bleeding time (decreased platelet aggregation)
Hepatic: Hepatic necrosis
Genitourinary: Urinary frequency
Renal: Uric acid stones, nephrotic syndrome
Overdosage Symptoms of overdose include nausea, vomiting, ataxia, respiratory depression, seizures
Toxicology Following GI decontamination, treatment is supportive only
Drug Interactions
Decreased effect of theophylline, verapamil; decreased uricosuric effects with salicylates, niacin
Increased effect of warfarin, tolbutamide
Risk of acetaminophen hepatotoxicity is increased, but therapeutic effects may be reduced
Mechanism of Action Inhibits renal tubular reabsorption of uric acid, thus promoting urinary excretion of uric acid and decreasing blood urate levels; also has antithrombic and platelet inhibitory effects
Pharmacokinetics
Absorption: Oral: Well absorbed
Protein binding: 98% to 99%
Half-life: 2.2-3 hours
Elimination: ~50% of dose appears in urine unchanged
Usual Dosage Geriatrics and Adults: Oral: 100-200 mg twice daily increasing to 400 mg twice daily, monitoring uric acid levels; decrease to 200 mg/day as a maintenance dose; see Special Geriatric Considerations
Monitoring Parameters Serum and urinary uric acid; CBC, renal function
Test Interactions Decreased uric acid (S)
Patient Information Take with food or milk; drink adequate fluids; avoid aspirin containing products
Additional Information This drug should only be used when other treatments for hyperuricemia or gout have failed or were not tolerated
Special Geriatric Considerations Since sulfinpyrazone loses its effectiveness when the Cl_{cr} is <50 mL/minute, its usefulness in the elderly is limited; see Additional Information
Dosage Forms
Capsule: 200 mg
Tablet: 100 mg

Sulfisoxazole (sul fi sox' a zole)
Brand Names Gantrisin®
Synonyms Sulfisoxazole Acetyl; Sulphafurazole
Therapeutic Class Antibiotic, Sulfonamide Derivative
Use Treatment of urinary tract infections, otitis media, *Chlamydia*; nocardiosis
Contraindications Hypersensitivity to any sulfa drug or any component; porphyria; patients with urinary obstruction
Precautions Use with caution in patients with G-6-PD deficiency (hemolysis may occur), hepatic or renal impairment; dosage modification required in patients with renal impairment; risk of crystalluria should be considered in patients with impaired renal function
Adverse Reactions
Central nervous system: Dizziness, headache, fever

Dermatologic: Kernicterus, rash, Stevens-Johnson syndrome, photosensitivity
Endocrine & metabolic: Folic acid deficiency (rare), thyroid function disturbance
Gastrointestinal: Nausea, vomiting, anorexia, diarrhea
Genitourinary: Crystalluria
Hematologic: Thrombocytopenia, leukopenia, agranulocytosis, aplastic anemia, hemolytic anemia, granulocytopenia
Hepatic: Jaundice, hepatitis, serum sickness-like reactions
Renal: Nephrotoxicity, hematuria
Miscellaneous: Hypersensitivity reactions

Overdosage Symptoms of overdose include drowsiness, dizziness, anorexia, abdominal pain, nausea, vomiting, hemolytic anemia, acidosis, jaundice

Drug Interactions Increased effect of tolbutamide, chlorpropamide, oral anticoagulants (displaced from protein binding sites); PABA (antagonizes the antibacterial activity of sulfas); thiopental

Mechanism of Action Interferes with bacterial growth by inhibiting bacterial folic acid synthesis through competitive antagonism of PABA

Pharmacokinetics
Absorption: Sulfisoxazole acetyl is hydrolyzed in the GI tract to sulfisoxazole which is readily absorbed
Protein binding: 85% to 88%
Metabolism: Metabolized in the liver by acetylation and glucuronide conjugation to inactive compounds
Half-life: 4-7 hours, prolonged with renal impairment
Time to peak: Following administration, peak serum levels occur within 2-3 hours
Elimination: Primarily in urine (95% within 24 hours), 40% to 60% as unchanged drug
In a single dose study, absorption and peak concentration were similar in elderly and younger subjects. In the elderly, half-life was prolonged and renal and nonrenal clearance decreased.

Usual Dosage
Pelvic inflammatory disease: 500 mg every 6 hours for 21 days; used in combination with ceftriaxone
Chlamydia trachomatis: 500 mg every 6 hours for 10 days

Geriatrics and Adults: Ophthalmic:
Ointment: Instill small amount to affected eye 1-3 times/day and at bedtime
Solution: Instill 1-2 drops to affected eye every 2-3 hours

Geriatrics: 2 g stat, 2-8 g/day every 6 hours; adjust dose for Cl_cr; single and 3-day dosing for urinary tract infections in the elderly are not reliable.

Adults: Oral: 2-4 g stat, 4-8 g/day in divided doses every 4-6 hours

Dosing interval in renal impairment:
Cl_{cr} 10-50 mL/minute: Administer every 8-12 hours
Cl_{cr} <10 mL/minute: Administer every 12-24 hours
>50% removed by hemodialysis

Monitoring Parameters Temperature, WBC, urine analysis and culture, appetite, mental status

Reference Range Therapeutic: 5-15 mg/dL; Toxic: >20 mg/dL (not routinely monitored)

Test Interactions False-positive protein in urine; false-positive urine glucose with Clinitest®

Patient Information Take with a glass of water on an empty stomach; avoid prolonged exposure to sunlight (wear sunscreen); report to physician any sore throat, mouth sores, rash, unusual bleeding, or fever; complete full course of therapy

Nursing Implications Give around-the-clock rather than 4 times/day, 3 times/day, etc (ie, 12-6-12-6, not 9-1-5-9) to promote less variation in peak and trough serum levels; maintain adequate fluid intake; watch for signs of adverse reactions

Additional Information Lipo Gantrisin® and Gantrisin® are not to be used interchangeably; routine alkalinization of urine is normally not required

Special Geriatric Considerations Sulfisoxazole is an effective anti-infective agent; most prescribers prefer the combination of sulfamethoxazole and trimethoprim for its dual mechanism of action; trimethoprim penetrates the prostate; adjust dose for renal function

Dosage Forms
Ophthalmic:
Ointment: 4% (3.75 g)
Solution: 4% (15 mL)
Syrup, as acetyl: 500 mg/5 mL (480 mL)
Tablet: 500 mg

References
Boisvert A, Barbeau G, and Belanger PM, "Pharmacokinetics of Sulfisoxazole in Young and Elderly Subjects," *Gerontology*, 1984, 30(2):125-31.

Sulfisoxazole Acetyl *see* Sulfisoxazole *on previous page*

Sulfisoxazole and Erythromycin see Erythromycin and Sulfisoxazole on page 265

Sulfisoxazole and Phenazopyridine (sul fi sox' zole)

Related Information

Phenazopyridine Hydrochloride on page 552

Sulfisoxazole on page 662

Brand Names Azo Gantrisin®

Therapeutic Class Antibiotic, Sulfonamide Derivative; Local Anesthetic, Urinary

Use Treatment of urinary tract infections and nocardiosis

Contraindications Porphyria, hypersensitivity to any sulfa drug or any component

Usual Dosage Oral: 4-6 tablets to start, then 2 tablets 4 times/day for 2 days, then continue with sulfisoxazole only

Test Interactions Increased creatinine

Special Geriatric Considerations Most combination products are best avoided in the elderly; for dose adjustment for renal function see Sulfisoxazole

Dosage Forms Tablet: Sulfisoxazole 500 mg and phenazopyridine 50 mg

Sulfoxaprim® see Co-trimoxazole on page 189

Sulfoxaprim® DS see Co-trimoxazole on page 189

Sulindac (sul in' dak)

Brand Names Clinoril®

Generic Available Yes

Therapeutic Class Analgesic, Non-narcotic; Anti-inflammatory Agent; Nonsteroidal Anti-inflammatory Agent (NSAID), Oral

Use Management of inflammatory disease, rheumatoid disorders; acute gouty arthritis, osteoarthritis, ankylosing spondylitis, acute painful shoulder, bursitis, tendonitis

Contraindications Hypersensitivity to sulindac, any component, aspirin or other nonsteroidal anti-inflammatory drugs (NSAIDs)

Warnings A potentially fatal hypersensitivity has occurred with sulindac; GI toxicity (bleeding, ulceration, perforation); CNS effects may occur (headaches, confusion, depression); hypersensitivity, anaphylactoid reactions (intermittent tolmetin use more often); renal function decline, acute renal insufficiency, interstitial nephritis, dysuria, cystitis, hematuria, nephrotic syndrome, hyperkalemia in acute renal insufficiency, hyponatremia, papillary necrosis, hepatic function impairment; elderly have increased risk for adverse reactions to NSAIDs; see Special Geriatric Considerations

Precautions Use with caution in patients with congestive heart failure, hypertension, decreased renal or hepatic function, history of GI disease (bleeding or ulcers), or those receiving anticoagulants; perform ophthalmologic evaluation for those who develop eye complaints during therapy (blurred vision, diminished vision, changes in color vision, retinal changes); NSAIDs may mask signs/symptoms of infections; photosensitivity reported

Adverse Reactions

Cardiovascular: Congestive heart failure, angina, hypertension, hypotension, fluid retention, arrhythmias, edema

Central nervous system: Headache, drowsiness, vertigo, dizziness, fatigue, hallucinations, confusion, depression, emotional lability, psychotic behavior, asthenia, pyrexia

Dermatologic: Rash, urticaria, angioedema, Stevens-Johnson syndrome, exfoliative dermatitis, ecchymosis, petechiae, purpura, bruising

Endocrine & metabolic: Hyperglycemia, hypoglycemia, hyperkalemia, gynecomastia, hyponatremia

Gastrointestinal: Dyspepsia, heartburn, nausea, diarrhea, constipation, flatulence, stomatitis, vomiting, abdominal pain, peptic ulcer, GI bleeding, GI perforation, gingival ulcers, pancreatitis, proctitis, paralytic ulcers, colitis, anorexia, weight loss

Genitourinary: Impotence, azotemia

Hematologic: Neutropenia, anemia, agranulocytosis, bone marrow suppression, hemolytic anemia, hemorrhage, inhibition of platelet aggregation

Hepatic: Hepatitis, elevated LFTs, cholestatic jaundice

Neuromuscular & skeletal: Involuntary muscle movements, muscle weakness, tremors

Ocular: Vision changes

Otic: Tinnitus

Renal: Dysuria, polyuria, pyuria, oliguria, anuria, acute renal failure

Respiratory: Exacerbation of asthma, dyspnea

Miscellaneous: Dry mucous membranes, thirst, sweating

Overdosage Symptoms include drowsiness, lethargy, disorientation, confusion, dizziness, numbness, paresthesia, nausea, vomiting, gastric irritation, abdominal pain, headache, tinnitus, sweating, blurred vision, muscle twitching, seizures, coma, acute renal failure, increased BUN and serum creatinine, hypotension, tachycardia, and metabolic acidosis

Toxicology Management of a nonsteroidal anti-inflammatory agent (NSAID) intoxication is primarily supportive and symptomatic. Fluid therapy is commonly effective in managing the hypotension that may occur following an acute NSAID overdose, except when this is due to an acute blood loss. Seizures tend to be very short-lived and often do not require drug treatment although recurrent seizures should be treated with I.V. diazepam. Since many of the NSAIDs undergo enterohepatic cycling, multiple doses of charcoal may be needed to reduce the potential for delayed toxicities.

Drug Interactions
DMSO or ASA may decrease sulindac serum concentration
May increase digoxin, methotrexate, and little effect on lithium serum concentrations or may decrease lithium levels
Aspirin may decrease NSAID serum concentrations
Other NSAIDs may increase adverse GI effects
Increased prothrombin time with anticoagulants
Decreased antihypertensive effects of ACE inhibitors, beta-blockers, and thiazide diuretics
Effects of loop diuretics may decrease
Increased response to sympathomimetics
Probenecid may increase toxicity of NSAIDs by increase in serum concentrations
Diuretics may increase risk of acute renal insufficiency; azotemia may be enhanced in elderly receiving loop diuretics

Mechanism of Action Inhibits prostaglandin synthesis, acts on the hypothalamus heat-regulating center to reduce fever, blocks prostaglandin synthetase action which prevents formation of the platelet-aggregating substance thromboxane A_2; decreases pain receptor sensitivity. Other proposed mechanisms of action are lysosomal stabilization, kinin and leukotriene production, alteration of chemotactic factors, and inhibition of neutrophil activation. This latter mechanism may be the most significant pharmacologic action to reduce inflammation.

Pharmacodynamics
Onset of anti-inflammatory action: Within 7 days
Maximum response: 2-3 weeks

Pharmacokinetics
Absorption: Oral: 90%; sulindac is a prodrug and therefore requires metabolic activation
Protein binding: >90%
Half-life:
  Parent: 7 hours
  Active metabolite: 18 hours
Requires hepatic metabolism to sulfide metabolite (active) for therapeutic effects
Metabolism: In the liver to sulfone metabolites (inactive)
Time to peak: Peak levels occur in 2-4 hours
Elimination: Principally in urine (50%) with some biliary excretion (25%)

Usual Dosage Geriatrics and Adults: Oral: 150-200 mg twice daily; not to exceed 400 mg/day; see Pharmacodynamics

Monitoring Parameters Monitor response (pain, range of motion, grip strength, mobility, ADL function), inflammation; observe for weight gain, edema; monitor renal function; observe for bleeding, bruising; evaluate gastrointestinal effects (abdominal pain, bleeding, dyspepsia); mental confusion, disorientation, CBC, serum, creatinine, BUN, liver function tests

Test Interactions Increased chloride (S), increased sodium (S)

Patient Information Serious gastrointestinal bleeding can occur as well as ulceration and perforation. Pain may or may not be present. Avoid aspirin and aspirin-containing products while taking this medication. If gastric upset occurs, take with food, milk, or antacid. If gastric adverse effects persist, contact physician. May cause drowsiness, dizziness, blurred vision, and confusion. Use caution when performing tasks which require alertness (eg, driving). Do not take for more than 3 days for fever or 10 days for pain without physician's advice.

Nursing Implications Observe for edema and fluid retention; monitor blood pressure; see Overdosage, Monitoring Parameters, Patient Information, and Special Geriatric Considerations

Additional Information Structurally similar to indomethacin but acts like aspirin; associated with the highest (one study) incidence of upper GI bleeds among NSAIDs; safest NSAID for use in mild renal impairment; maximum therapeutic response may not be realized for up to 3 weeks. There are no clinical guidelines to predict which NSAID will give which response in a particular patient. Trials with each must be initiated until response determined. Consider dose, patient convenience, and cost.

Special Geriatric Considerations Elderly are a high-risk population for adverse effects from nonsteroidal anti-inflammatory agents. As much as 60% of elderly who develop GI complications can develop peptic ulceration and/or hemorrhage asymptomatically. The concomitant use of H_2-blockers, omeprazole, and sucralfate is not effective as prophylaxis. Misoprostol is the only prophylactic agent proven effective. Also, concomitant disease and drug use contribute to the risk for GI adverse effects. Use lowest effective dose for shortest period possible. Consider renal function decline

(Continued)

Sulindac *(Continued)*

with age. Use of NSAIDs can compromise existing renal function especially when Cl_{cr} is $\leq$30 mL/minute. Tinnitus may be a difficult and unreliable indication of toxicity due to age-related hearing loss or eighth cranial nerve damage. CNS adverse effects such as confusion, agitation, and hallucination are generally seen in overdose or high-dose situations, but elderly may demonstrate these adverse effects at lower doses than younger adults.

Dosage Forms Tablet: 150 mg, 200 mg

References
Brooks PM, Day RO, "Nonsteroidal Anti-inflammatory Drugs – Differences and Similarities," *N Engl J Med*, 1991, 324(24):1716-25.

Clinch D, Banerjee AK, Ostick G, "Absence of Abdominal Pain in Elderly Patients With Peptic Ulcer," *Age Ageing*, 1984, 13(2):120-3.

Clive DM, Stoff JS, "Renal Syndromes Associated With Nonsteroidal Anti-inflammatory Drugs," *N Engl J Med*, 1984, 310(9):563-72.

Graham DY, "Prevention of Gastroduodenal Injury Induced by Chronic Nonsteroidal Anti-inflammatory Drug Therapy," *Gastroenterology*, 1989, 96(2 Pt 2 Suppl):675-81.

Gurwitz JH, Avarn J, Ross-Degan D, et al, "Nonsteroidal Anti-Inflammatory Drug-Associated Azotemia in the Very Old," *JAMA*, 1990, 264(4):471-5.

Knodel LC, "Preventing NSAID-Induced Ulcers: The Role of Misoprostol," *Consult Pharm*, 1989, 4:37-41.

Pounder R, "Silent Peptic Ulceration: Deadly Silence or Golden Silence?" *Gastroenterology*, 1989, 96:(2 Pt 2 Suppl)626-31.

Sulphafurazole *see* Sulfisoxazole *on page 662*

Sumatriptan Succinate *(soo' ma trip tan)*

Brand Names Imitrex®
Therapeutic Class Antimigraine Agent
Use Acute treatment of migraine with or without aura
Unlabeled use: Cluster headaches
Contraindications I.V. use; use in patients with ischemic heart disease or Prinzmetal angina, patients with signs or symptoms of ischemic heart disease, uncontrolled HTN, use with ergotamine derivatives, hypersensitivity to any component, management of hemiplegic or basilar migraine
Warnings Use with caution in elderly, patients with hepatic or renal impairment; may cause mild, transient elevation of blood pressure; may cause coronary vasospasm
Precautions Safety and efficacy in cluster headache not established; chest tightness has been reported commonly but rarely associated with EKG changes
Adverse Reactions
Cardiovascular: Transient elevation of blood pressure may occur
Central nervous system: Dizziness, drowsiness, headache, numbness
Dermatologic: Skin rashes
Gastrointestinal: Abdominal discomfort
Endocrine & metabolic: Hot flashes, polydipsia
Local: Injection site reaction, burning sensation
Neuromuscular & skeletal: Tightness in chest, neck pain, mouth discomfort, jaw discomfort, myalgia, tingling, weakness
Renal: Dysuria, renal calculus
Respiratory: Dyspnea
Miscellaneous: Thirst, dehydration, hiccups, dysmenorrhea, sweating
Overdosage Symptoms of overdose include tremor, coronary vasospasm, seizures, erythema of extremities, reduced respiratory rate, ataxia, cyanosis, mydriasis, paralysis
Toxicology Treatment is continued monitoring with general supportive care
Drug Interactions Increased toxicity: Ergot-containing drugs
Stability Store at 2°C to 20°C (36°F to 86°F); protect from light
Mechanism of Action Selective agonist for serotonin (5-HT, receptor) in cranial arteries to cause vasoconstriction and reduces sterile inflammation associated with antidromic neuronal transmission correlating with relief of migraine
Pharmacokinetics After S.C. administration:
Distribution: V_d: 50 L
Protein binding: 14% to 21%
Bioavailability: 97%
Half-life:
Distribution: 15 minutes
Terminal: 115 minutes
Time to peak serum concentration: 5-20 minutes
Elimination: In urine unchanged (22%), excreted as indole acetic acid metabolite (38%)
Usual Dosage Geriatrics and Adults: S.C.: 6 mg; a second injection may be administered at least 1 hour after the initial dose, but not more than 2 injections in a 24-hour period; see Special Geriatric Considerations
Monitoring Parameters Monitor blood pressure, signs and symptoms of coronary vasospasm, response (resolution of migraine)

Patient Information If pain or tightness in chest or throat occurs, notify physician; pain at injection site lasts <1 hour

Nursing Implications Do not administer I.V., may cause coronary vasospasm

Special Geriatric Considerations Use cautiously in elderly, particularly since many elderly have cardiovascular disease which would put them at risk for cardiovascular adverse effects; safety and efficacy in elderly (>65 years of age) have not been established; pharmacokinetic disposition is, however, similar to that in young adults

Dosage Forms Injection: 12 mg/mL (0.5 mL, 2 mL)

Sumycin® see Tetracycline on page 678

Superdophilus® [OTC] see Lactobacillus acidophilus and Lactobacillus bulgaricus on page 397

Suprax® see Cefixime on page 128

Suprofen (soo' pro fen)

Brand Names Profenal®

Therapeutic Class Analgesic, Non-narcotic; Anti-inflammatory Agent; Anti-inflammatory Agent, Ophthalmic; Nonsteroidal Anti-Inflammatory Agent (NSAID), Ophthalmic

Use Inhibition of intraoperative miosis

Contraindications Hypersensitivity to suprofen or any component; hypersensitivity to aspirin or other NSAIDs

Warnings Systemic effect of suprofen may occur when applied ocularly; this gives an increased potential for increased bleeding secondary to platelet inhibition

Precautions Most adverse reactions are generally seen with oral and parenteral dosing; however, caution should be used with ocular administration as systemic effects may occur. Use with caution in patients with congestive heart failure, hypertension, decreased renal or hepatic function, history of GI disease (bleeding or ulcers), or those receiving anticoagulants; perform ophthalmologic evaluation for those who develop eye complaints during therapy (blurred vision, diminished vision, changes in color vision, retinal changes); should be used with caution in patients with a history of herpes simplex, keratitis, and patients who might be affected by inhibition of platelet aggregation; slowing of corneal wound healing NSAIDs may mask signs/symptoms of infections; photosensitivity reported

Adverse Reactions
  Local: Transient stings and burning on instillation
  Ocular: Itching, allergy, pain, iritis, chemosis, discomfort, irritation, punctate epithelial staining

Toxicology Should solution be inadvertently drunk, have patient dilute with fluid intake; overdosage unusual with ophthalmic solution

Drug Interactions Reports of drug interactions not supported by animal studies; however, there are reports that acetylcholine and carbachol have been ineffective when used with suprofen and flurbiprofen

Mechanism of Action Inhibits prostaglandin synthesis by decreasing the activity of the enzyme, cyclo-oxygenase, which results in decreased formation of prostaglandin precursors; in animals, prostaglandins are mediators of intraocular inflammation; prostaglandins produce disruption of the blood-aqueous human barrier, increased vascular permeability, vasodilation, leukocytosis, and increased intraocular pressure (IOP)

Usual Dosage Geriatrics and Adults: Ophthalmic: Instill 2 drops into the conjunctival sac at 3, 2, and 1 hour prior to surgery; the day preceding surgery, instill 2 drops every 4 hours while awake

Monitoring Parameters Signs of inflammation and IOP

Patient Information May sting on instillation; do not touch dropper to eye; visual acuity may be decreased after administration; assess patient's or caregiver's ability to administer

Nursing Implications See Monitoring Parameters, Patient Information, and Special Geriatric Considerations

Special Geriatric Considerations Elderly may be sensitive to the systemic effects from ocular absorption; monitor closely; remove contact lenses before administering; assess ability to self-administer

Dosage Forms Solution, ophthalmic: 1% (2.5 mL)

References
Brooks PM, Day RO, "Nonsteroidal Anti-inflammatory Drugs – Differences and Similarities," N Engl J Med, 1991, 324(24):1716-25.

Clinch D, Banerjee AK, Ostick G, "Absence of Abdominal Pain in Elderly Patients With Peptic Ulcer," Age Ageing, 1984, 13:120-3.

Clive DM, Stoff JS, "Renal Syndromes Associated With Nonsteroidal Anti-inflammatory Drugs," N Engl J Med, 1984, 310(9):563-72.

Graham DY, "Prevention of Gastroduodenal Injury Induced by Chronic Nonsteroidal Anti-inflammatory Drug Therapy," Gastroenterology, 1989, 96(2 Pt 2 Suppl):675-81.

Knodel LC, "Preventing NSAID-Induced Ulcers: The Role of Misoprostol," Consult Pharm, 1989, 4:37-41.

(Continued)

Suprofen *(Continued)*

Pounder R, "Silent Peptic Ulceration: Deadly Silence or Golden Silence?" *Gastroenterology*, 1989, 96(2 Pt 2 Suppl):626-31.

Surfak® [OTC] *see* Docusate *on page 236*

Surmontil® *see* Trimipramine Maleate *on page 722*

Sus-Phrine® *see* Epinephrine *on page 256*

Sustaire® *see* Theophylline *on page 681*

Syllact® [OTC] *see* Psyllium *on page 610*

Symmetrel® *see* Amantadine Hydrochloride *on page 34*

Synacort® *see* Hydrocortisone *on page 351*

Synalar® *see* Fluocinolone Acetonide *on page 298*

Synalgos® [OTC] *see* Aspirin *on page 58*

Synemol® *see* Fluocinolone Acetonide *on page 298*

Synthroid® *see* Levothyroxine Sodium *on page 404*

Synthrox® *see* Levothyroxine Sodium *on page 404*

Syroxine® *see* Levothyroxine Sodium *on page 404*

Sytobex® *see* Cyanocobalamin *on page 192*

T_3/T_4 Liotrix *see* Liotrix *on page 410*

T_3 Thyronine Sodium *see* Liothyronine Sodium *on page 408*

T_4 Thyroxine Sodium *see* Levothyroxine Sodium *on page 404*

Tac™-3 *see* Triamcinolone *on page 710*

Tacrine Hydrochloride *(tak' reen)*
Brand Names Cognex®
Synonyms Tetrahydroaminoacrine; THA
Therapeutic Class Cholinergic Agent
Use Treatment of mild to moderate dementia of the Alzheimer's type
Contraindications Patients previously treated with the drug who developed jaundice and in those who are hypersensitive to tacrine or acridine derivatives
Warnings The use of tacrine has been associated with elevations in serum transaminases; serum transaminases (specifically ALT) must be monitored throughout therapy; see Monitoring Parameters for specific guidelines. Use extreme caution in patients with current evidence of a history of abnormal liver function tests; use caution in patients with bladder outlet obstruction, asthma, and sick sinus syndrome (tacrine may cause bradycardia). Tacrine may increase gastric acid secretion, therefore, closely monitor patients at increased risk for developing peptic ulcer disease.
Adverse Reactions
Central nervous system: Ataxia
Gastrointestinal: Diarrhea, nausea, vomiting, dyspepsia, anorexia
Hepatic: Elevated transaminases
Musculoskeletal: Myalgia
Note: In many of the studies comparing tacrine with placebo, there was a high incidence of physical complaints with placebo; overall frequency of adverse effects was 81% with tacrine and 75% with placebo
Toxicology General supportive measures; can cause a cholinergic crisis characterized by severe nausea, vomiting, salivation, sweating, bradycardia, hypotension, collapse, and convulsions; increased muscle weakness is a possibility and may result in death if respiratory muscles are involved
Tertiary anticholinergics, such as atropine, may be used as an antidote for overdosage. I.V. atropine sulfate titrated to effect is recommended; initial dose of 1-2 mg I.V. with subsequent doses based upon clinical response. Atypical increases in blood pressure and heart rate have been reported with other cholinomimetics when coadministered with quaternary anticholinergics such as glycopyrrolate.
Drug Interactions
Decreased effect of anticholinergics and potential decrease in tacrine effect
Increased effect of theophylline, cimetidine, succinylcholine, cholinesterase inhibitors, or cholinergic agonists; increased effect with cimetidine
Mechanism of Action A deficiency of cortical acetylcholine is thought to account for some of the symptoms of Alzheimer's disease; tacrine is a centrally acting reversible cholinesterase inhibitor; it presumably acts by slowing the degradation of acetylcholine thus elevating acetylcholine levels in the cerebral cortex
Pharmacokinetics
Absorption: Reduced with food
Protein binding: 55%
Metabolism: Extensive by cytochrome P-450 system; saturable at relatively low doses

Bioavailability, absolute: 17%

Half-life: 2-4 hours

No clinically relevant age-related changes in pharmacokinetics have been found

Usual Dosage Geriatrics and Adults: Initial: 10 mg 4 times/day; may increase by 40 mg/day every 6 weeks; maximum: 160 mg/day; best administered separate from meal times; see table.

Dose Adjustment Based Upon Transaminase Elevations

ALT	Regimen
≤3 x ULN*	Continue titration
>3 to ≤5 x ULN	Decrease dose by 40 mg/day, resume when ALT returns to normal
>5 x ULN	Stop treatment, may rechallenge upon return of ALT to normal

*ULN = upper limit of normal.

Patients with clinical jaundice confirmed by elevated total bilirubin (>3 mg/dL) should not be rechallenged with tacrine

Monitoring Parameters Serum transaminase levels (specifically ALT) weekly for at least the first 18 weeks, then monitor once every 3 months; for each dose increase, resume weekly monitoring for at least 6 weeks

Reference Range In clinical trials, serum concentrations >20 ng/mL were associated with a much higher risk of development of symptomatic adverse effects

Patient Information Effect of tacrine therapy is thought to depend upon its administration at regular intervals, as directed; take between meals if possible; if GI upset occurs, may take with meals; inform physician of the emergence of new events or any increase in the severity of existing adverse effects (those that occur upon initiation of therapy or an increase in dose, ie, nausea, vomiting, loose stools, diarrhea; and those that can occur later in therapy, ie, rash, jaundice, very light stools, or black stools); abrupt discontinuation of the drug or a large reduction in total daily dose (≥80 mg/day) may cause a decline in cognitive function and behavioral disturbances; unsupervised increases in the dose may also have serious consequences; do not change dose without consulting physician; be complaint with required liver tests

Nursing Implications See Monitoring Parameters and Usual Dosage

Special Geriatric Considerations Although tacrine is the only drug currently FDA-approved for the treatment of Alzheimer's disease, it is clearly not a cure. At least 25% of patients may not tolerate the drug and only 50% of patients demonstrate some improvement in symptoms or a slowing of deterioration. While worth a try in mild to moderate dementia of the Alzheimer's type, patients and their families must be counseled about the limitations of the drug and the importance of regular monitoring of liver function tests. No specific dosage adjustments are necessary due to age.

Dosage Forms Capsule: 10 mg, 20 mg, 30 mg, 40 mg

References

Crismon ML, "Tacrine: First Drug Approved for Alzheimer's Disease," *Ann Pharmacother*, 1994, 28(6):744-51.

Davis KL, Thal LJ, Gamzu ER, et al, "A Double-Blind, Placebo-Controlled Multicenter Study of Tacrine for Alzheimer's Disease," *N Engl J Med*, 1992, 327(18):1253-9.

Farlow M, Gracon SI, Hershey LA, et al, "A Controlled Trial of Tacrine in Alzheimer's Disease," *JAMA*, 1992, 268(18):2523-9.

Knapp MJ, Knopman DS, Solomon PR, et al, "A 30-Week Randomized Controlled Trial of High-Dose Tacrine in Patients With Alzheimer's Disease," *JAMA*, 1994, 271(13):985-91.

Tagamet® *see* Cimetidine *on page 165*

Talwin® *see* Pentazocine *on page 545*

Talwin® NX *see* Pentazocine *on page 545*

Tambocor® *see* Flecainide Acetate *on page 293*

Tamine® [OTC] *see* Brompheniramine and Phenylpropanolamine *on page 94*

Tamoxifen Citrate (ta mox' i fen)

Brand Names Nolvadex®

Generic Available No

Therapeutic Class Antineoplastic Agent, Hormone (Antiestrogen)

Use Palliative or adjunctive treatment of advanced breast cancer

Unlabeled use: Treatment of mastalgia, gynecomastia, male breast cancer, and pancreatic carcinoma; studies are currently underway to evaluate use of tamoxifen as chemosuppressive therapy in women at high risk for primary breast cancer

Contraindications Hypersensitivity to tamoxifen

Warnings Decreased visual acuity; retinopathy and corneal changes have been report-

(Continued)

Tamoxifen Citrate *(Continued)*

ed with use for more than 1 year at doses above recommended; hypercalcemia in patients with bone metastasis; hepatocellular carcinomas have been reported in animal studies; endometrial hyperplasia and polyps have occurred

Precautions Use with caution in patients with leukopenia, thrombocytopenia, and hyperlipidemia

Adverse Reactions

Cardiovascular: Edema

Central nervous system: Depression, headache

Dermatologic: Rash, pruritus vulvae

Endocrine & metabolic: Rarely hypercalcemia, hot flashes

Gastrointestinal: Nausea, vomiting

Neuromuscular & skeletal: Increased bone and tumor pain may occur at initiation of therapy which indicates a good tumor response and generally subsides rapidly

Overdosage Symptoms of overdose include hypercalcemia, edema

Toxicology General supportive care

Drug Interactions

Anticoagulants may have increased effect when used with tamoxifen

Bromocriptine increases serum concentrations of tamoxifen and N-desmethyl tamoxifen

Mechanism of Action Competitively binds to estrogen receptors on tumors and other tissue targets, producing a nuclear complex that decreases DNA synthesis and inhibits estrogen effects

Pharmacokinetics

Metabolism: In the liver

Half-life: 7 days

Time to peak: Oral: Peak serum levels occur within 4-7 hours

Elimination: In feces, with only small amounts appearing in urine; undergoes enterohepatic recycling

Usual Dosage Geriatrics and Adults: Oral: 10-20 mg twice daily (morning and evening)

Monitoring Parameters Monitor tumor, WBC, platelets

Test Interactions Transient increased serum calcium; T_4 elevations (no clinical evidence of hyperthyroidism)

Patient Information Report any vomiting that occurs after taking dose; women should be advised to notify their physician of vaginal bleeding or itching

Nursing Implications Monitor WBC and platelet counts

Additional Information "Hot flashes" may be countered by Bellergal-S® tablets; increase of bone pain usually indicates a good therapeutic response

Myelosuppressive effects:

WBC: Rare

Platelets: None

Onset (days): 7-10

Nadir (days): 14

Recovery (days): 21

Special Geriatric Considerations Studies have shown tamoxifen to be effective in the treatment of primary breast cancer in elderly women. Comparative studies with other antineoplastic agents in elderly women with breast cancer had more favorable survival rates with tamoxifen. Initiation of hormone therapy rather than chemotherapy is justified for elderly patients with metastatic breast cancer who are responsive.

Dosage Forms Tablet: 10 mg

References

Allan SG, Rodger A, Smyth JF, et al, "Tamoxifen as Primary Treatment of Breast Cancer in Elderly or Frail Patients: A Practical Management," *Br Med J [Clin Res]*, 1985, 290:358.

Taylor SG, Gelman RS, Falkson G, et al, "Combination Chemotherapy Compared to Tamoxifen as Initial Therapy for Stage IV Breast Cancer in Elderly Women," *Ann Intern Med*, 1986, 104:455-61.

Tapazole® *see* Methimazole *on page 454*

Taractan® *see* Chlorprothixene *on page 157*

TAT *see* Tetanus Antitoxin *on page 675*

Tavist® *see* Clemastine Fumarate *on page 171*

Tazidime® *see* Ceftazidime *on page 137*

TCN *see* Tetracycline *on page 678*

Tebamide® *see* Trimethobenzamide Hydrochloride *on page 720*

Tega-Cert® [OTC] *see* Dimenhydrinate *on page 227*

Tegopen® *see* Cloxacillin Sodium *on page 180*

Tegretol® *see* Carbamazepine *on page 117*

Telachlor® *see* Chlorpheniramine Maleate *on page 152*

Teldrin® [OTC] *see* Chlorpheniramine Maleate *on page 152*

Teline® *see* Tetracycline *on page 678*

Temaril® *see* Trimeprazine Tartrate *on page 719*

Temazepam (te maz' e pam)
Related Information
Antacid Drug Interactions *on page 764*
Anxiolytic/Hypnotic Use in Long-Term Care Facilities *on page 755-756*
Benzodiazepines Comparison *on page 802-803*
Brand Names Restoril®
Generic Available Yes
Therapeutic Class Benzodiazepine; Hypnotic; Sedative
Use Short-term treatment of insomnia
Restrictions C-IV
Contraindications Hypersensitivity to temazepam or any component, there may be cross-sensitivity with other benzodiazepines; severe uncontrolled pain, pre-existing CNS depression or narrow-angle glaucoma; sleep apnea
Precautions Use with caution in patients with mental impairment, reflex slowing, or the potential for drug dependence
Adverse Reactions
Central nervous system: Drowsiness, dizziness, confusion, sedation, ataxia, headache
Gastrointestinal: Dry mouth, constipation, diarrhea, nausea, vomiting
Neuromuscular & skeletal: Impaired coordination
Ocular: Blurred vision
Respiratory: Decreased respiratory rate, apnea, laryngospasm
Miscellaneous: Physical and psychological dependence with prolonged use
Overdosage Symptoms of overdose include somnolence, confusion, coma, and diminished reflexes
Toxicology Treatment for benzodiazepine overdose is supportive; rarely is mechanical ventilation required
Flumazenil has been shown to selectively block the binding of benzodiazepines to CNS receptors, resulting in a reversal of benzodiazepine-induced sedation; however, its use may not alter the course of overdose
Drug Interactions CNS depressants and alcohol may increase CNS adverse effects
Mechanism of Action Depresses all levels of the CNS, including the limbic and reticular formation, probably through the increased action of gamma-aminobutyric acid (GABA), which is a major inhibitory neurotransmitter in the brain
Pharmacodynamics Onset of hypnotic effect: 30 minutes to 1 hour; considered an intermediate acting benzodiazepine; studies have shown that the elderly are more sensitive to the effects of benzodiazepines as compared to younger adults
Pharmacokinetics
Protein binding: 96%
Metabolism: In the liver
Half-life: 3.5-18.4 hours (mean: 8.8 hours)
Time to peak: Oral: Peak serum levels occur at approximately 1.5 hours
Elimination: 80% to 90% in urine as inactive metabolites
Pharmacokinetics are not significantly affected by aging
Usual Dosage Oral may be taken 30 minutes before the desired onset of sleep

Geriatrics: Initial: 7.5 mg at bedtime; may need to increase to 15 mg
Adults: 15-30 mg at bedtime
Monitoring Parameters Respiratory, cardiovascular and mental status
Reference Range Therapeutic: 26 ng/mL after 24 hours
Patient Information Avoid alcohol and other CNS depressants; may cause daytime drowsiness; avoid activities needing good psychomotor coordination until CNS effects are known; may cause physical or psychological dependence; avoid abrupt discontinuation after prolonged use; may be taken 30 minutes before bedtime
Nursing Implications Provide safety measures (ie, side rails, night light, and call button); remove smoking materials from area; supervise ambulation
Additional Information Causes minimal change in REM sleep patterns; reformulation of the commercial product now allows for a faster onset
Special Geriatric Considerations Because of its lack of active metabolites, temazepam is recommended in the elderly when a benzodiazepine hypnotic is indicated; temazepam was recently (March 1993) marketed in a 7.5 mg capsule which would be appropriate initial dosing in the elderly; hypnotic use should be limited to 10-14 days; if insomnia persists, the patient should be evaluated for etiology; see Pharmacodynamics
Dosage Forms Capsule: 7.5 mg, 15 mg, 30 mg
References
Divoll M, Greenblatt DJ, Harmatz JS, et al, "Effect of Age and Gender on Disposition of Temazepam," *J Pharm Sci*, 1981, 70(10):1104-7.
Scharf MB, Berkowitz DV, and Brannen DE, "Effectiveness of Low-Dose Temazepam on Sleep Patterns in Geriatric Insomniac Subjects," *Consult Pharm*, 1993, 8(12):1367-73.

ALPHABETICAL LISTING OF DRUGS

Tempra® [OTC] *see* Acetaminophen *on page 13*
Tenex® *see* Guanfacine Hydrochloride *on page 335*
Tenormin® *see* Atenolol *on page 62*
Terazol® 7 *see* Terconazole *on page 674*

Terazosin (ter ay' zoe sin)
Brand Names Hytrin®
Generic Available No
Therapeutic Class Alpha-Adrenergic Blocking Agent, Oral
Use Management of mild to moderate hypertension; treatment of symptomatic benign prostatic hypertrophy (BPH)
Contraindications Hypersensitivity to terazosin, other alpha-adrenergic blockers, or any component
Warnings Can cause marked hypotension and syncope with sudden loss of consciousness with the first few doses. Anticipate a similar effect if therapy is interrupted for a few days, if dosage is increased rapidly, or if another antihypertensive drug is introduced.
Precautions Syncope and postural hypotension frequently occur with the first dose; use with caution in patients with confirmed or suspected coronary artery disease
Adverse Reactions
Cardiovascular: Orthostatic hypotension, syncope, palpitations, tachycardia, edema
Central nervous system: Dizziness, lightheadedness, nightmares, drowsiness, headache
Dermatologic: Rash
Gastrointestinal: Nausea, dry mouth
Genitourinary: Urinary frequency or incontinence
Neuromuscular & skeletal: Weakness
Miscellaneous: Nasal congestion, fluid retention
Overdosage Symptoms of overdose include hypotension, drowsiness, and shock
Toxicology Hypotension usually responds to I.V. fluids or Trendelenburg positioning. If unresponsive to these measures the use of a parenteral vasoconstrictor may be required (eg, norepinephrine 0.1-0.2 mcg/kg/minute titrated to response). Treatment is primarily supportive and symptomatic.
Drug Interactions Increased hypotensive effect with diuretics and other antihypertensive agents (especially beta-blockers)
Mechanism of Action An alpha₁-specific blocking agent with minimal alpha₂ effects; this allows peripheral postsynaptic blockade, with the resultant decrease in arterial tone, while preserving the negative feedback loop which is mediated by the peripheral presynaptic alpha₂-receptors

In BPH, terazosin relaxes the smooth muscle of the bladder neck, thus reducing bladder outlet obstruction
Pharmacokinetics
Absorption: Oral: Rapid
Protein binding: 90% to 95%
Metabolism: Extensive in the liver
Half-life: 9.2-12 hours; half-life is not significantly prolonged in elderly
Time to peak: Occurs within 60 minutes
Elimination: In feces (60%) and urine (40%)
Usual Dosage Geriatrics and Adults: Oral:
Hypertension: Initial: 1 mg at bedtime; slowly increase dose to achieve desired blood pressure, up to 20 mg/day; usual dose: 1-5 mg/day
Benign prostatic hypertrophy: Initial: 1 mg at bedtime, increasing as needed; most patients require 10 mg day; if no response after 4-6 weeks of 10 mg/day, may increase to 20 mg/day
Monitoring Parameters Blood pressure, standing and sitting/supine, urinary symptoms
Patient Information Report any gain of body weight; fainting sometimes occurs after the first dose, take first dose at bedtime; rise from sitting/lying carefully, may cause dizziness
Nursing Implications Syncope may occur usually within 90 minutes of the initial dose; administer initial dose at bedtime; assist patients with ambulation
Special Geriatric Considerations See Warnings and Nursing Implications; adverse reactions such as dry mouth and urinary problems can be particularly bothersome in the elderly
Dosage Forms Tablet: 1 mg, 2 mg, 5 mg, 10 mg

Terbinafine (ter' bin a feen)
Brand Names Lamisil®
Therapeutic Class Antifungal Agent, Topical
Use Topical antifungal for the treatment of tinea pedis (athlete's foot), tinea cruris (jock

672

itch), and tinea corporis (ring worm)

Unlabeled use: Cutaneous candidiasis and pityriasis versicolor

Contraindications Hypersensitivity to terbinafine or any component

Warnings For external use only

Adverse Reactions Local: Irritation, burning, itching, dryness

Stability Store at room temperature 5°C to 30°C (41°F to 86°F)

Mechanism of Action Synthetic alkylamine derivative which inhibits squalene epoxidases which is a key enzyme in sterol biosynthesis in fungi to result in a deficiency in ergosterol within fungal cell wall and result in fungal cell death

Pharmacokinetics

Absorption: Topical: Limited

Elimination: ~75% of cutaneously absorbed drug excreted in urine; 3.5% of administered dose recovered in urine and feces

Usual Dosage Geriatrics and Adults: Topical:

Athlete's foot: Apply to affected area twice daily for at least 1 week, not to exceed 4 weeks

Ringworm and jock itch: Apply to affected area once or twice daily for at least 1 week, not to exceed 4 weeks

Patient Information For external use only; not for oral, ophthalmic, or intravaginal use; if irritation or sensitivity occurs, discontinue use and notify physician

Special Geriatric Considerations No specific recommendations for use in the elderly

Dosage Forms Cream: 1% (15 g, 30 g)

Terbutaline Sulfate (ter byoo' ta leen)

Brand Names Brethaire®; Brethine®; Bricanyl®

Generic Available No

Therapeutic Class Adrenergic Agonist Agent; Beta-2-Adrenergic Agonist Agent; Bronchodilator

Use Bronchodilator in reversible airway obstruction and bronchial asthma

Contraindications Hypersensitivity to terbutaline or any component, cardiac arrhythmias associated with tachycardia, tachycardia caused by digitalis intoxication

Warnings Use caution in patients with unstable vasomotor symptoms, diabetes, hyperthyroidism, prostatic hypertrophy, or a history of seizures; also use caution in the elderly and those patients with cardiovascular disorders such as coronary artery disease, arrhythmias, and hypertension

Precautions Excessive or prolonged use may lead to tolerance; paradoxical bronchoconstriction may occur with excessive use, if it occurs, discontinue terbutaline immediately. Deaths have been reported after excessive use of sympathomimetics; though the exact cause is unknown, cardiac arrest after a severe asthmatic crisis is suspected.

Adverse Reactions

Cardiovascular: Tachycardia, palpitations, elevation or depression of blood pressure

Central nervous system: Nervousness, CNS stimulation, hyperactivity, insomnia

Gastrointestinal: GI upset

Neuromuscular: Tremors (may be more common in the elderly)

Overdosage Symptoms of overdose include hypertension, tachycardia, seizures, angina, hypokalemia, and tachyarrhythmias

Toxicology In cases of overdose, supportive therapy should be instituted, and prudent use of a cardioselective beta-adrenergic blocker (eg, atenolol or metoprolol) should be considered, keeping in mind the potential for induction of bronchoconstriction in an asthmatic individual. Dialysis has not been shown to be of value in the treatment of an overdose with this agent.

Drug Interactions

Decreased therapeutic effect: Beta-adrenergic blockers (eg, propranolol)

Increased therapeutic effect: Inhaled ipratropium → ↑ duration of bronchodilation, nifedipine → ↑ FEV-1

Increased toxicity (cardiovascular): MAO inhibitors, tricyclic antidepressants, sympathomimetic agents (eg, amphetamine, dopamine, dobutamine), inhaled anesthetics (eg, enflurane)

Stability Store injection at room temperature; protect from heat, light, and from freezing; use only clear solutions

Mechanism of Action Relaxes bronchial smooth muscle by action on $beta_2$-receptors with less effect on heart rate (minor $beta_1$ activity)

Pharmacodynamics S.C. doses are more bioavailable and of quicker onset than oral doses

Onset of action:

Oral: Within 30-45 minutes

Inhalation: 5-30 minutes

S.C.: Within 6-15 minutes

Duration of action:

Oral: 4-8 hours

(Continued)

Terbutaline Sulfate *(Continued)*

    Inhalation: 3-6 hours
    S.C.: 1.5-4 hours

Pharmacokinetics
    Protein binding: 25%
    Metabolism: In the liver to inactive sulfate conjugates
    Half-life: 11-16 hours
    Elimination: In urine

Usual Dosage Geriatrics and Adults:
    Oral: 2.5-5 mg/dose every 8 hours; maintenance: do not exceed 15 mg/24 hours
    S.C.: 0.25 mg/dose repeated in 15-30 minutes for one time only; a total dose of 0.5 mg
    should not be exceeded within a 4-hour period. **Note:** Side effects to S.C. dose are
    similar to epinephrine in severity.
    Inhalation: 2 puffs every 4-6 hours

Monitoring Parameters Pulmonary function, blood pressure, pulse

Patient Information Do not exceed recommended dosage; rinse mouth with water
following each inhalation to help with dry throat and mouth. Follow specific instructions accompanying inhaler. If more than one inhalation is necessary, wait at least 1
full minute between inhalations. May cause nervousness, restlessness, insomnia – if
these effects continue after dosage reduction, notify physician. Also notify physician
if palpitations, tachycardia, chest pain, muscle tremors, dizziness, headache, flushing, or if breathing difficulty persists.

Nursing Implications Parenteral form is only for S.C. use. Before using, the inhaler
must be shaken well; assess lung sounds, pulse, and blood pressure before administration and during peak of medication; observe patient for wheezing after administration, if this occurs, call physician

Special Geriatric Considerations Oral terbutaline should be avoided in the elderly
due to the increased incidence of adverse effects as compared to the inhaled form.
Elderly patients may find it useful to utilize a spacer device when using the metered
dose inhaler. Difficulty in using the inhaler often limits its effectiveness.

Dosage Forms
    Aerosol: 0.2 mg/actuation (10.5 g) (~300 inhalations)
    Injection: 1 mg/mL (1 mL)
    Tablet: 2.5 mg, 5 mg

Terconazole *(ter kone' a zole)*

Brand Names Terazol® 7
Synonyms Triaconazole
Therapeutic Class Antifungal Agent, Vaginal
Use Local treatment of vulvovaginal candidiasis
Adverse Reactions
    Central nervous system: Headache
    Dermatologic: Hives, rash
    Local: Irritation, burning, itching
    Neuromuscular & skeletal: Myalgia

Mechanism of Action Exact mechanism of action is unknown; it is proposed that terconazole disrupts fungal cell wall permeability

Pharmacokinetics Absorption: Extent of systemic absorption after vaginal administration may be dependent on the presence of a uterus; 5% to 8% in women who had a
hysterectomy versus 12% to 16% in nonhysterectomized women

Usual Dosage Geriatrics and Adults: One applicatorful in vagina at bedtime for 7 consecutive days

Monitoring Parameters Response to treatment

Patient Information Follow directions included with products; complete full course of
therapy; notify physician if irritating; use sanitary napkin to protect clothing

Nursing Implications Watch for local irritation; assist patient in administration, if necessary

Special Geriatric Considerations Assess patient's ability to self-administer, may be
difficult in patients with arthritis or limited range of motion

Dosage Forms Cream, vaginal: 0.4% (45 g)

References
    Drug Facts and Comparisons, St Louis, MO: 1989, 528-9.

Terfenadine *(ter fen' a deen)*

Brand Names Seldane®
Generic Available No
Therapeutic Class Antihistamine
Use Perennial and seasonal allergic rhinitis and other allergic symptoms including urti-
caria
Contraindications Hypersensitivity to terfenadine or any component
Warnings Rare cases of serious cardiovascular events (cardiac arrest, torsade de
pointes, Q-T prolongation, ventricular arrhythmias, death) have been reported in pa-

tients on terfenadine in the following situations: impaired liver function, concomitant use of macrolide antibiotics or ketoconazole or itraconazole, overdose (including single doses as low as 360 mg)

Adverse Reactions
Cardiovascular: See Warnings
Central nervous system: Sedation, fatigue, dizziness, nervousness, mental depression, insomnia, confusion, headache
Dermatologic: Rash
Gastrointestinal: Nausea, vomiting, weight gain, dry mouth
Hepatic: Elevation in liver enzymes
Neuromuscular & skeletal: Tremors, weakness
Respiratory: Cough, sore throat
Note: Minimal sedation and anticholinergic effects as compared to older antihistamines

Overdosage Symptoms of overdose include nausea, confusion, sedation, prolonged Q-T interval, torsade de pointes

Toxicology Lidocaine has been used successfully to treat cardiac arrhythmias; avoid type I antiarrhythmics, torsade may respond to I.V. magnesium. Patients should be carefully observed with EKG monitoring in cases of suspected overdose.

Drug Interactions Serious cardiac events have occurred with elevated terfenadine levels
Increased effect with pseudoephedrine
Increased toxicity with ketoconazole, itraconazole, fluconazole, metronidazole, miconazole, erythromycin, troleandomycin, azithromycin, clarithromycin, cimetidine, bepridil, psychotropics, probucol, astemizole, carbamazepine

Stability Keep away from direct sunlight

Mechanism of Action Competes with histamine for H_1-receptor sites on effector cells in the gastrointestinal tract, blood vessels, and respiratory tract; binds to lung receptors significantly greater than it binds to cerebellar receptors, resulting in a reduced sedative potential

Pharmacodynamics
Therapeutic effects and peak serum levels: Within 1-2 hours
Duration of antihistaminic effects: Up to 12 hours

Pharmacokinetics
Metabolism: Extensive first-pass; metabolized in the liver
Half-life: 16-22 hours
Time to peak: Oral:
Elimination: Primarily in feces and secondarily in urine

Usual Dosage Oral:
Geriatrics: 60 mg once or twice daily
Adults: 60 mg twice daily

Monitoring Parameters Relief of symptoms, mental status

Test Interactions Antigen skin testing procedures

Patient Information Drink plenty of water, may cause GI upset, take with food; do not exceed recommended dose; may cause drowsiness

Nursing Implications Give with food; see Monitoring Parameters

Special Geriatric Considerations Because of its low incidence of sedation and anticholinergic effects, terfenadine would be a rational choice in the elderly when an antihistamine is indicated; see Warnings

Dosage Forms Tablet: 60 mg

Terramycin® IV see Oxytetracycline Hydrochloride on page 531

Tessalon® Perles see Benzonatate on page 78

Tetanus and Diphtheria Toxoid see Diphtheria and Tetanus Toxoid on page 231

Tetanus Antitoxin (tet' n us)

Synonyms TAT

Therapeutic Class Antitoxin

Use Tetanus prophylaxis or treatment of active tetanus only when tetanus immune globulin (TIG) is not available; may be given concomitantly with tetanus toxoid adsorbed when immediate treatment is required, but active immunization is desirable

Contraindications Patients sensitive to equine-derived preparations

Warnings Tetanus antitoxin is not the same as tetanus immune globulin

Adverse Reactions
Dermatologic: Skin eruptions, erythema, urticaria
Local: Local pain, numbness
Neuromuscular & skeletal: Joint pain
Miscellaneous: Anaphylaxis, serum sickness may develop up to several weeks after injection in 10% of patients

Stability Refrigerate

Mechanism of Action Solution of concentrated globulins containing antitoxic antibodies obtained from horse serum after immunization against tetanus toxin

(Continued)

Tetanus Antitoxin *(Continued)*

Pharmacodynamics Protection from antitoxin lasts 15 days; this time is decreased in individuals who have received horse serum injections

Usual Dosage Geriatrics and Adults:

Prophylaxis (perform equine serum sensitivity tests): I.M., S.C.: >30 kg: 3000-5000 units

Treatment: Inject 10,000-40,000 units into wound; give 40,000-100,000 units I.V.; preferable to give part of I.V. dose I.M. or into wound; see Additional Information

Nursing Implications All patients should have sensitivity testing prior to starting therapy with tetanus antitoxin

Additional Information Tetanus immune globulin (Hyper-Tet®) is the preferred tetanus immunoglobulin for the treatment of active tetanus

Special Geriatric Considerations Tetanus is a rare disease in U.S. with <100 cases annually; 66% of cases occur in persons >50 years of age; protective tetanus and diphtheria antibodies decline with age; it is estimated that <50% of elderly are protected.

Elderly are at risk because:
Many lack proper immunization maintenance
Higher case fatality ratio
Immunizations are not available from childhood

Indications for vaccination:
Primary series with combined tetanus-diphtheria (Td) should be given to all elderly lacking a clean history of vaccination
Boosters should be given at 10-year intervals; earlier for wounds
Elderly are more likely to require tetanus immune globulin with infection of tetanus due to lower antibody titer

Dosage Forms Injection, equine: Not less than 400 units/mL in 5,000 and 20,000 unit vials

Tetanus Immune Globulin, Human

Related Information
Immunization Guidelines *on page 759-762*

Brand Names Hyper-Tet®

Synonyms TIG

Therapeutic Class Immune Globulin

Use Passive immunization against tetanus

Contraindications Hypersensitivity to tetanus immune globulin, thimerosal, or any immune globulin product or component; patients with IgA deficiency; I.V. administration

Warnings Have epinephrine 1:1000 available for anaphylactic reactions; do not give I.V.

Precautions TIG is preferred over tetanus antitoxin for passive immunity; tetanus antitoxin should only be used when TIG is unavailable due to high risk of adverse effects (ie, serum sickness); skin testing should not be done

Adverse Reactions
Central nervous system: Fever (mild), lethargy
Dermatologic: Hives, angioedema
Gastrointestinal: Nausea
Local: Pain, tenderness, erythema
Neuromuscular & skeletal: Muscle stiffness, myalgia
Respiratory: Chest tightness
Miscellaneous: Anaphylaxis reaction

Drug Interactions Never administer tetanus toxoid and TIG in same syringe (toxoid will be neutralized); toxoid may be given at a separate site

Stability Refrigerate at 2°C to 8°C (36°F to 46°F)

Mechanism of Action If given at time of injury, it will not interfere with primary immune response to tetanus toxoid given at a separate site

Pharmacokinetics Half-life (tetanus toxoids): 3.5-4.5 weeks

Usual Dosage Geriatrics and Adults: I.M.:
Prophylaxis of tetanus: 250 units
Treatment of tetanus: 3000-6000 units

Monitoring Parameters Monitor for hypersensitivity reactions

Patient Information Be aware of adverse reactions

Nursing Implications Do not administer I.V.

Additional Information Tetanus immune globulin is preferred over tetanus antitoxin for treatment of active tetanus

Special Geriatric Considerations Tetanus is a rare disease in U.S. with <100 cases annually; 66% of cases occur in persons >50 years of age; protective tetanus and diphtheria antibodies decline with age; it is estimated that <50% of elderly are protected.

Elderly are at risk because:
Many lack proper immunization maintenance

Higher case fatality ratio

Immunizations are not available from childhood

Indications for vaccination:

Primary series with combined tetanus-diphtheria (Td) should be given to all elderly lacking a clear history of vaccination

Boosters should be given at 10-year intervals; earlier for wounds

Elderly are more likely to require tetanus immune globulin with infection of tetanus due to lower antibody titer

Dosage Forms Injection: 250 units

Tetanus Toxoid Adsorbed

Related Information

Immunization Guidelines *on page 759-762*

Therapeutic Class Toxoid

Use Active immunity against tetanus

Contraindications Hypersensitivity to tetanus toxoid or any component; acute respiratory infections or other active infections

Warnings Not equivalent to tetanus toxoid fluid; the tetanus toxoid adsorbed is the preferred toxoid for immunization; do not use to treat active tetanus infections or use for immediate prophylaxis; allergic reactions, have epinephrine 1:1000 available for anaphylactic reactions

Precautions Avoid use in patients who receive immunosuppressive therapy or have immunodeficiency diseases; do not give I.V.

Adverse Reactions

Cardiovascular: Flushing, tachycardia, hypotension

Central nervous system: Malaise and transient fever, rarely neurological disturbances (radial nerve paralysis, difficulty swallowing), chills

Dermatologic: Urticaria, rash, pruritus

Local: Redness, warmth, edema, induration, tenderness

Neuromuscular & skeletal: Generalized aches, pains

Miscellaneous: Arthus-type hypersensitivity reactions have occurred rarely in patients >25 years of age and who have received multiple booster doses

Drug Interactions If primary immunization is started in individuals receiving an immunosuppressive agent, serologic testing may be needed to ensure adequate antibody response; chloramphenicol may interfere with response

Stability Refrigerate, do not freeze

Mechanism of Action Boosters are necessary every 10 years: 0.5 mL

Usual Dosage Geriatrics and Adults: I.M.: 0.5 mL in deltoid or midlateral thigh muscles; primary immunization requires 2 injections 4-8 weeks apart; give a third injection 6-12 months after second injection; boosters every 10 years

Patient Information Be aware of adverse reactions

Nursing Implications Inject intramuscularly in the area of the vastus lateralis (midthigh laterally) or deltoid

Additional Information Routine booster doses are recommended only every 10 years

Special Geriatric Considerations Tetanus is a rare disease in U.S. with <100 cases annually; 66% of cases occur in persons >50 years of age; protective tetanus and diphtheria antibodies decline with age; it is estimated that <50% of elderly are protected.

Elderly are at risk because:

Many lack proper immunization maintenance

Higher case fatality ratio

Immunizations are not available from childhood

Indications for vaccination:

Primary series with combined tetanus-diphtheria (Td) should be given to all elderly lacking a clean history of vaccination

Boosters should be given at 10-year intervals; earlier for wounds

Elderly are more likely to require tetanus immune globulin with infection of tetanus due to lower antibody titer

Dosage Forms Injection: Adsorbed: Tetanus 5 Lf units per 0.5 mL dose (0.5 mL, 5 mL); tetanus 10 Lf units per 2.5 mL dose (5 mL)

References

Bentley DW, "Vaccinations," *Clin Geriatr Med*, 1992, 8(4):745-60.
Gardner P and Schaffner W, "Immunization of Adults," *N Engl J Med*, 1993, 328(17):1252-8.

Tetanus Toxoid, Fluid

Related Information

Immunization Guidelines *on page 759-762*

Synonyms Tetanus Toxoid Plain

Therapeutic Class Toxoid

Use Active immunization against tetanus in adults

Contraindications Prior hypersensitivity reactions, neurological signs or symptoms

(Continued)

Tetanus Toxoid, Fluid *(Continued)*

after prior administrations; respiratory infections or other active infections or use for immediate prophylaxis; allergic reactions, have epinephrine 1:1000 available to treat anaphylactic reactions

Warnings For primary immunization, tetanus toxoid, absorbed is preferred; do not use to treat active infections

Precautions Concomitant immunosuppressive therapy, allergic reactions; do not give I.V.

Adverse Reactions
Cardiovascular: Flushing, tachycardia, hypotension
Central nervous system: Malaise and transient fever, chills, rarely neurological disturbances (radial nerve paralysis, difficulty swallowing)
Dermatologic: Urticaria, rash, pruritus
Local: Redness, warmth, edema, induration, tenderness
Neuromuscular & skeletal: Generalized aches, pains
Miscellaneous: Arthus-type hypersensitivity reactions have occurred rarely in patients >25 years of age and who have received multiple booster doses

Reactions rarely occur in patients receiving tetanus toxoid fluid intradermally

Drug Interactions If primary immunization is started in individuals receiving an immunosuppressive agent, serologic testing may be needed to ensure adequate antibody response; chloramphenicol may interfere with response

Stability Refrigerate, do not freeze

Usual Dosage Geriatrics and Adults: Inject 3 doses of 0.5 mL I.M. or S.C. at 4- to 8-week intervals with fourth dose given only 6-12 months after third dose; boosters every 10 years

Patient Information A nodule may be palpable at the injection site for a few weeks; be aware of adverse reactions

Nursing Implications Must not be used I.V.

Additional Information Tetanus toxoid, adsorbed is preferred for all basic immunizing and recall reactions because of more persistent antitoxin titer induction

Special Geriatric Considerations Tetanus is a rare disease in U.S. with <100 cases annually; 66% of cases occur in persons >50 years of age; protective tetanus and diphtheria antibodies decline with age; it is estimated that <50% of elderly are protected.

Elderly are at risk because:
Many lack proper immunization maintenance
Higher case fatality ratio
Immunizations are not available from childhood
Indications for vaccination:
Primary series with combined tetanus-diphtheria (Td) should be given to all elderly lacking a clean history of vaccination
Boosters should be given at 10-year intervals; earlier for wounds
Elderly are more likely to require tetanus immune globulin with infection of tetanus due to lower antibody titer

Dosage Forms Injection: Fluid: Tetanus 4 Lf units per 0.5 mL dose (7.5 mL); tetanus 5 Lf units per 0.5 mL dose (0.5 mL, 7.5 mL)

References
Gardner P and Schaffner W, "Immunization of Adults," *N Engl J Med*, 1993, 328(17):1252-8.

Tetanus Toxoid Plain *see Tetanus Toxoid, Fluid on previous page*

Tetraclear® [OTC] *see Tetrahydrozoline Hydrochloride on page 680*

Tetracycline *(tet ra sye' kleen)*
Related Information
Antacid Drug Interactions *on page 764*

Brand Names Achromycin®; Achromycin® V; Nor-tet®; Panmycin®; Robitet®; Sumycin®; Teline®; Tetracyn®; Tetralan®; Topicycline®

Synonyms TCN; Tetracycline Hydrochloride

Therapeutic Class Acne Products; Antibiotic, Ophthalmic; Antibiotic, Tetracycline Derivative; Antibiotic, Topical

Use Treatment of susceptible bacterial infections of both gram-positive and gram-negative organisms; also some unusual organisms including *Mycoplasma*, *Chlamydia*, and *Rickettsia*; may also be used for acne, exacerbations of chronic bronchitis, and treatment of gonorrhea and syphilis in patients that are allergic to penicillin

Contraindications Hypersensitivity to tetracycline or any component

Warnings Photosensitivity reaction may occur with this drug; avoid prolonged exposure to sunlight or tanning equipment; wear sunscreen

Precautions Outdated drug can cause nephropathy, throw away any unused medication

Adverse Reactions
Central nervous system: Pseudotumor cerebri, fever

Dermatologic: Rash, photosensitivity

Gastrointestinal: Nausea, vomiting, diarrhea, stomatitis, glossitis, antibiotic-associated pseudomembranous colitis

Hepatic: Hepatotoxicity

Neuromuscular & skeletal: Injury to growing bones and teeth

Renal: Renal damage

Miscellaneous: Hypersensitivity reactions, candidal superinfection, Fanconi-like syndrome

Overdosage Symptoms of overdose include photosensitivity, nausea, anorexia, diarrhea

Drug Interactions Calcium-, magnesium-, or aluminum-containing antacids and sodium bicarbonate (decreased tetracyclic absorption); iron, methoxyflurane, zinc, penicillins, cimetidine (decreased dissolution), oral anticoagulants, lithium (increased or decreased concentrations)

Food/Drug Interactions Do not take with food, take 1 hour before or 2 hours after meals

Stability Outdated tetracyclines have caused a Fanconi-like syndrome; reconstituted I.M. solution is stable for 24 hours at room temperature

Mechanism of Action Inhibits bacterial protein synthesis by binding with the 30S and possibly the 50S ribosomal subunit(s) of susceptible bacteria; may also cause alterations in the cytoplasmic membrane

Pharmacodynamics Bacteriostatic

Pharmacokinetics

Absorption:

Oral: 75%

I.M.: Poor with <60% of dose absorbed (the I.M. route is reserved for situations where oral therapy is not feasible)

Protein binding: 65%

Half-life: Normal renal function: 8-11 hours

Time to peak: Oral: Peak serum levels appear within 2-4 hours

Elimination: Primary route of elimination is the kidney, with 60% of a dose excreted as unchanged drug in urine; small amount appears in bile

Usual Dosage See manufacturer's and CDC's specific dosing recommendations by indication

Geriatrics and Adults:

Oral: 250-500 mg/dose every 6-12 hours

Ophthalmic:

Suspension: Instill 1-2 drops 2-4 times/day

Ointment: Instill every 2-12 hours

I.M.: 250-300 mg/day divided every 8-12 hours

I.V.: 250-500 mg every 12 hours; maximum: 500 mg every 6 hours

Slightly dialyzable (5% to 20%)

Administration Do not give I.M. injection I.V., or I.V. injection I.M. (specific products available for each). I.V. should be infused over at least 2 hours

Monitoring Parameters Temperature, WBC, cultures and sensitivity (if applicable), appetite, mental status

Reference Range Therapeutic: Not established; Toxic: >16 μg/mL

Test Interactions False-negative urine glucose with Clinistix®

Patient Information Take 1 hour before or 2 hours after meals with adequate amounts of fluid; avoid prolonged exposure to sunlight or sunlamps; avoid taking antacids, iron, or dairy products with tetracyclines

Nursing Implications See Administration

Additional Information Use of tetracycline in animal feed has caused emergence of resistant organisms

Tetracycline: Achromycin® V oral suspension, Sumycin® syrup, Tetralan® syrup

Tetracycline hydrochloride: Achromycin® injection, Achromycin® V capsule, Nor-tet® capsule, Panmycin® capsule, Robitet® capsule, Sumycin® capsule and tablet, Teline® capsule, Tetracyn® capsule, Tetralan® capsule

Special Geriatric Considerations The role of tetracycline has decreased because of the emergence of resistant organisms. Doxycycline is the tetracycline of choice when one is indicated because of its better GI absorption, less interactions with divalent cations, longer half-life, and the fact that the majority is cleared by nonrenal mechanisms

Dosage Forms

Capsule: 100 mg, 250 mg, 500 mg

Elixir: 80 mg/15 mL (15 mL, 30 mL, 473 mL, 946 mL)

Injection:

I.M.: 100 mg, 250 mg

I.V.: 250 mg, 500 mg

Ointment, ophthalmic: 1% (3.75 mg)

Solution, topical: 2.2 mg/mL (70 mL)

(Continued)

Tetracycline (Continued)

Suspension:
Ophthalmic: 1% (0.5 mL, 1 mL, 4 mL)
Oral: 125 mg/5 mL (60 mL, 480 mL)
Syrup: 80 mg/15 mL (15 mL, 30 mL, 120 mL); 150 mg/15 mL (480 mL)
Tablet: 250 mg, 500 mg

References

Yoshikawa TT, "Antimicrobial Therapy for the Elderly Patient," *J Am Geriatr Soc*, 1990, 38(12):1353-72.

Tetracycline Hydrochloride *see* Tetracycline *on page 678*

Tetracyn® *see* Tetracycline *on page 678*

Tetrahydroaminoacrine *see* Tacrine Hydrochloride *on page 668*

Tetrahydrozoline Hydrochloride (tet ra hye drozz' a leen)

Brand Names Collyrium Fresh® [OTC]; Eye-Zine® [OTC]; Murine® Plus [OTC]; Ocu Drop® [OTC]; Optigene® [OTC]; Soothe® [OTC]; Tetraclear® [OTC]; Tetra-Ide [OTC]; Tyzine®; Visine® [OTC]; Visine A.C.® [OTC]

Synonyms Tetryzoline

Generic Available Yes

Therapeutic Class Adrenergic Agonist Agent; Adrenergic Agonist Agent, Ophthalmic Nasal Agent, Vasoconstrictor; Ophthalmic Agent, Vasoconstrictor

Use Symptomatic relief of nasal congestion and conjunctival congestion

Contraindications Narrow-angle glaucoma, patients receiving MAO inhibitors, know hypersensitivity to tetrahydrozoline

Warnings Discontinue use prior to the use of anesthetics which sensitize the myocardium to the systemic effects of sympathomimetics

Precautions Use caution in patients with hypertension, diabetes, thyroid disorders heart disease, and asthma

Adverse Reactions

Cardiovascular: Tachycardia, palpitations, increased blood pressure, heart rate
Central nervous system: Headache
Local: Stinging, sneezing
Neuromuscular & skeletal: Tremors
Ocular: Blurred vision
Miscellaneous: Sweating

Overdosage Symptoms of overdose include CNS depression, hypothermia, bradycardia, cardiovascular collapse, coma

Toxicology Following initiation of essential overdose management, toxic symptom should be treated. The patient should be kept warm and monitored for alterations vital functions. Seizures commonly respond to diazepam (5-10 mg I.V. bolus in adul every 15 minutes if needed up to a total of 30 mg) or to phenytoin or phenobarbita

Drug Interactions MAO inhibitors can cause an exaggerated adrenergic response taken concurrently or within 21 days of discontinuing MAO inhibitors; beta-blocke can cause hypertensive episodes and increased risk of intracranial hemorrhage; a esthetics

Mechanism of Action Stimulates alpha-adrenergic receptors in the arterioles of th conjunctiva and the nasal mucosa to produce vasoconstriction

Pharmacodynamics

Onset of action: Intranasal: Decongestant effects occur within 4-8 hours
Duration: Ophthalmic vasoconstriction lasts 2-3 hours

Pharmacokinetics Absorption: Topical: Systemic absorption sometimes occurs

Usual Dosage Geriatrics and Adults:

Nasal congestion: Instill 2-4 drops or 3-4 sprays of 0.1% solution to the nasal mucos every 3-6 hours as needed

Conjunctival congestion: Instill 1-2 drops in each eye 2-4 times/day

Administration See Patient Information and package instructions

Monitoring Parameters Blood pressure, heart rate, symptom response

Patient Information Remove contact lenses before using in eye; do not use >7 hours; consult physician of changes in vision or visual acuity occur; do not excee recommended dose or duration to avoid rebound congestion

Nursing Implications Do not use for longer than 3-4 days without direct physician s pervision

Special Geriatric Considerations See Precautions and Usual Dosage; use with ca tion in patients with cardiovascular disease

Dosage Forms Solution:

Nasal: (Tyzine®): 0.05%, 0.1%
Ophthalmic:
Visine®: 0.05% (15 mL)
Visine A.C.®: 0.05% and zinc sulfate 0.25% (15 mL)

Tetra-Ide® **[OTC]** *see* Tetrahydrozoline Hydrochloride *on previous page*

Tetralan® *see* Tetracycline *on page 678*

Tetryzoline *see* Tetrahydrozoline Hydrochloride *on previous page*

T-Gen® *see* Trimethobenzamide Hydrochloride *on page 720*

T-Gesic® *see* Hydrocodone and Acetaminophen *on page 350*

THA *see* Tacrine Hydrochloride *on page 668*

Theo-24® *see* Theophylline *on this page*

Theobid® *see* Theophylline *on this page*

Theochron® *see* Theophylline *on this page*

Theoclear® L.A. *see* Theophylline *on this page*

Theo-Dur® *see* Theophylline *on this page*

Theolair™ *see* Theophylline *on this page*

Theon® *see* Theophylline *on this page*

Theophylline (thee off' i lin)
Related Information
Drug Levels Commonly Monitored Guidelines *on page 771-772*
Brand Names Accurbron®; Aerolate®; Aerolate III®; Aerolate JR®; Aerolate SR® S; Aquaphyllin®; Asmalix®; Bronkodyl®; Constant-T®; Duraphyl™; Elixicon®; Elixophyllin®; Elixophyllin® SR; LaBID®; Lixolin®; Lodrane®; Quibron®-T; Quibron®-T/SR; Respbid®; Slo-bid™; Slo-Phyllin®; Somophyllin®-CRT; Somophyllin®-T; Sustaire®; Theo-24®; Theobid®; Theochron®; Theoclear® L.A.; Theo-Dur®; Theolair™; Theon®; Theophyl-SR®; Theospan®-SR; Theo-Time®; Theovent®; Uniphyl®
Synonyms Theophylline Anhydrous
Generic Available Yes
Therapeutic Class Antiasthmatic; Bronchodilator; Theophylline Derivative
Use Bronchodilator in reversible bronchospasm due to asthma, chronic bronchitis, and emphysema
Contraindications Hypersensitivity to xanthines; peptic ulcer, uncontrolled seizure disorders, uncontrolled arrhythmias
Warnings May precipitate or worsen pre-existing arrhythmias
Precautions Use with caution in patients with peptic ulcer, hyperthyroidism, hypertension, and patients with compromised cardiac function; hepatic function, esophageal reflux disease, alcoholism, and elderly
Adverse Reactions Adverse reactions are uncommon at serum theophylline concentrations <20 µg/mL

Cardiovascular: Palpitations, sinus tachycardia, extrasystoles, hypotension, ventricular arrhythmias, flushing
Central nervous system: Irritability, restlessness, fever, headache, insomnia, seizures
Endocrine & metabolic: Hyperglycemia
Gastrointestinal: Nausea, vomiting, esophageal reflux, diarrhea, hematemesis, rectal bleeding, epigastric pain
Genitourinary: Diuresis
Neuromuscular & skeletal: Tremors, muscle twitching
Renal: Proteinuria
Respiratory: Tachypnea, respiratory arrest
Overdosage Symptoms of overdose include tachycardia, extrasystoles, nausea, vomiting, anorexia, tonic-clonic seizures, insomnia, circulatory failure; agitation, irritability, headache
Toxicology If seizures have not occurred, induce vomiting; ipecac syrup is preferred. Do not induce emesis in the presence of impaired consciousness. Repeated doses of charcoal have been shown to be effective in enhancing the total body clearance of theophylline. Do not repeat charcoal doses if an ileus is present. Charcoal hemoperfusion may be considered if the serum theophylline level exceed 40 mcg/mL, the patient is unable to tolerate repeat oral charcoal administrations, or if severe toxic symptoms are present. Clearance with hemoperfusion is better than clearance from hemodialysis. Administer a cathartic, especially if sustained release agents were used. Phenobarbital administered prophylactically may prevent seizures.
Drug Interactions
Changes in diet may affect the elimination of theophylline; theophylline may decrease the effects of phenytoin, lithium, and neuromuscular blocking agents
Theophylline increases the excretion of lithium; theophylline may have synergistic toxicity with sympathomimetics
Cimetidine, ranitidine, allopurinol, beta-blockers (nonspecific), erythromycin, influenza virus vaccine, corticosteroids, ephedrine, quinolones, thyroid hormones, oral contraceptives, amiodarone, troleandomycin, clindamycin, carbamazepine, isoniazid, loop diuretics, and lincomycin may increase theophylline concentrations

(Continued)

Theophylline *(Continued)*

Cigarette and marijuana smoking, rifampin, barbiturates, hydantoins, ketoconazole, sulfinpyrazone, sympathomimetics, isoniazid, loop diuretics, carbamazepine, and aminoglutethimide may decrease theophylline concentrations

Tetracyclines enhance toxicity and benzodiazepine's action may be antagonized; see table.

Factors Reported to Affect Theophylline Serum Levels

Decreased Theophylline Level	Increased Theophylline Level
Smoking (cigarettes, marijuana)	Hepatic cirrhosis
High protein/low carbohydrate diet	Cor pulmonale
Charcoal broiled beef	CHF
Phenytoin	Fever/viral illness
Phenobarbital	Propranolol
Carbamazepine	Allopurinol (>600 mg/d)
Rifampin	Erythromycin
I.V. isoproterenol	Cimetidine
	Troleandomycin
	Ciprofloxacin
	Oral contraceptives

Stability Store injection at room temperature; protect from heat and from freezing; use only clear solutions

Stability of parenteral admixture at room temperature (25°C): 30 days

Stability of parenteral admixture at refrigeration temperature (4°C): Do not refrigerate

Mechanism of Action Causes bronchodilatation, diuresis, CNS and cardiac stimulation, and gastric acid secretion by blocking phosphodiesterase which increases tissue concentrations of cyclic adenine monophosphate (cAMP) which in turn promotes catecholamine stimulation of lipolysis, glycogenolysis, and gluconeogenesis and induces release of epinephrine from adrenal medulla cells. Other proposed mechanisms include inhibition of extracellular adenosine, stimulation of endogenous catecholamines, antagonism of PGE_2 and $PGE_{2\alpha}$, mobilization of intracellular calcium, and increased sensitivity of beta-adrenergic receptors in reactive airways.

Pharmacokinetics

Absorption: Oral: Up to 100%, depending upon the formulation used

Distribution: V_d: 0.45 L/kg

Metabolism: In the liver by demethylation

Half-life: Varies from 3-15 hours in healthy adults (nonsmokers); 4-5 hours in smokers (1-2 packs/day); see table.

Half–life (h)	Patient Population
7–9	Normal healthy geriatrics/adults
18–24	Severe congestive heart failure
29	Cirrhosis

Time to peak: Peak plasma concentrations reached in 1-2 hours, 4 hours for sustained release

Elimination: In urine; adults excrete 10% in urine as unchanged drug

Usual Dosage See aminophylline for I.V. doses

Geriatrics and Adults:

Initial dosage recommendation: Loading dose (to achieve a serum level of about 10 mcg/mL; loading doses should be given using a rapidly absorbed oral product **not** a sustained release product):

If no theophylline has been administered in the previous 24 hours: 4-6 mg/kg theophylline

If theophylline has been administered in the previous 24 hours: Administer $\frac{1}{2}$ loading dose; 2-3 mg/kg theophylline can be given in emergencies when serum levels are not available

On the average, for every 1 mg/kg theophylline given, blood levels will rise 2 mcg/mL

Maintenance dose: See table.

Oral:

Nonsustained release: 16-20 mg/kg/day divided into 4 doses/day

Sustained release: 9-13 mg/kg/day divided into 2-3 doses/day

These recommendations, based on mean clearance rates for age or risk factors, were calculated to achieve a serum level of 10 mcg/mL. In healthy adults, a slow-release product can be used (9-13 mg/kg in divided dose). The total daily dose can be divided every 8-12 hours. Geriatrics should be started with a 25% reduction.

Maintenance Dose for Acute Symptoms

Population Group	Oral Theophylline (mg/kg/day)	I.V. Aminophylline
Healthy nonsmoking adults (including elderly patients)	10 (not to exceed 900 mg/day)	0.5 mg/kg/hour
Cardiac decompensation, cor pulmonale and/or liver dysfunction	5 (not to exceed 400 mg/day)	0.25 mg/kg/hour

*For continuous I.V. infusion divide total daily dose by 24 = mg/kg/hour.

Use ideal body weight for obese patients

Dose should be adjusted further based on serum levels. Guidelines for obtaining theophylline serum levels are shown in the table.

Guidelines for Obtaining Theophylline Serum Levels

Dosage Form	Time to Obtain Level
I.V. bolus	30 min after end of 30 min infusion
I.V. continuous infusion	12–24 h after initiation of infusion
P.O. liquid, fast–release tab	Peak: 1 h post a dose after at least 1 day of therapy Trough: Just before a dose after at least 1 day of therapy
P.O. slow–release product	Peak: 4 h post a dose after at least 1 day of therapy Trough: Just before a dose after at least 1 day of therapy

Monitoring Parameters Heart rate, CNS effects (insomnia, irritability); respiratory rate (COPD patients often have resting controlled respiratory rates in low 20's)

Reference Range

Sample size: 0.5-1 mL serum (red top tube)

Therapeutic: 10-20 μg/mL; Toxic: >20 μg/mL; some patients may have adequate clinical response with serum levels from 5-10 μg/mL

Timing of serum samples: If toxicity is suspected, obtain a level any time during a continuous I.V. infusion, or 2 hours after an oral dose; if lack of therapeutic is affected, draw a trough immediately before the next oral dose or intermittent I.V. dose

Test Interactions May elevate uric acid levels

Patient Information Oral preparations should be taken with a full glass of water; avoid drinking or eating large quantities of caffeine-containing beverages or food; take at regular intervals; take sustained release tablets whole; sustained release capsule forms may be opened and sprinkled on soft foods; do not chew beads; take with food if GI upset occurs; notify physician if nausea, vomiting, insomnia, nervousness, irritability, palpitations, seizures occur; do not change from one brand to another without consulting physician and pharmacist; do not change doses without consulting your physician

Nursing Implications Give oral and I.V. administration around-the-clock rather than 4 times/day, 3 times/day, etc (ie, 12-6-12-6, not 9-1-5-9) to promote less variation in peak and trough serum levels; do not crush sustained release drug products; do not crush enteric coated drug product; monitor vital signs, serum concentrations, and CNS effects (insomnia, irritability); encourage patient to drink adequate fluids (2 L/day) to decrease mucous viscosity in airways

Additional Information Saliva levels are approximately equal to 60% of plasma levels. Charcoal-broiled foods may increase elimination, reducing half-life by 50%; cigarette smoking may require an increase of dosage by 50% to 100%. Because different salts of theophylline have different theophylline content, various salts are equivalent. The following are percent content of theophylline for various salts:

Theophylline anhydrous: 100%
Theophylline monohydrate: 91%
Aminophylline anhydrous: 86%
Oxtriphylline: 64%

Most preparations are now labeled with actual milligram content delivered by the particular product.

Theophylline immediate release tablet/capsule: Bronkodyl®, Elixophyllin®, Quibron®-T, Slo-Phyllin®, Somophyllin®-T, Theolair™

Theophylline liquid: Accurbron®, Aerolate®, Aquaphyllin®, Asmalix®, Elixicon®, Elixophyllin®, Lixolin®, Theon®

(Continued)

683

Theophylline *(Continued)*

Theophylline timed release capsule: Aerolate III®, Aerolate JR®, Aerolate SR®, Elixophyllin® SR, Lodrane®, Slo-bid™ Gyrocaps®, Slo-Phyllin® Gyrocaps®, Somophyllin®-CRT, Theobid®, Theoclear® L.A., Theophyl-SR®, Theospan®-SR, Theospan®-SR

Theophylline timed release tablet: Constant-T®, Duraphyl™, LaBID®, Quibron®-T/S, Respbid®, Sustaire®, Theochron®, Theo-Dur®, Theolair™-SR, Theo-Time®, Uniphyl®

Special Geriatric Considerations Although there is a great intersubject variability for half-lives of methylxanthines (2-10 hours), elderly as a group have slower hepatic clearance. Therefore, use lower initial doses and monitor closely for response and adverse reactions. Additionally, elderly are at greater risk for toxicity due to concomitant disease (eg, CHF, arrhythmias), and drug use (eg, cimetidine, ciprofloxacin, etc); see Precautions and Drug Interactions

Dosage Forms

Capsule:
Immediate release: 100 mg, 200 mg
Sustained release (8-12 hours): 50 mg, 60 mg, 65 mg, 75 mg, 100 mg, 125 mg, 130 mg, 200 mg, 250 mg, 260 mg, 300 mg
Timed release:
12 hours: 50 mg, 75 mg, 125 mg, 130 mg, 200 mg, 250 mg, 260 mg
24 hours: 100 mg, 200 mg, 300 mg
Solution, oral: 80 mg/15 mL (15 mL, 30 mL, 500 mL); 150 mg/15 mL (480 mL)
Tablet: 125 mg, 250 mg
Tablet:
Immediate release: 100 mg, 125 mg, 200 mg, 250 mg, 300 mg
Sustained release: 100 mg, 200 mg, 300 mg
Timed release:
8-12 hours: 100 mg, 200 mg, 250 mg, 300 mg
8-24 hours: 100 mg, 200 mg, 250 mg, 300 mg, 500 mg
12-24 hours: 100 mg, 200 mg, 300 mg
24 hours: 400 mg

References

Kearney TE, Manoguerra AS, Curtis GP, et al, "Theophylline Toxicity and the Beta-Adrenergic System," *Ann Intern Med*, 1985, 102(6):766-9.

Mahler DA, Barlow PB, and Matthay RA, "Chronic Obstructive Pulmonary Disease," *Clin Geriatr Med*, 1986, 2(2):285-312.

Upton RA, "Pharmacokinetic Interactions Between Theophylline and Other Medication (Part I)," *Clin Pharmacokinet*, 1991, 20(1):66-80.

Theophylline Anhydrous see Theophylline *on page 681*

Theophylline Ethylenediamine see Aminophylline *on page 39*

Theophyl-SR® see Theophylline *on page 681*

Theospan®-SR see Theophylline *on page 681*

Theo-Time® see Theophylline *on page 681*

Theovent® see Theophylline *on page 681*

Thera-Flur® Gel see Fluoride *on page 299*

Theralax® [OTC] see Bisacodyl *on page 87*

Thermazene® see Silver Sulfadiazine *on page 644*

Thiamazole see Methimazole *on page 454*

Thioridazine *(thye oh rid' a zeen)*

Related Information
Antacid Drug Interactions *on page 764*
Antipsychotic Agents Comparison *on page 801*
Antipsychotic Medication Guidelines *on page 754*

Brand Names Mellaril®; Mellaril-S®

Synonyms Thioridazine Hydrochloride

Generic Available Yes

Therapeutic Class Antipsychotic Agent; Phenothiazine Derivative

Use Management of manifestations of psychotic disorders; depressive neurosis; alcohol withdrawal; nausea and vomiting; nonpsychotic symptoms associated with dementia in elderly; Tourette's syndrome; Huntington's chorea; spasmodic torticollis and Reye's syndrome; see Special Geriatric Considerations

Contraindications Severe CNS depression, hypersensitivity to thioridazine or any component; cross-sensitivity to other phenothiazines may exist; avoid use in patients with narrow-angle glaucoma, blood dyscrasias, severe liver or cardiac disease; subcortical brain damage; circulatory collapse; severe hypotension or hypertension

Warnings

Tardive dyskinesia: Prevalence rate may be 40% in elderly; elderly women especially at risk; embarrassment from dyskinesias may lead to greater social isolation; development of the syndrome and the irreversible nature are proportional to duration and total cumulative dose over time. May be reversible if diagnosed early in therapy; intermittent use of antipsychotics (not proven use) helps decrease total cumulative dose.

EPS: Extrapyramidal reactions are more common in elderly with up to 50% developing these reactions after age 60. These reactions may be more common in dementia patients. Drug-induced **Parkinson's syndrome** occurs often. Discontinuation usually resolves symptoms but may take weeks to months (12+) to clear. **Akathisia** is the most common EPS reaction in elderly. The symptoms of motor restlessness are difficult to diagnose in demented elderly; increased nervousness, assertiveness, restlessness with constant movement may indicate this adverse event. Consider decreasing dose if antipsychotic to treat as well as diagnose problem; usually see this reaction within 2-3 months of initiating antipsychotic drug.

Anticholinergic effects: These side effects most common with low potency antipsychotics (eg, thioridazine, chlorpromazine). CNS toxicity occurs more frequently and severely in elderly; increased confusion, memory loss, psychotic behavior, and agitation frequently occur as a consequence of anticholinergic effects to antipsychotic agents. Peripheral anticholinergic action troublesome to elderly; most peripheral anticholinergic effects last only 2-3 weeks; see Adverse Reactions.

Orthostatic hypotension: More common with low potency agents (eg, thioridazine, chlorpromazine, and clozapine) but of concern with all antipsychotic agents; orthostasis due to alpha-receptor blockade by antipsychotic agents. Elderly present many risk factors for orthostatic hypotension: blunted baroreceptor reflexes, decreased vascular tone, decreased vascular volume, and possible presence of cardiac diseases which result in decreased cardiac output.

Sedation: Common side effect with antipsychotic therapy; should not be used as a hypnotic unless insomnia is associated with target behavior symptoms treated with antipsychotic medications; see Special Geriatric Considerations. Anecdotal reports suggesting antipsychotic sedation in nonpsychotic patients is extremely unpleasant due to feelings of depersonalization, derealization, and dysphoria. Due to the long duration of action with antipsychotic drugs, these reactions may last up to 24 hours and result in decreased daytime function.

Cardiac toxicity: Life-threatening arrhythmias have occurred at therapeutic doses of antipsychotics. Thioridazine more commonly demonstrates EKG changes than other antipsychotics; suggested to use high potency antipsychotic agents (ie, haloperidol) in patients with cardiac conduction defects.

Precautions Use with caution in patients with severe cardiovascular disorder, seizures, and Parkinson's disease; benefits of therapy must be weighed against risks

Adverse Reactions
Cardiovascular: Orthostatic hypotension, tachycardia, arrhythmias, abnormal T waves with prolonged ventricular repolarization

Central nervous system: Sedation, drowsiness, restlessness, anxiety, extrapyramidal reactions, pseudoparkinsonian signs and symptoms, tardive dyskinesia, neuroleptic malignant syndrome, seizures, altered central temperature regulation

Dermatologic: Hyperpigmentation, pruritus, rash, photosensitivity

Endocrine & metabolic: Amenorrhea, galactorrhea, gynecomastia

Gastrointestinal: GI upset, dry mouth (problem for denture users), constipation, adynamic ileus, weight gain

Genitourinary: Urinary retention, overflow incontinence, priapism, impotence, sexual dysfunction (up to 60%)

Hematologic: Agranulocytosis, leukopenia (usually in patients with large doses for prolonged periods), thrombocytopenia, hemolytic anemia, eosinophilia

Hepatic: Cholestatic jaundice (rare)

Ocular: Retinal pigmentation, blurred vision

Miscellaneous: Anaphylactoid reactions

Overdosage Symptoms of overdose include deep sleep, coma, extrapyramidal symptoms, abnormal involuntary muscle movements, hypotension or hypertension; agitation, restlessness, fever, hypothermia or hyperthermia, seizures, cardiac arrhythmias, EKG changes

Toxicology Following initiation of essential overdose management, toxic symptom treatment and supportive treatment should be initiated. Hypotension usually responds to I.V. fluids or Trendelenburg positioning. If unresponsive to these measures the use of a parenteral inotrope may be required (eg, norepinephrine 0.1-0.2 mcg/kg/minute titrated to response). Do not use epinephrine. Seizures commonly respond to diazepam (I.V. 5-10 mg bolus in adults every 15 minutes if needed up to a total of 30 mg) or to phenytoin or phenobarbital. Also critical cardiac arrhythmias often respond to I.V. phenytoin (15 mg/kg up to 1 g), while other antiarrhythmics can be used. Neuroleptics often cause extrapyramidal symptoms (eg, dystonic reactions) requiring management with diphenhydramine 1-2 mg/kg up to a maximum of 50 mg I.M. or I.V. slow push followed by a maintenance dose for 48-72 hours. When these reactions are unresponsive to diphenhydramine, benztropine mesylate I.V. 1-2 mg may be effective. These agents are generally effective within 2-5 minutes.

(Continued)

Thioridazine *(Continued)*

Drug Interactions

Alcohol may increase CNS sedation

Anticholinergic agents may decrease pharmacologic effects; increase anticholinergic side effects; may enhance tardive dyskinesia

Aluminum salts may decrease absorption of phenothiazines

Barbiturates may decrease phenothiazine serum concentrations

Bromocriptine may have decreased efficacy when administered with phenothiazines

Guanethidine's hypotensive effect is decreased by phenothiazines

Lithium administration with phenothiazines may increase disorientation

Meperidine and phenothiazine coadministration increases sedation and hypotension

Methyldopa administration with phenothiazine (trifluoperazine) may significantly increase blood pressure

Norepinephrine, epinephrine have decreased pressor effect when administered with chlorpromazine; therefore, be aware of possible decreased effectiveness or when any phenothiazine is used

Phenytoin serum concentrations may increase or decrease with phenothiazines; tricyclic antidepressants may have increased serum concentrations with concomitant administration with phenothiazines

Propranolol administered with phenothiazines may increase serum concentrations of both drugs

Valproic acid may have increased half-life when administered with phenothiazines (chlorpromazine)

Stability Protect all dosage forms from light, clear or slightly yellow solutions may be used; should be dispensed in amber or opaque vials/bottles. Solutions may be diluted or mixed with fruit juices or other liquids but must be administered immediately after mixing; do not prepare bulk dilutions or store bulk dilutions.

Mechanism of Action Blocks postsynaptic mesolimbic dopaminergic D_1 and D_2 receptors in the brain; exhibits a strong alpha-adrenergic blocking and anticholinergic effect, depresses the release of hypothalamic and hypophyseal hormones; believed to depress the reticular activating system thus affecting basal metabolism, body temperature, wakefulness, vasomotor tone, and emesis

Pharmacokinetics

Absorption: May be affected by the inherent anticholinergic action on the gastrointestinal tissue causing variable absorption. Absorption from tablets is erratic with less variation seen with solutions. These agents are widely distributed in tissues with CNS concentrations exceeding that of plasma due to their lipophilic characteristics.

Protein binding: Antipsychotic agents are bound 90% to 99% to plasma proteins; highly bound to brain and lung tissue and other tissues with a high blood perfusion.

Time to peak: Oral absorption results in peak concentrations between 2-4 hours

Elimination: Occurs through hepatic metabolism (oxidation) where numerous active metabolites are produced; active metabolites excreted in urine; elimination half-lives of antipsychotics ranges from 20-40 hours which may be extended in elderly due to decline in oxidative hepatic reactions (phase I) with age.

The biologic effect of a single dose persists for 24 hours. When the patient has accommodated to initial side effects (sedation), once daily dosing is possible due to the long half-life of antipsychotics.

Steady-state plasma levels are achieved in 4-7 days; therefore, if possible, do not make dose adjustments more than once in a 7-day period. Due to the long half-lives of antipsychotics, as needed (PRN) use is ineffective since repeated doses are necessary to achieve therapeutic tissue concentrations in the CNS.

Usual Dosage Oral:

Geriatrics (nonpsychotic patient; dementia behavior): Initial: 10-25 mg 1-2 times/day; increase at 4- to 7-day intervals by 10-25 mg/day; increase dose intervals (qd, bid, etc) as necessary to control response or side effects. Maximum daily dose: 400 mg; gradual increases (titration) may prevent some side effects or decrease their severity.

Adults: Psychoses: Initial: 50-100 mg 3 times/day with gradual increments as needed and tolerated; maximum daily dose: 800 mg/day in 2-4 divided doses

Not dialyzable (0% to 5%)

Monitoring Parameters Orthostatic blood pressures; tremors, gait changes, abnormal movement in trunk, neck, buccal area or extremities; monitor target behaviors for which the agent is given

Reference Range Therapeutic: 1.0-1.5 μg/mL (SI: 2.7-4.1 μmol/L); Toxic: >10 μg/mL (SI: >27 μmol/L)

Test Interactions False-positives for phenylketonuria, urinary amylase, uroporphyrins, urobilinogen

Patient Information Oral concentrate must be diluted in 2-4 oz of liquid (water, fruit juice, carbonated drinks, milk, or pudding); do not take antacid within 1 hour of taking drug; avoid alcohol; avoid excess sun exposure (use sun block); may cause drowsiness, rise slowly from recumbent position; use of supportive stockings may help prevent orthostatic hypotension

Nursing Implications Dilute the oral concentrate with water or juice before administration; avoid skin contact with oral suspension or solution; may cause contact dermatitis; monitor orthostatic blood pressures 3-5 days after initiation of therapy or a dose increase; observe for tremor and abnormal movement or posturing (extrapyramidal symptoms)

Additional Information Oral formulations may cause stomach upset; may cause thermoregulatory changes

Thioridazine: Mellaril-S® oral suspension

Thioridazine hydrochloride: Mellaril® oral solution and tablet

Special Geriatric Considerations See Warnings

Many elderly patients receive antipsychotic medications for inappropriate nonpsychotic behavior. Before initiating antipsychotic medication, the clinician should investigate any possible reversible cause; any stress or stress from any disease can cause acute "confusion" or worsening of baseline nonpsychotic behavior. Most commonly acute changes in behavior are due to increases in drug dose or addition of new drug to regimen; fluid electrolyte loss; infections; and changes in environment.

Any changes in disease status in any organ system can result in behavior changes.

Dosage Forms

Concentrate, oral: 30 mg/mL (120 mL); 100 mg/mL (3.4 mL, 120 mL)

Suspension, oral: 25 mg/5 mL (480 mL); 100 mg/5 mL (480 mL)

Tablet: 10 mg, 15 mg, 25 mg, 50 mg, 100 mg, 150 mg, 200 mg

References

Peabody CA, Warner MD, Whiteford HA, et al, "Neuroleptics and the Elderly," *J Am Geriatr Soc*, 1987, 35(3):233-8.

Risse SC and Barnes R, "Pharmacologic Treatment of Agitation Associated With Dementia," *J Am Geriatr Soc*, 1986, 34(5):368-76.

Saltz BL, Woerner MG, Kane JM, et al, "Prospective Study of Tardive Dyskinesia Incidence in the Elderly," *JAMA*, 1991, 266(17):2402-6.

Seifert RD, "Therapeutic Drug Monitoring: Psychotropic Drugs," *J Pharm Pract*, 1984, 6:403-16.

Thioridazine Hydrochloride *see* Thioridazine *on page 684*

Thiothixene (thye oh thix' een)

Related Information

Antacid Drug Interactions *on page 764*

Antipsychotic Agents Comparison *on page 801*

Antipsychotic Medication Guidelines *on page 754*

Brand Names Navane®

Synonyms Tiotixene

Generic Available Yes

Therapeutic Class Antipsychotic Agent; Phenothiazine Derivative

Use Management of psychotic disorders; nonpsychotic symptoms associated with dementia in elderly, Tourette's syndrome, Huntington's chorea

Contraindications Hypersensitivity to thiothixene or any component; cross-sensitivity with other phenothiazines may exist; avoid use in patients with narrow-angle glaucoma, bone marrow depression, severe liver or cardiac disease; subcortical brain damage; circulatory collapse, severe hypotension or hypertension

Warnings

Tardive dyskinesia: Prevalence rate may be 40% in elderly; elderly women especially at risk; embarrassment from dyskinesias may lead to greater social isolation; development of the syndrome and the irreversible nature are proportional to duration and total cumulative dose over time. May be reversible if diagnosed early in therapy; intermittent use of antipsychotics (not proven use) helps decrease total cumulative dose.

EPS: Extrapyramidal reactions are more common in elderly with up to 50% developing these reactions after age 60. These reactions may be more common in dementia patients. Drug-induced **Parkinson's syndrome** occurs often. Discontinuation usually resolves symptoms but may take weeks to months (12+) to clear. **Akathisia** is the most common EPS reaction in elderly. The symptoms of motor restlessness are difficult to diagnose in demented elderly; increased nervousness, assertiveness, restlessness with constant movement may indicate this adverse event. Consider decreasing dose if antipsychotic to treat as well as diagnose problem; usually see this reaction within 2-3 months of initiating antipsychotic drug.

Anticholinergic effects: These side effects most common with low potency antipsychotics (eg, thioridazine, chlorpromazine). CNS toxicity occurs more frequently and severely in elderly; increased confusion, memory loss, psychotic behavior, and agitation frequently occur as a consequence of anticholinergic effects to antipsychotic agents. Peripheral anticholinergic action troublesome to elderly; most peripheral anticholinergic effects last only 2-3 weeks; see Adverse Reactions.

Orthostatic hypotension: More common with low potency agents (eg, thioridazine, chlorpromazine, and clozapine) but of concern with all antipsychotic agents; orthostasis due to alpha-receptor blockade by antipsychotic agents. Elderly pres-

(Continued)

Thiothixene *(Continued)*

ent many risk factors for orthostatic hypotension: blunted baroreceptor reflexes, decreased vascular tone, decreased vascular volume, and possible presence of cardiac diseases which result in decreased cardiac output.

Sedation: Common side effect with antipsychotic therapy; should not be used as a hypnotic unless insomnia is associated with target behavior symptoms treated with antipsychotic medications; see Special Geriatric Considerations. Anecdotal reports suggesting antipsychotic sedation in nonpsychotic patients is extremely unpleasant due to feelings of depersonalization, derealization, and dysphoria. Due to the long duration of action with antipsychotic drugs, these reactions may last up to 24 hours and result in decreased daytime function.

Cardiac toxicity: Life-threatening arrhythmias have occurred at therapeutic doses of antipsychotics. Thioridazine more commonly demonstrates EKG changes than other antipsychotics; suggested to use high potency antipsychotic agents (ie, haloperidol) in patients with cardiac conduction defects.

Precautions Watch for hypotension when administering I.M. or I.V.; use with caution in patients with cardiovascular disease, seizures, and Parkinson's disease; benefits of therapy must be weighed against risks of therapy

Adverse Reactions

Cardiovascular: Orthostatic hypotension, tachycardia, arrhythmias, abnormal T waves with prolonged ventricular repolarization

Central nervous system: Sedation, drowsiness, restlessness, anxiety, extrapyramidal reactions, pseudoparkinsonian signs and symptoms, tardive dyskinesia, neuroleptic malignant syndrome, seizures, altered central temperature regulation

Dermatologic: Hyperpigmentation, pruritus, rash, photosensitivity

Endocrine & metabolic: Amenorrhea, galactorrhea, gynecomastia

Gastrointestinal: GI upset, dry mouth (problem for denture users), constipation, adynamic ileus, weight gain

Genitourinary: Urinary retention, overflow incontinence, priapism, impotence, sexual dysfunction (up to 60%)

Hematologic: Agranulocytosis, leukopenia (usually in patients with large doses for prolonged periods), thrombocytopenia, hemolytic anemia, eosinophilia

Hepatic: Cholestatic jaundice (rare)

Ocular: Retinal pigmentation, blurred vision

Miscellaneous: Anaphylactoid reactions

EKG changes, retinal pigmentation are more common than with chlorpromazine

Overdosage Symptoms of overdose include deep sleep, coma, extrapyramidal symptoms, abnormal involuntary muscle movements, hypotension or hypertension; agitation, restlessness, fever, hypothermia or hyperthermia, seizures, cardiac arrhythmias, EKG changes

Toxicology Following initiation of essential overdose management, toxic symptom treatment and supportive treatment should be initiated. Hypotension usually responds to I.V. fluids or Trendelenburg positioning. If unresponsive to these measures the use of a parenteral inotrope may be required (eg, norepinephrine 0.1-0.2 mcg/kg/minute titrated to response). Do not use epinephrine. Seizures commonly respond to diazepam (I.V. 5-10 mg bolus every 15 minutes if needed up to a total of 30 mg) or to phenytoin or phenobarbital. Also critical cardiac arrhythmias often respond to I.V. phenytoin (15 mg/kg up to 1 g), while other antiarrhythmics can be used. Neuroleptics often cause extrapyramidal symptoms (eg, dystonic reactions) requiring management with diphenhydramine 1-2 mg/kg up to a maximum of 50 mg I.M. or I.V. slow push followed by a maintenance dose for 48-72 hours. When these reactions are unresponsive to diphenhydramine, benztropine mesylate I.V. 1-2 mg may be effective. These agents are generally effective within 2-5 minutes.

Drug Interactions

Alcohol may increase CNS sedation

Anticholinergic agents may decrease pharmacologic effects; increase anticholinergic side effects; may enhance tardive dyskinesia

Aluminum salts may decrease absorption of phenothiazines

Barbiturates may decrease phenothiazine serum concentrations

Bromocriptine may have decreased efficacy when administered with phenothiazines

Guanethidine's hypotensive effect is decreased by phenothiazines

Lithium administration with phenothiazines may increase disorientation

Meperidine and phenothiazine coadministration increases sedation and hypotension

Methyldopa administration with phenothiazine (trifluoperazine) may significantly increase blood pressure

Norepinephrine, epinephrine have decreased pressor effect when administered with chlorpromazine; therefore, be aware of possible decreased effectiveness or when any phenothiazine is used

Phenytoin serum concentrations may increase or decrease with phenothiazines; tricyclic antidepressants may have increased serum concentrations with concomitant administration with phenothiazines

Propranolol administered with phenothiazines may increase serum concentrations of both drugs

Valproic acid may have increased half-life when administered with phenothiazines (chlorpromazine)

Stability I.M. solution is stable for 12 months at room temperature; reconstituted powder is stable for 48 hours at room temperature

Mechanism of Action Blocks postsynaptic mesolimbic dopaminergic D_1 and D_2 receptors in the brain; exhibits a strong alpha-adrenergic blocking and anticholinergic effect, depresses the release of hypothalamic and hypophyseal hormones; believed to depress the reticular activating system thus affecting basal metabolism, body temperature, wakefulness, vasomotor tone, and emesis

Pharmacokinetics

Absorption: May be affected by the inherent anticholinergic action on the gastrointestinal tissue causing variable absorption. Absorption from tablets is erratic with less variation seen with solutions. These agents are widely distributed in tissues with CNS concentrations exceeding that of plasma due to their lipophilic characteristics.

Protein binding: Antipsychotic agents are bound 90% to 99% to plasma proteins; highly bound to brain and lung tissue and other tissues with a high blood perfusion.

Metabolism: Extensive in the liver

Half-life: >24 hours with chronic use

Time to peak: Oral absorption results in peak concentrations between 2-4 hours

Elimination: Occurs through hepatic metabolism (oxidation) where numerous active metabolites are produced; active metabolites excreted in urine; elimination half-lives of antipsychotics ranges from 20-40 hours which may be extended in elderly due to decline in oxidative hepatic reactions (phase I) with age.

The biologic effect of a single dose persists for 24 hours. When the patient has accommodated to initial side effects (sedation), once daily dosing is possible due to the long half-life of antipsychotics.

Steady-state plasma levels are achieved in 4-7 days; therefore, if possible, do not make dose adjustments more than once in a 7-day period. Due to the long half-lives of antipsychotics, as needed (PRN) use is ineffective since repeated doses are necessary to achieve therapeutic tissue concentrations in the CNS.

Usual Dosage

Geriatrics (nonpsychotic patients, dementia behavior): Initial: 1-2 mg 1-2 times/day; increase dose at 4- to 7-day intervals by 1-2 mg/day; increase dosing intervals (bid, tid, etc) as necessary to control response or side effects; maximum daily dose: 30 mg; gradual increases in dose may prevent some side effects or decrease their severity

Adults:

Oral: Initial: 2 mg 3 times/day, up to 20-30 mg/day; maximum: 60 mg/day

I.M.: 4 mg 2-4 times/day, increase dose gradually; usual: 16-20 mg/day; maximum: 30 mg/day; change to oral dose as soon as able

Not dialyzable (0% to 5%)

Monitoring Parameters Orthostatic blood pressures; tremors, gait changes, abnormal movement in trunk, neck, buccal area or extremities; monitor target behaviors for which the agent is given

Reference Range Serum concentration: 2-57 ng/mL; concentrations do not always correspond to response and are controversial; dose to response for efficacy and safety

Test Interactions Increased cholesterol (S), increased glucose; decreased uric acid (S)

Patient Information Oral concentrate must be diluted in 2-4 oz of liquid (water, fruit juice, carbonated drinks, milk, or pudding); do not take antacid within 1 hour of taking drug; avoid alcohol; avoid excess sun exposure (use sun block); may cause drowsiness, rise slowly from recumbent position; use of supportive stockings may help prevent orthostatic hypotension

Nursing Implications Store injection in the refrigerator; injection for intramuscular use only; dilute the oral concentrate with water or juice before administration; avoid skin contact with oral suspension or solution; may cause contact dermatitis; monitor orthostatic blood pressures 3-5 days after initiation of therapy or a dose increase; observe for tremor and abnormal movement or posturing (extrapyramidal symptoms)

Special Geriatric Considerations See Warnings

Many elderly patients receive antipsychotic medications for inappropriate nonpsychotic behavior. Before initiating antipsychotic medication, the clinician should investigate any possible reversible cause; any stress or stress from any disease can cause acute "confusion" or worsening of baseline nonpsychotic behavior. Most commonly acute changes in behavior are due to increases in drug dose or addition of new drug to regimen; fluid electrolyte loss; infections; and changes in environment.

Any changes in disease status in any organ system can result in behavior changes.

Dosage Forms

Capsule: 1 mg, 2 mg, 5 mg, 10 mg, 20 mg

Concentrate, oral, as hydrochloride: 5 mg/mL (30 mL, 120 mL)

Injection, as hydrochloride: 2 mg/mL (2 mL)

Powder for injection, as hydrochloride: 5 mg/mL (2 mL)

Thiuretic® *see* Hydrochlorothiazide *on page 347*

Thorazine® *see* Chlorpromazine Hydrochloride *on page 153*

Thyrar® *see* Thyroid *on next page*

Thyroglobulin (thye roe glob' yoo lin)

Brand Names Proloid®

Generic Available No

Therapeutic Class Thyroid Product

Use Replacement or supplemental therapy in hypothyroidism; pituitary TSH suppressants (thyroid nodules, thyroiditis, multinodular goiter, thyroid cancer), thyrotoxicosis, diagnostic suppression tests

Contraindications Recent myocardial infarction or thyrotoxicosis, uncomplicated by hypothyroidism; uncorrected adrenal insufficiency, hypersensitivity to active or extraneous constituents

Warnings Ineffective for weight reduction; high doses may produce serious or even life-threatening toxic effects particularly when used with some anorectic drugs; use cautiously in patients with pre-existing cardiovascular disease (angina, CHD), elderly since they may be more likely to have compromised cardiovascular function

Precautions Patients with angina pectoris or other cardiovascular disease; adrenal insufficiency, myxedema, diabetes mellitus and insipidus may have symptoms exaggerated or aggravated; thyroid replacement requires periodic assessment of thyroid status; TSH is the most reliable guide for evaluating adequacy of thyroid replacement dosage. TSH may be elevated during the first few months of thyroid replacement despite patients being clinically euthyroid. In cases where T_4 remains low and TSH is within normal limits, an evaluation of "free" (unbound) T_4 is needed to evaluate further increase in dosage. Chronic hypothyroidism predisposes patients to coronary artery disease.

Adverse Reactions

Cardiovascular: Palpitations, tachycardia, cardiac arrhythmias

Central nervous system: Nervousness, headache, insomnia, fever

Dermatologic: Hair loss

Gastrointestinal: Weight loss, increased appetite, diarrhea, abdominal cramps, vomiting

Neuromuscular & skeletal: Excessive bone loss with overtreatment (excess thyroid replacement), tremors

Miscellaneous: Heat intolerance, sweating

Overdosage Chronic excessive use results in signs and symptoms of hyperthyroidism, weight loss, nervousness, sweating, tachycardia, insomnia, heat intolerance, palpitations, vomiting, psychosis, fever, seizures, angina, arrhythmias, and CHF in those predisposed

Toxicology Reduce dose or temporarily discontinue therapy; normal hypothalamic-pituitary-thyroid axis will return to normal in 6-8 weeks; serum T_4 levels do not correlate well with toxicity; in massive acute ingestion, reduce GI absorption, give general supportive care; treat CHF with digitalis glycosides; excessive adrenergic activity (tachycardia) require propranolol 1-3 mg I.V. over 10 minutes or 80-160 mg orally/day; fever may be treated with acetaminophen

Drug Interactions

Cholestyramine and colestipol decrease the effect of orally administered thyroid replacement

Estrogens increase TBG, thereby decreasing effect of thyroid replacement

Anticoagulants may increase action

Beta-blocker effect is decreased when patients become euthyroid

Serum digitalis concentrations are reduced in hyperthyroidism or when hypothyroid patients are converted to a euthyroid state

Theophylline levels decrease when hypothyroid patients converted to a euthyroid state

Mechanism of Action The primary active compound is T_3 (tri-iodothyronine), which may be converted from T_4 (thyroxine); exact mechanism of action is unknown; however, it is believed the thyroid hormone exerts its many metabolic effects through control of DNA transcription and protein synthesis; involved in normal metabolism, growth, and development; promotes gluconeogenesis, increases utilization and mobilization of glycogen stores and stimulates protein synthesis, increases basal metabolic rate

Pharmacodynamics

Onset of therapeutic effects: May be seen in 3-5 days

Maximum effects: 4-6 weeks may be required for any given dose

Pharmacokinetics

Absorption: Oral: Erratic, 48% to 79%; T_3: 95% absorbed

Distribution: 80% of T_3 is derived from monodeiodination of T_4 in the periphery (liver, kidneys, other tissues)

Half-life: 6-7 days for T_4 and 1-2 days for T_3

Time to peak: Peak serum levels occur within 2-4 hours

Elimination: As conjugated forms in feces, bile

Usual Dosage Geriatrics and Adults (see Additional Information):

Initial: 15-30 mg; increase with 15 mg increments every 2-4 weeks; use 15 mg in patients with cardiovascular disease or myxedema

Maintenance dose: Usually 60-120 mg/day; monitor TSH and clinical symptoms

Thyroid cancer: Requires larger amounts than replacement therapy

Monitoring Parameters T_4, TSH, heart rate, blood pressure, clinical signs of hypo- and hyperthyroidism; TSH is the most reliable guide for evaluating adequacy of thyroid replacement dosage. TSH may be elevated during the first few months of thyroid replacement despite patients being clinically euthyroid. In cases where T_4 remains low and TSH is within normal limits, an evaluation of "free" (unbound) T_4 is needed to evaluate further increase in dosage.

Reference Range

TSH: 0.4-10 (for those ≥80 years) mIU/L

T_4: 4-12 μg/dL (SI: 51-154 nmol/L)

T_3 (RIA) (total T_3): 80-230 ng/dL (SI: 1.2-3.5 nmol/L)

T_4 free (Free T_4): 0.7-1.8 ng/dL (SI: 9-23 pmol/L)

Test Interactions Increased calcium (S); many drugs may have effects on thyroid function tests; para-aminosalicylic acid, aminoglutethimide, amiodarone, barbiturates, carbamazepine, chloral hydrate, clofibrate, colestipol, corticosteroids, danazol, diazepam, estrogens, ethionamide, fluorouracil, I.V. heparin, insulin, lithium, methadone, methimazole, mitotane, nitroprusside, oxyphenbutazone, phenylbutazone, PTU, perphenazine, phenytoin, propranolol, salicylates, sulfonylureas, and thiazides

Patient Information Do not change brands without physician's knowledge; report immediately to physician any chest pain, increased pulse, palpitations, heat intolerance, excessive sweating; do not stop use without physician's advice; replacement therapy will be for life; take as a single dose before breakfast

Nursing Implications Monitor pulse rate and blood pressure; see Precautions, Adverse Reactions, Toxicology, Monitoring Parameters, and Special Geriatric Considerations

Additional Information Contains levothyroxine and liothyronine in 2.5:1 ratio; 60 mg equivalent to 0.05-0.06 mg levothyroxine

Special Geriatric Considerations Thyroglobulin may contain variable amounts of T_3 and T_4 which may produce cardiac symptoms due to fluctuating serum concentrations of T_3 and T_4; should probably avoid use in elderly. Elderly do not have a change in serum thyroxine associated with aging; however, plasma T_3 concentrations are decreased 25% to 40% in elderly. There is not a compensatory rise in thyrotropin suggesting that lower T_3 is not reacted upon as a deficiency by the pituitary. This indicates a slightly lower than normal dosage of thyroid hormone replacement is usually sufficient in older patients than in younger adult patients. TSH must be monitored since insufficient thyroid replacement (elevated TSH) is a risk for coronary artery disease and excessive replacement (low TSH) may cause signs of hyperthyroidism and excessive bone loss. Some clinicians suggest that levothyroxine is the drug of choice for thyroid replacement; see Overdosage.

Dosage Forms Tablet: 30 mg, 65 mg, 100 mg, 130 mg, 200 mg, 325 mg

References

Helfand M and Crapo LM, "Monitoring Therapy in Patients Taking Levothyroxine," *Ann Intern Med*, 1990, 113(6):450-4.

Johnson DG and Campbell S, "Hormonal and Metabolic Agents," *Geriatric Pharmacology*, Bressler R and Katz MD, eds, New York, NY: McGraw-Hill, 1993, 427-50.

Sanders LR, "Pituitary, Thyroid, Adrenal and Parathyroid Diseases in the Elderly," *Geriatric Medicine*, 1990, 475-87.

Sawin CT, Geller A, Hershman JM, et al, "The Aging Thyroid. The Use of Thyroid Hormone in Older Persons," *JAMA*, 1989, 261(18):2653-5.

Watts NB, "Use of a Sensitive Thyrotropin Assay for Monitoring Treatment With Levothyroxine," *Arch Intern Med*, 1989, 149(2):309-12.

Thyroid (thye' roid)

Brand Names Armour® Thyroid; S-P-T; Thyrar®; Thyroid Strong®

Synonyms Desiccated Thyroid; Thyroid Extract

Generic Available Yes

Therapeutic Class Thyroid Product

Use Replacement or supplemental therapy in hypothyroidism; pituitary TSH suppressants (thyroid nodules, thyroiditis, multinodular goiter, thyroid cancer), thyrotoxicosis, diagnostic suppression tests

Contraindications Recent myocardial infarction or thyrotoxicosis, uncomplicated by hypothyroidism; uncorrected adrenal insufficiency, hypersensitivity to active or extraneous constituents

Warnings Ineffective for weight reduction; high doses may produce serious or even life-threatening toxic effects particularly when used with some anorectic drugs; use cautiously in patients with pre-existing cardiovascular disease (angina, CHD), elderly since they may be more likely to have compromised cardiovascular function

Precautions Patients with angina pectoris or other cardiovascular disease; adrenal insufficiency, myxedema, diabetes mellitus and insipidus may have symptoms exag-

(Continued)

Thyroid *(Continued)*

gerated or aggravated; thyroid replacement requires periodic assessment of thyroid status; TSH is the most reliable guide for evaluating adequacy of thyroid replacement dosage. TSH may be elevated during the first few months of thyroid replacement despite patients being clinically euthyroid. In cases where T_4 remains low and TSH is within normal limits, an evaluation of "free" (unbound) T_4 is needed to evaluate further increase in dosage. Chronic hypothyroidism predisposes patients to coronary artery disease.

Adverse Reactions
Cardiovascular: Palpitations, tachycardia, cardiac arrhythmias

Central nervous system: Nervousness, headache, insomnia, fever

Dermatologic: Hair loss

Gastrointestinal: Weight loss, increased appetite, diarrhea, abdominal cramps, vomiting

Neuromuscular & skeletal: Excessive bone loss with overtreatment (excess thyroid replacement), tremors

Miscellaneous: Heat intolerance, sweating

Overdosage Chronic excessive use results in signs and symptoms of hyperthyroidism, weight loss, nervousness, sweating, tachycardia, insomnia, heat intolerance, palpitations, vomiting, psychosis, fever, seizures, angina, arrhythmias, and CHF in those predisposed

Toxicology Reduce dose or temporarily discontinue therapy; normal hypothalamic-pituitary-thyroid axis will return to normal in 6-8 weeks; serum T_4 levels do not correlate well with toxicity; in massive acute ingestion, reduce GI absorption, give general supportive care; treat CHF with digitalis glycosides; excessive adrenergic activity (tachycardia) require propranolol 1-3 mg I.V. over 10 minutes or 80-160 mg orally/day; fever may be treated with acetaminophen

Drug Interactions
Cholestyramine and colestipol decrease the effect of orally administered thyroid replacement

Estrogens increase TBG, thereby decreasing effect of thyroid replacement

Anticoagulants may increase action

Beta-blocker effect is decreased when patients become euthyroid

Serum digitalis concentrations are reduced in hyperthyroidism or when hypothyroid patients are converted to a euthyroid state

Theophylline levels decrease when hypothyroid patients converted to a euthyroid state

Mechanism of Action The primary active compound is T_3 (tri-iodothyronine), which may be converted from T_4 (thyroxine) and then circulates throughout the body; exact mechanism of action is unknown; however, it is believed the thyroid hormone exerts its many metabolic effects through control of DNA transcription and protein synthesis; involved in normal metabolism, growth, and development; promotes gluconeogenesis, increases utilization and mobilization of glycogen stores and stimulates protein synthesis, increases basal metabolic rate

Pharmacodynamics
Onset of therapeutic effects: May be seen in 3-5 days

Maximum effects: 4-6 weeks may be required for any given dose

Pharmacokinetics
Absorption: T_4 is 48% to 79% absorbed; T_3 is 95% absorbed; desiccated thyroid contains thyroxine, liothyronine, and iodine (primarily bound); following absorption thyroxine is largely converted to liothyronine

Protein binding: 99% (bound to albumin, thyroxine-binding globulin, and thyroxin-binding prealbumin)

Metabolism: Liothyronine is metabolized in the liver, kidneys, and other tissues to inactive compounds

Half-life:

Liothyronine: 1-2 days

Thyroxine: 6-7 days

Elimination: In urine as conjugated forms

Usual Dosage Geriatrics and Adults (see Additional Information): Initial: 15-30 mg; increase with 15 mg increments every 2-4 weeks; use 15 mg in patients with cardiovascular disease or myxedema. Maintenance dose: Usually 60-120 mg/day; monitor TSH and clinical symptoms.

Thyroid cancer: Requires larger amounts than replacement therapy

Monitoring Parameters T_4, TSH, heart rate, blood pressure, clinical signs of hypo- and hyperthyroidism; TSH is the most reliable guide for evaluating adequacy of thyroid replacement dosage. TSH may be elevated during the first few months of thyroid replacement despite patients being clinically euthyroid. In cases where T_4 remains low and TSH is within normal limits, an evaluation of "free" (unbound) T_4 is needed to evaluate further increase in dosage

Reference Range
TSH 0.4-10 (for those $\geq$80 years) mIU/L

T$_4$: 4-12 µg/dL (51-154 mmol:/L)

T$_3$ (RIA) (total T$_3$): 80-230 ng/dL (1.2-3.5 mmol/L)

T$_4$ free (Free T$_4$): 0.7-1.8 ng/dL (9-23 pmol/L)

Test Interactions Increased calcium (S); many drugs may have effects on thyroid function tests; para-aminosalicylic acid, aminoglutethimide, amiodarone, barbiturates, carbamazepine, chloral hydrate, clofibrate, colestipol, corticosteroids, danazol, diazepam, estrogens, ethionamide, fluorouracil, I.V. heparin, insulin, lithium, methadone, methimazole, mitotane, nitroprusside, oxyphenbutazone, phenylbutazone, PTU, perphenazine, phenytoin, propranolol, salicylates, sulfonylureas, and thiazides

Patient Information Do not change brands without physician's knowledge; report immediately to physician any chest pain, increased pulse, palpitations, heat intolerance, excessive sweating; do not stop use without physician's advice; replacement therapy will be for life; take as a single dose before breakfast

Nursing Implications Monitor pulse rate and blood pressure; see Precautions, Adverse Reactions, Toxicology, Monitoring Parameters, Special Geriatric Considerations

Additional Information Equivalent levothyroxine dose: Thyroid USP 60 mg = levothyroxine 0.05-0.06 mg; liothyronine 15-37.5 mcg; liotrix 60 mg

Special Geriatric Considerations Desiccated thyroid contains variable amounts of T$_3$, T$_4$, and other tri-iodothyronine compounds which are more likely to cause cardiac signs and symptoms due to fluctuating levels; should avoid use in elderly for this reason; many clinicians consider levothyroxine to be the drug of choice

Dosage Forms Tablet: 15 mg, 30 mg, 60 mg, 120 mg, 180 mg, 300 mg

References

Helfand M and Crapo LM, "Monitoring Therapy in Patients Taking Levothyroxine," Ann Intern Med, 1990, 113(6):450-4.

Johnson DG and Campbell S, "Hormonal and Metabolic Agents," Geriatric Pharmacology, Bressler R and Katz MD, eds, New York, NY: McGraw-Hill, 1993, 427-50.

Sanders LR, "Pituitary, Thyroid, Adrenal and Parathyroid Diseases in the Elderly," Geriatric Medicine, 1990, 475-87.

Sawin CT, Geller A, Hershman JM, et al, "The Aging Thyroid. The Use of Thyroid Hormone in Older Persons," JAMA, 1989, 261(18):2653-5.

Watts NB, "Use of a Sensitive Thyrotropin Assay for Monitoring Treatment With Levothyroxine," Arch Intern Med, 1989, 149(2):309-12.

Thyroid Extract see Thyroid on page 691

Thyroid Strong® see Thyroid on page 691

Thyrolar® see Liotrix on page 410

Ticar® see Ticarcillin Disodium on next page

Ticarcillin and Clavulanic Acid (tye kar sill' in)

Brand Names Timentin®

Synonyms Ticarcillin Disodium and Clavulanate Potassium

Therapeutic Class Antibiotic, Penicillin

Use Treatment of infections of lower respiratory tract, urinary tract, skin and skin structures, bone and joint, and septicemia caused by susceptible organisms. Clavulanate expands activity of ticarcillin to include beta-lactamase producing strains of S. aureus, H. influenzae, Enterobacteriaceae, Pseudomonas, Klebsiella, Citrobacter, and Serratia

Contraindications Known hypersensitivity to ticarcillin, clavulanate, and any penicillin

Precautions Use with caution and modify dosage in patients with renal impairment; use with caution in patients with congestive heart failure due to high sodium load (~6 mEq/g); use with caution in patients with cephalosporin allergy

Adverse Reactions

Cardiovascular: Thrombophlebitis

Central nervous system: Seizures, headache, confusion, sedation, fever

Dermatologic: Rash

Endocrine & metabolic: Hypernatremia, hypokalemia, metabolic alkalosis

Gastrointestinal: Diarrhea, stomatitis

Hematologic: Inhibition of platelet aggregation, eosinophilia, leukopenia, decreased hemoglobin and hematocrit, prolongation of bleeding time, positive Coombs' test

Hepatic: Elevated AST, hepatitis

Renal: Acute interstitial nephritis

Miscellaneous: Hypersensitivity reactions, Jarisch-Herxheimer reactions

Toxicology Many beta-lactam-containing antibiotics have the potential to cause neuromuscular hyperirritability or convulsive seizures. Hemodialysis may be helpful to aid in the removal of the drug from the blood, otherwise most treatment is supportive or symptom directed.

Drug Interactions Aminoglycosides, bacteriostatic agents

Increased duration of neuromuscular blockers

Increased/prolonged levels with probenecid

Stability Reconstituted solution is stable for 6 hours at room temperature and 72 hours when refrigerated; for I.V. infusion in NS is stable for 24 hours at room temperature, 7 days when refrigerated, or 30 days when frozen; after freezing, thawed solution is sta-

(Continued)

Ticarcillin and Clavulanic Acid (Continued)

ble for 8 hours at room temperature; for I.V. infusion in D₅W solution is stable for 24 hours at room temperature, 3 days when refrigerated, or 7 days when frozen; after freezing, thawed solution is stable for 8 hours at room temperature; darkening of drug indicates loss of potency of clavulanate potassium; incompatible with sodium bicarbonate, aminoglycosides

Mechanism of Action Ticarcillin interferes with bacterial cell wall synthesis during active multiplication causing cell death and resultant bactericidal activity against susceptible bacteria; clavulanic acid prevents degradation of ticarcillin by binding to the active site on beta-lactamase

Pharmacokinetics

Distribution: Low concentrations of ticarcillin distribute into the CSF and increase when meninges are inflamed

Protein binding:

Ticarcillin: 45% to 65%

Clavulanic acid: 9% to 30%

Metabolism: Clavulanic acid is metabolized in the liver

Half-life:

Clavulanate: 66-90 minutes

Ticarcillin: 66-72 minutes in patients with normal renal function

Clavulanic acid does not affect the clearance of ticarcillin

Elimination: 45% of clavulanic acid is excreted unchanged in urine, whereas 60% to 90% of ticarcillin is excreted unchanged in urine

Removed by hemodialysis

Usual Dosage I.V.:

Geriatrics (based on ticarcillin): 3 g every 4-6 hours; adjust for renal function

Adults: 3.1 g (ticarcillin 3 g plus clavulanic acid 0.1 g) every 4-6 hours; maximum: 18-24 g/day; for urinary tract infections: 3.1 g every 6-8 hours

Dosing interval in renal impairment:

Cl_{cr} >60 mL/minute: Administer 3 g every 4 hours

Cl_{cr} 30-60 mL/minute: Administer 2 g every 4 hours

Cl_{cr} 10-30 mL/minute: Administer 2 g every 8 hours

Cl_{cr} <10 mL/minute: Administer 2 g every 12 hours

Dosing interval in hepatic/renal impairment: Cl_{cr} <10 mL/minute: Administer 2 g every 24 hours

Administration Infuse over 30 minutes; do not give I.M.

Monitoring Parameters Temperature, WBC, respiratory rate; culture and sensitivity (if applicable), mental status, appetite

Test Interactions Positive Coombs' test, false-positive urinary proteins

Nursing Implications See Administration

Additional Information Usually given for at least for 2 days after symptoms have disappeared

Special Geriatric Considerations When used as empiric therapy or for a documented pseudomonal pneumonia, it is best to combine with an aminoglycoside such as gentamicin or tobramycin; high sodium content may limit use in patients with congestive heart failure; adjust dose for renal function; see Precautions

Dosage Forms Powder for injection: Ticarcillin disodium 3 g and clavulanic acid 0.1 g per g (3.1 g)

Ticarcillin Disodium (tye kar sill' in)

Brand Names Ticar®

Therapeutic Class Antibiotic, Penicillin

Use Treatment of susceptible infections such as septicemia, acute and chronic respiratory tract infections, skin and soft tissue infections, and urinary tract infections due to susceptible strains of *Pseudomonas*, *Proteus*, and *Escherichia coli* and *Enterobacter*

Contraindications Hypersensitivity to ticarcillin or any component or penicillins

Precautions Use with caution in patients with congestive heart failure due to high sodium load (~6 mEq/g); dosage modification required in patients with impaired renal and/or hepatic function; use with caution in patients with a history of cephalosporin allergy

Adverse Reactions

Cardiovascular: Thrombophlebitis

Central nervous system: Seizures, headache, confusion, sedation, fever

Dermatologic: Rash

Endocrine & metabolic: Hypernatremia, hypokalemia, metabolic alkalosis

Gastrointestinal: Diarrhea, stomatitis

Hematologic: Inhibition of platelet aggregation, eosinophilia, leukopenia, neutropenia, bleeding diathesis, hemolytic anemia, positive Coombs' test, decreased hemoglobin and hematocrit

Hepatic: Elevated AST, hepatitis

Renal: Acute interstitial nephritis

Miscellaneous: Allergic reactions, Jarisch-Herxheimer reactions

Overdosage Symptoms of overdose include neuromuscular hypersensitivity, seizure

Toxicology Many beta-lactam-containing antibiotics have the potential to cause neuromuscular hyperirritability or convulsive seizures. Hemodialysis may be helpful to aid in the removal of the drug from the blood, otherwise most treatment is supportive or symptom directed.

Drug Interactions Aminoglycosides, bacteriostatic agents
Increased duration of neuromuscular blockers
Increased/prolonged levels with probenecid

Stability Reconstituted solution is stable for 72 hours at room temperature and 14 days when refrigerated; for I.V. infusion in NS or D_5W solution is stable for 72 hours at room temperature, 14 days when refrigerated or 30 days when frozen; after freezing, thawed solution is stable for 72 hours at room temperature or 14 days when refrigerated; incompatible with aminoglycosides

Mechanism of Action Interferes with bacterial cell wall synthesis during active multiplication causing cell death and resultant bactericidal activity against susceptible bacteria

Pharmacokinetics
Absorption: I.M.: 86%
Protein binding: 45% to 65%
Half-life: 66-72 minutes, prolonged with renal impairment and/or hepatic impairment
Time to peak: I.M.: Peak serum levels occur within 30-75 minutes
Elimination: Almost entirely in urine as unchanged drug and its metabolites with small amounts excreted in feces (3.5%); CNS distribution is low and increased when the meninges are inflamed

Usual Dosage Ticarcillin is generally given I.M. only for the treatment of uncomplicated urinary tract infections.

Geriatrics: I.V.: 3 g every 4-6 hours; adjust dosing interval for renal impairment

Adults: I.V.: 1-4 g every 4-6 hours

Dosing interval in renal impairment: I.V.:
Cl_{cr} >60 mL/minute: Administer 3 g every 4 hours
Cl_{cr} 30-60 mL/minute: Administer 2 g every 4 hours
Cl_{cr} 10-30 mL/minute: Administer 2 g every 8 hours
Cl_{cr} <10 mL/minute: Administer 2 g every 12 hours
Cl_{cr} <10 mL/minute with hepatic dysfunction: Administer 2 g every 24 hours
Peritoneal dialysis: Administer 3 g every 12 hours
Hemodialysis: Administer 2 g every 12 hours; follow each dialysis with 3 g
Moderately dialyzable (20% to 50%)

Administration Administer 1 hour apart from aminoglycosides; do not give I.M.

Monitoring Parameters Temperature, WBC, respiratory rate; cultures and sensitivity (if applicable), mental status, appetite

Test Interactions False-positive urinary or serum protein

Nursing Implications See Administration

Additional Information Sodium content of 1 g: 5.2 to 6.5 mEq; normally used with other antibiotics (ie, aminoglycosides)

Special Geriatric Considerations When used as empiric therapy or for documented pseudomonal pneumonia, it is best to combine with an aminoglycoside such as gentamicin or tobramycin; high sodium may limit use in patients with congestive heart failure; adjust dose for renal function; see Precautions

Dosage Forms Injection: 1 g, 3 g, 6 g, 20 g, 30 g

References
Brogden RN, Heel RC, Speight TM, et al, "Ticarcillin: A Review of Its Pharmacological Properties and Therapeutic Efficacy," *Drugs*, 1980, 20(5):325-52.
Yoshikawa TT, "Antimicrobial Therapy for the Elderly Patient," *J Am Geriatr Soc*, 1990, 38(12):1353-72.

Ticarcillin Disodium and Clavulanate Potassium *see* Ticarcillin and Clavulanic Acid *on page 693*

Ticlid® *see* Ticlopidine Hydrochloride *on this page*

Ticlopidine Hydrochloride
Brand Names Ticlid®
Generic Available No
Therapeutic Class Antiplatelet Agent
Use Reduction of risk of thrombotic stroke (fatal or nonfatal) in patients who have experienced stroke precursors or have had a completed thrombotic stroke

Unlabeled use (more study needed): Intermittent claudication, chronic arterial occlusion, subarachnoid hemorrhage, open heart surgery, coronary artery bypass grafts, and primary glomerulonephritis. **Note:** Because of the risk of neutropenia occurring with ticlopidine, reserve its use for those patients intolerant to aspirin.

(Continued)
695

Ticlopidine Hydrochloride (Continued)

Contraindications Hypersensitivity to ticlopidine; presence of hematopoietic disorders (ie, neutropenia, thrombocytopenia); hemostatic disorders; active pathological bleeding (ie, peptic ulcer or intracranial bleeding); severe liver impairment

Warnings Neutropenia, sometimes severe (ANC <450 neutrophils/mm^3), has been experienced by 0.9% to 2.4% of patients in two large clinical trials. The drop in ANC was in the first 3 weeks to 3 months of treatment. Discontinuation of the drug may be necessary; neutrophil counts should return to baseline in 1-3 weeks; see Monitoring Parameters.

Thrombocytopenia (platelet count <80,000 cells/mm^3) is rare, but can occur alone or in conjunction with neutropenia. If confirmed by clinical evaluation and laboratory findings, discontinue therapy. Rare case of pancytopenia and thrombotic thrombocytopenia purpura have been reported. Total cholesterol and triglyceride concentrations may be increased while the lipoprotein subfraction ratios remain unchanged.

Discontinue anticoagulant or fibrinolytic drug therapy before starting ticlopidine. Ticlopidine is not recommended for patients with severe hepatic disease and has not been studied in patients with severe renal function impairment. A dosage adjustment (decrease) may be necessary or the drug stopped if hemorrhagic or hematopoietic complications arise.

Precautions An increased risk of bleeding may be present in patients undergoing a surgical procedure who experience trauma or who have certain pathological conditions. When possible, discontinue ticlopidine 10-14 days prior to elective surgery. Prolonged bleeding time can be reversed in 2 hours following 20 mg I.V. methylprednisolone; oral steroids are also effective; platelet transfusion is another option.

Adverse Reactions
Dermatologic: Rash (>5%), pruritus, purpura
Gastrointestinal: Diarrhea, nausea, dyspepsia, GI pain vomiting, flatulence, anorexia
Hematologic: Bleeding disorders, neutropenia
Hepatic: Abnormal liver function tests (alkaline phosphatase and transaminase)

Overdosage In one case of intentional overdose, the only abnormalities reported were increased bleeding time and increased ALT.

Toxicology See Warnings and Precautions

Drug Interactions
Antacids decreased bioavailability
Cimetidine decreased ticlopidine clearance
Aspirin increased antiplatelet aggregation effects, coadministration is not recommended
Digoxin small decreased digoxin plasma concentrations
Theophylline increased half-life by ~50%

Mechanism of Action Ticlopidine is an inhibitor of platelet function with a mechanism which is different from other antiplatelet drugs. Ticlopidine results in a time and dose-dependent inhibition of platelet aggregation and release of granule constituents; this is accomplished through inhibition of ADP-induced platelet fibrinogen binding and further platelet-platelet interactions which are irreversible for life of the platelet. The drug significantly increases bleeding time. This effect may not be solely related to ticlopidine's effects on platelets. The prolongation of the bleeding time caused by ticlopidine is further increased by the addition of aspirin in *ex vivo* experiments. Although many metabolites of ticlopidine have been found, none have been shown to account for *in vivo* activity.

Pharmacodynamics
Onset of action: Within 6 hours
Peak effects: Oral: Achieved after 3-5 days of therapy
Because the duration of inhibition of platelet function corresponds to the normal life span of the platelet, these effects usually reverse 1-2 weeks after stopping the drug

Pharmacokinetics
Absorption: Following administration, 80% to 90% absorbed from GI tract with an average peak plasma steady-state concentration of 0.9 mg/mL ~2 hours after a 250 mg dose
Protein binding: 98% bound to plasma proteins, primarily albumin and lipoproteins, with ≤15% bound to alpha$_1$-acid glycoprotein
Metabolism: Metabolized in the liver extensively, principally by N-dealkylation and oxidation of the thiophene ring; four metabolites have been identified in humans
Half-life: 12-36 hours increasing to 4-5 days after continuous dosing; clearance decreases in older subjects; mean area under the serum concentration time curve was 2-3 times that in younger adults and trough levels were twice as high as compared to younger adults; at steady-state there were no significant differences in time to peak or elimination half-life between young and elderly subjects, but the average plasma concentration in the elderly was twice that of the younger group. It is unknown whether these differences are due to increased absorption, decreased clearance, or a change in plasma protein binding.
Elimination: <1% excreted unchanged in urine

Usual Dosage Oral:

Geriatrics: 250 mg twice daily with food; dosage in the elderly has not been determined; however, in two large clinical trials, the average age of subjects was 63 and 66 years; a dosage decrease may be necessary if bleeding abnormalities develop

Adults: 250 mg twice daily with food

Dosing in renal or hepatic impairment: Not established

Monitoring Parameters Signs of bleeding; CBC with differential every 2 weeks starting the second week through the third month of treatment; more frequent monitoring is recommended for patients whose absolute neutrophil counts have been consistently declining or are 30% less than baseline values. Liver function tests (alkaline phosphatase and transaminases) should be performed in the first 4 months of therapy if liver dysfunction is suspected.

Reference Range Serum levels do not correlate with clinical antiplatelet activity

Test Interactions Increased alkaline phosphatase, increased ALT, AST, slight increased bilirubin, decreased neutrophils

Patient Information Possibility of signs and symptoms of neutropenia, thrombocytopenia, and abnormal bleeding; comply with biweekly blood tests; report any symptoms of infection such as fever, chills, sore throat; report unusual bleeding; tell all physicians and dentists that you are on ticlopidine; take with food to minimize GI complaints

Nursing Implications Monitor for signs of bleeding, infection; administer with food

Special Geriatric Considerations See Pharmacokinetics and Usual Dosage. Because of the risk of neutropenia and its relative expense as compared with aspirin, ticlopidine should only be used in patients with a documented intolerance to aspirin.

Dosage Forms Tablet: 250 mg

References

Ito MK, Smith AR, and Lee ML, "Ticlopidine: A New Platelet Aggregation Inhibitor," *Clin Pharm*, 1992, 11(7):603-17.

Shah J, Teitelbaum P, Molony B, et al, "Single and Multiple Dose Pharmacokinetics of Ticlopidine in Young and Elderly Subjects," *Br J Clin Pharmacol*, 1991, 32:761-4.

Teitelbaum P, Gabzuda TG, Koretz SH, et al, "Pharmacokinetics of Ticlopidine Hydrochloride in Young and Old Normal Adult Subjects Following Single and Multiple Dosing," *J Pharm Sci*, 1987, 76:S99.

Ticon® *see* Trimethobenzamide Hydrochloride *on page 720*

TIG *see* Tetanus Immune Globulin, Human *on page 676*

Tigan® *see* Trimethobenzamide Hydrochloride *on page 720*

Tiject® *see* Trimethobenzamide Hydrochloride *on page 720*

Timentin® *see* Ticarcillin and Clavulanic Acid *on page 693*

Timolol Maleate (tye' moe lole)

Related Information

Beta-Blockers Comparison *on page 804-805*

Glaucoma Drug Therapy Comparison *on page 810*

Brand Names Blocadren®; Timoptic®

Therapeutic Class Beta-Adrenergic Blocker; Beta-Adrenergic Blocker, Ophthalmic

Use

Ophthalmic: Treatment of elevated intraocular pressure such as glaucoma or ocular hypertension

Oral: Treatment of hypertension and angina and reduce mortality following myocardial infarction, hypertrophic subaortic stenosis, and prophylaxis of migraine; treatment of the postmyocardial infarction patient

Contraindications Uncompensated congestive heart failure, cardiogenic shock, bradycardia or heart block, bronchial asthma, severe chronic obstructive pulmonary disease or history of asthma; hypersensitivity to beta-blocking agents

Warnings Severe CNS, cardiovascular and respiratory adverse effects have been seen following ophthalmic use; patients with a history of asthma, congestive heart failure, bradycardia, hyperthyroidism, or cerebral insufficiency appear to be at a higher risk; use cautiously in diabetes mellitus

Precautions Some products contain sulfites which can cause allergic reactions; diminished response over time; may increase muscle weaknesses; use with a miotic in angle-closure glaucoma; similar to other beta-blockers; use with caution in patients with decreased renal or hepatic function (dosage adjustment required); abrupt withdrawal of drug should be avoided; discontinuation should be accomplished over a 2-week tapering

Adverse Reactions

Cardiovascular: Bradycardia, arrhythmias, hypotension, syncope, congestive heart failure

Central nervous system: Dizziness, headache, confusion, mental depression, nightmares

Dermatologic: Rash

Endocrine: Blocks signs or symptoms of hypoglycemia

(Continued)

Timolol Maleate *(Continued)*

Gastrointestinal: Diarrhea, nausea

Ocular: Irritation, conjunctivitis, keratitis, visual disturbances, blepharitis

Respiratory: Bronchospasm, wheezing, dyspnea

Other adverse effects similar to other beta-blockers, alopecia, weakness

Overdosage Symptoms of overdose include severe hypotension, bradycardia, heart failure and bronchospasm

Toxicology Sympathomimetics (eg, epinephrine or dopamine), glucagon or a pacemaker can be used to treat the toxic bradycardia, asystole, and/or hypotension; initially, fluids may be the best treatment for toxic hypotension. For ophthalmic product, flush eye(s) with water or normal saline. Not significantly dialyzable.

Drug Interactions May cause bradycardia and asystole when also giving verapamil; has caused sinus bradycardia in one patient also taking quinidine; controversial when used with epinephrine; nonsteroidal anti-inflammatory agents, salicylates, sympathomimetics, thyroid hormones, insulins, lidocaine, calcium channel blockers, nifedipine, catecholamine-depleting drugs, clonidine, disopyramide, prazosin, theophylline, cimetidine

Mechanism of Action Blocks both beta$_1$-adrenergic and beta$_2$-adrenergic receptors, reduces intraocular pressure by most likely reducing aqueous humor production or possibly outflow; reduces blood pressure by blocking adrenergic receptors and decreasing sympathetic outflow, produces a negative chronotropic and inotropic activity through an unknown mechanism

Pharmacodynamics

Onset of action: Oral: Following administration hypotensive effects occur within 15-45 minutes

Peak effect: Within 30-150 minutes

Duration: ~4 hours; intraocular effects persist for 24 hours after ophthalmic instillation

Pharmacokinetics

Protein binding: 60%

Metabolism: Extensive in the liver; extensive first-pass effect

Half-life: 2-2.7 hours; half-life prolonged with reduced renal function

Elimination: Urinary (15% to 20% as unchanged drug)

Usual Dosage Geriatrics and Adults:

Ophthalmic: Initial: 0.25% solution, instill 1 drop twice daily; increase to 0.5% solution if response not adequate; decrease to 1 drop/day if controlled; do not exceed 1 drop twice daily of 0.5% solution

Oral:

Hypertension: Initial: 10 mg twice daily, increase gradually every 7 days, usual dosage: 20-40 mg/day in 2 divided doses; maximum: 60 mg/day

Prevention of myocardial infarction: 10 mg twice daily initiated within 1-4 weeks after infarction

Migraine: Initial: 10 mg twice daily; increase to maximum of 30 mg/day

Monitoring Parameters Intraocular pressure, heart rate, blood pressure, respiratory rate, funduscopic exam, visual field tests

Test Interactions Increased cholesterol (S), elevated glucose

Patient Information May sting on instillation; do not touch dropper to eye; visual acuity may be decreased after administration; distance vision may be altered; assess patient's or caregiver's ability to administer; apply gentle pressure to lacrimal sac during and immediately following instillation (1 minute) to avoid systemic absorption; stop drug if breathing difficulty occurs

Nursing Implications Monitor for signs of congestive heart failure, hypotension, respiratory difficulty (bronchospasm); use cautiously in diabetics receiving hypoglycemic agents; teach proper instillation of eye drops; see Monitoring Parameters

Additional Information Does not cause night blindness

Special Geriatric Considerations Due to alterations in the beta-adrenergic autonomic nervous system, beta-adrenergic blockade may result in less hemodynamic response than seen in younger adults. Studies indicate that despite decreased sensitivity to the chronotropic effects of beta blockade with age, there appears to be an increased myocardial sensitivity to the negative inotropic effect during stress (ie, exercise). Controlled trials have shown the overall response rate for propranolol to be only 20% to 50% in elderly populations. Therefore, all beta-adrenergic blocking drugs may result in a decreased response as compared to younger adults.

Dosage Forms

Solution, ophthalmic: 0.25% (2.5 mL, 5 mL, 10 mL, 15 mL)

Tablet: 5 mg, 10 mg, 20 mg

References

Kligman EW and Higbee MD, "Drug Therapy for Hypertension in the Elderly," *J Fam Pract*, 1989, 28(1):81-7.

Levison SP, "Treating Hypertension in the Elderly," *Clin Geriatr Med*, 1988, 4(1):1-12.

Passo MS, Palmer EA, and Van Buskirk EM, "Plasma Timolol in Glaucoma Patients," *Ophthalmology*, 1984, 91(11):1361-3.

Vestal RE, Wood AJ, and Shand DG, "Reduced Beta-Adrenoceptor Sensitivity in the Elderly," *Clin Pharmacol Ther*, 1979, 26(2):181-6.

Yin FC, Raizes, GS, Guarnieri T, et al, "Age-Associated Decrease in Ventricular Response to Haemo-dynamic Stress During Beta-Adrenergic Blockade," *Br Heart J*, 1978, 40(12):1349-55.

Timoptic® *see* Timolol Maleate *on page 697*

Tinactin® [OTC] *see* Tolnaftate *on page 705*

Tindal® *see* Acetophenazine Maleate *on page 18*

Tine Test *see* Tuberculin Purified Protein Derivative *on page 725*

Tine Test PPD® *see* Tuberculin Purified Protein Derivative *on page 725*

Tiotixene *see* Thiothixene *on page 687*

Titralac® Plus Liquid [OTC] *see* Calcium Salts (Oral) *on page 111*

TMP *see* Trimethoprim *on page 721*

TMP-SMX *see* Co-trimoxazole *on page 189*

Tobramycin (toe bra mye' sin)
Related Information
Aminoglycoside Dosing Guidelines *on page 753*
Drug Levels Commonly Monitored Guidelines *on page 771-772*
Brand Names Nebcin®; Tobrex®
Therapeutic Class Antibiotic, Aminoglycoside; Antibiotic, Ophthalmic
Use Treatment of documented or suspected *Pseudomonas aeruginosa* infection; infection with a nonpseudomonal enteric bacillus which is more sensitive to tobramycin than gentamicin based on susceptibility tests; empiric therapy in cystic fibrosis and immunocompromised patients; topically used to treat superficial ophthalmic infections caused by susceptible bacteria
Contraindications Hypersensitivity to tobramycin or other aminoglycosides
Warnings
Not intended for long-term therapy due to toxic hazards associated with extended administration; pre-existing renal insufficiency, vestibular or cochlear impairment, myasthenia gravis, hypocalcemia, conditions which depress neuromuscular transmission
I.M. & I.V.: Aminoglycosides are associated with significant nephrotoxicity or ototoxicity; the ototoxicity is directly proportional to the amount of drug given and the duration of treatment; tinnitus or vertigo are indications of vestibular injury and impending irreversible bilateral deafness; nephrotoxicity is associated with trough concentrations >2 mcg/mL and is usually reversible
Precautions Use with caution in patients with renal impairment; pre-existing auditory or vestibular impairment; and in patients with neuromuscular disorders; dosage modification required in patients with impaired renal function
Adverse Reactions
Cardiovascular: Thrombophlebitis
Central nervous system: Fever
Dermatologic: Allergic contact dermatitis, rash
Gastrointestinal: Diarrhea, pseudomembranous colitis
Neuromuscular & skeletal: Neuromuscular blockade
Ocular: Lacrimation, itching, edema of the eyelid, keratitis
Otic: Ototoxicity
Renal: Nephrotoxicity
Overdosage Symptoms of overdose include ototoxicity, nephrotoxicity, and neuromuscular toxicity
Toxicology The treatment of choice following a single acute overdose appears to be the maintenance of good urine output of at least 3 mL/kg/hour. Dialysis is of questionable value in the enhancement of aminoglycoside elimination. If required, hemodialysis is preferred over peritoneal dialysis in patients with normal renal function. Careful hydration may be all that is required to promote diuresis and therefore the enhancement of the drug's elimination.
Drug Interactions
Increased/prolonged effect: Depolarizing and nondepolarizing neuromuscular blocking agents
Increased toxicity: Concurrent use of amphotericin, vancomycin, or loop diuretics may increase nephrotoxicity
Stability Reconstituted solution is stable for 24 hours at room temperature and 96 hours when refrigerated; incompatible with penicillins
Mechanism of Action Interferes with bacterial protein synthesis by binding to 30S and 50S ribosomal subunits resulting in a defective bacterial cell membrane
Pharmacokinetics
Absorption: I.M.: Rapid and complete
Distribution: V_d: 0.2-0.3 L/kg
Half-life: 2-3 hours, directly dependent upon glomerular filtration rate; half-life (impaired renal function): 5-70 hours
(Continued)

Tobramycin (Continued)

Time to peak:
I.M.: Peak serum levels occur within 30-60 minutes
Following a 30-minute I.V. infusion, peak serum levels occur in 30 minutes
Elimination: With normal renal function, about 90% to 95% of dose is excreted in urine within 24 hours
The pharmacokinetics of the aminoglycosides are heterogeneous in the elderly. It is best to assume that clearance is reduced and half-life prolonged in the elderly, while volume of distribution is usually unchanged. The establishment of each patient's pharmacokinetic parameters is important for proper dosing in order to achieve an optimal therapeutic benefit and minimize the risks of toxicity. Following I.M. administration, the time to peak serum concentration was delayed in the elderly.

Usual Dosage Dosage should be based on an estimate of ideal body weight
Geriatrics: I.M., I.V.: 1.5-5 mg/kg/day in 1-2 divided doses

Adults: I.M., I.V.: 3-5 mg/kg/day in 3 divided doses or as indicated by adjustment for renal function

Renal dysfunction: 2 mg/kg (2-3 serum level measurements should be obtained after the initial dose to measure the half-life in order to determine the frequency of subsequent doses)

Ophthalmic: 1-2 drops every 4 hours; apply ointment 2-3 times/day; for severe infections apply ointment every 3-4 hours, or 2 drops every 30-60 minutes initially, then reduce to less frequent intervals
Dialyzable (50% to 100%)

Monitoring Parameters Draw peak concentrations 30 minutes after the end of a 30-minute infusion; the trough is drawn just before the next dose; urine output; serum BUN and creatinine, signs and symptoms of infection; culture and sensitivities

Reference Range
Therapeutic:
Peak: 5-10 μg/mL (SI: 11-21 μmol/L)
Trough: 1-1.5 μg/mL (SI: 2-3 μmol/L)
Toxic:
Peak: >12 μg/mL (SI: >21 μmol/L)
Trough: >2 μg/mL (SI: >9 μmol/L)

Test Interactions Increased protein; decreased magnesium

Patient Information Report symptoms of superinfection; for eye drops – no other eye drops 5-10 minutes before or after tobramycin

Nursing Implications Eye solutions: Allow 5 minutes between application of "multiple-drop" therapy; with I.M. or I.V. treatment, obtain drug levels after the third dose

Additional Information Should not be mixed with other drugs

Special Geriatric Considerations The aminoglycosides are an important therapeutic intervention for susceptible organisms and as empiric therapy in seriously ill patients. Their use is not without risk of toxicity; however, these risks can be minimized if initial dosing is adjusted for estimated renal function and appropriate monitoring is performed.

Dosage Forms
Injection, as sulfate: 10 mg/mL (2 mL); 40 mg/mL (1.5 mL, 2 mL)
Ophthalmic:
Ointment: 0.3% (3.5 g)
Solution: 0.3% (5 mL)
Powder for injection: 40 mg/mL (1.2 g); 30 mg/mL (1.2 g)

References
Bauer LA and Blouin RA, "Influence of Age on Tobramycin. Pharmacokinetics in Patients With Normal Renal Function," *Antimicrob Agents Chemother*, 1981, 20:587-9.
Matzke GR, Jameson JJ, and Halstenson CE, "Gentamicin Disposition in Young and Elderly Patients With Various Degrees of Renal Function," *J Clin Pharmacol*, 1987, 27(3):216-20.
Mayer PR, Brown CH, Carter RA, et al, "Intramuscular Tobramycin Pharmacokinetics in Geriatric Patients," *Drug Intell Clin Pharm*, 1986, 20:611-5.
Zaske DE, Irvine P, Strand LM, et al, "Wide Interpatient Variations in Gentamicin Dose Requirements for Geriatric Patients," *JAMA*, 1982, 248(23):3122-6.

Tobrex® see Tobramycin *on previous page*

Tocainide Hydrochloride (toe kay' nide)

Brand Names Tonocard®
Generic Available No
Therapeutic Class Antiarrhythmic Agent, Class IB
Use Suppress and prevent symptomatic life-threatening ventricular arrhythmias

Unlabeled use: Trigeminal neuralgia
Contraindications Second or third degree A-V block, hypersensitivity to tocainide o any component
Warnings Agranulocytosis, bone marrow suppression, leukopenia, neutropenia, aplas tic anemia, thrombocytopenia, septicemia, septic shock; fatalities secondary to blood

dyscrasias; pulmonary fibrosis, interstitial pneumonitis, fibrosing alveolitis, pneumonia, and pulmonary edema; may cause or exacerbate pre-existent arrhythmias; sudden death; use cautiously in patients with heart failure or poor cardiac reserve and in patients with renal or hepatic impairment

Precautions May exacerbate some arrhythmias; use with caution in congestive heart failure patients; administer with caution in patients with pre-existing bone marrow failure or cytopenia

Adverse Reactions
Cardiovascular: Hypotension, bradycardia, tachycardia, palpitations
Central nervous system: Vertigo, dizziness, paresthesia, confusion, hallucinations, nervousness, anxiety
Dermatologic: Rash, skin lesions
Gastrointestinal: Nausea, vomiting, diarrhea
Hematologic: Agranulocytosis, anemia, leukopenia, neutropenia
Neuromuscular & skeletal: Tremors
Ocular: Blurred vision
Otic: Tinnitus
Respiratory: Respiratory arrest
Miscellaneous: Sweating

Overdosage Symptoms of overdose include convulsions, confusion, altered mood, ataxia, paresthesia, congestive heart failure, cardiopulmonary depression; tremor may indicate maximum tolerable dose; also see GI side effects

Toxicology Toxicity is similar to that of lidocaine, but the effects are longer in duration. Bradycardia and asystole may be difficult to control with standard therapeutic agents. Temporary pacemaker insertion may be required. Provide general supportive care; gastric lavage and charcoal administration may be effective; treat seizures with I.V. diazepam or barbiturates.

Drug Interactions
Cimetidine decreases absorption of tocainide
Metoprolol, rifampin, allopurinol increases half-life of tocainide

Mechanism of Action Suppresses automaticity of conduction tissue, by increasing electrical stimulation threshold of ventricle, HIS-Purkinje system, and spontaneous depolarization of the ventricles during diastole by a direct action on the tissues; blocks both the initiation and conduction of nerve impulses by decreasing the neuronal membrane's permeability to sodium ions, which results in inhibition of depolarization with resultant blockade of conduction

Pharmacokinetics
Absorption: Oral: Extensive, 99% to 100%
Distribution: V_d: 1.62-3.2 L/kg
Protein binding: 10% to 20%
Metabolism: Metabolized in the liver to inactive metabolites; first-pass effect is negligible
Half-life: 11-14 hours, prolonged with renal and hepatic impairment with half-life increased to 23-27 hours
Time to peak: Peak serum levels occur within 30-160 minutes
Elimination: In urine (40% to 50% as unchanged drug)

Usual Dosage Geriatrics and Adults: Initial dose: 400 mg every 8 hours; increase to 1200-1800 mg/day in 3 divided doses; do not exceed 2400 mg/day; patients with hepatic and renal dysfunction may be controlled with doses <1200 mg/day; may be given in 2 divided doses if tolerated; food results in slower absorption and a 40% decrease in maximum serum concentration, but extent of absorption is unaltered

Moderately dialyzable (20% to 50%)

Monitoring Parameters Guide dose by clinical effect and EKG monitoring; periodically monitor CBC and liver function tests; monitor for tremor

Reference Range Therapeutic: 5-12 µg/mL (SI: 22-52 µmol/L)

Test Interactions Abnormal LFTs observed at initiation of drug

Patient Information Report any unusual bleeding, cough, tremor, palpitations, rash, bruising, chills, fever, sore throat, or any breathing difficulties; may cause drowsiness, nausea, vomiting, and diarrhea; notify physician if these adverse reactions persist or are severe; may take with food

Additional Information Known as "oral lidocaine"

Special Geriatric Considerations Tocainide may cause confusion; tremor indicates potential toxicity and should not be mistaken for age related changes; renal and phase I liver metabolism changes with age may affect clearance; monitor closely since half-life may be prolonged

Dosage Forms Tablet: 400 mg, 600 mg

References
Fenster PE and Nolan PE, "Antiarrhythmic Drugs," *Geriatric Pharmacology*, Bressler R and Katz MD, eds, New York, NY: McGraw-Hill, 1993, 6:105-49.

Tofranil® see Imipramine *on page 365*
Tofranil-PM® see Imipramine *on page 365*

Tolazamide (tole az' a mide)

Brand Names Ronase®; Tolinase®

Therapeutic Class Antidiabetic Agent; Hypoglycemic Agent, Oral; Sulfonylurea Agent

Use Adjunct to diet for the management of mild to moderately severe, stable, noninsulin-dependent (type II) diabetes mellitus

Contraindications Therapy of type I diabetes, hypersensitivity to sulfonylureas, diabetes complicated by ketoacidosis

Warnings False-positive response has been reported in patients with liver disease, severe malnutrition, acute pancreatitis, renal dysfunction

Adverse Reactions
Central nervous system: Headache, dizziness
Dermatologic: Rash, urticaria, photosensitivity
Endocrine & metabolic: Hypoglycemia
Gastrointestinal: Anorexia, nausea, vomiting, diarrhea, constipation, heartburn, epigastric fullness
Hematologic: Aplastic anemia, hemolytic anemia, bone marrow depression, thrombocytopenia, granulocytosis
Renal: Diuretic effect

Overdosage Symptoms of overdose include low blood sugar, tingling of lips and tongue, nausea, yawning, confusion, agitation, tachycardia, sweating, convulsions, stupor, and coma

Toxicology Intoxications with sulfonylureas can cause hypoglycemia and are best managed with glucose administration (oral for milder hypoglycemia or by injection in more severe forms)

Drug Interactions Monitor patient closely; large number of drugs interact with sulfonylureas including salicylates, anticoagulants, H_2 antagonists, TCA, MAO inhibitors, beta-blockers, thiazides

Mechanism of Action Stimulates insulin release from the pancreatic beta cells; reduces glucose output from the liver; insulin sensitivity is increased at peripheral target sites

Pharmacodynamics
Onset of action: Oral: Following administration, effects occur within 4-6 hours
Duration: 10-24 hours

Pharmacokinetics
Protein binding: >98% ionic/nonionic
Metabolism: Extensive in the liver to one active and three inactive metabolite
Half-life: 7 hours
Elimination: Renal

Usual Dosage Geriatrics and Adults: Oral: Initial: 100 mg/day; increase at 2- to 4-week intervals; maximum dose: 1000 mg; give as a single or twice daily dose (doses >500 mg/day twice daily)

Administration See Nursing Implications

Monitoring Parameters Fasting blood glucose; hemoglobin A_{1c}, or fructosamine

Reference Range Fasting blood glucose: Geriatrics: 100-150 mg/dL; Adults: 80-140 mg/dL

Test Interactions Decreased prothrombin time (S), decreased sodium (S)

Patient Information Tablets may be crushed; take drug at the same time each day; avoid alcohol; recognize signs and symptoms of hypoglycemia; avoid hypoglycemia, eat regularly, do not skip meals; carry a quick sugar source; medical alert bracelet

Nursing Implications Patients who are anorexic or NPO may need to have their dose held to avoid hypoglycemia

Additional Information Transferring a patient from one sulfonylurea to another does not require a priming dose; doses >1000 mg/day normally does not improve diabetic control

Special Geriatric Considerations Has not been studied in older patients, however, except for drug interactions it appears to have a safe profile and decline in renal function does not affect its pharmacokinetics. How "tightly" a geriatric patient's blood glucose should be controlled is controversial; however, a fasting blood sugar of <150 mg/dL is now an acceptable end point. Such a decision should be based on the patient's functional and cognitive status, how well they recognize hypoglycemic or hyperglycemic symptoms, and how to respond to them and their other disease states.

Dosage Forms Tablet: 100 mg, 250 mg, 500 mg

Tolbutamide (tole byoo' ta mide)

Brand Names Orinase®

Generic Available Yes

Therapeutic Class Antidiabetic Agent; Hypoglycemic Agent, Oral; Sulfonylurea Agent

Use Adjunct to diet for the management of mild to moderately severe, stable, noninsulin-dependent (type II) diabetes mellitus

Contraindications Diabetes complicated by ketoacidosis, therapy of type I diabetes, hypersensitivity to sulfonylureas

Precautions False-positive response has been reported in patients with liver disease, severe malnutrition, acute pancreatitis

Adverse Reactions
  Cardiovascular: Venospasm, thrombophlebitis
  Central nervous system: Headache, dizziness
  Dermatologic: Skin rash, hives, photosensitivity
  Endocrine & metabolic: Hypoglycemia, SIADH
  Gastrointestinal: Constipation, diarrhea, heartburn, anorexia, epigastric fullness
  Hematologic: Aplastic anemia, hemolytic anemia, bone marrow depression, thrombo-
    cytopenia, leukopenia
  Otic: Tinnitus
  Miscellaneous: Hypersensitivity reaction, disulfiram-like reactions

Overdosage Symptoms of overdose include low blood sugar, tingling of lips and tongue, nausea, yawning, confusion, agitation, tachycardia, sweating, convulsions, stupor, and coma

Drug Interactions
  Increased effects with salicylates, probenecid, MAO inhibitors, chloramphenicol, insu-
    lin, phenylbutazone, antidepressants, H_2 antagonists, and others
  Hypoglycemic effects may be decreased by beta-blockers, cholestyramine, hydan-
    toins, thiazides, rifampin, and others
  Ethanol may decrease the half-life of tolbutamide

Stability Use within 1 hour following reconstitution

Mechanism of Action Stimulates insulin release from the pancreatic beta cells; reduces glucose output from the liver; insulin sensitivity is increased at peripheral target sites, suppression of glucagon may also contribute

Pharmacodynamics
  Onset of hypoglycemic effect: 1 hour
  Duration: 6-24 hours; no apparent change in response with age

Pharmacokinetics
  Half-life, plasma: 4-25 hours
  Protein binding: 95% to 97% (principally to albumin) ionic/nonionic
  Metabolism/Elimination: Hepatic metabolism to hydroxymethyltolbutamide (mildly ac-
    tive) and carboxytolbutamide (inactive) both rapidly excreted renally, less 2% ex-
    creted in urine unchanged; metabolism does not appear to be affected by age
  Increased plasma concentrations and volume of distribution secondary to decreased
    albumin concentrations and less protein binding have been reported

Usual Dosage Oral:
  Geriatrics: Initial: 250 mg 1-3 times/day; usual: 500-2000 mg; maximum: 3 g/day
  Adults: Initial: 500-1000 mg 1-3 times/day; usual dose should not be more than 2 g/day
  Not dialyzable (0% to 5%)

Administration See Nursing Implications

Monitoring Parameters Fasting blood glucose, hemoglobin A_{1c}, or fructosamine

Reference Range Fasting blood glucose: Geriatrics: 100-150 mg/dL; Adults: 80-140 mg/dL

Test Interactions Increased protein; decreased prothrombin time (S), decreased sodium (S); false-positive proteinuria

Patient Information Fast the night before the test

Nursing Implications Patients who are anorexic or NPO may need to have their dose held to avoid hypoglycemia

Special Geriatric Considerations Because of its low potency and short duration, it is a useful agent in the elderly if drug interactions can be avoided, see Pharmacody-namics and Pharmacokinetics. How "tightly" a geriatric patient's blood glucose should be controlled is controversial; however, a fasting blood sugar of <150 mg/dL is now an acceptable end point. Such a decision should be based on the patient's functional and cognitive status, how well they recognize hypoglycemic or hyperglycemic symp-toms, and how to respond to them and their other disease states.

Dosage Forms Tablet: 250 mg, 500 mg

References
Miller AK, Adir J, and Vestal RE, "Effect of Age on the Pharmacokinetics of Tolbutamide in Man," *Pharmacologist*, 1977, 19:128.
Miller AK, Adir J, and Vestal RE, "Tolbutamide Binding to Plasma Proteins of Young and Old Human Subjects," *J Pharm Sci*, 1978, 67(8):1192-3.

Tolectin® see Tolmetin Sodium *on this page*
Tolinase® see Tolazamide *on previous page*

Tolmetin Sodium (tole' met in)
Brand Names Tolectin®
Generic Available No
Therapeutic Class Analgesic, Non-narcotic; Nonsteroidal Anti-inflammatory Agent (NSAID), Oral
Use Treatment of rheumatoid arthritis and osteoarthritis, juvenile rheumatoid arthritis, sunburn, mild to moderate pain
Contraindications Known hypersensitivity to tolmetin, any component, aspirin, or other nonsteroidal anti-inflammatory drugs (NSAIDs)
(Continued)

Tolmetin Sodium *(Continued)*

Warnings Anaphylactoid reactions have been reported in patients with intermittent use and aspirin sensitivity; GI toxicity (bleeding, ulceration, perforation); CNS effects may occur (headaches, confusion, depression); hypersensitivity, anaphylactoid reactions (intermittent tolmetin use more often); renal function decline, acute renal insufficiency, interstitial nephritis, dysuria, cystitis, hematuria, nephrotic syndrome, hyperkalemia in acute renal insufficiency, hyponatremia, papillary necrosis, hepatic function impairment; elderly have increased risk for adverse reactions to NSAIDs; see Special Geriatric Considerations

Precautions Use with caution in patients with congestive heart failure, hypertension, decreased renal or hepatic function, history of GI disease (bleeding or ulcers), or those receiving anticoagulants; perform ophthalmologic evaluation for those who develop eye complaints during therapy (blurred vision, diminished vision, changes in color vision, retinal changes); NSAIDs may mask signs/symptoms of infections; photosensitivity reported

Adverse Reactions

Cardiovascular: Congestive heart failure, angina, hypertension, hypotension, fluid retention, arrhythmias, edema

Central nervous system: Headache, drowsiness, vertigo, dizziness, fatigue, hallucinations, confusion, depression, emotional lability, psychotic behavior, asthenia, pyrexia

Dermatologic: Rash, urticaria, angioedema, Stevens-Johnson syndrome, exfoliative dermatitis, ecchymosis, petechiae, purpura, bruising

Endocrine & metabolic: Hyperglycemia, hypoglycemia, hyperkalemia, gynecomastia, hyponatremia

Gastrointestinal: Dyspepsia, heartburn, nausea, diarrhea, constipation, flatulence, stomatitis, vomiting, abdominal pain, peptic ulcer, GI bleeding, GI perforation, gingival ulcers, pancreatitis, proctitis, paralytic ulcers, colitis, anorexia, weight loss

Genitourinary: Impotence, azotemia

Hematologic: Neutropenia, anemia, agranulocytosis, bone marrow suppression, hemolytic anemia, hemorrhage, inhibition of platelet aggregation

Hepatic: Hepatitis, elevated LFTs, cholestatic jaundice

Neuromuscular & skeletal: Involuntary muscle movements, muscle weakness, tremors

Ocular: Vision changes

Otic: Tinnitus

Renal: Dysuria, polyuria, pyuria, oliguria, anuria, acute renal failure

Respiratory: Exacerbation of asthma, dyspnea

Miscellaneous: Dry mucous membranes, thirst, sweating

Overdosage Symptoms include drowsiness, lethargy, disorientation, confusion, dizziness, numbness, paresthesia, nausea, vomiting, gastric irritation, abdominal pain, headache, tinnitus, sweating, blurred vision, muscle twitching, seizures, coma, acute renal failure, increased BUN and serum creatinine, hypotension, tachycardia, and metabolic acidosis

Toxicology Management of a nonsteroidal anti-inflammatory agent (NSAID) intoxication is primarily supportive and symptomatic. Fluid therapy is commonly effective in managing the hypotension that may occur following an acute NSAID overdose, except when this is due to an acute blood loss. Seizures tend to be very short-lived and often do not require drug treatment although recurrent seizures should be treated with I.V. diazepam. Since many of the NSAIDs undergo enterohepatic cycling, multiple doses of charcoal may be needed to reduce the potential for delayed toxicities.

Drug Interactions

May increase digoxin, methotrexate, and lithium serum concentrations

Aspirin or other salicylates may decrease NSAID serum concentrations

Other NSAIDs may increase adverse GI effects

Increased prothrombin time with anticoagulants

Decreased antihypertensive effects of ACE inhibitors, beta-blockers, and thiazide diuretics

Effects of loop diuretics may decrease

Increased response to sympathomimetics

Probenecid may increase toxicity of NSAIDs by increase in serum concentrations

Diuretics may increase risk of acute renal insufficiency

Azotemia may be enhanced in elderly receiving loop diuretics

Mechanism of Action Inhibits prostaglandin synthesis, acts on the hypothalamus heat-regulating center to reduce fever, blocks prostaglandin synthetase action which prevents formation of the platelet-aggregating substance thromboxane A_2; decreases pain receptor sensitivity. Other proposed mechanisms of action for salicylate anti-inflammatory action are lysosomal stabilization, kinin and leukotriene production, alteration of chemotactic factors, and inhibition of neutrophil activation. This latter mechanism may be the most significant pharmacologic action to reduce inflammation.

Pharmacodynamics

Onset of analgesic action: 0.5-1 hour

Duration: 4-6 hours

Onset of anti-inflammatory action: Within 7 days; Maximum benefit: 1-2 weeks

Pharmacokinetics

Absorption: Oral: Well absorbed

Protein binding: >90%

Half-life: 1-2 hours

Time to peak: Peak serum levels occur within 30-60 minutes

Usual Dosage Geriatrics and Adults: Oral: 200-400 mg 3 times/day; usual dose: 600 mg to 1.8 g/day; maximum: 2 g/day

Monitoring Parameters Monitor response (pain, range of motion, grip strength, mobility, ADL function), inflammation; observe for weight gain, edema; monitor renal function; observe for bleeding, bruising; evaluate gastrointestinal effects (abdominal pain, bleeding, dyspepsia); mental confusion, disorientation, CBC, serum, creatinine, BUN, liver function tests

Test Interactions Increased protein

Patient Information Serious gastrointestinal bleeding can occur as well as ulceration and perforation. Pain may or may not be present. Avoid aspirin and aspirin-containing products while taking this medication. If gastric upset occurs, take with food, milk, or antacid. If gastric adverse effects persist, contact physician. May cause drowsiness, dizziness, blurred vision, and confusion. Use caution when performing tasks which require alertness (eg, driving). Do not take for more than 3 days for fever or 10 days for pain without physician's advice.

Nursing Implications Assess audiometric and ophthalmic exam before, during, and after treatment; see Overdosage, Patient Information, Monitoring Parameters, and Special Geriatric Considerations

Additional Information Only NSAID affected by food/milk, which decreases total bioavailability by 16%. If GI upset occurs with tolmetin, take with antacids other than sodium bicarbonate. Each 200 mg of tolmetin contains 0.8 mEq of sodium. There are no clinical guidelines to predict which NSAID will give response in a particular patient. Trials with each must be initiated until response determined. Consider dose, patient convenience, and cost.

Special Geriatric Considerations Elderly are a high-risk population for adverse effects from nonsteroidal anti-inflammatory agents. As much as 60% of elderly can develop peptic ulceration and/or hemorrhage asymptomatically. The concomitant use of H2-blockers, omeprazole, and sucralfate is not effective as prophylaxis. Misoprostol is the only prophylactic agent proven effective. Also, concomitant disease and drug use contribute to the risk for GI adverse effects. Use lowest effective dose for shortest period possible. Consider renal function decline with age. Use of NSAIDs can compromise existing renal function especially when Cl_{cr} is ≤30 mL/minute. Tinnitus may be a difficult and unreliable indication of toxicity due to age-related hearing loss or eighth cranial nerve damage. CNS adverse effects such as confusion, agitation, and hallucination are generally seen in overdose or high dose situations, but elderly may demonstrate these adverse effects at lower doses than younger adults.

Dosage Forms

Capsule: 400 mg

Tablet: 200 mg, 600 mg

References
Brooks PM, Day RO, "Nonsteroidal Anti-inflammatory Drugs – Differences and Similarities," *N Engl J Med*, 1991, 324(24):1716-25.

Clinch D, Banerjee AK, Ostick G, "Absence of Abdominal Pain in Elderly Patients With Peptic Ulcer," *Age Ageing*, 1984, 13:120-3.

Clive DM, Stoff JS, "Renal Syndromes Associated With Nonsteroidal Anti-inflammatory Drugs," *N Engl J Med*, 1984, 310(9):563-72.

Graham DY, "Prevention of Gastroduodenal Injury Induced by Chronic Nonsteroidal Anti-inflammatory Drug Therapy," *Gastroenterology*, 1989, 96(2 Pt 2 Suppl):675-81.

Gurwitz JH, Avarn J, Ross-Degan D, et al, "Nonsteroidal Anti-Inflammatory Drug-Associated Azotemia in the Very Old," *JAMA*, 1990, 264(4):471-5.

Knodel LC, "Preventing NSAID-Induced Ulcers: The Role of Misoprostol," *Consult Pharm*, 1989, 4:37-41.

Pounder R, "Silent Peptic Ulceration: Deadly Silence or Golden Silence?" *Gastroenterology*, 1989, 96(2 Pt 2 Suppl):626-31.

Tolnaftate (tole naf' tate)

Brand Names Absorbine® Antifungal [OTC]; Absorbine® Jock Itch [OTC]; Absorbine Jr.® Antifungal [OTC]; Aftate® [OTC]; Desenex® [OTC]; Genaspor® [OTC]; NP-27® [OTC]; Tinactin® [OTC]; Zeasorb-AF® [OTC]

Generic Available Yes

Therapeutic Class Antifungal Agent, Topical

Use Treatment of tinea pedis, tinea cruris, tinea corporis, tinea manuum, tinea versicolor infections

Contraindications Known hypersensitivity to tolnaftate; nail and scalp infections

Warnings Cream is not recommended for nail or scalp infections; keep from eyes; if no improvement within 4 weeks, treatment should be discontinued. Usually not effective alone for the treatment of infections involving hair follicles or nails.

(Continued)

Tolnaftate *(Continued)*

Adverse Reactions
Dermatologic: Pruritus, contact dermatitis
Local: Irritation, stinging

Mechanism of Action Distorts the hyphae and stunts mycelial growth in susceptible fungi

Pharmacodynamics Onset of action: Response may be seen 24-72 hours after initiation of therapy

Usual Dosage Geriatrics and Adults: Topical: Wash and dry affected area; apply 1-3 drops of solution or a small amount of cream or powder and rub into the affected areas 2-3 times/day for 2-4 weeks

Monitoring Parameters Resolution of skin infection

Patient Information Avoid contact with the eyes; apply to clean dry area; consult the physician if a skin irritation develops or if the skin infection worsens or does not improve after 10 days of therapy; does not stain skin or clothing

Nursing Implications Itching, burning, and soreness are usually relieved within 24-72 hours

Additional Information Usually not effective alone for the treatment of infections involving hair follicles or nails

Special Geriatric Considerations No specific recommendations for use in the elderly

Dosage Forms
Aerosol, topical:
Liquid: 1% (59.2 mL, 90 mL, 118.3 mL, 120 mL)
Powder: 1% (90 g, 100 g, 105 g, 150 g)
Cream: 1% (15 g, 30 g)
Gel, topical: 1% (15 g)
Powder, topical: 1% (45 g, 56.7 g, 67.5 g, 70.9 g, 90 g)
Solution, topical: 1% (10 mL, 15 mL)

Tolu-Sed® *see* Guaifenesin and Codeine *on page 332*

Tonocard® *see* Tocainide Hydrochloride *on page 700*

Topicycline® *see* Tetracycline *on page 678*

TOPV *see* Poliovirus Vaccine, Live, Trivalent *on page 575*

Toradol® *see* Ketorolac Tromethamine *on page 392*

Tornalate® *see* Bitolterol Mesylate *on page 91*

Torsemide

Brand Names Demadex®

Therapeutic Class Diuretic, Loop

Use Management of edema associated with congestive heart failure and hepatic or renal disease; used alone or in combination with antihypertensives in treatment of hypertension

Contraindications Hypersensitivity to torsemide or any component; allergy to sulfonamides may result in cross-hypersensitivity to torsemide

Warnings Loop diuretics are potent diuretics, excess amounts can lead to profound diuresis with fluid and electrolyte loss; close medical supervision and dose evaluation is required, particularly in the elderly

Adverse Reactions
Cardiovascular: Hypotension
Central nervous system: Dizziness, headache, encephalopathy
Dermatologic: Rash, photosensitivity
Endocrine & metabolic: Hyperglycemia, hypokalemia, hypochloremia, hyponatremia
Gastrointestinal: Cramps, nausea, vomiting
Genitourinary: Azotemia
Hepatic: Alteration of liver function test results
Neuromuscular & skeletal: Weakness
Otic: Impaired hearing
Renal: Decreased uric acid excretion, increased serum creatinine

Overdosage Symptoms of overdose include electrolyte depletion, volume depletion, hypotension, dehydration, circulatory collapse

Toxicology Following GI decontamination, treatment is supportive; hypotension responds to fluids and Trendelenburg position; replace electrolytes as necessary

Drug Interactions
Decreased effect: Indomethacin, other NSAIDs
Increased hypotensive effect: Other antihypertensives
Increased level of lithium
Increased risk of ototoxicity: Aminoglycosides, other loop diuretics, vancomycin
When given with digoxin, diuretic-induced hypokalemia increases the risk of digoxin toxicity

Mechanism of Action Inhibits reabsorption of sodium and chloride in the ascending loop of Henle and distal renal tubule, interfering with the chloride-binding cotransport system, thus causing increased excretion of water, sodium, chloride, magnesium, and calcium

Pharmacodynamics
Onset of diuresis: 30-60 minutes
Peak effect: 1-4 hours
Duration: ~6 hours

Pharmacokinetics
Absorption: Oral: Rapid
Protein binding: Plasma: ~97% to 99%
Metabolism: Hepatic by cytochrome P-450, 80%
Bioavailability: 80% to 90%
Half-life: 2-4; 7-8 hours in cirrhosis (dose modification appears unnecessary)
Elimination: 20% excreted unchanged in urine

Usual Dosage Geriatrics and Adults:
Oral: 5-10 mg once daily; if ineffective, may double dose until desired effect is achieved; in the treatment of hypertension, if 10 mg is insufficient, add an additional antihypertensive agent
I.V.: 10-20 mg/dose repeated in 2 hours as needed with a doubling of the dose with each succeeding dose until desired diuresis is achieved
Continues to be effective in patients with cirrhosis, no apparent change in dose is necessary

Administration Administer the I.V. dose slowly over 2 minutes

Monitoring Parameters Blood pressure, both standing and sitting/supine, serum electrolytes, weight, I & O; in high doses, monitor auditory function

Patient Information May be taken with food or milk; rise slowly from a lying or sitting position to minimize dizziness, lightheadedness or fainting; also use extra care when exercising, standing for long periods of time, and during hot weather; take in the morning

Nursing Implications See Monitoring Parameters; be alert to complaints about hearing difficulty; check patient for orthostasis

Additional Information 10-20 mg torsemide is approximately equivalent to:
Furosemide 40 mg
Bumetanide 1 mg

Special Geriatric Considerations Dosage adjustment in the elderly appears unnecessary; usual starting dose should be 5 mg

Dosage Forms
Injection: 10 mg/mL (2 mL, 5 mL)
Tablet: 5 mg, 10 mg, 20 mg, 100 mg

Totacillin® *see* Ampicillin *on page 51*

Trandate® *see* Labetalol Hydrochloride *on page 395*

Trandate® HCT *see* Labetalol and Hydrochlorothiazide *on page 395*

Transamine Sulphate *see* Tranylcypromine Sulfate *on this page*

Transdermal-NTG® *see* Nitroglycerin *on page 505*

Transderm-Nitro® *see* Nitroglycerin *on page 505*

Transderm Scop® *see* Scopolamine *on page 639*

Tranxene® *see* Clorazepate Dipotassium *on page 178*

Tranylcypromine Sulfate (tran ill sip' roe meen)
Brand Names Parnate®
Synonyms Transamine Sulphate
Generic Available No
Therapeutic Class Antidepressant, Monoamine Oxidase Inhibitor
Use Symptomatic treatment of depressed patients refractory to or intolerant to tricyclic antidepressants or electroconvulsive therapy
Contraindications Uncontrolled hypertension, known hypersensitivity to tranylcypromine, pheochromocytoma, congestive heart failure – patients <16 years of age, severe renal or hepatic impairment
Warnings Hypertensive crisis within several hours of ingestion of a contraindicated substance (tyramine-containing product)
Adverse Reactions
Cardiovascular: Hypotension, edema, hypertensive crises
Central nervous system: Drowsiness, hyperexcitability, insomnia
Dermatologic: Skin rash
Gastrointestinal: Dry mouth, constipation, weight gain
Genitourinary: Urinary retention, impotence
Hepatic: Hepatotoxicity (rare)
Ocular: Blurred vision
(Continued)

Tranylcypromine Sulfate *(Continued)*

Miscellaneous: Sweating, lupus-like reaction

Overdosage Symptoms of overdose include tachycardia, palpitations, muscle twitching, seizures, headache

Toxicology Competent supportive care is the most important treatment for an overdose with a monoamine oxidase (MAO) inhibitor. Both hypertension or hypotension can occur with intoxication. Hypotension may respond to I.V. fluids or vasopressors and hypertension usually responds to an alpha-adrenergic blocker (or phentolamine 5 mg I.V.) or nifedipine 10 mg; do not use parenteral reserpine. While treating the hypertension, care is warranted to avoid sudden drops in blood pressure, since this may worsen the MAO inhibitor toxicity. Muscle irritability and seizures often respond to diazepam, while hyperthermia is best treated antipyretics and cooling blankets. Cardiac arrhythmias are best treated with phenytoin or procainamide.

Drug Interactions

Decreased effect of antihypertensives

Increased toxicity with disulfiram (seizures), fluoxetine and other serotonin-active agents (eg, paroxetine, sertraline), TCAs (cardiovascular instability), meperidine (cardiovascular instability), phenothiazine (hypertensive crisis), sympathomimetics (hypertensive crisis), sumatriptan (hypothetical), CNS depressants, levodopa (hypertensive crisis), tyramine-containing foods (eg, aged foods), dextroamphetamine (psychosis)

Note: Many of these drug interactions can occur weeks after the MAO inhibitor has been stopped.

Food/Drug Interactions See Warnings and Patient Information

Mechanism of Action Inhibits the enzymes monoamine oxidase A and B which are responsible for the intraneuronal metabolism of norepinephrine and serotonin and increasing their availability to postsynaptic neurons; decreased firing rate of the locus ceruleus, reducing norepinephrine concentration in the brain; agonist effects of serotonin

Pharmacodynamics Onset of therapeutic effect: 2-3 weeks are required of continued dosing to obtain full effect

Pharmacokinetics

Half-life: 90-190 minutes

Time to peak: Oral: Peak serum levels occur within 2 hours

Elimination: In urine

Usual Dosage Geriatrics and Adults: Oral: 10 mg twice daily, increase to a maximum of 20-40 mg/day after 2 weeks

Administration Give second dose before 4 PM to avoid insomnia

Monitoring Parameters Blood pressure, heart rate, diet, mood and depressive symptoms, weight

Reference Range Inhibition of platelet monoamine oxidase ($\geq$80%) correlated with clinical response

Test Interactions Decreased glucose

Patient Information Tablets may be crushed; avoid alcohol; do not discontinue abruptly; avoid foods high in tyramine (eg, cheese [except cottage, ricotta, and cream], smoked or pickled fish, beef or chicken liver, dried sausage, fava or broad bean pods, yeast, vitamin supplements); change positions slowly; discuss list of drugs and foods to avoid with pharmacist or physician; take second dose no later than 4 PM to avoid insomnia

Nursing Implications Assist with ambulation during initiation of therapy; see Administration, Monitoring Parameters, and Drug Interactions

Additional Information Has a more rapid onset of therapeutic effect than other MAO inhibitors, but causes more severe hypertensive reactions

Special Geriatric Considerations The MAO inhibitors are effective and generally well tolerated by older patients; it is their potential interactions with tyramine- or tryptophan-containing foods (see Warnings) and other drugs (see Drug Interactions), and their effect on blood pressure that have limited their use. The MAO inhibitors are usually reserved for patients who do not tolerate or respond to the traditional "cyclic" or "second generation" antidepressants. Tranylcypromine is the preferred MAO inhibitor because its enzymatic-blocking effects are more rapidly reversed. The brain activity of monoamine oxidase increases with age and even more so in patients with Alzheimer's disease. Therefore, the MAO inhibitors may have an increased role in patients with Alzheimer's disease who are also depressed.

Dosage Forms Tablet: 10 mg

References

Georgotas A, Friedman E, McCarthy M, et al, "Resistant Geriatric Depression and Therapeutic Response to Monoamine-Oxidase Inhibitors," *Biol Psychiatry*, 1983, 18:195-205.

Goff DC and Jenike MA, "Treatment-Resistant Depression in the Elderly," *J Am Geriatr Soc*, 1986, 34(1):63-70.

Jenike MA, "MAO Inhibitors as Treatment for Depressed Patients With Primary Degenerative Dementia (Alzheimer's Disease)," *Am J Psychiatry* 1985, 142:763.

Trazodone (traz' oh done)

Related Information
Antidepressant Agents Comparison *on page 800*

Brand Names Desyrel®

Therapeutic Class Antidepressant

Use Treatment of depression

Contraindications Hypersensitivity to trazodone or any component

Warnings Monitor closely and use with extreme caution in patients with cardiac disease or arrhythmias

Precautions Cardiovascular effects may warrant EKG prior to initiation of treatment

Adverse Reactions Possesses fewer anticholinergic and cardiac adverse effects than tricyclic antidepressants

Cardiovascular: Postural hypotension (5%), arrhythmias
Central nervous system: Drowsiness (20% to 50%), sedation, dizziness, headache, insomnia, confusion, agitation, seizures, rarely extrapyramidal reactions
Gastrointestinal: Dry mouth (15% to 30%), constipation, nausea, vomiting
Hepatic: Hepatitis
Ocular: Blurred vision
Genitourinary: Prolonged priapism (1:6000), urinary retention (rare)
Neuromuscular & skeletal: Weakness

Overdosage Symptoms of overdose include drowsiness, vomiting, hypotension, tachycardia, incontinence, coma

Toxicology Following initiation of essential overdose management, toxic symptoms should be treated. Ventricular arrhythmias often respond to phenytoin 15-20 mg/kg with concurrent systemic alkalinization (sodium bicarbonate 0.5-2 mEq/kg I.V.). Arrhythmias unresponsive to this therapy may respond to lidocaine 1 mg/kg I.V. followed by a titrated infusion. Physostigmine (1-2 mg I.V. slowly) may be indicated in reversing cardiac arrhythmias that are due to vagal blockade or for anticholinergic effects. Seizures usually respond to diazepam I.V. boluses (5-10 mg, up to 30 mg). If seizures are unresponsive or recur, phenytoin or phenobarbital may be required.

Drug Interactions Trazodone may antagonize the antihypertensive effects of clonidine and methyldopa; may increase the serum concentrations of phenytoin or digoxin; effects may be additive with other CNS depressants; fluoxetine may increase trazodone serum concentration; may decrease the effect of anticoagulants

Mechanism of Action Traditionally believed to increase the synaptic concentration of serotonin in the central nervous system by inhibition of its reuptake by the presynaptic neuronal membrane. However, additional receptor effects have been found including desensitization of adenyl cyclase, down regulation of beta-adrenergic receptors, and down regulation of serotonin receptors

Pharmacodynamics Onset of therapeutic effects: May take 1-3 weeks to appear; 5-HT only

Pharmacokinetics
Protein binding: 85% to 95%
Metabolism: In the liver
Half-life: 4-7.5 hours, 2 compartment kinetics
Elimination: Geriatrics: 11.6 hours, nearly twice that of younger patients
Time to peak: Oral: Peak serum levels occur within 30-100 minutes, prolonged in the presence of food (up to 2.5 hours)
Elimination: Primarily in urine and secondarily in feces

Usual Dosage Oral:
Geriatrics: 25-50 mg at bedtime with 25-50 mg/day dose increase every 3 days for inpatients and weekly for outpatients, if tolerated; usual dose: 75-150 mg/day
Adults: Initial: 150 mg/day in 3 divided doses (may increase by 50 mg/day every 3-7 days); maximum: 600 mg/day

Monitoring Parameters Blood pressure, pulse, target symptoms

Reference Range Therapeutic: 0.5-2.5 μg/mL (SI: 1-6 μmol/L); not well established

Patient Information Take shortly after a meal or light snack, can be given as bedtime dose if drowsiness occurs; avoid alcohol; be aware of possible photosensitivity reaction; may cause painful erections; avoid sudden changes of position

Nursing Implications Use side rails on bed if administered to the elderly; observe patient's activity and compare with admission level; sitting and standing blood pressure and pulse

Additional Information Therapeutic effects may take up to 4 weeks to occur; therapy is normally maintained for several months after optimum response is reached to prevent recurrence of depression

Special Geriatric Considerations Very sedating, but little anticholinergic effects

Dosage Forms Tablet: 50 mg, 100 mg, 150 mg, 300 mg

References
Bayer AJ, Pathy MSJ, and Ankier SI, "Pharmacokinetic and Pharmacodynamic Characteristics of Trazodone in the Elderly," *Br J Clin Pharmacol*, 1983, 16:371-6.
Gerson SC, Plotkin DA, and Jarvik LF, "Antidepressant Drug Studies, 1964-1986: Empirical Evidence for Aging Patients," *J Clin Psychopharmacol*, 1988, 8(5):311-21.

Trecator®-SC *see* Ethionamide *on page 273*

Trendar® [OTC] *see* Ibuprofen *on page 360*

Trental® *see* Pentoxifylline *on page 547*

Triaconazole *see* Terconazole *on page 674*

Triafed® [OTC] *see* Triprolidine and Pseudoephedrine *on page 723*

Triam-A® *see* Triamcinolone *on this page*

Triamcinolone (trye am sin' oh lone)

Related Information

Antacid Drug Interactions *on page 764*

Corticosteroids Comparison, Topical *on page 809*

Brand Names Amcort®; Aristocort® Forte; Aristocort® Intralesional Suspension; Aristocort® Tablet; Aristospan®; Azmacort™; Cenocort®; Cenocort® Forte; Cinonide®; Flutex®; Kenacort® Syrup; Kenacort® Tablet; Kenalog® Injection; Tac™-3; Triam-A®; Triamolone®; Tri-Kort®; Trilog®; Trilone®; Trisoject®

Synonyms Triamcinolone Acetonide, Aerosol; Triamcinolone Acetonide, Parenteral; Triamcinolone Diacetate, Oral; Triamcinolone Diacetate, Parenteral; Triamcinolone Hexacetonide; Triamcinolone, Oral

Generic Available Yes

Therapeutic Class Anti-inflammatory Agent; Corticosteroid, Inhalant; Corticosteroid, Systemic; Corticosteroid, Topical (Medium Potency)

Use

Topical: Inflammatory dermatoses responsive to steroids. Inhalation: Control of bronchial asthma and related bronchospastic conditions

Systemic: Adrenocortical insufficiency, rheumatic disorders, allergic states, respiratory diseases, systemic lupus erythematosus, and other diseases requiring anti-inflammatory or immunosuppressive effects

Contraindications Known hypersensitivity to triamcinolone; systemic fungal infections; serious infections, except septic shock or tuberculous meningitis; primary treatment of acute episodes of asthma

Warnings Fatalities have occurred due to adrenal insufficiency in asthmatic patients during and after transfer from systemic corticosteroids to aerosol steroids; several months may be required for recovery from this syndrome; during this period, aerosol steroids do **not** provide the increased systemic steroid requirement needed to treat patients having trauma, surgery or infections

Precautions Use with caution in patients with hypothyroidism, cirrhosis, nonspecific ulcerative colitis and patients at increased risk for peptic ulcer disease; do not use occlusive dressings on weeping or exudative lesions and general caution with occlusive dressings should be observed; discontinue if skin irritation or contact dermatitis should occur; do not use in patients with decreased skin circulation; avoid the use of high potency steroids on the face

Adverse Reactions

Cardiovascular: Hypertension, edema, accelerated atherogenesis

Central nervous system: Euphoria, mental changes, headache, vertigo, seizures, psychoses, pseudotumor cerebri

Dermatologic: Folliculitis, hypertrichosis, acneiform eruption dermatitis, maceration, skin atrophy, acne, impaired wound healing, hirsutism, itching, hypopigmentation, hyperpigmentation

Endocrine & metabolic: Growth suppression, Cushing's syndrome, pituitary-adrenal axis suppression, alkalosis, glucose intolerance, hypokalemia, postmenopausal bleeding, hot flashes

Gastrointestinal: Peptic ulcer, nausea, vomiting, pancreatitis, oral candidiasis, dry throat, dry mouth

Local: Burning, irritation

Neuromuscular & skeletal: Muscle weakness, osteoporosis, fractures, aseptic necrosis of femoral and humeral heads, steroid myopathy

Ocular: Cataracts, glaucoma

Respiratory: Hoarseness, wheezing, cough

Miscellaneous: Increased susceptibility to infection, facial edema

Toxicology When consumed in excessive quantities for prolonged periods, systemic hypercorticism and adrenal suppression may occur; in those cases, discontinuation and withdrawal of the corticosteroid should be done judiciously

Drug Interactions

Steroids decrease the effect of anticholinesterases, isoniazid, salicylates, insulin, oral hypoglycemics

Decreased effect: Barbiturates, phenytoin, rifampin

Increased effect (hypokalemia) of potassium-depleting diuretics

Increased risk of digoxin toxicity (due to hypokalemia)

Increased effect: Estrogens, ketoconazole

Mechanism of Action Decreases inflammation by suppression of migration of polymorphonuclear leukocytes and reversal of increased capillary permeability; suppresses the immune system by reducing activity and volume of the lymphatic system; suppresses adrenal function at high doses

Pharmacodynamics Duration of action: Oral: 8-12 hours

Pharmacokinetics
 Time to peak: I.M.: Peak serum levels occur within 8-10 hours
 Half-life, biologic: 18-36 hours

Usual Dosage
 Geriatrics and Adults:
  Topical: Apply thin film 2-3 times/day
  Oral inhalation: 2 inhalations 3-4 times/day, not to exceed 16 inhalations/day
  Intra-articularly, intrasynovially, intralesionally: 2.5-40 mg, dose may be repeated when signs and symptoms recur
  Intra-articularly: 2-20 mg every 3-4 weeks as hexacetonide
  Intralesionally, sublesionally (as acetonide): Up to 1 mg per injection site and may be repeated one or more times weekly; multiple sites may be injected if they are 1 cm or more apart, not to exceed 30 mg

 Geriatrics: Systemically use the lowest effective daily dose

 Adults:
  Oral: 4-48 mg/day
  I.M.: Average dose: 40 mg once weekly
 See table.

Triamcinolone Dosing

	Acetonide	Diacetate	Hexacetonide
Intrasynovial	2.5–40 mg	5–40 mg	
Intralesional	2.5–40 mg	5–48 mg	Up to 0.5 mg per square inch of affected area
Sublesional	1–30 mg		
Systemic I.M.	2.5–60 mg/d	~40 mg/wk	20–100 mg
Intra-articular		5–40 mg	2–20 average
large joints	5–15 mg		10–20 mg
small joints	2.5–5 mg		2–6 mg
Tendon sheaths	10–40 mg		
Intradermal	1 mg/site		

Monitoring Parameters Blood pressure, blood glucose, electrolytes

Test Interactions Increases amylase (S), cholesterol (S), glucose, protein, sodium (S); decreases calcium (S), potassium (S), thyroxine (S)

Patient Information Report any change in body weight; do not discontinue or decrease the drug without contacting your physician; carry an identification card or bracelet advising that you are on steroids; may take with meals to decrease GI upset; take single daily dose in the morning; apply topical preparations in a thin layer. For the inhaler, follow instructions that accompany the product and do not exceed the recommended dose; notify physician if any signs of infection occur.

Nursing Implications Evaluate clinical response and mental status; may mask signs and symptoms of infection; inject I.M. dose deep in large muscle mass, avoid deltoid; avoid S.C. dose; apply topical products sparingly, do not occlude area unless desired; once daily doses should be given in the morning

Additional Information Systemic absorption may occur after topical application; 16 mg triamcinolone is equivalent to 100 mg cortisone (no mineralocorticoid activity)

Triamcinolone acetonide, aerosol: Azmacort™
Triamcinolone acetonide, parenteral: Cenocort®, Cinonide®, Kenalog® injection, Triam-A®, Tri-Kort®, Trilog®
Triamcinolone diacetate, oral: Aristocort® syrup, Kenacort® syrup
Triamcinolone diacetate, parenteral: Aristocort® intralesional, Amcort®, Aristocort® Forte, Cenocort® Forte, Triamolone®, Trilone®, Trisoject®
Triamcinolone hexacetonide: Aristospan®
Triamcinolone, oral: Aristocort® tablet, Kenacort® tablet

Special Geriatric Considerations Because of the risk of adverse effects, systemic corticosteroids should be used cautiously in the elderly, in the smallest possible dose, and for the shortest possible time. Azmacort™ (metered dose inhaler) comes with its own spacer device attached and may be easier to use in older patients.

Dosage Forms
 Aerosol:
  Oral inhalation: 100 mcg/metered spray (2 oz)
  Topical, as acetonide: 0.2 mg/2 second spray (23 g, 63 g)
 Cream, as acetonide: 0.025% (15 g, 60 g, 80 g, 240 g, 454 g); 0.1% (15 g, 30 g, 60 g, 80 g, 90 g, 120 g, 240 g); 0.5% (15 g, 20 g, 30 g, 240 g)
 (Continued)

711

Triamcinolone *(Continued)*

Injection, as acetonide: 10 mg/mL (5 mL); 40 mg/mL (1 mL, 5 mL, 10 mL)
Injection, as diacetate: 25 mg/mL (5 mL); 40 mg/mL (1 mL, 5 mL, 10 mL)
Injection, as hexacetonide: 5 mg/mL (5 mL); 20 mg/mL (1 mL, 5 mL)
Lotion, as acetonide: 0.025% (60 mL); 0.1% (15 mL, 60 mL)
Ointment, oral: 0.1% (5 g)
Ointment, topical, as acetonide: 0.025% (15 g, 30 g, 60 g, 80 g, 120 g, 454 g); 0.1%
   (15 g, 30 g, 60 g, 80 g, 120 g, 240 g, 454 g); 0.5% (15 g, 20 g, 30 g, 240 g)
Syrup: 2 mg/5 mL (120 mL); 4 mg/5 mL (120 mL)
Tablet: 1 mg, 2 mg, 4 mg, 8 mg

Triamcinolone Acetonide, Aerosol *see* Triamcinolone *on page 710*

Triamcinolone Acetonide, Parenteral *see* Triamcinolone *on page 710*

Triamcinolone and Nystatin *see* Nystatin and Triamcinolone
on page 514

Triamcinolone Diacetate, Oral *see* Triamcinolone *on page 710*

Triamcinolone Diacetate, Parenteral *see* Triamcinolone *on page 710*

Triamcinolone Hexacetonide *see* Triamcinolone *on page 710*

Triamcinolone, Oral *see* Triamcinolone *on page 710*

Triamolone® *see* Triamcinolone *on page 710*

Triamterene *(trye am' ter een)*
Brand Names Dyrenium®
Generic Available No
Therapeutic Class Diuretic, Potassium Sparing
Use Alone or in combination with other diuretics to treat edema and hypertension; decreases potassium excretion caused by kaliuretic diuretics
Contraindications Hyperkalemia, renal impairment, hypersensitivity to triamterene or any component; do not give to patients receiving spironolactone or amiloride
Precautions Use with caution in patients with severe hepatic encephalopathy and in patients with diabetes. Potassium excretion may be decreased in the elderly, increasing the risk of hyperkalemia with the use of triamterene.
Adverse Reactions
   Endocrine & metabolic: Hyperkalemia, electrolyte imbalance (decreased sodium, decreased magnesium, decreased bicarbonate, increased chloride, possibility of metabolic acidosis), hyperuricemia
   Gastrointestinal: Nausea, vomiting, diarrhea
   Genitourinary: Slight prerenal azotemia, slight alkalinization of urine
   Hematologic: Blood dyscrasias
   Hepatic: Abnormal liver function
   Renal: Nephrolithiasis
   Miscellaneous: Allergic reactions have been reported
Overdosage Symptoms of overdose include drowsiness, confusion, clinical signs of dehydration, electrolyte imbalance, and hypotension
Toxicology Ingestion of large amounts of potassium-sparing diuretics, may result in life-threatening hyperkalemia. This can be treated with I.V. glucose (dextrose 25% in water), with concurrent I.V. sodium bicarbonate (1 mEq/kg up to 44 mEq/dose). If needed, Kayexalate® oral or rectal solutions in sorbitol may also be used.
Drug Interactions
   Increased risk of hyperkalemia if given together with amiloride, spironolactone, angiotensin-converting enzyme (ACE) inhibitors, NSAIDs
   Increased toxicity of amantadine (possibly by decreasing its renal excretion)
Mechanism of Action Interferes with potassium/sodium exchange in the distal tubule
Pharmacodynamics
   Onset of action: Within 2-4 hours
   Duration: 7-9 hours
Pharmacokinetics
   Absorption: Oral: Unreliably absorbed
   Time to peak: One study found that peak levels in elderly were approximately twice those in younger patients
Usual Dosage Oral:
   Geriatrics: Initial: 50 mg/day; maximum: 100 mg/day in 1-2 divided doses
   Adults: 100-300 mg/day in 1-2 divided doses; maximum: 300 mg/day
Monitoring Parameters Blood pressure, serum electrolytes, renal function, weight, I & O
Test Interactions Interferes with fluorometric assay of quinidine
Patient Information Take in the morning; take the last dose of multiple doses no later than 6 PM unless instructed otherwise; take after meals; notify physician if weakness, headache or nausea occurs; avoid excessive ingestion of food high in potassium or use of salt substitute; may increase blood glucose; may impart a blue fluorescence color to urine

Nursing Implications Observe for hyperkalemia in geriatric patients and in patients with renal insufficiency; assess weight and I & O daily to determine weight loss
Special Geriatric Considerations Monitor serum potassium; see Precautions
Dosage Forms Capsule: 50 mg, 100 mg

Triamterene and Hydrochlorothiazide *see* Hydrochlorothiazide and Triamterene *on page 349*

Triavil® *see* Amitriptyline and Perphenazine *on page 43*

Triazolam (trye ay' zoe lam)
Related Information
Antacid Drug Interactions *on page 764*
Anxiolytic/Hypnotic Use in Long-Term Care Facilities *on page 755-756*
Benzodiazepines Comparison *on page 802-803*
Brand Names Halcion®
Generic Available No
Therapeutic Class Benzodiazepine; Hypnotic; Sedative
Use Short-term treatment of insomnia
Restrictions C-IV
Contraindications Hypersensitivity to triazolam, or any component, cross-sensitivity with other benzodiazepines may occur; severe uncontrolled pain; pre-existing CNS depression; narrow-angle glaucoma; sleep apnea
Warnings Abrupt discontinuance may precipitate withdrawal or rebound insomnia; anterograde amnesia has occurred with triazolam, generally it occurred with doses of 0.5 mg but it has also been reported with lower doses
Precautions Has potential for drug dependence and abuse; use with caution in patients with a potential for drug dependence
Adverse Reactions
Central nervous system: Drowsiness, ataxia, anterograde amnesia, confusion, dizziness, agitation, hallucinations, nightmares, headache
Gastrointestinal: Dry mouth, nausea, vomiting, constipation
Hepatic: Cholestatic jaundice
Neuromuscular & skeletal: Impaired coordination
Respiratory: Decreased respiratory rate, apnea, laryngospasm
Miscellaneous: Physical and psychological dependence may occur with prolonged use
Overdosage Symptoms of overdose include somnolence, confusion, coma, and diminished reflexes
Toxicology Treatment for benzodiazepine overdose is supportive; rarely is mechanical ventilation required
Flumazenil has been shown to selectively block the binding of benzodiazepines to CNS receptors, resulting in a reversal of benzodiazepine-induced sedation; however, its use may not alter the course of overdose
Drug Interactions Increased toxicity: CNS depressants, alcohol; macrolides may increase the bioavailability of triazolam
Mechanism of Action Benzodiazepines appear to potentiate the effects of GABA and other inhibitory neurotransmitters by binding to specific benzodiazepine-receptor sites in various areas of the CNS
Pharmacodynamics Hypnotic effects:
Onset of action: Within 15-30 minutes
Duration: 6-7 hours; studies have shown that the elderly are more sensitive to the effects of benzodiazepines as compared to younger adults
Pharmacokinetics
Distribution: V_d: 0.8-1.8 L/kg
Protein binding: 89%
Metabolism: Extensive in the liver
Half-life: 1.7-5 hours
Time to peak: In elderly, peak plasma concentrations and AUC are increased
Elimination: In urine as unchanged drug and metabolites; triazolam clearance is lower in elderly
Usual Dosage Oral:
Geriatrics: 0.0625-0.125 mg at bedtime
Adults: 0.125-0.25 mg at bedtime
Monitoring Parameters Respiratory, cardiovascular and mental status
Patient Information Avoid alcohol and other CNS depressants; may cause drowsiness; avoid activities needing good psychomotor coordination until CNS effects are known; may cause physical or psychological dependence; avoid abrupt discontinuation after prolonged use; **for short-term use only; do not exceed prescribed dose**
Nursing Implications Provide safety measures (ie, side rails, night light, call button); remove smoking materials from area; supervise ambulation
Additional Information Onset of action is rapid, patient should take triazolam right before going to bed

(Continued)

Triazolam *(Continued)*

Special Geriatric Considerations Due to the higher incidence of CNS adverse reactions and its short half-life, this benzodiazepine is not a drug of first choice; for short term only; see Warnings, Pharmacodynamics, and Pharmacokinetics

Dosage Forms Tablet: 0.125 mg, 0.25 mg

References
Greenblatt DJ, Harmatz JS, Shapiro L, et al, "Sensitivity to Triazolam in the Elderly," *N Engl J Med*, 1991, 324(24):1691-8.

Tribavirin *see* Ribavirin *on page 626*

Trichloroacetaldehyde Monohydrate *see* Chloral Hydrate *on page 146*

Tridil® *see* Nitroglycerin *on page 505*

Triethanolamine Polypeptide Oleate-Condensate

(trye eth a nole' a meen)

Brand Names Cerumenex® Otic

Generic Available No

Therapeutic Class Otic Agent, Cerumenolytic

Use Removal of ear wax (cerumen)

Contraindications Perforated tympanic membrane or otitis media, hypersensitivity to product or any component

Warnings Avoid undue exposure to peridural skin during administration and the flushing out of ear canal; discontinue if sensitization or irritation occurs

Adverse Reactions Local: Localized dermatitis, mild erythema and pruritus, severe eczematoid reactions involving the external ear and periauricular tissue

Mechanism of Action Emulsifies and disperses accumulated cerumen

Pharmacodynamics Onset of effect: Produces slight disintegration of very hard ear wax by 24 hours

Usual Dosage Geriatrics and Adults: Otic: Fill ear canal, insert cotton plug; allow to remain 15-30 minutes; flush ear with lukewarm water as a single treatment; if a second application is needed for unusually hard impactions, repeat the procedure

Monitoring Parameters Evaluate hearing before and after instillation of medication

Patient Information For external use in the ear only; warm to body temperature before using to improve effect; avoid touching dropper to any surface; hold ear lobe up and back; lie on your side or tilt the affected ear up for ease of administration; fill ear canal, let stand for 15-30 minutes, then flush

Nursing Implications Warm solution to body temperature before using; avoid undue exposure of the drug to the periauricular skin

Special Geriatric Considerations Avoid contact with hearing aids

Dosage Forms Solution, otic: 6 mL, 12 mL

Trifed® [OTC] *see* Triprolidine and Pseudoephedrine *on page 723*

Trifluoperazine Hydrochloride (trye floo oh per' a zeen)

Related Information
Antacid Drug Interactions *on page 764*
Antipsychotic Agents Comparison *on page 801*
Antipsychotic Medication Guidelines *on page 754*

Brand Names Stelazine®

Generic Available Yes

Therapeutic Class Antianxiety Agent; Antipsychotic Agent; Phenothiazine Derivative

Use Management of manifestations of psychotic disorders; depressive neurosis; alcohol withdrawal; nausea and vomiting; nonpsychotic symptoms associated with dementia in elderly, Tourette's syndrome; Huntington's chorea; spasmodic torticollis and Reye's syndrome; see Special Geriatric Considerations

Contraindications Hypersensitivity to trifluoperazine or any component, cross-sensitivity with other phenothiazines may exist; avoid use in patients with narrow-angle glaucoma, bone marrow depression, severe liver or cardiac disease; subcortical brain damage; circulatory collapse, severe hypotension or hypertension

Warnings

Tardive dyskinesia: Prevalence rate may be 40% in elderly; elderly women especially at risk; embarrassment from dyskinesias may lead to greater social isolation; development of the syndrome and the irreversible nature are proportional to duration and total cumulative dose over time. May be reversible if diagnosed early in therapy; intermittent use of antipsychotics (not proven use) helps decrease total cumulative dose.

EPS: Extrapyramidal reactions are more common in elderly with up to 50% developing these reactions after age 60. These reactions may be more common in dementia patients. Drug-induced **Parkinson's syndrome** occurs often. Discontinuation usually resolves symptoms but may take weeks to months (12+) to clear. **Akathisia** is the most common EPS reaction in elderly. The symptoms of motor restlessness are difficult to diagnose in demented elderly; increased nervousness, assertiveness, restlessness with constant movement may indicate this adverse event. Consider decreasing dose if antipsychotic to treat as well as diagnose problem; usually see this reaction within 2-3 months of initiating antipsychotic drug.

Anticholinergic effects: These side effects most common with low potency antipsychotics (eg, thioridazine, chlorpromazine). CNS toxicity occurs more frequently and severely in elderly; increased confusion, memory loss, psychotic behavior, and agitation frequently occur as a consequence of anticholinergic effects to antipsychotic agents. Peripheral anticholinergic action troublesome to elderly; most peripheral anticholinergic effects last only 2-3 weeks; see Adverse Reactions.

Orthostatic hypotension: More common with low potency agents (eg, thioridazine, chlorpromazine, and clozapine) but of concern with all antipsychotic agents; orthostasis due to alpha-receptor blockade by antipsychotic agents. Elderly present many risk factors for orthostatic hypotension: blunted baroreceptor reflexes, decreased vascular tone, decreased vascular volume, and possible presence of cardiac diseases which result in decreased cardiac output.

Sedation: Common side effect with antipsychotic therapy; should not be used as a hypnotic unless insomnia is associated with target behavior symptoms treated with antipsychotic medications; see Special Geriatric Considerations. Anecdotal reports suggesting antipsychotic sedation in nonpsychotic patients is extremely unpleasant due to feelings of depersonalization, derealization, and dysphoria. Due to the long duration of action with antipsychotic drugs, these reactions may last up to 24 hours and result in decreased daytime function.

Cardiac toxicity: Life-threatening arrhythmias have occurred at therapeutic doses of antipsychotics. Thioridazine more commonly demonstrates EKG changes than other antipsychotics; suggested to use high potency antipsychotic agents (ie, haloperidol) in patients with cardiac conduction defects.

Precautions Use with caution in patients with cardiovascular disease, seizures, and Parkinson's disease; benefits of therapy must be weighed against risks

Adverse Reactions

Cardiovascular: Hypotension (especially with I.V. use), orthostatic hypotension, tachycardia, arrhythmias, abnormal T waves with prolonged ventricular repolarization

Central nervous system: Sedation, drowsiness, restlessness, anxiety, extrapyramidal reactions, pseudoparkinsonian signs and symptoms, tardive dyskinesia, neuroleptic malignant syndrome, seizures, altered central temperature regulation

Dermatologic: Hyperpigmentation, pruritus, rash, photosensitivity

Endocrine & metabolic: Amenorrhea, galactorrhea, gynecomastia

Gastrointestinal: GI upset, dry mouth (problem for denture users), constipation, adynamic ileus, weight gain

Genitourinary: Urinary retention, overflow incontinence, priapism, impotence, sexual dysfunction (up to 60%)

Hematologic: Agranulocytosis, leukopenia (usually in patients with large doses for prolonged periods), thrombocytopenia, hemolytic anemia, eosinophilia

Hepatic: Cholestatic jaundice (rare)

Ocular: Blurred vision, retinal pigmentation is more common than with chlorpromazine

Miscellaneous: Anaphylactoid reactions

Overdosage Symptoms of overdose include deep sleep, coma, extrapyramidal symptoms, abnormal involuntary muscle movements, hypotension or hypertension; agitation, restlessness, fever, hypothermia or hyperthermia, seizures, cardiac arrhythmias, EKG changes

Toxicology Following initiation of essential overdose management, toxic symptom treatment and supportive treatment should be initiated. Hypotension usually responds to I.V. fluids or Trendelenburg positioning. If unresponsive to these measures the use of a parenteral inotrope may be required (eg, norepinephrine 0.1-0.2 mcg/kg/minute titrated to response). Do not use epinephrine. Seizures commonly respond to diazepam (I.V. 5-10 mg bolus every 15 minutes if needed up to a total of 30 mg) or to phenytoin or phenobarbital. Also critical cardiac arrhythmias often respond to I.V. phenytoin (15 mg/kg up to 1 g), while other antiarrhythmics can be used. Neuroleptics often cause extrapyramidal symptoms (eg, dystonic reactions) requiring management with diphenhydramine 1-2 mg/kg up to a maximum of 50 mg I.M. or I.V. slow push followed by a maintenance dose for 48-72 hours. When these reactions are unresponsive to diphenhydramine, benztropine mesylate I.V. 1-2 mg may be effective. These agents are generally effective within 2-5 minutes.

Drug Interactions

Alcohol may increase CNS sedation

Anticholinergic agents may decrease pharmacologic effects; increase anticholinergic side effects; may enhance tardive dyskinesia

Aluminum salts may decrease absorption of phenothiazines

Barbiturates may decrease phenothiazine serum concentrations

Bromocriptine may have decreased efficacy when administered with phenothiazines

Guanethidine's hypotensive effect is decreased by phenothiazines

(Continued)

Trifluoperazine Hydrochloride *(Continued)*

Lithium administration with phenothiazines may increase disorientation

Meperidine and phenothiazine coadministration increases sedation and hypotension

Methyldopa administration with phenothiazine (trifluoperazine) may significantly increase blood pressure

Norepinephrine, epinephrine have decreased pressor effect when administered with chlorpromazine; therefore, be aware of possible decreased effectiveness or when any phenothiazine is used

Phenytoin serum concentrations may increase or decrease with phenothiazines; tricyclic antidepressants may have increased serum concentrations with concomitant administration with phenothiazines

Propranolol administered with phenothiazines may increase serum concentrations of both drugs

Valproic acid may have increased half-life when administered with phenothiazines (chlorpromazine)

Stability Store injection at room temperature; protect from heat and from freezing; protect all dosage forms from light, clear or slightly yellow solutions may be used; should be dispensed in amber or opaque vials/bottles. Solutions may be diluted or mixed with fruit juices or other liquids but must be administered immediately after mixing; do not prepare bulk dilutions or store bulk dilutions.

Mechanism of Action Blocks postsynaptic mesolimbic dopaminergic D_1 and D_2 receptors in the brain; exhibits a strong alpha-adrenergic blocking and anticholinergic effect; depresses the release of hypothalamic and hypophyseal hormones; believed to depress the reticular activating system thus affecting basal metabolism, body temperature, wakefulness, vasomotor tone, and emesis

Pharmacokinetics

Absorption: May be affected by the inherent anticholinergic action on the gastrointestinal tissue causing variable absorption. Absorption from tablets is erratic with less variation seen with solutions. These agents are widely distributed in tissues with CNS concentrations exceeding that of plasma due to their lipophilic characteristics.

Protein binding: Antipsychotic agents are bound 90% to 99% to plasma proteins; highly bound to brain and lung tissue and other tissues with a high blood perfusion.

Half-life: >24 hours with chronic use

Time to peak: Oral absorption results in peak concentrations between 2-4 hours

Elimination: Occurs through hepatic metabolism (oxidation) where numerous active metabolites are produced; active metabolites excreted in urine; elimination half-lives of antipsychotics ranges from 20-40 hours which may be extended in elderly due to decline in oxidative hepatic reactions (phase I) with age.

Biologic effect of a single dose persists for 24 hours. When the patient has accommodated to initial side effects (sedation), once daily dosing is possible due to the long half-life of antipsychotics.

Steady-state plasma levels are achieved in 4-7 days; therefore, if possible, do not make dose adjustments more than once in a 7-day period. Due to the long half-lives of antipsychotics, as needed (PRN) use is ineffective since repeated doses are necessary to achieve therapeutic tissue concentrations in the CNS.

Usual Dosage Oral:

Geriatrics (nonpsychotic patients, dementia behavior): Initial: 0.5-1 mg 1-2 times/day; increase dose at 4- to 7-day intervals by 0.5-1 mg/day; increase dosing intervals (bid, tid, etc) as necessary to control response or side effects; maximum daily dose: 40 mg; gradual increases (titration) may prevent some side effects or decrease their severity

I.M.: Initial: 1 mg every 4-6 hours; increase at 1 mg increments; do not exceed 6 mg/day

Adults:

Psychoses:

Outpatients: 1-2 mg twice daily

Hospitalized or well supervised patients: Initial dose: 2-5 mg twice daily with optimum response in the 15-20 mg/day range; do not exceed 40 mg/day

Anxiety: 1-2 mg twice daily; maximum: 6 mg/day; therapy for anxiety should not exceed 12 weeks

I.M.: 1-2 mg every 4-6 hours; do not exceed 6 mg/day

Not dialyzable (0% to 5%)

Monitoring Parameters Orthostatic blood pressures; tremors, gait changes, abnormal movement in trunk, neck, buccal area or extremities; monitor target behaviors for which the agent is given

Test Interactions Increased cholesterol (S), increased glucose; decreased uric acid (S)

Patient Information Oral concentrate must be diluted in 2-4 oz of liquid (water, fruit juice, carbonated drinks, milk, or pudding); do not take antacid within 1 hour of taking drug; avoid alcohol; avoid excess sun exposure (use sun block); may cause drowsiness, rise slowly from recumbent position; use of supportive stockings may help prevent orthostatic hypotension

Nursing Implications Give I.M. injection deep in upper outer quadrant of buttock; watch for hypotension when administering I.M. or I.V.; dilute the oral concentrate with water or juice before administration; avoid skin contact with oral solution; may cause contact dermatitis; monitor orthostatic blood pressures 3-5 days after initiation of therapy or a dose increase; observe for tremor and abnormal movement or posturing (extrapyramidal symptoms)

Additional Information Do not exceed 6 mg/day for longer than 12 weeks when treating anxiety; drug-induced agitation, jitteriness, or insomnia may be confused with original anxious or psychotic symptoms

Special Geriatric Considerations See Warnings. Elderly are more susceptible to hypotension and neuromuscular reactions.

Many elderly patients receive antipsychotic medications for inappropriate nonpsychotic behavior. Before initiating antipsychotic medication, the clinician should investigate any possible reversible cause; any stress or stress from any disease can cause acute "confusion" or worsening of baseline nonpsychotic behavior. Most commonly acute changes in behavior are due to increases in drug dose or addition of new drug to regimen; fluid electrolyte loss; infections; and changes in environment. Any changes in disease status in any organ system can result in behavior changes.

Dosage Forms
Concentrate, oral: 10 mg/mL (60 mL)
Injection: 2 mg/mL (10 mL)
Tablet: 1 mg, 2 mg, 5 mg, 10 mg

Trifluorothymidine *see* Trifluridine *on this page*

Trifluridine (trye flure' i deen)
Brand Names Viroptic® Ophthalmic
Synonyms F_3T; Trifluorothymidine
Generic Available No
Therapeutic Class Antiviral Agent, Ophthalmic
Use Treatment of primary keratoconjunctivitis and recurrent epithelial keratitis caused by herpes simplex virus types I and II
Contraindications Known hypersensitivity to trifluridine or any component
Warnings Mild local irritation of conjunctiva and cornea may occur when instilled but usually transient effects
Adverse Reactions
Local: Burning, stinging
Ocular: Palpebral edema, epithelial keratopathy, keratitis, stromal edema, increased intraocular pressure
Miscellaneous: Hypersensitivity reactions, hyperemia
Stability Refrigerate at 2°C to 8°C (36°F to 46°F); storage at room temperature may result in a solution altered pH which could result in ocular discomfort upon administration and/or decreased potency
Mechanism of Action Interferes with viral replication by incorporating into viral DNA in place of thymidine, inhibiting thymidylate synthetase resulting in the formation of defective proteins
Pharmacokinetics Absorption: Ophthalmic instillation: Systemic absorption is negligible, while corneal penetration is adequate
Usual Dosage Geriatrics and Adults: Instill 1 drop into affected eye every 2 hours while awake, to a maximum of 9 drops/day, until re-epithelialization of corneal ulcer occurs; then use 1 drop every 4 hours for another 7 days; do **not** exceed 21 days of treatment; if improvement has not taken place in 7-14 days, consider another form of therapy
Monitoring Parameters Ophthalmologic exam (test for corneal staining with fluorescein or rose bengal)
Patient Information Notify physician if improvement is not seen after 7 days, condition worsens, or if irritation occurs; do not discontinue without notifying the physician, do not exceed recommended dosage
Nursing Implications Store in refrigerator
Special Geriatric Considerations Assess ability to self-administer
Dosage Forms Solution, ophthalmic: 1% (7.5 mL)

Trihexane® *see* Trihexyphenidyl Hydrochloride *on this page*

Trihexy® *see* Trihexyphenidyl Hydrochloride *on this page*

Trihexyphenidyl Hydrochloride (trye hex ee fen' i dill)
Brand Names Artane®; Trihexane®; Trihexy®
Synonyms Benzhexol Hydrochloride
Generic Available Yes: Tablet
Therapeutic Class Anticholinergic Agent; Anti-Parkinson's Agent
Use Adjunctive treatment of Parkinson's disease; also used in treatment of drug-induced extrapyramidal effects and acute dystonic reactions

(Continued)

Trihexyphenidyl Hydrochloride *(Continued)*

Contraindications Hypersensitivity to trihexyphenidyl or any component, patients with narrow-angle glaucoma; pyloric or duodenal obstruction, stenosing peptic ulcers; bladder neck obstructions; achalasia; myasthenia gravis

Precautions Use with caution in hot weather or during exercise. Elderly patients frequently develop increased sensitivity and require strict dosage regulation – side effects may be more severe in elderly patients with atherosclerotic changes. Use with caution in patients with tachycardia, cardiac arrhythmias, hypertension, hypotension, prostatic hypertrophy (especially in the elderly) or any tendency toward urinary retention, liver or kidney disorders and obstructive disease of the GI or GU tract. May exacerbate mental symptoms and precipitate a toxic psychosis when used to treat extrapyramidal reactions resulting from phenothiazines. When given in large doses or to susceptible patients, may cause weakness and inability to move particular muscle groups. Anticholinergic agents can aggravate tardive dyskinesia caused by neuroleptic agents.

Adverse Reactions

Cardiovascular: Tachycardia

Central nervous system: Drowsiness, nervousness, hallucinations, memory loss, coma **(the elderly may be at increased risk for confusion and hallucinations)**

Gastrointestinal: Nausea, vomiting, constipation, dryness of mouth

Genitourinary: Urinary hesitancy or retention

Ocular: Blurred vision, mydriasis

Miscellaneous: Heat intolerance

Overdosage Symptoms of overdose include CNS depression, confusion, nervousness, hallucinations, dizziness, blurred vision, nausea, vomiting, hyperthermia

Toxicology Anticholinergic toxicity is caused by strong binding of the drug to cholinergic receptors. Anticholinesterase inhibitors reduce acetylcholinesterase, the enzyme that breaks down acetylcholine and thereby allows acetylcholine to accumulate and compete for receptor binding with the offending anticholinergic. For anticholinergic overdose with severe life-threatening symptoms, physostigmine 1-2 mg S.C. or I.V., slowly may be given to reverse these effects.

Drug Interactions

Decreased effect of levodopa (decreased absorption); decreased effect with tacrine

Increased toxicity (central anticholinergic syndrome): Narcotic analgesics, phenothiazines, and other antipsychotics, tricyclic antidepressants, some antihistamines, quinidine, disopyramide

Mechanism of Action Thought to act by blocking excess acetylcholine at cerebral synapses; many of its effects are due to its pharmacologic similarities with atropine

Pharmacodynamics Peak effects: Within 60 minutes

Pharmacokinetics

Half-life: 5.6-10.2 hours

Time to peak: Oral: Peak serum levels occur within 60-90 minutes

Elimination: Primarily in urine

Usual Dosage Geriatrics and Adults:

Parkinsonism: 1 mg on first day, increase by 2 mg every 3-5 days as needed until a total of 6-10 mg/day (in 3-4 divided doses) is reached. If the patient is on concomitant levodopa therapy, the daily dose is reduced to 1-2 mg 3 times/day.

Drug-induced extrapyramidal reaction: 1 mg on first day, increase as needed; usual range: 5-15 mg/day in 3-4 divided doses

Monitoring Parameters Symptoms of EPS, Parkinson's, pulse, anticholinergic effects (ie, CNS, bowel and bladder function)

Patient Information Take after meals or with food if GI upset occurs; do not discontinue drug abruptly; notify physician if adverse GI effects, rapid or pounding heartbeat, confusion, eye pain, rash, fever or heat intolerance occurs. Observe caution when performing hazardous tasks or those that require alertness such as driving, as may cause drowsiness. Avoid alcohol and other CNS depressants. May cause dry mouth – adequate fluid intake or hard sugar-free candy may relieve. Difficult urination or constipation may occur – notify physician if effects persist; may increase susceptibility to heat stroke

Nursing Implications Tolerated best if given in 3 daily doses and with food; high doses may be divided into 4 doses, at meal times and at bedtime

Additional Information Incidence and severity of side effects are dose related; patients may be switched to sustained-action capsules when stabilized on conventional dosage forms

Special Geriatric Considerations Anticholinergic agents are generally not well tolerated in the elderly and their use should be avoided when possible; see Precautions and Adverse Reactions. In the elderly, anticholinergic agents should not be used as prophylaxis against extrapyramidal symptoms.

Dosage Forms

Capsule, sustained release: 5 mg

Elixir: 2 mg/5 mL (480 mL)

Tablet: 2 mg, 5 mg

References
Feinberg M, "The Problems of Anticholinergic Adverse Effects in Older Patients," *Drugs Aging*, 1993, 3(4):335-48.

Tri-Kort® *see* Triamcinolone *on page 710*

Trilafon® *see* Perphenazine *on page 549*

Trilisate® *see* Choline Magnesium Salicylate *on page 163*

Trilog® *see* Triamcinolone *on page 710*

Trilone® *see* Triamcinolone *on page 710*

Trimeprazine Tartrate (trye mep' ra zeen)

Related Information
Antacid Drug Interactions *on page 764*

Brand Names Temaril®

Synonyms Alimenazine Tartrate

Therapeutic Class Antihistamine; Phenothiazine Derivative

Use Perennial and seasonal allergic rhinitis and other allergic symptoms including urticaria

Contraindications Hypersensitivity to trimeprazine or any component, narrow-angle glaucoma, bladder neck obstruction, symptomatic prostate hypertrophy, asthmatic attacks, and stenosing peptic ulcer

Warnings Antihistamines are more likely to cause dizziness, excessive sedation, syncope, toxic confusion states, and hypotension in the elderly. Phenothiazine side effects (especially EPS) are more prone to develop in the elderly.

Precautions Use with caution in patients with cardiovascular disease, impaired liver function, asthma, sleep apnea, seizures, hypertensive crisis; avoid in patients with Reye's syndrome

Adverse Reactions
Cardiovascular: Postural hypotension
Central nervous system: Drowsiness, confusion, fatigue, excitation, extrapyramidal reactions with high doses
Dermatologic: Photosensitivity
Gastrointestinal: Dry mouth, constipation, increased appetite
Genitourinary: Urinary hesitancy or retention
Ocular: Blurred vision
Respiratory: Thickening of bronchial secretions

Overdosage Symptoms of overdose include deep sleep, coma, extrapyramidal symptoms, abnormal involuntary muscle movements, hypo- or hypertension

Toxicology Following initiation of essential overdose management, toxic symptom treatment and supportive treatment should be initiated. Hypotension usually responds to I.V. fluids or Trendelenburg positioning. If unresponsive to these measures the use of a parenteral vasopressor may be required (eg, norepinephrine 0.1-0.2 mcg/kg/minute titrated to response). Seizures commonly respond to diazepam (I.V. 5-10 mg bolus every 15 minutes if needed up to a total of 30 mg, I.V.) or to phenytoin or phenobarbital. Also critical cardiac arrhythmias often respond to I.V. phenytoin (15 mg/kg up to 1 g), while other antiarrhythmics can be used. Neuroleptics often cause extrapyramidal symptoms (eg, dystonic reactions) requiring management with diphenhydramine 1-2 mg/kg up to a maximum of 50 mg I.M. or I.V. slow push followed by a maintenance dose for 48-72 hours. When these reactions are unresponsive to diphenhydramine, benztropine mesylate I.V. 1-2 mg may be effective. These agents are generally effective within 2-5 minutes. Anticholinesterase inhibitors including physostigmine, neostigmine, pyridostigmine and edrophonium may be useful in treating life-threatening anticholinergic symptoms. Physostigmine 1-2 mg I.V., slowly may be given to reverse these effects.

Drug Interactions Increased effect/toxicity: CNS depressants, MAO inhibitors, alcohol

Mechanism of Action Blocks postsynaptic mesolimbic dopaminergic receptors in the brain; exhibits a strong alpha-adrenergic blocking effect and depresses the release of hypothalamic and hypophyseal hormones; competes with histamine for the H_1-receptor; reduces stimuli to the brainstem reticular system

Pharmacokinetics
Absorption: Well absorbed
Metabolism: Extensively hepatically metabolized largely to n-desalkyl metabolites
Bioavailability: Tablet: ~70%; the sustained release capsules give closely comparable serum and urinary levels
Half-life, elimination: 4.78 hours mean
Time to peak serum concentration:
Syrup: 3.5 hours
Tablet: 4.5 hours

Usual Dosage Oral:
Geriatrics: 2.5 mg twice daily
(Continued)

Trimeprazine Tartrate *(Continued)*

Adults: 2.5 mg 4 times/day (capsule: 5 mg every 12 hours)

Not dialyzable (0% to 5%)

Monitoring Parameters Relief of symptoms, mental status, blood pressure, EPS

Patient Information May cause drowsiness; avoid CNS depressants and alcohol

Additional Information Toxic manifestations normally appear between 4-10 weeks of therapy

Special Geriatric Considerations Because trimeprazine is a phenothiazine (and can, therefore, cause side effects such as extrapyramidal symptoms), it is not considered an antihistamine of choice in the elderly; see Warnings

Dosage Forms

Capsule, extended release: 5 mg

Syrup: 2.5 mg/5 mL

Tablet: 2.5 mg

Trimethobenzamide Hydrochloride (trye meth oh ben' za mide)

Brand Names Arrestin®; Bio-Gan®; Stemetic®; Tebamide®; T-Gen®; Ticon®; Tigan®; Tiject®

Generic Available Yes

Therapeutic Class Antiemetic

Use Control of nausea and vomiting (especially for long-term antiemetic therapy)

Contraindications Hypersensitivity to trimethobenzamide, benzocaine, similar local analgesics, or any component

Precautions Use in patients with acute vomiting should be **avoided**; electrolyte imbalance, gastroenteritis, dehydration, encephalitis, and CNS side effects have occurred when used in acute febrile illness

Adverse Reactions

Cardiovascular: Hypotension (especially with I.M. administration), coma

Central nervous system: Drowsiness, sedation, EPS symptoms, dizziness, seizures, convulsions, depression, disorientation (confusion), headache

Gastrointestinal: Diarrhea

Hematologic: Blood dyscrasias

Hepatic: Jaundice

Neuromuscular & skeletal: Opisthotonos, muscle cramps

Ocular: Blurred vision

Miscellaneous: Hypersensitivity skin reactions

Overdosage Symptoms of overdose include hypotension, seizures, CNS depression

Toxicology Following initiation of essential overdose management, toxic symptom treatment and supportive treatment should be initiated. Hypotension usually responds to I.V. fluids or Trendelenburg positioning. If unresponsive to these measures, the use of a parenteral inotrope may be required (eg, norepinephrine 0.1-0.2 mcg/kg/minute titrated to response). Seizures commonly respond to diazepam (I.V. 5-10 mg bolus every 15 minutes if needed up to a total of 30 mg) or to phenytoin or phenobarbital. Also critical cardiac arrhythmias often respond to I.V. phenytoin (15 mg/kg up to 1 g), while other antiarrhythmics can be used. Neuroleptics often cause extrapyramidal symptoms (eg, dystonic reactions) requiring management with diphenhydramine 1-2 mg/kg up to a maximum of 50 mg I.M. or I.V. slow push followed by a maintenance dose for 48-72 hours. When these reactions are unresponsive to diphenhydramine, benztropine mesylate I.V. 1-2 mg may be effective. These agents are generally effective within 2-5 minutes.

Stability Store injection at room temperature; protect from heat and from freezing; use only clear solutions

Mechanism of Action Acts centrally to inhibit the medullary chemoreceptor trigger zone; direct impulses to the vomiting center are not inhibited

Pharmacodynamics

Onset of antiemetic effects:

Oral: Within 10-40 minutes

I.M.: Within 15-35 minutes

Duration of action: Effects can persist for 3-4 hours

Usual Dosage Geriatrics and Adults:

Oral: 250 mg 3-4 times/day

I.M., rectal: 200 mg 3-4 times/day

Monitoring Parameters See Adverse Reactions

Patient Information May cause drowsiness

Nursing Implications Use only clear solution

Additional Information Note: Less effective than phenothiazines but may be associated with fewer side effects; rectal is ~60% absorbed

Special Geriatric Considerations No specific data for use in elderly has been established; see Adverse Reactions

Dosage Forms

Capsule: 100 mg, 250 mg

Injection: 100 mg/mL (2 mL, 20 mL)
Suppository: 100 mg, 200 mg

Trimethoprim (trye meth' oh prim)

Brand Names Proloprim®; Trimpex®

Synonyms TMP

Therapeutic Class Antibiotic, Miscellaneous

Use Treatment of uncomplicated urinary tract infections due to susceptible organisms (*Escherichia coli*, *Proteus mirabilis*, *Klebsiella pneumoniae*, *Enterobacter* sp, and co-agulase-negative *Staphylococcus* sp); acute exacerbations of chronic bronchitis

Contraindications Hypersensitivity to trimethoprim or any component, megaloblastic anemia due to folate deficiency

Precautions Use with caution in patients with impaired renal or hepatic function or with possible folate deficiency

Adverse Reactions

Central nervous system: Fever

Dermatologic: Rash (3% to 7%), pruritus, exfoliative dermatitis

Gastrointestinal: Nausea, vomiting, epigastric distress

Hematologic: Thrombocytopenia, neutropenia, leukopenia, megaloblastic anemia

Hepatic: Increased LFTS, cholestatic jaundice

Renal: BUN and serum creatinine (increase)

Overdosage Symptoms of overdose include bone marrow depression, nausea, vomiting, confusion, dizziness

Toxicology

Acute toxicity: Gastric lavage and supportive measures; acidification of urine increases renal elimination; hemodialysis is moderately effective

Chronic toxicity: Stop drug; give leucovorin 3-6 mg I.M. daily or 5-15 mg/day orally for 3 days or until normal hematopoiesis resumes

Drug Interactions Phenytoin increased serum concentration

Mechanism of Action Inhibits folic acid reduction to tetrahydrofolate, and thereby inhibits microbial growth

Pharmacokinetics

Absorption: Oral: Readily and extensively

Protein binding: 42% to 46%

Metabolism: Partially in the liver

Half-life: 8-14 hours, prolonged with renal impairment

Time to peak: Peak serum levels occur within 1-4 hours

Elimination: Significantly in urine (60% to 80% as unchanged drug); in elderly, the area under the curve and peak concentration have been reported to be greater compared to younger subjects

Usual Dosage Geriatrics and Adults: Oral: 100 mg every 12 hours or 200 mg every 24 hours for 10 days; longer treatment periods may be necessary for prostatitis (ie, 4-16 weeks)

Dosing interval in renal impairment:

Cl_{cr} 15-30 mL/minute: Administer 50 mg every 12 hours

Cl_{cr} <15 mL/minute: Not recommended

Moderately dialyzable (20% to 50%)

Monitoring Parameters Obtain culture and sensitivity results; repeat after treatment has concluded

Reference Range Therapeutic: Peak: 5-15 mg/L; Trough: 2-8 mg/L

Patient Information Complete full course of treatment; notify physician if sore throat, bleeding, or fever develops

Nursing Implications Watch for signs of bone marrow suppression such as fever, sore throat, or bleeding; tablets can be crushed

Special Geriatric Considerations Trimethoprim is often used in combination with sulfamethoxazole; it can be used alone in patients who are allergic to sulfonamides; adjust dose for renal function; see Pharmacokinetics and Usual Dosage.

Dosage Forms Tablet: 100 mg

References

Varoquaux O, Lajoie D, Gobert C, et al, "Pharmacokinetics of the Trimethoprim-Sulfamethoxazole Combination in the Elderly," *Br J Clin Pharmacol*, 1985, 20:575-81.

Trimethoprim and Sulfamethoxazole *see* Co-trimoxazole *on page 189*

Trimetrexate Glucuronate (tri me trex' ate)

Brand Names Neutrexin™

Therapeutic Class Antibiotic, Miscellaneous

Use Alternative therapy for the treatment of moderate-to-severe *Pneumocystis carinii* pneumonia (PCP) in immunocompromised patients, including patients with acquired immunodeficiency syndrome (AIDS), who are intolerant of, or are refractory to, co-trimoxazole therapy or for whom co-trimoxazole is contraindicated

Contraindications Previous hypersensitivity to trimetrexate or methotrexate, severe existing myelosuppression

(Continued)

721

Trimetrexate Glucuronate *(Continued)*

Warnings Must be administered with concurrent leucovorin to avoid potentially serious or life-threatening toxicities; leucovorin therapy must extend for 72 hours past the last dose of trimetrexate; use with caution in patients with mild myelosuppression, severe hepatic or renal dysfunction, hypoproteinemia, hypoalbuminemia, or previous extensive myelosuppressive therapies

Adverse Reactions
Central nervous system: Seizures, fever
Dermatologic: Rash
Gastrointestinal: Stomatitis, nausea, vomiting
Hematologic: Neutropenia, thrombocytopenia, anemia
Hepatic: Elevated liver function tests
Neuromuscular & skeletal: Peripheral neuropathy
Renal: Increased serum creatinine
Miscellaneous: Flu-like illness, hypersensitivity reactions

Drug Interactions
Decreased effect of pneumococcal vaccine
Increased toxicity (infection rates) of yellow fever vaccine

Stability Reconstituted I.V. solution is stable for 24 hours at room temperature or 7 days when refrigerated; intact vials should be refrigerated at 2°C to 8°C

Mechanism of Action Exerts an antimicrobial effect through potent inhibition of the enzyme dihydrofolate reductase (DHFR)

Pharmacokinetics
Distribution: V_d: 0.62 L/kg
Metabolism: Extensive in the liver
Half-life: 15-17 hours

Usual Dosage Geriatrics and Adults: I.V.: 45 mg/m^2 once daily over 60 minutes for 21 days; it is necessary to reduce the dose in patients with liver dysfunction, although no specific recommendations exist

Administration Reconstituted solution should be filtered (0.22 μM) prior to further dilution; final solution should be clear, hue will range from colorless to pale yellow; trimetrexate forms a precipitate instantly upon contact with chloride ion or leucovorin, therefore it should not be added to solutions containing sodium chloride or other anions; trimetrexate and leucovorin solutions **must** be administered separately; intravenous lines should be flushed with at least 10 mL of D$_5$W between trimetrexate and leucovorin

Monitoring Parameters Check and record patient's temperature daily
Lab tests:
Hematology (absolute neutrophil counts (ANC)), platelets
Renal functions (serum creatinine, BUN)
Hepatic function (ALT, AST, alkaline phosphatase)

Patient Information Report promptly any fever, rash, flu-like symptoms, numbness or tingling in the extremities, nausea, vomiting, abdominal pain, mouth sores, increased bruising or bleeding, black tarry stools

Nursing Implications Notify primary physician if there is:
Fever ≥103°F
Generalized rash
Seizures
Bleeding from any site
Uncontrolled nausea/vomiting
Laboratory abnormalities which warrant dose modification
Any other clinical adverse event or laboratory abnormality occurring in therapy which is judged as serious for that patient or which causes unexplained effects or concern

Initiate "Bleeding Precautions" for platelet counts ≤50,000/mm^3

Initiate "Infection Control Measures" for absolute neutrophil counts (ANC) ≤1000/mm^3

Additional Information Not a vesicant; methotrexate derivative

Special Geriatric Considerations No specific recommendations are available for the elderly; use with caution in patients with liver dysfunction; see Usual Dosage

Dosage Forms Injection: 25 mg

Trimipramine Maleate *(trye mi' pra meen)*

Related Information
Antidepressant Agents Comparison *on page 800*

Brand Names Surmontil®

Therapeutic Class Antidepressant, Tricyclic

Use Treatment of various forms of depression, often in conjunction with psychotherapy

Contraindications Narrow-angle glaucoma

Warnings To avoid cholinergic crisis do not discontinue abruptly in patients receiving long-term high dose therapy; some oral preparations contain tartrazine and injection contains sulfites both of which can cause allergic reactions

Precautions Use with caution in patients with cardiovascular disease, conduction disturbances, seizure disorders, urinary retention, hyperthyroidism or those receiving thyroid replacement; an EKG prior to the start of therapy is advised

Adverse Reactions
    Cardiovascular: Postural hypotension, arrhythmias, tachycardia, sudden death
    Central nervous system: Sedation, fatigue, insomnia, anxiety, impaired cognitive
        function, seizures have occurred occasionally, dizziness, headache
    Gastrointestinal: Dry mouth, constipation, increased appetite, unpleasant taste
    Genitourinary: Urinary retention
    Hematologic: Agranulocytosis, eosinophilia, may cause alterations in bleeding time
    Hepatic: Jaundice
    Neuromuscular & skeletal: Tremors, weakness
    Ocular: Blurred vision, increased intraocular pressure
    Miscellaneous: Allergic reactions
Overdosage Symptoms of overdose include agitation, confusion, hallucinations, urinary retention, hypothermia, hypotension, tachycardia
Toxicology Following initiation of essential overdose management, toxic symptoms should be treated. Ventricular arrhythmias often respond to phenytoin 15-20 mg/kg with concurrent systemic alkalinization (sodium bicarbonate 0.5-2 mEq/kg I.V.). Arrhythmias unresponsive to this therapy may respond to lidocaine 1 mg/kg I.V. followed by a titrated infusion. Physostigmine (1-2 mg I.V. slowly) may be indicated in reversing cardiac arrhythmias that are due to vagal blockade or for anticholinergic effects. Seizures usually respond to diazepam I.V. boluses (5-10 mg, up to 30 mg). If seizures are unresponsive or recur, phenytoin or phenobarbital may be required.
Drug Interactions
    May decrease or reverse effects of guanethidine and clonidine
    May increase effects of CNS depressants, adrenergic agents, anticholinergic agents
    With MAO inhibitors, hyperpyrexia, tachycardia, hypertension, seizures and death
        may occur; similar interactions as with other tricyclics may occur
Stability Solutions stable at a pH of 4-5; turns yellowish or reddish on exposure to light. Slight discoloration does not affect potency; marked discoloration is associated with loss of potency. Capsules stable for 3 years following date of manufacture.
Mechanism of Action Traditionally believed to increase the synaptic concentration of serotonin and/or norepinephrine in the central nervous system by inhibition of their reuptake by the presynaptic neuronal membrane. However, additional receptor effects have been found including desensitization of adenyl cyclase, down regulation of beta-adrenergic receptors, and down regulation of serotonin receptors.
Pharmacodynamics Onset of therapeutic effects: May take 1-3 weeks to appear; 5-HT >NE
Pharmacokinetics
    Protein binding: 95%
    Metabolism: Undergoes significant first-pass metabolism metabolized in the liver
    Half-life: 20-26 hours
    Time to peak: Oral: Therapeutic plasma levels occur within 6 hours
    Elimination: In urine
Usual Dosage Oral:
    Geriatrics: Initial: 25 mg at bedtime, increase by 25 mg/day every 3 days for inpatients and weekly for outpatients, as tolerated, to a maximum of 100 mg/day
    Adults: 50 mg/day as a single bedtime dose; maximum dose: 200 mg/day outpatients; 300 mg/day inpatients
Monitoring Parameters Blood pressure, pulse, target symptoms
Test Interactions Elevated glucose
Patient Information To prevent dizziness, avoid abrupt changes of position, may cause dry mouth, dizziness, blurred vision, constipation, sedation
Nursing Implications Monitor sitting and standing blood pressure and pulse
Additional Information May cause alterations in bleeding time
Special Geriatric Considerations Similar to doxepin in its side effect profile; has not been well studied in the elderly; very anticholinergic and, therefore, not considered a drug of first choice in the elderly when selecting an antidepressant
Dosage Forms Capsule: 25 mg, 50 mg, 100 mg

Trimox® see Amoxicillin Trihydrate on page 49

Trimpex® see Trimethoprim on page 721

Triofed® [OTC] see Triprolidine and Pseudoephedrine on this page

Triostat™ see Liothyronine Sodium on page 408

Triposed® [OTC] see Triprolidine and Pseudoephedrine on this page

Triprolidine and Pseudoephedrine (trye proe' li deen)
Related Information
    Pseudoephedrine on page 609
Brand Names Actagen® [OTC]; Actifed® [OTC]; Allerfrin® [OTC]; Allerphed® [OTC]; Aprodine® [OTC]; Cenafed® Plus [OTC]; Genac® [OTC]; Sudahist® [OTC]; Triafed® [OTC]; Trifed® [OTC]; Triofed® [OTC]; Triposed® [OTC]
Synonyms Pseudoephedrine and Triprolidine
Generic Available Yes
(Continued)

Triprolidine and Pseudoephedrine *(Continued)*

Therapeutic Class Antihistamine/Decongestant Combination

Use Temporary relief of nasal congestion, running nose, sneezing, itching of nose or throat and itchy, watery eyes due to common cold, hay fever or other upper respiratory allergies

Contraindications Narrow-angle glaucoma, bladder neck obstruction, asthmatic attacks, stenosing peptic ulcer, MAO inhibitor therapy, hypertension, coronary artery disease, hypersensitivity to pseudoephedrine, triprolidine or any component

Precautions Use with caution in patients with high blood pressure, heart disease, diabetes, asthma, thyroid disease, or prostatic hypertrophy

Adverse Reactions
Cardiovascular: Tachycardia, palpitations, arrhythmias
Central nervous system: Nervousness, excitability, dizziness, insomnia, drowsiness, headache
Gastrointestinal: Nausea, vomiting, dry mouth
Genitourinary: Difficult urination
Neuromuscular & skeletal: Tremors
Respiratory: Thickening of bronchial secretions

Overdosage Symptoms of overdose include hallucinations, CNS depression, seizures, death

Toxicology
There is no specific antidote for pseudoephedrine intoxication and the bulk of the treatment is supportive
Hyperactivity and agitation usually respond to reduced sensory input, however with extreme agitation haloperidol (2-5 mg I.M. for adults) may be required
Hyperthermia is best treated with external cooling measures, or when severe or unresponsive, muscle paralysis with pancuronium may be needed
Hypertension is usually transient and generally does not require treatment unless severe. For diastolic blood pressures >110 mm Hg, a nitroprusside infusion should be initiated.
Seizures usually respond to diazepam I.V. and/or phenytoin maintenance regimens

Drug Interactions
Decreased effect: Beta-blockers, methyldopa
Increased toxicity/effect: Tricyclic antidepressants, MAO inhibitors (increased blood pressure), sympathomimetics

Usual Dosage May dose according to **pseudoephedrine** component (4 mg/kg/day in divided doses 3-4 times/day)

Geriatrics and Adults:
Capsule, extended release: 1 capsule every 12 hours
Syrup: 10 mL
Tablet: 1 tablet 3-4 times/day; maximum: 4 tablets/day

Monitoring Parameters Relief of symptoms, blood pressure, pulse

Test Interactions Increased amylase, increased lipase

Patient Information Do not exceed recommended dosage; do not crush or chew extended release capsule

Nursing Implications Do not crush extended release capsule

Special Geriatric Considerations Use with caution in patients with cardiovascular disease; see Contraindications and Precautions; also see Pseudoephedrine monograph

Dosage Forms
Capsule: Triprolidine hydrochloride 2.5 mg and pseudoephedrine hydrochloride 60 mg
Capsule, extended release: Triprolidine hydrochloride 5 mg and pseudoephedrine hydrochloride 120 mg
Syrup: Triprolidine hydrochloride 1.25 mg and pseudoephedrine hydrochloride 30 mg per 5 mL
Tablet: Triprolidine hydrochloride 2.5 mg and pseudoephedrine hydrochloride 60 mg

TripTone® Caplets® [OTC] *see* Dimenhydrinate *on page 227*

Trisoject® *see* Triamcinolone *on page 710*

Tri-Statin® II Topical *see* Nystatin and Triamcinolone *on page 514*

Trisulfam® *see* Co-trimoxazole *on page 189*

Truphylline® *see* Aminophylline *on page 39*

Trypsin, Balsam Peru, and Castor Oil

Brand Names Granulex
Generic Available Yes
Therapeutic Class Protectant, Topical; Topical Skin Product
Use Treatment of decubitus ulcers, varicose ulcers, debridement of eschar, dehiscent wounds and sunburn

Warnings Do not spray on fresh arterial clots; avoid contact with eyes

Adverse Reactions Local: Itching or stinging may be associated with initial application

Mechanism of Action Trypsin is an enzymatic debriding agent. Peruvian balsam is a capillary bed stimulant and may have mild bactericidal action. Castor oil may improve epithelialization and act as a protective barrier.

Usual Dosage Geriatrics and Adults: Apply a minimum of twice daily or as often as necessary

Monitoring Parameters Size of the ulcer, skin integrity

Patient Information Avoid contact with eyes; for external use only; shake well before spraying

Nursing Implications Clean wound prior to application and at each redressing; shake well before spraying; hold can upright ~12" from area to be treated

Special Geriatric Considerations Preventive skin care should be instituted in all older patients at high risk for decubitus ulcers. Practical experience with Granulex has found that it is not as effective in debriding wounds as compared to other enzymatic products. Therefore, Granulex may be more appropriately used on stage 1 and 2 decubiti.

Dosage Forms Aerosol, topical: 4 oz

References
Chamberlain TM, Cali TJ, Cuzzell J, et al, "Assessment and Management of Pressure Sores in Long-Term Care Facilities," *Consult Pharm*, 1992, 7(12):1328-40.

T-Stat® see Erythromycin, Topical *on page 266*

Tuberculin Purified Protein Derivative

Brand Names Alplitest®; Aplisol®; Sclavo-PPD® Solution; Sclavo-Test-PPD®; Tine Test PPD®; Tubersol®

Synonyms Mantoux; PPD; Tine Test

Generic Available No

Therapeutic Class Diagnostic Agent, Skin Test

Use Skin test in diagnosis of tuberculosis, cell-mediated immunodeficiencies

Contraindications Tuberculin positive reactions; 250 TU strength should not be used for initial testing

Warnings Do not give I.V. or S.C.; epinephrine (1:1000) should be available to treat possible allergic reactions; skin test responsiveness may be suppressed during and after (up to 6 months) viral infections, vaccinations with live viral vaccines, and patients with tuberculosis, severe bacterial infections, malnutrition, malignant diseases or immunosuppression

Precautions Do not apply on hairy areas without adequate subcutaneous tissue or on acneiform skin; use extreme caution in patients with perceived active tuberculosis; positive test does not confirm diagnosis and further diagnostic procedures should be performed

Adverse Reactions
Dermatologic: Ulceration, necrosis
Local: Vesiculation, pain

Drug Interactions Reaction may be suppressed in patients receiving systemic corticosteroids, aminocaproic acid, or within 4-6 weeks following immunization with live or inactivated viral vaccines

Stability Refrigerate

Mechanism of Action Tuberculosis results in individuals becoming sensitized to certain antigenic components of the M tuberculosis organism. Culture extracts called tuberculins are contained in tuberculin skin test preparations. Upon intracutaneous injection of these culture extracts, a classic delayed (cellular) hypersensitivity reaction occurs. This reaction is characteristic of a delayed course (peak occurs >24 hours after injection, induration of the skin secondary to cell infiltration, and occasional vesiculation and necrosis). Delayed hypersensitivity reactions to tuberculin may indicate infection with a variety of nontuberculosis mycobacteria, or vaccination with the live attenuated mycobacterial strain of M bovis vaccine, BCG, in addition to previous natural infection with M tuberculosis.

Pharmacodynamics
Onset of action: Delayed hypersensitivity reactions to tuberculin usually occur within 5-6 hours following injection
Peak effect: Becomes maximal at 48-72 hours
Duration: Reactions subside over a few days

Usual Dosage Geriatrics and Adults: Intradermal: 0.1 mL about 4" below elbow; use $\frac{1}{4}$" to $\frac{1}{2}$" or 26- or 27-gauge needle; significant reactions are ≥5 mm in diameter

Interpretation of induration: Positive: ≥10 mm; inconclusive: 5-9 mm; negative: <5 mm

Administration Give intradermally; avoid subcutaneous injections

Monitoring Parameters Monitor for induration (48-72 hours), ulcerations, necrosis, vesiculations

Patient Information Return to physician or nurse for reaction interpretation at 48-72 hours

(Continued)

Tuberculin Purified Protein Derivative *(Continued)*

Nursing Implications Test dose: 0.1 mL intracutaneously; store in refrigerator; examine site at 48-72 hours after administration; whenever tuberculin is administered, a record should be made of the administration technique (Mantoux method, disposable multiple-puncture device), tuberculin used (OT or PPD), manufacturer and lot number of tuberculin used, date of administration, date of test reading, and the size of the reaction in millimeters (mm)

Special Geriatric Considerations Due to changes in the immune system with age, skin-test response may be delayed or reduced in magnitude; therefore when testing, use a 2-step test procedure; repeat test 2-4 weeks after reading first test dose; this elicits a "booster effect"

Dosage Forms Injection:
First test strength: 1 TU/0.1 mL (1 mL)
Intermediate test strength: 5 TU/0.1 mL (1 mL, 5 mL, 10 mL)
Second test strength: 250 TU/0.1 mL (1 mL)
Tine: 5 TU each test

References
Dutt AK and Stead WW, "Tuberculosis," *Clin Geriatr Med*, 1992, 8(4):761-75.

Tubersol® *see* Tuberculin Purified Protein Derivative *on previous page*

Tuinal® *see* Amobarbital and Secobarbital *on page 46*

Tums® E-X Extra Strength Tablet [OTC] *see* Calcium Salts (Oral) *on page 111*

Tums® [OTC] *see* Calcium Salts (Oral) *on page 111*

Tums® Extra Strength Liquid [OTC] *see* Calcium Salts (Oral) *on page 111*

Tusal® *see* Salicylates (Various Salts) *on page 633*

Tusstat® *see* Diphenhydramine Hydrochloride *on page 228*

Twice-A-Day® Nasal Solution [OTC] *see* Oxymetazoline Hydrochloride *on page 530*

Twilite® [OTC] *see* Diphenhydramine Hydrochloride *on page 228*

Tylenol® [OTC] *see* Acetaminophen *on page 13*

Tylenol® With Codeine *see* Acetaminophen and Codeine *on page 14*

Tylox® *see* Oxycodone and Acetaminophen *on page 528*

Typhoid Vaccine (tye' foid)

Related Information
Immunization Guidelines *on page 759-762*

Brand Names Vivotif Berna™

Therapeutic Class Vaccine, Inactivated Bacteria

Use Promotes active immunity to typhoid fever for patients exposed to typhoid carrier or foreign travel to typhoid fever endemic area

Contraindications Acute respiratory or other active infections, previous sensitivity to typhoid vaccine or enteric coated capsule; immunosuppressed patients

Precautions Immune deficiency conditions; vaccine does not protect all recipients

Adverse Reactions
Central nervous system: Malaise, headache, fever
Local: Tenderness, erythema, induration
Neuromuscular & skeletal: Myalgia

Overdosage No symptoms noted with oral capsule; can cause *S. typhi* shedding

Drug Interactions Simultaneous administration with other vaccines which cause local or systemic adverse effects should be avoided

Stability Refrigerate at 2°C to 8°C (36°F to 46°F); do not freeze; not viable at room temperature

Mechanism of Action >70% effective

Usual Dosage Geriatrics and Adults:
S.C.: 0.5 mL; repeat dose in 4 weeks (total immunization is 2 doses); booster: 0.5 mL S.C. or 0.1 mL intradermally at 3-year intervals
Primary immunization: Oral: 1 capsule on alternate days (every other day) for a total of 4 capsules; take 1 hour after meals with cold or lukewarm water
Booster: Repeat at 5-year intervals; use same schedule as for primary immunization (4 capsules)

Patient Information Oral capsule should be taken 1 hour before a meal with cold or lukewarm drink; systemic adverse effects may persist for 1-2 days

Nursing Implications Doses of vaccine are different between S.C. and intradermal; S.C. injection only should be used

Additional Information If >3 years elapse after vaccination, only booster is needed; do not need to repeat primary vaccination

Special Geriatric Considerations Vaccinating elderly is often overlooked; if no record of immunization can be recalled, repeat primary series

Dosage Forms
Capsule, enteric coated
Injection: 1.5 mL

References
Gardner P and Schaffner W, "Immunization of Adults," *N Engl J Med*, 1993, 328(17):1252-8.

Tyzine® *see* Tetrahydrozoline Hydrochloride *on page 680*

U-Cort™ *see* Hydrocortisone *on page 351*

Ultracef® *see* Cefadroxil Monohydrate *on page 125*

Ultralente *see* Insulin Preparations *on page 372*

Ultralente® Iletin®I *see* Insulin Preparations *on page 372*

Ultralente® Insulin (Beef) *see* Insulin Preparations *on page 372*

Ultralente® Purified Beef *see* Insulin Preparations *on page 372*

Unasyn® *see* Ampicillin Sodium and Sulbactam Sodium *on page 52*

Unilax® [OTC] *see* Docusate and Phenolphthalein *on page 238*

Unipen® *see* Nafcillin Sodium *on page 487*

Uniphyl® *see* Theophylline *on page 681*

Uni-Pro® [OTC] *see* Ibuprofen *on page 360*

Uni Tussin® [OTC] *see* Guaifenesin *on page 331*

Urabeth® *see* Bethanechol Chloride *on page 85*

Urea Peroxide *see* Carbamide Peroxide *on page 119*

Urecholine® *see* Bethanechol Chloride *on page 85*

Urex® *see* Methenamine *on page 452*

Urised® *see* Methenamine *on page 452*

Urispas® *see* Flavoxate *on page 292*

Uri-Tet® *see* Oxytetracycline Hydrochloride *on page 531*

Urodine® *see* Phenazopyridine Hydrochloride *on page 552*

Uro-KP-Neutral® *see* Potassium Phosphate and Sodium Phosphate *on page 580*

Uro-Mag® *see* Magnesium Oxide *on page 429*

Uroplus® DS *see* Co-trimoxazole *on page 189*

Uroplus® SS *see* Co-trimoxazole *on page 189*

Ursodeoxycholic Acid *see* Ursodiol *on this page*

Ursodiol (er' soe dye ole)
Brand Names Actigall™
Synonyms Ursodeoxycholic Acid
Generic Available No
Therapeutic Class Gallstone Dissolution Agent
Use Gallbladder stone dissolution in patients with radiolucent, noncalcified stones <20 mm in greatest diameter with an increased risk for surgical removal; safety beyond 2 years use is not established
Contraindications Not to be used with cholesterol, radiopaque, bile pigment stones, or stones larger than 20 mm in diameter; allergy to bile acids; chronic liver disease; patients who have very good reason for cholecystectomy for diseases which require this procedure (eg, cholangitis, biliary obstruction, gallstones, pancreatitis, etc)
Warnings Gallbladder stone dissolution may take several months of therapy; complete dissolution may not occur and recurrence of stones within 5 years has been observed in 50% of patients; use with caution in patients with a nonvisualizing gallbladder and those with chronic liver disease
Precautions Patients who develop abnormal liver tests during therapy should be closely monitored for worsening gallstone disease; discontinue if liver function tests persist in elevation
Adverse Reactions
Central nervous system: Fatigue, headache, depression, sleep difficulties
Dermatologic: Pruritus, rash, urticaria, dry skin, thinning hair
Gastrointestinal: Nausea, vomiting, dyspepsia, metallic taste, abdominal pain, biliary pain, constipation, cholecystitis, flatulence
Neuromuscular & skeletal: Myalgia, arthralgia, backache
Respiratory: Cough, rhinitis
Miscellaneous: Sweating
Overdosage Symptoms of overdose predominantly include diarrhea
(Continued)

ALPHABETICAL LISTING OF DRUGS

Ursodiol *(Continued)*

Toxicology No specific therapy for diarrhea and for overdose; give general supportive care

Drug Interactions Decreased effect with aluminum-containing antacids, cholestyramine, colestipol, clofibrate, oral contraceptives (estrogens)

Mechanism of Action Decreases the cholesterol content of bile and bile stones by reducing the secretion of cholesterol from the liver and the fractional reabsorption of cholesterol by the intestines

Pharmacokinetics

Metabolism: Undergoes extensive enterohepatic recycling; following hepatic conjugation and biliary secretion, the drug is hydrolyzed to active ursodiol, where it is recycled or transformed to lithocholic acid by colonic microbial flora

Half-life: 100 hours

Elimination: In feces via bile

Usual Dosage Geriatrics and Adults: Oral: 8-10 mg/kg/day in 2-3 divided doses; use beyond 24 months is not established; obtain ultrasound images at 6-month intervals for the first year of therapy; 30% of patients have stone recurrence after dissolution

Monitoring Parameters ALT, AST at initiation, 1 and 3 months and every 6 months thereafter, sonogram

Patient Information Frequent blood work necessary to follow drug effects; report any persistent nausea, vomiting, abdominal pain

Nursing Implications See Adverse Reactions and Special Geriatric Considerations

Special Geriatric Considerations No specific clinical studies in elderly; would recommend starting at lowest recommended dose with scheduled monitoring

Dosage Forms Capsule: 300 mg

Uticort® *see* Betamethasone *on page 82*

Utimox® *see* Amoxicillin Trihydrate *on page 49*

Valadol® [OTC] *see* Acetaminophen *on page 13*

Valdrene® *see* Diphenhydramine Hydrochloride *on page 228*

Valergen® *see* Estradiol *on page 269*

Valisone® *see* Betamethasone *on page 82*

Valium® *see* Diazepam *on page 211*

Valproate Semisodium *see* Valproic Acid and Derivatives *on this page*

Valproate Sodium *see* Valproic Acid and Derivatives *on this page*

Valproic Acid *see* Valproic Acid and Derivatives *on this page*

Valproic Acid and Derivatives *(val proe' ik)*

Related Information

Antacid Drug Interactions *on page 764*

Drug Levels Commonly Monitored Guidelines *on page 771-772*

Brand Names Depakene®; Depakote®

Synonyms Dipropylacetic Acid; Divalproex Sodium; DPA; 2-Propylpentanoic Acid; 2-Propylvaleric Acid; Valproate Semisodium; Valproate Sodium; Valproic Acid

Generic Available Yes

Therapeutic Class Anticonvulsant, Miscellaneous

Use Management of simple and complex absence seizures; mixed seizure types; myoclonic and generalized tonic-clonic (grand mal) seizures; may be effective in partial seizures

Unlabeled use: Treatment of atypical absence, myoclonic, and grand mal seizures; treatment of bipolar affective disorder and incontinence following ileoanal anastomosis; aggressive behavior associated with dementia

Contraindications Hypersensitivity to valproic acid or derivatives or any component; hepatic dysfunction and hepatic disease

Warnings Hepatic failure resulting in fatalities has occurred in patients; monitor patients closely for appearance of malaise, loss of seizure control, weakness, facial edema, anorexia, jaundice and vomiting; hepatotoxicity has been reported after days to 6 months of therapy

Precautions May cause severe thrombocytopenia, bleeding; hyperammonemia in absence of abnormal LFTs or mental changes may occur; valproic acid may interact with other anticonvulsants; see Drug Interactions; carcinogenicity reported in animals (fibrosarcoma, pulmonary adenomas), but no such data in humans

Adverse Reactions

Central nervous system: Drowsiness, ataxia, irritability, confusion, restlessness, sedation, hyperactivity, headache, malaise, dizziness, depression, psychosis, aggression

Dermatologic: Alopecia, erythema multiforme, rash, transient hair loss, bruising

Endocrine & metabolic: Hyperammonemia, abnormal thyroid tests, parotid gland swelling

728

Gastrointestinal: Nausea, vomiting, indigestion, diarrhea, abdominal cramps, constipation, anorexia, weight loss, weight gain, pancreatitis

Hematologic: Thrombocytopenia, prolongation of bleeding time, leukopenia, eosinophilia, bone marrow suppression, hemorrhage

Hepatic: Transient elevated liver enzymes, liver failure, lymphocytosis

Neuromuscular & skeletal: Asterixis, dysarthria, incoordination, weakness, tremors

Ocular: Diplopia, "spots before eyes"

Miscellaneous: Peripheral edema

Overdosage Symptoms of overdose include coma, deep sleep, motor restlessness, asterixis, visual hallucinations

Toxicology Supportive treatment is necessary; naloxone has been used to reverse CNS depressant effects, but may block action of other anticonvulsants

Drug Interactions

Valproic acid may displace phenytoin and diazepam from protein binding sites. Aspirin may displace valproic acid from protein binding sites which may result in toxicity. Valproic acid may significantly increase phenobarbital serum concentrations in patients receiving phenobarbital or primidone. Valproic acid may inhibit the metabolism of phenytoin.

Phenobarbital, primidone, phenytoin and carbamazepine may decrease serum levels of valproic acid

Food may delay absorption but does not affect extent absorbed

Mechanism of Action Causes increased availability of gamma-aminobutyric acid (GABA), an inhibitory neurotransmitter, to brain neurons or may enhance the action of GABA or mimic its action at postsynaptic receptor sites; valproate may also inhibit catabolism of GABA; potentiate postsynaptic GABA response, have direct membrane stabilization effect possibly by effecting potassium channel operation

Pharmacokinetics

Protein binding: 80% to 90% (dose dependent)

Metabolism: Extensive in the liver

Half-life (adults): 8-17 hours, increased half-life in patients with liver disease

Time to peak: Oral: Peak serum levels occur within 1-4 hours; 3-5 hours after divalproex (enteric coated)

Elimination: 2% to 3% excreted unchanged in urine

Usual Dosage Geriatrics and Adults:

Oral: Initial: 10-15 mg/kg/day in 1-3 divided doses; increase by 5-10 mg/kg/day at weekly intervals until therapeutic levels are achieved; maintenance: 30-60 mg/kg/day in 2-3 divided doses; twice daily administration most frequent; see Additional Information

Rectal: Dilute syrup 1:1 with water for use as a retention enema; loading dose: 17-20 mg/kg one time; maintenance: 10-15 mg/kg/dose every 8 hours

Not dialyzable (0% to 5%)

Monitoring Parameters Monitor serum concentrations; observe for side effects and obtain LFTs and CBC during first 6 months of therapy

Reference Range

Therapeutic: 50-100 μg/mL (SI: 350-690 μmol/L); Toxic: >200 μg/mL (SI: >1390 μmol/L)

Seizure control may improve at levels >100 μg/mL (SI: 690 μmol/L), but toxicity may occur at levels of 100-150 μg/mL (SI: 690-1040 μmol/L)

Test Interactions False-positive result for urine ketones; possible alterations in thyroid function tests

Patient Information Take with food or milk; do not chew, break or crush the tablet or capsule; do not administer with carbonated drinks; report any sore throat, fever, or fatigue

Nursing Implications Do not crush enteric coated drug product or capsules; see Monitoring Parameters

Additional Information Tremors may indicate overdosage. The most frequent side effects to valproic acid use are anorexia, vomiting, and nausea; taking doses with meals or changing to the enteric coated product may reduce these side effects

Sodium content of valproate sodium syrup (5 mL): 23 mg (1 mEq)

Divalproex sodium: Depakote®

Valproate sodium: Depakene® syrup

Valproic acid: Depakene® capsule

Special Geriatric Considerations No specific data available for use in elderly; see Warnings, Additional Information

Dosage Forms

Capsule, as valproic acid: 250 mg

Capsule, sprinkle: 125 mg

Syrup, as sodium valproate: 250 mg/5mL (5 mL, 50 mL, 480 mL)

Tablet, enteric coated, delayed release, as divalproex sodium: 125 mg, 250 mg, 500 mg

References

Dreifuss FE, Santilli N, Langer DH, et al, "Valproic Acid Hepatic Fatalities: A Retrospective Review," Neurology, 1987, 37(3):379-85.

(Continued)

Valproic Acid and Derivatives *(Continued)*

Mazure CM, Druss BG, and Cellar JS, "Valproate Treatment of Older Psychotic Patients With Organic Mental Syndromes and Behavioral Dyscontrol," *JAGS*, 1992, 40:914-6.

Mellow AM, Solano-Lopez C, and Davis S, "Sodium Valproate in the Treatment of Behavioral Disturbance in Dementia," *J Geriatr Psychiatr Neurol*, 1993, 6:205-9.

Valrelease® *see Diazepam on page 211*

Vancenase® *see Beclomethasone Dipropionate on page 75*

Vancenase® AQ *see Beclomethasone Dipropionate on page 75*

Vanceril® *see Beclomethasone Dipropionate on page 75*

Vancocin® *see Vancomycin Hydrochloride on this page*

Vancoled® *see Vancomycin Hydrochloride on this page*

Vancomycin Hydrochloride (van koe mye' sin)
Related Information
Drug Levels Commonly Monitored Guidelines *on page 771-772*
Brand Names Lyphocin®; Vancocin®; Vancoled®; Vancor®
Generic Available Yes
Therapeutic Class Antibiotic, Miscellaneous
Use Treatment of patients with the following infections or conditions: treatment of infections due to documented or suspected methicillin-resistant *S. aureus* or beta-lactam resistant coagulase negative *Staphylococcus*; treatment of serious or life-threatening infections (ie, endocarditis, meningitis) due to documented or suspected staphylococcal or streptococcal infections in patients who are allergic to penicillins and/or cephalosporins; empiric therapy of infections associated with central lines, VP shunts, vascular grafts, prosthetic heart valves; treatment of febrile granulocytopenic patient who has not responded after 48 hours to antibiotic treatment directed at gram-negative rod infections; used orally for staphylococcal enterocolitis or for antibiotic-associated pseudomembranous colitis produced by *C. difficile*
Contraindications Hypersensitivity to vancomycin or any component; avoid in patients with previous hearing loss
Precautions Use with caution in patients with renal impairment or those receiving other nephrotoxic or ototoxic drugs; dosage modification required in patients with impaired renal function
Adverse Reactions
Cardiovascular: Tachycardia, hypotension
Central nervous system: Fever, chills
Dermatologic: Erythema multiforme-like reaction with intense pruritus, rash involving face, neck, upper trunk, urticaria, macular skin rash, back and upper arms (red neck or red man syndrome)
Gastrointestinal: Nausea (oral), bitter taste
Hematologic: Neutropenia, eosinophilia, thrombocytopenia
Local: Phlebitis
Otic: Ototoxicity
Renal: Nephrotoxicity
Toxicology There is no specific therapy for an overdosage with vancomycin. Care is symptomatic and supportive in nature. Peritoneal filtration and hemofiltration have been shown to reduce the serum concentration of vancomycin.
Drug Interactions Anesthetic agents, aminoglycosides (may increase risk of nephrotoxicity and ototoxicity), nondepolarizing muscle relaxants
Stability After the oral or parenteral solution is reconstituted, refrigerate and discard after 14 days; after further dilution, the parenteral solution is stable, at room temperature, for 24 hours
Mechanism of Action Inhibits bacterial cell wall synthesis by blocking glycopeptide polymerization through binding tightly to D-alanyl-D-alanine portion of cell wall precursor; also inhibits RNA synthesis
Pharmacokinetics
Absorption:
Oral: Poor
I.M.: Erratic
Protein binding: 10%
Half-life: Biphasic: Terminal: Adults: 5-11 hours, half-life prolonged significantly with reduced renal function
Time to peak: Following completion of I.V. infusion, peak serum levels occur within 45-65 minutes
Elimination: As unchanged drug in urine (80% to 90%); oral doses are excreted primarily in feces
Geriatrics: Volume of distribution has been reported to be decreased 44% while total clearance decreased by 23% and the terminal half-life increased to 12 hours
Usual Dosage Initial dosage recommendation: I.V.:
Geriatrics: Best to individualize therapy; dose (mg/kg/24 hours) = $(0.227 \times Cl_{cr}) + 5.67$

Cl$_{cr}$ male: (140 - age) divided by serum creatinine
Cl$_{cr}$ female: Cl$_{cr}$ male x 0.85
The calculated dose should be divided and given as specified in the following dosing intervals based upon Cl$_{cr}$:
Cl$_{cr}$ >65 mL/minute: Administer every 8 hours
Cl$_{cr}$ 40-65 mL/minute: Administer every 12 hours
Cl$_{cr}$ 20-39 mL/minute: Administer every 24 hours
Cl$_{cr}$ 10-19 mL/minute: Administer every 48 hours
Not dialyzable (0% to 5%)

Adults: With normal renal function: 0.5 g every 6 hours or 1 g every 12 hours

Renal dysfunction, end stage renal disease, or on dialysis: 10-20 mg/kg; subsequent dosages and frequency of administration are best determined by measurement of serum levels and assessment of renal insufficiency

Geriatrics and Adults: Intrathecal: 20 mg/day

C. difficile colitis: Geriatrics and Adults: Oral: 125-500 mg every 6-8 hours for 7-10 days; no dosage adjustment necessary for renal impairment

Monitoring Parameters Peak and trough vancomycin levels, serum BUN and creatinine, hearing, culture and sensitivity results, I.V. site; signs of Red Man's syndrome

Reference Range
Therapeutic:
Depends on MIC of organism being treated, usually peak: 20-35 µg/mL (SI: 20-35 mg/L)
Trough: 5-10 µg/mL (SI: 5-10 mg/L)
Toxic: >80-100 µg/mL (SI: 80-100 mg /L)

Patient Information Report pain at infusion site, dizziness, fullness or ringing in ears with I.V. use; nausea or vomiting with oral use

Nursing Implications Obtain drug levels after the third dose; peaks are drawn 30 minutes to 3 hours after the completion of a 1-hour infusion; troughs are obtained just before the next dose; slow I.V. infusion rate to ≥2 hours if maculopapular rash appears on face, neck, thorax, trunk, and upper extremities; dosage modification required in patients with impaired renal function; do not give antidiarrheal products to patients on oral vancomycin; do not give I.M.

Special Geriatric Considerations As a result of age-related changes in renal function and volume of distribution, accumulation, and toxicity are a risk in the elderly; see Pharmacokinetics and Adverse Reactions; hence, careful monitoring and dosing adjustment is necessary

Dosage Forms
Capsule: 125 mg, 250 mg
Powder for oral solution: 1 g, 10 g
Powder for injection: 500 mg, 1 g, 2 g, 5 g, 10 g

References
Cutler NR, Narang PK, Lesko LJ, et al, "Vancomycin Disposition: The Importance of Age," *Clin Pharmacol Ther*, 1984, 36(6):803-10.
Rodvold KA, Blum RA, Fischer JH, et al, "Vancomycin Pharmacokinetics in Patients With Various Degrees of Renal Function," *Antimicrob Agents Chemother*, 1988, 32(6):848-52.

Vancor® *see* Vancomycin Hydrochloride *on previous page*
Vantin® *see* Cefpodoxime Proxetil *on page 135*
Vapo-Iso® *see* Isoproterenol *on page 380*
Vaponefrin® *see* Epinephrine *on page 256*

Varicella-Zoster Immune Globulin (Human)
Related Information
Immunization Guidelines *on page 759-762*
Synonyms VZIG
Therapeutic Class Immune Globulin
Use Passive immunization of susceptible immunodeficient patients after exposure to varicella
Contraindications Allergic response to gamma globulin or anti-immunoglobulin; sensitivity to thimerosal; persons with IgA deficiency; do not administer to patients with thrombocytopenia or coagulopathies
Warnings Do not give I.V.; caution in patients with sensitivity to human immunoglobulin preparations
Precautions Skin test should not be performed to determine if patient is sensitive to agent
Adverse Reactions
Central nervous system: Lethargy, fever, chills
Dermatologic: Urticaria, angioedema
Gastrointestinal: Nausea
Local: Pain, redness, swelling
Neuromuscular & skeletal: Muscle stiffness, tenderness, myalgia
(Continued)

Varicella-Zoster Immune Globulin (Human) *(Continued)*

Respiratory: Chest tightness

Drug Interactions Live virus vaccines; do not give immune globulin within 3 months of immunization

Stability Refrigerate at 2°C to 8°C (36°F to 46°F)

Usual Dosage I.M. (do not inject I.V.): Administer by deep injection in the gluteal muscle or in another large muscle mass. Inject 125 units/10 kg (22 pounds); maximum dose: 625 units (5 vials); minimum dose: 125 units; do not give fractional doses.

Patient Information Be aware of adverse reactions

Nursing Implications Administer as soon as possible after presumed exposure; do not inject I.V.; administer by deep I.M. injection into gluteal muscle or other large muscle; administer entire contents of each vial; see Usual Dosage

Special Geriatric Considerations VZIG provides passive immunity for those susceptible to varicella; neoplastic disease, immunosuppressed elderly, or institutionalized who are exposed to other patients with varicella; CDC provides specific guidelines for use. Live attenuated vaccine is available but not approved in U.S. Age is the most important risk factor for reactivation of varicella zoster; persons <50 years of age have incidence of 2.5 cases per 1000, whereas those 60-79 have 6.5 cases per 1000 and those >80 years have 10 cases per 1000

Dosage Forms Injection: 125 units of antibody in single dose vials

Vascor® *see* Bepridil *on page 81*

Vasocidin® *see* Sodium Sulfacetamide and Prednisolone Acetate *on page 652*

VasoClear® [OTC] *see* Naphazoline Hydrochloride *on page 492*

Vasocon-A® *see* Naphazoline and Antazoline *on page 491*

Vasocon Regular® *see* Naphazoline Hydrochloride *on page 492*

Vasoderm® *see* Fluocinonide *on page 299*

Vasoderm-D® *see* Fluocinonide *on page 299*

Vasodilan® *see* Isoxsuprine Hydrochloride *on page 384*

Vasopressin *(vay soe press' in)*

Brand Names Pitressin®; Pitressin® Tannate in Oil

Synonyms Antidiuretic Hormone; 8-Arginine Vasopressin; Vasopressin Tannate

Therapeutic Class Antidiuretic Hormone Analog; Hormone, Posterior Pituitary

Use Treatment of diabetes insipidus; prevention and treatment of postoperative abdominal distention; differential diagnosis of diabetes insipidus

Unlabeled use: Adjunct in the treatment of GI hemorrhage and esophageal varices

Contraindications Hypersensitivity to vasopressin or any component; chronic nephritis with nitrogen retention

Warnings I.V. infiltration may lead to severe vasoconstriction and localized tissue necrosis; also gangrene of extremities, tongue, and ischemic colitis

Precautions Use with caution in patients with seizure disorders, migraine, asthma, vascular disease, renal disease, cardiac disease (may precipitate anginal pain or myocardial infarction)

Adverse Reactions

Cardiovascular: Pounding in the head, increased blood pressure, bradycardia, arrhythmias, venous thrombosis, vasoconstriction with higher doses, angina, cardiac arrest

Central nervous system: Vertigo, fever

Dermatologic: Urticaria

Endocrine & metabolic: Water intoxication

Gastrointestinal: Abdominal cramps, nausea, vomiting, flatus

Neuromuscular & skeletal: Tremors

Respiratory: Wheezing

Miscellaneous: Sweating

Overdosage Symptoms of overdose include drowsiness, weight gain, confusion, listlessness

Toxicology Restrict fluids and withdraw vasopressin until polyuria; may require treatment with osmotic diuretics or furosemide

Drug Interactions Lithium, epinephrine, demeclocycline, heparin, and alcohol block antidiuretic activity to varying degrees; carbamazepine, chlorpropamide, phenformin, urea and fludrocortisone potentiate antidiuretic response

Stability Store injection at room temperature; protect from heat and from freezing; use only clear solutions

Mechanism of Action Increases cyclic adenosine monophosphate (cAMP) which increases water permeability at the renal tubule resulting in decreased urine volume and increased osmolality; causes peristalsis by directly stimulating the smooth muscle in the GI tract

Pharmacodynamics

Nasal:
   Onset of action: 1 hour
   Duration: 3-8 hours

Parenteral: Duration of action:
   Aqueous: 2-8 hours
   Tannate: 24-72 hours

Pharmacokinetics Destroyed by trypsin in GI tract, must be administered parenterally or intranasally

Nasal:
   Metabolism: In the liver and kidneys
   Half-life: 15 minutes
   Elimination: In urine
Parenteral:
   Metabolism: Most of dose is metabolized by liver and kidney
   Half-life: 10-20 minutes
   Elimination: 5% of S.C. dose (aqueous) is excreted unchanged in urine after 4 hours

Usual Dosage Geriatrics and Adults:

Diabetes insipidus:
   I.M., S.C. (tannate form): Highly variable dosage; titrated based upon serum and urine sodium and osmolality in addition to fluid balance and urine output: 5-10 units 2-4 times/day as needed
   Continuous infusion: Initial: 0.5 milliunit/kg/hour (0.0005 unit/kg/hour); titrate up to 2 milliunits/kg/hour; maximum: 10 milliunits/kg/hour

Abdominal distention: I.M.: 5 units stat, 10 units every 3-4 hours

GI hemorrhage: I.V. continuous infusion: Initial: 0.2-0.4 unit/minute, then titrate dose as needed

Monitoring Parameters EKG, serum and urine sodium, urine output, fluid input and output, urine specific gravity, urine and serum osmolality

Reference Range Plasma: 0-2 pg/mL (SI: 0-2 ng/L) if osmolality <285 mOsm/L; 2-12 pg/mL (SI: 2-12 ng/L) if osmolality >290 mOsm/L

Test Interactions Decreased sodium (S)

Patient Information If nausea, abdominal cramping, or blanching of the skin occurs, take 1-2 glasses of water with each dose

Nursing Implications Before withdrawing a dose, vasopressin tannate in oil should be shaken thoroughly to obtain a uniform suspension; vasopressin tannate in oil must not be administered I.V.; monitor fluid I & O; watch for signs of I.V. infiltration and gangrene

Special Geriatric Considerations Elderly patients should be cautioned not to increase their fluid intake beyond that sufficient to satisfy their thirst in order to avoid water intoxication and hyponatremia; under experimental conditions, the elderly have shown to have a decreased responsiveness to vasopressin with respect to its effects on water homeostasis

Dosage Forms
Injection: 20 units/mL (0.5 mL, 1 mL)
Injection, as tannate (in oil): 5 units/mL (1 mL)

References
Lindeman RD, Lee TD Jr, Yiengst MJ, et al, "Influence of Age, Renal Disease, Hypertension, Diuretics, and Calcium on the Antidiuretic Responses to Suboptimal Infusions of Vasopressin," *J Lab Clin Med*, 1966, 68(2):206-23.
Miller JH and Shock NW, "Age Differences in the Renal Tubular Response to Antidiuretic Hormone," *J Gerontol*, 1953, 8:446-50.

Vasopressin Tannate see Vasopressin *on previous page*

Vasosulf® see Sodium Sulfacetamide and Phenylephrine *on page 651*

Vasotec® see Enalapril *on page 250*

V-Cillin K® see Penicillin V Potassium *on page 543*

Veetids® see Penicillin V Potassium *on page 543*

Velosef® see Cephradine *on page 145*

Veltane® see Brompheniramine Maleate *on page 95*

Venlafaxine

Related Information
   Antidepressant Agents Comparison *on page 800*
Brand Names Effexor®
Therapeutic Class Antidepressant
Use Treatment of depression
Contraindications Hypersensitivity to venlafaxine or any component; patients receiving MAO inhibitors within the past 14 days; MAO inhibitors should not be initiated within 7 days of discontinuing venlafaxine

(Continued)

Venlafaxine (Continued)

Precautions Sustained hypertension (increased diastolic blood pressure) which is dose related, reduced clearance in persons with impaired renal or hepatic impairment; use with caution in patients with a history of mania, history of seizures; taper dose when discontinuing after therapy of 1 week or longer

Adverse Reactions
Cardiovascular: Hypertension, tachycardia
Central nervous system: Headache, somnolence, dizziness, insomnia, nervousness, anxiety
Gastrointestinal: Nausea, dry mouth, constipation, anorexia, diarrhea, vomiting
Genitourinary: Abnormal ejaculation/orgasm, impotence (men)
Neuromuscular & skeletal: Tremors, weakness
Ocular: Blurred vision
Miscellaneous: Sweating

Overdosage Symptoms of overdosage include somnolence, convulsions, coma, mild sinus tachycardia

Toxicology In overdose, maintain adequate airway and oxygenation and other supportive measures and symptomatic treatment; removal of venlafaxine from the gastrointestinal tract may be achieved with activated charcoal, emesis, or gastric lavage; hemodialysis, hemoperfusion, exchange transfusion, and forced diuresis will not remove substantial amounts of venlafaxine due to its large volume of distribution; monitor cardiac rhythm and vital signs

Drug Interactions Cimetidine reduced the clearance of venlafaxine and increased its serum concentration; MAO inhibitors; see Precautions

Mechanism of Action Venlafaxine and its metabolite o-desmethylvenlafaxine inhibits the reuptake of serotonin and norepinephrine and weakly inhibits the reuptake of dopamine

Pharmacodynamics Onset of action: 1-3 weeks; 5 HT = NE

Pharmacokinetics
Absorption: 92% to 100%; not affected by food
Distribution: V_d: 7.5 L/kg
Protein binding, plasma: 27% to 30%
Metabolism: Major active metabolite o-desmethylvenlafaxine (OVD); 2 less active metabolites; metabolic pathway (first-pass) are saturable
Peak concentration: 1.8-3 hours
Half-life (prolonged in renal and hepatic impairment):
Venlafaxine: 5 hours
OVD: 11 hours
Elimination: 1% to 10% excreted unchanged in urine; 30% OVD, 26% conjugated OVD, and 27% other metabolites
Not readily dialyzed

Usual Dosage When discontinuing this medication, it is imperative to taper the dose; if venlafaxine is used >6 weeks, the dose should be tapered over 2 weeks when discontinuing its use

Geriatrics: No specific recommendations, but may be best to start lower at 25-50 mg twice daily and increase as tolerated by 25 mg/dose
Adults: Oral: 75 mg/day, administered in 2 or 3 divided doses, taken with food; dose may be increased to 150 mg/day up to 225-375 mg/day

Dosing adjustment in renal impairment: Reduce dose by 25% in mild-moderate impairment (Cl_{cr} 10-70 mL/minute); reduce dose by 50% and hold dose until a dialysis in dialysis patients

Dosing adjustment in hepatic impairment: Reduce dose by 50% or more

Administration May be administered with food; if switching from a MAO inhibitor to venlafaxine, allow 2 weeks "washout" period before starting venlafaxine; allow 7 days "wash out" if switching venlafaxine therapy to a MAO inhibitor

Monitoring Parameters Signs and symptoms of depression, weight; blood pressure

Reference Range Not established

Test Interactions Increase in serum cholesterol (mean: 3 mg/dL)

Patient Information Use caution when driving or operating machinery; advise physician and pharmacist of any changes or additions in drug therapy; avoid alcohol; notify physician of rash or any other adverse event; may cause dry mouth, increased blood pressure

Nursing Implications See Monitoring Parameters

Special Geriatric Considerations Has not been studied exclusively in the elderly, however, its low anticholinergic activity, minimal sedation, and hypotension makes this a potentially valuable antidepressant in treating elderly with depression. No dose adjustment is necessary for age alone, additional studies are necessary; adjust dose for renal function in elderly; see Usual Dosage.

Dosage Forms Tablet: 25 mg, 37.5 mg, 50 mg, 75 mg, 100 mg

Venoglobulin®-I see Immune Globulin on page 366

Ventolin® *see* Albuterol *on page 24*

Verapamil Hydrochloride (ver ap' a mill)
Related Information
Calcium Channel Blocking Agents Comparison *on page 806-807*
Brand Names Calan®; Calan® SR; Isoptin®; Isoptin® SR; Verelan®
Synonyms Iproveratril Hydrochloride
Generic Available Yes
Therapeutic Class Antianginal Agent; Antiarrhythmic Agent, Class IV; Calcium Channel Blocker
Use Angina (vasospastic, chronic stable, and unstable), hypertension; I.V. for supraventricular tachyarrhythmias (PSVT, atrial fibrillation, atrial flutter)

Unlabeled use: Migraine headache, cardiomyopathy, incontinence
Contraindications Sinus bradycardia; advanced heart block; ventricular tachycardia; cardiogenic shock, hypotension, congestive heart failure; hypersensitivity to verapamil or any component, hypersensitivity to calcium channel blockers and adenosine; atrial fibrillation or flutter associated with accessory conduction pathways; not to be given within a few hours of I.V. beta-blocking agents
Warnings Monitor EKG and blood pressure closely in patients receiving I.V. therapy; hypotension, congestive heart failure; cardiac conduction defects, PVCs, idiopathic hypertrophic subaortic stenosis; may cause platelet inhibition; do not abruptly withdraw (chest pain); hepatic dysfunction, renal function impairment, increased angina, decreased neuromuscular transmission with Duchenne's muscular dystrophy; increased intracranial pressure with cranial tumors; elderly may have greater hypotensive effect
Precautions Sick sinus syndrome, severe left ventricular dysfunction, congestive heart failure, hepatic or renal impairment, hypertrophic cardiomyopathy (especially obstructive), concomitant therapy with beta-blockers or digoxin, edema
Adverse Reactions
Cardiovascular: Hypotension, bradycardia, first, second, or third degree A-V block, worsening heart failure, palpitations, congestive heart failure, myocardial infarction, angina, tachycardia
Central nervous system: Dizziness, headache, fatigue, seizures (occasionally with I.V. use), lightheadedness, psychotic symptoms, insomnia, paresthesia, asthenia
Gastrointestinal: Constipation (more of a problem in elderly), nausea, abdominal discomfort, diarrhea, dry mouth
Hepatic: Increase in hepatic enzymes
Ocular: Blurred vision
Respiratory: May precipitate insufficiency of respiratory muscle function in Duchenne muscular dystrophy
Miscellaneous: Peripheral edema
Overdosage Symptoms of overdose include heartblock, hypotension, asystole, nausea, weakness, dizziness, drowsiness, confusion and slurred speech; profound bradycardia and occasionally hyperglycemia
Toxicology Ipecac-induced emesis can hypothetically worsen calcium antagonist toxicity, since it can produce vagal stimulation. The potential for seizures precipitously following acute ingestion of large doses of a calcium antagonist may also contraindicate the use of ipecac. Supportive and symptomatic treatment, including I.V. fluids and Trendelenburg positioning, should be initiated as intoxication may cause hypotension. Although calcium (calcium chloride I.V. 1-2 g over 5-10 minutes with repeats as needed) has been used as an "antidote" for acute intoxications, there is limited experience to support its routine use and should be reserved for those cases where definite signs of myocardial depression are evident. Heart block may respond to isoproterenol, glucagon, atropine and/or calcium although a temporary pacemaker may be required.
Drug Interactions
Increased cardiovascular adverse effects with beta-adrenergic blocking agents, digoxin, quinidine, and disopyramide
Verapamil may increase serum concentrations of digoxin, quinidine, carbamazepine, prazosin, and cyclosporine necessitating a decrease in dosage
Phenobarbital and rifampin may decrease verapamil serum concentrations by increased hepatic metabolism
Avoid combination with disopyramide, discontinue disopyramide 48 hours before starting therapy, do not restart until 24 hours after verapamil has been discontinued
May interfere with lithium control
May increase pharmacologic action of theophylline
Stability Store injection at room temperature; protect from heat and from freezing; use only clear solutions; compatible in solutions of pH of 3-6, but may precipitate in solutions having a pH of ≥ 6
Mechanism of Action Inhibits calcium ion from entering the "slow channels" or select voltage-sensitive areas of vascular smooth muscle and myocardium during depolarization; produces a relaxation of coronary vascular smooth muscle and coronary vasodilation; increases myocardial oxygen delivery in patients with vasospastic angina
(Continued)

Verapamil Hydrochloride *(Continued)*

Pharmacodynamics
Duration:
 Oral: 6-8 hours; elderly have greater hypotensive effect than younger adults
 I.V.: 10-20 minutes
Peak effects:
 Oral (nonsustained tablets): 2 hours
 I.V.: 1-5 minutes

Pharmacokinetics
Protein binding: 90%
Metabolism: In the liver; extensive first-pass effect
Bioavailability: Oral: 20% to 30%
Half-life (single dose) (adults): 2-8 hours, increased up to 12 hours with multiple dosing; elderly have increased half-life: 7-8 hours; increased half-life with hepatic cirrhosis
Elimination: 70% in urine (3% to 4% as unchanged drug), and 16% in feces

Usual Dosage Geriatrics and Adults:
Oral: 120-480 mg/24 hours divided 3-4 times/day
 Sustained release:
  Geriatrics: 120 mg/day; adjust dose after 24 hours by increases of 120 mg/day; when switching from immediate release forms, total daily dose may remain the same
  Adults: 240 mg/day
I.V.: 5-10 mg (0.075-0.15 mg/kg); may repeat 10 mg (0.15 mg/kg) 15-30 minutes after the initial dose if needed and if patient tolerated initial dose

Not dialyzable (0% to 5%)

Monitoring Parameters Heart rate, blood pressure, signs and symptoms of congestive heart failure

Reference Range Therapeutic: 50-200 ng/mL (SI: 100-410 nmol/L) for parent; under normal conditions norverapamil concentration is the same as parent drug; Toxic: >90 µg/mL

Patient Information Sustained release products should be taken with food and not crushed; limit caffeine intake; avoid alcohol; notify physician if angina pain is not reduced when taking this drug, irregular heartbeat, shortness of breath, swelling, dizziness, constipation, nausea, or hypotension occur; do not stop therapy without advice of physician

Nursing Implications Help patient with ambulation; monitor blood pressure closely; give around-the-clock rather than 4 times/day, 3 times/day, etc (ie, 12-6-12-6, not 9-1-5-9) to promote less variation in peak and trough serum levels; I.V. rate of infusion is over 2 minutes; do not crush sustained release drug product

Additional Information Incidence of adverse reactions is most common with I.V. administration; discontinue disopyramide 48 hours before starting therapy, do not restart therapy until 24 hours after verapamil has been discontinued

Special Geriatric Considerations Elderly may experience a greater hypotensive response; constipation may be more of a problem in elderly; calcium channel blockers are no more effective in elderly than other therapies; however, they do not cause significant CNS effects which is an advantage over some antihypertensive agents; generic verapamil products which are bioequivalent in young adults may not be bioequivalent in elderly; use generics cautiously; see Pharmacodynamics

Dosage Forms
Capsule: 120 mg
Capsule, sustained release: 120 mg, 180 mg, 240 mg
Injection: 2.5 mg/mL (2 mL, 4 mL)
Tablet: 40 mg, 80 mg, 120 mg
Tablet, sustained release: 120 mg, 180 mg, 240 mg

References
Carter BL, Noyes MA, and Demmler RW, "Difference in Serum Concentrations of and Responses to Generic Verapamil in the Elderly," *Pharmacotherapy*, 1993, 13(4):359-68.

Verazinc® [OTC] *see* Zinc Sulfate *on page 742*

Verelan® *see* Verapamil Hydrochloride *on previous page*

Vermizine® *see* Piperazine Citrate *on page 570*

Versed® *see* Midazolam Hydrochloride *on page 472*

V-Gan® *see* Promethazine Hydrochloride *on page 599*

Vibramycin® *see* Doxycycline *on page 243*

Vibra-Tabs® *see* Doxycycline *on page 243*

Vicks® Formula 44® *see* Dextromethorphan *on page 209*

Vicks® Sinex® Nasal Solution [OTC] *see* Phenylephrine Hydrochloride *on page 557*

Vicks Sinex® Long-Acting Nasal Solution [OTC] *see* Oxymetazoline
Hydrochloride *on page 530*

Vicks Vatronol® *see* Ephedrine Sulfate *on page 255*

Vicodin® *see* Hydrocodone and Acetaminophen *on page 350*

Vidarabine (vye dare' a been)
Brand Names Vira-A® Injection; Vira-A® Ophthalmic
Synonyms Adenine Arabinoside; Ara-A; Arabinofuranosyladenine
Generic Available No
Therapeutic Class Antiviral Agent, Ophthalmic; Antiviral Agent, Parenteral
Use Treatment of acute keratoconjunctivitis and epithelial keratitis due to herpes simplex virus; herpes simplex encephalitis; neonatal herpes simplex virus infections; herpes zoster in immunosuppressed patients; reduces mortality from herpes simplex encephalitis from 70% to 28%; definitive diagnosis of herpes simplex conjunctivitis should be made before instituting ophthalmic therapy
Contraindications Hypersensitivity to vidarabine or any component
Warnings Administration requires dilution in large fluid volumes; use with caution in patients at risk of fluid overload (cerebral edema) and in patients with impaired renal function; reduce dosage in patients with severe renal insufficiency
Adverse Reactions
Cardiovascular: Thrombophlebitis
Central nervous system: Ataxia, disorientation, depression, agitation
Dermatologic: Rash
Endocrine & metabolic: Hypokalemia, SIADH
Gastrointestinal: Anorexia, nausea, vomiting, diarrhea, weight loss
Hematologic: Decreased WBC and platelets
Hepatic: Increase in AST and total bilirubin
Local: Burning, lacrimation, pain
Neuromuscular & skeletal: Myoclonus, tremors, weakness
Ocular: Keratitis, photophobia, foreign body sensation, uveitis, stromal edema, blurred vision
Overdosage Symptoms of overdose include bone marrow depression, thrombocytopenia, leukopenia with doses >20 mg/kg/day
Toxicology Treatment is supportive only
Drug Interactions Increased vidarabine toxicity with allopurinol (possible)
Stability Do **not** refrigerate diluted I.V. solution; constituted solutions remain stable for 2 weeks at room temperature; however, should be diluted just prior to administration and used within 48 hours
Stability of parenteral admixture at room temperature (25°C): 2 days
Mechanism of Action Inhibits viral DNA synthesis by blocking DNA polymerase
Pharmacokinetics
Absorption: Oral, I.M., S.C.: Poor
Distribution: Crosses into the CNS
Protein binding: 20% to 30% (vidarabine) and 0% to 3% (ara-hypoxanthine)
Metabolism: Following administration rapidly deaminated to ara-hypoxanthine (active)
Half-life: Adults: 1.5 hours
Ara-hypoxanthine: Normal renal function: 3.3 hours
Elimination: In urine as unchanged drug (1% to 3%) and the active metabolite (40% to 53%)
Usual Dosage Geriatrics and Adults:
I.V.: 15 mg/kg/day as a 12-hour or longer infusion for 10 days
Dosing adjustment in renal impairment: Cl$_{cr}$ <10 mL/minute: Administer 75% of normal dose
Ophthalmic: Keratoconjunctivitis: Instill ½" of ointment in lower conjunctival sac 5 times/day every 3 hours while awake until complete re-epithelialization has occurred, then twice daily for an additional 7 days
Administration Do not give I.M. or S.C.; administer I.V. solution through an in-line 0.22 or 0.45 micron filter; administer by slow I.V. infusion over 12-24 hours
Monitoring Parameters CBC with platelet count, renal function tests, liver function tests, hemoglobin, and hematocrit
Patient Information Do not use eye make-up when on this medication for ophthalmic infection; use sunglasses if photophobic reaction occurs; may cause blurred vision; notify physician if improvement not seen after 7 days or if condition worsens
Nursing Implications See Administration
Special Geriatric Considerations See Warnings and Usual Dosage; assess ability to self-administer ophthalmic ointment; no specific recommendations for use in the elderly
Dosage Forms
Injection, suspension: 200 mg/mL [base 187.4 mg] (5 mL)
Ointment, ophthalmic, as monohydrate: 3% [30 mg/g = 28 mg/g base] (3.5 g)

ALPHABETICAL LISTING OF DRUGS

Videx® *see* Didanosine *on page 216*

Viosterol *see* Ergocalciferol *on page 259*

Vira-A® Injection *see* Vidarabine *on previous page*

Vira-A® Ophthalmic *see* Vidarabine *on previous page*

Virazole® Aerosol *see* Ribavirin *on page 626*

Viroptic® Ophthalmic *see* Trifluridine *on page 717*

Visine A.C.® [OTC] *see* Tetrahydrozoline Hydrochloride *on page 680*

Visine® L.R. Ophthalmic [OTC] *see* Oxymetazoline Hydrochloride *on page 530*

Visine® [OTC] *see* Tetrahydrozoline Hydrochloride *on page 680*

Visken® *see* Pindolol *on page 566*

Vistaril® *see* Hydroxyzine *on page 356*

Vistazine® *see* Hydroxyzine *on page 356*

Vita-C® [OTC] *see* Ascorbic Acid *on page 57*

Vitamin B$_3$ *see* Niacin *on page 498*

Vitamin B$_3$ *see* Niacinamide *on page 499*

Vitamin B$_6$ *see* Pyridoxine Hydrochloride *on page 613*

Vitamin B$_{12}$ *see* Cyanocobalamin *on page 192*

Vitamin C *see* Ascorbic Acid *on page 57*

Vitamin D$_2$ *see* Ergocalciferol *on page 259*

Vitamin K$_1$ *see* Vitamin K and Menadiol *on this page*

Vitamin K$_4$ *see* Vitamin K and Menadiol *on this page*

Vitamin K and Menadiol

Brand Names AquaMEPHYTON®; Konakion®; Mephyton®

Synonyms Menadiol and Vitamin K; Methylphytyl Napthoquinone; Phylloquinone; Phytomenadione; Phytonadione; Vitamin K$_1$; Vitamin K$_4$

Therapeutic Class Vitamin, Water Soluble

Use Prevention and treatment of hypoprothrombinemia caused by drug-induced or anticoagulant-induced vitamin K deficiency, and nutritional vitamin K deficiency

Contraindications Hypersensitivity to phytonadione, menadiol, or any component

Warnings Ineffective in hereditary hypoprothrombinemia, hypoprothrombinemia caused by severe liver disease; giving high doses may depress prothrombin concentration in hepatic disease; menadiol is ineffective in treatment of oral anticoagulant-induced hypoprothrombinemia; phytonadione is the treatment of choice; deaths have occurred with I.V. phytonadione; the reaction is of the hypersensitivity type; avoid I.V. use unless other routes are not possible

Precautions Severe reactions resembling anaphylaxis or hypersensitivity have occurred rarely during or immediately after I.V. administration (even with proper dilution and rate of administration); restrict I.V. administration for emergency use only. Use cautiously in asthmatic and atrophic patients due to possibility of sulfite sensitivity.

Adverse Reactions I.V. administration see Warnings and Precautions
  Cardiovascular: Transient flushing reaction, rarely hypotension, cyanosis
  Central nervous system: Rarely dizziness
  Dermatologic: Rash, urticaria
  Gastrointestinal: GI upset with oral administration, dysgeusia
  Local: Swelling and tenderness at injection site
  Respiratory: Dyspnea
  Miscellaneous: Anaphylaxis, sweating

Overdosage Symptoms of overdose include decreased liver function, hemolytic anemia, prolonged PT

Toxicology Not described

Drug Interactions
  Oral anticoagulant effects are antagonized by vitamin K
  Mineral oil decreases absorption of oral vitamin K

Stability Protect injection from light at all times; may be autoclaved

Mechanism of Action Promotes liver synthesis of clotting factors (II, VII, IX, X); however, the exact mechanism as to this stimulation is unknown. Menadiol is a water soluble form of vitamin K; phytonadione has a more rapid and prolonged effect than menadione; menadiol sodium diphosphate (K$_4$) is half as potent as menadione (K$_3$)

Pharmacodynamics Coagulation factors increase within 6-12 hours after oral doses, within 1-2 hours following parenteral administration; after parenteral administration, patient may become normal after 12-14 hours; phytonadione controls hemorrhage in 3-6 hours

Pharmacokinetics
  Absorption: Orally from the intestines in the presence of bile
  Metabolism: Rapid in the liver

Elimination: In bile and urine

Usual Dosage I.V. route should be restricted for emergency use only with phytonadione

Geriatrics and Adults: Treatment of oral anticoagulant overdose:
Phytonadione: Oral, I.M., I.V., S.C.: 2.5-10 mg/dose; up to 25 mg initially; further doses should be determined by prothrombin time response or clinical condition; may repeat in 6-8 hours if given by I.M., I.V., S.C. route; may repeat 12-48 hours after oral route

Vitamin K deficiency: Due to drugs, malabsorption or decreased synthesis of vitamin K:
Oral: 5-25 mg/24 hours
I.M., I.V.: 10 mg

Minimum daily requirement (not well established): 0.03 mcg/kg/day

Menadiol:
Oral:
Hypoprothrombinemia due to obstructive jaundice and biliary fistulas: 5 mg/day
Hypoprothrombinemia secondary to salicylates or antibacterials: 5-10 mg/day
I.M., I.V., S.C.: 5-15 mg 1-2 times/day

Monitoring Parameters Monitor PT and PTT

Test Interactions Decreased prothrombin time (S); menadione has caused false elevations of urinary 17-hydroxycorticosteroids

Patient Information Do not take doses in excess of RDA without physician's advice

Nursing Implications I.V. administration: Dilute in normal saline, D$_5$W or D$_5$NS and infuse slowly; rate of infusion should not exceed 1 mg/minute. **This route should be used only if administration by another route is not feasible for phytonadione;** see Warnings. I.V. administration should not exceed 1 mg/minute; for I.V. infusion, dilute in PF (preservative free) D$_5$W or normal saline.

Additional Information Phytonadione is more effective and is preferred to other vitamin K preparations in the presence of impending hemorrhage; oral absorption depends on the presence of bile salts; injection contains benzyl alcohol 0.9% as preservative; monitor PT and PTT

Special Geriatric Considerations See Usual Dosage

Dosage Forms
Injection:
Aqueous colloidal: 2 mg/mL (0.5 mL); 10 mg/mL (1 mL, 2.5 mL, 5 mL)
Aqueous (I.M.): 2 mg/mL (0.5 mL); 10 mg/mL (1 mL); 37.5 mg/mL (menadiol sodium diphosphate only) (2 mL)
Tablet: 5 mg

Vivactil® see Protriptyline Hydrochloride on page 608

Vivotif Berna™ see Typhoid Vaccine on page 726

V-Lax® [OTC] see Psyllium on page 610

Voltaren® see Diclofenac Sodium on page 212

Voltaren® Ophthalmic Solution see Diclofenac Sodium on page 212

Voxsuprine® see Isoxsuprine Hydrochloride on page 384

VZIG see Varicella-Zoster Immune Globulin (Human) on page 731

Warfarin Sodium (war' far in)
Brand Names Carfin®; Coumadin®; Panwarfin®; Sofarin®
Generic Available Yes: Tablet
Therapeutic Class Anticoagulant
Use Prophylaxis and treatment of venous thrombosis, pulmonary embolism and thromboembolic disorders; atrial fibrillation with embolism and as an adjunct in the prophylaxis of systemic embolism after myocardial infarction

Unlabeled use: Prevention of recurrent transient ischemic attacks and to reduce risk of recurrent myocardial infarction

Contraindications Hypersensitivity to warfarin or any component; severe liver or kidney disease; open wounds; uncontrolled bleeding; GI ulcers; neurosurgical procedures; malignant hypertension

Warnings Concomitant use with vitamin K may decrease anticoagulant effect; monitor carefully; concomitant use with ethacrynic acid, indomethacin, mefenamic acid, phenylbutazone, or aspirin increases warfarin's anticoagulant effect and may cause severe GI irritation

Precautions Do not switch brands once desired therapeutic response has been achieved

Adverse Reactions
Central nervous system: Fever
Dermatologic: Skin lesions, alopecia
Gastrointestinal: Anorexia, nausea, vomiting, diarrhea
Hematologic: Hemorrhage

(Continued)

739

Warfarin Sodium *(Continued)*

Respiratory: Hemoptysis

Overdosage Symptoms of overdose include internal or external hemorrhage, hematuria

Toxicology Avoid emesis and lavage to avoid the possible trauma and incidental bleeding. When a large or chronic ingestion occurs vitamin K_1 (phytonadione) should be administered 10-15 mg I.M./I.V.; when hemorrhaging occurs whole blood or plasma transfusions can help control bleeding by replacing clotting factors

Drug Interactions Amiodarone, metronidazole, anabolic steroids, chloral hydrate, clofibrate, disulfiram, nonsteroidal anti-inflammatory agents, chloramphenicol, cimetidine, salicylates, streptokinase, urokinase, sulfonamides, ketoconazole, sucralfate, phenylbutazone, quinolones, corticosteroids, erythromycin, omeprazole, isoniazid, phenytoin may increase the effects of warfarin; alcohol, cholestyramine, sucralfate, barbiturates, trazodone, carbamazepine, rifampin, and estrogens may decrease the effects of warfarin; caution must be observed when any drug is added to or deleted from the therapeutic regimen of a patient receiving warfarin

Mechanism of Action Interferes with hepatic synthesis of vitamin K-dependent coagulation factors (II, VII, IX, X)

Pharmacodynamics

Onset of action: Following rapid oral absorption, anticoagulation effects occur within 36-72 hours

Peak effect: Within 5-7 days; the elderly are more sensitive to the effects of warfarin and usually respond to a lower mg/day dose

Pharmacokinetics

Metabolism: In the liver

Half-life: 42 hours, highly variable among individuals

The pharmacokinetics of warfarin have not been shown to be altered by aging

Usual Dosage Oral:

Geriatrics: Usual maintenance dose: 2-5 mg/day

Adults: 5-15 mg/day for 2-5 days, then adjust dose according to results of prothrombin time; usual maintenance dose range: 2-10 mg/day

Monitoring Parameters Prothrombin time (PT), PT ratio, international normalization ratio (INR); stool guaiac for blood; hemoglobin, hematocrit

Reference Range See table.

Indication	PT Ratio	INR
Acute MI	1.3-1.5	2-3
Atrial fibrillation	1.3-1.5	2-3
Mechanical prosthetic valves	1.5-2	3-4.5
Pulmonary embolism treatment	1.3-1.5	2-3
Systemic embolism prevention	1.3-1.5	2-3
recurrent	1.5-2	3-4.5
Tissue heart valve	1.3-1.5	2-3
Valvular heart disease	1.3-1.5	2-3
Venous thrombosis prophylaxis (high risk surgery) treatment	1.3-1.5	2-3

Adapted from American College of Chest Physicians and National Heart, Lung, and Blood Institute.

Patient Information Do not take with food; report any signs of bleeding; avoid hazardous activities; use soft tooth brush; urine may turn red/orange; carry Medi-Alert® ID identifying drug usage; consult physician and dentist before dental procedures; be sure of other drugs (aspirin and alcohol) and foods to avoid; report any bleeding, red or dark urine, red or tarry black stools to physician at once

Nursing Implications Avoid all I.M. injections; monitor patient for signs and symptoms of bleeding

Special Geriatric Considerations See Drug Interactions, Pharmacodynamics,and Usual Dosage. Before committing an elderly patient to long-term anticoagulation therapy, their risk for bleeding complications secondary to falls, drug interactions, living situation, and cognitive status should be considered. The risk for bleeding complications decreases with the duration of therapy and has been associated with increased age.

Dosage Forms Tablet: 2 mg, 2.5 mg, 5 mg, 7.5 mg, 10 mg

References

Gurwitz JH, Avorn J, Ross-Degnan D, et al, "Aging and the Anticoagulant Response to Warfarin Therapy," *Ann Intern Med*, 1992, 116(11):901-4.

Redwood M, Taylor C, Bain BJ, et al, "The Association of Age With Dosage Requirement for Warfarin," *Age Ageing*, 1991, 20(3):217-20.

Shepherd AM, Hewick DS, Moreland TA, et al, "Age as a Determinant of Sensitivity to Warfarin," *Br J Clin Pharmacol*, 1977, 4(3):315-20.

4-Way® Long Acting Nasal Solution [OTC] *see* Oxymetazoline Hydrochloride *on page 530*

Wehamine® *see* Dimenhydrinate *on page 227*

Wellbutrin® *see* Bupropion *on page 98*

Westcort® *see* Hydrocortisone *on page 351*

Westrim® LA [OTC] *see* Phenylpropanolamine Hydrochloride *on page 559*

White Mineral Oil *see* Mineral Oil *on page 473*

Wigraine® *see* Ergotamine *on page 261*

Wincillin®-VK *see* Penicillin V Potassium *on page 543*

WinGel® [OTC] *see* Aluminum Hydroxide and Magnesium Hydroxide *on page 29*

Wintomylon® *see* Nalidixic Acid *on page 489*

Wyamycin® *see* Erythromycin *on page 263*

Wycillin® *see* Penicillin G Procaine, Aqueous *on page 541*

Wydase® *see* Hyaluronidase *on page 344*

Wygesic® *see* Propoxyphene and Acetaminophen *on page 604*

Wymox® *see* Amoxicillin Trihydrate *on page 49*

Wytensin® *see* Guanabenz Acetate *on page 333*

Xanax® *see* Alprazolam *on page 27*

Xero-Lube® [OTC] *see* Saliva Substitute *on page 636*

X-Prep® Liquid [OTC] *see* Senna *on page 641*

Xylocaine® *see* Lidocaine Hydrochloride *on page 406*

Yodoxin® *see* Iodoquinol *on page 375*

Zantac® *see* Ranitidine Hydrochloride *on page 623*

Zarontin® *see* Ethosuximide *on page 275*

Zaroxolyn® *see* Metolazone *on page 464*

Zeasorb-AF® [OTC] *see* Tolnaftate *on page 705*

Zebeta® *see* Bisoprolol Fumarate *on page 89*

Zefazone® *see* Cefmetazole Sodium *on page 129*

Zestril® *see* Lisinopril *on page 412*

Zetran® *see* Diazepam *on page 211*

Zidovudine (zye doe' vue deen)

Brand Names Retrovir®

Synonyms Azidothymidine; AZT; Compound S

Generic Available No

Therapeutic Class Antiviral Agent, Oral; Antiviral Agent, Parenteral

Use Management of patients with HIV infections who have had at least one episode of *Pneumocystis carinii* pneumonia or who have CD4 cell counts of ≤500/mm³; patients who have HIV-related symptoms or who are asymptomatic with abnormal laboratory values indicating HIV-related immunosuppression

Contraindications Life-threatening hypersensitivity to zidovudine or any component

Warnings Is often associated with hematologic toxicity including granulocytopenia and severe anemia requiring transfusions; zidovudine has been shown to be carcinogenic in rats and mice

Precautions Use with caution in patients with impaired renal or hepatic function; reduce dosage or interrupt therapy in patients with anemia and/or granulocytopenia and myopathy

Adverse Reactions

Central nervous system: Malaise, dizziness, asthenia, manic syndrome, seizures, confusion, fever, severe headache, insomnia

Dermatologic: Rash

Gastrointestinal: Nausea

(Continued)

Zidovudine *(Continued)*

Hematologic: Granulocytopenia, thrombocytopenia, pancytopenia, anemia

Hepatic: Cholestatic hepatitis

Neuromuscular & skeletal: Myalgia, tremors

In pancytopenia and anemia, dosage reduction or discontinuation of drug may be required

Overdosage Symptoms of overdose include ataxia, granulocytopenia

Toxicology Erythropoietin, thymidine, and cyanocobalamin have been used experimentally to treat zidovudine-induced hematopoietic toxicity, yet none are presently specified as the agent of choice.

Drug Interactions Acyclovir, coadministration with other drugs metabolized by glucuronidation increased toxicity of either drug, acetaminophen, cimetidine, indomethacin, lorazepam, aspirin; probenecid may inhibit glucuronidation and decrease renal clearance; the risk of nephrotoxicity may be increased when taken with zidovudine

Mechanism of Action Zidovudine is a thymidine analog which interferes with the HIV viral RNA dependent DNA polymerase resulting in inhibition of viral replication

Pharmacokinetics

Absorption: Oral: Well absorbed, 66% to 70%

Protein binding: 25% to 38%

Metabolism: Extensive first-pass; metabolized in the liver via glucuronidation to inactive metabolites

Half-life, terminal: 60 minutes

Time to peak: Oral: Peak serum levels occur within 30-90 minutes

Elimination: Urinary excretion (63% to 95%); following oral administration, 72% to 74% of drug is excreted in urine as metabolites and 14% to 18% as unchanged drug; following I.V. administration, 45% to 60% is excreted in urine as metabolites and 18% to 29% as unchanged drug; significant penetration into the CSF

Usual Dosage Geriatrics and Adults:

Oral:

Asymptomatic infection: 100 mg every 4 hours while awake (500 mg/day)

Symptomatic HIV infection: Initial: 200 mg every 4 hours (1200 mg/day), then after 1 month, 100 mg every 4 hours (600 mg/day)

I.V.: 1-2 mg/kg/dose every 4 hours

Monitoring Parameters CBC with differential every 2 weeks

Patient Information Take 30 minutes before or 1 hour after a meal with a glass of water; take zidovudine exactly as prescribed and that administration every 4 hours means dosing around-the-clock; limit use of acetaminophen containing analgesics

Nursing Implications Monitor complete blood count and platelet count at least every 2 weeks; observe for appearance of opportunistic infections

Additional Information Does not reduce risk of transmitting HIV infections

Special Geriatric Considerations Has not been studied exclusively in the elderly; no dosage adjustments are recommended based upon age

Dosage Forms

Capsule: 100 mg

Injection: 10 mg/mL (20 mL)

Syrup: 50 mg/5 mL (240 mL)

References

Fischl MA, Richman DD, Hansen N, et al, "The Safety and Efficacy of Zidovudine (AZT) in the Treatment of Subjects With Mildly Symptomatic Human Immunodeficiency Virus Type 1 (HIV) Infection. A Double-Blind, Placebo-Controlled Trial. The AIDS Clinical Trials Group," *Ann Intern Med*, 1990, 112(10):727-37.

Volberding PA, Lagakos SW, Koch MA, et al, "Zidovudine in Asymptomatic Human Immunodeficiency Virus Infection. A Controlled Trial in Persons With Fewer Than 500 CD4-Positive Cells per Cubic Millimeter. The AIDS Clinical Trials Group of the National Institute of Allergy and Infectious Diseases," *N Engl J Med*, 1990, 322(14):941-9.

Zinacef® *see* Cefuroxime *on page 141*

Zinca-Pak® *see* Zinc Sulfate *on this page*

Zincate® *see* Zinc Sulfate *on this page*

Zinc Sulfate (zink)

Brand Names Eye-Sed® [OTC]; Orazinc® [OTC]; Verazinc® [OTC]; Zinca-Pak®; Zincate®

Generic Available Yes

Therapeutic Class Mineral, Oral; Trace Element, Parenteral

Use Zinc supplement (oral and parenteral); may improve wound healing in those who are deficient (pressure sores)

Contraindications Hypersensitivity to any component

Warnings Do not use undiluted by direct injection into a peripheral vein because of potential for phlebitis, tissue irritation and potential to increase renal loss of minerals from a bolus injection

Adverse Reactions
Central nervous system: Restlessness, dizziness
Gastrointestinal: Nausea, vomiting, gastric ulcers, diarrhea

Overdosage Symptoms of overdose include profuse sweating, decreased consciousness, blurred vision, tachycardia, hypothermia, hyperamylasemia, hypotension, pulmonary edema, diarrhea, vomiting, jaundice, oliguria; impaired lymphocyte and polymorphonuclear leukocyte function and a decrease in high density lipoproteins has been reported with excessive supplementation in healthy persons

Toxicology Emesis should be instituted following ingestion of zinc sulfate except when there is evidence of mucosal burns, instead dilute rapidly with milk or water. Calcium disodium edetate or dimercaprol can be very effective at binding zinc. Supportive care should always be instituted.

Drug Interactions Decreased effect of penicillamine and iron; decreased absorption of some fluoroquinolones, tetracyclines, and iron

Food/Drug Interactions Bran products, dairy products reduce zinc absorption

Stability Store oral liquid (injectable used orally) in refrigerator

Mechanism of Action Provides for normal growth and tissue repair, is a cofactor for more than 70 enzymes; ophthalmic astringent and weak antiseptic due to precipitation of protein and clearing mucus from outer surface of the eye

Pharmacokinetics
Absorption: Zinc and its salts are poorly absorbed from the gastrointestinal tract (20% to 30%)
Elimination: In feces with only traces appearing in urine

Usual Dosage Geriatrics and Adults: Oral: Zinc deficiency: 110-220 mg zinc sulfate (25-50 mg elemental zinc)/dose 3 times/day

Monitoring Parameters Skin integrity

Reference Range Serum: 50-150 µg/dL (<20 µg/dL as solid test with dermatitis followed by alopecia)

Patient Information Take with food if GI upset occurs, but avoid foods high in calcium, phosphorous or phytate (high fiber foods)

Nursing Implications Give with food if GI upset occurs; avoid foods high in calcium or phosphorus; injection must be diluted before use; refrigerate suspension

Additional Information Zinc acetate can be used as an alternative to zinc sulfate in patients who cannot tolerate the gastrointestinal irritant effects of the sulfate salt

Special Geriatric Considerations May be useful to promote wound healing in patients with pressure sores

Dosage Forms
Capsule: 110 mg, 220 mg
Injection: 1 mg/mL (10 mL, 30 mL); 4 mg/mL (10 mL); 5 mg/mL (5 mL, 10 mL)
Solution, ophthalmic: 0.217% (15 mL)
Tablet: 66 mg, 200 mg

Zithromax™ see Azithromycin on page 71

Zocor™ see Simvastatin on page 645

Zofran® see Ondansetron on page 518

Zolicef® see Cefazolin Sodium on page 127

Zoloft™ see Sertraline Hydrochloride on page 643

Zolpidem Tartrate (zole pi' dem)
Brand Names Ambien™
Therapeutic Class Hypnotic; Sedative
Use Short-term treatment of insomnia
Restrictions C-IV
Warnings Closely monitor elderly or debilitated patients for impaired cognitive or motor performance
Precautions Administer with caution to depressed patients; tolerance and withdrawal symptoms are not seen, but caution should be used in patients with a history of drug dependence
Adverse Reactions
Central nervous system: Headache, drowsiness, dizziness
Gastrointestinal: Nausea, diarrhea
Neuromuscular & skeletal: Myalgia
Overdosage Symptoms of overdose include impairment of consciousness, coma
Toxicology Treatment for zolpidem overdose is supportive. Monitor for hypotension and CNS depression; flumazenil may be useful in reversing the hypnotic effects.
Drug Interactions Increased effect/toxicity with alcohol, CNS depressants
Mechanism of Action Structurally dissimilar to benzodiazepines, however, has much or all of its actions explained by its effects on benzodiazepine (BZD) receptors, especially the omega-1 receptor; retains hypnotic and much of the anxiolytic properties of the BZD, but has reduced effects on skeletal muscle and seizure threshold.

(Continued)

Zolpidem Tartrate *(Continued)*

Pharmacodynamics
Onset of action: 30 minutes
Duration: 6-8 hours

Pharmacokinetics
Absorption: Rapid
Protein binding: 92%
Metabolism: Hepatic to inactive metabolites
Half-life: 2-2.6 hours, in cirrhosis increased to 9.9 hours; in elderly, maximum AUC and half-life are increased

Usual Dosage Oral (duration of therapy should be limited to 7-10 days):
Geriatrics: 5 mg immediately before bedtime
Adults: 10 mg immediately before bedtime; maximum dose: 10 mg

Dosing adjustment in hepatic impairment: Decrease dose to 5 mg
Not dialyzable

Monitoring Parameters Mental status

Reference Range 80-150 ng/mL

Patient Information Avoid alcohol and other CNS depressants while taking this medication; for fastest onset, take on an empty stomach; may cause drowsiness

Nursing Implications Patients may require assistance with ambulation; lower doses in the elderly are usually effective; institute safety measures; give on an empty stomach

Additional Information Zolpidem causes less disturbances in sleep stages as compared to benzodiazepines; time spent in sleep stages 3 and 4 are maintained; zolpidem decreases sleep latency

Special Geriatric Considerations In doses >5 mg, there was subjective evidence of impaired sleep on the first post-treatment night; there have been no reports of increased hypotension and/or falls in the elderly with this drug; can be considered an alternative to benzodiazepines when a hypnotic is indicated; see Pharmacokinetics and Additional Information

Dosage Forms Tablet: 5 mg, 10 mg

ZORprin® *see* Aspirin *on page 58*

Zostrix®-HP *see* Capsaicin *on page 114*

Zostrix® [OTC] *see* Capsaicin *on page 114*

Zosyn™ *see* Piperacillin Sodium and Tazobactam Sodium *on page 569*

Zovirax® *see* Acyclovir *on page 21*

Zurinol® *see* Allopurinol *on page 26*

Zydone® *see* Hydrocodone and Acetaminophen *on page 350*

Zyloprim® *see* Allopurinol *on page 26*

Zymenol® [OTC] *see* Mineral Oil *on page 473*

APPENDIX

ABBREVIATIONS COMMONLY USED
IN MEDICAL ORDERS

Abbreviation	From	Meaning
aa̅, aa	ana	of each
ac	ante cibum	before meals or food
ad	ad	to, up to
a.d.	aurio dextra	right ear
ad lib	ad libitum	at pleasure
AM	ante meridiem	morning
amp		ampul
amt		amount
aq	aqua	water
a.s.	aurio sinister	left ear
ASAP		as soon as possible
a.u.	aures utrae	each ear
bid	bis in die	twice daily
bm		bowel movement
bp		blood pressure
BSA		body surface area
c̄	cum	with
cap	capsula	capsule
cm		centimeter
comp	compositus	compound
cont		continue
d	dies	day
d/c		discontinue
disp	dispensa	dispense
elix	elixir	elixir
ex aq		in water
FDA		Food and Drug Administration
g	gramma	gram
gr	granum	grain
gtt	gutta	a drop
h	hora	hour
hs	hora somni	at bedtime
I.M.		intramuscular
I.V.		intravenous
kg		kilogram
L		liter
mcg		microgram
mEq		milliequivalent
mg		milligram
mL		milliliter
mm		millimeter
NF		National Formulary
no.	numerus	number
noc	nocturnal	in the night
non rep	non repetatur	do not repeat, no refills
NPO		nothing by mouth
o.d.	oculus dexter	right eye
o.s.	oculus sinister	left eye
o.u.	oculo uterque	each eye
pc	post cibos	after meals
per		through or by
PM	post meridiem	afternoon or evening
P.O.	per os	by mouth
P.R.	per rectum	rectally
prn	pro re nata	as needed
q		every
qd		every day
qh	quiaque hora	every hour
qid	quater in die	four times a day
qod		every other day
qs	quantum sufficiat	a sufficient quantity
qs ad		a sufficient quantity to make
qty		quantity
Rx	recipe	take, a recipe
rep	repetatur	let it be repeated
s̄	sine	without
S.C.		subcutaneous

(continued)

Abbreviation	From	Meaning
sig	signa	label, or let it be printed
sol	solutio	solution
ss	semis	one-half
stat	statim	at once, immediately
supp	suppositorium	suppository
syr	syrupus	syrup
tab	tabella	tablet
tal		such
tid	ter in die	three times a day
tr, tinct	tincture	tincture
tsp		teaspoonful
ung	unguentum	ointment
USAN		United States Adopted Names
USP		United States Pharmacopeia
u.d., ut dict	ut dictum	as directed
v.o.		verbal order
w.a.		while awake

BODY SURFACE AREA OF ADULTS

BODY SURFACE AREA OF ADULTS

HEIGHT	BODY SURFACE AREA	WEIGHT
CM 200 — 79 IN 78 195 — 77 76 190 — 75 74 185 — 73 72 180 — 71 70 175 — 69 68 170 — 67 66 165 — 65 64 160 — 63 62 155 — 61 60 150 — 59 58 145 — 57 56 140 — 55 54 135 — 53 52 130 — 51 50 125 — 49 48 120 — 47 46 115 — 45 44 110 — 43 42 105 — 41 40 CM 100 — 30 IN	$2.80\ M^2$ 2.70 2.60 2.50 2.40 2.30 2.20 2.10 2.00 1.95 1.90 1.85 1.80 1.75 1.70 1.65 1.60 1.55 1.50 1.45 1.40 1.35 1.30 1.25 1.20 1.15 1.10 1.05 1.00 0.95 0.90 $0.86\ M^2$	KG 150 — 330 LB 145 — 320 140 — 310 135 — 300 130 — 290 125 — 280 120 — 270 260 115 — 250 110 — 240 105 — 230 100 — 220 95 — 210 90 — 200 85 — 190 80 — 180 170 75 — 160 70 — 150 65 — 140 60 — 130 55 — 120 50 — 110 105 45 — 100 95 40 — 90 85 80 35 — 75 70 KG 30 — 66 LB

A straight edge is placed from the patient's height in the left column to his weight in the right column and this intersection on the body surface area column indicates his body surface area.

From the formula of Du Bois and Du Bois, *Arch Intern Med*, 17, 863 (1916): $S = W^{0.425} \times H^{0.725} \times 71.84$ or $\log S = \log W \times .425 + \log H^7 \times 0.725 + 1.8564$ (S = body surface in cm^2, W^7 = weight

Cautionary note: With increased age, height may decrease due to kyphotic changes which may make the surface area in the nomogram inaccurate. Since obtaining height in elderly is rather difficult and/or innacurate, some clinicians use: $BSA = 0.06\ (BW_{kg}^{0.805})$

IDEAL BODY WEIGHT CALCULATION

Adults (18 years and older)

IBW (male)   = 50 + (2.3 x height in inches over 5 feet)
IBW (female) = 45.5 + (2.3 x height in inches over 5 feet)
*IBW is in kg.

CREATININE CLEARANCE ESTIMATING METHODS
IN PATIENTS WITH STABLE RENAL FUNCTION

The following formulas provide an acceptable estimate of the patient's creatinine clearance except when:

a.   patient's serum creatinine is changing rapidly (either up or down)

b.   patients are markedly emaciated

In these situations (a and b above), certain assumptions have to be made.

a.   In patients with rapidly rising serum creatinines (ie, >0.5-0.7 mg/dL/day), it is best to assume that the patient's creatinine clearance is probably <10 mL/minute.

b.   In emaciated patients, although their actual creatinine clearance is less than their calculated creatinine clearance (because of decreased creatinine production), it is not possible to easily predict how much less.

Adults   (18 years and older)

Method 1: (Cockroft DW and Gault MH, *Nephron*, 1976, 16:31-41)

Estimated creatinine clearance (Cl_{cr}):
        (mL/min)

$$\text{Male} = \frac{(140 - \text{age})\ \text{IBW (kg)}}{72 \times \text{serum creatinine}}$$

$$\text{Female} = \text{Estimated } Cl_{cr} \text{ male} \times 0.85$$

Note: The use of the patient's ideal body weight (IBW) is recommended for the above formula except when the patient's actual body weight is less than ideal. Use of the IBW is especially important in obese patients.

Method 2: (Jelliffe RW, *Ann Intern Med*, 1973, 79:604)

Estimated creatinine clearance (Cl_{cr}):
        (mL/min/1.73 m^2)

$$\text{Male} = \frac{98 - 0.8\ (\text{age} - 20)}{\text{serum creatinine}}$$

$$\text{Female} = \text{Estimated } Cl_{cr} \text{ male} \times 0.90$$

APOTHECARY-METRIC CONVERSIONS

Exact Equivalents

1 gram (g) = 15.43 grains	0.1 mg = 1/600 gr
1 milliliter (mL) = 16.23 minims	0.12 mg = 1/500 gr
1 minim (℥) = 0.06 milliliter	0.15 mg = 1/400 gr
1 grain (gr) = 64.8 milligrams	0.2 mg = 1/300 gr
1 ounce (℥) = 31.1 grams	0.3 mg = 1/200 gr
1 fluid ounce (fl℥) = 29.57 mL	0.4 mg = 1/150 gr
1 pint (pt) = 473.2 mL	0.5 mg = 1/120 gr
1 ounce (oz) = 28.35 grams	0.6 mg = 1/100 gr
1 pound (lb) = 453.6 grams	0.8 mg = 1/80 gr
1 kilogram (kg) = 2.2 pound	1 mg = 1/65 gr
1 quart (qt) = 946.4	

Approximate Equivalents*

Liquids	Solids
1 teaspoonful = 5 mL	¼ grain = 15 mg
1 tablespoonful = 15 mL	½ grain = 30 mg
	1 grain = 60 mg
	1½ grain = 100 mg
	5 grains = 300 mg
	10 grains = 600 mg

*Use exact equivalents for compounding and calculations requiring a high degree of accuracy.

POUNDS-KILOGRAMS CONVERSION

1 pound = 0.45359 kilograms
1 kilogram = 2.2 pounds

TEMPERATURE CONVERSION

Celsius to Fahrenheit = (°C x 9/5) + 32 = °F
Fahrenheit to Celsius = (°F - 32) x 5/9 = °C

MILLIMOLE AND MILLIEQUIVALENT CALCULATIONS

Definitions

mole = gram molecular weight of a substance (aka molar weight)

millimole (mM) = milligram molecular weight of a substance (a millimole is 1/1000 of a mole)

equivalent weight = gram weight of a substance which will combine with or replace one gram (one mole) of hydrogen; an equivalent weight can be determined by dividing the molar weight of a substance by its ionic valence

milliequivalent (mEq) = milligram weight of a substance which will combine with or replace one milligram (one millimole) of hydrogen (a milliequivalent is 1/1000 of an equivalent)

Calculations

moles $= \dfrac{\text{weight of a substance (grams)}}{\text{molecular weight of that substance (grams)}}$

millimoles $= \dfrac{\text{weight of a substance (milligrams)}}{\text{molecular weight of that substance (milligrams)}}$

equivalents = moles x valence of ion

milliequivalents = millimoles x valence of ion

moles $= \dfrac{\text{equivalents}}{\text{valence of ion}}$

millimoles $= \dfrac{\text{milliequivalents}}{\text{valence of ion}}$

millimoles = moles x 1000

milliequivalents = equivalents x 1000

Note: Use of equivalents and milliequivalents is valid only for those substances which have fixed ionic valences (eg, sodium, potassium, calcium, chlorine, magnesium bromine, etc). For substances with variable ionic valences (eg, phosphorous), a reliable equivalent value cannot be determined. In these instances, one should calculate millimoles (which are fixed and reliable) rather than milliequivalents.

MILLIEQUIVALENTS FOR SELECTED IONS

Approximate Milliequivalents — Weights of Selected Ions

Salt	mEq/g Salt	mg Salt/mEq
Calcium carbonate ($CaCO_3$)	20	50
Calcium chloride ($CaCl_2 \cdot 2H_2O$)	14	73
Calcium gluconate (Ca gluconate$_2 \cdot 1H_2O$)	4	224
Calcium lactate (Ca lactate$_2 \cdot 5H_2O$)	6	154
Magnesium sulfate ($MgSO_4$)	16	60
Magnesium sulfate ($MgSO_4 \cdot 7H_2O$)	8	123
Potassium acetate (K acetate)	10	98
Potassium chloride (KCl)	13	75
Potassium citrate (K_3 citrate $\cdot 1H_2O$)	9	108
Potassium iodide (KI)	6	166
Sodium bicarbonate ($NaHCO_3$)	12	84
Sodium chloride (NaCl)	17	58
Sodium citrate (Na_3 citrate $\cdot 2H_2O$)	10	98
Sodium iodide (NaI)	7	150
Sodium lactate (Na lactate)	9	112
Zinc sulfate ($ZnSO_4 \cdot 7H_2O$)	7	144

Valences and Approximate Weights of Selected Ions

Substance	Electrolyte	Valence	Ionic Wt
Calcium	Ca^{++}	2	40
Chloride	Cl^-	1	35.5
Magnesium	Mg^{++}	2	24
Phosphate	PO_4^{---}	3	95*
	HPO_4^{--}	2	96
	$H_2PO_4^-$	1	97
Potassium	K^+	1	39
Sodium	Na^+	1	23
Sulfate	SO_4^{--}	2	96*

*The atomic weight of phosphorus is 31, and of sulfur is 32.

AMINOGLYCOSIDE DOSING GUIDELINES

Aminoglycosides	Usual Loading Dose (mg/kg)	Expected Peak Serum Levels (mcg/mL)
Tobramycin Gentamicin	1.5-2	4-10
Amikacin Kanamycin	5-7.5	15-30

Percentage of Loading Dose Required*
for Dosage Interval Selected

Cl_{cr} (mL/min)	Half-Life (h)	8 h %	12 h %	24 h %
90	3.1	84		
80	3.4	80	91	
70	3.9	76	88	
60	4.5	71	84	
50	5.3	65	79	
40	6.5		72	92
30	8.4		63	86
25	9.9		57	81
20	11.9			75
17	13.6			70
15	15.1			67
12	17.9			61
10*	20.4			56
7	25.9			47
5	31.5			41
2	46.8			30
0	69.3			21

*Sarubbi FA and Hull JH, "Amikacin Serum Concentrations: Predictions of Levels and Dosage Guidelines," *Ann Intern Med*, 1978, 89:612-8.

Patients >65 years of age should not receive initial aminoglycoside maintenance dosing more often than every 12 hours.

ANTIPSYCHOTIC MEDICATION GUIDELINES

Appropriate indications for use of antipsychotic medications are outlined in the Health Care Finance Administration's Omnibus Reconciliation Act (OBRA) of 1987. In addition to psychotic disorders, specific nonpsychotic behavior is identified for antipsychotic treatment. Specifically, behavior associated with organic mental syndromes (nonpsychotic behavior) is indicated:

> agitated psychotic symptoms (biting, kicking, hitting, scratching, assertive and belligerent behavior, sexual aggressiveness) that presents a danger to themselves or others or interferes with family and/or staff's ability to provide care (ADLs)
>
> psychotic symptoms (hallucinations, delusions, paranoia)
>
> continuous (24-hour) crying out and screaming

Behavior less responsive to antipsychotic therapy includes:

> repetitive, bothersome behavior (ie, pacing, wandering; repeated statements or words; calling out; fidgeting)
>
> poor self care
>
> unsociability
>
> indifference to surroundings
>
> uncooperative behavior
>
> restlessness
>
> impaired memory
>
> anxiety
>
> depression
>
> insomnia

If antipsychotic therapy is to be used for one or more of these symptoms **only**, then the use of antipsychotic agents is inappropriate. Antipsychotics may worsen these symptoms, especially symptoms of sedation and lethargy as well as enhance "confusion" due to their anticholinergic properties.

Selection of an antipsychotic agent should be based upon side effect profile since all antipsychotic agents are equally effective at equivalent doses. Coadministration of two or more antipsychotics does not have any pharmacologic basis or clinical advantage. Coadministration of two or more antipsychotic agents does not improve clinical response and increases the potential for side effects.

Once behavior control is obtained, assess patient to determine if precipitating event (stress from drugs, fluid/electrolyte changes, infection, changes in environment) has been resolved or patient has accommodated to their environment or situation. Determine whether antipsychotic can be decreased in dose or tapered off by monitoring selected target symptoms for which the antipsychotic therapy was initiated. OBRA '87 act requires attempts at dose reduction within a 6-month period unless documented as to why this cannot be done. Identifying target symptoms is essential for adequate monitoring. Due to side effects, intermittent use (not PRN) is preferable; ie, only when patient has behavior warranting use of these agents.

ANXIOLYTIC/HYPNOTIC USE IN LONG-TERM CARE FACILITIES

One of the regulations regarding medication use in long-term care facilities concerns "unnecessary drugs." The regulation states, "Each resident's drug regimen must be free from unnecessary drugs." Recently, the Health Care Financing Administration (HCFA) issued the final interpretive guidelines on this regulation. The following is a summary of these guidelines as they pertain to anxiolytic/hypnotic agents.

A. Long-Acting Benzodiazepines

Long-acting benzodiazepine drugs should not be used in residents unless an attempt with a shorter-acting drug has failed. If they are used, the doses must be no higher than the listed dose, unless higher doses are necessary for maintenance or improvement in the resident's functional status. Daily use should be less then 4 continuous months unless an attempt at a gradual dose reduction is unsuccessful. Residents on diazepam for seizure disorders or for the treatment of tardive dyskinesia are exempt from this restriction. Residents on clonazepam for bipolar disorder, tardive dyskinesia, nocturnal myoclonus, or seizure disorder are also exempt. Residents on long-acting benzodiazepines should have a gradual dose reduction at least twice within 1 year before it can be concluded that the gradual dose reduction is "clinically contraindicated."

Long-Acting Benzodiazepines

Generic	Brand	Maximum Daily Geriatric Dose (mg)
Chlordiazepoxide	Librium®	20
Clonazepam	Klonopin™	1.5
Clorazepate	Tranxene®	15
Diazepam	Valium®	5
Flurazepam	Dalmane®	15
Prazepam	Centrax®	15
Quazepam	Doral®	7.5

B. Benzodiazepine or Other Anxiolytic/Sedative Drugs

Anxiolytic/sedative drugs should be used for purposes other than sleep induction only when other possible causes of the resident's distress have been ruled out and the use results in maintenance or improvement in the resident's functional status. Daily use should not exceed 4 continuous months unless an attempt at gradual dose reduction has failed. Anxiolytics should only be used for generalized anxiety disorder, dementia with agitated states that either endangers the resident or others, or is a source of distress or dysfunction; panic disorder, or symptomatic anxiety associated with other psychiatric disorders. The dose should not exceed those listed below unless a higher dose is needed as evidenced by the resident's response. Gradual dosage reductions should be attempted at least twice within 1 year before it can be concluded that a gradual dose reduction is "clinically contraindicated."

Short-Acting Benzodiazepines

Generic	Brand	Maximum Daily Geriatric Dose (mg)
Alprazolam	Xanax®	0.75
Halazepam	Paxipam®	40
Lorazepam	Ativan®	2
Oxazepam	Serax®	30

Other Anxiolytic and Sedative Drugs

Generic	Brand	Maximum Daily Geriatric Dose (mg)
Chloral hydrate	Noctec®, etc	750
Diphenhydramine	Benadryl®	50
Hydroxyzine	Atarax®, Vistaril®	50

Note: Chloral hydrate, diphenhydramine, and hydroxyzine are not necessarily drugs of choice for treatment of anxiety disorders. HCFA lists them only in the event of their possible use.

C. Drugs Used for Sleep Induction

Drugs for sleep induction should only be used when all possible reasons for insomnia have been ruled out (ie, pain, noise, caffeine). The use of the drug must result in the maintenance or improvement of the resident's functional status. Daily use of a hypnotic should not exceed 10 consecutive days unless an attempt at a gradual dose reduction is unsuccessful. The dose should not exceed those listed below unless a higher dose has been deemed necessary. Gradual dose reductions should be attempted at least three times within 6 months before it can be concluded that a gradual dose reduction is "clinically contraindicated."

Hypnotic Drugs

Generic	Brand	Daily Geriatric Dose (mg)
Alprazolam*	Xanax®	0.25
Chloral hydrate	Noctec®	500
Diphenhydramine	Benadryl®	25
Estazolam	ProSom™	0.5
Halazepam*	Paxipam®	20
Hydroxyzine	Atarax®, Vistaril®	50
Lorazepam*	Ativan®	1
Oxazepam*	Serax®	15
Temazepam	Restoril®	15
Triazolam	Halcion®	0.125

*Not officially indicated as a hypnotic agent.

Note: Chloral hydrate, diphenhydramine, and hydroxyzine are not necessarily drugs of choice for sleep disorders. HCFA lists them only in the event of their possible use.

D. Miscellaneous Hypnotic/Sedative/Anxiolytic Drugs

The initiation of the following medications should not occur in any dose in any resident. Residents currently using these drugs or residents admitted to the facility while using these drugs should receive gradual dose reductions. Newly admitted residents should have a period of adjustment before attempting reduction. Dose reductions should be attempted at least twice within 1 year before it can be concluded that it is "clinically contraindicated."

Examples of Barbiturates

Generic	Brand
Amobarbital	Amytal®
Amobarbital/Secobarbital	Tuinal®
Butabarbital	Butisol Sodium®
Combinations	Fiorinal®, etc
Pentobarbital	Nembutal®
Secobarbital	Seconal™

Miscellaneous Hypnotic/Sedative/Anxiolytic Agents

Generic	Brand
Ethchlorvynol	Placidyl®
Glutethimide	Doriden®
Meprobamate	Equanil®, Miltown®
Methyprylon	Noludar®
Paraldehyde	Paral®

FEDERAL OBRA REGULATIONS
RECOMMENDED MAXIMUM DOSES

Hypnotics
Should not be used for more than 10 continuous days

Drug	Brand Name	Usual Max Single Dose for Age ≥65	Usual Max Single Dose
Amobarbital	Amytal®	150 mg	300 mg
Butabarbital	Butisol®	100 mg	200 mg
Chloral hydrate	Noctec®	750 mg	1500 mg
Flurazepam	Dalmane®	15 mg	30 mg
Glutethimide	Doriden®	500 mg	1000 mg
Triazolam	Halcion®	0.25 mg	0.5 mg
Pentobarbital	Nembutal®	100 mg	200 mg
Methprylon	Noludar®	200 mg	400 mg
Ethchlorvynol	Placidyl®	500 mg	1000 mg
Temazepam	Restoril®	15 mg	30 mg
Secobarbital	Seconal®	100 mg	200 mg

Antipsychotics

Drug	Brand Name	Usual Max Daily Dose for Age ≥65	Usual Max Daily Dose	Daily Oral Dose for Residents With Organic Mental Syndromes
Chlorpromazine	Thorazine®	800 mg	1600 mg	75 mg
Haloperidol	Haldol®	50 mg	100 mg	4 mg
Loxapine	Loxitane®	125 mg	250 mg	10 mg
Thioridazine	Mellaril®	400 mg	800 mg	75 mg
Molindone	Moban®	112 mg	225 mg	10 mg
Thiothixene	Navane®	30 mg	60 mg	7 mg
Fluphenazine	Prolixin®	20 mg	40 mg	7 mg
Mesoridazine	Serentil®	250 mg	500 mg	25 mg
Trifluoperazine	Stelazine®	40 mg	80 mg	8 mg
Chlorprothixene	Taractan®	800 mg	1600 mg	75 mg
Acetophenazine	Tindal®	150 mg	300 mg	20 mg
Perphenazine	Trilafon®	32 mg	64 mg	8 mg
Trifluopromazine	Vesprin®	100 mg	200 mg	—

Anxiolytics

Drug	Brand Name	Usual Daily Dose for Age ≥65	Usual Daily Dose for Age <65
Lorazepam	Ativan®	3 mg	6 mg
Prazepam	Centrax®	30 mg	60 mg
Diazepam	Valium®	20 mg	60 mg
Chlordiazepoxide	Librium®	40 mg	100 mg
Meprobamate	Miltown®	600 mg	1600 mg
Halazepam	Paxipam®	80 mg	160 mg
Oxazepam	Serax®	60 mg	90 mg
Clorazepate	Tranxene®	30 mg	60 mg
Alprazolam	Xanax®	2 mg	4 mg

Antidepressants

Drug	Brand Name	Usual Max Daily Dose for Age ≥65	Usual Max Daily Dose
Doxepin	Adapin® Sinequan®	150 mg	300 mg
Amitriptyline	Elavil®	150 mg	300 mg
Amoxapine	Asendin®	200 mg	400 mg
Nortriptyline	Aventyl® Pamelor®	75 mg	150 mg
Trazodone	Desyrel®	300 mg	600 mg
Imipramine	Tofranil®	150 mg	300 mg
Maprotiline	Ludiomil®	150 mg	300 mg
Desipramine	Norpramin® Pertofrane®	150 mg	300 mg
Trimipramine	Surmontil®	150 mg	300 mg
Protriptyline	Vivactil®	30 mg	60 mg

IMMUNIZATION GUIDELINES

Table 1. **Dosage and Administration Guidelines for Vaccines Available in the United States**

Vaccine	Dosage	Route of Administration	Type
DT	0.5 mL	I.M.	Toxoids
Td	0.5 mL	I.M.	Toxoids
DTP	0.5 mL	I.M.	Diphtheria and tetanus toxoids with killed *B. pertussis* organisms
Haemophilus B conjugate vaccine	0.5 mL	I.M.	
ProHIBit® (PRP-D), manufactured by Connaught Laboratories	0.5 mL	I.M.	Polysaccharide (diphtheria toxoid conjugate)
HibTITER® (HbOC)†, manufactured by Praxis Biologicals	0.5 mL	I.M.	Oligosaccharide (diphtheria CRM$_{197}$ protein conjugate)
Hepatitis B,¶		I.M., S.C. in individuals at risk of hemorrhage	Yeast recombinant-derived inactivated viral antigen
Geriatrics and Adults			
Recombivax HB® (MSD)	10 mcg (1 mL)		
Engerix-B® (SKF)	20 mcg (1 mL)		
Dialysis patients and immunosuppressed patients			
Recombivax HB® (MSD)	>11 y, 40 mcg (2 mL); use special dialysis formulation and give as two 1 mL doses at different sites		
Engerix-B® (SKF)	>11 y, 40 mcg (2 mL); give as two 1 mL doses at different sites		
Influenza			
Geriatrics and Adults	0.5 mL (1 dose)	Only one dose needed for annual updates	Inactivated virus subvirion (split) (contraindicated in patients allergic to chicken eggs)
Measles	0.5 mL	S.C.	Live virus (contraindicated in patients with anaphylactic allergy to neomycin)

High-risk areas: Two doses (first dose at 12 months with MMR; second dose as above)

Vaccine	Dosage	Route of Administration	Type
Meningococcal	0.5 mL	S.C.	Polysaccharide
MMR•	0.5 mL	S.C.	Live virus
MR	0.5 mL	S.C.	Live virus
Mumps	0.5 mL	S.C.	Live virus
Pneumococcal polyvalent	0.5 mL (≥2 y)	I.M. or S.C. (I.M. preferred)	Polysaccharide
Poliovirus (OPV) trivalent	0.5 mL	Oral	Live virus
Poliovirus (IPV),**, †† trivalent	0.5 mL	S.C.	Inactivated virus

APPENDIX

Vaccine	Dosage	Route of Administration	Type
Rabies	1 mL	I.M.‡‡, ID§§	Inactivated virus
Rubella	0.5 mL (≥12 mo)¶¶	S.C.	Live virus
Tetanus (adsorbed)##	0.5 mL	I.M.	Toxoid
Tetanus (fluid)	0.5 mL	I.M., S.C.	Toxoid
Yellow fever	0.5 mL⟜	S.C.	Live attenuated virus

†The conjugate (HbCV) vaccine is preferred over the polysaccharide (HbPV) vaccine.

¶Engerix-B® — an alternate schedule for postexposure prophylaxis or more rapid induction using four doses at 0, 1, 2, and 12 months can be used.

**The primary series consists of 3 doses. The first two doses should be administered at an interval of 8 weeks. The third dose should be given at least 6 and preferably 12 months after the second dose. When polio vaccine is given to persons >18 years, IPV should be given.

•See measles.

††IPV is indicated for unimmunized or partially immunized patients with compromised immunity; HIV infection; unimmunized adults or adults at future risk of exposure to poliomyelitis; household contacts of an immunodeficient individual.

‡‡I.M. injection can be given into the deltoid muscle. Repeat doses are given on days 3, 7, 14, and 28 postexposure.

§§For pre-exposure prophylaxis against rabies for high-risk individuals, 1 mL I.M. or 0.1 mL intradermal is administered on days 0, 7, and 21 (or 28). Both I.M. and I.D. dosage forms are available.

¶¶As MMR in a two-dose schedule.

##Adsorbed preferred to fluid toxoid because of longer lasting immunity.

⟜9 months of age living in or traveling to endemic areas. Contraindicated in patients who have had an anaphylactic reaction to eggs.

Note: For each vaccine, check the manufacturer's package insert for specific product information since preparations may change from time to time.

References:
ACIP, General Recommendations on Immunization, MMWR 1989, 38:205-14, 219-27.

Table 2. **Guidelines for Spacing Live and Killed Antigen Administration**

Antigen Combinations	Recommended Minimum Interval Between Doses
≥2 killed antigens	None. May be given simultaneously or at any interval between doses.
Killed and live antigens	None. May be given simultaneously or at any interval between doses. (Exception: Concurrent administration of cholera and yellow fever vaccines should be avoided. Separate these vaccines by at least 3 weeks.)
≥2 live antigens	4 weeks minimum interval if not administered simultaneously. (Recent receipt of OPV is not a contraindication to MMR.) Vaccines associated with systemic reactions (cholera and parenteral typhoid or influenza and DTP in young children) should be given on separate occasions.

Table 3. **Passive Immunization Agents — Immune Globulins**

Immune Globulin	Dosage	Route
Hepatitis B (H-BIG®)		I.M.
percutaneous inoculation	0.06 mL/kg/dose (within 24 hours) (5 mL max)	
perinatal	0.5 mL/dose (within 12 hours of birth)	
sexual exposure	0.06 mL/kg/dose (within 14 days of contact) (5 mL max)	
Immune globulin (IG)		I.M.*
hepatitis A prophylaxis	0.02 mL/kg/dose (as soon as possible or within 2 weeks after exposure) (single exposure)	
	0.06 mL/kg/dose (>3 months or continuous exposure) repeat every 4-6 months	
hepatitis B	0.06 mL/kg/dose (H-BIG should be used)	
hepatitis C	0.06 mL/kg/dose (percutaneous exposure)	
measles†	0.25 mL/kg/dose (max 15 mL/dose) (within 6 days of exposure)	
	0.5 mL/kg/dose (max 15 mL/dose) (immunocompromised children)	
Rabies‡	20 IU/kg/dose (within 3 days)	
Tetanus (serious, contaminated, wounds; <3 previous tetanus vaccine doses)	250-500 units/dose	I.M.
Varicella-zoster (VZIG)	Within 48 hours but not later than 96 hours after exposure	I.M.¶
	0-10 kg 125 units = 1 vial	
	10.1-20 kg 250 units = 2 vials	
	20.1-30 kg 375 units = 3 vials	
	30.1-40 kg 500 units = 4 vials	
	>40 kg 625 units = 5 vials	

*Deep I.M. in the gluteal region for large doses only. Deltoid muscle or the anterolateral aspect of the thigh are preferred sites for injection. No greater than 5 mL/site in adults; maximum dose: 20 mL at one time.
†IG prophylaxis may not be indicated in a patient who has received IGIV within 3 weeks of exposure.
‡½ of dose used to infiltrate the wound with the remaining ½ of dose given I.M. Rabies immune globulin is not recommended in previously HDCV immunized patients.
¶No greater than 2.5 mL of VZIG/one injection site. Doses >2.5 mL should be divided and administered at different sites.

Table 4. **Guidelines for Spacing the Administration of Immune Globulin (IG) Preparations and Vaccines**

Immunobiologic Combinations	Recommended Minimum Interval Between Doses
Simultaneous Administration	
IG and killed antigen	None. May be given simultaneously at different sites or at any time between doses.
IG and live antigen	Should generally not be given simultaneously. If unavoidable to do so, give at different sites and revaccinate or test for seroconversion in 3 months. Example: MMR should not be given to patients who have received immune globulin within the previous 3 months.

Nonsimultaneous Administration

First	Second	
IG	Killed antigen	None
Killed antigen	IG	None
IG	Live antigen	6 weeks, and preferably 3 months
Live antigen	IG	2 weeks

*The live virus vaccines, OPV and yellow fever are exceptions to these recommendations. Either vaccine may be administered simultaneously or any time before or after IG without significantly decreasing antibody response.

SODIUM CONTENT OF SELECTED MEDICINALS

Name and Dosage Unit*	Sodium mg	mEq
Antibiotics		
Amikacin sulfate, 1 g	29.9	1.3
Aminosalicylate sodium, 1 g	109	4.7
Ampicillin, suspension 250 mg/5 mL, 5 mL	10	0.4
Ampicillin sodium, 1 g	66.7	3
Azlocillin sodium, 1 g	50	2.2
Carbenicillin disodium 382 mg (tablet)	22	1
Cefazolin sodium, 1 g	47	2
Cefotaxime sodium, 1 g	30.5	2.2
Cefoxitin sodium, 1 g	53	2.3
Ceftriaxone sodium, 1 g	83	3.6
Cefuroxime, 1 g	54.2	2.4
Chloramphenicol sodium succinate, 1 g	51.8	2.3
Dicloxacillin, 250 mg (capsule)	13	0.6
Dicloxacillin, suspension 65 mg/5 mL	27	1.2
Erythromycin ethyl succinate, suspension 200 mg/5 mL	29	1.3
Erythromycin Base Filmtab®, 250 mg	70	3
Methicillin sodium, 1 g	66.7	2.9
Metronidazole, 500 mg I.V.	322	14
Mezlocillin sodium, 1 g	42.6	1.9
Moxalactam sodium, 1 g	88	3.8
Nafcillin sodium, 1 g	66.7	2.9
Nitrofurantoin, suspension 25 mg/5 mL	7	0.3
Penicillin G potassium, 1,000,000 units I.V.	7.6	0.3
Penicillin G sodium, 1,000,000 units I.V.	46	2
Penicillin V potassium, suspension, 250 mg/5 mL	38	1.7
Piperacillin sodium, 1 g	42.6	1.8
Ticarcillin disodium, 1 g	119.6	5.2
Antacids, Liquid (content per 5 mL)		
Amphojel®	<2.3	<0.1
ALternaGEL®	2	0.1
Basaljel®	2.4	0.1
Extra Strength Maalox®-Plus	0.65	~0.05
Gaviscon®	13	0.57
Maalox®	1.3	0.06
Tums E-X™	<4.8	<0.2
Sodium Content of Miscellaneous Medicinals		
Acetazolamide sodium, 500 mg	47.2	2.05
Chlorothiazide sodium, 500 mg	57.5	2
Cisplatin, 10 mg	35.4	1.54
Edetate calcium disodium, 1 g	122	5.3
Fleet® Enema, 4.5 oz	5000†	218
Fleet® Phospho®-Soda, 20 mL	2217	96.4
Hydrocortisone sodium succinate, 1 g	47.5	2.07
Hypaque® M 75%, injection, 20 mL	200	8.7
Hypaque® M 90%, injection, 20 mL	220	9.6
Metamucil® Instant Mix (orange)	6	0.27
Methotrexate sodium, 100 mg vial	20	0.86
Methotrexate sodium, 100 mg vial (low sodium)	15	0.65
Naproxen sodium, 250 mg (tablet)	23	1
Neutra-Phos®, capsule and 75 mL reconstituted solution	164	7.13
Oragrafin® (capsule)	19	0.8
Pentobarbital sodium, 50 mg/mL, 1 mL vial	5	0.2
Phenobarbital sodium, 65 mg, 1 mL vial	6	0.3
Phenytoin sodium, 1 g	88	3.8
Promethazine expectorant, 5 mL	53	2.3
Shohl's solution modified, 1 mL	23	1
Sodium ascorbate, 500 mg acid equivalent	65.3	2.84
Sodium bicarbonate, 50 mL 8.4%	1150	50
Sodium nitroprusside, 50 mg	7.8	0.34
Sodium polystyrene sulfonate, 1 g	94.3‡	4.1
Thiopental sodium, 1 g	86.8	3.8
Valproate sodium, 250 mg/5 mL, 5 mL	23	1

*Product formulations and hence sodium content are subject to change by the manufacturer.
†Average systemic absorption 250-300 mg.
‡Total sodium content. Only about 33% is liberated in clinical use.

ANTACID DRUG INTERACTIONS

Drug	Aluminum Salts	Calcium Salts	Magnesium Salts	Magnesium Aluminum Combinations
			Antacid	
Allopurinol	↓			
Benzodiazepines	↑		↓	↓
Calcitriol			x*	x*
Captopril				↓
Cimetidine				↓
Corticosteroids	↓		↓	↓
Dicumarol			↑	
Diflunisal	↓			
Digoxin	↓		↓	
Iron	↓	↓	↓	↓
Isoniazid	↓			
Ketoconazole				↓
Levodopa				↑
Nitrofurantoin			↓	
Penicillamine	↓		↓	↓
Phenothiazines	↓		↓	↓
Phenytoin		↓		↓
Quinidine		↑	↑	↑
Quinolones				↓
Ranitidine	↓			↓
Salicylates		↓		↓
Sodium polystyrene sulfonate	x†		x†	x†
Tetracyclines	↓	↓	↓	↓
Valproic acid				↑

Pharmacologic effect increased (↑) or decreased (↓) by antacids.
*Concomitant use in patients on chronic renal dialysis may lead to hypermagnesemia.
†Concomitant use may cause metabolic alkalosis in patients with renal failure.

APPENDIX

FEVER DUE TO DRUGS

Allopurinol	Iodides	Phenytoin
Aminosalicylic acid	Isoniazid	Procainamide
Antihistamines	Methyldopa	Propylthiouracil
Barbiturates	Penicillins	Quinidine
Cephalosporins	Phenolphthalein	Sulfonamides

Abstracted from Harrison's *Principles of Internal Medicine*, 12 ed, Wilson JD, ed, New York, NY: McGraw-Hill Book Co, 1991 and Tabor PA, "Drug-Induced Fever," *Drug Intell Clin Pharm*, 1986, 20:413-20.

DISCOLORATION OF FECES DUE TO DRUGS

Black
Acetazolamide
Alcohols
Alkalies
Aluminum hydroxide
Aminophylline
Amphetamine
Amphotericin
Anticoagulants
Aspirin
Barium
Betamethasone
Bismuth
Charcoal
Chloramphenicol
Chlorpropamide
Clindamycin
Corticosteroids
Cortisone
Cyclophosphamide
Cytarabine
Dicumarol
Digitalis
Ethacrynic acid
Fenoprofen
Ferrous salts
Floxuridine
Fluorides
Fluorouracil
Halothane
Heparin
Hydralazine
Hydrocortisone
Ibuprofen
Indomethacin
Iodine drugs
Iron salts
Levarterenol
Levodopa
Manganese
Mefenamic acid
Melphalan
Methylprednisolone
Methotrexate
Methylene blue

Black (continued)
Nitrates
Oxyphenbutazone
Paraldehyde
Phenacetin
Phenolphthalein
Phenylbutazone
Phenylephrine
Phosphorous
Potassium salts
Prednisolone
Procarbazine
Pyrivinium
Reserpine
Salicylates
Sulfonamides
Tetracycline
Thallium
Theophylline
Thiotepa
Triamcinolone
Warfarin

Blue
Chloramphenicol
Methylene blue

Dark Brown
Dexamethasone

Gray
Colchicine

Green
Indomethacin
Iron
Medroxyprogesterone

Greenish Gray
Oral antibiotics
Oxyphenbutazone
Phenylbutazone

Light Brown
Anticoagulants

Orange-Red
Phenazopyridine
Rifampin

Pink
Anticoagulants
Aspirin
Heparin
Oxyphenbutazone
Phenylbutazone
Salicylates

Red
Anticoagulants
Aspirin
Heparin
Oxyphenbutazone
Phenolphthalein
Phenylbutazone
Pyrvinium
Salicylates
Tetracycline syrup

Red-Brown
Oxyphenbutazone
Phenylbutazone
Rifampin

Tarry
Ergot preparations
Ibuprofen
Salicylates
Warfarin

White/Speckling
Aluminum hydroxide
Antibiotics (oral)
Indocyanine green

Yellow
Senna

Yellow-Green
Senna

Adapted from Drugdex® — Drug Consults, Micromedex, Vol 62, Rocky Mountain Drug Consultation Center, Denver, CO: January, 1995.

DISCOLORATION OF URINE DUE TO DRUGS

Black
Cascara
Ferrous salts
Iron dextran
Levodopa
Methocarbamol
Methyldopa
Naphthalene
Phenacetin
Phenols
Quinine
Sulfonamides

Blue
Anthraquinone
DeWitts pills
Indigo blue
Indigo carmine
Methocarbamol
Methylene blue
Nitrofurans
Resorcinol
Triamterene

Blue-Green
Amitriptyline
Anthraquinone
DeWitt's pills
Doan's® pills
Indigo blue
Indigo carmine
Methylene blue
Resorcinol

Brown
Anthraquinone dyes
Cascara
Chloroquine
Danthron
Furazolidone
Levodopa
Methocarbamol
Methyldopa
Metronidazole
Nitrofurans
Nitrofurantoin
Phenacetin
Phenols
Primaquine
Quinine
Rifampin
Senna
Sodium diatrizoate
Sulfonamides

Brown-Black
Methocarbamol
Methyldopa
Metronidazole
Nitrates
Nitrofurans
Phenacetin
Povidone iodine
Quinine
Senna

Dark
Aminosalicylic acid
Cascara
Furazolidone
Levodopa

Dark *(cont)*
Metronidazole
Nitrites
Phenacetin
Phenol
Primaquine
Quinine
Resorcinol
Riboflavin
Senna

Green
Amitriptyline
Anthraquinone
Chlorophyll, water soluble
DeWitts pills
Indigo blue
Indigo carmine
Indomethacin
Methocarbamol
Methylene blue
Nitrofurans
Phenols
Resorcinol
Suprofen

Green-Yellow
DeWitt's pills
Methylene blue

Milky
Phosphates

Orange
Chlorzoxazone
Dihydroergotamine
    mesylate
Heparin sodium
Phenazopyridine
Phenindione
Rifampin
Sulfasalazine
Warfarin

Orange-Red
Chlorzoxazone
Doxidan
Phenazopyridine
Rifampin

Orange-Red-Brown
Warfarin

Orange-Yellow
Fluorescein sodium
Rifampin
Sulfasalazine

Pink
Aminopyrine
Anthraquinone dyes
Cascara
Danthron
Deferoxamine
Merbromin
Methyldopa
Phenolphthalein
Phenothiazines
Phensuximide
Phenytoin
Salicylates
Senna

Purple
Phenophthalein

Red
Anthraquinone
Cascara
Daunorubicin
Deferoxamine
Dihydroergotamine
    mesylate
Dimethylsulfoxide
DMSO
Doxorubicin
Heparin
Ibuprofen
Methyldopa
Oxyphenbutazone
Phenacetin
Phenazopyridine
Phenolphthalein
Phenothiazines
Phensuximide
Phenylbutazone
Phenytoin
Rifampin
Senna

Red-Brown
Cascara
Deferoxamine
Methyldopa
Oxyphenbutazone
Phenacetin
Phenolphthalein
Phenothiazines
Phenylbutazone
Phenytoin
Quinine
Senna

Red-Purple
Chlorzoxazone
Ibuprofen
Phenacetin
Senna

Rust
Cascara
Chloroquine
Metronidazole
Nitrofurantoin
Phenacetin
Riboflavin
Senna
Sulfonamides

Yellow
Nitrofurantoin
Phenacetin
Riboflavin
Sulfasalazine

Yellow-Brown
Bismuth
Cascara
Chloroquine
DeWitt's pills
Methylene blue
Metronidazole
Nitrofurantoin
Primaquine
Quinacrine

Yellow-Brown *(cont)*
Senna
Sulfonamides

Yellow-Pink
Cascara

Yellow-Pink *(cont)*
Senna

Adapted from Drugdex® — Drug Consults, Micromedex, Vol 62, Rocky Mountain Drug Consultation Center, Denver, CO: January, 1995.

HEMATOLOGIC ADVERSE EFFECTS OF DRUGS

Drug	Red Cell Aplasia	Thrombo-cytopenia	Neutro-penia	Pancyto-penia	Hemolysis
Acetazolamide		+	+	+	
Allopurinol			+		
Amiodarone	+				
Amphotericin B				+	
Amrinone		+ +			
Asparaginase		+ + +	+ + +	+ + +	+ +
Barbiturates		+		+	
Benzocaine					+ +
Captopril			+ +		+
Carbamazepine		+ +	+		
Cephalosporins			+		+ +
Chloramphenicol		+	+ +	+ + +	
Chlordiazepoxide			+	+	
Chloroquine		+			
Chlorothiazides		+ +			
Chlorpropamide	+	+ +	+	+ +	+
Chlortetracycline				+	
Chlorthalidone			+		
Cimetidine		+	+ +	+	
Codeine		+			
Colchicine				+	
Cyclophosphamide		+ + +	+ + +	+ + +	+
Dapsone					+ + +
Desipramine		+ +			
Digitalis		+			
Digitoxin		+ +			
Erythromycin		+			
Estrogen		+		+	
Ethacrynic acid			+		
Fluorouracil		+ + +	+ + +	+ + +	+
Furosemide		+	+		
Gold salts	+	+ + +	+ + +	+ + +	
Heparin		+ +		+	
Ibuprofen			+		+
Imipramine			+ +		
Indomethacin		+	+ +	+	
Isoniazid		+		+	
Isosorbide dinitrate					+
Levodopa					+ +
Meperidine		+			
Meprobamate		+	+	+	
Methimazole			+ +		
Methyldopa		+ +			+ + +
Methotrexate		+ + +	+ + +	+ + +	+ +
Methylene blue					+
Metronidazole			+		
Nalidixic acid					+

(continued)

Drug	Red Cell Aplasia	Thrombo-cytopenia	Neutro-penia	Pancyto-penia	Hemolysis
Naproxen				+	
Nitrofurantoin			+ +		+
Nitroglycerine		+			
Penicillamine		+ +	+		
Penicillins		+	+ +	+	+ + +
Phenazopyridine					+ + +
Phenothiazines		+	+ +	+ + +	+
Phenylbutazone		+	+ +	+ + +	+
Phenytoin		+ +	+ +	+ +	+
Potassium iodide		+			
Prednisone		+			
Primaquine					+ + +
Procainamide			+		
Procarbazine		+	+ +	+ +	+
Propylthiouracil		+	+ +	+	+
Quinidine		+ + +	+		
Quinine		+ + +	+		
Reserpine		+			
Rifampicin		+ +	+		+ + +
Spironolactone			+		
Streptomycin		+		+	
Sulfamethoxazole with trimethoprim			+		
Sulfonamides	+	+ +	+ +	+ +	+ +
Sulindac	+	+	+	+	
Tetracyclines		+			+
Thioridazine			+ +		
Tolbutamide		+ +	+	+ +	
Triamterene					+
Valproate	+				
Vancomycin			+		

+ = rare or single reports.
+ + = occasional reports.
+ + + = substantial number of reports.

Adapted from D'Arcy PF and Griffin JP, eds, *Iatrogenic Diseases*, New York, NY: Oxford University Press, 1986, 128-30.

ANTIDOTE CHART

Antidote	Poison/Drug	Indications/Symptoms
Acetylcysteine	Acetaminophen	• Unknown quantity was ingested and <24 h have elapsed since the time of ingestion • >7.5 g ingested acutely • Serum acetaminophen >140 mcg/mL at 4 h postingestion • Ingested dose >140 mg/kg
Amyl nitrite, sodium nitrite, sodium thiosulfate	Cyanide	• Begin treatment at the first sign of toxicity if cyanide exposure is known or strongly suspected
Antivenin polyvalent	Pit viper bites (rattlesnake, cottonmouth, copperhead)	• History of envenomation by a pit viper and experiencing mild moderate, or severe symptoms **Mild:** Local swelling (progressive), pain, no systemic systems **Moderate:** Ecchymosis and swelling beyond the bite site, some systemic symptoms, and/or lab changes **Severe:** Profound edema involving entire extremity, cyanosis, serious systemic involvement, significant lab changes
Atropine	Organophosphate and carbamate insecticides	• Myoclonic seizures, severe hallucinations, weakness, arrhythmias, excessive salivation, involuntary urination and defecation
Calcium EDTA (Versenate®)	Lead	• Symptomatic patients or asymptomatic children with blood levels >50 mcg/dL
Calcium gluconate	Hydrofluoric acid (HF)	• Calcium gluconate gel 2.5% for dermal exposure of HF of <20% concentration • SC injections or intra-arterial administration of calcium gluconate for dermal exposures of concentrations >20% or failure to respond to gel
Deferoxamine (Desferal®)	Iron	• Serum iron >350 mcg/dL or unable to obtain SI in a reasonable time and patient has signs and symptoms consistent with iron toxicity
Digoxin immune fab (Digibind®)	Digoxin	• Serious cardiac arrhythmias, progressive bradyarrhythmias, second or third degree heart block unresponsive to atropine, serum digoxin level >10 ng/mL or potassium levels >5 mEq/L
Dimercaprol (BAL in oil)	Arsenic	• Any symptoms of arsenic toxicity
	Lead	• All patients with symptoms, or asymptomatic children with blood levels 70 mcg/dL
	Mercury	• Serious, acute toxicity with inorganic mercury salts
Ethanol	Ethylene glycol or methanol	• Ethylene glycol or methanol blood levels >20 mg/dL or blood levels not readily available and suspected ingestion of toxic amounts, or any symptomatic patient with a history of ethylene glycol or methanol ingestion
Flumazenil (Mazicon®)	Benzodiazepines	• Complete or partial reversal of the sedative effects of benzodiazepines in cases where they were used in general anesthesia or for sedation for diagnostic or therapeutic procedures
Naloxone	Opiates (heroin, morphine, etc)	• Respiratory depression ± coma from unknown cause, or from opioid overdose
Physostigmine (Antilirium®)	Atropine and anticholinergics	• Myoclonic seizures, hypertension, severe arrhythmias, hallucinations
Phytonadione (Vitamin K₁)	Warfarin	• Large acute ingestion of warfarin rodenticides or chronic exposure, or greater than normal prothrombin time
Pralidoxime (Protopam®)	Organophosphate insecticide	• An adjunct to atropine therapy for treatment of profound muscle weakness, respiratory depression, muscle twitching and cholinergic syndrome
Pyridoxine (Vitamin B₆)	Isoniazid	• Unknown overdose or ingested amount >80 mg/kg
Succimer (Chemet®)	Lead (unlabeled use: mercury, arsenic)	• Blood lead levels >45 mcg/dL • Symptoms of lead poisoning • Unlabeled: other heavy metal poisoning

DRUG LEVELS COMMONLY MONITORED GUIDELINES

Drug	When to Sample	Therapeutic Levels	Usual Half-Life	Potentially Toxic Levels
Antibiotics				
Gentamicin	30 min after 30 min infusion Trough: <0.5 h before next dose	Peak: 4–10 mcg/mL Trough: <2 mcg/mL	2 h	Peak: >12 mcg/mL Trough: >2 mcg/mL
Tobramycin			2 h	
Amikacin		Peak: 20–35 mcg/mL Trough: <8 mcg/mL	2 h	Peak: >35 mcg/mL Trough: >8 mcg/mL
Vancomycin	Peak: 1 h after 1 h infusion Trough: <0.5 h before next dose	Peak: 30–40 mcg/mL Trough: 5–10 mcg/mL	6–8 h	Peak: >80 mcg/mL Trough: >13 mcg/mL
Anticonvulsants				
Carbamazepine	Trough: just before next oral dose In combination with other anticonvulsants	4–12 mcg/mL 4–8 mcg/mL	15–20 h	>12 mcg/mL
Ethosuximide	Trough: just before next oral dose	40–100 mcg/mL	30–60 h	>100 mcg/mL
Phenobarbital	Trough: just before next dose	15–40 mcg/mL	40–120 h	>40 mcg/mL
Phenytoin Free phenytoin	Trough: just before next dose Draw at same time as total level	10–20 mcg/mL 1–2 mcg/mL	Concentration dependent	>20 mcg/mL
Primidone	Trough: just before next dose (Note: Primidone is metabolized to phenobarb, order levels separately)	5–12 mcg/mL	10–12 h	>12 mcg/mL
Valproic acid	Trough: just before next dose	50–100 mcg/mL	5–20 h	>100 mcg/mL
Bronchodilators				
Aminophylline (I.V.)	18–24 h after starting or changing a maintenance dose given as a constant infusion	10–20 mcg/mL	Nonsmoking adult: 8 h smoking adults: 4 h	>20 mcg/mL
Theophylline (P.O.)	Peak levels: not recommended Trough level: just before next dose	10–20 mcg/mL		

(continued)

Drug	When to Sample	Therapeutic Levels	Usual Half–Life	Potentially Toxic Levels
Cardiovascular Agents				
Digoxin	Trough: just before next dose (levels drawn earlier than 6 h after a dose will be artificially elevated)	0.5–2 ng/mL	36 h	>2 ng/mL
Lidocaine	Steady–state levels are usually achieved after 6–12 h	1.2–5.0 mcg/mL	1.5 h	>6 mcg/mL
Procainamide	Trough: just before next oral dose I.V.: 6–12 h after infusion started Combined procainamide plus NAPA	4–10 mcg/mL NAPA: 6–10 h 5–30 mcg/mL	Procain: 2.7–5 h >30 (NAPA + procain)	>10 mcg/mL
Quinidine	Trough: just before next oral dose	2–5 mcg/mL	6 h	>10 mcg/mL
Other Agents				
Amitriptyline plus nortriptyline	Trough: just before next dose	100–250 ng/mL		
Nortriptyline	Trough: just before next dose	50–150 ng/mL		
Lithium	Trough: just before next dose	0.6–1.6 mEq/mL	18–20 h	>3 mEq/mL
Imipramine plus desipramine	Trough: just before next dose	150–250 ng/mL		
Desipramine	Trough: just before next dose	125–160 ng/mL		
Methotrexate	By protocol	<0.5 μmol/L after 48 h		
Cyclosporine	Trough: just before next dose	Highly variable Renal: 50–250 ng/mL (RIA) Hepatic: 150–400 ng/mL		

NORMAL LABORATORY VALUES FOR ADULTS

CHEMISTRY

Lab Test		Normal Values	Lab Test		Normal Values
Chemistry, Routine			**Thyroid Function**		
Albumin		3.5-5.0 g/dL	FTI (free thyroxine index)		4.5-12.0
Bilirubin, conjugated		0-0.2 mg/dL	T_3 resin uptake		25%-35%
Bilirubin, total		0.2-1.2 mg/dL	T_3 (tri-iodothyronine)		70-200 ng/dL
Blood urea nitrogen		8-23 mg/dL	T_4 (thyroxine)		4.0-11.0 μg/dL
Calcium		8.4-10.3 mg/dL			
Creatinine		0.5-1.2 mg/dL	**Others**		
Glucose		65-110 mg/dL	Ammonia, plasma		20-60 μg/dL
Phosphorus		2.8-4.5 mg/dL	Amylase, serum		44-128 units/L
Protein, total		6.0-8.0 g/dL	Calcium, ionized		4.6-5.2 mg/dL
Uric acid	male	3.5-7.2 mg/dL	Cholesterol		140-230 mg/dL
	female	2.6-6.5 mg/dL	Iron, serum		50-170 μg/dL
			Lactate, serum		1.4-3.9 mEq/L
Electrolytes			Lipase		10-208 units/L
Chlorides		100-110 mEq/L	Magnesium		1.5-2.5 mg/dL
CO_2		23-31 mEq/L	Oncotic pressure		22-28 mm Hg
Potassium		3.5-5.0 mEq/L	Osmolality		280-300 mOsm/kg
Sodium		136-146 mEq/L	Serum ferritin	male	25-400 ng/mL
Anion gap		5-14 mEq/L		female	10-150 ng/mL
			TIBC		270-390 μg/dL
Enzymes			Triglycerides		50-150 mg/dL
Alk phos	male	34-110 units/L			
	female	24-100 units/L			
ALT		5-35 units/L			
AST		5-35 units/L			
CPK	male	0-206 units/L			
	female	0-175 units/L			
LDH		50-200 units/L			

HEMATOLOGY

Hematocrit	male	40%-52%	Sed rate	male	0-10 mm/h
	female	35%-47%	(Westergren)	female	0-20 mm/h
Hemoglobin	male	13.5-17.5 g/dL	WBC count		4.5-11.0 10^3/mm^3
	female	11.5-16.0 g/dL	WBC differential		
MCH		27-34 pg	Bands		2%-8%
MCV		82-100 fL	Basophils		0%-2%
Platelet count		150-450 10^3/mm^3	Eosinophils		0%-4%
RBC count	male	4.5-5.9 10^6/mm^3	Lymphocytes		20%-45%
	female	4.0-4.9 10^6/mm^3	Monocytes		2%-8%
Reticulocyte count		0.5%-1.5%	Neutrophils		40%-70%

BLOOD GASES

	Arterial	Venous
Base excess	-3.0 to +3.0 mEq/L	-5.0 to +5.0 mEq/L
HCO_3	18-25 mEq/L	18-25 mEq/L
O_2 saturation	90-98%	60-85%
pCO_2	34-45 mm Hg	35-52 mm Hg
pH	7.35-7.45	7.32-7.42
pO_2	80-95 mm Hg	30-48 mm Hg
TCO_2	23-29 mEq/L	24-30 mEq/L

Weight/Volume Equivalents

1 mg/dL = 10 mcg/mL   1 ppm = 1 mg/L
1 mg/dL = 1 mg%   1 mcg/mL = 1 mg/L

APPENDIX

The effects of aging on laboratory parameters has not been fully elucidated. While some alterations in values have been associated with increased age, no reference values have been established for the elderly. The following changes may be seen in elderly patients:

Alkaline phosphatase	↑
Albumin	↓
Uric acid	↑ (possible)
Creatinine clearance	↓
BUN	↑
ESR	↑
WBC	↓
Mg++	↓
Hemoglobin	↓
Urine Spec Gravity	↓
2-hour postprandial blood glucose	↑

References

Cavalieri TA, Chopra A, and Bryman PN, "When Outside the Norm Is Normal: Interpreting Lab Data in the Aged," *Geriatrics*, 1992, 47(5):66-70.

Fraser CG, "Age-Related Changes in Laboratory Test Results, Clinical Implications," *Drugs & Aging*, 1993, 3(3):246-57.

Hodkinson HM, "Alterations of Laboratory Findings," *Principles of Geriatric Medicine and Gerontology*, 2nd ed, Hazzard WR, Andres R, Bierman EL, et al, eds, New York, NY: McGraw-Hill, 1990, 241-6.

Kelso T, "Laboratory Values in the Elderly, Are They Different?" *Emergency Med Clin N Am*, 1990, 8(2):241-54.

ALLERGIC SKIN REACTIONS TO DRUGS

Skin eruptions are the most common clinically observed form of drug "allergy". Cutaneous manifestations of hypersensitivity may include pruritus, urticaria, and angioedema; maculopapular, morbilliform, or erythematous rashes; erythema multiforme; eczema; erythema nodosum; photosensitivity reactions; and fixed drug eruptions. The most severe drug-related reactions are exfoliative dermatitis and vesiculobullous eruptions such as the Stevens-Johnson syndrome and toxic epidermal necrolysis (Lyell's syndrome). This table lists the incidence of drugs associated with cutaneous manifestations reported in 22,227 consecutive medical inpatients in the Boston Collaborative Drug Surveillance Program.

Drug	Reaction per 1000 Recipients
Sulfamethoxazole and trimethoprim	59
Ampicillin	52
Semisynthetic penicillins	36
Blood, whole human	35
Corticotropin	28
Erythromycin	23
Sulfisoxazole	17
Penicillin G	16
Gentamicin sulfate	16
Practolol	16
Cephalosporins	13
Quinidine	13
Plasma protein fraction	12
Dipyrone	11
Mercurial diuretics	9.5
Nitrofurantoin	9.1
Packed RBCs	8.1
Heparin	7.7
Chloramphenicol	6.8
Trimethobenzamide	6.6
Phenazopyridine	6.5
Methenamine	6.4
Nitrazepam	6.3
Barbiturates	4.7
Glutethimide	4.5
Indomethacin	4.4
Chlordiazepoxide	4.2
Metoclopramide	4.0
Diazepam	3.8
Propoxyphene	3.4
Isoniazid	3.0
Guaifenesin and theophylline	2.9
Nystatin	2.9
Chlorothiazide	2.8
Furosemide	2.6
Isophane insulin suspension	1.3
Phenytoin	1.1
Phytonadione	0.9
Flurazepam	0.5
Chloral hydrate	0.2

Reference

Patterson R and Anderson J, "Allergic Reactions to Drugs and Biologic Agents", *JAMA*, 1982, 248:2637-45.

SKIN TESTS FOR DELAYED HYPERSENSITIVITY

Candida 1:100
> Dose = 0.1 mL intradermally
> Can be used as a control antigen.

Coccidioidin 1:100
> Dose = 0.1 mL intradermally
> (apply with PPD **and** a control antigen)
> Mercury derivative used as a preservative for spherulin.

Histoplasmin 1:100
> Dose = 0.1 mL intradermally
> (yeast derived)

Multitest CMI (Candida, diphtheria toxoid, tetanus toxoid, Streptococcus, old tuberculin, Trichophyton, Proteus antigen, and negative control)
> Press loaded unit into the skin with sufficient pressure to puncture the skin and allow adequate penetration of all points

Mumps 40 cfu per mL
> Dose = 0.1 mL intradermally
> (contraindicated in patients allergic to eggs, egg products, or thimerosal)

Purified Protein Derivative 5 TU (PPD Mantoux Tuberculin)
> Dose = 0.1 mL intradermally
> A positive immune response is 5 mm or more of induration. Tuberculin positive patients must have an induration of 10 mm or more

Tetanus Toxoid 1:5
> Dose = 0.1 mL intradermally
> Can be used as a control antigen.

Tine Test
> Indication: Survey and screen for exposure to tuberculosis (grasp forearm firmly; stretch the skin of the volar surface tightly; apply the tines to the selected site; press for at least 1 second so that a circular halo impression is left on the skin)

General Information

1. Intradermal skin tests should be injected in the flexor surface of the forearm.

2. A pale wheal 6-10 mm in diameter should form over the needle tip as soon as the injection is administered. If no bleb forms, the injection must be repeated.

3. Space skin tests at least 2 inches apart to prevent reactions from overlapping.

4. Read skin tests for diameter of induration and presence of erythema at 24, 48, and 72 hours. After injection, maximal responses usually occur at 48 hours. Maximal responses to mumps or coccidioidin may occur at 24 hours.

5. False-negative results may occur in patients with malnutrition, viral infections, febrile illnesses, immunodeficiency disorders, severe disseminated infections, uremia, patients who have received immunosuppressive therapy (steroids, antineoplastic agents), patients who have received a recent live attenuated virus vaccine (MMR, measles), or subdermal injection of the antigen.

6. False-positive results may occur in patients sensitive to ingredients in the skin test solution such as thimerosal, due to cross sensitivity between similar antigens, or with improper interpretation of skin test.

7. Side effects are pain, blisters, extensive erythema and necrosis at the injection site.

   *Emergency equipment and epinephrine should be readily available to treat severe allergic reactions that may occur.

8. With initial PPD skin testing, the elderly frequently exhibit anergy; therefore, the 2-step PPD is recommended. For example, if initial PPD is negative, repeat test with 5 TU PPD 2-4 weeks later.

Recommended Interpretation of Skin Test Reactions

Reaction	Local Reaction	
	After Intradermal Injections of Antigens	After Dinitrochlorobenzene
1+	Erythema >10 mm and/or induration >1-5 mm	Erythema and/or induration covering <½ area of dose site
2+	Induration 6-10 mm	Induration covering >½ area of dose site
3+	Induration 11-20 mm	Vesiculation and induration at dose site or spontaneous flare at days 7-14 at the site
4+	Induration >20 mm	Bulla or ulceration at dose site or spontaneous flare at days 7-14 at the site

References

Ahmed AR and Blose DA, "Delayed-Type Hypersensitivity Skin Testing, A Review," *Arch Dermatol*, 1983, 119:934-45.

Gordon EG, Krouse HA, Kinney JL, et al, "Delayed Cutaneous Hypersensitivity in Normals: Choice of Antigens and Comparison to *in vitro* Assays of Cell-Mediated Immunity," *J Allergy Clin Immunol*, 1983, 72:487-94.

Sokal JE, "Measurement of Delayed Skin-Test Responses," *N Engl J Med*, 1975, 293:501-2.

OVERDOSE AND TOXICOLOGY INFORMATION*

Drug or Drug Class	Signs/Symptoms	Treatment/Comments
Acetaminophen	Generally asymptomatic	Assess severity of ingestion; adult doses ≥140 mg/kg are thought to be toxic. Obtain serum concentration ≥4 hours post ingestion and use acetaminophen nomogram to evaluate need for acetylcysteine. Gastric decontamination within 2-4 hours after ingestion. May administer activated charcoal for one dose, this may decrease absorption of acetylcysteine if given within one hour of acetylcysteine. For unknown ingested quantities and for significant ingestion give acetylcysteine orally (diluted 1:4 with juice or carbonated beverage); initial: 140 mg/kg then give 70 mg/kg every 4 hours for 17 doses.

Acetaminophen (μg/mL plasma)

500 —
200 —
150 —
100 —
50 —
10 —
5 —
1 —

Probable hepatic toxicity

Possible hepatic toxicity

Hepatic toxicity unlikely   25%

4 8 12 16 20 24

Hours after ingestion

The Rumack-Matthew nomogram, relating expected severity of liver toxicity to serum acetaminophen concentrations. (From Smilkstein MJ et al, *Ann Emerg Med*, 1991, 10:1058.)

Drug or Drug Class	Signs/Symptoms	Treatment/Comments
Alpha-adrenergic blocking agents	Hypotension, drowsiness	Give activated charcoal, additional treatment is symptomatic; use I.V. fluids, dopamine, or norepinephrine to treat hypotension. Epinephrine may worsen hypotension due to beta effects.
Aminoglycosides	Ototoxicity, nephrotoxicity, neuromuscular toxicity	Hemodialysis or peritoneal dialysis may be useful in patients with decreased renal function; calcium may reverse the neuromuscular toxicity.
Anticholinergics, antihistamines	Coma, hallucinations, delirium, tachycardia, dry skin, urinary retention, dilated pupils	For life-threatening arrhythmias or seizures. Adults: 2 mg/dose physostigmine, may repeat 1-2 mg in 20 minutes and give 1-4 mg slow I.V. over 5-10 minutes if signs and symptoms recur (relatively contraindicated if QRS >0.1 msec).
Anticholinesterase agents	Nausea, vomiting, diarrhea, miosis, CNS depression, excessive salivation, excessive sweating, muscle weakness	Suction oral secretions, decontaminate skin, atropinize patient; atropine dose must be individualized Adults: Initial atropine dose: 1 mg; titrate dose upward; pralidoxime (2-PAM) may need to be added for moderate to severe intoxications.

*As for all overdoses and toxic ingestions, provide airway, breathing, and cardiac support, call local Poison Control Center; use appropriate general poisoning management and give general supportive therapy when needed (eg, I.V. fluids, blood pressure support, control seizures, etc). Consult more specific toxicology reference (eg, Poisondex®) for further information.

(continued)

Drug or Drug Class	Signs/Symptoms	Treatment/Comments
Barbiturates	Respiratory depression, circulatory collapse, bradycardia, hypotension, hypothermia, slurred speech, confusion, coma	Repeated oral doses of activated charcoal given every 3-6 hours will increase clearance. Adults: 30-60 g Assure GI motility, adequate hydration, and renal function. Urinary alkalinization with I.V. sodium bicarbonate will increase renal elimination of longer acting barbiturates (eg, phenobarbital)
Benzodiazepines	Respiratory depression, apnea (after rapid I.V.), hypoactive reflexes, hypotension, slurred speech, unsteady gait, coma	Dialysis is of limited value; support blood pressure and respiration until symptoms subside. Flumazenil: Initial dose: 0.2 mg given I.V. over 30 seconds. If further response is desired after 30 seconds, give 0.3 mg over another 30 seconds. Further doses of 0.5 mg can be given over 30 seconds at 1-minute intervals up to a total of 3 mg.
Beta-adrenergic blockers	Hypotension, bronchospasm, bradycardia, hypoglycemia, seizures	Activated charcoal; treat symptomatically; glucagon, atropine, isoproterenol, dobutamine, or cardiac pacing may be needed to treat bradycardia, conduction defects, or hypotension
Carbamazepine	Dizziness, drowsiness, ataxia, involuntary movements, opisthotonos, seizures, nausea, vomiting, agitation, nystagmus, coma, urinary retention, respiratory depression, tachycardia, arrhythmias	Use supportive therapy, general poisoning management as needed; use repeated oral doses of activated charcoal given every 3-6 hours to decrease serum concentrations; charcoal hemoperfusion may be needed; treat hypotension with I.V. fluids, dopamine, or norepinephrine, monitor EKG; diazepam may control convulsions but may exacerbate respiratory depression
Cardiac glycosides	Hyperkalemia may develop rapidly and result in life-threatening cardiac arrhythmias, progressive bradyarrhythmias, second or third degree heart block unresponsive to atropine, ventricular fibrillation, asystole	Obtain serum drug level, induce emesis or perform gastric lavage; give activated charcoal to reduce further absorption; atropine may reverse heart block, digoxin immune fab (digoxin specific antibody fragments) is used in serious cases, each 40 mg of digoxin immune fab binds with 0.6 mg of digoxin
Heparin	Severe hemorrhage	1 mg of protamine sulfate will neutralize approximately 90 units of heparin sodium (bovine) or 115 units of heparin sodium (porcine) or 100 units of heparin calcium (porcine)
Hydantoin derivatives	Nausea, vomiting, nystagmus, slurred speech, ataxia, coma	Gastric lavage or emesis; repeated oral doses of activated charcoal may increase clearance of phenytoin. Use 0.5-1 g/kg (30-60 g/dose) activated charcoal every 3-6 hours until nontoxic serum concentration is obtained; assure adequate GI motility, supportive therapy
Iron	Lethargy, nausea, vomiting, green or tarry stools, hypotension, weak rapid pulse, metabolic acidosis, shock, coma, hepatic necrosis, renal failure, local GI erosions	If immediately after ingestion and not already vomiting, give ipecac or lavage with saline solution; give deferoxamine mesylate I.V. at 15 mg/kg/hour in cases of severe poisoning (serum Fe >350 mcg/mL) until the urine color is normal, the patient is asymptomatic or a maximum daily dose of 8 g is reached; urine output should be maintained >2 mL/kg/hour to avoid hypovolemic shock
Isoniazid	Nausea, vomiting, blurred vision, CNS depression, intractable seizures, coma, metabolic acidosis	Control seizures with diazepam, give pyridoxine I.V. equal dose to the suspected overdose of isoniazid or up to 5 g empirically; give activated charcoal

(continued)

Drug or Drug Class	Signs/Symptoms	Treatment/Comments
Nonsteroidal anti-inflammatory drugs	Dizziness, abdominal pain, sweating, apnea, nystagmus, cyanosis, hypotension, coma, seizures (rarely)	Induce emesis; give activated charcoal via NG tube; provide symptomatic and supportive care
Opioids and morphine analogs	Respiratory depression, miosis, hypothermia, bradycardia, circulatory collapse, pulmonary edema, apnea	Establish airway and adequate ventilation; give naloxone 0.4 mg and titrate to a maximum of 10 mg; additional doses may be needed every 20-60 minutes. May need to institute continuous infusion, as duration of action of opiates can be longer than duration of action of naloxone
Phenothiazines	Deep, unarousable sleep, anticholinergic symptoms, extrapyramidal signs, diaphoresis, rigidity, tachycardia, cardiac dysrhythmias, hypotension	Activated charcoal; do **not** dialyze; use I.V. benztropine mesylate 1-2 mg/dose slowly over 3-6 minutes for extrapyramidal signs; use I.V. fluids and norepinephrine to treat hypotension; avoid epinephrine which may cause hypotension due to phenothiazine-induced alpha-adrenergic blockade and unopposed epinephrine B_2 action; use benzodiazepines for seizure management and to decrease rigidity
Salicylates	Nausea, vomiting, respiratory alkalosis, hyperthermia, dehydration, hyperapnea, tinnitus, headache, dizziness, metabolic acidosis, coma	Induce emesis or gastric lavage immediately; give several doses of activated charcoal, rehydrate and use sodium bicarbonate to correct metabolic acidosis and enhance renal elimination by alkalinizing the urine; give supplemental potassium after renal function has been determined to be adequate. Monitor electrolytes; obtain stat serum salicylate level and follow
Tricyclic antidepressants	Agitation, confusion, hallucinations, urinary retention, hypothermia, hypotension, tachycardia, arrhythmias, seizures	Give activated charcoal ± lavage; use sodium bicarbonate for QRS >0.1 msec; I.V. fluids and norepinephrine may be used for hypotension; benzodiazepines may be used for seizure management
Warfarin	Internal or external hemorrhage, hematuria	For moderate overdoses, give oral, S.C., or I.D., or slow I.V. (I.V. associated with anaphylactoid reactions) phytonadione; usual dose: 2.5-10 mg, adjust per prothrombin time; for severe hemorrhage, give fresh frozen plasma or whole blood
Xanthine derivatives	Vomiting, abdominal pain, bloody diarrhea, tachycardia, extrasystoles, tachypnea, tonic/clonic seizures	Give activated charcoal orally; repeated oral doses of activated charcoal increase clearance; use 0.5-1 g/kg (30-60 g/dose) of activated charcoal every 1-4 hours (depending on the severity of ingestion) until nontoxic serum concentrations are obtained. Assure adequate GI motility, supportive therapy; charcoal hemoperfusion or hemodialysis can also be effective in decreasing serum concentrations and should be used if the serum concentration approaches 90-100 mcg/mL in acute overdoses

NEUTRALIZING CAPACITY OF COMMONLY USED ANTACIDS

Antacid*	Neutralizing Capacity†	Volume to Give 80 mEq of Neutralizing Capacity (mL)
Ducon®[1,3,6]	7.04	11.4
Maalox® TC[1,6,10]	4.2	19
Mylanta®-II[1,6,10]	4.14	19.3
Delcid®[1,6]	4.1	19.5
Titralac®[1,9]	3.87	20.7
Camalox®[1,3,6]	3.59	22.3
Gelusil-II®[1,6,10]	3	26.7
Basaljel® ES[1]	2.9	27.6
Aludrox®[1,6]	2.81	28.5
Maalox®[1,6]	2.58	31
Creamalin®[1,6]	2.57	31.1
Di-Gel®[1,6,10]	2.45	32.7
Mylanta®[1,6,10]	2.38	33.6
Silain®-Gel[1,6,10]	2.31	34.6
Maalox® Plus[1,6,10]	2.3	34.8
Marblen®[1,3,5,7,8]	2.28	35.1
Wingel®[1,6]	2.25	35.6
Gelusil-M®[1,6,8]	2.23	35.9
Riopan®[1,6]	2.21	36.2
Gelusil®[1,6,10]	2.2	36.4
Amphojel®[1]	1.93	41.5
Riopan Plus®[1,6,10]	1.8	44.4
A-M-T[1,8]	1.79	44.7
Kolantyl® Gel[1,6,11,12]	1.69	47.3
Trisogel®[1,8]	1.65	48.5
Malcogel®[1,8]	1.59	50.3
Robalate®[13]	1.13	70.3
Phosphaljel®[2]	0.42	190.5

*Ingredients

1. Aluminum hydroxide
2. Aluminum phosphate
3. Calcium carbonate
4. Calcium hydroxide
5. Magnesium carbonate
6. Magnesium hydroxide
7. Magnesium phosphate
8. Magnesium trisilicate
9. Glycine
10. Simethicone
11. Methyl cellulose
12. Bentyl
13. Dihydroxyaluminum aminoacetate

†Neutralizing capacity — based on an *in vitro* test where an mEq of antacid is defined by the mEq of HCl is required to keep the antacid suspension at pH = 3 for 2 hours.

Adapted from Fordtran JS, et al, *N Engl J Med*, 1975, 288(18):923 and Drake and Hollander, *Ann Intern Med*, 1981, 94:215.

Penicillins, Penicillin-Related Antibiotics & Other Antibiotics

KEY TO TABLE

A — Recommended drug therapy

B — Alternate drug therapy

C — Organism is usually or always sensitive to this agent

D — Organism portrays variable sensitivity to this agent

(Blank) This drug should not be used for this organism or insufficient data is available

GRAM-POSITIVE AEROBES

		Listeria monocytogenes (Bacilli)	Corynebacterium jeikeium	Corynebacterium sp.	Streptococcus, Viridans Group (Cocci)	Streptococcus pneumoniae	Streptococcus bovis (Group D)	Enterococcus sp. (Group D)	Streptococcus agalactiae (Group B)	Streptococcus pyogenes (Group A)	Staph. epidermidis Methicillin-Resistant	Staph. epidermidis Methicillin-Susceptible	Staph. aureus Methicillin-Resistant	Staph. aureus Methicillin-Susceptible
Penicillins	Amoxicillin				C	C	C		C	C				
	Ampicillin	A			C	C	C	A	C	C				
	Penicillin G	A	B	B	A	A	A	A	A	A				
	Penicillin V				C	C	C	C	C	C				
	Azlocillin													
	Mezlocillin				D	C	D	D	C	C				
	Piperacillin				D	C	D	C	C	C				
	Ticarcillin				D	C	D		C	C				
	Cloxacillin				D							A		A
	Dicloxacillin				D							A		A
	Methicillin				D							A		A
	Nafcillin				D							A		A
	Oxacillin				D							A		A
Penicillin-Related Antibiotics	Amoxicillin/Clavulanate	C			C	C	C	C	C	C		C		C
	Ampicillin/Sulbactam	C			C	C	C	C	C	C		C		C
	Ticarcillin/Clavulanate				C	C	C	D	C	C		C		C
	Aztreonam													
	Imipenem/Cilastatin				C	C	C	D	C	C		C		C
	Piperacillin/Tazobactam				C	C	C	C	C	C		C		C
Other Antibiotics	Chloramphenicol	C				B		D						
	Clindamycin		D	D	C	D			C	C		B		B
	Co-trimoxazole	B			C						B	C	B	C
	Metronidazole													
	Rifampin			D							A	C	A	C
	Sulfonamides													
	Tetracyclines	C			C	C		C					A	D
	Vancomycin	D	A		B	B	B	B	B	B	A	B	A	B
UTI Agents	Indanyl Carbenicillin							D						
	Nitrofurantoin							D						

Penicillins, Penicillin-Related Antibiotics & Other Antibiotics

KEY TO TABLE

A Recommended drug therapy

B Alternate drug therapy

C Organism is usually or always sensitive to this agent

D Organism portrays variable sensitivity to this agent

(Blank) This drug should not be used for this organism or insufficient data is available

| | | GRAM-NEGATIVE AEROBES | | | | | | | | | | | |
| | | Enteric bacilli | | | | | | | | | | Cocci | | |
Class	Drug	Yersinia enterocolitica	Shigella sp.	Serratia sp.	Salmonella sp.	Proteus sp.	Proteus mirabilis	Klebsiella pneumoniae	Escherichia coli	Enterobacter sp.[1]	Citrobacter sp.[1]	Neisseria meningitidis	Neisseria gonorrhoeae	Moraxella (Branhamella) catarrhalis
Penicillin	Amoxicillin				B		A		C			C	D	
Penicillin	Ampicillin	A			B		A		A			C	D	
Penicillin	Penicillin G											A	D	
Penicillin	Penicillin V												D	
Penicillin	Azlocillin													
Penicillin	Mezlocillin			A		B	C	B	C	A	A		D	
Penicillin	Piperacillin			A		B	C	B	C	A	A		D	
Penicillin	Ticarcillin			A		B	C	D	C	A	A		D	
Penicillin	Cloxacillin													
Penicillin	Dicloxacillin													
Penicillin	Methicillin													
Penicillin	Nafcillin													
Penicillin	Oxacillin													
Penicillin-Related Antibiotics	Amoxicillin/Clavulanate				C		C	C	C			C	C	A
Penicillin-Related Antibiotics	Ampicillin/Sulbactam	C			C		C	C	C			C	C	C
Penicillin-Related Antibiotics	Ticarcillin/Clavulanate			A	C	B	C	B	C	A	A	C	C	C
Penicillin-Related Antibiotics	Aztreonam			B	C	C	C	B	C	A	C		C	C
Penicillin-Related Antibiotics	Imipenem/Cilastatin			B	C	B	C	B	C	B	B	D	C	C
Penicillin-Related Antibiotics	Piperacillin/Tazobactam			A	C	B	C	B	C	A	A	C	C	C
Other Antibiotics	Chloramphenicol	C			B				C			B		
Other Antibiotics	Clindamycin													
Other Antibiotics	Co-trimoxazole	C	A	C	B	C	B	C	A	C	C			A
Other Antibiotics	Metronidazole													
Other Antibiotics	Rifampin											D		
Other Antibiotics	Sulfonamides		C			C		C	C	C		D		
Other Antibiotics	Tetracyclines	C	C					C	C		D		C	B	C
Other Antibiotics	Vancomycin													
UTI Agents	Indanyl Carbenicillin			C		C	C	C	C	C	C			
UTI Agents	Nitrofurantoin							C	C	C	C			

[1] *Citrobacter freundii, Citrobacter diversus, Enterobacter cloacae* and *Enterobacter aerogenes* often have significantly different antibiotic sensitivity patterns. Speciation and susceptibility testing are particularly important

Penicillins, Penicillin-Related Antibiotics & Other Antibiotics

KEY TO TABLE

A Recommended drug therapy

B Alternate drug therapy

C Organism is usually or always sensitive to this agent

D Organism portrays variable sensitivity to this agent

(Blank) This drug should not be used for this organism or insufficient data is available

Class	Antibiotic	Vibrio cholerae	Xanthomonas maltophilia	Pseudomonas aeruginosa	Pasteurella multocida	Legionella pneumophila	Haemophilus influenzae	Haemophilus ducreyi	Gardnerella vaginalis	Campylobacter jejuni	Brucella sp.	Bordetella pertussis	Acinetobacter sp.
Penicillin	Amoxicillin				C		B		C				
	Ampicillin				C		B		B	D			
	Penicillin G				A								
	Penicillin V				C								
	Azlocillin												
	Mezlocillin			A	C		D						A
	Piperacillin			A	C		D						A
	Ticarcillin			A	C		D						A
	Cloxacillin												
	Dicloxacillin												
	Methicillin												
	Nafcillin												
	Oxacillin												
Penicillin-Related Antibiotics	Amoxicillin/Clavulanate				B		B	B	C				C
	Ampicillin/Sulbactam				B		C	C	C				C
	Ticarcillin/Clavulanate		B	A	C		C						A
	Aztreonam			C			C						B
	Imipenem/Cilastatin			A			C						B
	Piperacillin/Tazobactam			A	C		C						A
Other Antibiotics	Chloramphenicol	C			C		B			C	C		
	Clindamycin								C	C			
	Co-trimoxazole	A	A				A	B			B	A	
	Metronidazole									A			
	Rifampin					A	D					A	
	Sulfonamides				C			C		C			
	Tetracyclines	A			C		C	C		A	C		
	Vancomycin												
UTI Agents	Indanyl Carbenicillin			D									C
	Nitrofurantoin												

784

Penicillins, Penicillin-Related Antibiotics & Other Antibiotics

KEY TO TABLE

A — Recommended drug therapy

B — Alternate drug therapy

C — Organism is usually or always sensitive to this agent

D — Organism portrays variable sensitivity to this agent

(Blank) This drug should not be used for this organism or insufficient data is available

		OTHERS									ANAEROBES			
											Gram -	Gram +		
		Treponema pallidum	Leptospira sp.	Borrelia burgdorferi (Lyme disease)	Rickettsia sp.	Ureaplasma urealyticum	Mycoplasma pneumoniae	Chlamydia trachomatis	Chlamydia psittaci	Chlamydia pneumoniae (TWAR)	Bacteroides sp.	Streptococcus, anaerobic	Clostridium perfringens	Clostridium difficile[2]
Penicillin	Amoxicillin			B							D	C	D	
	Ampicillin			B							C	C	D	
	Penicillin G	A	A	B							C	A	A	
	Penicillin V	C	C	B							C	C	C	
	Azlocillin													
	Mezlocillin										C	C	C	
	Piperacillin										C	C	C	
	Ticarcillin										C	C	C	
	Cloxacillin													
	Dicloxacillin													
	Methicillin													
	Nafcillin													
	Oxacillin													
Penicillin-Related Antibiotics	Amoxicillin/Clavulanate										C	C	C	
	Ampicillin/Sulbactam										C	C	C	
	Ticarcillin/Clavulanate										C	C	C	
	Aztreonam													
	Imipenem/Cilastatin										C	C	B	
	Piperacillin/Tazobactam										C	C	C	
Other Antibiotics	Chloramphenicol				A						C	C	C	D
	Clindamycin										A	B	B	
	Co-trimoxazole													
	Metronidazole										A	D	A	A
	Rifampin													
	Sulfonamides							D						
	Tetracyclines	B	B	A	A	A	A	A	B	B	D	C	C	
	Vancomycin											B		B
UTI Agents	Indanyl Carbenicillin													
	Nitrofurantoin													

[2] Vancomycin is effective orally only.

Cephalosporins, Aminoglycosides, Macrolides & Quinolones

KEY TO TABLE

- **A** Recommended drug therapy
- **B** Alternate drug therapy
- **C** Organism is usually or always sensitive to this agent
- **D** Organism portrays variable sensitivity to this agent
- **(Blank)** This drug should not be used for this organism or insufficient data is available

GRAM-POSITIVE AEROBES

Class	Drug	Listeria monocytogenes[a]	Corynebacterium jeikeium	Corynebacterium sp.	Streptococcus, Viridans Group	Streptococcus pneumoniae	Streptococcus bovis (Group D)	Enterococcus sp. (Group D)	Streptococcus pyogenes (Group A)	Streptococcus agalactiae (Group B)	Staph. epidermidis: Methicillin-Resistant[a]	Staph. epidermidis: Methicillin-Susceptible	Staph. aureus: Methicillin-Resistant[a]	Staph. aureus: Methicillin-Susceptible
1st Generation	Cefadroxil				B	B	C		B	B		B		B
1st Generation	Cefazolin				B	B	C		B	B		B		B
1st Generation	Cephalexin				B	B	C		B	B		B		B
1st Generation	Cephalothin				B	B	C		B	B		B		B
1st Generation	Cephapirin				B	B	C		B	B		B		B
1st Generation	Cephradine				B	B	C		B	B		B		B
2nd Generation and others	Cefaclor				C	C	C		C	C		D		D
2nd Generation and others	Cefamandole				C	C	C		C	C		C		C
2nd Generation and others	Cefmetazole				C	C	C		C	C		D		D
2nd Generation and others	Cefonicid				C	C	C		C	C		D		D
2nd Generation and others	Cefotetan				C	C	C		C	C		D		D
2nd Generation and others	Cefoxitin				C	C	C		C	C		D		D
2nd Generation and others	Cefpodoxime Proxetil				C	C	C		C	C		D		D
2nd Generation and others	Cefprozil				C	C	D		C	C				D
2nd Generation and others	Cefuroxime				C	C	C		C	C		D		D
2nd Generation and others	Cefuroxime Axetil				C	C			C	C		C		C
2nd Generation and others	Loracarbef				C	C	D		C	C		C		C
3rd Generation	Cefixime				D	D			C	C				
3rd Generation	Cefoperazone				D	D	C		C	C		D		D
3rd Generation	Cefotaxime				D	D	C		C	C		D		D
3rd Generation	Ceftazidime				D		D		D	D				
3rd Generation	Ceftizoxime				D	D	C		C	C		D		D
3rd Generation	Ceftriaxone				C	C	C		C	C		D		D
Aminoglycosides	Amikacin	C	C				D	D						
Aminoglycosides	Gentamicin	A	B		A		D	A			A	D	A	D
Aminoglycosides	Netilmicin	C	C					C						
Aminoglycosides	Streptomycin						D	C						
Aminoglycosides	Tobramycin	C	C					D						D
Macrolides	Azithromycin	C			C	C			C	C				C
Macrolides	Clarithromycin	C			C	C			C	C				C
Macrolides	Erythromycin	C	C	A	C	B			B	B				C
Quinolones	Lomefloxacin		D		D	D	D	D	D	D	D	D	D	D
Quinolones	Ciprofloxacin		D		D	D	D	D	D	D	D	D	D	D
Quinolones	Norfloxacin							D	D					
Quinolones	Ofloxacin		D		D	D	D	D	D	D	D	D	D	D

Cephalosporins, Aminoglycosides, Macrolides & Quinolones

KEY TO TABLE

A Recommended drug therapy

B Alternate drug therapy

C Organism is usually or always sensitive to this agent

D Organism portrays variable sensitivity to this agent

(Blank) This drug should not be used for this organism or insufficient data is available

Class	Drug	Vibrio cholerae	Xanthomonas maltophilia	Pseudomonas aeruginosa	Pasteurella multocida	Legionella pneumophila	Haemophilus influenzae	Haemophilus ducreyi	Campylobacter jejuni	Gardnerella vaginalis	Brucella sp.	Bordetella pertussis	Acinetobacter sp.
1st Generation	Cefadroxil						D						
	Cefazolin						D						
	Cephalexin						D						
	Cephalothin						D						
	Cephapirin						D						
	Cephradine						D						
2nd Generation and others	Cefaclor						B						
	Cefamandole				C		B						
	Cefmetazole				D		C						
	Cefonicid						C						
	Cefotetan				D		C						
	Cefoxitin				D		C						
	Cefpodoxime Proxetil						B						
	Cefprozil						B						
	Cefuroxime						B						
	Cefuroxime Axetil				D		B						
	Loracarbef						B						
3rd Generation	Cefixime						A						D
	Cefoperazone		D	D	C		A		C				D
	Cefotaxime			D	C				C				A
	Ceftazidime			D	A				C				A
	Ceftizoxime			D	C				C				A
	Ceftriaxone			D	C				A				A
Aminoglycosides	Amikacin			C	A				C	C			C
	Gentamicin			C	A				C	C	C		C
	Netilmicin			C	A				C	C			C
	Streptomycin										C		
	Tobramycin			C	A				C	C			C
Macrolides	Azithromycin					D	B	C	C		C	C	
	Clarithromycin					D	B	C			C	C	
	Erythromycin					D	A		C		A	A	
Quinolones	Lomefloxacin	C	C	D	C		C	C	D	B	C		D
	Ciprofloxacin	C	B	A	C	B	C	B	C	B	C		C
	Norfloxacin			C						B			D
	Ofloxacin	C	B	D	C	C	C	C	C	C	B	C	C

Cephalosporins, Aminoglycosides, Macrolides & Quinolones

KEY TO TABLE

A Recommended drug therapy

B Alternate drug therapy

C Organism is usually or always sensitive to this agent

D Organism portrays variable sensitivity to this agent

(Blank) This drug should not be used for this organism or insufficient data is available

	Drug	Treponema pallidum	Leptospira sp.	Borrelia burgdorferi (Lyme disease)	Rickettsia sp.	Ureaplasma urealyticum	Mycoplasma pneumoniae	Chlamydia trachomatis	Chlamydia pneumoniae (TWAR)	Chlamydia psittaci	Bacteroides sp. (Gram −)	Streptococcus, anaerobic (Gram +)	Clostridium perfringens	Clostridium difficile [2]
1st Generation	Cefadroxil											B		
	Cefazolin											B		
	Cephalexin											B		
	Cephalothin											B		
	Cephapirin											B		
	Cephradine											B		
2nd Generation and others	Cefaclor													
	Cefamandole													
	Cefmetazole										C	C	C	
	Cefonicid													
	Cefotetan										B	C	C	
	Cefoxitin										B	C	C	
	Cefpodoxime Proxetil													
	Cefprozil													
	Cefuroxime											C	C	
	Cefuroxime Axetil													
	Loracarbef													
3rd Generation	Cefixime													
	Cefoperazone												D	
	Cefotaxime		C								D	C	C	
	Ceftazidime												D	
	Ceftizoxime		C								D	C	C	
	Ceftriaxone	C	A									C		
Aminoglycosides	Amikacin													
	Gentamicin													
	Netilmicin													
	Streptomycin													
	Tobramycin													
Macrolides	Azithromycin	D		C			B	C	C	C		D	D	
	Clarithromycin	D		D			B	C	C	C		D	D	
	Erythromycin	D		C		A	A	A	A	A		D	D	
Quinolones	Lomefloxacin					D	D	D						
	Ciprofloxacin				D	D	D	D						
	Norfloxacin													
	Ofloxacin					D	D	D	C					

[2] Vancomycin is effective orally only.

Cephalosporins, Aminoglycosides, Macrolides & Quinolones

KEY TO TABLE

- **A** Recommended drug therapy
- **B** Alternate drug therapy
- **C** Organism is usually or always sensitive to this agent
- **D** Organism portrays variable sensitivity to this agent
- (Blank) This drug should not be used for this organism or insufficient data is available

Class	Drug	Yersinia enterocolitica	Shigella sp.	Serratia sp.	Salmonella sp.	Proteus sp.	Proteus mirabilis	Klebsiella pneumoniae	Escherichia coli	Enterobacter sp.	Citrobacter sp.[1]	Neisseria meningitidis	Neisseria gonorrhoeae	Moraxella (Branhamella) catarrhalis
1st Generation	Cefadroxil						A	A	B					D
1st Generation	Cefazolin						A	A	B					D
1st Generation	Cephalexin						A	A	B					D
1st Generation	Cephalothin						A	A	B					D
1st Generation	Cephapirin						A	A	B					D
1st Generation	Cephradine						A	A	B					D
2nd Generation and others	Cefaclor						C	A	B				C	B
2nd Generation and others	Cefamandole					D	C	A	B				C	B
2nd Generation and others	Cefmetazole	D	C	C		D	C	A	B				C	B
2nd Generation and others	Cefonicid						C	A	B				C	B
2nd Generation and others	Cefotetan	C	C	C		D	C	A	B				C	B
2nd Generation and others	Cefoxitin				D	D	C	A	B				C	B
2nd Generation and others	Cefpodoxime Proxetil						C	A	B				C	B
2nd Generation and others	Cefprozil		C				C	D	B				C	B
2nd Generation and others	Cefuroxime	C	C			D	C	A	B				C	B
2nd Generation and others	Cefuroxime Axetil						C	A	B			C	C	B
2nd Generation and others	Loracarbef						C	C	B				C	B
3rd Generation	Cefixime		C	C		C	C	A	A				C	B
3rd Generation	Cefoperazone		B	A	A	A	C	A	A	A	A			B
3rd Generation	Cefotaxime	A	B	A	A	A	C	A	A	A	A	B	C	B
3rd Generation	Ceftazidime		B	A		A	C	A	A	A	A			B
3rd Generation	Ceftizoxime	A	B	A	A	A	C	A	A	A	A	B	C	B
3rd Generation	Ceftriaxone	A	B	A	A	A	C	A	A	A	A	B	A	B
Aminoglycosides	Amikacin	A		C			C	C	C	C	C			
Aminoglycosides	Gentamicin	A	D	C	D	C	C	C	C	C	C			
Aminoglycosides	Netilmicin	A	D	C	D	C	C	C	C	C	C			
Aminoglycosides	Streptomycin													
Aminoglycosides	Tobramycin	A		C	D	C	C	C	C	C	C			
Macrolides	Azithromycin												C	C
Macrolides	Clarithromycin												C	C
Macrolides	Erythromycin												D	C
Quinolones	Lomefloxacin	C	C	C	C	C	C	C	C	C	D	C	C	C
Quinolones	Ciprofloxacin	C	B	C	B	C	C	C	C	C	C	C	A	C
Quinolones	Norfloxacin	C	C	C	C	C	C	C	C	C	C	C		
Quinolones	Ofloxacin	C	C	C	C	C	C	C	C	C	C	C	A	C

Header: GRAM-NEGATIVE AEROBES — Enteric bacilli; Cocci

[1] Citrobacter freundii, Citrobacter diversus, Enterobacter cloacae and Enterobacter aerogenes often have significantly different antibiotic sensitivity patterns. Speciation and susceptibility testing are particularly important

PREVENTION OF BACTERIAL ENDOCARDITIS

Recommendations by the American Heart Association
(*JAMA*, December 12, 1990, 264:22)

Table 1. **Cardiac Conditions***

Endocarditis Prophylaxis Recommended

Prosthetic cardiac valves, including bioprosthetic and homograft valves

Previous bacterial endocarditis, even in the absence of heart disease

Most congenital cardiac malformations

Rheumatic and other acquired valvular dysfunction, even after valvular surgery

Hypertrophic cardiomyopathy

Mitral valve prolapse with valvular regurgitation

Endocarditis Prophylaxis Not Recommended

Isolated secundum atrial septal defect

Surgical repair without residua beyond 6 months of secundum atrial septal defect, ventricular septal defect, or patent ductus arteriosus

Previous coronary artery bypass graft surgery

Mitral valve prolapse without valvular regurgitation†

Physiologic, functional, or innocent heart murmurs

Previous Kawasaki disease without valvular dysfunction

Previous rheumatic fever without valvular dysfunction

Cardiac pacemakers and implanted defibrillators

---

*This table lists selected conditions but is not meant to be all-inclusive.

†Individuals who have a mitral valve prolapse associated with thickening and/or redundancy of the valve leaflets may be at increased risk for bacterial endocarditis, particularly men who are 45 years of age or older.

Table 2. **Dental or Surgical Procedures***

Endocarditis Prophylaxis Recommended

Dental procedures known to induce gingival or mucosal bleeding, including professional cleaning

Tonsillectomy and/or adenoidectomy

Surgical operations that involve intestinal or respiratory mucosa

Bronchoscopy with a rigid bronchoscope

Sclerotherapy for esophageal varices

Esophageal dilatation

Gallbladder surgery

Cystoscopy

Urethral dilatation

Urethral catheterization if urinary tract infection is present†

Urinary tract surgery if urinary tract infection is present†

Prostatic surgery

Incision and drainage of infected tissue†

Vaginal hysterectomy

Vaginal delivery in the presence of infection†

Endocarditis Prophylaxis Not Recommended‡

Dental procedures not likely to induce gingival bleeding, such as simple adjustment of orthodontic appliances or fillings above the gum line

Injection of local intraoral anesthetic (except intraligamentary injections)

Shedding of primary teeth

Tympanostomy tube insertion

Endotracheal intubation

Bronchoscopy with a flexible bronchoscope, with or without biopsy

Cardiac catheterization

Endoscopy with or without gastrointestinal biopsy

Cesarean section

In the absence of infection (for urethral catheterization, dilatation and curettage, uncomplicated vaginal delivery, therapeutic abortion, sterilization procedures, or insertion or removal of intrauterine devices

---

*This table lists selected conditions but is not meant to be all-inclusive.

†In addition to prophylactic regimen for genitourinary procedures, antibiotic therapy should be directed against the most likely bacterial pathogen.

‡In patients who have prosthetic heart valves, a previous history of endocarditis, or surgically constructed systemic-pulmonary shunts or conduits, physicians may choose to administer prophylactic antibiotics even for low-risk procedures that involve the lower respiratory, genitourinary, or gastrointestinal tracts.

Table 3. **Recommended Standard Prophylactic Regimen for Dental, Oral, or Upper Respiratory Tract Procedures in Patients Who Are at Risk***

Drug	Dosing Regimen
Standard Regimen	
Amoxicillin	3 g orally 1 hour before procedure; then 1.5 g 6 hours after initial dose
Amoxicillin/Penicillin-Allergic Patients	
Erythromycin or Clindamycin	Erythromycin ethylsuccinate, 800 mg, or erythromycin stearate, 1 g, orally 2 hours before procedure; then half the dose 6 hours after initial dose 300 mg orally 1 hour before procedure and 150 mg 6 hours after initial dose

*Includes those with prosthetic heart valves and other high-risk patients.

Table 4. **Alternate Prophylactic Regimens for Dental, Oral, or Upper Respiratory Tract Procedures in Patients Who Are at Risk**

Drug	Dosing Regimen
Patients Unable to Take Oral Medications	
Ampicillin	Intravenous or intramuscular administration of ampicillin, 2 g, 30 minutes before procedure; then intravenous or intramuscular administration of ampicillin, 1 g or oral administration of amoxicillin, 1.5 g, 6 hours after initial dose
Ampicillin/Amoxicillin/Penicillin-Allergic Patients Unable to Take Oral Medications	
Clindamycin	Intravenous administration of 300 mg 30 minutes before procedure and an intravenous or oral administration of 150 mg 6 hours after initial dose
Patients Considered High Risk and Not Candidates for Standard Regimen	
Ampicillin, gentamicin, and amoxicillin	Intravenous or intramuscular administration of ampicillin, 2 g, plus gentamicin, 1.5 mg/kg (not to exceed 80 mg), 30 minutes before procedure; followed by amoxicillin, 1.5 g, orally 6 hours after initial dose; alternatively, the parenteral regimen may be repeated 8 hours after initial dose
Ampicillin/Amoxicillin/Penicillin-Allergic Patients Considered High Risk	
Vancomycin	Intravenous administration of 1 g over 1 hour, starting 1 hour before procedure; no repeated dose necessary

Table 5. **Regimens for Genitourinary/Gastrointestinal Procedures**

Drug	Dosing Regimen
Standard Regimen	
Ampicillin, gentamicin, and amoxicillin	Intravenous or intramuscular administration of ampicillin, 2 g plus gentamicin, 1.5 mg/kg (not to exceed 80 mg), 30 minutes before procedure; followed by amoxicillin, 1.5 g orally 6 hours after initial dose; alternatively, the parenteral regimen may be repeated once 8 hours after initial dose
Ampicillin/Amoxicillin/Penicillin-Allergic Patient Regimen	
Vancomycin and gentamicin	Intravenous administration of vancomycin, 1 g over 1 hour plus intravenous or intramuscular administration of gentamicin, 1.5 mg/kg (not to exceed 80 mg), 1 hour before procedure; may be repeated once 8 hours after initial dose
Alternate Low-Risk Patient Regimen	
Amoxicillin	3 g orally 1 hour before procedure: then 1.5 g 6 hours after initial dose

TABLETS THAT CANNOT BE CRUSHED OR ALTERED

There are a variety of reasons for crushing tablets or capsule contents prior to administering to the patient. Patients may have nasogastric tubes which do not permit the administration of tablets or capsules; an oral solution for a particular medication may not be available from the manufacturer or readily prepared by pharmacy; patients may have difficulty swallowing capsules or tablets; or mixing of powdered medication with food or drink may make the drug more palatable.

Generally, medications which should not be crushed fall into one of the following categories.

- **Extended-Release Products**. The formulation of some tablets is specialized as to allow the medication within it to be slowly released into the body. This is sometimes accomplished by centering the drug within the core of the tablet, with a subsequent shedding of multiple layers around the core. Wax melts in the GI tract. Slow-K® is an example of this. Capsules may contain beads which have multiple layers which are slowly dissolved with time.

- **Medications Which Are Irritating to the Stomach**. Tablets which are irritating to the stomach may be enteric-coated which delays release of the drug until the time when it reaches the small intestine. Enteric-coated aspirin is an example of this.

- **Foul Tasting Medication**. Some drugs are quite unpleasant to taste so the manufacturer coats the tablet in a sugar coating to increase its palatability. By crushing the tablet, this sugar coating is lost and the patient tastes the unpleasant tasting medication.

- **Sublingual Medication**. Medication intended for use under the tongue should not be crushed. While it appears to be obvious, it is not always easy to determine if a medication is to be used sublingually. Sublingual medications should indicate on the package that they are intended for sublingual use.

- **Effervescent Tablets**. These are tablets which, when dropped into a liquid, quickly dissolve to yield a solution. Many effervescent tablets, when crushed, lose their ability to quickly dissolve.

Recommendations

1. It is not advisable to crush certain medications.

2. Consult individual monographs prior to crushing capsule or tablet.

3. If crushing a tablet or capsule is contraindicated, consult with your pharmacist to determine whether an oral solution exists or can be compounded.

Oral Dosage Forms That Should Not Be Crushed

Drug Product	Dosage Forms	Reasons/Comments
Accutane®	Capsule	Mucous membrane irritant
Acutrim®	Tablet	Slow release
Adalat® CC	Tablet	Slow release
Aerolate® SR, JR, III	Capsule	Slow release*†
Afrinol® Repetabs®	Tablet	Slow release
Anaplex SR	Capsule	Slow release
Ansaid®	Tablet	Taste‖
Allerest® 12-Hour	Caplet	Slow release
Artane® Sequels®	Capsule	Slow release*†
Arthritis Bayer Time Release	Capsule	Slow release
Asacol®	Tablet	Slow release
ASA Enseals®	Tablet	Enteric-coated
Asbron G® Inlay	Tablet	Multiple compressed tablet†
Aspirin Delayed-Release	Tablet	Enteric-coated
Atrohist Plus	Tablet	Slow release*
Atrohist Sprinkle	Capsule	Slow release
Azulfidine® EN-tabs®	Tablet	Enteric-coated
Baros	Tablet	Effervescent tablet¶
Betachron E-R	Capsule	Slow release
Betapen®-VK	Tablet	Taste‖
Biphetamine	Capsule	Slow release

(continued)

Drug Product	Dosage Forms	Reasons/Comments
Bisacodyl	Tablet	Enteric-coated‡
Bisco-Lax®	Tablet	Enteric-coated‡
Bontril SR	Capsule	Slow release
Breonesin®	Capsule	Liquid filled§
Brexin® LA	Capsule	Slow release
Bromfed®	Capsule	Slow release†
Bromfed-PD®	Capsule	Slow release†
Calan® SR	Tablet	Slow release♦
Cama Arthritis Pain Reliever	Tablet	Multiple compressed tablet
Carbiset-TR®	Tablet	Slow release
Cardizem®	Tablet	Slow release
Cardizem® CD	Capsule	Slow release*
Cardizem® SR	Capsule	Slow release*
Carter's Little Pills®	Tablet	Enteric-coated
Cefal Filmtab®	Tablet	Enteric-coated
Charcoal Plus	Tablet	Enteric-coated
Chloral Hydrate	Capsule	Note: Product is in liquid form within a special capsule†
Chlorphedrine SR	Capsule	Slow release
Chlorpheniramine Maleate Time Release	Capsule	Slow release
Chlor-Trimeton® 12-Hour Allergy	Tablet	Slow release†
Choledyl® SA	Tablet	Slow release†
Chromagen®	Capsule	Taste‖
Cipro™	Tablet	Taste‖
Cleocin®	Capsule	Taste†‖
Codimal-LA®	Capsule	Slow release
Codimal-LA® Half	Capsule	Slow release
Colace®	Capsule	Taste‖
Comhist® LA	Capsule	Slow release*
Compazine® Spansule®	Capsule	Slow release†
Congess SR, JR	Capsule	Slow release
Contac®	Capsule	Slow release*
Cotazym-S®	Capsule	Enteric-coated*
Creon®	Capsule	Enteric-coated*
Creon® 10 Minimicrospheres	Capsule	Enteric-coated*
Creon® 25	Capsule	Enteric-coated*
Dallergy®	Capsule	Slow release†
Dallergy-D®	Capsule	Slow release
Dallergy-JR®	Capsule	Slow release
Deconamine® SR	Capsule	Slow release†
Deconsal® II	Tablet	Slow release
Deconsal® Sprinkle	Capsule	Slow release*
Demazin® Repetabs®	Tablet	Slow release†
Depakene® ta>Capsule	Slow-release-mucous membrane irritant†	
Depakote®	Capsule	Enteric-coated
Desoxyn® Gradumets®	Tablet	Slow release
Desyrel®	Tablet	Taste‖
Dexatrim® Max Strength	Tablet	Slow release
Dexedrine® Spansule®	Capsule	Slow release
Diamox® Sequels®	Capsule	Slow release
Dilacor™ XR	Capsule	Slow release
Dilatrate SR	Capsule	Slow release
Dimetane® Extentab®	Tablet	Slow release†
Disobrom®	Tablet	Slow release
Disophrol® Chronotab®	Tablet	Slow release
Dital	Capsule	Slow release
Docusate	Capsule	Liquid filled§
Docusate with Casanthranol	Capsule	Liquid filled§
Donnatal® Extentab®	Tablet	Slow release†
Donnazyme	Tablet	Enteric-coated
Doxidan® liquigels	Capsule	Liquid filled§
Drisdol®	Capsule	Liquid filled§
Drixoral®	Tablet	Slow release†
Drixoral® Sinus	Tablet	Slow release
Dulcolax®	Tablet	Enteric-coated‡
Dura-Vent®	Tablet	Slow release
Dura-Vent®/A	Capsule	Slow release
Dura-Vent®/DA	Tablet	Slow release
Dura-Tap/PD®	Capsule	Slow release

(continued)

Drug Product	Dosage Forms	Reasons/Comments
Duratuss	Tablet	Slow release♦
Easprin®	Tablet	Enteric-coated
Ecotrin®	Tablet	Enteric-coated
E.E.S.® 400	Tablet	Enteric-coated†
Efidac/24®	Tablet	Slow release
Elixophyllin® SR	Capsule	Slow release*†
E-Mycin®	Tablet	Enteric-coated
Endafed®	Capsule	Slow release
Entex® LA	Tablet	Slow release†
Entex® PSE	Tablet	Slow release†
Entozyme	Tablet	Enteric-coated
Equanil®	Tablet	Taste‖
Ergostat®	Tablet	Sublingual form•
Eryc®	Capsule	Enteric-coated*
Ery-Tab®	Tablet	Enteric-coated
Erythrocin® Stearate	Tablet	Enteric-coated
Erythromycin Base	Tablet	Enteric-coated
Eskalith® CR	Tablet	Slow release
Fedahist® TimeCaps®	Capsule	Slow release†
Feldene®	Capsule	Mucous membrane irritant
Fenesin™	Tablet	Slow release
Feocyte	Tablet	Slow release
Feosol®	Tablet	Enteric-coated†
Feosol® Spansule®	Capsule	Slow release*†
Ferrous Gluconate	Tablet	Film-coated
Feratab®	Tablet	Enteric-coated†
Fergon®	Tablet	May cause excessive GI upset
Fero-Grad 500® mg	Tablet	Slow release
Fero-Gradumet®	Tablet	Slow release
Ferralet® SR	Tablet	Slow release
Feverall™ Sprinkle Caps	Capsule	Taste*
		Note: Capsule contents intended to be placed in a teaspoonful of water or soft food.
Fumatinic	Capsule	Slow release
Gastrocrom®	Capsule	Note: Contents should be dissolved in water for administration.
Geocillin®	Tablet	Taste
Gris-PEG®	Tablet	Note: Crushing may result in precipitation as larger particles.
Guaifed	Capsule	Slow release
Guaifed-PD	Capsule	Slow release
Guaimax-D	Tablet	Slow release
Halfprin	Tablet	Enteric coated
Humabid® DM	Tablet	Slow release
Humabid® DM Sprinkle	Capsule	Slow release*
Humabid® LA	Tablet	Slow release
Humabid® Sprinkle	Capsule	Slow release*
Hydergine® LC	Capsule	Note: Product is in liquid form within a special capsulet††
Hydergine® Sublingual	Tablet	Sublingual route†
Hytakerol®	Capsule	Liquid filled§†
Iberet®	Tablet	Slow release†
Iberet-500®	Tablet	Slow release†
Ilotycin®	Tablet	Enteric-coated
Imdur™	Tablet	Slow release♦
Inderal® LA	Capsule	Slow release
Inderide® LA	Capsule	Slow release
Indocin® SR	Capsule	Slow release*†
Ionamin®	Capsule	Slow release
Isoclor® Timesule®	Capsule	Slow release†
Isoptin® SR	Tablet	Slow release
Isordil® Sublingual	Tablet	Sublingual form•
Isordil® Tembid®	Tablet	Slow release
Isosorbide Dinitrate Sublingual	Tablet	Sublingual form•
Isosorbide Dinitrate SR	Tablet	Slow release
Isuprel® Glossets®	Tablet	Sublingual form•
K+® 8	Tablet	Slow release†
K+® 10	Tablet	Slow release†

(continued)

Drug Product	Dosage Forms	Reasons/Comments
Kaon-Cl® 6.7 mEq	Tablet	Slow release†
Kaon-Cl® 10	Tablet	Slow release†
K + Care®	Tablet	Effervescent tablet†¶
K-Dur®	Tablet	Slow release♦
Klor-Con®	Tablet	Slow release†
Klor-Con®/EF	Tablet	Effervescent tablet†¶
Klorvess®	Tablet	Effervescent tablet†¶
Klotrix®	Tablet	Slow release†
K-Lyte®	Tablet	Effervescent tablet¶
K-Lyte/Cl®	Tablet	Effervescent tablet¶
K-Tab®	Tablet	Slow release†
Levsinex® TimeCaps®	Capsule	Slow release
Macrobid®	Capsule	Slow release
Meprospan®	Capsule	Slow release*
Mestinon® Timespan®	Tablet	Slow release†
MI-Cebrin	Tablet	Enteric-coated
MI-Cebrin T	Tablet	Enteric-coated
Micro-K®	Capsule	Slow release*†
Motrin®	Tablet	Taste†‖
Motrin® IB	Tablet	Taste†‖
Motrin® IB-sinus	Tablet	Taste†‖
MS Contin®	Tablet	Slow release†
MSC Triaminic®	Tablet	Enteric-coated
Naldecon®	Tablet	Slow release†
Nasabid™	Capsule	Slow release
Nasatab LA	Tablet	Slow release
Nico 400	Capsule	Slow release
Nicobid®	Capsule	Slow release
Nitro-Bid®	Capsule	Slow release*
Nitrocine® TimeCaps®	Capsule	Slow release
Nitroglyn®	Capsule	Slow release*
Nitrong®	Tablet	Slow release
Nitrostat®	Tablet	Sublingual route•
Nolamine®	Tablet	Slow release
Nolex® LA	Tablet	Slow release
Norflex®	Tablet	Slow release
Norpace® CR	Capsule	Slow release form within a special capsule
Novafed®	Capsule	Slow release
Novafed® A	Capsule	Slow release
Optilets-500® Filmtab®	Tablet	Enteric-coated
Optilets-M-500® Filmtab®	Tablet	Enteric-coated
Oragrafin®	Capsule	Note: Product is in liquid form within a special capsule
Ordrine® SR	Capsule	Slow release
Oramorph SR™	Tablet	Slow release†
Ornade® Spansule®	Capsule	Slow release
Oruvail®	Capsule	Slow release
Pabalate	Tablet	Enteric-coated
Pabalate SF	Tablet	Enteric-coated
Pancrease®	Capsule	Enteric-coated*
Pancrease® MT	Capsule	Enteric-coated*
Panmycin®	Capsule	Taste
Papaverine Sustained Action	Capsule	Slow release
Pathilon® Sequels®	Capsule	Slow release*
Pavabid® Plateau	Capsule	Slow release*
PBZ-SR®	Tablet	Slow release†
Pentasa®	Capsule	Slow release
Perdiem®	Granules	Wax coated
Peritrate® SA	Tablet	Slow release♦
Permitil® Chronotab®	Tablet	Slow release†
Phazyme®	Tablet	Slow release
Phazyme® 95	Tablet	Slow release♦
Phenergan®	Tablet	Taste†‖
Phyllocontin®	Tablet	Slow release
Plendil®	Tablet	Slow release
Pneumonist®	Tablet	Slow release†
Polaramine® Repetabs®	Tablet	Slow release†
Prelu-2®	Capsule	Slow release
Prilosec™	Capsule	Slow release
Pro-Banthine®	Tablet	Taste
Procainamide HCl SR	Tablet	Slow release
Procan® SR	Tablet	Slow release

(continued)

Drug Product	Dosage Forms	Reasons/Comments
Procardia®	Capsule	Delays absorption§#
Procardia XL®	Tablet	Slow release Note: AUC is unaffected.
Pronestyl-SR®	Tablet	Slow release
Proventil® Repetabs®	Tablet	Slow release†
Prozac®	Capsule	Slow release*
Quadra-Hist®	Tablet	Slow release
Quibron®-T SR	Tablet	Slow release†
Quinaglute® Dura-Tabs®	Tablet	Slow release
Quinalan® Lanatabs®	Tablet	Slow release
Quinalan® SR	Tablet	Slow release
Quinidex® Extentabs®	Tablet	Slow release
Respaire® SR	Capsule	Slow release
Respid®	Tablet	Slow release
Ritalin-SR®	Tablet	Slow release
Robimycin® Robitab®	Tablet	Enteric-coated
Rondec-TR®	Tablet	Slow release†
Roxanol SR™	Tablet	Slow release†
Ru-Tuss®	Tablet	Slow release
Ru-Tuss® DE	Tablet	Slow release
Seldane-D®	Tablet	Slow release
Sinemet® CR	Tablet	Slow release♦
Singlet®	Tablet	Slow release
Slo-bid™ Gyrocaps®	Capsule	Slow release*
Slo-Niacin®	Tablet	Slow release
Slo-Phyllin GG®	Capsule	Slow release†
Slo-Phyllin® Gyrocaps®	Capsule	Slow release*†
Slow FE®	Tablet	Slow release†
Slow-K®	Tablet	Slow release†
Slow-Mag®	Tablet	Slow release
Sorbitrate® SA	Tablet	Slow release
Sorbitrate® Sublingual	Tablet	Sublingual route
Sparine®	Tablet	Taste‖
S-P-T	Capsule	Note: Liquid gelatin thyroid suspension.
Stamoist E	Tablet	Slow release
Stamoist LA	Tablet	Slow release
Sudafed® 12-Hour	Caplet	Slow release†
Surfak® Liquigels	Capsule	Liquid filled§
Tavist-D®	Tablet	Multiple compressed tablet
Teldrin®	Capsule	Slow release*
Temaril® Spansule®	Capsule	Slow release†
Tepanil® Tentab®	Tablet	Slow release
Tessalon® Perles	Capsule	Slow release
Theo-24®	Tablet	Slow release†
Theobid®	Capsule	Slow release*†
Theobid® Jr	Capsule	Slow release*†
Theoclear® L.A	Capsule	Slow release†
Theochron®	Tablet	Slow release
Theo-Dur®	Tablet	Slow release† ♦
Theo-Dur® Sprinkle	Capsule	Slow release*†
Theo-Sav	Tablet	Slow release♦
Theolair™ SR	Tablet	Slow release†
Theovent®	Capsule	Slow release†
Theox®	Tablet	Slow release
Therapy Bayer	Caplet	Enteric-coated
Thorazine® Spansule®	Capsule	Slow release
Toprol XL®	Tablet	Slow release♦
Touro A&H®	Capsule	Slow release*
Touro EX®	Tablet	Slow release♦
Touro LA®	Tablet	Slow release♦
T-Phyl®	Tablet	Slow release
Trental®	Tablet	Slow release
Triaminic®	Tablet	Enteric-coated†
Triaminic-12® Tablet	Slow release†	
Trilafon® Repetabs®	Tablet	Slow release†
Trinalin® Repetabs®	Tablet	Slow release
Tuss-LA®	Tablet	Slow release
Tuss-Ornade® Spansule®	Capsule	Slow release
ULR-LA®	Tablet	Slow release
Unicap®	Capsule	Liquid filled§
Uniphyl®	Tablet	Slow release

(continued)

Drug Product	Dosage Forms	Reasons/Comments
Valrelease®	Capsule	Slow release
Vanex® Forte	Caplet	Slow release
Vantin®	Tablet	Taste†‖
Verelan®	Capsule	Slow release*
Volmax®	Tablet	Slow release†
Wyamycin® S	Tablet	Slow release
Wygesic®	Tablet	Taste
Zephrex LA®	Tablet	Slow release
ZORprin®	Tablet	Slow release
Zymase®	Capsule	Enteric-coated

Adapted from Mitchell JF and Pawlicki KS, "Oral Solid Dosage Forms That Should Not Be Crushed: 1994 Revision," *Hosp Pharm*, 1994, 29(7):666-75.

*Capsule may be opened and the contents taken without crushing or chewing; soft food such as applesauce or pudding may facilitate administration; contents may generally be administered via nasogastric tube using an appropriate fluid provided entire contents are washed down the tube.

†Liquid dosage forms of the product are available; however, dose, frequency of administration, and manufacturers may differ from that of the solid dosage form.

‡Antacids and/or milk may prematurely dissolve the coating of the tablet.

§Capsule may be opened and the liquid contents removed for administration.

‖The taste of this product in a liquid form would likely be unacceptable to the patient; administration via nasogastric tube should be acceptable.

¶Effervescent tablets must be dissolved in the amount of diluent recommended by the manufacturer.

#If the liquid capsule is crushed or the contents expressed, the active ingredient will be, in part, absorbed sublingually.

•Tablets are made to disintegrate under the tongue.

♦Tablet is scored.

COMPARISON
CHARTS

ANTIDEPRESSANT AGENTS COMPARISON

Drug	Class	Therapeutic Drug Conc (ng/mL)	Anticholinergic Side Effects	Sedation	Orthostatic Hypotension	Usual Adult Daily Dose (mg)
Amitriptyline	TCA	100–250	+ + + +	+ + + +	+ +	75–300
Amoxapine	TCA	20–100*	+ + +	+ +	+	150–600
Bupropion	Aminoketone	50–100†	+ +	+ +	+	225–450
Clomipramine	TCA	330–800*†	+ + +	+ + +	+ +	100–250
Desipramine	TCA	115–160	+	+	+	75–300
Doxepin	TCA	>110	+ +	+ + +	+ +	75–300
Fluoxetine	SSRI	*†	+/-	+/-	+/-	20–80
Fluvoxamine	SSRI	-	(-)	(-/+)	(-)	20–80
Imipramine	TCA	150–250†	+ +	+ +	+ + +	75–300
Maprotiline	Teracyclic	*	+ +	+ +	+	75–225
Nortriptyline	TCA	50–150	+ +	+ +	+	75–300
Paroxetine	SSRI	-	(-)	+/-	(-)	10–50
Protriptyline	TCA	100–200	+ + +	+	+	15–60
Sertraline	SSRI	-	(-)	+/-	(-)	50–200
Trazodone	Triazolopyridine	900–2100*	+	+ +	+ +	150–600
Trimipramine	TCA	Not established	+ +	+ + +	+ +	75–300
Venlafaxine	Phenyl-Ethyl-Amine	-	(-)	(-)	(-)	75–325

TCA = tricyclic antidepressant.
*Drug concentration in the serum correlates poorly with clinical response.
†Levels represent a combination of parent compound and active metabolites.

ANTIPSYCHOTIC AGENTS COMPARISON

Antipsychotic Agent	Equivalent Dosages (approx) (mg)	Usual Adult Daily Maintenance Dose (mg)	Sedation (Incidence)	Extrapyramidal Side Effects	Anticholinergic Side Effects	Cardiovascular Side Effects	Orthostatic Hypotension
Acetophenazine	20	60–120	Moderate	High	Low	Low	Low
Chlorpromazine	100	200–1000	High	Moderate	Moderate	Moderate/high	High
Chlorprothixene	100	75–600	High	Moderate	Moderate	Low/moderate	Moderate
Clozapine	50	50–400	High	Low	High	High	High
Fluphenazine	2	5–40	Low	High	Low	Low	Low
Haloperidol	2	5–40	Low	High	Low	Low	Low
Loxapine	10	25–100	Moderate	High	Low	Low	Moderate
Mesoridazine	50	30–400	High	Low	High	Moderate	Moderate
Molindone	15	25–100	Low	High	Low	Low	Low
Perphenazine	10	16–48	Low	High	Low	Low	Low
Pimozide	0.3–0.5	1–10	Moderate	High	Moderate	Moderate	Moderate
Promazine	200	40–1200	Moderate	Moderate	High	Moderate	Moderate
Risperidone	–	4–16	Low	None/low	Low	Low	Low
Thioridazine	100	200–800	High	Low	High	Moderate/high	High
Thiothixene	5	5–40	Low	Moderate	Low	Low/moderate	Low
Trifluoperazine	5	10–40	Low	High	Low	Low	Low

BENZODIAZEPINES COMPARISON

	Peak Blood Levels (oral)	Protein Binding %	Major Active Metabolite	t½ (parent) Adults	t½* (metabolite) Adults	Adult Oral Dosage Range	Geriatric Oral Dosage Range
Anxiolytic							
Alprazolam (Xanax®)	1–2 h	80	No	12–15 h	—	0.75–4 mg/d	0.25–0.75 mg/d
Chlordiazepoxide (Librium®)	2–4 h	90–98	Yes	5–30 h	24–96 h	15–100 mg/d	10–20 mg/d†
Clorazepate (Tranxene®)	1 h	ND‡	Yes	Not significant	50–100 h	15–60 mg/d	7.5–15 mg/d†
Diazepam (Valium®)	1–2 h	98	Yes	20–50 h	50–100 h	6–40 mg/d	1–5 mg/d†
Halazepam (Paxipam®)	1–3 h	ND‡	Yes	14 h	50–100 h	60–160 mg/d	20–40 mg/d
Lorazepam (Ativan®)	0.5–3 h	85	No	10–20 h	—	2–6 mg/d	0.5–2 mg/d
Oxazepam (Serax®)	2–4 h	86–99	No	5–20 h	—	30–120 mg/d	10–30 mg/d
Prazepam (Centrax®)	6 h	ND‡	Yes	1 h	50–100 h	20–60 mg/d	10–15 mg/d†

(continued)

	Peak Blood Levels (oral)	Protein Binding %	Major Active Metabolite	t½ (parent) Adults	t½* (metabolite) Adults	Adult Oral Dosage Range	Geriatric Oral Dosage Range
Sedative/Hypnotic							
Estazolam (ProSom™)	2 h	93	No	10-24 h	—	1-2 mg	0.5-1 mg
Flurazepam (Dalmane®)	0.5-2 h	97	Yes	Not significant	40-114 h	15-30 mg	15 mg†
Quazepam (Doral®)	2 h	>95	Yes	25-41 h	40-114 h	7.5-15 mg	7.5 mg†
Temazepam (Restoril®)	2-3 h	96	No	9.5-12 h	—	7.5-30 mg	7.5-15 mg
Triazolam (Halcion®)	0.5-2 h	89-94	No	1.7-5 h	—	0.125-0.5 mg	0.0625-0.125 mg
Miscellaneous							
Clonazepam (Klonopin®)	1-2 h	86	No	18-50 h	—	1.5-20 mg/d	0.5-1.5 mg/d

* = significant metabolite.
†Not recommended for use in geriatric patients.
‡No specific data available, but all benzodiazepines are highly protein bound.

Abstracted from Micromedex, Inc.

BETA-BLOCKERS COMPARISON

Agent	Adrenergic Receptor Blocking Activity	Lipid Solubility	Half-life (h)	Primary (Secondary) Route of Elimination	Starting Oral Daily Dose
Acebutolol (Sectral®)	beta₁	Low	3-4	Hepatic (renal)	400 mg
Atenolol (Tenormin®)	beta₁	Low	6-9*	Renal (hepatic)	50 mg
Betaxolol (Kerlone®)	beta₁	Low	14-22	Hepatic (renal)	20 mg
Bisoprolol (Zebeta®)	beta₁	Low	9-12	Renal/ hepatic	2.5-5 mg
Carteolol (Cartrol®)	beta₁ beta₂	Low	6	Renal (biliary)	15 mg
Esmolol (Brevibloc®)	beta₁	Low	0.15	Red blood cell	NA
Labetalol (Trandate® Normodyne®)	alpha₁ beta₁ beta₂	Moderate	5.5-8	Renal (hepatic)	200 mg
Metoprolol (Lopressor®)	beta₁	Moderate	3-7	Hepatic/ renal	50 mg
Nadolol (Corgard®)	beta₁ beta₂	Low	20-24	Renal	320 mg

*Half-life increased to 16-27 h in creatinine clearances of 15-35 mL/min and >27 h in Cl$_{cr}$ <15 mL/min.
Note: For specific geriatric information, see individual monographs.

(continued)

Agent	Adrenergic Receptor Blocking Activity	Lipid Solubility	Half-life (h)	Primary (Secondary) Route of Elimination	Starting Oral Daily Dose
Penbutolol (Levatol®)	beta$_1$ beta$_2$	High	5	Hepatic (renal)	20 mg
Pindolol (Visken®)	beta$_1$ beta$_2$	Moderate	3–4†	Hepatic/ renal	20 mg
Propranolol (Inderal®, various)	beta$_1$ beta$_2$	High	3–5	Hepatic	80 mg
Propranolol long-acting (Inderal-LA®)	beta$_1$ beta$_2$	High	9–18	Hepatic	80 mg
Sotalol (Betapace®)	beta$_1$ beta$_2$	Low	7–18	Renal (hepatic)	80 mg
Timolol (Blocadren®)	beta$_1$ beta$_2$	Low to moderate	4	Hepatic (renal)	20 mg

†Half-life variable: 7–15 h.
Note: All beta$_1$ selective agents will inhibit beta$_2$ receptors at higher doses.

CALCIUM CHANNEL BLOCKING AGENTS COMPARISON

	Amlodipine	Bepridil	Diltiazem	Felodipine	Isradipine	Nicardipine	Nifedipine	Nimodipine	Verapamil
Absorption (%)	—	99-100	40	99-100	90-95	35	60-75	13	20-35
Protein binding	93	>99	High	>99	95	Very high	Very high	Very high	High
Half-life	30-50 h	24 h	6-8 h	11-16 h	8 h	2-4 h	5 h	1-2 h	Oral: One dose: 2.8-7.4 h Rep dose: 4.5-12 h I.V. (biphasic) Short phase: 4 min Long phase: 2-5 h
Onset of action	—	60 min	Oral: 60 min	2-5 h	2 h	20 min	Oral: 10-20 min	20 min	Oral: 30 min I.V.: 1-5 min
Peak	6-12 h	2-3 h	Oral: 2-3 h	2.5-5 h	1.5 h	0.5-2 h	Oral: 0.5-6 h	<1 h	Oral: 1-2 h Oral. ext release: 5-7 h I.V.: 2 h
Duration of action	—	24 h	Ext release: 12 h Tablet: 6-8 h	24 h	12 h	8 h	12-24 h	4-6 h	Oral. ext release: 24 h Tablet: 8-10 h I.V.: 2 h
Elimination	Hepatic 90% Renal 10%	Hepatic/biliary almost 100%	Biliary/renal 96%-98% (2%-4% unchanged)	Hepatic 99% Renal <0.5%	Hepatic/biliary 100%	Renal 60% Biliary/fecal 35%	Renal 80% Biliary/fecal 20%	Renal 60% Biliary/fecal 35%	Renal 70% Biliary/fecal 9%-16%

(continued)

	Amlodipine	Bepridil	Diltiazem	Felodipine	Isradipine	Nicardipine	Nifedipine	Nimodipine	Verapamil
Actions									
contractility	↓	↓	↓	↓	0	↓	↓	↓	↓↓
heart rate	±	↓	↓	↓	±	↓	↓	↓	↓
cardiac output	↓	0	↓	↓	↓	↑↓	↓	↓	↓↑
peripheral vascular resistance	↓↓↓	↓	↓	↓↓↓	↓↓↓	↓↓↓	↓↓↓	↓↓	↓↓
Side effects									
constipation	–	+	+	+	–	–	+	–	+
dizziness	+	++	+	++	++	+	++	+	+
flushing	++	–	++	++	+	++	++	–	–
headache	++	++	+	++	++	+	++	+	+
nausea	+	++	+	+	+	+	++	+	+

+ + = most frequent
+ = less frequent
– = rare
± = negligible effect
0 = no effect

807

CORTICOSTEROIDS COMPARISON, SYSTEMIC

Relative Potencies and Equivalent Doses of Corticosteroids
(Glucocorticoid potency compared to hydrocortisone "mg" for "mg" basis)

Compound	Gluco-corticoid Potency	Mineralo-corticoid Potency	Equivalent Dose (mg)	Duration* of Action
Cortisone (Cortone®) 　Injection: 50 mg/mL suspension 　Tablet: 5 mg	0.8	+ +	25	S
Dexamethasone (Decadron®, 　Dexone®, Hexadrol®) 　Elixir: 0.5 mg/5 mL 　Injection: 4 mg/mL 　Intensol: 1 mg/mL 　Tablet: 0.25 mg, 0.5 mg, 　　0.75 mg, 1 mg, 1.5 mg, 　　2 mg, 4 mg	25-30	0	0.75	L
Fludrocortisone (Florinef®) 　Tablet: 0.1 mg	10	+ + + + +		I
Hydrocortisone (Cortef®) 　Injection: 50 mg/mL 　Suspension: 10 mg/5 mL 　Tablet: 5 mg, 10 mg, 20 mg	1	+ +	20	S
Methylprednisolone (Medrol®, 　Solu-Medrol®, Depo-Medrol®) 　Injection: 40 mg, 125 mg, 　　500 mg, 1 g 　Injection, suspension: 　　80 mg/mL 　Tablet: 2 mg, 4 mg, 16 mg, 　　24 mg	5	0	4	I
Prednisolone (Delta-Cortef®, 　Prelone™ Syrup, Pediapred®) 　Liquid: 5 mg/5 mL 　Syrup: 15 mg/5 mL 　Tablet: 5 mg	4	+	5	I
Prednisone (Deltasone®, Liquid 　Pred™, Orasone®) 　Liquid: 5 mg/5 mL 　Tablet: 1 mg, 2.5 mg, 5 mg, 　　10 mg, 20 mg, 50 mg	4	+	5	I

* S = Short, 8-12 h biologic activity

I = Intermediate, 12-36 h biologic activity

L = Long, 36-54 h biologic activity

CORTICOSTEROIDS COMPARISON, TOPICAL

The following topical corticosteroid preparations are grouped in order of potency.

Drug/Dosage Form	Brand Name
I Super Potency	
Clobetasol propionate 0.05% cream and ointment	Temovate®
Betamethasone dipropionate 0.05% cream and ointment	Diprolene®
Halobetasol propionate 0.05% cream and ointment	Ultravate™
Diflorasone diacetate 0.05% (optimized) ointment	Psorcon®
II Higher Potency	
Amcinonide 0.1% ointment	Cyclocort®
Betamethasone dipropionate 0.05% (optimized) cream	Diprolene® AF
Betamethasone dipropionate 0.05% ointment	Diprosone®, Maxivate®
Mometasone furoate 0.1% ointment	Elocon®
Diflorasone diacetate 0.05% ointment	Florone®, Maxiflor®
Halcinonide 0.1% cream	Halog®
Fluocinonide 0.05% ointment	Lidex®
Fluocinonide 0.05% cream	Lidex®
Desoximetasone 0.05% gel	Topicort®
Desoximetasone 0.25% cream	Topicort®
Desoximetasone 0.25% ointment	Topicort®
Fluocinonide 0.05% gel	Lidex®
III High Potency	
Triamcinolone acetonide 0.5% ointment	Aristocort®, Kenalog®
Fluticasone propionate 0.005% ointment	Cutivate™
Amcinonide 0.1% cream	Cyclocort®
Amcinonide 0.1% lotion	Cyclocort®
Betamethasone dipropionate 0.05% cream	Diprosone®, Maxivate®
Diflorasone diacetate 0.05% cream	Florone®, Maxiflor®
Fluocinonide 0.05% cream	Lidex®-E
Betamethasone valerate 0.01% ointment	Valisone®
IV Mid-Potency	
Triamcinolone acetonide 0.1% ointment	Aristocort®, Kenalog®
Flurandrenolide 0.05% ointment	Cordran®
Mometasone furoate 0.1% cream	Elocon®
Fluocinolone acetonide 0.025% ointment	Synalar®
Hydrocortisone valerate 0.2% ointment	Westcort®
V Mid-Potency	
Flurandrenolide 0.05% cream	Cordran®
Fluticasone propionate 0.05% cream	Cutivate™
Betamethasone dipropionate 0.05% lotion	Diprosone®
Triamcinolone acetonide 0.1% lotion	Aristocort®, Kenalog®
Hydrocortisone butyrate 0.1% cream	Locoid®
Fluocinolone acetonide 0.025% cream	Synalar®
Betamethasone valerate 0.1% cream	Valisone®
Hydrocortisone valerate 0.2% cream	Westcort®
VI Low Potency	
Alclometasone dipropionate 0.05% ointment	Aclovate®
Alclometasone dipropionate 0.05% cream	Aclovate®
Triamcinolone acetonide 0.1% cream	Aristocort®, Kenalog®
Fluocinolone acetonide 0.025% cream	Synalar®
Fluocinolone acetonide 0.01% solution	Synalar®
Betamethasone valerate 0.1% lotion	Valisone®
Desonide 0.05% cream	DesOwen®, Tridesilon®
VII Lowest Potency	
Hydrocortisone acetate	Hytone®
Dexamethasone phosphate	Decaderm®

GLAUCOMA DRUG THERAPY COMPARISON

	Ophthalmic Agent	Strengths Available	Reduces Aqueous Humor Production	Increases Aqueous Humor Outflow	Average Duration of Action
Mydriatics	**Sympathomimetics**				
	Dipivefrin	0.1%	Significant	Moderate	12 h
	Epinephrine	0.25–2%	Significant	Moderate	18 h
	Beta-blockers				
	Betaxolol	0.5%	Significant	Some activity	12 h
	Levobunolol	0.5%	Significant	Some activity	18 h
	Metipranolol	0.3%	Significant	Some activity	18 h
Miscellaneous	Timolol	0.25–0.5%	Significant	Some activity	18 h
	Carbonic Anhydrase Inhibitors				
	Acetazolamide	125–250 mg	Significant	No data	10 h
	Methazolamide	50 mg	Significant	No data	14 h
	Cholinesterase Inhibitors				
	Demecarium	0.125–0.25%	No data	Significant	7 d
	Echothiophate	0.03–0.25%	No data	Significant	2 wk
	Isoflurophate	0.025%	No data	Significant	2 wk
	Physostigmine	0.25–0.5%	No data	Significant	24 h
Miotics	**Direct Acting**				
	Acetylcholine	1%	Some activity	Significant	14 min
	Carbachol	0.75–3%	Some activity	Significant	8 h
	Pilocarpine	0.25–10%	Some activity	Significant	5 h

*All miotic drugs significantly affect accommodation.

NARCOTIC AGONIST COMPARATIVE PHARMACOLOGY

Drug	Analgesic	Antitussive	Constipation	Respiratory Depression	Sedation	Emesis	Physical Dependence
Phenanthrenes							
Codeine	+	+++	+	+	+	+	+
Hydrocodone	+	+++		+			+
Hydromorphone	++	+++	+	++	+	+	++
Levorphanol	++	++	++	++	++	+	++
Morphine	++	+++	++	++	++	++	++
Oxycodone	++	+++	++	++	++	++	++
Oxymorphone	++	+	++	+++		+++	+++
Phenylpiperidines							
Fentanyl	++			+		+	++
Meperidine	++	+	+	++	+		++
Diphenylheptanes							
Methadone	++	++	++	++	++	++	+
Propoxyphene	+			+	+	++	+

PHARMACOKINETICS OF
NARCOTIC AGONIST ANALGESICS

Drug	Onset (min)	Peak (h)	Duration (h)	Adult t½ (h)	Average Dosing Interval (h)		Equianalgesic Doses* (mg)	
							I.M.	P.O.
Buprenorphine†	15	1	4–8	2–3	6		0.3	NA
Butorphanol†	<10	0.5–1	3–5	2.5–3.5	3	(3–6)	2–3	NA
Codeine	15–30	0.5–1	4–6	3–4	3	(3–6)	120	200
Fentanyl	7–8	ND	1–2	1.5–6	1	(0.5–2)	0.1	NA
Hydrocodone	ND	ND	4–6	3.3–4.4			ND	ND
Hydromorphone	15–30	0.5–1	4–6	2–4	4	(3–6)	1.5	7.5
Levorphanol	30–90	0.5–1	4–8	12–16	12		2	4
Meperidine	10–45	0.5–1	2–4	3–4	3	(2–4)	75	300
Methadone	30–60	0.5–1	4–6 (acute) >8 (chronic)	15–30	8	(6–12)	10	20
Morphine	15–60	0.5–1	3–6	2–4	4	(3–6)	10	60
Nalbuphine†	<15	1	3–6	5		3–6	10	NA
Oxycodone (P.O.)	15–30	0.5–1	4–6	3–4	4	(3–6)	NA	30
Oxymorphone	5–15	0.5–1	3–6	ND		4–6	1	10‡
Pentazocine†	15–20	0.25–1	3–4	2–3	3	(3–6)	30	150
Propoxyphene (P.O.)	30–60	2–2.5	4–6	3.5–15	6	(4–8)	ND	130§–200¶

ND = no data available.   NA = not applicable.
*Based on acute, short-term use. Chronic administration may alter pharmacokinetics and decrease the oral parenteral dose ratio. The morphine oral–parenteral ratio decreases to ~1.5–2.5:1 upon chronic dosing.
†Has partial antagonist activity.
‡Rectal.
§HCl salt.
¶Napsylate salt.

THERAPEUTIC CATEGORY
INDEX

THERAPEUTIC CATEGORY INDEX

(Continued)

THERAPEUTIC CATEGORY INDEX

THERAPEUTIC CATEGORY INDEX

ANTIFUNGAL AGENT, SYSTEMIC

ANTIFUNGAL AGENT, TOPICAL

ANTIFUNGAL AGENT, VAGINAL

ANTIHEMOPHILIC AGENT

ANTIHISTAMINE

ANTIHISTAMINE, INHALATION

ANTIHISTAMINE/DECONGESTANT COMBINATION

ANTIHYPERTENSIVE

ANTIHYPOGLYCEMIC AGENT

ANTIHYPERTENSIVE, COMBINATION

ANTI-INFECTIVE AGENT, ORAL

ANTI-INFLAMMATORY AGENT

(Continued)

THERAPEUTIC CATEGORY INDEX

(Continued)

(Continued)

(Continued)

NOTES

NOTES

HEALTH SCIENCES LIBRARY
EDMONTON GENERAL HOSPITAL

NOTES

PHARM-EGH
HEALTH SCIENCES LIBRARY
EDMONTON GENERAL HOSPITAL
95-11702-09